NCLEX-PN® Questions & Answers

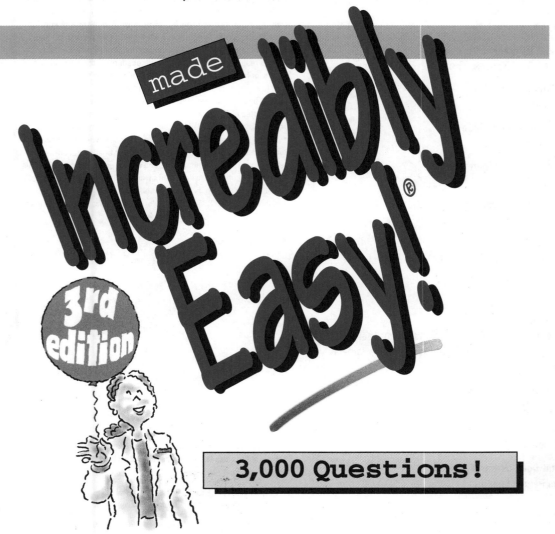

made

Incredibly Easy!®

3rd edition

3,000 Questions!

Wolters Kluwer | Lippincott Williams & Wilkins
Health

Philadelphia · Baltimore · New York · London
Buenos Aires · Hong Kong · Sydney · Tokyo

Staff

Executive Publisher
Judith A. Schilling McCann, RN, MSN

Editorial Director
David Moreau

Clinical Director
Joan M. Robinson, RN, MSN

Art Director
Mary Ludwicki

Electronic Project Manager
John Macalino

Editorial Project Manager
Gabrielle Mosquera

Clinical Project Manager
Lorraine M. Hallowell, RN, BSN, RVS

Editors
Karen Comerford, Margaret Eckman, Diane Labus

Clinical Editor
Pamela Kovach, RN, BSN

Copy Editors
Kimberly Bilotta (supervisor), Scotti Cohn, Jeannine Fielding, Shana Harrington, Dorothy P. Terry, Pamela Wingrod

Designer
Georg W. Purvis IV

Illustrator
Bot Roda

Digital Composition Services
Diane Paluba (manager), Joyce Rossi Biletz, Donna Morris

Associate Manufacturing Manager
Beth J. Welsh

Editorial Assistants
Karen J. Kirk, Jeri O'Shea, Linda K. Ruhf

Indexer
Barbara Hodgson

PNQAIE3011008-030311

Library of Congress Cataloging-in-Publication Data

NCLEX-PN questions & answers made incredibly easy ! —3rd ed.
      p. ; cm.
   Includes index.
   1. Practical nursing—Examinations, questions, etc. 2. National Council Licensure Examination for Practical/Vocational Nurses—Study guides. I. Lippincott Williams & Wilkins. II. Title: NCLEX-PN questions and answers made incredibly easy.
   [DNLM: 1. Nursing, Practical—United States—Examination Questions. WY 18.2 N3365 2009]
RT62.N377 2009
610.73'076—dc22
ISBN13 978-0-7817-9919-5
ISBN10 0-7817-9919-8   2008030418

Contents

Part IV Maternal-neonatal care

Part V Care of the child

Part VI Coordinated care

Appendices and index

Advisory board

Contributors and consultants

Carol Allred, RN, MSN, BC
Allied Health Director
Uintah Basin Applied Technology College
Roosevelt, Utah

Kimberly S. Amos, RN, BSN, RT(R)
Practical Nursing Instructor
Isothermal Community College
Spindale, N.C.

Barbara C. Anderson, RN, BSN, MEd
Director
Virginia Beach School of Practical Nursing
Virginia Beach, Va.

Kathleen Bredberg, RN, MSN
Director, Vocational Nursing Program
Grayson County College
Denison, Tex.

Karen M. Brown, RNC, BSN, MS, EdD
Associate Dean of Instruction
Kirtland Community College
Roscommon, Mich.

Cheryl Bruno-Mofu, RN
Nursing Professor
Palo Verde College
Blythe, Calif.

Tammy Bryant, RN, BSN
Program Director—LPN Program
Southwest Georgia Technical College
Thomasville

Carol Carroll, RN, MSN
Instructor
Uintah Basin Applied Technology College
Roosevelt, Utah

Patricia L. Clowers, APRN, MSN
Director of Nursing
East Mississippi Community College
Mayhew

Marsha L. Conroy, RN, MSN, APN
Nurse Educator
Cuyahoga Community College
Cleveland
Indiana Wesleyan University
Marion, Ind.

Kim Cooper, RN, MSN
Nursing Department Chair
Ivy Tech Community College
Terre Haute, Ind.

Donna S. Davis, RN, BSN
Nursing Instructor
Giles County Technology Center
Pearisburg, Va.

Mary Davis, RN, MSN
Practical Nursing Instructor
Valdosta Technical Community College
Valdosta, Ga.

Doreen DeAngelis, RN, MSN
Nursing Instructor
Penn State University, Fayette Campus
Uniontown, Pa.

Cheryl DeGraw, RN, MSN, CRNP, CNE
Nursing Instructor
Florence-Darlington Technical College
Florence, S.C.

Erica Fooshee, RN, MSN
Nursing Instructor
Pensacola (Fla.) Junior College

Linda J. Franklin, RN, BSN
Practical Nursing Instructor
Meridian Technology Center
Stillwater, Okla.

Shirley Lyon Garcia, RN, BSN
Adjunct Nursing Faculty, PNE
McDowell Technical Community College
Marion, N.C.

Ruth Howell, BSN, MEd
Director, Practical Nursing Program
Tri County Technology Center
Bartlesville, Okla.

Kynthia James, RN, MSN
Instructor
Southwest Georgia Technical College
Thomasville

Noel C. Piano, RN, MS
Coordinator/Instructor
Lafayette School of Practical Nursing
Williamsburg, Va.
Adjunct Faculty
Thomas Nelson Community College
Hampton, Va.

Kristi Robinia, RNC, MSN
Program Coordinator for Practical Nursing
Northern Michigan University
Marquette

Ora V. Robinson, RN, PhD
Assistant Professor
California State University San Bernardino

Kendra S. Seiler, MSN
Nursing Instructor
Rio Hondo College
Whittier, Calif.

Catherine Shields, RN, BSN
Practical Nursing Instructor
Ocean County Vocational Technical School
Toms River, N.J.

Betty E. Sims, RN, MSN, FRE
Director of Nursing Education
Coastal Bend College
Beeville, Tex.

Brigitte Thiele, RN, BSN
Coordinator of Practical Nursing Education
Kennett Career and Technology Center
Kennett, Mo.

Laura Travis, RN, BSN
Health Careers Coordinator
Tennessee Technology Center at Dickson

Julie A. Will, RN, MSN
Chair, School of Health Sciences
Ivy Tech Community College of Indiana
Terre Haute, Ind.

Hollace Yowler, RN, MSN
Associate Professor
Ivy Tech Community College of Indiana
Madison, Ind.

Not another boring foreword

If you're like most nursing students I know, you're too busy attending classes, going to clinicals, and preparing for NCLEX to have the time to wade through a foreword that uses pretentious terms and umpteen dull paragraphs to get to the point. So let's cut right to the chase! Here's why this book is so terrific:

1. It will teach you all the important things you need to know about preparing for and passing the NCLEX. (And it will leave out all the fluff that wastes your time.)
2. It will help you remember what you've learned.
3. It will make you smile as it enhances your knowledge and skills.

Don't believe me? Try these features on for size:

• Reliable NCLEX preparation guidelines and hundreds of test-taking hints and strategies
• About 3,000 NCLEX-style questions to test your knowledge in all areas tested on the real exam
• A two-column format with questions on the left and answers and rationales on the right
• All information based on the latest test blueprint.

See? I told you! And that's not all. Look for me and my friends in the margins throughout this book. We'll be there to explain key concepts, provide important hints, and offer reassurance. Oh, and if you don't mind, we'll be spicing up the pages with a bit of humor along the way, to teach and entertain in a way that no other resource can.

I hope you find this book helpful. Best of luck on the exam and throughout your career!

Joy

Part I Surviving the NCLEX®

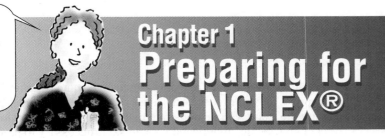

> It may seem obvious, but one of the best ways to prepare for the NCLEX—or any important exam—is to understand exactly what you're facing.

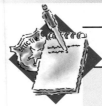

Just the facts

In this chapter, you'll learn:

♦ why you must take the NCLEX®

♦ specific information about taking the exam by computer

♦ strategies to use when answering exam questions

♦ common mistakes and how to avoid them.

NCLEX basics

Passing the National Council Licensure Examination (NCLEX®) is an important landmark in your career as a nurse. The first step on your way to passing the NCLEX exam is to understand what it is and how it's administered.

> Preparing for your licensing exam is a key step in your nursing career.

NCLEX structure

The NCLEX is a test written by nurses who, like most of your nursing instructors, have a master's degree and clinical expertise in a particular area. Only one small difference distinguishes nurses who write NCLEX questions: they're trained to write questions in a style particular to the NCLEX.

If you've completed an accredited nursing program, you've already taken numerous tests written by nurses with backgrounds and experiences similar to those of the nurses who write for this exam. The test-taking experience you've already gained will help you pass the exam. So your review should be just that—a review.

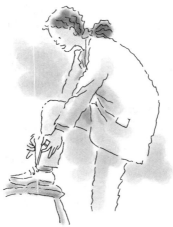

What's the point?

The exam is designed for one purpose: to determine whether it's appropriate for you to receive a license to practice as a nurse. By passing the exam, you demonstrate that you possess the minimum level of knowledge, understanding, and skills necessary to practice nursing safely.

Mix 'em up

In nursing school, you probably took courses organized according to the medical model. Courses were separated into such subjects as medical-surgical, pediatric, maternal-neonatal, and psychiatric nursing. In contrast, the NCLEX is integrated, meaning that different subjects are mixed together.

As you answer NCLEX questions, you may encounter patients in any stage of life, from neonatal to geriatric. These patients—*clients,* in NCLEX lingo—may be of any background, may be completely well or extremely ill, and may have any of various disorders.

Client needs, front and center

The exam draws questions from four categories of client needs that were developed by the National Council of State Boards of Nursing (NCSBN), the organization that sponsors and manages the exam. *Client needs categories* ensure that many topics appear on every examination.

The NCSBN developed client needs categories after conducting a work-study analysis of new nurses. All aspects of nursing care observed in the study were broken down into four categories. Two categories were broken down further into subcategories. (See *Client needs categories.*)

The whole kit and caboodle

The categories and subcategories are used to develop the exam's *test plan,* the content guidelines for the distribution of test questions. Question-writers and the people who put the examination together use the test plan and client needs categories to make sure that a full spectrum of nursing content is covered in the exam. Client needs categories appear in most exam review and question-and-answer books, including this one.

Now you see 'em, now you don't

As a test-taker, you don't have to concern yourself with client needs categories. You'll see these categories for each question and answer in this book, but they'll be invisible on the actual exam.

Client needs categories

Each question on the NCLEX is assigned a category based on client needs. This chart lists client needs categories and subcategories and the percentages of each type of question that appear on the examination.

Category	Subcategories	Percentage of NCLEX questions
Safe, effective care environment	Coordinated care	12% to 18%
	Safety and infection control	8% to 14%
Health promotion and maintenance	—	7% to 13%
Psychosocial integrity	—	8% to 14%
Physiological integrity	Basic care and comfort	11% to 17%
	Pharmacological therapies	9% to 15%
	Reduction of risk potential	10% to 16%
	Physiological adaptation	11% to 17%

Testing by computer

Like many standardized tests today, the exam is administered by computer. That means you won't be filling in empty circles, sharpening pencils, or erasing frantically. It also means that you must become familiar with computer tests if you aren't already. Fortunately, the skills required to take the exam on a computer are simple enough to allow you to focus on the questions, not the keyboard.

Q&A

Depending on the question format, when you take the test, you'll be presented with a question and four or more possible answers, a blank space in which to enter your answer, a figure on which you must click to select the correct area, a series of charts or exhibits to view in order to select the correct response, or items you must prioritize by dragging and dropping them in place.

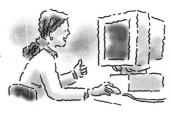

You're reacting to me!

Feeling smart? Think hard!

The exam is a *computer-adaptive test*. This means that the computer reacts to your answers, supplying more difficult questions if you answer correctly and slightly easier questions if you answer incorrectly. Each test is thus uniquely adapted to the individual test-taker.

Onscreen calculations

During the test you may use an onscreen calculator to calculate medication dosages. You'll be shown how to use the calculator during the tutorial before the test begins.

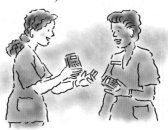

We passed the exam and we're still using calculators!

There's no going back

When you take the exam, the computer will show you only one question at a time on the screen. Take a reasonable amount of time to answer each question. After your answer is recorded, you can't go back to review the question or to change your answer. You can't skip a question either—they must all be answered.

A matter of time

You have a great deal of flexibility with the time you spend on individual questions. The examination lasts a maximum of 5 hours, however, so don't waste time. If you fail to answer a set number of questions within 5 hours, the computer will determine that you lack minimum competency.

Time is of the essence

The 5-hour period includes a brief tutorial, two scheduled optional breaks, and any unscheduled breaks you may take. The computer will alert you to the first optional break at 2 hours into the exam and the second at 3½ hours into the exam.

Most students have plenty of time to complete the test, so take as much time as you need to get the answer right without wasting time. Keep moving at a decent pace to help you maintain concentration, but don't forget to take your allotted breaks.

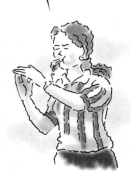

Time out! The student calls a 10-minute rest period. Time remaining…

Difficult items = Good news

If you find as you progress through the test that the questions seem to be increasingly difficult, it's a good sign. The more questions you answer correctly, the more difficult the questions become.

Some students, however, knowing that questions get progressively harder, focus on the degree of difficulty of subsequent questions to try to figure out if they're answering questions correctly. Avoid the temptation to do this because it may get you off track. Stay focused on selecting the best answer for each question that's put before you.

I'm free!

The computer test finishes when one of these events occurs:
• You demonstrate minimum competency, according to the computer program.

• You demonstrate a lack of minimum competency, according to the computer program.
• You've answered the maximum number of questions (205 total questions).
• You've used the maximum time allowed (5 hours).

Unlocking the NCLEX mystery

In 2003, the NCSBN added alternate-format items to the exam. However, most of the questions on the exam are the traditional four-option, multiple-choice items with only one correct answer. Regardless of the type, certain strategies can help you understand and answer any question.

Alternate formats

The first type of alternate-format item is the *multiple-response, multiple-choice question*. Unlike a traditional multiple-choice question, each multiple-response, multiple-choice question can have more than one correct answer for every question and it may contain more than four possible answer options. You'll recognize this type of question because it will ask you to select *all* answers that apply—not just the *best* answer (as may be requested in the more traditional multiple-choice questions). (See *Sample NCLEX questions,* pages 8 and 9.)

All *or* nothing

Keep in mind that, for each multiple-response, multiple-choice question, you *must select one or more than one response* and you *must select all correct answers* for the item to be counted as correct. There's no partial credit in scoring these items.

Don't go blank!

The second type of alternate-format item is the *fill-in-the-blank question*. These questions require you to provide the answer yourself, rather than select it from a list of options. For these questions, you must perform a calculation and type your answer (a number, without any words, commas, or spaces) in the blank space provided after the question.

Drag and drop

Another type of alternate-format item is the *drag-and-drop question*. This type of question will present you with a list of options that require you to click and drag each item into the correct ascending order or sequence. You must use all the options.

Sample NCLEX questions

Sometimes, getting used to the format is as important as knowing the material. Try your hand at these sample questions and you'll have a leg up when you take the real test!

Sample four-option, multiple-choice question

A client's arterial blood gas (ABG) results are as follows: pH, 7.16; $Paco_2$, 80 mm Hg; Pao_2, 46 mm Hg; HCO_3^-, 24 mEq/L; Sao_2, 81%. This ABG result represents which condition?

1. Metabolic acidosis
2. Metabolic alkalosis
3. Respiratory acidosis
4. Respiratory alkalosis

   Correct answer: 3

Sample multiple-response, multiple-choice question

The nurse is caring for a 45-year-old married woman who has undergone hemicolectomy for colon cancer. The woman has two children. Which concepts about families should the nurse keep in mind when providing care for this client? Select all that apply:

1. Illness in one family member can affect all members.
2. Family roles don't change because of illness.
3. A family member may have more than one role at a time in the family.
4. Children typically aren't affected by adult illness.
5. The effects of an illness on a family depend on the stage of the family's life cycle.
6. Changes in sleeping and eating patterns may be signs of stress in a family.

   Correct answer: 1, 3, 5, 6

Sample "hot-spot" question

An elderly client has a history of aortic stenosis. Identify the area where the nurse should place the stethoscope to best hear the murmur.

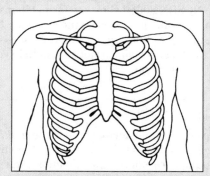

Correct answer:

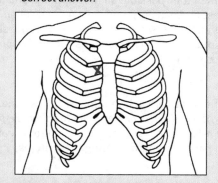

Sample fill-in-the-blank calculation question

An infant who weighs 8 kg is to receive ampicillin (Omnipen) 25 mg/kg I.V. every 6 hours. How many milligrams should the nurse administer per dose? Record your answer using a whole number.

_____ mg

   Correct answer: 200

Sample NCLEX questions (continued)

Sample drag-and-drop question

When teaching an antepartum client about the passage of the fetus through the birth canal during labor, the nurse describes the cardinal mechanisms of labor. Place these events in ascending chronological order. Use all the options.

Unordered options

1. Flexion
2. External rotation
3. Descent
4. Expulsion
5. Internal rotation
6. Extension

Correct answer:

Ordered options

3. Descent
1. Flexion
5. Internal rotation
6. Extension
2. External rotation
4. Expulsion

Sample chart/exhibit question

A preschooler is being admitted to the hospital and isolation precautions need to be implemented. Based on the progress note below, which isolation precautions would be used for this client?

Progress notes

11/8/08 1100	5-year-old with varicella admitted with high fever, dehydration, and pruritic rash on face and trunk with lesions in all stages. See graphic record for vital signs. I.V. started in ⒧ arm. Isolation precautions instituted. ———— ———— J. Trump, RN

☐ **1.** Standard precautions

☐ **2.** Airborne precautions

☐ **3.** Droplet precautions

☐ **4.** Contact precautions

Correct answer: 2

Master that mouse!

The fourth type of alternate-format item is a question that asks you to identify an area on an illustration or graphic. For these so-called *"hot-spot" questions*, the computerized exam will ask you to place your cursor and click over the correct area on an illustration. Try to be as precise as possible when marking the location. As with the fill-in-the-blank questions, the identification questions on the computerized exam may require extremely precise answers for them to be considered correct.

Show me the facts!

The fifth type of alternate-format item is the *chart/exhibit* format. Here you'll be given a problem, then a series of small screens containing additional information you'll need in order to answer the question. By clicking on the Tab button, you can access each screen in turn. Your answer can then be chosen from four multiple-choice answer options.

The standard is still the standard

The NCSBN hasn't yet established a percentage of alternate-format items to be administered to each candidate. In fact, your exam may contain only one alternate-format item. So relax; the standard, four-option, multiple-choice format questions make up most of the test.

Understanding the question

Exam questions are commonly lengthy. As a result, it's easy to become overloaded with information. To focus on the question and avoid becoming overwhelmed, apply these proven strategies for answering the exam questions:
• Determine what the question is asking.
• Determine relevant facts about the client.
• Rephrase the question in your mind.
• Choose the best option(s) or answer to enter.

Determine what the question is asking

Read the question twice. If the answer isn't apparent, rephrase the question in simpler, more personal terms. Breaking down the question into easier, less intimidating terms may help you focus more accurately on the correct answer.

Give it a try

For example, a question might be, "A 20-year-old female with cystic fibrosis has a small-bowel obstruction. She's admitted to the medical-surgical unit for treatment, which involves placement of an intestinal tube connected to intermittent suction. Which nursing intervention would be most effective for this client?"

The options for this question—each numbered from 1 to 4—may include:
1. Record intake and output accurately.
2. Turn the client from side to side, as prescribed.
3. Give the client sips of water to facilitate passage of the tube through the bowel.
4. Add antacids to the intestinal tube to reduce bowel reaction.

Hocus, focus on the question

Read the question again, ignoring all details except what's being asked. Focus on the last line of the question. It asks you to select the *most* effective nursing intervention for this client.

> Focusing on what the question is really asking can help you choose the correct answer.

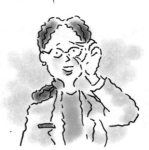

Determine what facts about the client are relevant

Next, sort out the relevant client information. Start by asking whether the information provided about the client is *not* relevant. For instance, do you need to know that the client has been admitted to the medical-surgical unit? Probably not; her care plan won't be affected by her location in the hospital.

Determine what you *do* know about the client. In the example, you know that:
- she's a 20-year-old female
- she has a small-bowel obstruction
- she has cystic fibrosis (a fact that may be relevant).

Rephrase the question

After you've determined relevant information about the client and the question being asked, consider rephrasing the question to make it more clear. Eliminate jargon, and put the question in simpler, more personal terms.

Here's how you might rephrase the question in the example: "My client has a small-bowel obstruction. She requires placement of an intestinal tube, which will be connected to intermittent suction. She's 20 years old and has a history of cystic fibrosis. Which nursing intervention would be most effective for this client?"

Choose the best option

Armed with all the information you now have, it's time to select an option. You know that the client will have an intestinal tube placed and connected to intermittent suction. You know that while the tube is being advanced into the intestine, the client will lie quietly on her right side for about 2 hours to promote the tube's passage, eliminating option 2. You also know that nothing but normal saline solution should be instilled into the intestinal tube, a fact that eliminates option 4. In addition, you know it isn't likely that the client will be permitted anything by mouth, eliminating option 3.

By process of elimination, option 1, *Record intake and output accurately,* is the best option because monitoring fluid balance is the *most* effective nursing intervention for this client.

> Don't spend your time chasing after irrelevant facts and details. Determine what's most essential to the client's situation and proceed from there.

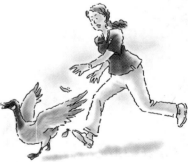

When more than one option seems correct

What if you encounter a standard-format question for which two or more options appear correct? Such questions are fairly common and usually include a key word or phrase that can help point you in the right direction. Reread the question carefully, and look for one of these commonly used words or phrases:
- most appropriate

- best
- first
- last
- next
- most helpful
- most suitable.

After eliminating any obviously incorrect options, begin prioritizing or ranking the remaining choices with the key word in mind. Then choose the best or most appropriate answer from the remaining ones, keeping in mind that only one answer can be correct.

Note that key terms and phrases have been highlighted throughout the question-and-answer section appearing later in this book. Check out the underlined words and phrases that serve as hints for you.

Key strategies

Regardless of the type of question, four key strategies will help you determine the correct answer for each question. (See *Strategies for success.*) These strategies are:

- considering the nursing process
- referring to Maslow's hierarchy of needs
- reviewing patient safety
- reflecting on principles of therapeutic communication.

Strategies for success

Keeping a few main strategies in mind as you answer each exam question can help ensure greater success. These four strategies are critical for answering exam questions correctly:

- If the question asks what you should do in a situation, use the nursing process to determine which step in the process would be next.
- If the question asks what the client needs, use Maslow's hierarchy to determine which need to address first.
- If the question indicates that the client doesn't have an urgent physiologic need, focus on the patient's safety.
- If the question involves communicating with a patient, use the principles of therapeutic communication.

Nursing process

One of the ways to answer a question is to apply the nursing process. Steps in the nursing process include:

- data collection
- planning
- implementation
- evaluation.

First things first

The nursing process may provide insights that help you analyze a question. According to the nursing process, data collection comes before planning, which comes before implementation, which comes before evaluation.

You're halfway to the correct answer when you encounter a four-option, multiple-choice question that asks you to collect data and then provides two data collection options and two implementation options. You can immediately eliminate the implementation options, which then gives you, at worst, a 50-50 chance of selecting the correct answer. Use this sample question to apply the nursing process:

A client returns from an endoscopic procedure during which he was sedated. Before offering the client food, which action should the nurse take?
1. Monitor the client's respiratory status.
2. Check the client's gag reflex.
3. Place the client in a side-lying position.
4. Have the client drink a few sips of water.

Collect data before intervening

According to the nursing process, the nurse must collect client data before performing an intervention. Does the question indicate that data has been properly collected? No, it doesn't. Therefore, you can eliminate options 3 and 4 because they're both interventions.

That leaves options 1 and 2, both of which demonstrate data collection. Your nursing knowledge should tell you the correct answer—in this case, option 2. The sedation required for an endoscopic procedure may impair the client's gag reflex, so you would check gag reflex before giving food to the client to reduce the risk of aspiration and airway obstruction.

Final elimination

Why not select option 1, monitoring the client's respiratory status? You might select this option, but the question is specifically asking about offering the client food, an action that wouldn't be taken if the client's respiratory status was at all compromised. In this case, you're making a judgment based on the phrase, "Before offering the client food." If the question was trying to test your knowledge of respiratory depression following an endoscopic procedure, it probably wouldn't mention a function—such as giving food to a client—that clearly occurs only after the client's respiratory status has been stabilized.

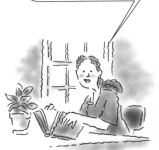

Say it 1,000 times: Studying is fun... studying is fun... studying is fun...

Maslow's hierarchy

Knowledge of Maslow's hierarchy of needs can be a vital tool for establishing priorities on the examination. Maslow's theory states that physiologic needs are the most basic human needs of all. Only after physiologic needs have been met can safety concerns be addressed. Only after safety concerns are met can concerns involving love and belonging be addressed, and so forth. Apply the principles of Maslow's hierarchy of needs to this sample question:

A client complains of severe pain 2 days after surgery. Which action should the nurse perform first?
1. Offer reassurance to the client that he'll feel less pain tomorrow.
2. Allow the client time to verbalize his feelings.
3. Check the client's vital signs.

4. Administer an analgesic.

Phys before psych

In this example, two of the options—3 and 4—address physiologic needs. Options 1 and 2 address psychosocial concerns. According to Maslow, physiologic needs must be met before psychosocial needs, so you can eliminate options 1 and 2.

Final elimination

Now, use your nursing knowledge to choose the best answer from the two remaining options. In this case, option 3 is correct because the client's vital signs should be checked before administering an analgesic (data collection before intervention). When prioritizing according to Maslow's hierarchy, remember your ABCs—airway, breathing, circulation—to help you further prioritize. Check for a patent airway before addressing breathing. Check breathing before checking the health of the cardiovascular system.

One caveat...

Just because an option appears on the exam doesn't mean it's a viable choice for the client referred to in the question. Always examine your choice in light of your knowledge and experience. Ask yourself, "Does this choice make sense for this client?" Allow yourself to eliminate choices—even ones that might normally take priority—if they don't make sense for a particular client's situation.

Client safety

Client safety takes a high priority on the exam.

As you might expect, client safety takes high priority on the exam. You'll encounter many questions that can be answered by asking yourself, "Which answer will best ensure the safety of this client?" Use client safety criteria for situations involving laboratory values, drug administration, or nursing care procedures.

Client 1st, equipment 2nd

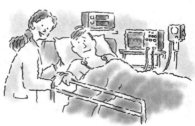

You may encounter a question in which some options address the client and others address the equipment. When in doubt, select an option relating to the client; never place equipment before a client.

For instance, suppose a question asks what the nurse should do first when entering a client's room where an infusion pump alarm is sounding. If two options deal with the infusion pump, one with the infusion tubing, and another with the client's catheter insertion site, select the one relating to the client's catheter insertion site. Always check the client first; the equipment can wait.

Therapeutic communication

Some exam questions focus on the nurse's ability to communicate effectively with the client. Therapeutic communication incorporates verbal or nonverbal responses and involves:

- listening to the client
- understanding the client's needs
- promoting clarification and insight about the client's condition.

Room for improvement

Like other exam questions, those dealing with therapeutic communication require choosing the best response. First, eliminate options that indicate the use of poor therapeutic communication techniques, such as those in which the nurse:

- tells the client what to do without regard for the client's feelings or desires (the "do this" response)
- asks a question that can be answered "yes" or "no," or with another one-syllable response
- seeks reasons for the client's behavior
- implies disapproval of the client's behavior
- offers false reassurances
- attempts to interpret the client's behavior rather than allowing the client to verbalize his own feelings
- offers a response that focuses on the nurse, not the client.

Ah, that's better!

When answering exam questions, look for responses that:

- allow the client time to think and reflect
- encourage the client to talk
- encourage the client to describe a particular experience
- reflect that the nurse has listened to the client such as through paraphrasing the client's response.

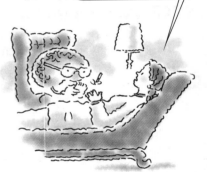

So you're saying that the correct response will likely be one that encourages talking and sharing feelings? I think I've had a major breakthrough, doctor.

Avoiding pitfalls

Even the most knowledgeable students can get tripped up on certain exam questions. (See *A tricky question*, page 16.) Students commonly cite three areas that can be difficult for unwary test-takers:

  knowing the difference between NCLEX and the "real world"

  delegating care

  knowing laboratory values.

A tricky question

The exam occasionally asks a particular kind of question called the "further teaching" question, which involves client-teaching situations. These questions can be tricky. You'll have to choose the response that suggests that the client hasn't learned the correct information. Here's an example:

A client undergoes a total hip replacement. Which statement by the client indicates that he requires further teaching?

1. "I'll need to keep several pillows between my legs at night."
2. "I'll need to remember not to cross my legs. It's such a bad habit."
3. "The occupational therapist is showing me how to use a 'sock puller' to help me get dressed."
4. "I don't know if I'll be able to get off that low toilet seat at home by myself."

The answer you should choose here is option 4 because it indicates that the client has a poor understanding of the precautions required after a total hip replacement and that he needs further teaching. Remember: If you see the phrase *further teaching* or *further instruction,* you're looking for a wrong answer by the client.

NCLEX versus the real world

Some students who take the exam have extensive practical experience in health care. For example, many test-takers have worked as nursing assistants. In that capacity, test-takers may have been exposed to less than optimum clinical practice and may carry those experiences over to the exam.

However, the NCLEX is a textbook examination—not a test of clinical skills. Take the exam with the understanding that what happens in the real world may differ from what the exam and your nursing school say should happen.

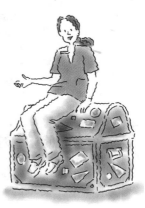

Remember, this is an exam, not the real world.

Don't take shortcuts

If you've had practical experience in health care, you may know a quicker way to perform a procedure or tricks to get by when you don't have the right equipment. Situations such as staff shortages may force you to improvise. On the exam, such scenarios can lead to trouble. Always check your practical experiences against textbook nursing care, taking care to select the response that follows the textbook.

Delegating care

On the exam, you may encounter questions that assess your ability to delegate care. Delegating care involves coordinating the efforts of other health care workers to provide effective care for your client. On the exam, you may be asked to assign duties to:
• nursing assistants

• other support staff.

In addition, you'll be asked to decide when to notify a registered nurse, a physician, a social worker, or another hospital staff member. In each case, you'll have to decide when, where, and how to delegate.

Should's and shouldn'ts

As a general rule, it's okay to delegate actions that involve stable clients or standard, unchanging procedures. Bathing, feeding, dressing, and transferring clients are examples of procedures that can be delegated.

Be careful not to delegate complicated or complex activities. In addition, don't delegate activities that involve data collection, evaluation, or your own nursing judgment. On the exam and in the real world, these duties fall squarely on your shoulders. Make sure that you take primary responsibility for collecting client data and evaluating the client and for making decisions about the client's care. Never hand off those responsibilities to someone with less training.

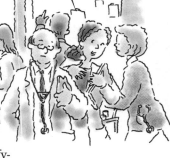

You can delegate tasks or refer to the physician, but remember that this exam wants to see the nurse at work!

Calling in reinforcements

Deciding when to notify a registered nurse, a physician, a social worker, or another hospital staff member is an important element of nursing care. On the exam, however, choices that involve notifying the physicians are usually incorrect. Remember that this exam wants to see you, the nurse, at work.

If you're sure the correct answer is to notify the physician, make sure that the client's safety has been addressed before notifying a physician or another staff member. On the exam, the client's safety has a higher priority than notifying other health care providers.

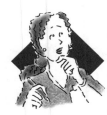

Quick quiz

1. Because the exam is a computer-adaptive test, the computer provides questions according to:

1. the number of questions you answer correctly.
2. a random selection of questions in specific client needs categories.
3. a strict pattern established after studying the responses of new nurses.
4. a standardized order established for the exam given on that particular date.

Answer: 1. The exam is a computer-adaptive test, meaning that the computer reacts to the answers you give, supplying more difficult questions if you answer correctly and slightly easier questions if you answer incorrectly.

2.   According to the nursing process, which of the following should be a nurse's first priority?
1.   Developing a care plan for a newly admitted client
2.   Following a physician's order to administer an antibiotic
3.   Repositioning a patient to prevent skin breakdown
4.   Monitoring a postoperative client's respiratory status

Answer: 4. According to the nursing process, a nurse's first priority is to collect client data before performing interventions (option 2 and 3) or planning (option 1).

3.   When answering an exam question that focuses on the nurse's ability to communicate with the client, which type of communication is involved?
1.   Verbal only
2.   Therapeutic
3.   Nonverbal only
4.   Nontherapeutic

Answer: 2. Therapeutic communication incorporates verbal and nonverbal responses and involves listening to the client.

4.   When answering an exam question, which client priority should the nurse take care of first?
1.   Notifying the physician
2.   Addressing the client's safety
3.   Calling the social worker
4.   Ensuring client privacy

Answer: 2. Make sure the client's safety has been addressed before notifying the physician or another staff member, and before attending to matters of privacy. On the exam, the client's safety has a higher priority than these other options.

Scoring

☆☆☆   If you answered all four questions correctly, wowsa, wowsa, wowsa! You're ready for the exam!

☆☆   If you answered three questions correctly, super! You've got a handle on the exam!

☆   If you answered fewer than three questions correctly, take it easy, kiddo! By the time you finish working with this book, you'll be so ready for the exam that you won't be able to *stand* it. *That's* how ready you'll be. Promise.

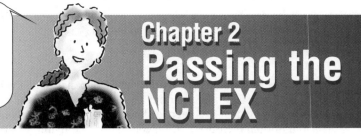

Pssst! Here's my secret formula for passing the NCLEX: Develop a creative study plan that includes sufficient scheduled study time, get plenty of rest and regular exercise, and believe in yourself!

Chapter 2
Passing the NCLEX

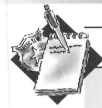

Just the facts

In this chapter, you'll learn:

♦ how to properly prepare for the NCLEX

♦ tips to maintain concentration during difficult study times

♦ how to make more effective use of your time

♦ creative studying strategies to enhance your learning

♦ the advantages of taking NCLEX practice tests.

Study preparations

If you're like most people preparing to take the NCLEX, you're probably feeling nervous, anxious, or concerned. Keep in mind that most test-takers pass the first time around.

Passing the test won't happen by accident, however; you'll need to prepare carefully and efficiently. To help jump-start your preparations:

• determine your strengths and weaknesses
• create a study schedule
• set realistic goals
• find an effective study space
• find creative ways to study
• think positively.

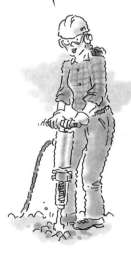

Studying for the exam can seem overwhelming until you break it down into manageable parts.

Strengths and weaknesses

Most students recognize that, even at the end of their nursing studies, they know more about some topics than others. Because the exam covers a broad range of material, you should make some decisions about how intensively you'll review each topic.

Making a list...

Base those decisions on a list. Divide a sheet of paper in half vertically. On one side, list topics you think you know well. On the other side, list topics you feel less secure about. Pay no attention if one side is longer than the other. When you're done studying, you'll feel strong in every area.

...checking it twice

To make sure that your list reflects a comprehensive view of all the areas you studied in school, look at the contents page in the front of this book. For each topic listed, place it in the "know well" column or "needs review" column. Separating content areas this way shows immediately which topics need less or more study time.

Scheduling study time

Most people can identify a period of the day when they feel most alert; that's their best time to study. If you feel most alert and energized in the morning, for example, set aside sections of time in the morning for topics that need a lot of review. Then use the evening to study topics for which you just need some refreshing. The opposite is true as well; if you're more alert in the evening, study difficult topics at that time.

The great countdown

Set up a basic schedule for studying. Using a calendar or organizer, determine how much time remains before you take the exam. (See *2 to 3 months before the NCLEX*.) Fill in the remaining days with specific times and topics to be studied. For example, you might schedule the respiratory system on a Tuesday morning and the GI system that afternoon. Remember to schedule difficult topics during your most alert times.

Keep in mind that you shouldn't fill each day with studying. Be realistic and set aside time for normal activities. Try to allow ample study time before the exam and then stick to the schedule.

Realistic goals

Part of creating a schedule means setting realistic goals. You no doubt studied a great deal in nursing school, and by now you have a sense of your own capabilities. Ask yourself, "How much can I cover in a day?" Set that amount of time aside and then stay on task. You'll feel better about yourself—and your chances of passing the exam—when you meet your goals regularly.

---

2 to 3 months before the NCLEX

With 2 to 3 months remaining before you plan to take the NCLEX examination, take these steps:
• Establish a study schedule. Set aside ample time to study, but also leave time for social activities, exercise, family and personal responsibilities, and other matters.
• Become knowledgeable about the exam, its content, the types of questions it asks, and the testing format.
• Begin studying your notes, texts, and other study materials.
• Answer some exam practice questions to help you identify strengths and weaknesses as well as to become familiar with NCLEX-style questions.

Optimum study time

When you were creating your schedule, you might have asked yourself, "How long should I study? One hour at a stretch? Two hours? Three?" To make the best use of your study time, you'll need to know what works best for you.

From beginning to end

Experts are divided about the optimum length of study time. Some say you should study no more than 1 hour at a time several times per day. Their reasoning: You remember the material you study at the beginning and end of a session best, and tend to remember less material studied in the middle of the session.

Other experts say you should hold longer study sessions because you lose time in the beginning, when you're just getting warmed up, and again at the end, when you're cooling down. Therefore, say those experts, a long, concentrated study period will allow you to cover more material.

To thine own self be true

So what's the answer? It doesn't matter as long as you determine what's best for you. At the beginning of your licensing exam study schedule, try study periods of varying lengths. Pay close attention to those that seem more successful.

Remember that you're a trained nurse who's competent at collecting data. Think of yourself as a client, and collect data about your own progress. Then implement the strategy that works best for you.

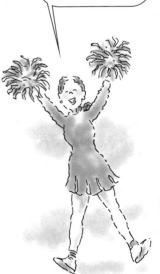

Approach your studying with enthusiasm, sincerity, and determination. It also helps to be awake!

Study space

Find a space conducive to effective learning. Whatever you do, don't study with a television or loud radio on in the room. Instead, find an inviting study space that:
• is located in a quiet, convenient place, away from normal traffic patterns
• contains a solid chair that encourages good posture (Avoid studying in bed; you'll be more likely to fall asleep and not accomplish your goals.)
• has comfortable, soft lighting with which you can see clearly without eye strain
• has a temperature between 65° and 70° F
• contains flowers or green plants, familiar photos or paintings, and easy access to soft, instrumental background music.

Accentuate the positive

Consider taping positive messages around your study space. Make signs with words of encouragement, such as, "You can do it!" "Keep studying!" and "Remember the goal!" These upbeat messages can help keep you going when your attention begins to waver.

Maintaining concentration

When you're faced with reviewing the amount of information covered by the exam, it's easy to become distracted and lose your concentration. When you lose concentration, you make less effective use of valuable study time. To stay focused, keep these tips in mind:

• Alternate the order of the subjects you study during the day to add variety. Try alternating between topics you find most interesting and those you find least interesting.
• Approach your studying with enthusiasm, sincerity, and determination.
• After you've decided to study, begin immediately. Don't let anything interfere with your thought processes after you've begun.
• Concentrate on accomplishing one task at a time, to the exclusion of everything else.
• Don't try to do two things at once, such as studying and watching television or conversing with friends.
• Work continuously without interruption for a while, but don't study for such a long period that the whole experience becomes grueling or boring.
• Allow time for periodic breaks to give yourself a change of pace. Use these breaks to ease your transition into studying a new topic.
• When studying in the evening, wind down from your studies slowly. Don't progress directly from studying to sleeping.

Taking care of yourself

Maintaining physical and mental health is critical for success in taking the exam. Never neglect your physical and mental well-being in favor of longer study hours. (See *4 to 6 weeks before the NCLEX.*)

A few simple rules

You can increase your likelihood of passing the test by following these simple health rules:
• Get plenty of rest. You can't think deeply or concentrate for long periods when you're tired.
• Eat nutritious meals. Maintaining your energy level is impossible when you're undernourished.
• Exercise regularly. Regular exercise helps you work harder and think more clearly. As a result,

---

4 to 6 weeks before the NCLEX

With 4 to 6 weeks remaining before your planned NCLEX examination date, take these steps:
• Focus on areas of weakness. That way, you'll have time to review these areas again before the test date.
• Find a study partner or form a study group.
• Take a practice test to gauge your skill level early.
• Take time to eat, sleep, exercise, and socialize to avoid burnout.

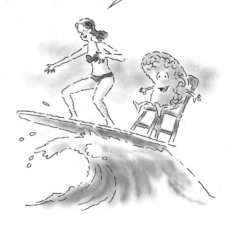

Kowabonga! Regular exercise helps you work harder and think more clearly.

you'll study more efficiently and increase the likelihood of your success.

Memory powers, activate!

Active studying can renew your powers of concentration. If you're having trouble concentrating but would rather push through than take a break, try making your studying more active by reading aloud. By reading review material aloud to yourself, you're engaging your ears as well as your eyes—and making studying a more active process. Hearing the material aloud also fosters memory and subsequent recall.

You can also rewrite in your own words a few of the more difficult concepts you're reviewing. Explaining these concepts in writing forces you to think through the material and can jump-start your memory.

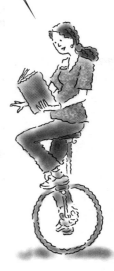

Studying getting dull? Get creative and liven it up.

Creative studying

Even when you study in a perfect study space and concentrate better than ever, studying for the exam can get a little, well, dull. Even people with terrific study habits occasionally feel bored or sluggish. That's why it's important to have some creative tricks in your study bag to liven up your studying during these down times.

Creative studying doesn't have to be hard work. It simply involves making efforts to alter your study habits a bit. Some techniques that might help include making use of short study sessions, studying with a partner or group, and creating flash cards or other audiovisual study tools.

Quick study

We all have spaces in our day that might otherwise be dead time. (See *1 week before the NCLEX.*) These are perfect times to review for the exam but not to cover new material because, by the time you get deep into new material, your time will be over. Always keep some flash cards or a small notebook handy for situations when you have a few extra minutes.

You'll be amazed how many short sessions you can find in a day and how much you can review in 5 minutes. These occasions offer short stretches of time you can use for studying:

• eating breakfast
• waiting for or riding on a train or bus
• waiting in line at the bank, post office, bookstore, or other places.

1 week before the NCLEX

With 1 week remaining before the NCLEX examination, take these steps:
• Take a review test to measure your progress.
• Record key ideas and principles on note cards or audiotapes.
• Rest, eat well, and avoid thinking about the examination during non-study times.
• Treat yourself to one special event. You've been working hard, and you deserve it!

Study partners

Studying with a partner or group of students can be an excellent way to energize your studying. Working with a partner allows you to test each other on the material and can provide a welcome break from solitary studying. Your partner also can give you encouragement and motivation to keep you moving toward your goal. Perhaps most important, working with a partner can provide a welcome break from solitary studying.

You can do it!

You are such a great motivator!

The perfect partner

Exercise some care when choosing a study partner or assembling a study group. A partner who doesn't fit your needs won't help you make the most of your study time. Look for a partner who:
• possesses similar goals. For example, someone taking the exam at approximately the same date who feels the same sense of urgency as you do might make an excellent partner.
• possesses roughly the same level of knowledge. Tutoring someone can sometimes help you learn, but partnering should be give-and-take so both partners can gain knowledge.
• can study without excess chatting or interruptions. Socializing is an important part of creative study but, remember, you still have to pass the exam—so stay serious!

Audiovisual tools

Using CD-ROMs, flash cards, and other audiovisual tools fosters retention and makes learning and reviewing fun.

CD-ROM—it's the bomb!

CD-ROMs provide an audiovisual format that allows the learner to apply her knowledge and receive immediate feedback. CD-ROMs present nursing information and case studies and simulate clinical situations through an interactive medium. These products are available on many nursing topics. You'll even find CD-ROMs that specifically address exam preparation and include sample test questions.

Better late than never

If you weren't required to use CD-ROMs during your nursing education, this is a great time to start. Check the library of your nursing school for CD-ROMs to borrow or use on the premises, or purchase your own online or at your local bookstore or school's bookstore.

Flash Gordon? No, it's Flash Card!

Flash cards can provide you with an excellent study tool. The process of writing material on a flash card will help you remember it. In addition, flash cards are small and portable, making them perfect for those 5-minute slivers of time that show up during the day.

Creating a flash card should be fun. Use magic markers, highlighters, and other colorful tools to make them visually stimulating. The more effort you put into creating your flash cards, the better you'll remember the material written on the cards.

Picture this!

Flowcharts, drawings, diagrams, and other image-oriented study aids can also help you learn material more effectively. Substituting images for text can be a great way to give your eyes a break and recharge your brain. Remember to use vivid colors to make your creations visually engaging.

The ears have it

If you learn more effectively when you hear information rather than see it, consider recording key ideas using a handheld tape recorder. Recording information helps promote memory because you say the information aloud when taping and then listen to it when playing it back. Like flash cards, tapes are portable and perfect for those short study periods during the day. (See *The day before the NCLEX*.)

Check your attitude

Positive thinking is more than a cliché for a greeting card; it's a bonafide technique for enhancing your chances of success.

Saying is believing

As the clock ticks down to that all-important moment, think about all the hard work you've done and all the material you've learned. Tell yourself that you're ready and that you can do it. You might even want to plan a post-examination celebration. Giving yourself some well-deserved words of encouragement will help you walk into the testing room with a positive, confident attitude.

> ### The day before the NCLEX
>
> With 1 day before the NCLEX examination, take these steps:
> • Drive to the test site, review traffic patterns, and find out where to park. If your route to the test site takes you through heavy traffic or if you're expecting bad weather, set aside extra time to ensure prompt arrival.
> • Do something relaxing during the day.
> • Rest, eat well, and avoid dwelling on the exam during nonstudy periods.
> • Call a supportive friend or relative for some last-minute words of encouragement.
> • Avoid classmates who may be nervous or excessively jittery about the exam because they'll only increase your anxiety.

Practice questions

Practice questions should be an important part of your study strategy. They can improve your studying by helping you review material and familiarize yourself with the exact style of questions you'll encounter on the exam.

Never put off 'til tomorrow

Consider working through some practice questions as soon as you begin studying for the exam. For example, you might try a half-dozen questions from each chapter in this book.

If you do well, you probably know the material contained in that chapter fairly well and can spend less time reviewing that particular topic. If you have trouble with the questions, spend extra study time on that topic.

I'm getting there

Practice questions also can provide an excellent means of marking your progress. Don't worry if you have trouble answering the first few practice questions you try; you'll need time to adjust to the way the questions are asked. Eventually you'll become accustomed to the question format and you'll begin to focus more on the questions themselves.

If you make practice questions a regular part of your study regimen, you'll be able to notice areas in which you're improving. You can then adjust your study time accordingly.

Practice makes perfect

As you near the examination date, continue to do practice questions, but also set aside time to take an entire NCLEX practice test. (We've included four at the back of this book.) That way, you'll know exactly what to expect. The more you know ahead of time, the better you're likely to do on the exam.

Note that 85 questions is the minimum number of questions you'll be asked on the actual examination. By tackling larger practice tests, you'll increase your confidence, build test-taking endurance, and strengthen the concentration skills that enable you to succeed on the exam. (See *The day of the NCLEX*.)

The day of the NCLEX

On the day of the NCLEX examination, take these steps:
- Get up early.
- Wear comfortable clothes, preferably with layers, so you can adjust to fit the room temperature.
- Leave your house early.
- Arrive at the test site early.
- Avoid looking at your notes as you wait for your test computer.
- Listen carefully to the instructions given before entering the test room.
- Stay confident and positive, and have faith in yourself.

   Good luck!

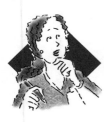

Quick quiz

1. The best time to study is:
1. in the morning.
2. early in the evening.
3. late at night.
4. when you feel most alert and free from distractions.

Answer: 4. Study when you're most alert and free from distractions. If you feel most alert and energized in the morning, for example, set aside sections of time in the morning for topics that need a lot of review.

2. The temperature of the ideal study area should be between:
1. 60º and 65º F.
2. 65º and 70º F.
3. 70º and 75º F.
4. 75º and 80º F.

Answer: 2. The ideal study area has a temperature between 65º and 70º F.

3. To help you maintain concentration during long study periods, recommended study strategies include:
1. studying the topics you find most interesting first, then the topics you find least interesting.
2. studying the topics you find least interesting first, then the topics you find most interesting.
3. alternating the order of the subjects you study during the day.
4. studying topics sequentially, regardless of your interest level.

Answer: 3. Alternating the order of the subjects you study during the day adds variety to your study, helps you remain focused, and makes the most of your study time.

4. When selecting a study partner, choose one who:
1. possesses similar goals as you.
2. is more knowledgeable than you are and able to tutor you on all study material.
3. is highly social and will keep you entertained.
4. isn't as knowledgeable as you are so you can tutor him.

Answer: 1. A partner who doesn't fit your needs won't help you make the most of your study time. Look for a partner who possesses similar goals to yours, possesses about the same level of knowledge as you, and won't spend too much time socializing.

Scoring

☆☆☆   If you answered all four questions correctly, that's *it!* We're calling the testing center right now. You're *ready!*

☆☆   If you answered three questions correctly, outstanding! All you need now is a snack before the test, and you'll be rarin' to go!

☆   If you answered fewer than three questions correctly, fear not. You've got NCLEX *success* written all over your future!

Part II Care of the adult

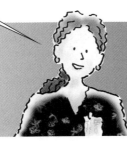

If you'd like to rummage through a Web site dedicated to cardiovascular disorders, check out the American Heart Association's www.americanheart.org. Go for it!

Chapter 3
Cardiovascular disorders

1. Which artery primarily feeds the anterior wall of the heart?
  1. Circumflex artery
  2. Internal mammary artery
  3. Left anterior descending artery
  4. Right coronary artery

2. When do coronary arteries primarily receive blood flow?
  1. During cardiac standstill
  2. During diastole
  3. During expiration
  4. During systole

3. A nurse is screening clients for their risk of developing cardiovascular disease. The nurse should consider at <u>greatest</u> risk the client who's a:
  1. non-Hispanic white male.
  2. non-Hispanic African-American female.
  3. Mexican-American male.
  4. non-Hispanic African-American male.

4. Which condition <u>most commonly</u> results in coronary artery disease (CAD)?
  1. Atherosclerosis
  2. Diabetes mellitus
  3. Myocardial infarction (MI)
  4. Renal failure

5. A 47-year-old male with a family history of premature heart disease is diagnosed with atherosclerosis. The nurse explains that blood flow is impeded through which mechanism?
  1. Plaque obstructing the veins
  2. Plaque obstructing the arteries
  3. Blood clots forming outside the vessel wall
  4. Hardened vessels dilating to allow blood to flow through

CN: Client needs category   CNS: Client needs subcategory   CL: Cognitive level

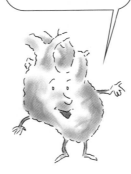

Different arteries supply my different sections with the blood I need to stay healthy.

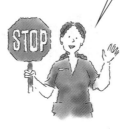

Stop and think! Although all of the answers relate to CAD, only one answer is correct.

1. 3. The left anterior descending artery is the primary source of blood for the anterior wall of the heart. The circumflex artery supplies the lateral wall, the internal mammary artery supplies the breastbone and mammary structures, and the right coronary artery supplies the inferior wall of the heart.
CN: Physiological integrity; CNS: Physiological adaptation; CL: Knowledge

2. 2. Although the coronary arteries may receive a minute portion of blood during systole, most of the blood flow to coronary arteries is supplied during diastole. Blood doesn't flow during cardiac standstill. Breathing patterns are irrelevant to blood flow.
CN: Physiological integrity; CNS: Physiological adaptation; CL: Knowledge

3. 2. A non-Hispanic African-American female has the highest risk of developing cardiovascular disease. A non-Hispanic white male and a non-Hispanic African-American male both have higher risks than the Mexican-American male, who has the lowest risk.
CN: Health promotion and maintenance; CNS: None; CL: Analysis

4. 1. Atherosclerosis, or plaque formation, is the leading cause of CAD. Diabetes mellitus is a risk factor for CAD, but isn't the most common cause. Renal failure doesn't cause CAD, but the two conditions are related. MI is commonly a result of CAD.
CN: Physiological integrity; CNS: Physiological adaptation; CL: Analysis

5. 2. Arteries, not veins, provide coronary blood flow. Atherosclerosis is a direct result of plaque formation in arteries. Hardened vessels can't dilate properly and, therefore, constrict blood flow.
CN: Physiological integrity; CNS: Physiological adaptation; CL: Comprehension

6. Which risk factor for coronary artery disease can be controlled?
1. Advancing age
2. Cigarette smoking
3. Heredity
4. Gender

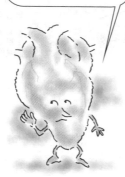

No thanks. I quit smoking years ago.

7. Exceeding which serum total cholesterol level significantly increases the risk of coronary artery disease (CAD)?
1. 100 mg/dl
2. 150 mg/dl
3. 175 mg/dl
4. 200 mg/dl

8. Which action is the <u>first</u> priority of care for a client exhibiting signs and symptoms of coronary artery disease?
1. Decrease anxiety.
2. Enhance myocardial oxygenation.
3. Administer sublingual nitroglycerin.
4. Educate the client about his symptoms.

9. Medical treatment of coronary artery disease (CAD) includes which procedure?
1. Cardiac catheterization
2. Coronary artery bypass surgery
3. Oral medication administration
4. Percutaneous transluminal coronary angioplasty (PTCA)

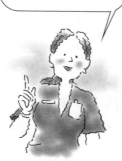

Conservative methods of treatment should always be your first course of action.

10. A diagnostic cardiac catheterization reveals prolonged occlusion of the right coronary artery in a 62-year-old male client. In which area of the heart would this have produced an infarction?
1. Anterior
2. Apical
3. Inferior
4. Lateral

6. 2. Cigarette smoking is a lifestyle change that involves behavior modification. Aging and gender aren't modifiable risk factors for developing coronary artery disease. Heredity refers to our genetic makeup and isn't modifiable at this time.
CN: Physiological integrity; CNS: Reduction of risk potential; CL: Analysis

7. 4. Total cholesterol levels above 200 mg/dl are considered excessive. They require dietary restriction and, perhaps, medication. The other levels listed are all below the nationally accepted levels for cholesterol and carry a lesser risk for CAD.
CN: Physiological integrity; CNS: Reduction of risk potential; CL: Comprehension

8. 2. Enhancing myocardial oxygenation is always the first priority when a client exhibits signs or symptoms of cardiac compromise. Without adequate oxygen, the myocardium suffers damage. Sublingual nitroglycerin dilates the coronary vessels to increase blood flow, but its administration isn't the first priority. Although educating the client and decreasing anxiety are important in care delivery, neither are priorities when a client is compromised.
CN: Physiological integrity; CNS: Physiological adaptation; CL: Application

9. 3. Oral medication administration is a noninvasive, medical treatment for CAD. Cardiac catheterization isn't a treatment, but a diagnostic tool. Coronary artery bypass surgery and PTCA are invasive, surgical treatments.
CN: Physiological integrity; CNS: Physiological adaptation; CL: Analysis

10. 3. The right coronary artery supplies the right ventricle, or the inferior portion of the heart. Therefore, prolonged occlusion could produce an infarction in that area. The right coronary artery doesn't supply the anterior portion (left ventricle), lateral portion (some of the left ventricle and the left atrium), or the apical portion (left ventricle) of the heart.
CN: Physiological integrity; CNS: Physiological adaptation; CL: Analysis

CN: Client needs category   CNS: Client needs subcategory   CL: Cognitive level

11. Which of the following is the <u>most common</u> symptom of myocardial infarction (MI)?
1. Chest pain
2. Dyspnea
3. Edema
4. Palpitations

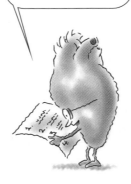

I may experience many symptoms during a heart attack, but which one are you most likely to see?

11. 1. The most common symptom of an MI is chest pain resulting from deprivation of oxygen to the heart. Dyspnea is the second most common symptom, related to an increase in the metabolic needs of the body during an MI. Edema is a later sign of heart failure, commonly seen after an MI. Palpitations may result from reduced cardiac output, producing arrhythmias.

CN: Safe, effective care environment; CNS: Coordinated care; CL: Analysis

12. Which landmark is the correct one for obtaining an apical pulse?
1. Left fifth intercostal space, midaxillary line
2. Left fifth intercostal space, midclavicular line
3. Left second intercostal space, midclavicular line
4. Left seventh intercostal space, midclavicular line

12. 2. The correct landmark for obtaining an apical pulse is the left fifth intercostal space in the midclavicular line. This is the point of maximum impulse and the location of the left ventricle. The left second intercostal space in the midclavicular line is where pulmonic sounds are auscultated. Normally, heart sounds aren't heard in the midaxillary line or the seventh intercostal space in the midclavicular line.

CN: Physiological integrity; CNS: Basic care and comfort; CL: Application

13. Which system is the most likely origin of pain the client describes as knifelike chest pain that increases in intensity with inspiration?
1. Cardiac
2. GI
3. Musculoskeletal
4. Pulmonary

13. 4. Pulmonary pain is generally described by these symptoms. Musculoskeletal pain only increases with movement. Cardiac and GI pains don't change with respiration.

CN: Physiological integrity; CNS: Physiological adaptation; CL: Analysis

14. A male client is hospitalized to rule out an acute myocardial infarction (MI); he has a normal lactate dehydrogenase level and an elevated creatine kinase (CK-MB) level. The nurse enters the client's room and finds him pacing the floor. Which statement by the nurse would be <u>most appropriate</u> in this situation?
1. "You've had a heart attack. Get back in bed."
2. "You seem upset. Why don't you get into bed and, if you wish, we can talk for a while."
3. "You sure have a lot of energy; do you want to play cards?"
4. "Your physician doesn't want you up. Would you please get back into your bed?"

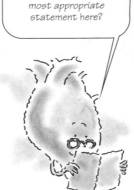

What should be the most appropriate statement here?

14. 2. Given the laboratory data, especially the elevated CK-MB level, the nurse should realize that the client probably had an MI and that he needs to lie down and rest his heart. However, the nurse should also realize the need to respond to the client's emotional distress by acknowledging his feelings and offering to discuss the situation. Telling the client that he had a heart attack would be giving a medical diagnosis that hasn't yet been made and would also be practicing outside the scope of nursing. A comment about his energy level acknowledges the client's pacing, but not his underlying concerns. Stating the physician's preferences attempts to impose authority to control the client's behavior. It doesn't acknowledge the client's distress.

CN: Psychosocial integrity; CNS: None; CL: Application

15. Which blood test is <u>most indicative</u> of cardiac damage?

1. Arterial blood gas (ABG) levels
2. Complete blood count (CBC)
3. Complete chemistry
4. Creatine kinase isoenzymes (CK-MB)

15. 4. CK-MB isoenzymes are present in the blood after a myocardial infarction. These enzymes spill into the plasma when cardiac tissue is damaged. ABG levels are obtained to review respiratory function, a CBC is obtained to review blood counts, and a complete chemistry is obtained to review electrolytes.

CN: Health promotion and maintenance; CNS: None; CL: Analysis

16. What's the primary reason for administering morphine to a client with a myocardial infarction?

1. To sedate the client
2. To decrease the client's pain
3. To decrease the client's anxiety
4. To decrease oxygen demand on the client's heart

16. 4. Morphine is administered because it decreases myocardial oxygen demand. Morphine will also decrease pain and anxiety while causing sedation, but it isn't primarily given for those reasons.

CN: Physiological integrity; CNS: Pharmacological therapies; CL: Application

17. Which condition is the <u>most</u> direct cause of a myocardial infarction (MI)?

1. Smoking two packs of cigarettes per day
2. Inflammation of the coronary arteries
3. Coronary artery thrombosis
4. Coronary artery vasospasm

17. 3. Coronary artery thrombosis causes an occlusion of the artery, leading to MI. Smoking is the leading modifiable risk factor for developing coronary heart disease. Vasospasm and inflammation of the coronary arteries may contribute to the development of coronary heart disease but aren't direct causes.

CN: Physiological integrity; CNS: Physiological adaptation; CL: Analysis

I'm commonly prescribed as a supplement to furosemide. Do you know what I am?

18. A 74-year-old female client with heart failure and 2+ pitting edema is prescribed furosemide (Lasix). Due to the effects of furosemide, what supplemental medication would the nurse expect to see ordered for this client?

1. Chloride
2. Digoxin
3. Potassium
4. Sodium

18. 3. Supplemental potassium is given with furosemide because of the potassium loss that occurs as a result of this diuretic. Chloride and sodium aren't lost during diuresis. Digoxin acts to increase contractility, but isn't given routinely with furosemide.

CN: Physiological integrity; CNS: Pharmacological therapies; CL: Analysis

19. Which finding would be a metabolic change occurring after a myocardial infarction (MI)?

1. Slowing of impulses through the atrioventricular (AV) node
2. Increased platelet aggregation
3. Decreased left ventricular ejection fraction
4. Increased serum glucose and free fatty acid protein levels

19. 4. Glucose and fatty acids are metabolites whose levels increase after an MI. Slow conduction of impulses through the AV node is an electrophysiologic change. Hematologic changes affect the blood cells and platelets. Ejection fraction measures the mechanical pumping action of the heart.

CN: Physiological integrity; CNS: Physiological adaptation; CL: Analysis

CN: Client needs category   CNS: Client needs subcategory   CL: Cognitive level

20. Which complication is indicated by a third heart sound (S_3)?
1. Ventricular dilation
2. Systemic hypertension
3. Aortic valve malfunction
4. Increased atrial contractions

20. 1. An S_3 sound occurs when the ventricles are resistant to filling and is heard just after S_2 when the atrioventricular valves open. Increased atrial contraction or systemic hypertension can result in a fourth heart sound. Aortic valve malfunction is heard as a murmur.

CN: Health promotion and maintenance; CNS: None; CL: Analysis

21. After an anterior wall myocardial infarction (MI), which problem is indicated by auscultation of crackles in the lungs?
1. Left-sided heart failure
2. Pulmonic valve malfunction
3. Right-sided heart failure
4. Tricuspid valve malfunction

21. 1. The left ventricle is responsible for most of the cardiac output. An anterior wall MI may result in a decrease in left ventricular function. When the left ventricle doesn't function properly, resulting in left-sided heart failure, fluid accumulates in the interstitial and alveolar spaces in the lungs and causes crackles. Pulmonic and tricuspid valve malfunction causes right-sided heart failure.

CN: Physiological integrity; CNS: Physiological adaptation; CL: Analysis

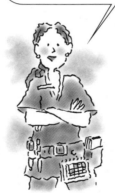

The most common tool is usually the most accurate.

22. A 52-year-old client is admitted to the emergency department with chest discomfort, diaphoresis, and nausea. Suspecting possible myocardial infarction (MI), the nurse would expect the physician to order which common diagnostic test to quickly determine myocardial damage?
1. Cardiac catheterization
2. Cardiac enzymes
3. Echocardiogram
4. Electrocardiogram (ECG)

22. 4. ECG is the quickest, most accurate, and most widely used tool to diagnose MI. Cardiac enzymes also are used to diagnose MI, but the results can't be obtained as quickly. An echocardiogram is used most widely to view myocardial wall function after an MI has been diagnosed. Cardiac catheterization is an invasive study for determining coronary artery disease.

CN: Safe, effective care environment; CNS: Coordinated care; CL: Application

23. What's the <u>first</u> intervention for a client experiencing myocardial infarction (MI)?
1. Administering morphine
2. Administering oxygen
3. Administering sublingual nitroglycerin
4. Obtaining an electrocardiogram (ECG)

23. 2. Administering supplemental oxygen to the client is the first priority of care. The myocardium is deprived of oxygen during an infarction, so additional oxygen is administered to assist in oxygenation and prevent further damage. Morphine and sublingual nitroglycerin are also used to treat MI, but they're more commonly administered after the oxygen. An ECG is the most common diagnostic tool used to evaluate MI.

CN: Physiological integrity; CNS: Pharmacological therapies; CL: Application

24. A client has been diagnosed with left-sided heart failure. Which symptoms should the nurse expect to see? Select all that apply.
1. Syncope
2. Orthopnea
3. Jugular vein distention (JVD)
4. Peripheral edema
5. S_3 heart gallop
6. Nocturia

24. 1, 2, 5. Left-sided heart failure causes decreased cardiac output and increases pulmonary congestion. Decreased cardiac output may cause a decrease in cerebral perfusion, resulting in syncope. Orthopnea is caused by pulmonary congestion. Development of an S_3 gallop is caused by the left atria attempting to fill the distended left ventricle. JVD, peripheral edema, and nocturia are all observed with right-sided heart failure.
CN: Physiological integrity; CNS: Physiological adaptation; CL: Application

25. Which drug class protects the ischemic myocardium by decreasing catecholamines and sympathetic nerve stimulation?
1. Beta-adrenergic blockers
2. Calcium channel blockers
3. Opioids
4. Nitrates

We're a class act when it comes to protecting the myocardium.

25. 1. Beta-adrenergic blockers work by decreasing catecholamines and sympathetic nerve stimulation. They protect the myocardium, helping to reduce the risk of another infarction by decreasing the heart's workload. Calcium channel blockers reduce workload by decreasing the heart rate and dilating arteries. Opioids reduce myocardial oxygen demand. Nitrates reduce myocardial oxygen consumption and decrease blood pressure.
CN: Physiological integrity; CNS: Pharmacological therapies; CL: Application

26. A 47-year-old female client who recently experienced a myocardial infarction (MI) is admitted to the hospital. A nurse who's aware of the most common complication of an MI would monitor this client closely for which condition?
1. Cardiogenic shock
2. Heart failure
3. Arrhythmias
4. Pericarditis

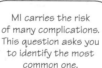

MI carries the risk of many complications. This question asks you to identify the most common one.

26. 3. Arrhythmias, caused by oxygen deprivation to the myocardium, are the most common complication of an MI. Cardiogenic shock, another complication of MI, is defined as the end stage of left ventricular dysfunction. The condition occurs in approximately 15% of clients with MI. Because the pumping function of the heart is compromised by an MI, heart failure is the second most common complication. Pericarditis most commonly results from a bacterial or viral infection.
CN: Physiological integrity; CNS: Physiological adaptation; CL: Application

27. With which disorder is jugular vein distention (JVD) <u>most prominent</u>?
1. Abdominal aortic aneurysm
2. Heart failure
3. Myocardial infarction (MI)
4. Pneumothorax

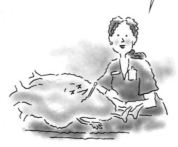

27. 2. Elevated venous pressure, exhibited as JVD, indicates the heart's failure to pump. This isn't a symptom of abdominal aortic aneurysm or pneumothorax. An MI, if severe enough, can progress to heart failure; however, in and of itself, an MI doesn't cause JVD.
CN: Physiological integrity; CNS: Physiological adaptation; CL: Analysis

CN: Client needs category   CNS: Client needs subcategory   CL: Cognitive level

28. Which drug class causes dilation of the coronary arteries, decreases afterload, reduces cardiac contractility, and slows the heart rate?
1. Positive inotropic agents
2. Nitrates
3. Beta-adrenergic blockers
4. Calcium channel blockers

28. 4. Calcium channel blockers inhibit calcium influx through the coronary arteries, causing arterial dilation and decreasing peripheral vascular resistance, which reduces afterload. Impulse conduction is slowed when calcium flow into cardiac cells is inhibited and contractility is decreased. Positive inotropics slow heart rate, but they increase contractility and cardiac output. Nitrates dilate the coronary arteries but don't slow the heart rate. Beta-adrenergic blockers decrease the heart rate and reduce myocardial oxygen demand.
CN: Physiological integrity; CNS: Pharmacological therapies; CL: Analysis

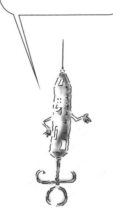

Keep in mind that digoxin strengthens myocardial contraction.

29. A nurse is about to administer digoxin to a client with heart failure. Which parameter should the nurse check before administering the medication?
1. Apical pulse
2. Blood pressure
3. Radial pulse
4. Respiratory rate

29. 1. An apical pulse is essential for accurately assessing the client's heart rate before administering digoxin. The apical pulse is the most accurate pulse point in the body. Blood pressure is usually only affected if the heart rate is too low, in which case the nurse would withhold digoxin. The radial pulse can be affected by cardiac and vascular disease and, therefore, won't always accurately depict the heart rate. Digoxin has no effect on respiratory function.
CN: Physiological integrity; CNS: Pharmacological therapies; CL: Application

30. A client is admitted with sinus bradycardia, nausea, and anorexia, and reports blurred and yellow vision disturbances. Toxicity of which drug is <u>most</u> likely responsible for all of these symptoms?
1. Digoxin (Lanoxin)
2. Atenolol (Tenormin)
3. Benazepril (Lotensin)
4. Diltiazem (Cardizem)

30. 1. Digoxin toxicity typically causes bradycardia, nausea, anorexia, and yellow vision disturbances. Benazepril is used in hypertension and doesn't cause bradycardia. Calcium channel blockers such as diltiazem and beta-adrenergic blockers such as atenolol can cause bradycardia, but don't cause yellow vision disturbances.
CN: Physiological integrity; CNS: Pharmacological therapies; CL: Application

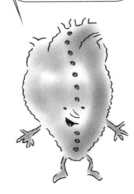

It's important to know my right from my left, especially when we're talking about heart failure.

31. A 61-year-old client is newly diagnosed with left-sided heart failure. Which sign <u>most commonly</u> associated with this type of heart failure would the nurse expect to find when assessing this client?
1. Crackles
2. Arrhythmias
3. Hepatic engorgement
4. Hypotension

31. 1. Crackles in the lungs are a classic sign of left-sided heart failure. These sounds are caused by fluid backing up into the pulmonary system. Arrhythmias can be associated with right- and left-sided heart failure. Hepatic engorgement is associated with right-sided heart failure. Left-sided heart failure causes hypertension secondary to an increased workload on the system.
CN: Physiological integrity; CNS: Physiological adaptation; CL: Application

32. In which disorder would a nurse expect to assess sacral edema in a bedridden client?
1. Diabetes mellitus
2. Pulmonary emboli
3. Renal failure
4. Right-sided heart failure

32. 4. Sacral, or dependent, edema is secondary to right-sided heart failure. The most accurate area on the body to assess dependent edema in a bedridden client is the sacral area. Diabetes mellitus, pulmonary emboli, and renal disease aren't directly linked to sacral edema.
CN: Physiological integrity; CNS: Physiological adaptation; CL: Analysis

33. Which symptom might a client with right-sided heart failure exhibit?
1. Adequate urine output
2. Polyuria
3. Oliguria
4. Polydipsia

33. 3. Inadequate deactivation of aldosterone by the liver after right-sided heart failure leads to fluid retention, which causes oliguria. Adequate urine output, polyuria, and polydipsia aren't associated with right-sided heart failure.
CN: Physiological integrity; CNS: Physiological adaptation; CL: Application

34. A nurse is monitoring an adult client taking atenolol (Tenormin). Which assessment finding would indicate a potential complication associated with atenolol?
1. Baseline blood pressure of 166/88 mm Hg followed by a blood pressure of 138/74 mm Hg after two doses of medication
2. Baseline resting heart rate of 106 beats/minute followed by a resting heart rate of 88 beats/minute after two doses of medication
3. Development of audible expiratory wheezes
4. Serum potassium level of 4.2 mEq/L

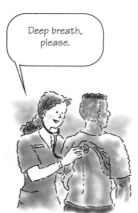

Deep breath, please.

34. 3. Audible wheezing may indicate serious bronchospasm, especially in clients with asthma or obstructive pulmonary disease. Decreases in blood pressure and heart rate are expected outcomes when beta-adrenergic blockers are administered. A serum potassium level of 4.2 mEq/L is within normal limits.
CN: Physiological integrity; CNS: Pharmacological therapies; CL: Analysis

35. Stimulation of the sympathetic nervous system produces which response?
1. Bradycardia
2. Tachycardia
3. Hypotension
4. Decreased myocardial contractility

35. 2. Stimulation of the sympathetic nervous system causes tachycardia, or an increase in heart rate. This response causes an increase in contractility, which compensates for the response. The other symptoms listed are related to the parasympathetic nervous system, which is responsible for slowing the heart rate.
CN: Physiological integrity; CNS: Physiological adaptation; CL: Knowledge

36. Which condition is most closely associated with weight gain, nausea, and a decrease in urine output?
1. Angina pectoris
2. Cardiomyopathy
3. Left-sided heart failure
4. Right-sided heart failure

36. 4. Weight gain, nausea, and a decrease in urine output are secondary effects of right-sided heart failure. Cardiomyopathy is usually identified as a symptom of left-sided heart failure. Left-sided heart failure causes primarily pulmonary symptoms rather than systemic ones. Angina pectoris doesn't cause weight gain, nausea, or a decrease in urine output.
CN: Physiological integrity; CNS: Physiological adaptation; CL: Application

CN: Client needs category CNS: Client needs subcategory CL: Cognitive level

37. A nurse receives a report on a client who has been diagnosed with an abdominal aortic aneurysm (AAA). Given her knowledge of the condition, the nurse would expect the client to have which underlying disease?
 1. Atherosclerosis
 2. Diabetes mellitus
 3. Chronic obstructive pulmonary disease
 4. Renal failure

38. In which area is an abdominal aortic aneurysm most commonly located?
 1. Distal to the iliac arteries
 2. Distal to the renal arteries
 3. Adjacent to the aortic arch
 4. Proximal to the renal arteries

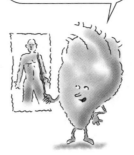

Location, location, location. It's all about location.

39. A client with pulmonary edema is given digoxin. What's digoxin's <u>most</u> direct and beneficial effect on myocardial contraction in the failing heart?
 1. Decreases cardiac output
 2. Decreases ventricular emptying capacity
 3. Increases circulating blood volume
 4. Slows conduction of impulses through the atrioventricular (AV) node

40. A client is admitted with acute pulmonary edema. What signs and symptoms should the nurse expect to find when collecting data on this client?
 1. Weight gain, abdominal distention, peripheral edema, jugular vein distention (JVD), tachycardia, and restlessness
 2. Apprehension and restlessness, cough with frothy pink sputum, moist gurgling respirations with tachypnea, and orthopnea
 3. Exertional dyspnea, cough with mucopurulent sputum, prolonged expiration with wheezing and crackles, and orthopnea
 4. Sharp chest pain that worsens on inspiration, dyspnea, cyanosis, and tachycardia

37. 1. Atherosclerosis is linked to 75% of all AAAs. Plaque damages the wall of the artery and weakens it, causing an aneurysm. Although the other conditions are related to the development of aneurysm, none is a direct cause.
CN: Health promotion and maintenance; CNS: None; CL: Analysis

38. 2. The portion of the aorta distal to the renal arteries is more prone to aneurysm formation due to increased pressure as it divides into the iliac arteries. The aorta is proximal to the iliac arteries. There's no area adjacent to the aortic arch, which bends into the thoracic (descending) aorta. Aortic aneurysms proximal to the renal ateries are uncommon.
CN: Physiological integrity; CNS: Physiological adaptation; CL: Knowledge

39. 4. Digoxin's physiologic effect on the heart slows impulse conduction through the AV node. Digoxin increases cardiac output and ventricular emptying capacity. Digoxin also promotes diuresis, thereby decreasing the circulating blood volume.
CN: Physiological integrity; CNS: Pharmacological therapies; CL: Analysis

40. 2. Apprehension and restlessness with frothy pink sputum and moist breath sounds are typical findings in clients with acute pulmonary edema. Weight gain, edema, and JVD are signs and symptoms of right-sided heart failure. Exertional dyspnea and mucopurulent sputum are typical of emphysema. Chest pain that worsens with inspiration, dyspnea, cyanosis, and tachycardia is a typical sign of acute pulmonary embolism.
CN: Physiological integrity; CNS: Physiological adaptation; CL: Analysis

CN: Client needs category   CNS: Client needs subcategory   CL: Cognitive level

41. A client who's being treated for unilateral lower extremity deep vein thrombophlebitis is being discharged. Which statement indicates to the nurse that additional discharge teaching is needed?

1. "I should elevate my legs when sitting and should get up and walk around periodically."
2. "I need to take my warfarin (Coumadin) exactly the way my physician ordered it."
3. "Tight compression hose rolled down behind the knee won't fall down, and improves the circulation in my legs."
4. "I should contact my physician immediately if I have frequent nosebleeds, bleeding from my gums, oozing from minor cuts, or if I see blood in my urine."

I think I need to explain further...

41. 3. Rolling the hose down behind the knee indicates improperly fitting hose that will impede venous return and cause venous stasis. Support hose should be smooth from the toes to the end of the hose. Elevating the legs while sitting promotes venous return. Warfarin must be taken exactly as prescribed and the client must monitor himself for potential bleeding.
CN: Physiological integrity CNS: Reduction of risk potential; CL: Application

42. A male client is admitted to the emergency department with a pulsating sensation in his abdomen and an audible bruit. The physician suspects that the client may have an abdominal aortic aneurysm (AAA). Which diagnostic test would the nurse expect the physician to order first to provide a definitive diagnosis?

1. Abdominal X-ray
2. Arteriogram
3. Computed tomography (CT) scan
4. Ultrasound

42. 4. Ultrasound is a noninvasive, cost-effective method of determining the presence of an AAA with 95% accuracy. Arteriograms and CT scans are more expensive, require the use of contrast agents and radiation, and are riskier to the client. An abdominal aneurysm would only be visible on an X-ray if it were calcified.
CN: Health promotion and maintenance; CNS: None; CL: Application

43. Which complication is of <u>greatest concern</u> when caring for a preoperative client with an abdominal aortic aneurysm?

1. Hypertension
2. Aneurysm rupture
3. Cardiac arrhythmias
4. Diminished pedal pulses

First things first. This question is asking you to prioritize, once again.

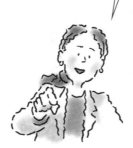

43. 2. Rupture of the aneurysm is a life-threatening emergency and is of the greatest concern for the nurse caring for this type of client. Hypertension should be avoided and controlled because it can cause the weakened vessel to rupture. Diminished pedal pulses, a sign of poor circulation to the lower extremities, are associated with an aneurysm but aren't life-threatening. Cardiac arrhythmias aren't directly linked to an aneurysm.
CN: Physiological integrity; CNS: Basic care and comfort; CL: Analysis

44. Which blood vessel layer may be damaged in a client with an aneurysm?

1. Externa
2. Interna
3. Media
4. Interna and media

44. 3. The factor common to all types of aneurysms is a damaged media. The media has more smooth muscle and less elastic fibers, so it's more capable of vasoconstriction and vasodilation. The interna and externa are generally not damaged in an aneurysm.
CN: Physiological integrity; CNS: Physiological adaptation; CL: Knowledge

45. Which precaution should a nurse take when caring for a client with a myocardial infarction who has received a thrombolytic agent?
1. Avoid puncture wounds.
2. Monitor potassium level.
3. Maintain a supine position.
4. Encourage fluids.

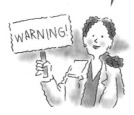

Be aware of all precautions that relate to your client's condition.

WARNING!

45. 1. Thrombolytic agents are declotting agents that place the client at risk for hemorrhage from puncture wounds. All unnecessary needle sticks and invasive procedures should be avoided. The potassium level should be monitored in all cardiac clients, not just those receiving a thrombolytic agent. Although no specific position is required, most cardiac clients seem more comfortable in semi-Fowler's position. The client's fluid balance must be carefully monitored, so it may be inappropriate to encourage fluids at this time.
CN: Physiological integrity; CNS: Reduction of risk potential; CL: Application

46. Which condition is linked to more than 50% of clients with an abdominal aortic aneurysm?
1. Diabetes mellitus
2. Hypertension
3. Peripheral vascular disease
4. Syphilis

46. 2. Continuous pressure on the vessel walls from hypertension causes the walls to weaken and an aneurysm to occur. Atherosclerotic changes can occur with peripheral vascular diseases and are linked to aneurysms, but the link isn't as strong as it is with hypertension. Only 1% of clients with syphilis experience an aneurysm. Diabetes mellitus isn't directly linked to aneurysm.
CN: Health promotion and maintenance; CNS: None; CL: Comprehension

47. Which arrhythmia is the most likely cause of sudden cardiac death?
1. Atrial fibrillation
2. Ventricular fibrillation
3. Atrial tachycardia
4. Ventricular bigeminy

47. 2. Ventricular fibrillation is the arrhythmia most commonly associated with sudden cardiac death. Atrial fibrillation is associated with irregular heart rates; atrial tachycardia is associated with heart rates of over 100 beats/minute. Ventricular bigeminy is associated with ventricular irritability but not sudden cardiac death.
CN: Physiological integrity; CNS: Reduction of risk potential; CL: Application

48. A nurse is caring for a client with a 7-cm infrarenal abdominal aortic aneurysm. The computed tomography (CT) scan indicates that the aneurysm may be leaking. When collecting data on the client, the nurse should be alert for which signs and symptoms? Select all that apply.
1. Constant, severe lower back pain
2. Constant, "tearing" abdominal pain
3. Hypotension
4. Increased red blood cell (RBC) count
5. Weak or absent bilateral leg pulses
6. Intermittent severe lower back pain

48. 1, 2, 3, 5. Severe, constant lower back or constant, "tearing" abdominal pain indicates a leaking or ruptured aneurysm as blood enters the abdominal cavity and retroperitoneal space. The client's blood pressure and RBC count will fall as he becomes hypovolemic from hemorrhage. Diminished blood flow through the iliac and femoral arteries causes weak or absent bilateral leg pulses. Pain from a leaking or ruptured aneurysm is constant.
CN: Physiological integrity; CNS: Reduction of risk potential; CL: Application

49. A nurse is caring for a female client who has a known 3-cm infrarenal abdominal aortic aneurysm (AAA). Which statements accurately characterize this disorder? Select all that apply.
1. AAA occurs more commonly above the level of the renal artery origins.
2. AAA occurs more commonly in men than women.
3. AAA is rarely linked to genetic factors.
4. A client with an AAA may also have "blue toe syndrome."
5. A 3-cm AAA rarely causes symptoms such as back pain.

50. A nurse reviews the chart of a new client who recently underwent an abdominal aortic aneurysm resection. It's suspected that a hereditary disease is linked to his condition. Which hereditary disease most closely linked to aneurysms would the nurse expect to find in the client's medical records?
1. Cystic fibrosis
2. Lupus erythematosus
3. Marfan syndrome
4. Myocardial infarction (MI)

51. Which treatment is the <u>definitive</u> one for a ruptured aneurysm?
1. Antihypertensive medication administration
2. Aortogram
3. Beta-adrenergic blocker administration
4. Surgical intervention

52. A client is diagnosed with a 4.5-cm infrarenal abdominal aortic aneurysm (AAA). Which statements should the nurse include when teaching the client about the disease? Select all that apply.
1. Controlling blood pressure and lipid levels is beneficial in slowing aneurysm expansion.
2. An AAA will be monitored for expansion every 6 to 12 months.
3. Smoking has no effect on the rate of aneurysm expansion.
4. Genetic factors influence the development of AAA.
5. All AAAs need to be repaired as soon as they are identified.

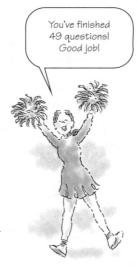

You've finished 49 questions! Good job!

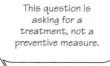

This question is asking for a treatment, not a preventive measure.

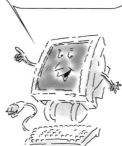

49. 2, 4, 5. AAA is more than twice as common in men as women and up to 28% of these clients have a first-degree family member with an AAA. Small AAAs (< 4 cm) are commonly identified coincidentally and are usually asymptomatic. Larger AAAs may be lined with an intraluminal thrombus, and "blue toe syndrome" occurs when the thrombus from the aneurysm microembolizes to the foot.
CN: Physiological integrity; CNS: Reduction of risk potential; CL: Analysis

50. 3. Marfan syndrome results in the degeneration of the elastic fibers of the aortic media. Therefore, clients with the syndrome are more likely to develop an aneurysm. Although cystic fibrosis is hereditary, it hasn't been linked to aneurysms. Lupus erythematosus isn't hereditary. MI is neither hereditary nor a disease.
CN: Health promotion and maintenance; CNS: None; CL: Analysis

51. 4. When the vessel ruptures, surgery is the only intervention that can repair it. Administration of antihypertensive medications and beta-adrenergic blockers can help control hypertension, reducing the risk of rupture. An aortogram is a diagnostic tool used to detect an aneurysm.
CN: Physiological integrity; CNS: Basic care and comfort; CL: Application

52. 1, 2, 4. Multiple factors lead to arterial wall damage and aneurysm formation. These include heredity, atherosclerosis, infection, smoking, and hypertension. Clients with AAAs of 4 to 5.4 cm should be monitored for expansion of the aneurysm using ultrasound or computed tomography scan every 6 to 12 months. The average aneurysm expansion rate is 10% per year but the rate of expansion is highly individual; many AAAs remain stable without expansion for many years.
CN: Physiological integrity; CNS: Physiological adaptation; CL: Application

CN: Client needs category   CNS: Client needs subcategory   CL: Cognitive level

53. A client is being discharged home with a diagnosis of hypertrophic cardiomyopathy. Which statement by the client demonstrates that he understands the disease process?
1. "I should start a vigorous aerobic exercise program to strengthen my heart function."
2. "Since this is a heredity disorder, my family members should probably be evaluated for similar symptoms."
3. "Exercise or exertion of any kind could kill me. I should have a caretaker to perform my activities of daily living."
4. "I should keep a journal of my symptoms and take my prescribed medications only when I have symptoms."

54. Septal involvement occurs in which type of cardiomyopathy?
1. Congestive
2. Dilated
3. Hypertrophic
4. Restrictive

55. Which recurring condition most commonly occurs in clients with cardiomyopathy?
1. Heart failure
2. Diabetes mellitus
3. Myocardial infarction (MI)
4. Pericardial effusion

56. Which statement by the client indicates that he understands how to monitor himself while taking warfarin (Coumadin)?
1. "I should use a soft toothbrush."
2. "I shouldn't worry if I see a lot of bruises as my blood thins."
3. "I should adjust my diet to eat less protein."
4. "I should use a safety razor to shave."

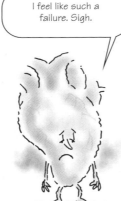

I feel like such a failure. Sigh.

53. 2. Hypertrophic cardiomyopathy is a heredity disease in which the heart muscle is abnormally thick and asymmetrical. In young clients, especially athletes, the first symptom may be sudden death during strenuous exercise. Strenuous physical exertion is restricted because it may precipitate arrhythmias or sudden cardiac death. The client is usually encouraged to perform normal activities of daily living after discussing restrictions with his physician. Medications, such as beta-adrenergic blockers, calcium channel blockers, and antiarrhythmics, are usually prescribed and should be taken daily to help prevent complications.
CN: Physiological integrity; CNS: Physiological adaptation; CL: Analysis

54. 3. In hypertrophic cardiomyopathy, hypertrophy of the ventricular septum—not the ventricle chambers—is apparent. This abnormality isn't seen in other types of cardiomyopathy.
CN: Physiological integrity; CNS: Physiological adaptation; CL: Knowledge

55. 1. Because the structure and function of the heart muscle is affected, heart failure most commonly occurs in clients with cardiomyopathy. MI results from atherosclerosis. Pericardial effusion is most predominant in clients with pericarditis. Diabetes mellitus is unrelated to cardiomyopathy.
CN: Physiological integrity; CNS: Physiological adaptation; CL: Comprehension

56. 1. A soft toothbrush will help prevent bleeding from friable gum tissue. Increased bruising should be reported to the physician. Dietary adjustments include consuming consistent amounts of dark green, leafy vegetables, which are high in vitamin K, but don't include protein restriction. Electric razors are recommended to reduce the risk of cutting the skin.
CN: Physiological integrity; CNS: Pharmacological therapies; CL: Application

CN: Client needs category   CNS: Client needs subcategory   CL: Cognitive level

57. A nurse is caring for a client with cardiac tamponade. Which signs and symptoms should the nurse watch for? Select all that apply.
  1. Paradoxical chest movement
  2. Tracheal deviation
  3. Pulsus paradoxus
  4. Widening pulse pressure
  5. Narrowing pulse pressure
  6. Muffled heart sounds

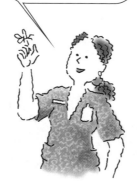

Remember. This question requires more than one answer.

57. 3, 5, 6. Pulsus paradoxus is a symptom of cardiac tamponade caused by a marked decrease in cardiac output that results in a diminished pulse and decreased blood pressure during inspiration. Narrowing pulse pressure and muffled heart sounds are additional signs of cardiac tamponade. Paradoxical chest movement occurs with flail chest. Tracheal deviation is seen with tension pneumothorax. Widening pulse pressure is found in increased intracranial pressure.
CN: Physiological integrity; CNS: Physiological adaptation; CL: Application

58. A nurse is planning care for a client with heart failure. Which nursing diagnosis should receive priority?
  1. Ineffective tissue perfusion (cardiopulmonary, renal) related to sympathetic response to heart failure
  2. Imbalanced nutrition: Less than body requirements related to rapid tiring while feeding
  3. Anxiety related to unknown nature of illness
  4. Decreased cardiac output related to decreased pumping ability

58. 4. The primary nursing diagnosis for a client with heart failure is *Decreased cardiac output related to pumping ability. Ineffective tissue perfusion, Imbalanced nutrition,* and *Anxiety* don't take priority over decreased cardiac output. The client's heart must produce cardiac output sufficient to meet the body's metabolic demands.
CN: Physiological integrity; CNS: Physiological adaptation; CL: Application

59. A nurse is caring for a 59-year-old male client diagnosed with myocardial infarction (MI). The purpose of giving nitrates to a client who has had an MI is to:
  1. relieve pain.
  2. dilate coronary arteries.
  3. relieve headaches caused by other medications.
  4. calm and relax the client.

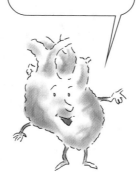

It's important to know what nitrates do.

59. 2. Nitrates dilate the arteries, allowing oxygen to continue flowing to the heart. Nitrates can cause headaches but don't relieve pain and don't calm or relax the client.
CN: Physiological integrity; CNS: Pharmacological therapies; CL: Application

60. Which drug class is most widely used in the treatment of cardiomyopathy?
  1. Antihypertensives
  2. Beta-adrenergic blockers
  3. Calcium channel blockers
  4. Nitrates

60. 2. By decreasing the heart rate and contractility, beta-adrenergic blockers improve myocardial filling and cardiac output, which are primary goals in the treatment of cardiomyopathy. Antihypertensives aren't usually indicated because they would decrease cardiac output in clients who are commonly already hypotensive. Calcium channel blockers are sometimes used for the same reasons as beta-adrenergic blockers; however, they aren't as effective as beta-adrenergic blockers and cause increased hypotension. Nitrates aren't used because of their dilating effects, which would further compromise the myocardium.
CN: Physiological integrity; CNS: Pharmacological therapies; CL: Comprehension

CN: Client needs category   CNS: Client needs subcategory   CL: Cognitive level

61. The telemetry monitor technician notifies the nurse that her client has sinus bradycardia with a heart rate of 42 beats/minute. What should the nurse do <u>first</u>?

1. Immediately review the client's current medical regimen to see if he has been taking beta-adrenergic blockers or calcium channel blockers.
2. Obtain a 12-lead electrocardiogram (ECG).
3. Notify the client's physician.
4. Check the client's level of consciousness (LOC), obtain vital signs, and assess the client for symptoms.

62. Which condition is associated with a predictable level of pain that occurs as a result of physical or emotional stress?

1. Anxiety
2. Stable angina
3. Unstable angina
4. Variant angina

63. One hour after returning from having a cardiac catheterization through a percutaneous femoral access site, a client calls the nurse to report that there's something wet under his buttocks. Upon entering the client's room, what step should the nurse take <u>first</u>?

1. Reinforce the groin dressing.
2. Obtain vital signs.
3. Help the client to sit up so the wet area can be visualized.
4. Apply gloves and assess the femoral access site.

64. Which characteristic should a nurse expect to see on a normal cardiac rhythm strip obtained from an adult client?

1. PR interval of greater than 0.24 second
2. Heart rate of 88 beats/minute
3. Two P waves preceding each QRS complex
4. QRS complexes greater than 0.16 second that vary in configuration

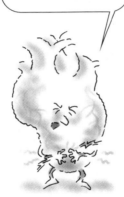

Stress can be a real pain in the heart.

61. 4. The first priority is to gather data by assessing the client's LOC, obtaining vital signs, and determining the presence or absence of symptoms. Calling the physician and reviewing the medication record are necessary actions but not priorities. Obtaining a 12-lead ECG may be necessary but isn't the priority.
CN: Physiological integrity; CNS: Physiological adaptation; CL: Analysis

62. 2. The pain of stable angina is predictable in nature, builds gradually, and quickly reaches maximum intensity. Anxiety generally isn't described as painful. Unstable angina doesn't always need a trigger, is more intense, and lasts longer than stable angina. Variant angina usually occurs at rest—not as a result of exertion or stress.
CN: Physiological integrity; CNS: Physiological adaptation; CL: Analysis

63. 4. Observing standard precautions and assessing the femoral access site for potential bleeding is the first priority. Reinforcing the groin dressing may be necessary after the site is assessed. Obtaining vital signs isn't the priority at this time. After a femoral puncture, the client is usually prescribed complete bed rest with his affected leg straight and immobilized for 2 to 4 hours to reduce the risk of bleeding.
CN: Physiological integrity; CNS: Physiological adaptation; CL: Application

64. 2. The normal adult heart rate is between 60 and 100 beats/minute. The normal PR interval is 0.12 to 0.20 second. In a normal cardiac cycle, there should be one P wave preceding each QRS complex. A normal QRS complex should be less than 0.10 second.
CN: Physiological integrity; CNS: Reduction of risk potential; CL: Application

65. Which type of angina is most closely associated with an impending myocardial infarction (MI)?
   1. Angina decubitus
   2. Chronic stable angina
   3. Nocturnal angina
   4. Unstable angina

66. When a client experiences chest pain during an acute anginal episode, the nurse should expect which form of nitroglycerin to be administered <u>first</u>?
   1. Nitroglycerin I.V. drip at 10 mcg/minute
   2. Application of 2″ (5 cm) of nitroglycerin paste to the chest wall
   3. Metered buccal nitroglycerin spray, 0.4 mg/spray
   4. Transdermal nitroglycerin patch, 0.2 mg/hour

67. Which statement by an adult client who has had a fasting lipoprotein profile indicates that further teaching is needed?
   1. "Changing my diet has really helped! Now my LDL cholesterol level is 98 mg/dl."
   2. "My total cholesterol level is optimal! It used to be 350 and now it's 250 mg/dl."
   3. "My HDL cholesterol level is 60 mg/dl and that helps lower my risk of coronary heart disease."
   4. "Even though my lipoprotein profile is normal this year, I know I'll need another one 5 years from now."

68. Which diagnostic test result is <u>most</u> consistent with a diagnosis of angina?
   1. Troponin level greater than 1.5 ng/ml
   2. Creatine kinase isoenzymes (CK-MB) level of 45%
   3. 12-lead electrocardiogram (ECG) with depressed, inverted, or downward slope to the T waves in leads II, III, and aV_F
   4. Transthoracic echocardiogram that shows a left ventricular ejection fraction of 30%

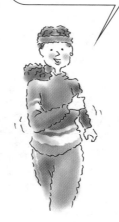

You're more than halfway finished! Keep going!

65. 4. Unstable angina progressively increases in frequency, intensity, and duration and is related to an increased risk of MI within 3 to 18 months. Angina decubitus, chronic stable angina, and nocturnal angina aren't associated with an increased risk of MI.
CN: Physiological integrity; CNS: Physiological adaptation; CL: Knowledge

66. 3. Sublingual or buccal nitroglycerin is the route of choice to quickly reduce myocardial oxygen demand and dilate coronary arteries. I.V. nitroglycerin is usually begun after a trial of sublingual or buccal spray nitroglycerin has proved unsuccessful in relieving the client's symptoms. Nitroglycerin paste and transdermal patches may be administered later because they have slower actions.
CN: Physiological integrity; CNS: Pharmacological therapies; CL: Analysis

67. 2. The National Cholesterol Education Program classifies a total cholesterol of 240 mg/dl or more as high. LDL cholesterol levels of 100 mg/dl or less and HDL cholesterol levels 60 mg/dl or more are optimal. Adults should have a fasting lipoprotein profile every 5 years beginning at age 20.
CN: Physiological integrity; CNS: Reduction of risk potential; CL: Analysis

68. 3. The 12-lead ECG with abnormal T waves indicates ischemia. Elevated troponin and CK-MB levels indicate myocardial infarction, not ischemia. A decreased ejection fraction indicates heart failure.
CN: Physiological integrity; CNS: Reduction of risk potential; CL: Analysis

CN: Client needs category   CNS: Client needs subcategory   CL: Cognitive level

69. Which result is the primary treatment goal for angina?
 1. Reversal of ischemia
 2. Reversal of infarction
 3. Reduction of stress and anxiety
 4. Reduction of associated risk factors

70. A 59-year-old female client is experiencing chest pain at rest that's unresponsive to nitroglycerin. The physician diagnoses unstable angina and alerts the nurse that the client will require treatment with immediate <u>surgical</u> intervention. Which treatment is most suitable?
 1. Cardiac catheterization
 2. Echocardiogram
 3. Nitroglycerin
 4. Percutaneous transluminal coronary angioplasty (PTCA)

71. Which intervention should be the first priority for a client experiencing chest pain while walking?
 1. Sitting the client down
 2. Getting the client back to bed
 3. Obtaining an electrocardiogram (ECG)
 4. Administering sublingual nitroglycerin

72. A 58-year-old male with heart failure is experiencing tachycardia, decreased blood pressure, and decreased peripheral pulses. The nurse interprets these symptoms as indicating which condition?
 1. Anaphylactic shock
 2. Cardiogenic shock
 3. Distributive shock
 4. Myocardial infarction (MI)

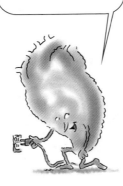

Pay attention. This info could really shock you!

69. 1. Reversal of ischemia is the primary goal, achieved by reducing oxygen consumption and increasing oxygen supply. An infarction is permanent and can't be reversed. Reduction of associated risk factors, such as stress and anxiety, is a progressive, long-term treatment goal that has cumulative effects. Reduction of these factors will decrease the risk of angina, but this usually isn't an immediate goal.
CN: Physiological integrity; CNS: Physiological adaptation; CL: Comprehension

70. 4. PTCA can alleviate the blockage and restore blood flow and oxygenation. An echocardiogram is a noninvasive diagnostic test. Nitroglycerin is an oral medication. Cardiac catheterization is a diagnostic tool, not a treatment.
CN: Physiological integrity; CNS: Physiological adaptation; CL: Application

71. 1. The initial priority is to decrease the oxygen consumption; this would be achieved by sitting the client down. An ECG can be obtained after the client is sitting down. After the ECG, sublingual nitroglycerin would be administered. When the client's condition is stabilized, he can return to bed.
CN: Physiological integrity; CNS: Basic care and comfort; CL: Application

72. 2. Cardiogenic shock is related to ineffective pumping of the heart and is an acute and serious complication of heart failure. Anaphylactic shock results from an acute allergic reaction. Distributive shock results from changes in the intravascular volume distribution and is usually associated with increased cardiac output. An MI isn't a shock state but can lead to cardiogenic shock; however, an MI is usually associated with chest pain.
CN: Physiological integrity; CNS: Physiological adaptation; CL: Analysis

CN: Client needs category   CNS: Client needs subcategory   CL: : Cognitive level

73. Which condition most commonly causes cardiogenic shock?
1. Acute myocardial infarction (MI)
2. Coronary artery disease (CAD)
3. Decreased hemoglobin level
4. Hypotension

This question is asking you to distinguish between the causes and the symptoms of shock.

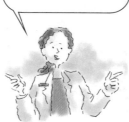

73. 1. Of all clients with an acute MI, 15% suffer cardiogenic shock secondary to the myocardial damage and decreased function. CAD causes MI. Hypotension is the result of a reduced cardiac output produced by the shock state. A decreased hemoglobin level is a result of bleeding.
CN: Physiological integrity; CNS: Reduction of risk potential; CL: Knowledge

74. A nurse is analyzing laboratory results for a client admitted with a possible myocardial infarction (MI). Which result would be used to rule out an MI?
1. Total white blood cell (WBC) count of 15,000/mm³
2. Troponin level of less than 0.2 ng/ml
3. Total red blood cell (RBC) count of 4.7 million/mm³
4. Mean corpuscular hemoglobin (MCH) of 27 pg/cell

74. 2. Cardiac troponins are proteins that exist in cardiac muscle and are released with cardiac muscle injury. A troponin level of less than 0.2 ng/ml is considered normal. An elevated WBC count (15,000/mm³) is seen in many disease processes and with severe infarcts but doesn't specifically indicate MI. A total RBC count of 4.7 million/mm³ is within normal limits for males and females, but isn't used to rule out an MI. MCH is an RBC index providing information about the hemoglobin concentration of RBCs and isn't used to rule out an MI.
CN: Physiological integrity; CNS: Reduction of risk potential; CL: Analysis

75. The nurse is taking the health history of a 49-year-old female client, when the client mentions that her heart sometimes seems to race. The nurse should be especially vigilant to monitor this client for which life-threatening cardiac arrhythmia?
1. Ventricular fibrillation (VF)
2. Ventricular tachycardia (VT)
3. Premature ventricular contractions (PVCs)
4. Premature atrial contractions (PACs)

75. 1. VF is a life-threatening arrhythmia. It occurs when the ventricle fibrillates, failing to fully contract and pump blood through the heart. VT, PVCs, and PACs aren't life-threatening.
CN: Health promotion and maintenance; CNS: None; CL: Application

76. Which factor would be <u>most useful</u> in detecting a client's risk of developing cardiogenic shock?
1. Decreased heart rate
2. Decreased cardiac index
3. Decreased blood pressure
4. Decreased cerebral blood flow

76. 2. The cardiac index, a figure derived by dividing the cardiac output by the client's body surface area, is used to identify whether the cardiac output is meeting a client's needs. Decreased cerebral blood flow, blood pressure, and heart rate are less useful in detecting the risk of cardiogenic shock.
CN: Physiological integrity; CNS: Physiological adaptation; CL: Analysis

77. Which symptom is one of the <u>earliest</u> signs of cardiogenic shock?
1. Tachycardia
2. Decreased urine output
3. A fourth heart sound (S₄)
4. Altered level of consciousness

77. 4. Initially, the decrease in cardiac output results in a decrease in cerebral blood flow that causes restlessness, agitation, or confusion. Tachycardia, decreased urine output, and an S₄ heart sound are all later signs of shock.
CN: Physiological integrity; CNS: Basic care and comfort; CL: Application

CN: Client needs category   CNS: Client needs subcategory   CL: Cognitive level

78. Which diagnostic study can determine when cellular metabolism becomes anaerobic and when pH decreases?
1. Arterial blood gas (ABG) analysis
2. Complete blood count (CBC)
3. Electrocardiogram (ECG)
4. Lung scan

79. Which of the following is the initial treatment goal for cardiogenic shock?
1. To correct hypoxia
2. To prevent infarction
3. To correct metabolic acidosis
4. To increase myocardial oxygen supply

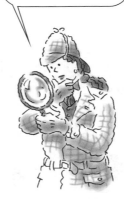

When answering questions, look for phrases such as *most commonly*.

80. Which drug is <u>most commonly</u> used to treat cardiogenic shock?
1. Dopamine (Intropin)
2. Enalapril (Vasotec)
3. Furosemide (Lasix)
4. Metoprolol (Lopressor)

81. Which instrument is used as a diagnostic and monitoring tool for determining the severity of a shock state?
1. Arterial line
2. Indwelling urinary catheter
3. Intra-aortic balloon pump (IABP)
4. Pulmonary artery (PA) catheter

78. 1. ABG levels reflect cellular metabolism and indicate hypoxia. A CBC is performed to determine various constituents of venous blood. An ECG shows the electrical activity of the heart. A lung scan is performed to view the lungs' function.
CN: Health promotion and maintenance; CNS: None; CL: Analysis

79. 4. A balance must be maintained between oxygen supply and demand. In a shock state, the myocardium requires more oxygen. If it can't get more oxygen, the shock worsens. Increasing the oxygen will also help correct metabolic acidosis and hypoxia. Infarction typically causes the shock state, so prevention isn't an appropriate goal for this condition.
CN: Physiological integrity; CNS: Physiological adaptation; CL: Comprehension

80. 1. Dopamine, a sympathomimetic drug, improves myocardial contractility and blood flow through vital organs by increasing perfusion pressure. Enalapril is an angiotensin-converting enzyme inhibitor that directly lowers blood pressure. Furosemide is a diuretic and doesn't have a direct effect on contractility or tissue perfusion. Metoprolol is a beta-adrenergic blocker that slows the heart rate and lowers blood pressure, neither of which is a desired effect in the treatment of cardiogenic shock.
CN: Physiological integrity; CNS: Pharmacological therapies; CL: Application

81. 4. A PA catheter is used to give accurate pressure measurements within the heart, which aids in determining the course of treatment. An arterial line is used to directly assess blood pressure continuously. An indwelling urinary catheter is used to drain the bladder. An IABP is an assistive device used to rest the damaged heart.
CN: Physiological integrity; CNS: Pharmacological therapies; CL: Knowledge

CN: Client needs category CNS: Client needs subcategory CL: Cognitive level

82. During a local wellness fair, a nurse takes some clients' blood pressures. Which client is <u>most</u> at risk for the diagnosis of essential (primary) hypertension?
1. A 35-year-old pregnant female with a blood pressure of 126/80 mm Hg
2. A 72-year-old female with a blood pressure of 142/88 mm Hg
3. A 44-year-old male with end-stage renal failure and a blood pressure of 130/70 mm Hg
4. A 76-year-old male with a systolic blood pressure of 136 mm Hg

83. Which sound will be heard during the <u>first</u> phase of Korotkoff's sounds?
1. Disappearance of sounds
2. Faint, clear tapping sounds
3. A murmur or swishing sound
4. Soft, muffling sounds

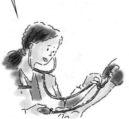

Listen carefully and note the first sound you hear.

84. Which parameter is the major determinant of diastolic blood pressure?
1. Baroreceptors
2. Cardiac output
3. Renal function
4. Vascular resistance

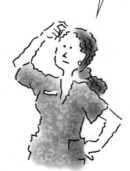

Chemoreceptors? Chemoreceptors? What's all this talk about chemoreceptors?

85. Which statement by a client indicates to the nurse that the client understands the role of chemoreceptors in regulating blood pressure?
1. "Chemoreceptors in my neck sense when my blood pressure is too low."
2. "Chemoreceptors in my neck sense when my blood pressure is too high."
3. "Chemoreceptors in my brain sense when my pulse rate is too low."
4. "Chemoreceptors in my brain sense when my pulse rate is too high."

82. 2. Hypertension is defined by the Seventh Report of the Joint National Committee on Prevention, Detection, Evaluation and Treatment of High Blood Pressure as a sustained systolic blood pressure of 140 mm Hg or a diastolic blood pressure of 90 mm Hg. Secondary hypertension is attributed to an identifiable medical diagnosis, such as pregnancy-induced hypertension or renovascular disease. The 76-year-old male has prehypertension, which is defined as systolic blood pressure of 120 to 139 mm Hg or a diastolic pressure of 80 to 89 mm Hg.
CN: Physiological integrity; CNS: Reduction of risk potential; CL: Analysis

83. 2. In phase I, auscultation produces a faint, clear tapping sound that gradually increases in intensity. Phase II produces a murmur sound, and precedes Phase III, the phase marked by an increased intensity of sound. Phase IV produces a muffling sound that gives a soft blowing noise. Phase V, the final phase, is marked by the disappearance of sounds.
CN: Physiological integrity; CNS: Basic care and comfort; CL: Application

84. 4. Vascular resistance is the impedance of blood flow by the arterioles that most predominantly affects the diastolic pressure. Baroreceptors are nerve endings that are embedded in the blood vessels and respond to the stretching of vessel walls. They don't directly affect diastolic blood pressure. Cardiac output determines systolic blood pressure. Renal function helps control blood volume and indirectly affects diastolic blood pressure.
CN: Physiological integrity; CNS: Physiological adaptation; CL: Knowledge

85. 1. Chemoreceptors respond to a decrease in blood pressure by stimulating sympathetic nervous system activity. The receptors don't respond to the other conditions.
CN: Physiological integrity; CNS: Reduction of risk potential; CL: Analysis

CN: Client needs category CNS: Client needs subcategory CL: Cognitive level

86. A nurse knows that the kidneys play an important role in regulating blood pressure. When hypertension occurs, which responses by the kidneys help normalize blood pressure?
1. The kidneys retain sodium and excrete water.
2. The kidneys excrete sodium and excrete water.
3. The kidneys retain sodium and retain water.
4. The kidneys excrete sodium and retain water.

87. Which hormone is responsible for raising arterial pressure and promoting venous return?
1. Angiotensin I
2. Angiotensin II
3. Epinephrine
4. Renin

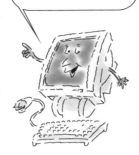

Don't get too tense to answer this question. (Oh, I'm just two, er, too clever for words.)

88. Which term is used to describe persistently elevated blood pressure with an unknown cause that accounts for approximately 90% of hypertension cases?
1. Accelerated hypertension
2. Malignant hypertension
3. Primary hypertension
4. Secondary hypertension

89. When obtaining a health history from a client admitted with hypertension, the nurse should expect the client to report which symptom?
1. Blurred vision
2. Epistaxis
3. Headache
4. Peripheral edema

86. 2. The kidneys respond to a rise in blood pressure by excreting sodium and excess water. This affects systolic blood pressure by regulating blood volume. Retaining sodium or water would only further increase blood pressure. Sodium and water must travel across the kidney membrane together; one can't travel without the other.
CN: Physiological integrity; CNS: Physiological adaptation; CL: Application

87. 2. Angiotensin II, triggered by angiotensin I, is responsible for vasoconstriction, thereby increasing arterial blood pressure. Angiotensin I is the hormone that causes angiotensin II to respond. Epinephrine directly stimulates the sympathetic nervous system and increases the heart rate. Renin produces angiotensin I when triggered by reduced blood flow.
CN: Physiological integrity; CNS: Physiological adaptation; CL: Knowledge

88. 3. Characterized by a progressive, usually asymptomatic blood pressure increase over several years, primary hypertension is the most common type. Malignant hypertension, also known as *accelerated hypertension,* is rapidly progressive and uncontrollable and causes a rapid onset of complications. Secondary hypertension occurs secondary to a known, potentially correctable cause.
CN: Physiological integrity; CNS: Reduction of risk potential; CL: Analysis

89. 3. An occipital headache is typical of hypertension owing to increased pressure in the cerebral vasculature. Blurred vision (due to arteriolar changes in the eye) and epistaxis (nosebleed) are far less common than headache, but can also be diagnostic signs. Peripheral edema can occur from an increase in sodium and water retention, but it's usually a latent sign.
CN: Physiological integrity; CNS: Physiological adaptation; CL: Analysis

CN: Client needs category   CNS: Client needs subcategory   CL: Cognitive level

90. The diaphragm of the stethoscope is typically placed over which artery to obtain a blood pressure measurement?
1. Brachial
2. Brachiocephalic
3. Radial
4. Ulnar

91. Which statement explains why furosemide (Lasix) is administered to treat hypertension?
1. It dilates peripheral blood vessels.
2. It decreases sympathetic cardioacceleration.
3. It inhibits the angiotensin-converting enzyme.
4. It inhibits reabsorption of sodium and water in the loop of Henle.

92. The hypothalamus responds to a decrease in blood pressure by secreting which substance?
1. Angiotensin
2. Antidiuretic hormone (ADH)
3. Epinephrine
4. Renin

93. Which statement by the nurse accurately explains the need for a client with hypertension to obtain an annual eye exam?
1. "By examining your corneas, an ophthalmologist can visualize microvascular hemorrhages in your eyes."
2. "By examining the fovea in your eyes, an ophthalmologist can visualize microvascular venous occlusions in your eyes."
3. "By examining the retina in your eyes, an ophthalmologist can detect changes in the arteries in your eyes."
4. "By examining the sclera of your eyes, an ophthalmologist can detect changes in the arteries in your eyes."

90. 1. The brachial artery is typically used because of its easy accessibility and location. The brachiocephalic artery isn't accessible for blood pressure measurement. The radial and ulnar arteries can be used in extraordinary circumstances, but the measurement may not be as accurate.
CN: Physiological integrity; CNS: Basic care and comfort; CL: Application

91. 4. Furosemide is a loop diuretic that inhibits sodium and water reabsorption in the loop of Henle, thereby causing a decrease in blood pressure. Vasodilators cause dilation of peripheral blood vessels, directly relaxing vascular smooth muscle and decreasing blood pressure. Adrenergic blockers decrease sympathetic cardioacceleration and decrease blood pressure. Angiotensin-converting enzyme inhibitors decrease blood pressure due to their action on angiotensin.
CN: Physiological integrity; CNS: Pharmacological therapies; CL: Comprehension

92. 2. ADH acts on the renal tubules to promote water retention, which increases blood pressure. Angiotensin, epinephrine, and renin aren't stored in the hypothalamus, but they all help to increase blood pressure.
CN: Physiological integrity; CNS: Physiological adaptation; CL: Knowledge

93. 3. The retina is the only site in the body where arteries can be seen without invasive techniques. Changes in the retinal arteries signal similar damage to vessels elsewhere. The cornea is the nonvascular, transparent, fibrous coat where the iris can be seen. The fovea is the point of central vision. The sclera is the fibrous tissue that forms the outer protective covering over the eyeball.
CN: Health promotion and maintenance; CNS: None; CL: Application

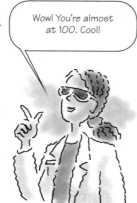

Wow! You're almost at 100. Cool!

94. A client is admitted for right leg vein ligation and stripping for varicose veins. Nursing interventions for this client postoperatively should include:
1. educating the client to elevate his legs when he's sitting.
2. educating the client to remain inactive until healing is complete.
3. applying knee-high stockings over his dressing.
4. applying ice to dressings to decrease swelling.

95. Which factor causes <u>primary</u> varicose veins?
1. Hypertension
2. Pregnancy
3. Thrombosis
4. Trauma

96. Which client statement given during a review of systems interview is consistent with the diagnosis of varicose veins?
1. "My legs feel tired and have a dull ache, especially when I walk or stand for long periods."
2. "I have severe foot pain that awakens me but it gets better if I dangle my foot off the edge of the bed."
3. "My legs become numb and get weaker the farther I walk."
4. "After I walk ½ mile (1,320 feet) I get severe calf pain that goes away when I rest."

97. A client with a family history of varicose veins is concerned about developing varicosities. Which statement by the nurse reflects an understanding of where varicosities are most likely to occur?
1. "With your family history, it's important to increase water and fiber intake."
2. "With your family history, your best defense is regular exercise such as walking."
3. "Be sure to include upper body weight lifting in a regular exercise routine."
4. "Be sure to drink cranberry juice to promote renal health."

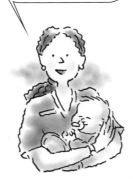

Oooh, I love babies. But not the varicose veins that go with being pregnant!

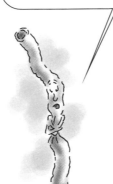

Maybe if I stay awake all night I'll feel better.

94. 1. Postoperative nursing interventions must focus on maintaining peripheral circulation and venous return. Elevating the legs and early ambulation are encouraged to facilitate venous return. Applying knee-high stockings and ice would constrict circulation.
CN: Physiological integrity; CNS: Reduction of risk potential; CL: Application

95. 2. Primary varicose veins have a gradual onset and progressively worsen. In pregnancy, the expanding uterus and increased vascular volume impede blood return to the heart. Hypertension has no role in varicose vein formation. Thrombosis and trauma cause valvular incompetence and are secondary causes.
CN: Health promotion and maintenance; CNS: None; CL: Comprehension

96. 1. Fatigue, aching, and pressure are classic symptoms of varicose veins, secondary to increased blood volume and edema. Severe foot pain that awakens the client and severe calf pain after walking that's relieved with rest are symptoms of decreased peripheral arterial blood flow. Numbness and weakness that increase as the client walks are consistent with spinal stenosis.
CN: Physiological integrity; CNS: Physiological adaptation; CL: Analysis

97. 2. Varicosities most commonly occur in the saphenous veins of the legs. Increasing water and fiber intake are interventions for hemorrhoids, which are varicosities located outside the anal sphincter. Varicosities don't develop in the arms or renal veins.
CN: Physiological integrity; CNS: Reduction of risk potential; CL: Application

CN: Client needs category   CNS: Client needs subcategory   CL: Cognitive level

98. Which condition is caused by increased hydrostatic pressure and chronic venous stasis?
1. Venous occlusion
2. Cool extremities
3. Nocturnal calf muscle cramps
4. Diminished blood supply to the feet

99. Which activity should a client with varicose veins <u>avoid</u>?
1. Exercise
2. Leg elevations
3. Prolonged lying
4. Wearing tight clothing

100. Which noninvasive diagnostic test demonstrates the backward flow of blood through incompetent venous valves?
1. Venous duplex Doppler ultrasonography
2. Ascending venography
3. Descending venography
4. Segmental pulse volume recordings

101. Which signs and symptoms are produced by posthrombotic deep vein changes in the legs?
1. Pallor and severe pain
2. Severe pain and edema
3. Edema and pigmentation
4. Absent hair growth and pigmentation

102. Which statement by a client indicates that he understands the surgical procedure to remove varicose veins?
1. "The surgeon will tie off a large vein in my leg and then remove it."
2. "The surgeon will use a laser to prevent further varicose veins."
3. "A piece of vein will be removed and then used to replace my blocked artery."
4. "A cold solution will be infused to shrink the vein."

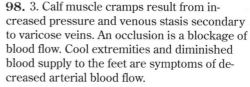

Congratulations! You've finished 100 questions. You're almost there!

98. 3. Calf muscle cramps result from increased pressure and venous stasis secondary to varicose veins. An occlusion is a blockage of blood flow. Cool extremities and diminished blood supply to the feet are symptoms of decreased arterial blood flow.
CN: Health promotion and maintenance; CNS: None; CL: Analysis

99. 4. Tight clothing, especially below the waist, increases vascular volume and impedes blood return to the heart. Exercise, leg elevations, and lying down usually relieve symptoms of varicose veins.
CN: Health promotion and maintenance; CNS: None; CL: Comprehension

100. 1. Venous duplex ultrasound is a noninvasive method that visualizes veins and measures the speed, direction, and pattern of blood flow in real time. Ascending and descending venography are invasive tests of the veins that use injected contrast medium and ionizing radiation. Segmental pulse volume recordings are noninvasive tests of the peripheral arteries.
CN: Health promotion and maintenance; CNS: None; CL: Application

101. 3. Blood clots in the deep veins of the leg typically cause permanent damage to the venous valves. Incompetent valves lead to impaired venous return, and edema and pigmentation result from venous stasis. Severe pain, pallor, and absent hair growth are symptoms of an altered arterial blood flow.
CN: Physiological integrity; CNS: Physiological adaptation; CL: Comprehension

102. 1. Ligation and stripping surgically removes varicose veins. The use of laser ablation therapy won't prevent further varicose veins from developing. Veins can be used to create bypasses for blocked arteries but this isn't a treatment for varicose veins. Infusion of a cold solution isn't used to treat varicose veins.
CN: Physiological integrity; CNS: Physiological adaptation; CL: Analysis

CN: Client needs category   CNS: Client needs subcategory   CL: Cognitive level

103. Which treatment is recommended for postoperative management of a client who has undergone ligation and stripping?
1. Sitting
2. Bed rest
3. Ice packs
4. Thigh-high elastic leg compression

103. 4. Thigh-high elastic leg compression helps venous return to the heart, thereby decreasing venous stasis. Sitting and bed rest are contraindicated because both promote decreased blood return to the heart and venous stasis. Although ice packs would help reduce edema, they would also cause vasoconstriction and impede blood flow.
CN: Physiological integrity; CNS: Basic care and comfort; CL: Application

104. Which client is most at risk for developing deep vein thrombosis (DVT)?
1. A 62-year-old female recovering from a total hip replacement
2. A 35-year-old female 2 days postpartum
3. A 33-year-old male runner with Achilles tendonitis
4. An ambulatory 70-year-old male who's recovering from pneumonia

104. 1. DVT is more common in immobilized clients who have had surgical procedures such as total hip replacement. Pregnancy can cause varicose veins, which can lead to venous stasis, but it isn't a primary cause of DVT. Clients who are recovering from an injury or pneumonia may have decreased mobility but these clients don't have the highest risk of developing DVT.
CN: Physiological integrity; CNS: Reduction of risk potential; CL: Analysis

105. Which complication of lower extremity deep vein thrombosis is manifested by dyspnea, chest pain, and diminished breath sounds?
1. Hemothorax
2. Pneumothorax
3. Pulmonary embolism
4. Pulmonary hypertension

I'll answer this question after I've had my nap.

105. 3. A pulmonary embolism is a thrombus that forms in a vein, travels to the lungs, and lodges in the pulmonary vasculature. *Hemothorax* refers to blood in the pleural space. Pneumothorax is caused by an opening in the pleura. Pulmonary hypertension is an increase in pulmonary artery pressure, which increases the workload of the right ventricle.
CN: Physiological integrity; CNS: Physiological adaptation; CL: Analysis

106. Which term refers to the condition of blood coagulating faster than normal, causing thrombin and other clotting factors to multiply?
1. Embolus
2. Hypercoagulability
3. Venous stasis
4. Venous wall injury

106. 2. Hypercoagulability is the condition of blood coagulating faster than normal, causing thrombin and other clotting factors to multiply. This condition, along with venous stasis and venous wall injury, accounts for the formation of deep vein thrombosis. An embolus is a blood clot or fatty globule that forms in one area and is carried through the bloodstream to another area.
CN: Physiological integrity; CNS: Physiological adaptation; CL: Comprehension

CN: Client needs category CNS: Client needs subcategory CL: Cognitive level

107. Which subjective description of pain should a nurse expect from a client with lower-extremity deep vein thrombosis (DVT)?
1. "I had severe, cramping pain in my right calf that began suddenly as I was walking."
2. "My right leg became warm and painful and there was a hard, red streak running up my thigh."
3. "I felt a burning sensation all over my right leg."
4. "My lower leg below my knee is red and tender and I think I have a fever."

108. Which treatment should be included in the discharge treatment plan for a client with deep vein thrombosis (DVT)?
1. Application of heat
2. Bed rest
3. Exercise
4. Leg elevation

109. Which term best describes the findings on cautious palpation of the vein in typical superficial thrombophlebitis?
1. Dilated
2. Knotty
3. Smooth
4. Tortuous

110. A client is admitted with a venous ulcer of his medial right ankle. What other signs and symptoms should the nurse expect to see? Select all that apply.
1. Hyperpigmentation below the right knee
2. Lipodermatosclerosis of the right leg below the knee
3. Right foot toe ulcers with eschar
4. Paleness of the right leg when raised above the level of the heart
5. Dependent rubor of the right foot
6. Swelling of the right leg below the knee

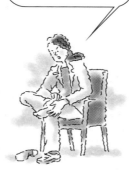

This question is asking you to characterize the type of pain experienced during lower extremity deep vein thrombosis.

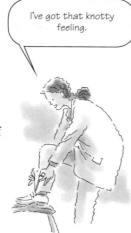

I've got that knotty feeling.

107. 1. DVT is associated with deep leg pain of sudden onset that's caused by venous outflow obstruction. Erythema and pain with a palpable cord is seen with superficial thrombophlebitis. A burning sensation is associated with an alteration in nerve tissue. Redness and tenderness of the lower leg with fever suggest cellulitis.
CN: Physiological integrity; CNS: Basic care and comfort; CL: Analysis

108. 4. Leg elevation alleviates the pressure caused by thrombosis and occlusion by assisting venous return. The application of heat would dilate the vessels and pool blood in the area of the thrombus, increasing the risk of further thrombus formation. Bed rest adds to venous stasis, thereby increasing the risk of thrombosis formation. When DVT is diagnosed, exercise isn't recommended until the clot has resolved.
CN: Physiological integrity; CNS: Basic care and comfort; CL: Comprehension

109. 2. The knotty feeling is secondary to the emboli adhering to the vein wall. Varicose veins may be described as dilated, tortuous, and soft. Normal veins feel smooth and soft.
CN: Physiological integrity; CNS: Physiological adaptation; CL: Application

110. 1, 2, 6. Hyperpigmentation (caused by red blood cells leaking into the skin), lipodermatosclerosis (fibrotic skin changes), and leg swelling are caused by venous hypertension. Toe ulcers with gangrenous changes, skin pallor with elevation, and dependent rubor are all signs of severe peripheral arterial occlusive disease.
CN: Physiological integrity; CNS: Reduction of risk potential; CL: Analysis

111. A 57-year-old client with a history of diabetes mellitus complains of a cramplike pain in his calves during his morning walks. When he tells the nurse that his pain subsides after resting briefly, the nurse tells him that he may be experiencing intermittent claudication. How would the nurse most accurately explain the cause of this condition?
1. Inadequate cardiac output
2. Elevated leg position
3. Dependent leg position
4. Inadequate muscle oxygenation

112. Which medical treatment should be administered to treat intermittent claudication?
1. Analgesics
2. Warfarin (Coumadin)
3. Heparin
4. Pentoxifylline (Trental)

113. Which <u>oral</u> medication is administered to prevent further thrombus formation?
1. Warfarin (Coumadin)
2. Heparin
3. Furosemide (Lasix)
4. Metoprolol (Lopressor)

114. Which position would best aid breathing in a client with acute pulmonary edema?
1. Lying flat in bed
2. Left side-lying
3. High Fowler's position
4. Semi-Fowler's position

115. Which blood gas abnormality is <u>initially</u> most suggestive of pulmonary edema?
1. Anoxia
2. Hypercapnia
3. Hyperoxygenation
4. Hypocapnia

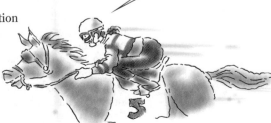

111. 4. When a muscle is deprived of oxygen, it produces pain much like that of angina. Inadequate cardiac output would cause heart failure. Leg position neither alleviates nor aggravates the condition.
CN: Physiological integrity; CNS: Physiological adaptation; CL: Application

112. 4. Pentoxifylline decreases blood viscosity, increases red blood cell flexibility, and improves flow through small vessels. Analgesics are administered for pain relief. Warfarin and heparin are anticoagulants.
CN: Physiological integrity; CNS: Pharmacological therapies; CL: Knowledge

113. 1. Warfarin prevents vitamin K from synthesizing certain clotting factors. This oral anticoagulant can be given long-term. Heparin is a parenteral anticoagulant that interferes with coagulation by readily combining with antithrombin; it can't be given by mouth. Neither furosemide nor metoprolol affect anticoagulation.
CN: Physiological integrity; CNS: Pharmacological therapies; CL: Application

114. 3. High Fowler's position facilitates breathing by reducing venous return. Lying flat and side-lying positions worsen breathing and increase the heart's workload. Semi-Fowler's position won't reduce the workload of the heart as well as high Fowler's position will.
CN: Physiological integrity; CNS: Basic care and comfort; CL: Comprehension

115. 4. In an attempt to compensate for the increased work of breathing due to hyperventilation, carbon dioxide (CO_2) decreases, causing hypocapnia. If the condition persists, CO_2 retention occurs and hypercapnia results. Although oxygenation is relatively low, the client isn't anoxic. Hyperoxygenation would result if the client was given oxygen in excess. However, secondary to fluid buildup, the client would have a low oxygenation level.
CN: Physiological integrity; CNS: Physiological adaptation; CL: Analysis

CN: Client needs category CNS: Client needs subcategory CL: Cognitive level

116. A nurse is caring for a 78-year-old female client with sick sinus syndrome who's awaiting permanent pacemaker placement. Given this client's risk of decreased cardiac output, what assessment findings would indicate that she's experiencing an initial drop in cardiac output?
1. Decreased blood pressure
2. Altered level of consciousness (LOC)
3. Decreased blood pressure and diuresis
4. Increased blood pressure and fluid volume

117. Which action is the priority response to a client coughing up pink, frothy sputum?
1. Suctioning the client
2. Administering sublingual nitroglycerin
3. Administering oxygen at 40% to 100%
4. Placing the client in a side-lying position

118. A 66-year-old male client has experienced an episode of acute pulmonary edema. Fearful of a repeated episode, the client asks what precautions he should take. The nurse should instruct the client to:
1. limit calorie intake.
2. restrict carbohydrates.
3. measure weight twice per day.
4. call the physician if he gains more than 3 lb (1.4 kg) in 1 day.

119. A nurse knows that a 45-year old client with severe hypertension will experience increased workload of the heart due to:
1. increased afterload.
2. increased cardiac output.
3. increased preload.
4. overload of the heart.

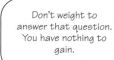

Don't weight to answer that question. You have nothing to gain.

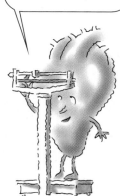

116. 4. The body compensates for a decrease in cardiac output with a rise in blood pressure due to the stimulation of the sympathetic nervous system, and an increase in fluid volume as the kidneys retain sodium and water. Blood pressure doesn't initially drop in response to the compensatory mechanism of the body. Alteration in LOC will occur only if decreased cardiac output persists.
CN: Physiological integrity; CNS: Physiological adaptation; CL: Analysis

117. 3. Production of pink, frothy sputum is a classic sign of acute pulmonary edema. The priority intervention is to promote oxygenation; the nurse should then administer oxygen and then suction the client if needed. Administering sublingual nitroglycerin will increase myocardial blood flow and might also be ordered but it isn't the first priority. The client should be positioned in high Fowler's position to promote expansion of the lungs.
CN: Physiological integrity; CNS: Physiological adaptation; CL: Application

118. 4. Gaining 3 lb in 1 day is indicative of fluid retention that would increase the heart's workload, thereby putting the client at risk for acute pulmonary edema. Restricting carbohydrates wouldn't affect fluid status. The body needs carbohydrates for energy and healing. Limiting calorie intake doesn't influence fluid status. The client must be weighed in the morning after the first urination. If the client is weighed later in the day, the finding wouldn't be accurate because of fluid intake during the day.
CN: Physiological integrity; CNS: Reduction of risk potential; CL: Application

119. 1. *Afterload* refers to the resistance normally maintained by the aortic and pulmonic valves, the condition and tone of the aorta, and the resistance offered by the systemic and pulmonary arterioles. Hypertension increases afterload as the left ventricle has to work harder to eject blood against vasoconstriction. Cardiac output is the amount of blood expelled from the heart per minute. Preload is the volume of blood in the ventricle at the end of diastole. *Overload* refers to an abundance of circulating volume and can contribute to hypertension.
CN: Physiological integrity; CNS: Physiological adaptation; CL: Analysis

120. After a client recovers from an episode of acute pulmonary edema, the nurse teaches him that enalapril maleate (Vasotec) has been ordered for which reason?
1. To decrease overload by promoting diuresis
2. To increase contractility of the heart
3. To decrease contractility of the heart
4. To decrease workload of the heart

121. A 71-year-old male has a potassium level of 3.2 mEq/L. The nurse knows that the client will be advised to alter his diet by:
1. increasing his intake of bananas and oranges.
2. avoiding intake of bananas and oranges.
3. increasing his intake of oatmeal and apples.
4. avoiding intake of oatmeal and apples.

122. Which statement by a nurse to the health care aide <u>best</u> explains the need to promptly report changes in respiratory rate for a client diagnosed with heart failure?
1. "Pulmonary edema, a life-threatening condition, can develop in minutes."
2. "Severe acute respiratory syndrome (SARS) is a common complication of heart failure."
3. "Pneumonia is a consequence of inadequate ventilation with heart failure."
4. "Pneumothorax, a life-threatening condition, can develop in minutes."

123. A 56-year-old female is having a consultation about possible circulation problems. Which information should the nurse provide about varicosities?
1. They're located only in the calves of the legs.
2. They become stronger as the walls of the vessels hold the blood.
3. They're caused by incompetent arteries.
4. They're veins that have become dilated and lost their elasticity.

Don't let this test become a grind. You're thisclose to being finished.

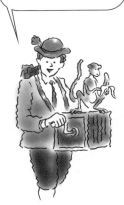

120. 4. Enalapril maleate is an angiotensin-converting enzyme inhibitor that reduces blood pressure and decreases the workload of the heart. Diuretics are given to decrease circulating fluid volume. Inotropic agents increase cardiac contractility. Negative inotropic agents decrease cardiac contractility.
CN: Physiological integrity; CNS: Pharmacological therapies; CL: Application

121. 1. A normal serum potassium blood level is 3.5 to 5 mEq/L in older adult clients. Bananas and oranges are high in potassium. Oatmeal and apples are high in fiber.
CN: Health promotion and maintenance; CNS: None; CL: Application

122. 1. Pulmonary edema, a life-threatening complication of heart failure, can develop in minutes, secondary to a sudden fluid shift from the pulmonary vasculature to the lungs' interstitial alveoli. SARS and pneumonia are caused by infections. Pneumothorax is a collection of air or gas in the pleural space, causing the lung to collapse.
CN: Physiological integrity; CNS: Reduction of risk potential; CL: Application

123. 4. Varicosities are veins that become dilated and lose their elasticity. They can be located in the lower extremities, esophagus, or rectal area and are caused by incompetant venous valves, not arteries.
CN: Physiological integrity; CNS: Reduction of risk potential; CL: Application

CN: Client needs category CNS: Client needs subcategory CL: Cognitive level

124. Which action should a nurse take when administering a new blood pressure medication to a client?
1. Administer the medication to the client without explanation.
2. Inform the client of the new drug only if he asks about it.
3. Inform the client of the new medication, its name, use, and the reason for the change.
4. Administer the medication and inform the client that the physician will explain the medication later.

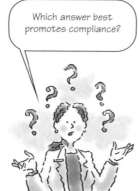

Which answer best promotes compliance?

124. 3. Informing the client about the medication, its use, and the reason for the change is important to the care of the client. Teaching the client about his treatment regimen promotes compliance. The other responses are inappropriate.
CN: Safe, effective care environment; CNS: Safety and infection control; CL: Application

125. A 52-year-old client with a history of hypertension has just had a total hip replacement. The physician orders hydrochlorothiazide 35 mg oral solution by mouth, once per day. The label on the solution reads hydrochlorothiazide 50 mg/5 milliliters. To administer the correct dose, how many milliliters should the nurse pour? Record your answer using one decimal place.

_____ml

125. 3.5. The correct formula to calculate a drug dosage is:
    dose on hand/quantity on hand = dose desired/X.
In this example, the equation is:
    50 mg/5 ml = 35 mg/X
    X = 3.5 ml.
CN: Physiological integrity; CNS: Pharmacological therapies; CL: Application

126. A nurse is assessing a client who's at risk for cardiac tamponade due to chest trauma sustained in a motorcycle accident. What's the client's pulse pressure if his blood pressure is 108/82 mm Hg? Record your answer using a whole number.

_____ mm Hg

126. 26. Pulse pressure is the difference between systolic and diastolic pressures. Normally, systolic pressure exceeds diastolic pressure by about 40 mm Hg. Narrowed pulse pressure, a difference of less than 30 mm Hg, is a sign of cardiac tamponade.
CN: Physiological integrity; CNS: Physiological adaptation; CL: Application

127. A 40-year-old client is admitted with a diagnosis of new-onset atrial fibrillation. To obtain an accurate pulse count, the nurse counts the apical heart rate. Identify the area where the nurse should place the stethoscope to best hear the apical rate.

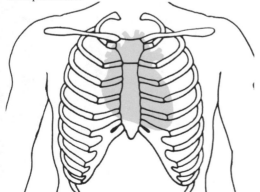

127.

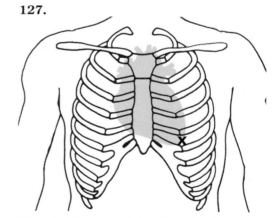

The apical heart rate is best heard at the point of maximal impulse, which is generally in the fifth intercostal space at the midclavicular line.
CN: Health promotion and maintenance; CNS: None; CL: Application

CN: Client needs category   CNS: Client needs subcategory   CL: Cognitive level

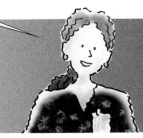

This challenging chapter covers HIV infection, AIDS, rheumatoid arthritis, DIC, and lots of other complex disorders. You can handle it, though; I know you can.

Chapter 4
Hematologic & immune disorders

1. Which nutritional teaching should a nurse provide a client who has acquired immunodeficiency syndrome (AIDS)? Select all that apply.
1. Thoroughly cook meats and poultry.
2. Choose foods low in fat.
3. Choose foods low in calories.
4. Weigh yourself weekly.
5. Eat small, frequent meals.

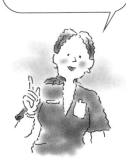

More than one answer may be correct. Be careful to choose the best answer.

2. Which client situation would carry the highest risk of human immunodeficiency virus (HIV) transmission?
1. A client with urinary incontinence
2. A trauma victim requiring frequent suctioning of oral secretions because of his inability to swallow
3. A malnourished client with bleeding gums and open lesions of his oral mucous membranes
4. A client with acute diarrhea

3. Immediately after giving an injection, a nurse is accidentally stuck with the needle when a client becomes agitated. When is the best time for the employer to test the nurse for human immunodeficiency virus antibodies to determine if she became infected as a result of the needle stick?
1. Immediately and then again in 6 weeks, at 3 months, and at 6 months
2. Immediately and then again in 3 months and at 6 months
3. In 2 weeks and then again in 6 months
4. In 2 weeks and then again in 1 year

1. 1, 2, 5. To prevent food-borne illness, all meat and poultry should be cooked thoroughly. It's necessary to avoid foods high in fats because drugs used to treat AIDS may cause hyperlipidemia. Consuming small, frequent meals consisting of high-calorie, nutrient-dense food will help improve overall nutrition. Daily weights are important in determining patterns of weight loss.
CN: Health promotion and maintenance; CNS: None; CL: Application

2. 3. Although HIV has been found in urine, saliva, and feces, it's most easily transmitted via blood, semen, and vaginal secretions. Open oral lesions and bleeding gums provide a portal for transmission of the virus.
CN: Health promotion and maintenance; CNS: None; CL: Analysis

3. 1. The employer will want to test the nurse immediately to determine whether a preexisting infection is present, and then again in 6 weeks, at 3 months, and at 6 months to detect seroconversion as a result of the needle stick. Waiting until 3 months may delay treatment and the client may seroconvert sooner. Waiting 2 weeks to perform the first test is too late to detect preexisting infection. Postexposure antibody formation may take 2 weeks to 6 months.
CN: Health promotion and maintenance; CNS: None; CL: Application

CN: Client needs category   CNS: Client needs subcategory   CL: Cognitive level

4. Which blood test is used <u>first</u> to identify a response to human immunodeficiency virus (HIV) infection?
1. Western blot
2. CD4⁺ T-cell count
3. Erythrocyte sedimentation rate
4. Enzyme-linked immunosorbent assay (ELISA)

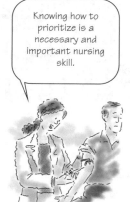

Knowing how to prioritize is a necessary and important nursing skill.

5. The nurse would instruct a client with human immunodeficiency virus who has frequent bouts of diarrhea to avoid consuming:
1. milk.
2. red licorice.
3. chicken soup.
4. broiled meat.

6. Which dietary recommendation may help the client with rheumatoid arthritis reduce inflammation?
1. Consume more salmon.
2. Drink vitamin D–fortified milk.
3. Increase red meat consumption.
4. Consume more spinach

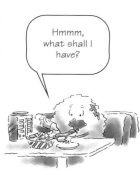

Hmmm, what shall I have?

7. Which nonsteroidal anti-inflammatory drug (NSAID) is most <u>commonly</u> used to treat rheumatoid arthritis?
1. leflunomide (Arava)
2. etanercept (Enbrel)
3. Ibuprofen
4. Methotrexate (Trexall)

4. 4. The ELISA is the first screening test for HIV. A Western blot test confirms a positive ELISA. Other blood tests that support the diagnosis of HIV include CD4⁺ and CD8⁺ counts, complete blood cell counts, immunoglobulin levels, p24 antigen assay, and quantitative ribonucleic acid assays.
CN: Health promotion and maintenance; CNS: None; CL: Knowledge

5. 1. Clients with chronic diarrhea may develop intolerance to lactose, which may worsen the diarrhea. Although red licorice may be eaten, black licorice should be avoided. Other foods that the client should avoid include fatty foods, other lactose-containing foods, caffeine, and sugar. Chicken soup and broiled meat may be consumed.
CN: Physiological integrity; CNS: Reduction of risk potential; CL: Application

6. 1. Salmon is high in omega-3 fatty acids. The therapeutic effect of fish oil suppresses inflammatory mediator production (such as prostaglandins); how it works is unknown. Iron-rich foods, such as spinach and red meats, are recommended to decrease the anemia associated with rheumatoid arthritis. Calcium and vitamin D found in milk may help reduce bone resorption.
CN: Physiological integrity; CNS: Physiological adaptation; CL: Application

7. 3. Ibuprofen, fenoprofen, naproxen, piroxicam, and indomethacin are NSAIDs used for clients with rheumatoid arthritis. Leflunomide, etanercept, and methotrexate are disease-modifying antirheumatic drugs. They help to decrease the development of bone erosion and narrowing of the joint spaces.
CN: Physiological integrity; CNS: Pharmacological therapies; CL: Knowledge

8. Which statement by a client would indicate the need for further teaching regarding safer sex practices?

1. "I should use plenty of oil-based lubricant to prevent latex condom tearing."
2. "I should inspect the condom for damage or defects before I use it."
3. "I must check the expiration date on the package before using the condom."
4. "Latex condoms are the best choice for preventing the spread of HIV."

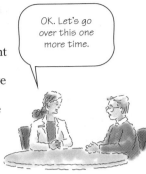

OK. Let's go over this one more time.

8. 1. Water-based lubricants should be used; oil- or petroleum-based products can damage latex condoms. Latex condoms or polyurethane (if the client has a latex allergy) condoms have been proven to decrease the spread of human immunodeficiency virus (HIV). Checking for damaged, defective, or expired condoms ensures the integrity of the condoms and decreases the likelihood of HIV transmission.

CN: Health promotion and maintenance; CNS: None; CL: Analysis

9. Which client is most at risk for developing rheumatoid arthritis?

1. A 25-year-old Asian female
2. A 44-year-old Native-American female
3. A 65-year-old African-American female
4. A 70-year-old African-American male

9. 2. The peak onset for rheumatoid arthritis is between ages 30 and 60. It's three times more common in women than in men. Native-Americans have a higher incidence than any other ethnic group.

CN: Health promotion and maintenance; CNS: None; CL: Analysis

10. Which instruction would be appropriate when teaching a client with human immunodeficiency virus who's at high risk for altered oral mucous membranes?

1. "Brush your teeth frequently with a firm toothbrush."
2. "Use mouthwash that contains an astringent agent."
3. "Be sure to heat all your food."
4. "Lubricate your lips."

10. 4. Lubricating the lips will keep them moist and prevent cracking. A firm toothbrush would damage already sensitive gums. An astringent would be painful, as would foods that are too hot.

CN: Physiological integrity; CNS: Reduction of risk potential; CL: Application

11. A pregnant female client has just been diagnosed with human immunodeficiency virus (HIV) infection. Which action would <u>decrease</u> the risk of HIV transmission to the fetus or infant during the course of pregnancy, labor, and delivery?

1. Using a scalp monitor only in the final stages of labor
2. Allowing the infant to breast-feed only after the mother's nipples have been disinfected with an antimicrobial agent
3. Reinforcing client teaching regarding the importance of continuing antiretroviral therapy throughout her pregnancy
4. Withholding zidovudine (Retrovir) therapy until the infant has blood testing to determine the presence of HIV antibodies

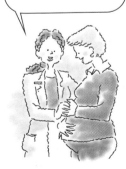

With pregnancy questions, you need to be concerned about the client and the infant.

11. 3. Maintaining antiretroviral therapy throughout pregnancy decreases the risk of fetal HIV infection to less than 4%; compliance with therapy should be continually evaluated and reinforced. Scalp monitoring at anytime during labor and delivery causes impaired skin integrity and increases the likelihood of HIV transmission. HIV has been found in breast milk and infants shouldn't be breast-fed. Zidovudine is given to infants of HIV-positive mothers beginning immediately after birth and for 6 weeks to decrease the risk of HIV transmission to the infant.

CN: Health promotion and maintenance; CNS: None; CL: Analysis

CN: Client needs category   CNS: Client needs subcategory   CL: Cognitive level

12. Which group or factor is linked to higher morbidity and mortality in human immunodeficiency virus (HIV)–infected clients?
1. Homosexual males
2. Lower socioeconomic levels
3. Treatment in a large teaching hospital
4. Treatment by a physician who specializes in HIV infection

13. After teaching a client about rheumatoid arthritis, which statement indicates the client understands the disease process?
1. "It will get better and worse again."
2. "Once it clears up, it will never come back."
3. "I'll definitely have to have surgery for this."
4. "It will never get any better than it is right now."

14. Which medication would be prescribed first for a client with rheumatoid arthritis?
1. Aspirin
2. Cyclophosphamide (Cytoxan)
3. Ferrous sulfate
4. Prednisone

The word first is a clue!

15. A nurse should be aware of the many complications that may occur as a result of human immunodeficiency virus (HIV) infection. Which client situation suggests that the client has acquired immunodeficiency syndrome (AIDS) wasting syndrome?
1. A 34-year-old male with oral pain, dysphagia, and yellow-white plaques in his mouth and throat
2. A 42-year-old female with recurrent vaginitis causing intense itching and white thick vaginal discharge
3. A 52-year-old male with impaired memory, hallucinations, loss of balance, and personality changes
4. A 46-year-old female who has lost 12% of her body weight, with weakness, fever, and chronic diarrhea for the past 35 days

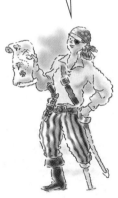

12. 2. Morbidity and mortality have been associated with lower socioeconomic status, receiving care in a community hospital or by a physician without much experience with HIV infection, or lack of access to adequate health care.
CN: Physiological integrity; CNS: Physiological adaptation; CL: Analysis

13. 1. The client with rheumatoid arthritis needs to understand it's a somewhat unpredictable disease characterized by periods of exacerbation and remission. There's no cure, but symptoms can be managed at times. Surgery may be indicated in some cases, but not always.
CN: Psychosocial integrity; CNS: None; CL: Application

14. 1. Nonsteroidal anti-inflammatory drugs (NSAIDs), such as aspirin, are considered first-line therapy by some physicians. Cytoxan may be used in cases of severe synovitis, rather than as first-line therapy. Ferrous sulfate isn't used to treat rheumatoid arthritis. Prednisone may be used to control inflammation when NSAIDs aren't tolerated.
CN: Physiological integrity; CNS: Pharmacological therapies; CL: Application

15. 4. AIDS wasting syndrome is diagnosed when there's a loss of 10% or more of body weight and the presence of one or more of the following for more than 30 days: fever, weakness, and at least two loose stools daily. Oral pain with visible yellow-white plaques and vaginitis with a white, cottage cheese-like discharge suggest infection with *Candida albicans*. Impaired intellect and motor functioning indicate HIV infection of the central nervous system with AIDS dementia complex.
CN: Physiological integrity; CNS: Physiological adaptation; CL: Analysis

CN: Client needs category   CNS: Client needs subcategory   CL: Cognitive level

16. Which blood component is decreased in anemia?
1. Erythrocytes
2. Granulocytes
3. Leukocytes
4. Platelets

17. A middle-aged client arrives at the emergency department complaining of chest and stomach pain. He also reports passing black stools for 1 month. Which intervention should the nurse institute <u>first</u>?
1. Give nasal oxygen.
2. Take his vital signs.
3. Begin cardiac monitoring.
4. Draw blood for laboratory analysis.

18. A physician evaluates a client who arrived at the emergency department with chest and stomach pain and a report of black, tarry stools for several months. Which order would the nurse anticipate for the client?
1. Cardiac monitoring, oxygen, creatine kinase (CK) and lactate dehydrogenase (LD) levels
2. Prothrombin time (PT), partial thromboplastin time (PTT), fibrinogen and fibrin split product values
3. Electrocardiogram (ECG), complete blood count, testing for occult blood, comprehensive serum metabolic panel
4. EEG, alkaline phosphatase and aspartate aminotransferase (AST) levels, basic serum metabolic panel

19. What's the goal when medications are prescribed to treat rheumatoid arthritis?
1. To cure the disease
2. To prevent osteoporosis
3. To control inflammation
4. To encourage bone regeneration

20. A nurse in a family health clinic is caring for a female client with anemia. The nurse recognizes that the client:
1. needs to restrict activity as much as possible.
2. should be encouraged to eat foods high in calcium.
3. needs to have activities spaced to allow for rest periods.
4. should be supervised when ambulating.

CN: Client needs category   CNS: Client needs subcategory   CL: Cognitive level

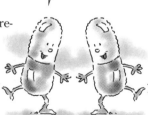

Make sure you know the action of a drug before you administer it.

16. 1. Anemia is defined as a decreased number of erythrocytes. Leukopenia is a decreased number of leukocytes. Thrombocytopenia is a decreased number of platelets. Granulocytopenia is a decreased number of granulocytes.
CN: Health promotion and maintenance; CNS: None; CL: Knowledge

17. 2. The nurse should collect data first; vital signs will show whether the client is hemodynamically stable. Monitoring his heart rhythm may be indicated based on the nurse's findings. Giving nasal oxygen and drawing blood require a physician's order and wouldn't be part of data collection.
CN: Physiological integrity; CNS: Physiological adaptation; CL: Application

18. 3. An ECG evaluates the complaint of chest pain, laboratory tests determine anemia, and the stool test for occult blood determines blood in the stools. Cardiac monitoring, oxygen, and CK and LD levels are appropriate for a primary cardiac problem. A basic metabolic panel and alkaline phosphatase and AST levels assess liver function. PT, PTT, fibrinogen, and fibrin split products are measured to verify bleeding dyscrasias. An EEG evaluates the brain's electrical activity.
CN: Physiological integrity; CNS: Reduction of risk potential; CL: Analysis

19. 3. The goal of medications in the treatment of rheumatoid arthritis is to control inflammation. There's no cure for rheumatoid arthritis. Rheumatoid arthritis causes bone erosion at the joints, not osteoporosis. Medications aren't available to replace bone lost through erosion.
CN: Physiological integrity; CNS: Pharmacological therapies; CL: Comprehension

20. 3. Clients with anemia fatigue easily and need rest between activities to conserve energy. Activities don't need to be severely restricted for clients with anemia. The client needs to eat food that's high in iron, such as lean red meat and fortified breakfast cereal, not calcium. The client doesn't need close supervision when walking.
CN: Physiological integrity; CNS: Physiological adaptation; CL: Application

21. A client with anemia may be tired due to a tissue deficiency of which substance?
1. Carbon dioxide
2. Factor VIII
3. Oxygen
4. T-cell antibodies

So, where do you stem from?

22. Which factor would be <u>most likely</u> to cause anemia?
1. Immobility
2. Diabetes mellitus
3. Medications
4. Rhinovirus infection

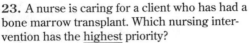

23. A nurse is caring for a client who has had a bone marrow transplant. Which nursing intervention has the <u>highest</u> priority?
1. Assisting the client with daily hygiene needs
2. Listening to the client's breath sounds every 2 hours to detect congestion
3. Palpating the client's pulses every 2 hours
4. Administering pain medication as necessary to promote rest and comfort

24. In community health and epidemiologic studies, which definition of disease prevalence is correct?
1. The number of individuals affected by a particular disease at a specific time
2. The rate at which individuals without a specific disease develop that disease
3. The proportion of individuals affected by the disease who live for a particular period
4. The proportion of individuals without the disease who eventually develop the disease within a specific period

21. 3. Anemia stems from a decreased number of red blood cells and the resulting deficiency of oxygen in body tissues. Clotting factors, such as factor VIII, relate to the body's ability to form blood clots and aren't related to anemia, nor is carbon dioxide or T-cell antibodies.
CN: Physiological integrity; CNS: Physiological adaptation; CL: Application

22. 3. Medications may cause changes in the bone marrow, leading to anemias. Anemia isn't caused by immobility or a rhinovirus infection, which causes the common cold. Diabetes is a chronic disease characterized by disturbances in carbohydrate, protein, and fat metabolism.
CN: Health promotion and maintenance; CNS: None; CL: Comprehension

23. 2. The two major complications of bone marrow transplantation are bleeding and infection. Listening to the client's breath sounds frequently, comparing them to his baseline, and reporting any congestion immediately help prevent complications due to infection. Although hygiene and comfort needs should be addressed, these don't take priority over assessing for infection. Collecting data for potentially impaired peripheral circulation isn't a priority for clients after a bone marrow transplant.
CN: Physiological integrity; CNS: Reduction of risk potential; CL: Application

24. 1. Prevalence is the number of individuals affected by the disease at a specific time. Risk is the proportion of individuals without the disease who develop the disease within a particular period. Incidence rate is the rapidity with which individuals without the disease contract it. Survival is the proportion of individuals affected by the disease who live for a particular length of time.
CN: Health promotion and maintenance; CNS: None; CL: Analysis

25. Which client has the highest risk of developing anemia?
1. A client with a colostomy following colon resection
2. A client with gastric esophageal reflux disease (GERD)
3. A client who has had a gastrectomy
4. A client with frequent bouts of dumping syndrome

26. A nurse has instructed a client about taking his oral liquid iron preparation prescribed for his anemia. Which statement by the client indicates that he needs additional teaching?
1. "I should take the iron with an antacid to prevent gastric distress."
2. "I expect my stools to be dark green or black."
3. "I should rinse my mouth with water after taking the iron."
4. "I should add the iron to juice and drink it with a straw."

27. A nurse is caring for a 41-year-old male with rheumatoid arthritis. The nurse plans to ambulate the client:
1. when the client first awakens in the morning.
2. after returning from physical therapy.
3. after the client has a bath.
4. just before the noontime meal.

28. For which condition is a client who has just had a total hip replacement most at risk?
1. Anemia
2. Polycythemia
3. Purpura
4. Thrombocytopenia

29. Which term describes a decreased number of platelets?
1. Thrombectomy
2. Thrombocytopenia
3. Thrombocytopathy
4. Thrombocytosis

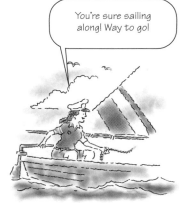

You're sure sailing along! Way to go!

25. 3. Lack of intrinsic factor following gastrectomy would cause pernicious anemia due to the client's inability to absorb vitamin B_{12}. The presence of a colostomy, GERD, or dumping syndrome would not place a client at risk for developing anemia.
CN: Physiological integrity; CNS: Physiological adaptation; CL: Application

26. 1. Antacids will interfere with absorption of iron and should be avoided. Dark green or black stools are a commonly occurring adverse effect of iron supplements. Both rinsing his mouth after swallowing liquid iron and drinking the liquid iron through a straw will help the client prevent discoloration of his teeth from contact with the iron preparation.
CN: Physiological integrity; CNS: Pharmacological therapies; CL: Application

27. 3. Warmth and the movement of the extremities during a bath eases the stiffness and pain of rheumatoid arthritis. Ambulation when the client first awakens is the worst time because pain and stiffness are greatest after long periods of immobility. The client may be too tired to walk soon after returning from therapy. There's no relationship between eating and ease of ambulation in rheumatoid arthritis.
CN: Physiological integrity; CNS: Basic care and comfort; CL: Comprehension

28. 1. Surgery is a risk factor for anemia. Polycythemia can occur from severe hypoxia due to congenital heart and pulmonary disease. Purpura and thrombocytopenia may result from decreased bone marrow production of platelets and doesn't result from surgery.
CN: Physiological integrity; CNS: Reduction of risk potential; CL: Application

29. 2. Thrombocytopenia is a decreased number of platelets. Thrombocytosis is an excess number of platelets, and thrombocytopathy is platelet dysfunction. Thrombectomy is the surgical removal of a thrombus.
CN: Physiological integrity; CNS: Physiological adaptation; CL: Knowledge

CN: Client needs category   CNS: Client needs subcategory   CL: Cognitive level

30. Which signs and symptoms are classic for thrombocytopenia?
1. Weakness and fatigue
2. Dizziness and vomiting
3. Bruising and petechiae
4. Light-headedness and nausea

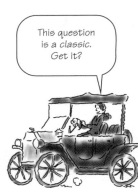

This question is a classic. Get it?

31. Which explanation about the action of heparin should the nurse provide to a client who has just started taking the drug?
1. It slows the time it takes the blood to clot.
2. It stops the blood from clotting.
3. It thins the blood.
4. It dissolves clots in the arteries of the heart.

32. The physician orders a bone marrow biopsy and a platelet transfusion for a client with a bleeding disorder. The nurse knows the platelets will be administered:
1. immediately following the bone marrow biopsy.
2. 1 to 2 hours before the bone marrow biopsy.
3. immediately before the start of the bone marrow biopsy.
4. slowly during the bone marrow biopsy.

33. A 70-year-old female client with cancer and iron deficiency anemia is on iron replacement therapy. Which statement indicates the client has a good understanding of her medication?
1. "I'll always take the iron supplement on an empty stomach."
2. "I'll take the iron supplement with orange juice."
3. "When I take liquid iron, I should swish it in my mouth before swallowing."
4. "Iron supplements might change my stools to a lighter color."

30. 3. Platelets are necessary for clot formation, so petechiae and bruising are signs of a decreased number of platelets. Weakness and fatigue are signs of anemia. Light-headedness, nausea, dizziness, and vomiting are *not* usual signs of thrombocytopenia.
CN: Health promotion and maintenance; CNS: None; CL: Analysis

31. 1. Heparin prolongs the time needed for blood to clot; however, it doesn't thin the blood. If given in large doses, heparin may stop the blood from clotting; however, this isn't why heparin is usually given. Heparin doesn't dissolve clots.
CN: Physiological integrity; CNS: Pharmacological therapies; CL: Application

32. 3. Administering platelets immediately before beginning an invasive procedure increases the number of circulating platelets and therefore provides the greatest protection from potential hemorrhage. Administering platelets following the procedure may have some benefit but isn't as effective and may not prevent hemorrhage. Administering platelets too early may result in fewer circulating platelets during the procedure. Platelets are fragile and are administered as rapidly as the client can tolerate to minimize their destruction.
CN: Physiological integrity; CNS: Reduction of risk potential; CL: Analysis

33. 2. Taking iron with orange juice or ascorbic acid enhances absorption. Taking iron after meals or a snack, rather than on an empty stomach, decreases GI upset. Liquid iron can permanently stain the teeth. The client should use a straw to swallow the liquid. Iron will turn the client's stools dark and tarry, not lighter.
CN: Physiological integrity; CNS: Pharmacological therapies; CL: Knowledge

34. A pregnant woman arrives at the emergency department with abruptio placentae at 34 weeks' gestation. She's at risk for which blood dyscrasia?
1. Thrombocytopenia
2. Idiopathic thrombocytopenic purpura (ITP)
3. Disseminated intravascular coagulation (DIC)
4. Heparin-associated thrombosis and thrombocytopenia (HATT)

35. Which statement by a client with sickle cell disease indicates further teaching is needed to reinforce the therapeutic regimen?
1. "I should avoid vacationing or traveling in areas of high altitude."
2. "Cigarette smoking can cause a sickle cell crisis."
3. "I should drink 4 to 6 liters of fluids each day."
4. "I should take one baby aspirin daily to help prevent sickle cell crisis."

36. A client with thrombocytopenia, secondary to leukemia, develops epistaxis. The nurse should instruct the client to:
1. lie supine with his neck extended.
2. sit upright, leaning slightly forward.
3. blow his nose and then put lateral pressure on it.
4. hold his nose while bending forward at the waist.

37. Which laboratory test, besides a platelet count, is best for confirming the diagnosis of essential thrombocytopenia?
1. Bleeding time
2. Complete blood count (CBC)
3. Immunoglobulin (Ig) G level
4. Prothrombin time (PT) and International Normalized Ratio (INR)

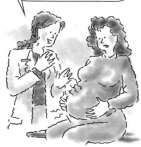

At 34 weeks, this patient is suffering from abruptio placentae and may be at risk for...

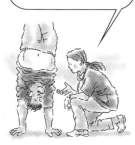

I'm pretty sure this isn't one of the options for question 36!

34. 3. Abruptio placentae is a cause of DIC because of activation of the clotting cascade after hemorrhage. Thrombocytopenia results from decreased bone marrow production. ITP can result in DIC, but not because of abruptio placentae. A client with abruptio placentae wouldn't receive heparin and, as a result, wouldn't be at risk for HATT.
CN: Physiological integrity; CNS: Reduction of risk potential; CL: Application

35. 4. Aspirin inhibits platelet aggregation and won't help prevent sickle cell crisis. Hydroxyurea is prescribed for some people to help prevent sickle cell crisis. High altitudes increase oxygen demand and therefore can also precipitate a crisis. Tobacco, alcohol, and dehydration can precipitate a sickle cell crisis and should be avoided.
CN: Health promotion and maintenance; CNS: None; CL: Analysis

36. 2. The upright position, leaning slightly forward, avoids increasing the vascular pressure in the nose and helps the client avoid aspirating blood. Lying supine won't prevent aspiration of blood. Nose blowing can dislodge any clotting that has occurred. Bending at the waist increases vascular pressure and promotes bleeding rather than stopping it.
CN: Physiological integrity; CNS: Physiological adaptation; CL: Application

37. 1. After a platelet count, the best test to determine thrombocytopenia is bleeding time. The platelet count is decreased and bleeding time is prolonged. IgG assays are nonspecific, but may help determine the diagnosis. A CBC shows the hemoglobin levels, hematocrit, and white blood cell values. PT and INR evaluate the effect of warfarin (Coumadin) therapy.
CN: Physiological integrity; CNS: Physiological adaptation; CL: Application

38. A nurse is documenting care for a client with iron deficiency anemia. Which nursing diagnosis is most appropriate?
1. Impaired gas exchange
2. Deficient fluid volume
3. Ineffective airway clearance
4. Ineffective breathing pattern

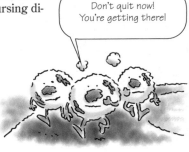

Don't quit now! You're getting there!

39. Which organs are part of the immune system?
1. Paranasal sinuses and pharynx
2. Adrenals and kidneys
3. Lymph nodes and thymus
4. Pancreas and liver

40. Which statement is an example of passive acquired immunity?
1. A child receives the necessary immunizations before beginning school.
2. After having chickenpox, a teenager is unlikely to get the disease again.
3. A nurse who was accidentally exposed to hepatitis B virus from a needle stick receives hepatitis B immune globulin.
4. An adult develops shingles.

41. T cells are involved in which type of immunity?
1. Humoral immunity
2. Cell-mediated immunity
3. Antigen-mediated immunity
4. Immunoglobulin-mediated immunity

38. 1. Iron is necessary for hemoglobin synthesis. Hemoglobin is responsible for oxygen transport in the body. Iron deficiency anemia causes subnormal hemoglobin levels, which impair tissue oxygenation and warrants a nursing diagnosis of *Impaired gas exchange*. Iron deficiency anemia doesn't cause a deficient fluid volume and is less directly related to ineffective airway clearance and ineffective breathing pattern than it is to ineffective gas exchange.
CN: Physiological integrity; CNS: Physiological adaptation; CL: Analysis

39. 3. The immune system includes the lymph nodes, thymus, and spleen. The paranasal sinuses and pharynx are part of the respiratory system. The adrenals are endocrine organs. Kidneys belong to the genitourinary system. The liver and pancreas are part of the GI system.
CN: Physiological integrity; CNS: Physiological adaptation; CL: Knowledge

40. 3. Immune globulin provides a temporary immunity that's passively acquired. Antibodies from one person are recovered and administered to another person to help prevent that person from being infected. Since the recipient's immune system didn't make the antibodies, the immunity is considered to be passively acquired. Immunizations and actual disease processes such as chickenpox cause the body to manufacture antibodies against future exposure to these specific antigens; this is called *active immunity*. Active immunity produces antibodies that are either permanent or longer lasting than passively acquired immunity. Shingles develops when latent varicella zoster virus is activated. Varicella zoster is the virus that causes chickenpox.
CN: Physiological integrity; CNS: Reduction of risk potential; CL: Application

41. 2. T cells are responsible for cell-mediated immunity, in which the T cells respond directly to the antigen. B cells are responsible for humoral or immunoglobulin-mediated immunity. There's no antigen-mediated immunity.
CN: Physiological integrity; CNS: Physiological adaptation; CL: Knowledge

42. Following a kidney transplantation, a client is prescribed a combination of medications that includes steroids and cyclosporine (Gengraf). Which patient teaching should the nurse reinforce?

1. Avoid eating home-canned foods.
2. Avoid being in crowds, especially when known contagions have been identified as a public health concern.
3. If symptoms of bleeding occur, such as petechiae, dark stools, bleeding gums, or easy bruising, stop the medications immediately and seek medical care.
4. Take acetaminophen(Tylenol) if temperature rises above 101° F (38.3° C).

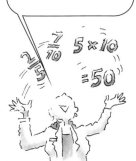

Congratulations! You're more than one-half finished!

42. 2. The client should avoid situations in which infections can be transmitted because his ability to resist pathogens is diminished. Steroids impair the immune system and cyclosporine is given to suppress the immune response to decrease the chance of transplant organ rejection. Home-canned foods should be boiled for 20 minutes and inspected before being consumed, but generally pose no greater risk of infection than commercially canned foods. Steroids and cyclosporine aren't associated with bleeding tendencies and should never be stopped abruptly. Even mild febrile episodes should be reported immediately because the client's immune system is impaired, and taking medications such as acetaminophen could mask the presence of serious infections.
CN: Physiological integrity; CNS: Pharmacological therapies; CL: Application

43. Which client is <u>most</u> at risk for developing Hodgkin's disease?

1. A 38-year-old male with a recent history of infectious mononucleosis who has a sister with Hodgkin's disease
2. A 28-year-old male with obesity, hypertension, and hyperlipidemia
3. A 50-year-old female in a same-sex, monogamous relationship who has a maternal aunt with Hodgkin's disease
4. A 68-year-old male who required multiple blood transfusions during a splenectomy following a car accident

43. 1. Clients who are at risk for developing Hodgkin's disease include males ages 15 to 40 and older than age 55 who have a sibling with the disease. Clients who have had an illness caused by Epstein-Barr virus, who have a compromised immune system, or who are on long-term steroid therapy are also at risk. Obesity, hypertension, dyslipidemia, monogamous same-sex relationships, and multiple blood transfusions don't increase a client's risk of Hodgkin's disease. There's no evidence that having another relative, other than a sibling, with Hodgkin's disease increases the risk of the disease.
CN: Physiological integrity; CNS: Physiological adaptation; CL: Application

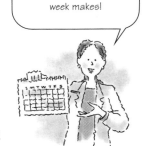

What a difference a week makes!

44. What's the life span for normal platelets?
1. 1 to 3 days
2. 3 to 5 days
3. 7 to 10 days
4. 3 to 4 months

44. 3. The life span of a normal platelet is 7 to 10 days. However, in idiopathic thrombocytopenia, the platelet life span is reduced to 1 to 3 days.
CN: Physiological integrity; CNS: Physiological adaptation; CL: Knowledge

45. What's the normal life span for healthy red blood cells (RBCs)?
1. 60 days
2. 90 days
3. 120 days
4. 240 days

45. 3. A healthy RBC lives for about 120 days.
CN: Physiological integrity; CNS: Physiological adaptation; CL: Knowledge

CN: Client needs category   CNS: Client needs subcategory   CL: Cognitive level

46. Which statement indicates that a client with thrombocytopenia understands the function of platelets in her body?
1. "Platelets regulate acid-base balance."
2. "Platelets regulate the immune response."
3. "Platelets protect the body from infection."
4. "Platelets stop bleeding when arteries and veins are injured."

46. 4. Platelets clump together to plug small breaks in blood vessels. They also initiate the clotting cascade by releasing thromboplastin, which (in the presence of calcium) converts prothrombin into thrombin. Platelets don't perform the other functions.
CN: Physiological integrity; CNS: Reduction of risk potential; CL: Application

47. A 43-year-old female client is undergoing treatment for colon cancer. The physician documents thrombocytopenia on the client's diagnosis list. What observations can the nurse expect?
1. Diarrhea
2. Thin, brittle hair
3. Bruises on the skin
4. Urinary urgency

47. 3. With thrombocytopenia, there's an abnormal decrease in the number of blood platelets, which can result in bruises and bleeding. The client may have constipation, but usually not diarrhea. Thin, brittle hair isn't a sign of thrombocytopenia, but could be a sign of hypothyroidism. Urinary urgency could be a sign of urinary tract infection, but not thrombocytopenia.
CN: Physiological integrity; CNS: Reduction of risk potential; CL: Application

48. A client involved in a motor vehicle collision arrives in the emergency department unconscious and severely hypotensive. He's suspected to have several fractures (pelvis and legs). Which parenteral fluid is the best choice for his current condition?
1. Whole blood
2. Normal saline solution
3. Lactated Ringer's solution
4. Packed red blood cells (RBCs)

Don't worry about your accident. We've packed you with helpful things!

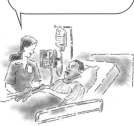

48. 4. In a trauma situation, the first blood product given is unmatched (O negative) packed RBCs. Fresh frozen plasma is commonly used to replace clotting factors. Normal saline or lactated Ringer's solution is used to increase volume and blood pressure, but too much colloid will hemodilute the blood and won't improve oxygen-carrying capacity, whereas RBCs would.
CN: Physiological integrity; CNS: Physiological adaptation; CL: Application

49. A nurse is monitoring a 17-year-old male client who's receiving a blood transfusion for volume replacement. The client complains of itching about 20 minutes after the infusion begins. The nurse should:
1. report the symptom so that the infusion can be stopped immediately.
2. call the physician immediately.
3. give the client oral diphenhydramine (Benadryl) and continue to monitor the client's symptoms.
4. do nothing because itching is a normal response to a blood transfusion.

49. 1. Itching is a sign of an adverse reaction, so the nurse must report the symptom immediately so that the infusion can be stopped. The physician should be called, but only after the infusion has been stopped and the client is assessed. No medications should be administered without first reporting the symptom and having the infusion stopped.
CN: Physiological integrity; CNS: Reduction of risk potential; CL: Application

50. A client with systemic lupus erythematosus (SLE) has a nursing diagnosis of *Disturbed body image*. Which nursing interventions would be most appropriate for this diagnosis? Select all that apply.
1. Encourage the client to ask questions about the disease process.
2. Provide the client with information regarding hair-loss support groups.
3. Allow for frequent rest periods during the day.
4. Instruct the client to use sunscreen and avoid prolonged sun exposure.
5. Withhold corticosteroid medications.
6. Instruct the patient to report any rashes, petechiae, ulcers, or bruising

51. Systemic lupus erythematosus (SLE) primarily attacks which tissue?
1. Connective
2. Heart
3. Lung
4. Nerve

52. Which symptom is most commonly an early indication of stage I Hodgkin's disease?
1. Pericarditis
2. Night sweats
3. Splenomegaly
4. Persistent hypothermia

53. Which statement shows that a client needs more education about the cause of an exacerbation of systemic lupus erythematosus (SLE)?
1. "I need to stay away from sunlight."
2. "I don't have to worry if I get strep throat."
3. "I need to work on managing stress in my life."
4. "I don't have to worry about changing my diet."

50. 2, 4, 6. SLE can cause patchy alopecia and sun exposure can result in rashes. Vasculitis from SLE can cause petechiae, ulcers and bruising. All of these conditions may lead to disturbed body image. Encouraging clients to learn about the disease process and explore their feelings improves their coping skills. Frequent rest periods help clients deal with the fatigue and pain that occur with SLE. Corticosteroids are the treatment of choice for clients with SLE.
CN: Psychosocial integrity; CNS: None; CL: Application

51. 1. SLE is a chronic, inflammatory, autoimmune disorder that primarily affects connective tissue. It also affects the skin and kidneys and may affect the pulmonary, cardiac, neural, and renal systems.
CN: Physiological integrity; CNS: Physiological adaptation; CL: Knowledge

52. 2. In stage I, symptoms include a single enlarged lymph node (usually), unexplained fever, night sweats, malaise, and generalized pruritus. Although splenomegaly may be present in some clients, night sweats are generally more prevalent. Pericarditis isn't associated with Hodgkin's disease. Persistent hypothermia is associated with Hodgkin's disease, but isn't an early sign.
CN: Health promotion and maintenance; CNS: None; CL: Knowledge

53. 2. Infection may cause an exacerbation of SLE. Other factors that can precipitate an exacerbation are immunizations, sunlight exposure, and stress. A client's diet doesn't exacerbate SLE.
CN: Health promotion and maintenance; CNS: None; CL: Application

54. Which sign or symptom reported by a client with systemic lupus erythematosus (SLE) alerts the nurse that he may be experiencing a life-threatening complication?
1. Joint pain
2. Foamy urine
3. Butterfly rash on face
4. Fever

55. A 73-year-old female client is about to receive a blood transfusion to treat severe anemia. She asks the nurse how long the procedure will take. The nurse explains that the treatment takes:
1. 8 hours.
2. at least 12 hours.
3. at least 24 hours.
4. no longer than 4 hours.

56. Which statement by a nurse accurately explains the need for a client who's being treated with hydroxychloroquine (Plaquenil) for systemic lupus erythromatosus to have an ophthalmologic examination every 6 months?
1. "Hydroxychloroquine can cause damage to the retinas of your eyes."
2. "Dry eye syndrome is a common side effect of hydroxychloroquine."
3. "Hydroxychloroquine has been known to cause cataract formation."
4. "The pressure in your eyes must be measured to see if you're developing glaucoma."

57. Which symptom is a classic sign of systemic lupus erythematosus (SLE)?
1. Vomiting
2. Weight loss
3. Difficulty urinating
4. Superficial rash over the cheeks and nose

58. Which laboratory test results support the diagnosis of systemic lupus erythematosus (SLE)?
1. Elevated serum complement level
2. Thrombocytosis, elevated sedimentation rate
3. Pancytopenia, positive antinuclear antibody (ANA) titer
4. Leukocytosis, elevated blood urea nitrogen (BUN) and creatinine levels

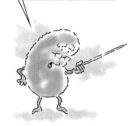

My life is difficult enough. I don't need any more complications.

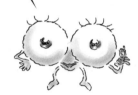

I just heard that hydroxychloroquine can really cause problems for me.

54. 2. Foamy urine indicates proteinuria and is associated with kidney damage, which is a life-threatening complication of SLE. Joint pain, rashes, and fever are all common symptoms of SLE but aren't life-threatening.
CN: Physiological integrity; CNS: Physiological adaptation; CL: Application

55. 4. The American Association of Blood Banks recommends that blood or blood components should be transfused within 4 hours. If they aren't, they should be divided and stored appropriately in the blood bank. Any length of time over 4 hours would compromise the integrity of the transfusion components.
CN: Safe, effective care environment; CNS: Safety and infection control; CL: Application

56. 1. Hydroxychloroquine can cause retinal damage and clients should have ophthalmologic examinations every 6 months. Dry eye syndrome, cataract formation, and glaucoma are all diseases of the eye but aren't associated with hydroxychloroquine use.
CN: Physiological integrity; CNS: Pharmacological therapies; CL: Analysis

57. 4. Although all these symptoms can be signs of SLE, the classic sign is the butterfly rash over the cheeks and nose.
CN: Physiological integrity; CNS: Physiological adaptation; CL: Knowledge

58. 3. Laboratory findings for clients with SLE usually show pancytopenia, positive ANA titer, and decreased serum complement levels. Clients may have elevated BUN and creatinine levels from nephritis, but the increase does *not* indicate SLE. Thrombocytosis and elevated sedimentation rate usually indicate polyarteritis nodosa, not SLE.
CN: Physiological integrity; CNS: Physiological adaptation; CL: Application

59. Which laboratory value is expected for a client recently diagnosed with chronic lymphocytic leukemia?
1. Elevated erythrocyte sedimentation rate (ESR)
2. Uncontrolled proliferation of granulocytes
3. Thrombocytopenia and increased lymphocytes
4. Elevated aspartate aminotransferase (AST) and alanine aminotransferase (ALT) levels

60. A nurse receives laboratory results for a hospitalized, 48-year-old female client who has acute leukemia. Referring to the provided laboratory slip, which result requires immediate reporting by the nurse?
1. RBC count
2. Hemoglobin
3. Hematocrit
4. Platelet count

Laboratory results

Laboratory test	Results
Red blood cell (RBC) count	4 million/mm³
White blood cell (WBC) count	13,000/mm³
Hemoglobin	12.2 g/dl
Hematocrit	35%
Platelet count	14,500/mm³

61. According to a standard staging classification of Hodgkin's disease, which criteria reflect stage II?
1. Involvement of extralymphatic organs or tissues
2. Involvement of a single lymph node region or structure
3. Involvement of two or more lymph node regions or structures
4. Involvement of lymph node regions or structures on both sides of the diaphragm

62. Which signs and symptoms would indicate involvement of upper chest and neck lymph nodes in a client with Hodgkin's disease?
1. Fever, weight loss, and night sweats
2. Bone pain and jaundice
3. Cough, dysphagia, and stridor
4. Weight loss and malaise

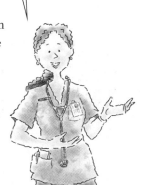

To answer question 62, you should be familiar with the signs and symptoms of Hodgkin's disease and their causes.

59. 3. Chronic lymphocytic leukemia shows a proliferation of small abnormal mature B lymphocytes and decreased antibody response. Thrombocytopenia is also commonly present. Uncontrolled proliferation of granulocytes occurs in myelogenous leukemia. AST, ALT, and ESR values are *not* affected.
CN: Physiological integrity; CNS: Physiological adaptation; CL: Knowledge

60. 4. Platelet count 14,500/mm³. A platelet count below 20,000/mm³ is considered a life-threatening situation and generally requires medical treatment of immediate platelet transfusions. The RBC count, hemoglobin, and hematocrit level are lower than normal but don't require immediate intervention if the client is asymptomatic. The WBC count is slightly elevated and would be expected in leukemia.
CN: Physiological integrity; CNS: Physiological adaptation; CL: Analysis

61. 3. Stage II involves two or more lymph node regions. Stage I involves only one lymph node region; stage III involves nodes on both sides of the diaphragm; and stage IV involves extralymphatic organs or tissues.
CN: Physiological integrity; CNS: Physiological adaptation; CL: Knowledge

62. 3. Enlarged lymph nodes of the neck and upper chest can produce such symptoms as cough, dysphagia, and stridor due to pressure and obstruction of the structures of the respiratory system and esophagus. Although fever, weight loss, night sweats, and malaise are also seen with Hodgkin's disease, these symptoms aren't directly related to enlargement of neck and chest lymph nodes. Bone pain and jaundice may indicate bone and liver metastasis.
CN: Physiological integrity; CNS: Physiological adaptation; CL: Application

63. When protective isolation isn't indicated, which activity is recommended for a client receiving chemotherapy?
1. Bed rest
2. Activity as tolerated
3. Walk to bathroom only
4. Out of bed for brief periods

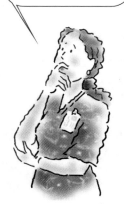

Let's see...I know I remember reading about this somewhere.

64. A nurse is teaching a client with serious allergies how to prevent death from anaphylaxis. Which recommendation is <u>most appropriate</u> for this client?
1. Dry-mop all hardwood floors.
2. Wear a medical identification bracelet or necklace at all times.
3. Have carpet installed in every room of the house.
4. Advise family and friends not to visit during the winter.

65. Which nursing intervention is <u>most appropriate</u> for a client with multiple myeloma?
1. Monitoring respiratory status
2. Balancing rest and activity
3. Restricting fluid intake
4. Preventing bone injury

66. Which food should a client with leukemia avoid?
1. White bread
2. Raw carrot sticks
3. Stewed apples
4. Well-done steak

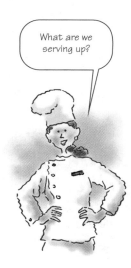

What are we serving up?

67. A client with leukemia has neutropenia. Which function must be frequently monitored?
1. Blood pressure
2. Bowel sounds
3. Heart sounds
4. Breath sounds

63. 2. It's important that the client be able to engage in activities that are of interest and to maintain as much independence and autonomy as possible. Bed rest isn't necessary, nor is it necessary to limit the client's activity to only walks to the bathroom or out of bed for brief periods.
CN: Health promotion and maintenance; CNS: None; CL: Application

64. 2. If the client becomes unconscious or can't report allergies, medical identification jewelry could provide that information and help health care providers intervene and treat anaphylaxis as soon as possible. The client should wet-mop hardwood floors because dry-mopping scatters dust, which can trigger allergies. The client should minimize the amount of carpet in the home because carpet traps allergens, such as dust and dirt. Unless the client is ill, the nurse may encourage visits by family and friends to promote healthy social interaction.
CN: Health promotion and maintenance; CNS: None; CL: Comprehension

65. 4. When caring for a client with multiple myeloma, the nurse should focus on relieving pain, preventing bone injury and infection, and maintaining hydration. Monitoring respiratory status and balancing rest and activity are appropriate interventions for any client. To prevent such complications as pyelonephritis and renal calculi, the nurse should keep the client well hydrated, not restrict the client's fluid intake.
CN: Safe, effective care environment; CNS: Safety and infection control; CL: Application

66. 2. A low-bacteria diet would be indicated, which excludes raw fruits and vegetables.
CN: Health promotion and maintenance; CNS: None; CL: Application

67. 4. Pneumonia—viral and fungal—is a common cause of death in clients with neutropenia, so frequent assessment of respiratory rate and breath sounds is required. Although assessing blood pressure, bowel sounds, and heart sounds is important, it won't help detect pneumonia.
CN: Physiological integrity; CNS: Physiological adaptation; CL: Application

CN: Client needs category   CNS: Client needs subcategory   CL: Cognitive level

68. Which process removes excess white blood cells (WBCs) from the body?
1. Erythrapheresis
2. Granulapheresis
3. Leukapheresis
4. Plasmapheresis

69. Which client is at <u>highest</u> risk for developing multiple myeloma?
1. A 20-year-old Asian female
2. A 30-year-old White male
3. A 50-year-old Hispanic female
4. A 60-year-old Black male

70. Which substance has <u>abnormal</u> values in multiple myeloma?
1. Immunoglobulins
2. Platelets
3. Red blood cells (RBCs)
4. White blood cells (WBCs)

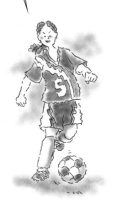

Forget the weights. Keep an eye on those "abs."

71. For which condition is a client with multiple myeloma monitored?
1. Hypercalcemia
2. Hyperkalemia
3. Hypernatremia
4. Hypermagnesemia

72. Which are the <u>most</u> common signs and symptoms of hypercalcemia?
1. Fatigue, muscle weakness, confusion, constipation
2. Diarrhea, oliguria, headaches
3. Tremors, tetany, bradycardia, hypotension
4. Hallucinations, fainting, headaches, blurred vision

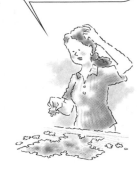

I'm feeling hyper. I know this piece goes somewhere.

73. A client with multiple myeloma has developed hypercalcemia. Which nursing intervention has <u>highest</u> priority?
1. Protecting the client from trauma
2. Elevating the head of bed 45 degrees
3. Carefully monitoring fluid intake and output
4. Providing a quiet, darkened room

68. 3. Leukapheresis is the removal of excess WBCs. Plasmapheresis is the filtering of the plasma. There are no processes called granulapheresis or erythrapheresis.
CN: Physiological integrity; CNS: Basic care and comfort; CL: Knowledge

69. 4. Multiple myeloma is more common in middle-aged and older male clients (two-thirds are older than age 65) and is twice as common in Blacks as Whites. Asians have the lowest incidence.
CN: Health promotion and maintenance; CNS: None; CL: Comprehension

70. 1. Multiple myeloma is characterized by an overproduction of immunoglobulins and multiple tumors throughout the skeleton, which results in significant bone marrow loss and hard bone tissue. This produces pancytopenia and osteoporosis. Platelet counts and RBC and WBC levels aren't usually affected in clients with multiple myeloma.
CN: Health promotion and maintenance; CNS: None; CL: Knowledge

71. 1. Calcium is released when bone is destroyed. This causes an increase in serum calcium levels. Multiple myeloma doesn't affect potassium, sodium, or magnesium levels.
CN: Physiological integrity; CNS: Physiological adaptation; CL: Application

72. 1. Common signs and symptoms of hypercalcemia include fatigue, muscle weakness, confusion, and constipation. Hallucinations, headaches, and hypertension are less common symptoms. Diarrhea, oliguria, fainting, and blurred vision aren't associated with hypercalcemia. Tremors, tetany, and cardiac arrhythmias are associated with hypocalcemia.
CN: Physiological integrity; CNS: Physiological adaptation; CL: Application

73. 3. Hypercalcemia may lead to renal dysfunction. By carefully monitoring fluid intake and output, the nurse would be alert to decreased urine output. All clients should be protected from trauma. Elevating the head of the bed is an intervention for impaired ventilation, gastroesophageal reflux disease, and increased intracranial pressure. A quiet, dark room commonly used to decrease sensory stimulus for clients who have meningitis or preeclampsia.
CN: Physiological integrity; CNS: Reduction of risk potential; CL: Application

CN: Client needs category   CNS: Client needs subcategory   CL: Cognitive level

74. The neurologic complications of multiple myeloma usually involve which body system?
   1. Brain
   2. Spinal column
   3. Autonomic nervous system
   4. Parasympathetic nervous system

74. 2. Back pain or paresthesia in the lower extremities may indicate impending spinal cord compression from a spinal tumor. This should be recognized and treated promptly because progression of the tumor may result in paraplegia. The other options, which reflect parts of the nervous system, aren't usually affected by multiple myeloma.
CN: Physiological integrity; CNS: Physiological adaptation; CL: Application

75. Which intervention should be stressed when teaching about multiple myeloma?
   1. Maintaining bed rest
   2. Enforcing fluid restriction
   3. Drinking 3 qt (3 L) of fluid daily
   4. Keeping the lower extremities elevated

75. 3. The client needs to drink 3 to 5 qt (3 to 5 L) of fluid each day to dilute calcium and uric acid and thereby reduce the risk of renal dysfunction. Walking is encouraged to prevent further bone demineralization. The lower extremities don't need to be elevated.
CN: Physiological integrity; CNS: Basic care and comfort; CL: Application

76. Although a client's physiologic response to a health crisis is important to the health outcome, which nursing intervention <u>must</u> also be addressed?
   1. Teaching the family how to care for the client
   2. Helping the client effectively cope with the crisis
   3. Maintaining I.V. access, medications, and diet
   4. Teaching the client basic information about the illness

76. 2. Although all of the answers are important in the care of the client, if the individual can't cope with the emotional, spiritual, and psychological aspects of his crisis, the other components of care may be less effective as well.
CN: Psychosocial integrity; CNS: None; CL: Application

77. To promote healing of a laceration, which intervention is correct?
   1. Elevating the body part
   2. Monitoring blood pressure
   3. Applying a pressure dressing and heat
   4. Applying a pressure dressing and ice pack

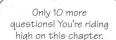

Only 10 more questions! You're riding high on this chapter.

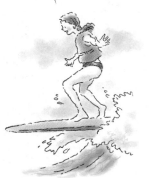

77. 4. Pressure dressings help clotting by promoting the localization of microorganisms and the development of meshwork for repair and healing. Ice decreases blood flow to the site, slowing the bleeding. Heat increases blood flow to the site, increasing the bleeding. Monitoring blood pressure is important when the individual is bleeding, but does nothing to promote clotting. Elevating the body part helps reduce edema, but doesn't directly promote healing.
CN: Physiological integrity; CNS: Physiological adaptation; CL: Application

CN: Client needs category   CNS: Client needs subcategory   CL: Cognitive level

78. An elderly client has a wound that isn't healing normally. Interventions should be based on which principle or test result?
1. Laboratory test results
2. Kidney function test results
3. Poor wound healing expected as part of the aging process
4. Diminished immune function interfering with ability to fight infection

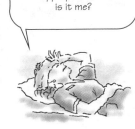

Is this question appropriate, or is it me?

79. Which response to an antigen is an appropriate, therapeutic, immune system response?
1. Widespread histamine release
2. Autoimmune response
3. Inflammation and increased body temperature
4. Antibody production by T cells

80. Which intervention has the most impact in delaying the development of acquired immunodeficiency syndrome (AIDS) once a client has been infected with human immunodeficiency virus (HIV)?
1. Monthly plasmapharesis
2. Eating a balanced, nutritious diet
3. Compliance with the complete therapeutic regimen
4. Getting adequate rest and sleep

81. Which condition or factor may cause an acquired immune deficiency?
1. Age
2. Genetics
3. Environment
4. Medical treatments

78. 4. Immune function is important in the healing process, and diminished response may slow or prevent the healing process from taking place. Although immune function declines with age, there are healthy behaviors that will enhance the elderly individual's response to tissue trauma (nutrition, exercise). Kidney function and laboratory results are important, but are *not* solely responsible for health outcomes.
CN: Physiological integrity; CNS: Physiological adaptation; CL: Analysis

79. 3. Temperature elevations and activation of the inflammatory response are normal immune system responses to detected antigens. Widespread histamine release is an exaggerated response that can lead to anaphylaxis. An autoimmune response is one in which the immune system forms antibodies against the body's own tissues, resulting in disease. Antibodies are produced by B cells, not T cells.
CN: Physiological integrity; CNS: Reduction of risk potential; CL: Application

80. 3. Compliance with the complete therapeutic regimen includes adhering to a healthy lifestyle, taking prescribed medications, and reducing risks from other infections and is the most important intervention in delaying the onset of AIDS. Eating a balanced diet and getting adequate rest and sleep are part of the overall therapeutic regimen. Plasmapharesis isn't a treatment for HIV/AIDS.
CN: Health promotion and maintenance; CNS: None; CL: Analysis

81. 4. Immune deficiencies may result from medical treatments, such as medications, radiation, or transplants. Immune function may decline with age, but it isn't considered the cause of acquired immune deficiency. Genetics and environment haven't been shown to be factors in acquired immune deficiency.
CN: Physiological integrity; CNS: Physiological adaptation; CL: Analysis

82. Which statement best explains the reason for using stress management with clients?
1. Everyone is stressed.
2. It has become an accepted practice.
3. Eastern health practices have shown its effectiveness.
4. Prolonged psychological stress may contribute to the development of physical illness.

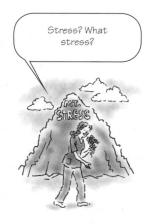

Stress? What stress?

82. 4. Psychological and emotional stress stimulate the central nervous system, increasing the levels of corticotropin and cortisol, which results in harmful effects on immune, cardiac, neural, and endocrine function. Although stress management may be a common therapy for stressed individuals and Eastern countries may promote its use, nursing interventions need to focus on research-based rationales for intervention. Many people report high levels of stress, but not everyone would claim to be stressed.
CN: Psychosocial integrity; CNS: None; CL: Knowledge

83. Which additional physician order should a nurse anticipate for a client who has been prescribed corticosteroids?
1. Perform blood glucose checks every 6 hours.
2. Restrict fluids to 1,000 ml in 24 hours.
3. Administer lactulose 40 g in 4 oz of water daily.
4. Obtain serum platelet counts with hemoglobin and hematocrit levels every 12 hours.

83. 1. Corticosteroids cause elevated blood glucose levels; insulin may be necessary to maintain normal blood glucose levels. Corticosteroids can cause edema but fluid restrictions are generally unnecessary unless the client also has renal or cardiac disease. Lactulose is given for constipation and to treat hepatic encephalopathy. Hematologic studies, such as platelet counts, hemoglobin, and hematocrit levels, aren't usually necessary when monitoring clients undergoing corticosteroid therapy.
CN: Physiological integrity; CNS: Pharmacological therapies; CL: Application

84. During the recovery phase of a surgical client's hospitalization, a nurse notes that the client's immune status appears to be altered. Although there's no obvious rationale for the immunocompromise, which area should be further investigated?
1. Nutrition
2. Acquired immune disorder
3. Family history of immune problems
4. Personal history of substance abuse or use

84. 4. Substance abuse, including alcohol consumption and tobacco or marijuana use, influences immunocompetence and overall health status. Although nutrition is important for immunocompetence, it would be part of the client's daily assessment. A family history would have been assessed initially. Assessing the client for an acquired immune disorder would be a joint effort with the physician and wouldn't be conducted independently.
CN: Psychosocial integrity; CNS: None; CL: Application

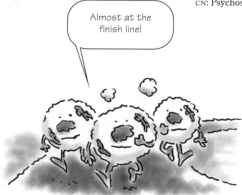

Almost at the finish line!

85. The nurse is using the Z-track method of I.M. injection to administer iron dextran to a client with iron deficiency anemia. Which techniques should the nurse use to give this injection? Select all that apply:
1. Confirm the client's identity before administering the iron dextran.
2. Inject the iron dextran into the deltoid muscle.
3. Change the needle after drawing up the iron dextran.
4. Before inserting the needle, displace the skin laterally by pulling it away from the injection site.
5. Inject the iron dextran after aspirating for a blood return.
6. After removing the needle, massage the injection site.

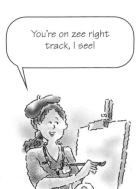

You're on zee right track, I see!

86. The nurse is assisting in planning care for a client with human immunodeficiency virus (HIV). Which statement by the nurse indicates her understanding of HIV transmission? Select all that apply:
1. "I'll wear a gown, a mask, and gloves with all client contact."
2. "I don't need to wear any personal protective equipment due to decreased risk of occupational exposure."
3. "I'll wear a mask if the client has a cough caused by an upper respiratory infection."
4. "I'll wear a mask, a gown, and gloves when splashing of body fluids is likely."
5. "I'll wash my hands after client care."

85. 1, 3, 4, 5. Before administering any medication, the nurse confirms the client's identity. After drawing up iron dextran, she removes the first needle and attaches a second needle to prevent tracking the medication through the subcutaneous tissue when the needle is inserted. To administer the injection by Z-track method, the nurse first displaces the skin laterally by pulling it away from the injection site. The nurse should aspirate for a blood return before administering iron dextran; if no blood appears, the medication may be injected. Iron dextran should be administered into the large dorsogluteal muscle only. After injecting iron dextran, the nurse shouldn't massage the site because this could force the medication into the subcutaneous tissue.
CN: Physiological integrity; CNS: Pharmacological therapies; CL: Application

86. 4, 5. Standard precautions include wearing gloves for known or anticipated contact with blood, body fluids, tissue, mucous membranes, and nonintact skin. If the task or procedure may result in splashing or splattering of blood or body fluids to the face, the nurse should wear a mask and goggles or a face shield. If the task or procedure may result in splashing or splattering of blood or body fluids, the nurse should wear a fluid-resistant gown or apron. The nurse should wash her hands before and after client care and after removing gloves. A gown, a mask, and gloves aren't necessary for all client care unless contact with body fluids, tissue, mucous membranes, and nonintact skin is expected. Nurses have an increased, not decreased, risk of occupational exposure to blood-borne pathogens. HIV isn't transmitted in sputum unless blood is present.
CN: Safe, effective care environment; CNS: Safety and infection control; CL: Application

87. The nurse is preparing a client with systemic lupus erythematosus (SLE) for discharge. Which instructions should the nurse include in the teaching plan? Select all that apply:
1. Stay out of direct sunlight.
2. Refrain from limiting activity between flare-ups.
3. Monitor body temperature.
4. Taper the corticosteroid dosage as ordered by the physician when symptoms are under control.
5. Apply cold packs to relieve joint pain and stiffness.

87. 1, 3, 4. The client with SLE should stay out of direct sunlight and avoid other sources of ultraviolet light because they may precipitate severe skin reactions and exacerbate the disease. The client should monitor his temperature, because fever can signal an exacerbation, which he should report to the physician. Corticosteroids must be tapered gradually once symptoms are relieved because they can suppress the function of the adrenal glands. Stopping corticosteroids abruptly can cause adrenal insufficiency, a potentially life-threatening condition. Fatigue can cause a flare-up of SLE; encourage clients to pace activities and plan for rest periods. The client should apply heat, not cold, to relieve joint pain. Cold packs may aggravate Raynaud's phenomenon, which commonly occurs in clients with SLE.
CN: Physiological integrity; CNS: Reduction of risk potential; CL: Application

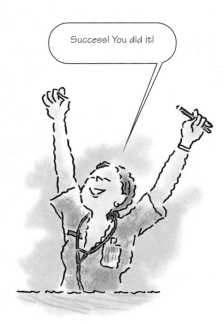

Success! You did it!

CN: Client needs category   CNS: Client needs subcategory   CL: Cognitive level

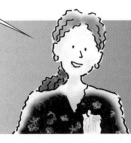

Chapter 5
Respiratory disorders

1. Clients with chronic illnesses are <u>more likely</u> to get pneumonia when which situation is present?
   1. Dehydration
   2. Group living
   3. Malnutrition
   4. Severe periodontal disease

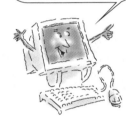

In question 1, the word *chronic* is a hint for finding the correct answer.

2. Which pathophysiological mechanism that occurs in the lung parenchyma allows pneumonia to develop?
   1. Atelectasis
   2. Bronchiectasis
   3. Effusion
   4. Inflammation

3. Which organism most commonly causes community-acquired pneumonia in adults?
   1. *Haemophilus influenzae*
   2. *Klebsiella pneumoniae*
   3. *Streptococcus pneumoniae*
   4. *Staphylococcus aureus*

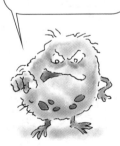

Pssst. Yeah. I'm talking to you. You'd better strep lively—er, I mean, step lively. Got it?

4. An elderly client with pneumonia commonly exhibits which symptom first?
   1. Altered mental status and dehydration
   2. Fever and chills
   3. Hemoptysis and dyspnea
   4. Pleuritic chest pain and cough

1. 2. Clients with chronic illness generally have poor immune systems. Typically, residing in group living situations increases the chance of disease transmission. Adequate fluid intake, adequate nutrition, and proper oral hygiene help maintain normal defenses and can reduce the incidence of getting such diseases as pneumonia.
CN: Physiological integrity; CNS: Physiological adaptation; CL: Comprehension

2. 4. The common feature of all types of pneumonia is an inflammatory pulmonary response to the offending organism or agent. Atelectasis and bronchiectasis indicate a collapse of a portion of the airway that doesn't occur in pneumonia. An effusion is an accumulation of excess pleural fluid in the pleural space, which may be a secondary response to pneumonia.
CN: Physiological integrity; CNS: Physiological adaptation; CL: Knowledge

3. 3. Pneumococcal or streptococcal pneumonia, caused by *S. pneumoniae,* is the most common cause of community-acquired pneumonia. *H. influenzae* is the most common cause of infection in children. *Klebsiella* species is the most common gram-negative organism found in the hospital setting. *S. aureus* is the most common cause of hospital-acquired pneumonia.
CN: Physiological integrity; CNS: Physiological adaptation; CL: Knowledge

4. 1. Fever, chills, hemoptysis, dyspnea, cough, and pleuritic chest pain are the common symptoms of pneumonia, but elderly clients may first exhibit only an altered mental status and dehydration due to a blunted immune response.
CN: Physiological integrity; CNS: Physiological adaptation; CL: Application

CN: Client needs category   CNS: Client needs subcategory   CL: Cognitive level

5. When auscultating the chest of a client with pneumonia, the nurse would expect to hear which sounds over areas of consolidation?
1. Bronchial
2. Bronchovesicular
3. Tubular
4. Vesicular

6. A diagnosis of pneumonia is typically achieved by which diagnostic test?
1. Arterial blood gas (ABG) analysis
2. Chest X-ray
3. Blood cultures
4. Sputum culture and sensitivity

7. A client with pneumonia has a nursing diagnosis of *Ineffective airway clearance related to increased secretions and ineffective cough.* Which intervention would facilitate effective coughing?
1. Lying in semi-Fowler's position
2. Sipping water, hot tea, or coffee
3. Inhaling and exhaling from pursed lips
4. Using thoracic breathing

8. On entering the room of a client with chronic obstructive pulmonary disease (COPD), the nurse notices that the client is receiving oxygen at 4 L/minute by way of a nasal cannula. The nurse's actions should be based on which statement?
1. The flow rate is too high.
2. The flow rate is too low.
3. The flow rate is correct.
4. The client shouldn't receive oxygen.

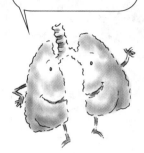

For question 5, think of where you normally hear each type of breath sound.

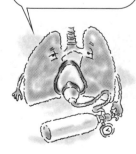

Oxygen therapy is beneficial for clients with COPD—just watch the flow rate.

5. 1. Chest auscultation reveals bronchial breath sounds over areas of consolidation. Bronchovesicular breath sounds are normal over midlobe lung regions, tubular sounds are commonly heard over large airways, and vesicular breath sounds are commonly heard in the bases of the lung fields.
CN: Physiological integrity; CNS: Physiological adaptation; CL: Application

6. 2. Chest X-ray will show the presence of lung infiltrates, which confirms the diagnosis. ABG analysis will determine the extent of hypoxia present due to the pneumonia, and blood cultures will help determine if the infection is systemic. Sputum culture and sensitivity will identify the organism causing the pneumonia, but it isn't always possible to obtain an adequate specimen.
CN: Physiological integrity; CNS: Physiological adaptation; CL: Application

7. 2. Sips of water, hot tea, or coffee may stimulate coughing. The best position is sitting in a chair with the knees flexed and the feet placed firmly on the floor. The client should inhale through the nose and exhale through pursed lips. Diaphragmatic, not thoracic, breathing helps to facilitate coughing.
CN: Physiological integrity; CNS: Basic care and comfort; CL: Application

8. 1. The administration of oxygen at 1 to 2 L/minute by way of a nasal cannula is recommended for clients with COPD: therefore, a rate of 4 L/minute is too high. The normal mechanism that stimulates breathing is a rise in blood carbon dioxide. Clients with COPD retain blood carbon dioxide, so their mechanism for stimulating breathing is a low blood oxygen level. High levels of oxygen may cause hypoventilation and apnea. Oxygen delivered at 1 to 2 L/minute should aid in oxygenation without causing hypoventilation. Oxygen therapy is the only therapy that has been demonstrated to be life-preserving for patients with COPD.
CN: Safe, effective care environment; CNS: Safety and infection control; CL: Application

CN: Client needs category   CNS: Client needs subcategory   CL: Cognitive level

9. A client has been treated with antibiotic therapy for right lower-lobe pneumonia for 10 days and will be discharged today. Which physical finding would lead the nurse to believe it's <u>appropriate</u> to discharge this client?
1. Continued dyspnea
2. Fever of 102° F (38.9° C)
3. Respiratory rate of 32 breaths/minute
4. Normal vesicular breath sounds in right base

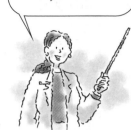

Make sure your answer responds to the question asked.

10. A 20-year-old client is being treated for pneumonia. He has a persistent cough and complains of severe pain on coughing. What type of instruction could be given to help the client <u>reduce</u> the discomfort he is having?
1. "Hold in your cough as much as possible."
2. "Place the head of your bed flat to help with coughing."
3. "Restrict fluids to help decrease the amount of sputum."
4. "Splint your chest wall with a pillow when you cough."

11. An elderly client with pneumonia has a nursing diagnosis of *Ineffective airway clearance*. Which intervention would be <u>most</u> appropriate?
1. Monitoring the need for suctioning every hour
2. Suctioning every hour
3. Suctioning once per shift
4. Asking the physician for an order to suction

12. A nurse is working in a walk-in clinic. She has been alerted that there's an outbreak of tuberculosis (TB). Which client entering the clinic <u>today</u> is most likely to have TB?
1. A 16-year-old female high school student
2. A 33-year-old day-care worker
3. A 43-year-old homeless man with a history of alcoholism
4. A 54-year-old businessman

Consider your current clients and choose the most likely response.

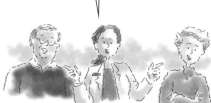

9. 4. If the client still has pneumonia, the breath sounds in the right base will be bronchial, not the normal vesicular breath sounds. If the client still has dyspnea, fever, and increased respiratory rate, the client should be reexamined by the physician before discharge because he may have another source of infection or still have pneumonia.
CN: Physiological integrity; CNS: Physiological adaptation; CL: Analysis

10. 4. Showing this client how to splint his chest wall will help decrease discomfort when coughing. Holding in his coughs will only increase his pain. Placing the head of the bed flat may increase the frequency of his cough and require more respiratory effort; a 45-degree angle may help him cough more efficiently and with less pain. Increasing fluid intake will help thin his secretions, making it easier for him to clear them. Promoting fluid intake is appropriate in this situation.
CN: Physiological integrity; CNS: Physiological adaptation; CL: Application

11. 1. Suctioning should be performed only when necessary, based on the client's condition at the time of assessment. Suctioning is a nursing procedure and doesn't require a physician's order.
CN: Physiological integrity; CNS: Basic care and comfort; CL: Application

12. 3. Clients who are economically disadvantaged, malnourished, and have reduced immunity, such as a client with a history of alcoholism, are at extremely high risk for developing TB. A high school student, a businessman, and a day-care worker probably have a much lower risk of contracting TB.
CN: Physiological integrity; CNS: Physiological adaptation; CL: Comprehension

CN: Client needs category   CNS: Client needs subcategory   CL: Cognitive level

13. Tuberculosis (TB) is a communicable disease transmitted by which method?
  1. Sexual contact
  2. Using dirty needles
  3. Using an infected person's eating utensils
  4. Inhaling droplets exhaled from an infected person

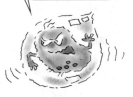

This droplet transmission stuff sure beats the subway!

13. 4. The TB bacillus is airborne and carried in droplets exhaled by an infected person who is coughing, sneezing, laughing, or singing. Sexual contact and dirty needles don't spread the TB bacillus, but may spread other communicable diseases. It's never advisable to use dirty utensils, but if cleaned normally, it isn't necessary to dispose of eating utensils used by someone infected with TB.
CN: Physiological integrity; CNS: Physiological adaptation; CL: Knowledge

14. An adult client is being screened in the clinic for tuberculosis. He reports having negative purified protein derivative (PPD) test results in the past. The nurse performs a PPD test on his right forearm. When should he return to have the test read?
  1. Immediately
  2. In 24 hours
  3. In 48 hours
  4. In 1 week

14. 3. PPD tests should be read in 48 to 72 hours. If read too early or too late, the results won't be accurate.
CN: Health promotion and maintenance; CNS: None; CL: Knowledge

15. The right forearm of a client who had a purified protein derivative (PPD) test for tuberculosis (TB) is reddened and raised about 5 mm where the test was given. This PPD would be read as having which result?
  1. Indeterminate
  2. Needs to be redone
  3. Negative
  4. Positive

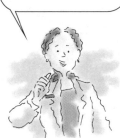

Don't be so negative! I'm sure you'll get this one right!

15. 3. This test would be classed as negative. A 5-mm raised area would be a positive result if a client had recent close contact with someone diagnosed with or suspected of having infectious TB. Follow-up should be done with this client, and a chest X-ray should be ordered. The test can be redone in 6 months to see if the client's test results change. If the PPD test is reddened and raised 10 mm or more, it's considered positive according to the Centers for Disease Control and Prevention. *Indeterminate* isn't a term used to describe results of a PPD test.
CN: Health promotion and maintenance; CNS: None; CL: Knowledge

16. A client with a primary tuberculosis (TB) infection can expect to develop which condition?
  1. Active TB within 2 weeks
  2. Active TB within 1 month
  3. A fever requiring hospitalization
  4. A positive skin test

16. 4. A primary TB infection occurs when the bacillus has successfully invaded the entire body after entering through the lungs. At this point, the bacilli are walled off and skin tests read positive. However, all but infants and immunosuppressed people will remain asymptomatic. The general population has a 10% risk of developing active TB over their lifetime, often because of a break in the body's immune defenses. The active stage shows the classic symptoms of TB: fever, hemoptysis, and night sweats.
CN: Physiological integrity; CNS: Physiological adaptation; CL: Application

CN: Client needs category   CNS: Client needs subcategory   CL: Cognitive level

17. A client was infected with tuberculosis (TB) bacillus 10 years ago but never developed the disease. He's now being treated for cancer. The client begins to develop signs of TB. This is known as which type of infection?
1. Active infection
2. Primary infection
3. Superinfection
4. Tertiary infection

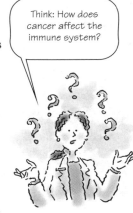

Think: How does cancer affect the immune system?

18. A client has active tuberculosis (TB). Which symptom will he exhibit?
1. Chest and lower back pain
2. Chills, fever, night sweats, and hemoptysis
3. Fever higher than 104° F (40° C) and nausea
4. Headache and photophobia

19. Which diagnostic test is definitive for tuberculosis?
1. Chest X-ray
2. Mantoux skin test
3. Sputum culture
4. Tuberculin skin test

20. A client with a positive Mantoux skin test result will be sent for a chest X-ray. Why is this done?
1. To confirm the diagnosis
2. To determine if a repeat skin test is needed
3. To determine the extent of lesions
4. To determine if this is a primary or secondary infection

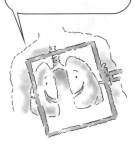

Tell me why I'm supposed to be here again?

21. A chest X-ray shows a client's lungs to be clear. His tuberculin Mantoux skin test is positive, with 10 mm of induration. His previous test was negative. These test results are possible because of which reason?
1. He had tuberculosis (TB) in the past and no longer has it.
2. He was successfully treated for TB but skin tests always stay positive.
3. He is a "seroconverter," meaning the TB has gotten to his bloodstream.
4. He is a "tuberculin converter," which means he has been infected with TB since his last skin test.

17. 1. Some people carry dormant TB infections that may develop into active disease. In addition, primary sites of infection containing TB bacilli may remain latent for years and then activate when the client's resistance is lowered, as when a client is being treated for cancer. There's no such thing as tertiary infection, and superinfection doesn't apply in this case.
CN: Physiological integrity; CNS: Physiological adaptation; CL: Application

18. 2. Typical signs and symptoms are chills, fever, night sweats, and hemoptysis. Clients with TB typically have low-grade fevers, not higher than 102° F (38.9° C). Chest pain may be present from coughing, but isn't usual. Nausea, headache, and photophobia aren't usual TB symptoms.
CN: Physiological integrity; CNS: Physiological adaptation; CL: Application

19. 3. Skin tests may be falsely positive or falsely negative. Lesions in the lung may not be big enough to be seen on X-ray. The sputum culture for *Mycobacterium tuberculosis* is the only method of confirming the diagnosis.
CN: Physiological integrity; CNS: Physiological adaptation; CL: Knowledge

20. 3. If the lesions are large enough, the chest X-ray will show their presence in the lungs. Sputum culture confirms the diagnosis. There can be false-positive and false-negative skin test results. A chest X-ray can't determine if this is a primary or secondary infection.
CN: Physiological integrity; CNS: Physiological adaptation; CL: Application

21. 4. A tuberculin converter's skin test will be positive, meaning he's been exposed to and infected with TB and now has a cell-mediated immune response to the skin test. The client's blood and X-ray results may stay negative. It doesn't mean the infection has advanced to the active stage. Because his X-ray is negative, he should be monitored every 6 months to see if he develops changes in his chest X-ray or pulmonary examination. Being a seroconverter doesn't mean the TB has gotten into his bloodstream; it means it can be detected by a blood test.
CN: Physiological integrity; CNS: Physiological adaptation; CL: Application

CN: Client needs category CNS: Client needs subcategory CL: Cognitive level

22. A client with a positive skin test for tuberculosis (TB) isn't showing signs of active disease. To help prevent the development of active TB, the client should be treated with isoniazid, 300 mg daily, for how long?
1. 10 to 14 days
2. 2 to 4 weeks
3. 3 to 6 months
4. 9 to 12 months

23. A client with a productive cough, chills, and night sweats is suspected of having active tuberculosis (TB). The physician should take which action?
1. Admit him to the hospital in respiratory isolation.
2. Prescribe isoniazid, and tell him to go home and rest.
3. Give a tuberculin skin test, and tell him to come back in 48 hours to have it read.
4. Give a prescription for isoniazid, 300 mg daily for 2 weeks, and send him home.

24. A client is diagnosed with active tuberculosis and started on triple antibiotic therapy. What signs and symptoms would the client show if therapy is <u>inadequate</u>?
1. Decreased shortness of breath
2. Improved chest X-ray
3. Nonproductive cough
4. Positive acid-fast bacilli in a sputum sample after 2 months of treatment

25. Which instruction should the nurse give a client about his active tuberculosis (TB)?
1. "It's okay to miss a dose every day or two."
2. "If adverse effects occur, stop taking the medication."
3. "Only take the medication until you feel better."
4. "You must comply with the medication regimen to treat TB."

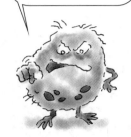

Think about TB's resistant strains.

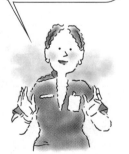

Read question 24 carefully! It's easy to miss the two little letters in front of "adequate."

22. 4. Because of the increasing incidence of resistant strains of TB, the disease must be treated for up to 24 months in some cases, but treatment typically lasts from 9 to 12 months. Isoniazid is the most common medication used for the treatment of TB, but other antibiotics are added to the regimen to obtain the best results.
CN: Physiological integrity; CNS: Pharmacological therapies; CL: Application

23. 1. This client is showing signs and symptoms of active TB and, because of the productive cough, is highly contagious. He should be admitted to the hospital and placed in respiratory isolation, and three sputum cultures should be obtained to confirm the diagnosis. He would most likely be given isoniazid and two or three other antitubercular antibiotics until the diagnosis is confirmed, and then isolation and treatment would continue if the cultures were positive for TB. After 7 to 10 days, three more consecutive sputum cultures will be obtained. If they're negative, he would be considered noncontagious and may be sent home, although he'll continue to take the antitubercular drugs for 9 to 12 months.
CN: Physiological integrity; CNS: Physiological adaptation; CL: Application

24. 4. Continuing to have acid-fast bacilli in the sputum after 2 months indicates continued infection. The other choices would all indicate improvement.
CN: Physiological integrity; CNS: Physiological adaptation; CL: Application

25. 4. The regimen may last up to 24 months. It's essential that the client comply with therapy during that time or resistance will develop. At no time should he stop taking the medications without his physician's approval.
CN: Physiological integrity; CNS: Physiological adaptation; CL: Analysis

26. A client diagnosed with active tuberculosis (TB) would be hospitalized primarily for which reason?
1. To evaluate his condition
2. To determine his compliance
3. To prevent spread of the disease
4. To determine the need for antibiotic therapy

27. A client is admitted with chronic obstructive pulmonary disease (COPD). Which signs and symptoms are characteristic of COPD? Select all that apply:
1. Decreased respiratory rate
2. Dyspnea on exertion
3. Barrel chest
4. Shortened expiratory phase
5. Clubbed fingers and toes
6. Fever

28. Which assessment finding would help confirm a diagnosis of asthma in a child suspected of having the disorder?
1. Circumoral cyanosis
2. Increased forced expiratory volume
3. Inspiratory and expiratory wheezing
4. Normal breath sounds

29. A 22-year-old female client is experiencing a new-onset asthmatic attack. Which position is best for this client?
1. High Fowler's
2. Left side-lying
3. Right side-lying
4. Supine with pillows under each arm

30. A client with acute asthma showing inspiratory and expiratory wheezes and a decreased forced expiratory volume should be treated <u>immediately</u> with which class of medication?
1. Beta-adrenergic blockers
2. Bronchodilators
3. Inhaled steroids
4. Oral steroids

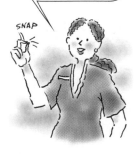

You make these questions look like a snap!

SNAP

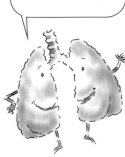

Listen to how we sound—any changes from normal are clues.

26. 3. The client with active TB is highly contagious until three consecutive sputum cultures are negative, so he's put in respiratory isolation in the hospital. Assessment of his physical condition, need for antibiotic therapy, and determinations of compliance aren't considered primary reasons for hospitalization in this case.
CN: Physiological integrity; CNS: Physiological adaptation; CL: Application

27. 2, 3, 5. Typical findings for clients with COPD include dyspnea on exertion, a barrel chest, and clubbed fingers and toes. Clients with COPD are usually tachypneic with a prolonged expiratory phase. Fever isn't associated with COPD, unless an infection is also present.
CN: Physiological integrity; CNS: Physiological adaptation; CL: Comprehension

28. 3. Inspiratory and expiratory wheezes are typical findings in asthma. Circumoral cyanosis may be present in extreme cases of respiratory distress. The nurse would expect the client to have a decreased forced expiratory volume because asthma is an obstructive pulmonary disease. Breath sounds will be "tight" sounding or markedly decreased; they won't be normal.
CN: Physiological integrity; CNS: Physiological adaptation; CL: Analysis

29. 1. The best position is high Fowler's, which helps lower the diaphragm and facilitates passive breathing and thereby improves air exchange. A side-lying position won't facilitate the client's breathing. A supine position increases the breathing difficulty of an asthmatic client.
CN: Physiological integrity; CNS: Physiological adaptation; CL: Application

30. 2. Bronchodilators are the first line of treatment for asthma because bronchoconstriction is the cause of reduced airflow. Inhaled or oral steroids may be given to reduce the inflammation but aren't used for emergency relief. Beta-adrenergic blockers aren't used to treat asthma and can cause bronchoconstriction.
CN: Physiological integrity; CNS: Pharmacological therapies; CL: Application

CN: Client needs category   CNS: Client needs subcategory   CL: Cognitive level

31. A 19-year-old client comes to the emergency department with acute asthma. His respiratory rate is 44 breaths/minute, and he appears in acute respiratory distress. Which action should be taken <u>first</u>?
1. Take a full medical history.
2. Give a bronchodilator by nebulizer.
3. Apply a cardiac monitor to the client.
4. Provide emotional support to the client.

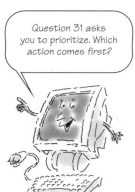

Question 31 asks you to prioritize. Which action comes first?

31. 2. The client having an acute asthma attack needs to increase oxygen delivery to the lung and body. Nebulized bronchodilators open airways and increase the amount of oxygen delivered. It may not be necessary to place the client on a cardiac monitor because he's only 19 years old, unless he has a medical history of cardiac problems. First, resolve the acute phase of the attack; then obtain a full medical history to determine the cause of the attack and how to prevent attacks in the future.
CN: Physiological integrity; CNS: Physiological adaptation; CL: Application

32. A client is found to be allergic to Chinese food, which causes acute asthma. Which instruction should the nurse give the client?
1. "Only eat Chinese food once per month."
2. "Use your inhalers before eating Chinese food."
3. "Avoid Chinese food because it's a trigger for you."
4. "Determine other causes, because Chinese food wouldn't cause such a violent reaction."

32. 3. If the trigger of an acute asthma attack is known, this trigger should always be avoided. Food is typically a trigger for an acute asthma attack, and using an inhaler before eating wouldn't prevent an attack.
CN: Physiological integrity; CNS: Reduction of risk potential; CL: Application

33. Which nursing activity requires greater caution when performed on a client with chronic obstructive pulmonary disease (COPD)?
1. Administering opioids for pain relief
2. Increasing the client's fluid intake
3. Monitoring the client's cardiac rhythm
4. Assisting the client with coughing and deep breathing

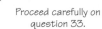

Proceed carefully on question 33.

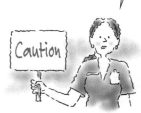

Caution

33. 1. Opioids suppress the respiratory center in the medulla. Both COPD and pneumonia cause alterations in gas exchange; any further problems with oxygenation could result in respiratory failure and cardiac arrest. Increasing the fluid intake would help to thin the client's secretions. Although the nurse would need to monitor the intake and output and watch for signs of heart failure, this isn't as critical as administering opioids. The cardiac rhythm provides an indication of the client's myocardial oxygenation; it should be a part of the nurse's regular assessment. Helping with coughing and deep breathing should be included in the plan of care. The only caution would be to assess for possible rupture of emphysematous alveolar sacs and pneumothorax.
CN: Physiological integrity; CNS: Physiological adaptation; CL: Application

34. The term "blue bloater" refers to which condition?
1. Acute respiratory distress syndrome (ARDS)
2. Asthma
3. Chronic obstructive bronchitis
4. Emphysema

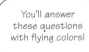

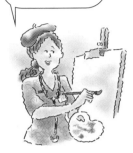

You'll answer these questions with flying colors!

34. 3. Clients with chronic obstructive bronchitis appear bloated; they have large barrel chests and peripheral edema, cyanotic nail beds and, at times, circumoral cyanosis. Clients with asthma don't exhibit characteristics of chronic disease. Clients with emphysema appear pink and cachectic, and clients with ARDS are acutely short of breath and frequently need intubation for mechanical ventilation and large amounts of oxygen.
CN: Physiological integrity; CNS: Physiological adaptation; CL: Application

35. The term "pink puffer" refers to the client with which condition?
1. Acute respiratory distress syndrome (ARDS)
2. Asthma
3. Chronic obstructive bronchitis
4. Emphysema

35. 4. Because of the large amount of energy it takes to breathe, clients with emphysema are usually cachectic. They're pink and, they usually breathe through pursed lips, hence the term "puffer." Clients with asthma don't have any particular characteristics. Clients with chronic obstructive bronchitis are bloated and cyanotic in appearance, and clients with ARDS are usually acutely short of breath.
CN: Physiological integrity; CNS: Physiological adaptation; CL: Application

36. A 66-year-old client has marked dyspnea at rest, is thin, and uses accessory muscles to breathe. He's tachypneic, with a prolonged expiratory phase. He has no cough. He leans forward with his arms braced on his knees to support his chest and shoulders for breathing. This client has symptoms of which respiratory disorder?
1. Acute respiratory distress syndrome (ARDS)
2. Asthma
3. Chronic obstructive bronchitis
4. Emphysema

36. 4. These are classic signs and symptoms of a client with emphysema. Clients with asthma are acutely short of breath during an attack and appear very frightened. Clients with bronchitis are bloated and cyanotic in appearance, and clients with ARDS are acutely short of breath and require emergency care.
CN: Physiological integrity; CNS: Physiological adaptation; CL: Application

37. It's highly recommended that clients with asthma, chronic bronchitis, and emphysema have Pneumovax and flu vaccinations for which reason?
1. All clients are recommended to have these vaccines.
2. These vaccines produce bronchodilation and improve oxygenation.
3. These vaccines help reduce the tachypnea these clients experience.
4. Respiratory infections can cause severe hypoxia and possibly death in these clients.

Give it a shot! Which illnesses am I susceptible to?

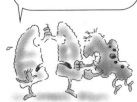

37. 4. It's highly recommended that clients with respiratory disorders be given vaccines to protect against respiratory infection. Infections can cause respiratory failure, and these clients may need to be intubated and mechanically ventilated. The vaccines have no effect on respiratory rate or bronchodilation.
CN: Health promotion and maintenance CNS: None; CL: Application

CN: Client needs category   CNS: Client needs subcategory   CL: Cognitive level

38. Exercise has which effect on clients with asthma, chronic bronchitis, and emphysema?
1. It enhances cardiovascular fitness.
2. It improves respiratory muscle strength.
3. It reduces the number of acute attacks.
4. It worsens respiratory function and is discouraged.

39. Clients with chronic obstructive bronchitis are given diuretic therapy. Which reason best explains why?
1. Reducing fluid volume reduces oxygen demand.
2. Reducing fluid volume improves clients' mobility.
3. Reducing fluid volume reduces sputum production.
4. Reducing fluid volume improves respiratory function.

40. Which best describes pleural effusion?
1. The collapse of alveoli
2. The collapse of a bronchiole
3. Fluid in the alveolar space
4. The accumulation of fluid between the linings of the pleural space

41. A client with emphysema should receive only enough supplemental oxygen to maintain his Pao_2 at 60 mm Hg or higher, or he may lose his hypoxic drive. Which statement is correct about hypoxic drive?
1. The client doesn't notice he needs to breathe.
2. The client breathes only when his oxygen levels climbs above a certain point.
3. The client breathes only when his oxygen levels dip below a certain point.
4. The client breathes only when his carbon dioxide level dips below a certain point.

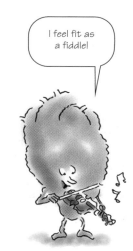

I feel fit as a fiddle!

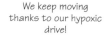

We keep moving thanks to our hypoxic drive!

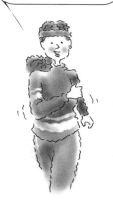

38. 1. Exercise can improve cardiovascular fitness and help the client tolerate periods of hypoxia better, perhaps reducing the risk of heart attack. Most exercise has little effect on respiratory muscle strength, and these clients can't tolerate the type of exercise necessary to do this. Exercise won't reduce the number of acute attacks. In some instances, exercise may be contraindicated. The client should check with his physician before starting any exercise program.
CN: Health promotion and maintenance; CNS: None; CL: Application

39. 1. Reducing fluid volume reduces the workload of the heart, which reduces oxygen demand and, in turn, reduces the respiratory rate. Sputum may get thicker and make it harder to clear airways. Reducing fluid volume won't improve respiratory function but may improve oxygenation. Reducing fluid volume may reduce edema and improve mobility a little, but exercise tolerance will still be poor.
CN: Physiological integrity; CNS: Physiological adaptation; CL: Application

40. 4. Pleural fluid normally seeps continually into the pleural space from the capillaries lining the parietal pleura and is reabsorbed by the visceral pleural capillaries and lymphatics. Any condition that interferes with either the secretion or drainage of this fluid will lead to a pleural effusion. The collapse of alveoli or a bronchiole has no particular name. Fluid within the alveolar space can be caused by heart failure or acute respiratory distress syndrome.
CN: Physiological integrity; CNS: Physiological adaptation; CL: Application

41. 3. Clients with emphysema breathe when their oxygen levels drop to a certain level; this is known as the *hypoxic drive*. Clients with emphysema and chronic obstructive pulmonary disease take a breath when they've reached this low oxygen level. They don't take a breath when their levels of carbon dioxide are higher than normal, as do those with healthy respiratory physiology. If too much oxygen is given, the client has little stimulus to take another breath. His carbon dioxide levels climb, he loses consciousness, and respiratory arrest occurs.
CN: Physiological integrity; CNS: Physiological adaptation; CL: Application

CN: Client needs category   CNS: Client needs subcategory   CL: Cognitive level

42. Teaching for a client with chronic obstructive pulmonary disease should include which topic?
 1. How to listen to his own lungs
 2. How to decrease his fluid intake
 3. How to treat respiratory infections without going to the physician
 4. How to recognize the signs of an impending respiratory infection

43. Which respiratory disorder is most common in the first 24 to 48 hours after surgery?
 1. Atelectasis
 2. Bronchitis
 3. Pneumonia
 4. Pneumothorax

44. Which measure can reduce or prevent the incidence of atelectasis in a postoperative client?
 1. Chest physiotherapy
 2. Mechanical ventilation
 3. Reducing oxygen requirements
 4. Use of an incentive spirometer

45. Emergency treatment of a client in status asthmaticus includes which drug class?
 1. Inhaled beta-adrenergic agents
 2. Inhaled corticosteroids
 3. I.V. beta-adrenergic agents
 4. Oral corticosteroids

46. Which treatment goal is <u>best</u> for the client with status asthmaticus?
 1. To avoid intubation
 2. To determine the cause of the attack
 3. To improve exercise tolerance
 4. To reduce secretions

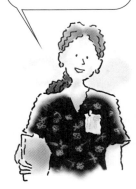

You're one-third finished with this chapter. Way to go!

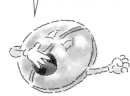

It's a tough job but somebody's got to do it!

42. 4. Respiratory infection in clients with a respiratory disorder can be fatal. It's important that the client understands how to recognize the signs and symptoms of an impending respiratory infection. The client can't listen to his own lungs effectively. The client should be taught to increase his fluid intake to help thin secretions. If the client has signs and symptoms of an infection, he should contact his physician at once to obtain prompt treatment.
CN: Physiological integrity; CNS: Reduction of risk potential; CL: Application

43. 1. Atelectasis develops when there's interference with the normal negative pressure that promotes lung expansion. Clients in the postoperative phase typically guard their breathing because of pain and positioning, which causes hypoxia. It's uncommon for any of the other respiratory disorders to develop after surgery.
CN: Physiological integrity; CNS: Physiological adaptation; CL: Application

44. 4. Using an incentive spirometer requires the client to take deep breaths and promotes lung expansion. Chest physiotherapy helps mobilize secretions but won't prevent atelectasis. Reducing oxygen requirements or placing someone on mechanical ventilation doesn't affect the development of atelectasis.
CN: Physiological integrity; CNS: Basic care and comfort; CL: Application

45. 1. Inhaled beta-adrenergic agents help promote bronchodilation, which improves oxygenation. I.V. beta-adrenergic agents can be used but have to be monitored because of their greater systemic effects. They're typically used when the inhaled beta-adrenergic agents don't work. Corticosteroids are slow acting, so their use won't reduce hypoxia in the acute phase.
CN: Physiological integrity; CNS: Pharmacological therapies; CL: Application

46. 1. Inhaled beta-adrenergic agents, I.V. corticosteroids, and supplemental oxygen are used to reduce bronchospasm, improve oxygenation, and avoid intubation. Improvement in exercise tolerance and determining the trigger for the client's attack are later goals. Typically, secretions aren't a problem in status asthmaticus.
CN: Physiological integrity; CNS: Physiological adaptation; CL: Application

CN: Client needs category   CNS: Client needs subcategory   CL: Cognitive level

47. A client was given morphine for pain. He's sleeping and his respiratory rate is 4 breaths/minute. If action isn't taken quickly, he might have which reaction?
1. Asthma attack
2. Respiratory arrest
3. Seizure
4. Wake up on his own

48. Which additional data should immediately be gathered to determine the status of a client with a respiratory rate of 4 breaths/minute?
1. Arterial blood gas (ABG) levels and breath sounds
2. Level of consciousness and a pulse oximetry value
3. Breath sounds and reflexes
4. Pulse oximetry value and heart sounds

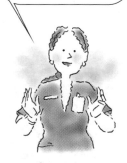

Ask yourself: "Which collected data would help first, and which could wait?"

49. A client is in danger of respiratory arrest following the administration of an opioid analgesic. An arterial blood gas analysis is obtained. The nurse would expect the $Paco_2$ to be which value?
1. 15 mm Hg
2. 30 mm Hg
3. 40 mm Hg
4. 80 mm Hg

50. A client needs to have a chest tube inserted in the right upper chest. Which action is part of the nurse's role?
1. The nurse isn't needed
2. Preparing the chest tube drainage system
3. Bringing the chest X-ray to the client's room
4. Inserting the chest tube

51. Clients at high risk for respiratory failure include those with which diagnosis?
1. Breast cancer
2. Cervical sprains
3. Fractured hip
4. Guillain-Barré syndrome

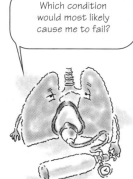

Which condition would most likely cause me to fail?

47. 2. Opioids suppress the respiratory center in the medulla and can cause respiratory arrest if given in large quantities. It's unlikely he'll have an asthma attack or a seizure or wake up on his own.
CN: Physiological integrity; CNS: Pharmacological therapies CL: Application

48. 2. First, the nurse should attempt to rouse the client, because this should increase the client's respiratory rate. Then a spot pulse oximetry check should be done and breath sounds should be checked. The physician should be notified immediately of the findings. He'll probably order an ABG to determine specific carbon dioxide and oxygen levels. Heart sounds and reflexes will be checked after these initial actions are completed.
CN: Physiological integrity; CNS: Physiological adaptation; CL: Comprehension

49. 4. A client about to go into respiratory arrest will have inefficient ventilation and will be retaining carbon dioxide. The value expected would be around 80 mm Hg. All other values are lower than normal.
CN: Physiological integrity; CNS: Physiological adaptation; CL: Analysis

50. 2. The nurse must anticipate that a drainage system is required and assemble it before the insertion so that the tube can be directly connected to the drainage system. The chest X-ray doesn't need to be brought to the client's room. A physician will insert the chest tube.
CN: Physiological integrity; CNS: Physiological adaptation; CL: Application

51. 4. Guillain-Barré syndrome is a progressive neuromuscular disorder that can affect the respiratory muscles and cause respiratory failure. The other conditions typically don't affect the respiratory system.
CN: Physiological integrity; CNS: Physiological adaptation; CL: Analysis

52. A client has started a new drug for hypertension. Thirty minutes after he takes the drug, he develops chest tightness and becomes short of breath and tachypneic. He has a decreased level of consciousness. These signs indicate which condition?
1. Asthma attack
2. Pulmonary embolism
3. Hypersensitivity to the medication
4. Rheumatoid arthritis

53. Emergency treatment for a client with impending anaphylaxis secondary to hypersensitivity to a drug should include which action first?
1. Administer oxygen.
2. Insert an I.V. catheter.
3. Obtain a complete blood count (CBC).
4. Take vital signs.

54. Following the initial care of a client with asthma and impending anaphylaxis from hypersensitivity to a drug, the nurse should take which step next?
1. Administer beta-adrenergic blockers.
2. Administer bronchodilators.
3. Obtain serum electrolyte levels.
4. Have the client lie flat in the bed.

55. A 19-year-old client went to a party, took "some pills," and drank beer. He's brought to the emergency department because he won't wake up. When collecting data from him, the nurse would expect to find which reaction?
1. Hyperreflexive reflexes
2. Muscle spasms
3. Shallow respirations
4. Tachypnea

56. When an unconscious client has been diagnosed with probable drug overdose complicated by alcohol ingestion, the nurse knows that the priority intervention is to:
1. administer I.V. fluids.
2. administer I.V. naloxone (Narcan).
3. continue close monitoring of vital signs.
4. draw blood for a drug screen.

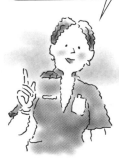

First things first. Set your priorities properly.

52. 3. These signs indicate a hypersensitivity to the new medication, leading to anaphylaxis and respiratory failure. An asthma attack is characterized by wheezing. A client with pulmonary embolism typically has chest pain with inspiration and hypoxemia. Rheumatoid arthritis doesn't cause respiratory symptoms.
CN: Physiological integrity; CNS: Pharmacological therapies; CL: Analysis

53. 1. Giving oxygen would be the best first action in this case. Vital signs then should be checked and the physician immediately notified. If the client doesn't already have an I.V. catheter, one may be inserted now if anaphylactic shock is developing. Obtaining a CBC would not help the emergency situation.
CN: Physiological integrity; CNS: Pharmacological therapies; CL: Application

54. 2. Bronchodilators would help open the client's airway and improve his oxygenation status. Beta-adrenergic blockers aren't indicated in the management of asthma because they may cause bronchospasm. Obtaining laboratory values wouldn't be done on an emergency basis, and having the client lie flat in bed could worsen the client's ability to breathe.
CN: Physiological integrity; CNS: Physiological adaptation; CL: Application

55. 3. The client probably can't be roused from the combination of pills and alcohol he has taken. This has probably caused him to breathe shallowly, which, if action isn't taken immediately, could lead to respiratory arrest. The nurse wouldn't expect to find tachypnea and doesn't have enough information about which drugs he took to expect muscle spasms or hyperreflexia.
CN: Physiological integrity; CNS: Physiological adaptation; CL: Application

56. 2. If the client took opioids, giving naloxone could reverse the effects and awaken the client. I.V. fluids will most likely be administered, and he'll be closely monitored over a period of several hours to several days. A drug screen should be drawn in the emergency department, but results may not come back for several hours.
CN: Physiological integrity; CNS: Physiological adaptation; CL: Application

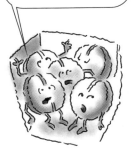

Hey! There are too many of us! What should we do first?

CN: Client needs category   CNS: Client needs subcategory   CL: Cognitive level

57. An unconscious client who overdosed on an opioid receives naloxone (Narcan) to reverse the overdose. After he awakens, which action by the nurse would be the best?
1. Feed the client.
2. Teach the client about the effects of taking pills and alcohol together.
3. Discharge the client from the hospital.
4. Admit the client to a psychiatric facility.

58. A 45-year-old male client is brought to the hospital with smoke inhalation due to a house fire. What's the nurse's <u>first</u> priority for this client?
1. Checking the oral mucous membranes
2. Checking for any burned areas
3. Obtaining a medical history
4. Ensuring a patent airway

59. In a client with smoke inhalation, the nurse would expect to hear which breath sound?
1. Crackles
2. Decreased breath sounds
3. Inspiratory and expiratory wheezing
4. Upper airway rhonchi

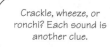

Crackle, wheeze, or ronchi? Each sound is another clue.

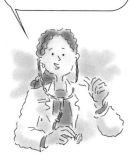

60. A client is receiving oxygen by way of a nasal cannula at a rate of 2 L/minute. How should the oxygen flow meter be set?
1. The bottom of the ball should sit on top of the line marked "2."
2. The top of the ball should sit below the line marked "2."
3. The line marked "2" should cut the ball in half.
4. Any part of the ball should touch the line marked "2."

61. Which statement <u>best</u> describes what happens to the alveoli in acute respiratory distress syndrome (ARDS)?
1. Alveoli are overexpanded.
2. Alveoli increase perfusion.
3. Alveolar spaces are filled with fluid.
4. Alveoli improve gaseous exchange.

57. 2. This client needs information about the dangers of combining pills and alcohol. Discharge at this point is inappropriate. Unless the client was trying to commit suicide, admission to a psychiatric facility isn't necessary. It may not be advisable to feed the client at first, in case his level of consciousness decreases again, increasing the possibility of aspiration.
CN: Physiological integrity; CNS: Physiological adaptation; CL: Application

58. 4. The nurse's first priority is to make sure the airway is open and the client is breathing. Checking the mucous membranes and burned areas is important but not as vital as maintaining a patent airway. Obtaining a medical history can be pursued after ensuring a patent airway.
CN: Physiological integrity; CNS: Physiological adaptation; CL: Application

59. 1. In smoke inhalation, the most frequently heard sounds are crackles throughout the lung fields. Decreased breath sounds or inspiratory and expiratory wheezing is associated with asthma, and rhonchi are heard when there's sputum in the airways.
CN: Physiological integrity; CNS: Physiological adaptation; CL: Application

60. 3. The oxygen flow rate is set by centering the indicator on the line marked "2."
CN: Safe, effective care environment; CNS: Safety and infection control; CL: Knowledge

61. 3. In ARDS, the alveolar membranes are more permeable and the spaces are fluid-filled. The fluid interferes with gas exchange and reduces perfusion.
CN: Physiological integrity; CNS: Physiological adaptation; CL: Knowledge

62. A 69-year-old client develops acute shortness of breath and progressive hypoxia requiring mechanical ventilation after repair of a fractured right femur. The hypoxia was <u>probably</u> caused by which condition?
　　1. Asthma attack
　　2. Atelectasis
　　3. Bronchitis
　　4. Fat embolism

63. The nurse is caring for a client with a fracture of the right femur caused by a skiing accident. Which is an early sign of fat emboli?
　　1. Abdominal cramping
　　2. Fatty stools
　　3. Confusion
　　4. Numbness in the right foot

64. If a client with a fat embolism continues to be hypoxic following respiratory therapy, the nurse knows that oxygen demand can be reduced by:
　　1. administering diuretics.
　　2. administering neuromuscular blockers.
　　3. placing the head of the bed flat.
　　4. administering bronchodilators.

65. Positive end-expiratory pressure (PEEP) therapy has which effect on the heart?
　　1. Bradycardia
　　2. Tachycardia
　　3. Increased blood pressure
　　4. Reduced cardiac output

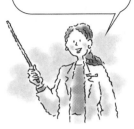

Several answers may seem correct, but the word probably points to the best one.

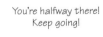

You're halfway there! Keep going!

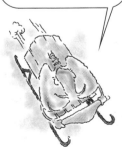

62. 4. Long bone fractures are correlated with fat emboli, which cause shortness of breath and hypoxia. It's unlikely the client has developed asthma or bronchitis without a previous history. He could develop atelectasis, but it typically doesn't produce progressive hypoxia.
CN: Physiological integrity; CNS: Physiological adaptation; CL: Application

63. 3. Irritation and confusion are signs of hypoxia, which is caused by the fat emboli traveling to the lungs and producing an inflammatory response in the lung tissue. Abdominal cramping may be a sign of abdominal distention and constipation caused by immobility. Fatty stools occur with pancreatitis. Numbness may be secondary to neurovascular impairment.
CN: Physiological integrity; CNS: Physiological adaptation; CL: Application

64. 2. Neuromuscular blockers cause skeletal muscle paralysis, reducing the amount of oxygen used by the restless skeletal muscles. This should improve oxygenation. Bronchodilators may be used, but they typically don't have enough of an effect to reduce the amount of hypoxia present. The head of the bed should be partially elevated to facilitate diaphragm movement, and diuretics can be administered to reduce pulmonary congestion. However, bronchodilators, diuretics, and head elevation would improve oxygen delivery, not reduce oxygen demand.
CN: Physiological integrity; CNS: Physiological adaptation; CL: Application

65. 4. PEEP reduces cardiac output by increasing intrathoracic pressure and reducing the amount of blood delivered to the left side of the heart, thereby reducing cardiac output. It doesn't affect heart rate, but a decrease in cardiac output may reduce blood pressure, commonly causing a compensatory tachycardia.
CN: Physiological integrity; CNS: Physiological adaptation; CL: Application

66. Occasionally, clients with acute respiratory distress syndrome are placed in the prone position. How does this position help the client?
1. It improves cardiac output.
2. It makes the client more comfortable.
3. It prevents skin breakdown.
4. It recruits more alveoli.

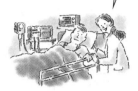

It's important to know which values to monitor.

67. Which condition could lead to acute respiratory distress syndrome (ARDS)?
1. Appendicitis
2. Massive trauma
3. Receiving conscious sedation
4. Right meniscus injury

68. A nurse is monitoring the progress of a client with acute respiratory distress syndrome (ARDS). Which data best indicate that the client's condition is improving?
1. Arterial blood gas (ABG) values are normal.
2. The bronchoscopy results are negative.
3. The client's blood pressure has stabilized.
4. The sputum and sensitivity culture shows no growth in bacteria.

69. A nurse has advised a client's family that they shouldn't increase the oxygen flow rate. Which rationale is most correct for not increasing the oxygen level on a client when it isn't needed?
1. Extra oxygen may cause the client to breathe too rapidly.
2. Oxygen toxicity may reduce the amount of functional alveolar surface area.
3. Increased oxygen may decrease carbon dioxide levels and cause apnea.
4. Increasing the oxygen level may cause pulmonary barotrauma.

In question 70, break kyphoscoliosis down to find its meaning—and a clue.

70. Which effect can thoracic kyphoscoliosis have on lung function?
1. Improves lung expansion
2. Obstructs lung deflation
3. Reduces alveolar compression during expiration
4. Restricts lung expansion

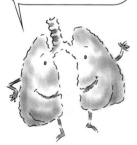

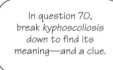

66. 4. Turning the client to the prone position may recruit new alveoli in the posterior region of the lung and improve oxygenation status. Cardiac output shouldn't be affected by the prone position. Skin breakdown can still occur over the new pressure points. Generally the client is obtunded when this measure is used. If not, he should be well-sedated.
CN: Physiological integrity; CNS: Physiological adaptation; CL: Application

67. 2. In a client with massive trauma, the tissues lining the alveoli and pulmonary capillaries are injured directly or indirectly, increasing the permeability of protein and fluid and leading to the development of hypoxemia and ARDS. Appendicitis, unless it causes overwhelming sepsis, won't lead to ARDS. Injuries to the meniscus and conscious sedation don't lead to ARDS.
CN: Physiological integrity; CNS: Physiological adaptation; CL: Application

68. 1. Normal ABG values would indicate that the client's oxygenation has improved. ARDS is characterized by hypoxia, so the bronchoscopy and sputum culture results have no bearing on the improvement of ARDS. Increased blood pressure isn't relative to the client's respiratory condition.
CN: Physiological integrity; CNS: Physiological adaptation; CL: Analysis

69. 2. Oxygen toxicity causes direct pulmonary trauma, reducing the amount of alveolar surface area available for gaseous exchange, which results in increased carbon dioxide levels and decreased oxygen uptake. Excessive oxygen therapy may eliminate hypoxic respiratory drive, causing the patient to breathe too slowly or even to stop breathing. Pulmonary barotrauma is caused by high lung pressures, not excessive oxygenation.
CN: Physiological integrity; CNS: Physiological adaptation; CL: Application

70. 4. Thoracic kyphoscoliosis causes lung compression, restricts lung expansion, and results in more rapid and shallow respiration. It doesn't cause obstruction or reduce alveolar compression during expiration. It also doesn't improve lung expansion because of the compression.
CN: Physiological integrity; CNS: Physiological adaptation; CL: Application

CN: Client needs category   CNS: Client needs subcategory   CL: Cognitive level

71. A 24-year-old client comes into the clinic complaining of right-sided chest pain and shortness of breath. He reports that it started suddenly. The nurse's data collection should include:
1. auscultation of breath sounds.
2. chest X-ray.
3. echocardiogram.
4. electrocardiogram.

72. A client presents with shortness of breath and absent breath sounds on the right side, from the apex to the base. Which condition would best explain this?
1. Acute asthma
2. Chronic bronchitis
3. Pneumonia
4. Spontaneous pneumothorax

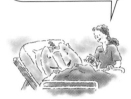

Listening to breath sounds sure helps diagnose a lot of conditions, doesn't it?

73. Which treatment would the nurse expect for a client with spontaneous pneumothorax?
1. Antibiotics
2. Bronchodilators
3. Chest tube placement
4. Hyperbaric chamber

74. A client is receiving emergency care following a motor vehicle collision. The physician has diagnosed a left pneumothorax. Which sign would typically be present when the client's lungs were auscultated?
1. Absence of breath sounds over the left lung field
2. Crackles one-third up the posterior lung fields
3. Wheezing on expiration throughout the lung fields
4. Clear breath sounds bilaterally

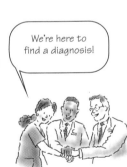

We're here to find a diagnosis!

75. A nurse is reviewing data on a client suspected of having a pneumothorax. Which data would confirm the diagnosis?
1. Auscultation of breath sounds
2. Chest X-ray results
3. Client can't use incentive spirometer
4. Client is experiencing dyspnea

71. 1. Because he's short of breath, auscultation of the lungs will indicate normal or abnormal breath sounds. He may need a chest X-ray and an electrocardiogram, but they require a physician's order. An endocardiogram also requires a physician's order and may be necessary if a pulmonary embolus is suspected.
CN: Physiological integrity; CNS: Physiological adaptation; CL: Application

72. 4. Spontaneous pneumothorax occurs when the client's lung collapses, causing an acute decrease in the amount of functional lung used in oxygenation, resulting in shortness of breath with absent breath sounds. A client with an asthma attack would present with wheezing breath sounds, and bronchitis would be indicated by auscultating rhonchi. Bronchial breath sounds over the area of consolidation would indicate pneumonia.
CN: Physiological integrity; CNS: Physiological adaptation; CL: Application

73. 3. The only way to reexpand the lung is to place a chest tube on the right side so the air in the pleural space can be removed and the lung reexpanded. Antibiotics and bronchodilators would have no effect on lung reexpansion, nor would the hyperbaric chamber.
CN: Physiological integrity; CNS: Physiological adaptation; CL: Application

74. 1. Pneumothorax can occur as a result of trauma where the pleurae separating the lung from the chest wall are damaged, allowing air to enter the pleural space. This air causes the lung to collapse, resulting in absent breath sounds.
CN: Physiological integrity; CNS: Physiological adaptation; CL: Application

75. 2. A chest X-ray will show the area of collapsed lung if pneumothorax is present as well as the volume of air in the pleural space. Listening to breath sounds won't confirm a diagnosis. The client wouldn't do well with an incentive spirometer at this time. A client may experience dyspnea for many reasons besides a pneumothorax.
CN: Physiological integrity; CNS: Physiological adaptation; CL: Application

CN: Client needs category   CNS: Client needs subcategory   CL: Cognitive level

76. A nurse is assisting the physician with placement of a chest tube in a client who has experienced chest trauma. Upon insertion of the chest tube, the nurse observes serosanguineous drainage in the collection chamber. Which explanation <u>best</u> describes what caused this type of drainage from the chest tube insertion?

1. The physician didn't insert the chest tube correctly.
2. It is normal for the drainage to be serosanguineous.
3. An artery was disrupted when the chest tube was inserted.
4. The client has experienced a hemothorax instead of a pneumothorax.

77. A hospitalized client needs a central venous access device inserted. The physician places the device in the subclavian vein. Shortly afterward, the client develops shortness of breath and appears restless. Which action would the nurse take <u>first</u>?

1. Administer a sedative.
2. Advise the client to calm down.
3. Auscultate breath sounds.
4. Check to see if the client can have medication.

78. Which measure would be ordered for a client who recently had a central venous access device inserted and who now appears short of breath and anxious?

1. Chest X-ray
2. Electrocardiogram
3. Laboratory tests
4. Sedation

79. Based on the following progress note, the arterial blood gas results indicate which condition?

Progress notes	
10/04/08 2200	Client states, "I'm having trouble breathing." Vital signs: T, 98° F; HR, 102 beats/minute; RR, 28 and shallow. Bilateral breath sounds with crackles lower 1/3 posterior lungs. Client confused to time and place. Arterial blood gases obtained by L. Smith, R.T., from right radial artery. Results: pH, 7.16; Paco₂ 80 mm Hg; Pao₂, 46 mm Hg; HCO3−, 24 mEg/L; Sao2 81%————————Barbara Smith, R.N.

1. Metabolic acidosis
2. Metabolic alkalosis
3. Respiratory acidosis
4. Respiratory acidosis

When I'm in distress, what should you do first?

76. 4. Because of the traumatic cause of injury, the client has a hemothorax, in which blood collection causes the collapse of the lung. The placement of the chest tube will drain the blood from the space and reexpand the lung. There's a slight chance of nicking an intercostal artery during insertion, but it's fairly unlikely if the person placing the chest tube has been trained. The initial chest X-ray would help confirm whether there was blood in the pleural space or just air.

CN: Physiological integrity; CNS: Physiological adaptation; CL: Application

77. 3. Because this is an acute episode, listen to the client's lungs to see if anything has changed. Don't give this client medication, especially sedatives, if he's having trouble breathing as they may decrease respirations further. Give the client emotional support, and contact the physician who placed the central venous access.

CN: Safe, effective care environment; CNS: Coordinated care; CL: Application

78. 1. Inserting an I.V. catheter in the subclavian vein can result in a pneumothorax, so a chest X-ray should be done. If it's negative, then other tests should be done but they aren't appropriate as the first intervention.

CN: Health promotion and maintenance; CNS: None; CL: Knowledge

79. 3. The pH is less than 7.35, which is acidemic and eliminates metabolic and respiratory alkalosis as possibilities. Because the Paco₂ is high at 80 mm Hg and the metabolic measure, HCO₃⁻, is normal, the client has respiratory acidosis.

CN: Physiological integrity; CNS: Physiological adaptation; CL: Analysis

CN: Client needs category   CNS: Client needs subcategory   CL: Cognitive level

80. When monitoring the closed chest drainage system of a client who has just returned from a lobectomy, the nurse must ensure which of the following?
1. The fluid in the water-seal chamber rises from inspiration and falls with expiration.
2. The tubing remains looped below the level of the bed.
3. The drainage chamber doesn't drain more than 100 ml in 8 hours.
4. The suction-control chamber bubbles vigorously when connected to suction.

81. When a chest tube is accidentally dislodged from a client, which intervention should the nurse perform <u>first</u>?
1. Notify the physician.
2. Wipe the chest tube with alcohol and reinsert.
3. Cover the chest tube insertion site opening with petroleum gauze, and apply pressure.
4. Auscultate the lung fields for breath sounds.

82. A nurse plans to assist with removal of a chest tube. Which step should be the nurse's <u>priority</u> for this procedure?
1. Provide the results of the most recent chest X-ray for the physician to review before removal.
2. Make sure that the physician orders arterial blood gas analysis before removal.
3. Disconnect the drainage system from the chest tube before the tube's removal.
4. Teach the client that chest tube removal is typically a pain-free procedure.

83. Which of the following is the <u>number one cause</u> of lung cancer?
1. Genetics
2. Occupational exposure
3. Smoking a pipe
4. Smoking cigarettes

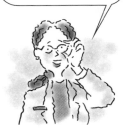

What do I expect to see after a chest tube insertion?

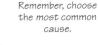

Remember, choose the *most common* cause.

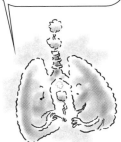

80. 1. Rise and fall of the water-seal chamber immediately after surgery indicates patency of the chest tube drainage system. The tubing should be coiled on the bed, without dependent loops, to promote drainage. Up to 500 ml of drainage can occur in the first 24 hours after surgery. Gentle bubbling is indicated after surgery to prevent excessive evaporation.
CN: Physiological integrity; CNS: Physiological adaptation; CL: Application

81. 3. If a chest tube is accidentally dislodged, immediately cover the insertion site opening with petroleum gauze and apply pressure to prevent air from entering the chest and causing tension pneumothorax. Next, notify the physician. It isn't appropriate to attempt to reinsert the chest tube. Auscultation of the lungs may be important but isn't the priority.
CN: Physiological integrity; CNS: Physiological adaptation; CL: Application

82. 1. A chest X-ray should be done before chest tube removal to ensure that the client's lung has remained expanded after suction was discontinued. Pulse oximetry would be sufficient and is the more commonly used method to track oxygenation. Disconnecting the drainage system before the chest tube is removed could cause tension pneumothorax. The client may require analgesia before chest tube removal to minimize discomfort.
CN: Physiological integrity; CNS: Physiological adaptation; CL: Application

83. 4. As many as 85% of clients with lung cancer smoke cigarettes. Cigarette smoke contains several organ-specific carcinogens. There may be a genetic predisposition for the development of cancer. Occupational hazards such as pollutants can cause cancer. Pipe smokers inhale less often and tend to develop cancers of the lip and mouth.
CN: Physiological integrity; CNS: Physiological adaptation; CL: Application

CN: Client needs category   CNS: Client needs subcategory   CL: Cognitive level

84. A nurse is preparing to reinforce the teaching plan for a client who has recently been diagnosed with squamous cell carcinoma of the left lung. Which statement by the nurse is correct?
   1. "You have a slow-growing cancer that rarely spreads."
   2. "In terms of prognosis, you may have only a few months to live."
   3. "Squamous cell cancer is a very rapid-growing cancer."
   4. "The cancer has generally metastasized by the time the diagnosis is made."

84. 1. Squamous cell carcinoma of the lung is a slow-growing, rarely metastasizing type of cancer. It has the best prognosis of all lung cancer types.
CN: Physiological integrity; CNS: Physiological adaptation; CL: Analysis

85. Warning signs and symptoms of lung cancer include persistent cough, bloody sputum, dyspnea, and which other symptom?
   1. Dizziness
   2. Generalized weakness
   3. Hypotension
   4. Recurrent pleural effusions

85. 4. Recurring episodes of pleural effusions can be caused by the tumor and should be investigated. Dizziness, hypotension, and generalized weakness aren't typically considered warning signals but may occur in advanced stages of cancer.
CN: Physiological integrity; CNS: Physiological adaptation; CL: Application

86. Which laboratory test value is elevated in clients who smoke and therefore can't be used as a general indicator of cancer?
   1. Acid phosphatase level
   2. Serum calcitonin level
   3. Alkaline phosphatase level
   4. Carcinoembryonic antigen level

That's no smoke screen in question 86. Think about the risks of smoking.

86. 4. Because the level of carcinoembryonic antigen is elevated in clients who smoke, it can't be used as a general indicator of cancer. However, the carcinoembryonic antigen level is helpful in monitoring cancer treatment because it usually falls to normal within 1 month if treatment is successful. An elevated acid phosphatase level may indicate prostate cancer. An elevated alkaline phosphatase level may reflect bone metastasis. An elevated serum calcitonin level usually signals thyroid cancer.
CN: Physiological integrity; CNS: Physiological adaptation; CL: Knowledge

87. A definitive diagnosis of lung cancer is obtained by which evaluation?
   1. Bronchoscopy
   2. Chest X-ray
   3. Computerized tomography of the chest
   4. Surgical biopsy

87. 4. Only surgical biopsy with cytologic examination of the cells can give a definitive diagnosis of the type of cancer. Bronchoscopy gives positive results in only 30% of the cases. Chest X-ray and computerized tomography can identify location but don't diagnose the type of cancer.
CN: Physiological integrity; CNS: Physiological adaptation; CL: Application

CN: Client needs category   CNS: Client needs subcategory   CL: Cognitive level

88. Which statements are true about staging lung cancer tumors? Select all that apply.
1. Staging describes the severity of the cancer.
2. Staging helps the physician plan appropriate treatment.
3. Staging systems don't change over time.
4. Surgical biopsy with cytologic cell examination is the only data collection method used to perform staging.
5. Staging helps to determine whether the cancer has spread to distant areas of the body.

89. Which intervention is the key to increasing the survival rates of clients with lung cancer?
1. Early bronchoscopy
2. Early detection
3. High-dose chemotherapy
4. Smoking cessation

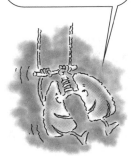

Tell me. Am I being upstaged—or staged—here?

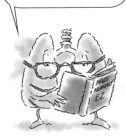

No, it isn't a trick question...the answer is pretty obvious if you look in the right spot.

90. A nurse is assigned to care for a client with a chest tube and observes that there's constant bubbling in the water seal chamber of the closed drainage system. Which explanation best describes this observation?
1. Constant bubbling indicates that the tube is working correctly.
2. Constant bubbling indicates that there's a loose connection.
3. Constant bubbling indicates that the suction rate is too high.
4. Constant bubbling indicates that the suction rate is too low.

91. A client has been diagnosed with lung cancer and requires a wedge resection. How much of the lung is removed?
1. One entire lung
2. A lobe of the lung
3. A small, localized area near the surface of the lung
4. A segment of the lung, including a bronchiole and its alveoli

88. 1, 2, 5. Staging describes the extent and severity of the cancer and helps the physician determine the most appropriate therapy. Staging systems continue to evolve as cancer is better understood. Multiple data collection methods, such as laboratory results, physical examinations, and imaging results, are used to determine the stage of a cancer.
CN: Physiological integrity; CNS: Physiological adaptation; CL: Analysis

89. 2. Detecting cancer early when the cells may be premalignant and potentially curable would be most beneficial. However, a tumor must be 1 cm in diameter before it's detectable on a chest X-ray, so this is difficult. If the cancer is detected early, a bronchoscopy may help identify cell type. Smoking cessation won't reverse the process but may prevent further decompensation.
CN: Health promotion and maintenance; CNS: None; CL: Application

90. 2. Constant bubbling in the water seal chamber indicates that there's a leak or loose connection between the client and the water seal chamber. The amount of suction affects the suction control chamber, not the water seal chamber.
CN: Physiological integrity; CNS: Physiological adaptation; CL: Application

91. 3. A very small area of tissue close to the surface of the lung is removed in a wedge resection. A segment of the lung is removed in a segmental resection, a lobe is removed in a lobectomy, and an entire lung is removed in a pneumonectomy.
CN: Physiological integrity; CNS: Physiological adaptation; CL: Application

92. When a client has a lobectomy, what fills the space where the lobe was?

1. The space stays empty.
2. The surgeon fills the space with a gel.
3. The lung space fills up with serous fluid.
4. The remaining lobe or lobes overexpand to fill the space.

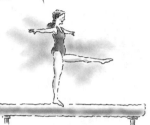

Consider: What would keep everything in balance?

92. 4. The remaining lobe or lobes overexpand slightly to fill the space previously occupied by the removed tissue. The diaphragm is carried higher on the operative side to further reduce the empty space. The surgeon doesn't use gel to fill the space. Serous fluid overproduction would compress the remaining lobes and diminish their function, and also possibly cause a mediastinal shift. The space can't remain "empty," because truly empty would imply a vacuum, which would interfere with the intrathoracic pressure changes that allow breathing.
CN: Physiological integrity; CNS: Physiological adaptation; CL: Application

93. If a client requires a pneumonectomy, what fills the area of the thoracic cavity?

1. The space remains filled with air only.
2. The surgeon fills the space with a gel.
3. Serous fluid fills the space and consolidates the region.
4. The tissue from the other lung grows over to the other side.

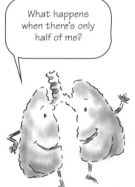

What happens when there's only half of me?

93. 3. Serous fluid fills the space and eventually consolidates, preventing extensive mediastinal shift of the heart and remaining lung. There's no gel that can be placed in the pleural space. The tissue from the other lung can't cross the mediastinum, although a temporary mediastinal shift exists until the space is filled. Air can't be left in the space.
CN: Physiological integrity; CNS: Physiological adaptation; CL: Application

94. During a pneumonectomy, the phrenic nerve on the surgical side is typically cut to cause hemidiaphragm paralysis. Why is this done?

1. Paralyzing the diaphragm reduces oxygen demand.
2. Cutting the phrenic nerve is a mistake during surgery.
3. The client isn't using that lung to breathe any longer.
4. Paralyzing the diaphragm reduces the space left by the pneumonectomy.

94. 4. Because the hemidiaphragm is a muscle that doesn't contract when paralyzed, an uncontracted hemidiaphragm remains in an "up" position, which reduces the space left by the pneumonectomy. Serous fluid has less space to fill, thus reducing the extent and duration of mediastinal shift after surgery. Although it's true that the client no longer needs the hemidiaphragm on the operative side to breathe, this alone wouldn't be sufficient justification for cutting the phrenic nerve. Paralyzing the hemidiaphragm doesn't significantly decrease total-body oxygen demand.
CN: Physiological integrity; CNS: Physiological adaptation; CL: Application

Here's another test-taking hint for you!

95. Which is the <u>primary</u> goal of surgical resection for lung cancer?

1. Remove the tumor and all surrounding tissue.
2. Remove the tumor and as little surrounding tissue as possible.
3. Remove all the tumor and any collapsed alveoli in the same region.
4. Remove as much of the tumor as possible, without removing any alveoli.

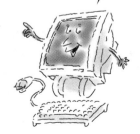

95. 2. The goal of surgical resection is to remove the cancerous lung tissue that has tumor in it while preserving as much surrounding tissue as possible. It may be necessary to remove alveoli and bronchioles, but care is taken to remove only what's absolutely necessary.
CN: Physiological integrity; CNS: Physiological adaptation; CL: Application

CN: Client needs category   CNS: Client needs subcategory   CL: Cognitive level

96. Which position is contraindicated when caring for a client who has had a pneumonectomy for lung cancer?
 1. Semi-Fowler's
 2. Lying on the nonoperative side
 3. Reverse Trendelenburg's
 4. Prone

97. A nurse performing preoperative teaching for a client who will be undergoing surgery should focus primarily on which area?
 1. Deciding if the client should have surgery
 2. Providing emotional support to the client and family
 3. Providing detailed explanations of the surgery to the client and family
 4. Providing general information, answering questions, and offering emotional support to the client and family

98. How is a benign lung tumor treated?
 1. With radiation only
 2. With chemotherapy only
 3. Left alone unless symptoms are present
 4. Removed, involving the least possible amount of tissue

99. In the client with terminal lung cancer, the focus of nursing care is on which nursing intervention?
 1. Providing emotional support
 2. Providing nutritional support
 3. Providing pain control
 4. Preparing the client's will

100. Which statement best defines a pulmonary embolism?
 1. It's a blood clot that originates in the lung.
 2. It's a blood clot that has occluded an alveolus.
 3. It's a blood clot that has occluded a bronchiole.
 4. It's a blood clot that has occluded a pulmonary blood vessel.

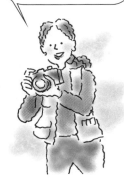

The nurse does a lot of teaching but, in this case, what would be the main focus?

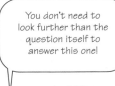

You don't need to look further than the question itself to answer this one!

96. 2. A client who has undergone a pneumonectomy doesn't have a chest tube in place. Lying the client on his operative side or on his back prevents fluid from draining into his unaffected lung and promotes maximum ventilation.
CN: Physiological integrity; CNS: Reduction of risk potential; CL: Application

97. 4. The nurse's role is to provide general information about the client's surgery, explain his preoperative and postoperative care, and offer emotional support. The nurse's role isn't to decide whether the client should have surgery. Providing only emotional support isn't sufficient. If the client has questions that require detailed explanations of the surgery, he should be referred to his surgeon.
CN: Physiological integrity; CNS: Physiological adaptation; CL: Application

98. 4. The tumor is removed to prevent further compression of lung tissue as the tumor grows, which could lead to respiratory decompensation. If for some reason it can't be removed, then chemotherapy or radiation may be used to try to shrink the tumor.
CN: Physiological integrity; CNS: Physiological adaptation; CL: Application

99. 3. The client with terminal lung cancer may have extreme pleuritic pain and should be treated to reduce his discomfort. Preparing the client and his family for the impending death is also important but shouldn't be the primary focus until pain is under control. Nutritional support may be provided, but as the terminal phase advances, the client's nutritional needs greatly decrease. Nursing care doesn't focus on helping the client prepare a will.
CN: Physiological integrity; CNS: Physiological adaptation; CL: Application

100. 4. A pulmonary embolism is a blood clot or some other material that, having originated in one area of the body, travels through the bloodstream and lodges in the pulmonary arteries. It doesn't originate in a pulmonary artery. An embolism remains in the bloodstream and isn't in the bronchial tree, the "air side" of the lung architecture; therefore, it isn't in the bronchiole or the alveoli.
CN: Physiological integrity; CNS: Physiological adaptation; CL: Application

CN: Client needs category   CNS: Client needs subcategory   CL: Cognitive level

101. Which of the following is the <u>most common</u> origin for a pulmonary embolism?
1. Amniotic fluid
2. Bone marrow
3. Septic thrombi
4. Venous thrombi

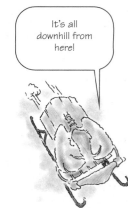

It's all downhill from here!

102. Which client is at <u>highest</u> risk for developing a pulmonary embolism?
1. An ambulatory client with an inflammatory joint disease
2. An ambulatory client who has type 1 diabetes
3. A healthy client who's 6 months pregnant
4. A client who has fractures of his pelvis and right femur

103. Which intervention to prevent pulmonary embolism after lower extremity surgery is <u>best</u>?
1. Early ambulation
2. Frequent chest X-rays to find a pulmonary embolism
3. Frequent lower extremity venous scans
4. Intubation of the client

104. At 8 a.m., the nurse assesses a client who's scheduled for surgery at 10 a.m. During the assessment, the nurse observes dyspnea, a nonproductive cough, and back pain. What should the nurse do <u>next</u>?
1. Check to see that the chest X-ray was done yesterday, as ordered.
2. Check the serum electrolyte levels and complete blood count (CBC).
3. Make sure that the physician is immediately notified of these findings.
4. Sign the preoperative checklist for this client.

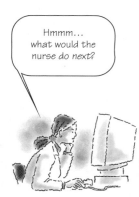

Hmmm... what would the nurse do next?

101. 4. Venous thrombi in the thigh and pelvis are the most common sources for pulmonary emboli. Clients who are immobile form clots from this source. When dislodged, the clots are carried through the bloodstream and lodge in the pulmonary vasculature. The other options are also sources, but not the most common.
CN: Physiological integrity; CNS: Physiological adaptation; CL: Application

102. 4. Thrombosis formation is caused by abnormalities in blood flow, vein wall integrity, and blood coagulation. The client with pelvic and femur fractures will be immobilized and probably have edema, which leads to venous stasis and predisposes him to the development of deep vein thrombosis. A pulmonary embolus commonly arises from clots in the deep veins of the legs that break off and travel to the pulmonary arteries. The risk of developing venous thrombosis isn't as high with the other conditions.
CN: Physiological integrity; CNS: Physiological adaptation; CL: Application

103. 1. Early ambulation helps reduce pooling of blood, which reduces the tendency of the blood to form a clot that could then dislodge. None of the other measures will prevent pulmonary embolism from forming.
CN: Physiological integrity; CNS: Physiological adaptation; CL: Application

104. 3. The nurse should make sure that the physician is immediately notified of the findings because dyspnea, a nonproductive cough, and back pain may signal a change in the client's respiratory status. The nurse should check any ordered tests (such as chest X-ray, serum electrolyte levels, and CBC) after notifying the physician because they may help explain the change in the client's condition. The nurse should sign the preoperative checklist *after* notifying the physician of the client's condition and learning the physician's decision on whether to proceed with surgery.
CN: Safe, effective care environment; CNS: Coordinated care; CL: Application

105. When a client's ventilation is impaired, the body retains which substance?
1. Sodium bicarbonate
2. Carbon dioxide
3. Nitrous oxide
4. Oxygen

106. When a client has a pulmonary embolism, he may develop chest pain caused by which condition?
1. Costochondritis
2. Myocardial infarction
3. Pleuritic pain
4. Referred pain from the pelvis

107. Which symptom would a nurse most likely observe <u>first</u> in a client with an acute pulmonary embolism?
1. Distended jugular veins
2. Bradycardia
3. Dyspnea
4. Nonproductive cough

108. Hemoptysis may be present in the client with a pulmonary embolism because of which reason?
1. Alveolar damage in the infarcted area
2. Involvement of major blood vessels in the occluded area
3. Loss of lung parenchyma
4. Loss of lung tissue

109. A client with a large pulmonary embolism will have an arterial blood gas analysis performed to determine the extent of hypoxia. Which acid-base disorder may be present?
1. Metabolic acidosis
2. Metabolic alkalosis
3. Respiratory acidosis
4. Respiratory alkalosis

Here's a hint for question 106: think about what causes the condition.

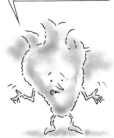

Something is throwing us off balance. Be sure to take a deep breath before answering this one.

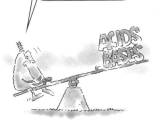

105. 2. When ventilation is impaired, the body retains carbon dioxide. Sodium bicarbonate is used to treat acidosis. Nitrous oxide, which has analgesic and anesthetic properties, commonly is administered before minor surgical procedures. When ventilation is impaired, the body doesn't retain oxygen. Instead, the tissues use oxygen, and carbon dioxide is the end result.
CN: Physiological integrity; CNS: Physiological adaptation; CL: Knowledge

106. 3. Pleuritic pain is caused by the inflammatory reaction of the lung parenchyma to the pulmonary embolism. The pain isn't associated with myocardial infarction, costochondritis, or referred pain from the pelvis to the chest.
CN: Physiological integrity; CNS: Physiological adaptation; CL: Application

107. 3. Dyspnea is usually the first symptom of pulmonary embolus because the thrombus prevents gas exchange in the pulmonary arterial bed. If the embolus is large enough, the client may then develop right ventricular failure with such symptoms as distended jugular veins, tachycardia, and circulatory collapse. He may also have hemoptysis.
CN: Physiological integrity; CNS: Physiological adaptation; CL: Analysis

108. 1. The infarcted area produces alveolar damage that can lead to the production of bloody sputum, sometimes in large amounts. There's a loss of lung parenchyma and subsequent scar tissue formation.
CN: Physiological integrity; CNS: Physiological adaptation; CL: Application

109. 4. A client with a large pulmonary embolism will have a large region of lung tissue unavailable for perfusion. This causes the client to hyperventilate and blow off large amounts of carbon dioxide, which crosses the unaffected alveolar-capillary membrane more readily than does oxygen, resulting in respiratory alkalosis.
CN: Physiological integrity; CNS: Physiological adaptation; CL: Application

110. A ventilation-perfusion scan is frequently performed to diagnose a pulmonary embolism. This test provides what type of information?
1. Amount of perfusion present in the lung
2. Extent of the occlusion and amount of perfusion lost
3. Location of the pulmonary embolism
4. Location and size of the pulmonary embolism

111. Which test definitively diagnoses a pulmonary embolism?
1. Arterial blood gas (ABG) analysis
2. Computed tomography scan
3. Pulmonary angiogram
4. Ventilation-perfusion scan

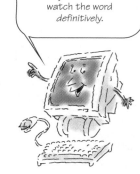

In question 111... watch the word *definitively.*

112. A client with pulmonary embolism has received a thrombolytic medication. Which teaching point should the nurse reinforce with this client and his family?
1. The medication was given to break apart the blood clot blocking the pulmonary artery.
2. The medication is taken orally and will thin the blood.
3. The medication will prevent future clots from forming.
4. The medication will help the client to breathe by dilating bronchial tubes.

110. 2. The ventilation-perfusion scan provides information on the extent of occlusion caused by the pulmonary embolism and the amount of lung tissue involved in the area not perfused.
CN: Physiological integrity; CNS: Physiological adaptation; CL: Application

111. 3. Pulmonary angiogram is used to definitively diagnose a pulmonary embolism. A catheter is passed through the circulation to the region of the occlusion; the region can be outlined with an injection of contrast medium and viewed by fluoroscopy. This shows the location of the clot, as well as the extent of the perfusion defect. Computed tomography scan can show the location of infarcted or ischemic tissue. ABG levels can define the amount of hypoxia present. The ventilation-perfusion scan can report whether there's a ventilation-perfusion mismatch present and define the amount of tissue involved.
CN: Physiological integrity; CNS: Physiological adaptation; CL: Application

112. 1. A thrombolytic medication is given I.V. to break apart or dissolve blood clots. It isn't given orally, doesn't prevent future clots from forming, and has no effect on the bronchial tubes.
CN: Physiological integrity; CNS: Pharmacological therapies; CL: Application

113. Following a pulmonary embolism, a client is placed on I.V. heparin. The client asks the nurse about the purpose of the heparin. Which statement by the nurse is the correct explanation of the purpose of heparin therapy?

1. "Heparin will dissolve the clot in your lungs."
2. "Heparin will slow the development of any more clots."
3. "Heparin will prevent pieces of the clot from breaking off and going to your lung."
4. "Heparin will dissolve any circulating clots."

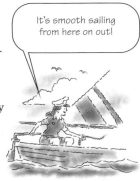

It's smooth sailing from here on out!

113. 2. Heparin is an anticoagulant and is administered to slow thrombus formation. Fibrinolytic medications dissolve clots. Heparin won't prevent clots from embolizing or dissolve circulating clots.

CN: Physiological integrity; CNS: Pharmacological therapies; CL: Application

114. A client who was hospitalized for pulmonary embolism is being discharged on warfarin (Coumadin) therapy. Which teaching by the nurse about warfarin therapy is correct?

1. It inhibits the formation of blood clots.
2. It's given to continue to reduce the size of the pulmonary embolism.
3. It will reduce blood pressure and prevent venous stasis.
4. Coagulation studies to monitor bleeding times will be necessary every 6 months.

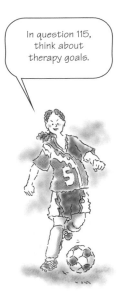

In question 115, think about therapy goals.

114. 1. Warfarin inhibits clot formation by interfering with clotting factors that are dependent on vitamin K. Warfarin doesn't dissolve clots and won't reduce the size of the pulmonary embolus. It doesn't reduce blood pressure and won't prevent venous stasis. Coagulation studies will be performed every 2 to 4 weeks while the client is receiving warfarin.

CN: Physiological integrity; CNS: Physiological adaptation; CL: Application

115. The goal of oxygen therapy for a client with a pulmonary embolism is to obtain which value?

1. $Paco_2$ above 40 mm Hg
2. $Paco_2$ below 40 mm Hg
3. Pao_2 above 60 mm Hg
4. Pao_2 below 60 mm Hg

115. 3. The goal of oxygen therapy for a client with a pulmonary embolism is to have a Pao_2 greater than 60 mm Hg on an Fio_2 of 40% or less. The normal range of the $Paco_2$ is 35 to 45 mm Hg. In the absence of other pathologic states, it should reach normal levels before the Pao_2 does on room air because carbon dioxide crosses the alveolar-capillary membrane with greater ease.

CN: Physiological integrity; CNS: Physiological adaptation; CL: Application

116. A client is receiving oxygen via a nasal cannula at 2 L/minute. What percentage of oxygen concentration is coming through the cannula?

1. 23% to 30%
2. 30% to 40%
3. 40% to 60%
4. 50% to 75%

116. 1. The percentage of oxygen concentration as it passes out of the nasal cannula at 2 L/minute is 23% to 30%. The oxygen concentration via cannula at 3 to 5 L/minute is 30% to 40%. A simple mask at 6 to 8 L/minute delivers 40% to 60% of oxygen. A partial rebreather mask at 8 to 11 L/minute delivers 50% to 75% of oxygen.

CN: Psychological integrity CNS: Reduction of risk potential; CL: Comprehension

CN: Client needs category   CNS: Client needs subcategory   CL: Cognitive level

117. A client with a pulmonary embolism typically has chest pain and apprehension. Which of the following would be the best treatment method?
1. Analgesics
2. Guided imagery
3. Positioning the client on the left side
4. Providing emotional support

Watch for clues for what you're treating.

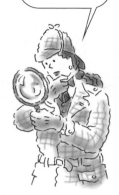

118. A client with a pulmonary embolism may have an umbrella-like filter placed in the vena cava for which reason?
1. The filter prevents further clot formation.
2. The filter collects clots so they don't go to the lung.
3. The filter break up clots into insignificantly small pieces.
4. The filter contains anticoagulants that are slowly released, dissolving any clots.

119. A client with a pulmonary embolism may need an embolectomy, which involves which action?
1. Removal of an embolism in the lower extremity
2. Extracting the embolism from the lung by bronchoscopy
3. Surgical removal of the embolism source in the pelvis
4. Surgical removal of the embolism in the pulmonary vasculature

120. Nursing management of a client with a pulmonary embolism focuses on which action?
1. Assessing oxygenation status
2. Monitoring the oxygen delivery device
3. Monitoring for other sources of clots
4. Determining whether the client requires another ventilation-perfusion scan

117. 1. After the pulmonary embolism has been diagnosed and the amount of hypoxia determined, chest pain and the accompanying apprehension can be treated with analgesics. The nurse must monitor respiratory status frequently. Guided imagery and providing emotional support can be used as alternatives. Positioning the client on the left side when a pulmonary embolism is suspected may prevent a clot that has extended through the capillaries and into the pulmonary veins from breaking off and traveling through the heart into the arterial circulation, leading to a massive stroke.
CN: Physiological integrity; CNS: Physiological adaptation; CL: Application

118. 3. The umbrella-like filter is placed in a client at high risk for the formation of more clots that could potentially become pulmonary emboli. The filter breaks the clots into small pieces that won't significantly occlude the pulmonary vasculature. The filter doesn't release anticoagulants and doesn't prevent further clot formation. The filter doesn't collect the clots, because if it did, it would have to be emptied periodically, causing the client to require surgery in the future.
CN: Physiological integrity; CNS: Physiological adaptation; CL: Application

119. 4. If the pulmonary embolism is large and doesn't respond to treatment, surgical removal may be necessary to restore perfusion to the area of the lung. This is rarely done because of the associated high mortality risk. It's impossible to remove a pulmonary embolism through bronchoscopy because the defect isn't in the bronchial tree. A thrombectomy can be performed at other sources of clots, but when a pulmonary embolism has already occurred, it would have little effect on oxygenation.
CN: Physiological integrity; CNS: Physiological adaptation; CL: Application

120. 1. Nursing management of a client with a pulmonary embolism focuses on assessing oxygenation status and ensuring treatment is adequate. If the client's status begins to deteriorate, it's the nurse's responsibility to contact the physician and attempt to improve oxygenation. Monitoring for other clot sources and ensuring the oxygen delivery device is working properly are other nursing responsibilities, but they aren't the focus of care.
CN: Physiological integrity; CNS: Physiological adaptation; CL: Application

CN: Client needs category   CNS: Client needs subcategory   CL: Cognitive level

121. Pulse oximetry gives what type of information about the client?
1. Amount of carbon dioxide in the blood
2. Amount of oxygen in the blood
3. Percentage of hemoglobin carrying oxygen
4. Respiratory rate

122. What effect does hemoglobin amount have on oxygenation status?
1. It has no effect.
2. More hemoglobin reduces the client's respiratory rate.
3. Low hemoglobin levels cause reduced oxygen-carrying capacity.
4. Low hemoglobin levels cause increased oxygen-carrying capacity.

123. How does positive end-expiratory pressure (PEEP) improve oxygenation?
1. It provides more oxygen to the client.
2. It opens up bronchioles and allows oxygen to get in the lungs.
3. It opens up collapsed alveoli and helps keep them open.
4. It adds pressure to the lung tissue during inhalation.

124. Which statement best explains how opening up collapsed alveoli improves oxygenation?
1. Alveoli need oxygen to live.
2. Alveoli have no effect on oxygenation.
3. Collapsed alveoli increase oxygen demand.
4. Gaseous exchange occurs in the alveolar membrane.

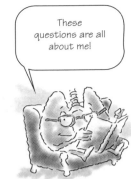

These questions are all about me!

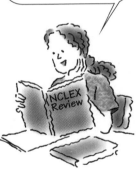

To answer question 122, think about hemoglobin's role.

121. 3. Pulse oximetry determines the percentage of hemoglobin carrying oxygen. This doesn't ensure that the oxygen being carried through the bloodstream is actually being taken up by the tissue. Pulse oximetry doesn't provide information about the amount of oxygen or carbon dioxide in the blood or the client's respiratory rate.
CN: Physiological integrity; CNS: Physiological adaptation; CL: Application

122. 3. Hemoglobin carries oxygen to all tissues in the body. If the hemoglobin level is low, the amount of oxygen-carrying capacity is also low. More hemoglobin will increase oxygen-carrying capacity and thus increase the total amount of oxygen available in the blood. If the client has been tachypneic during exertion, or even at rest, because oxygen demand is higher than the available oxygen content, then an increase in hemoglobin may decrease the respiratory rate to normal levels.
CN: Physiological integrity; CNS: Physiological adaptation; CL: Application

123. 3. PEEP delivers positive pressure to the lung at the end of expiration. This helps open collapsed alveoli and helps them stay open so gas exchange can occur in these newly opened alveoli, improving oxygenation. The bronchioles don't participate in gas exchange except to act as a conduit for inspired and expired air. The alveolar walls are rigid enough; they generally don't collapse. PEEP doesn't directly add pressure to the lung tissue or provide more oxygen to the client.
CN: Physiological integrity; CNS: Physiological adaptation; CL: Application

124. 4. Gaseous exchange occurs in the alveolar membrane, so if the alveoli collapse, no exchange occurs. Collapsed alveoli receive oxygen, as well as other nutrients, from the bloodstream. Collapsed alveoli have no effect on oxygen demand, though by decreasing the surface area available for gas exchange, they decrease oxygenation of the blood.
CN: Physiological integrity; CNS: Physiological adaptation; CL: Application

125. Continuous positive airway pressure can be provided through an oxygen mask to improve oxygenation in hypoxic clients by which method?

1. The mask provides 100% oxygen to the client.
2. The mask provides continuous air that the client can breathe.
3. The mask provides pressurized oxygen so the client can breathe more easily.
4. The mask provides pressurized oxygen at the end of expiration to open collapsed alveoli.

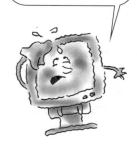

Whew! Just a few more questions to go!

125. 3. The mask provides pressurized oxygen continuously through both inspiration and expiration. By providing a client with pressurized oxygen, the client has less resistance to overcome in taking in his next breath, making it easier to breathe. The mask can be set to deliver any amount of oxygen needed. Pressurized oxygen delivered at the end of expiration is positive end-expiratory pressure, not continuous positive airway pressure.
CN: Physiological integrity; CNS: Physiological adaptation; CL: Application

126. The nurse is caring for a client with pneumonia. The physician orders 600 mg of ceftriaxone (Rocephin) oral suspension to be given once per day. The medication label indicates that the strength is 125 mg/5 ml. How many milliliters of medication should the nurse pour to administer the correct dose? Record your answer using a whole number.

_____ ml

126. 24. To calculate drug dosages, use the formula:

Dose on hand/Quantity on hand = Dose desired/X.

In this case, 125 mg/5 ml = 600 mg/X.
Therefore, X = 24 ml.
CN: Physiological integrity; CNS: Pharmacological therapies; CL: Application

127. The nurse is caring for a client who's scheduled for a bronchoscopy. Which interventions should the nurse perform to prepare the client for this procedure? Select all that apply:

1. Explain the procedure.
2. Withhold food and fluids for 2 hours before the test.
3. Provide a clear liquid diet for 6 to 12 hours before the test.
4. Confirm that a signed informed consent form has been obtained.
5. Ask the client to remove his dentures.
6. Administer a sedative.

127. 1, 4, 5, 6. All procedures must be explained to the client in order to obtain informed consent and to reduce anxiety. A signed informed consent form is required for all invasive procedures. Dentures need to be removed for bronchoscopy because they may become dislodged during the procedure. A sedative is given to relax the client. Food and fluids are restricted for 6 to 12 hours before the test to avoid the risk of aspiration during the procedure.
CN: Physiological integrity; CNS: Reduction of risk potential; CL: Application

128. A client is admitted to the progressive care unit with an arterial line for continuous measurement of systolic, diastolic, and mean blood pressures. The nurse is evaluating the waveform. Identify the area that indicates that the aortic valve has closed.

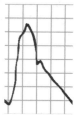

Hurray! You did it! Maybe we can take a break and get a little snack?

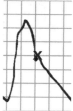

128.

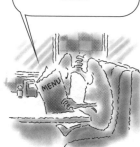

When the pressure in the ventricle is less than the pressure in the aortic root, the aortic valve closes. This event appears as a small notch on the waveform's downside.
CN: Physiological integrity; CNS: Reduction of risk potential; CL: Comprehension

CN: Client needs category   CNS: Client needs subcategory   CL: Cognitive level

Stroke, subdural hematoma, laminectomy—they're all here in this comprehensive chapter on neurosensory disorders in adults. I've got a sixth sense you're going to do great!

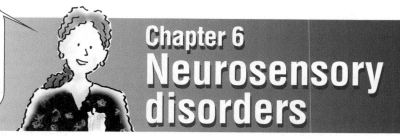

Chapter 6
Neurosensory disorders

1. An elderly client had a stroke and can see only the nasal visual field on one side and the temporal portion on the opposite side. Which term correctly describes this condition?
1. Astereognosis
2. Homonymous hemianopsia
3. Oculogyric crisis
4. Receptive aphasia

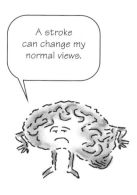

A stroke can change my normal views.

2. A client had an embolic stroke. Which condition places a client at risk for thromboembolic stroke?
1. Atrial fibrillation
2. Bradycardia
3. Deep vein thrombosis (DVT)
4. History of myocardial infarction (MI)

3. A heparin infusion at 1,500 units/hour is ordered for a 65-year-old client with a stroke in evolution. The infusion contains 25,000 units of heparin in 500 ml of saline solution. How many milliliters per hour should be given?
1. 15 ml/hour
2. 30 ml/hour
3. 45 ml/hour
4. 50 ml/hour

4. Which medication may be prescribed to prevent a thromboembolic stroke ?
1. Acetaminophen
2. Streptokinase
3. Ticlopidine
4. Methylprednisolone

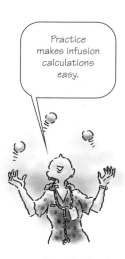

Practice makes infusion calculations easy.

1. 2. Homonymous hemianopsia describes the loss of visual field on the nasal side and the opposite temporal side due to damage of the optic nerves. Receptive aphasia is the inability to understand words or word meaning. Oculogyric crisis, a fixed position of the eyeballs that can last for minutes or hours, occurs in response to antipsychotic medications. Astereognosis is the inability to identify common objects through touch.
CN: Physiological integrity; CNS: Physiological adaptation; CL: Application

2. 1. Atrial fibrillation occurs with the irregular and rapid discharge from multiple ectopic atrial foci that causes quivering of the atria without atrial systole. This asynchronous atrial contraction predisposes to mural thrombi, which may embolize, leading to a stroke. Bradycardia, past MI, or DVT won't lead to arterial embolization.
CN: Physiological integrity; CNS: Physiological adaptation; CL: Application

3. 2. An infusion prepared with 25,000 units of heparin in 500 ml of saline solution yields 50 units of heparin per milliliter of solution. The equation is set up as 50 units times X (the unknown quantity) equals 1,500 units/hour; X equals 30 ml/hour.
CN: Physiological integrity; CNS: Pharmacological therapies; CL: Application

4. 3. Ticlopidine inhibits platelet aggregation and is used to prevent thromboembolic stroke. Aspirin, not acetaminophen, interferes with platelet aggregation. Streptokinase is a medication used with evolving myocardial infarctions and dissolves clots. Methylprednisolone is a steroid with anticoagulant properties.
CN: Physiological integrity; CNS: Pharmacological therapies; CL: Application

5. To maintain airway patency during a stroke in evolution, which nursing intervention is appropriate?
 1. Thicken all dietary liquids.
 2. Restrict dietary and parenteral fluids.
 3. Place the client in the supine position.
 4. Have tracheal suction available at all times.

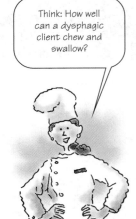

Think: How well can a dysphagic client chew and swallow?

6. For a client with a stroke, what criteria must be fulfilled before the client is fed?
 1. The gag reflex returns.
 2. Speech returns to normal.
 3. Cranial nerves III, IV, and VI are intact.
 4. The client swallows small sips of water without coughing.

7. Which diet would be least likely to lead to aspiration in a client who had a stroke with residual dysphagia?
 1. Clear liquid
 2. Full liquid
 3. Mechanical soft
 4. Thickened liquid

8. A 77-year-old client had a thromboembolic right brain stroke; his left arm is swollen. Which condition commonly causes swelling after a stroke?
 1. Elbow contracture secondary to spasticity
 2. Loss of muscle contraction decreasing venous return
 3. Deep vein thrombosis (DVT) due to immobility of the ipsilateral side
 4. Hypoalbuminemia due to protein escaping from an inflamed glomerulus

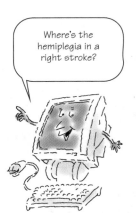

Where's the hemiplegia in a right stroke?

9. After a brain stem infarction, a nurse would observe for which condition?
 1. Aphasia
 2. Bradypnea
 3. Contralateral hemiplegia
 4. Numbness and tingling of the face or arm

5. 4. Because of a potential loss of gag reflex and potential altered level of consciousness, the client should be kept in Fowler's or a semiprone position with tracheal suction available at all times. Unless heart failure is present, restricting fluids isn't indicated. Thickening dietary liquids isn't done until the gag reflex returns or the stroke has evolved and the deficit can be assessed.
CN: Physiological integrity; CNS: Reduction of risk potential; CL: Application

6. 1. An intact gag reflex shows a properly functioning cranial nerve IX (glossopharyngeal). A nurse shouldn't offer food or fluids without assessing for intact gag reflexes. Cranial nerves III, IV, and VI evaluate eye movement and accommodation. Speech may be normal while the gag reflex is absent.
CN: Physiological integrity; CNS: Reduction of risk potential; CL: Application

7. 4. Thickened liquids are easiest to form into a bolus and swallow. Clear and full liquids are amorphous and can't easily form a bolus. A mechanical soft diet may be too hard to chew and too dry to swallow when dysphagia is present.
CN: Physiological integrity; CNS: Reduction of risk potential; CL: Application

8. 2. In clients with hemiplegia or hemiparesis, loss of muscle contraction decreases venous return and may cause swelling of the affected extremity. Stroke isn't linked to protein loss. DVT may develop in clients with a stroke but is more likely in the lower extremities. Contractures, or bony calcifications, may occur with stroke but don't appear with swelling.
CN: Physiological integrity; CNS: Physiological adaptation; CL: Analysis

9. 2. The brain stem contains the medulla and the vital cardiac, vasomotor, and respiratory centers. A brain stem infarction leads to vital sign changes such as bradypnea. Numbness, tingling in the face or arm, contralateral hemiplegia, and aphasia may occur with a stroke.
CN: Physiological integrity; CNS: Physiological adaptation; CL: Application

10. Which condition is a risk factor for the development of cataracts?
1. History of frequent streptococcal throat infections
2. Maternal exposure to rubella during pregnancy
3. Increased intraocular pressure
4. Prolonged use of steroidal anti-inflammatory agents

11. A client who had cataract surgery should be told to call his physician if which condition is present?
1. Blurred vision
2. Eye pain
3. Glare
4. Itching

12. Clear fluid is draining from the nose of a client who had a head trauma 3 hours ago. This may indicate which condition?
1. Basilar skull fracture
2. Cerebral concussion
3. Cerebral palsy
4. Sinus infection

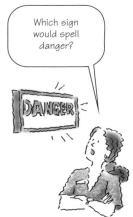

Which sign would spell danger?

13. A 19-year-old client with a mild concussion is discharged from the emergency department. Before discharge, he complains of a headache. When offered acetaminophen, his mother tells the nurse the headache is severe and could her son have something stronger. Which response by the nurse is appropriate?
1. "Your son had a mild concussion; acetaminophen is strong enough."
2. "Aspirin is avoided because of the danger of Reye's syndrome in children or young adults."
3. "Opioids are avoided after a head injury because they may hide a worsening condition."
4. "Stronger medications, such as aspirin, may lead to vomiting, which increases intracranial pressure (ICP)."

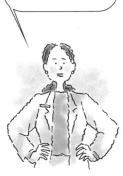

Help your client understand why certain medications may not be appropriate.

10. 4. Corticosteroid use, aging, exposure to ultraviolet light or radiation, and diabetes are risk factors for cataracts.
CN: Health promotion and maintenance; CNS: None; CL: Application

11. 2. Pain shouldn't be present after cataract surgery. The client should be told that the other symptoms might be present.
CN: Physiological integrity; CNS: Physiological adaptation; CL: Comprehension

12. 1. Clear fluid draining from the ear or nose of a client may mean a cerebrospinal fluid leak, which is common in basilar skull fractures. Concussion is associated with a brief loss of consciousness, sinus infection is associated with facial pain and pressure with or without nasal drainage, and cerebral palsy is associated with nonprogressive paralysis present since birth.
CN: Physiological integrity; CNS: Physiological adaptation; CL: Analysis

13. 3. Opioids may mask changes in the level of consciousness that indicate increased ICP and shouldn't be given. Saying acetaminophen is strong enough ignores the mother's question and therefore isn't appropriate. Aspirin is contraindicated in conditions that may cause bleeding, such as trauma, and for children or young adults with viral illnesses because of the danger of Reye's syndrome. Aspirin isn't a stronger analgesic than acetaminophen.
CN: Physiological integrity; CNS: Reduction of risk potential; CL: Application

CN: Client needs category   CNS: Client needs subcategory   CL: Cognitive level

14. A client admitted to the hospital with a sub-arachnoid hemorrhage (SAH) complains of severe headache, nuchal rigidity, and projectile vomiting. The nurse knows lumbar puncture (LP) would be contraindicated in this client in which circumstance?
  1. Continued vomiting
  2. Increased intracranial pressure (ICP)
  3. Mechanical ventilation needed
  4. Anticipated blood in the cerebrospinal fluid

14. 2. Sudden removal of cerebrospinal fluid results in pressures lower in the lumbar area than the brain and favors herniation of the brain; therefore, LP is contraindicated with increased ICP. Vomiting may be caused by reasons other than increased ICP; therefore, LP isn't strictly contraindicated. Blood in the cerebrospinal fluid is diagnostic for SAH and was obtained before signs and symptoms of increased ICP. An LP may be performed on clients needing mechanical ventilation.
CN: Physiological integrity; CNS: Physiological adaptation; CL: Application

15. A client with head trauma develops a urine output of 300 ml/hour, dry skin, and dry mucous membranes. Which nursing intervention is <u>most appropriate</u> to perform immediately?
  1. Evaluate urine specific gravity.
  2. Anticipate treatment for renal failure.
  3. Provide emollients to the skin to prevent breakdown.
  4. Slow the I.V. fluids and notify the physician.

15. 1. Urine output of 300 ml/hour may indicate diabetes insipidus, which is failure of the pituitary to produce antidiuretic hormone. This may occur with increased intracranial pressure and head trauma; the nurse evaluates for low urine specific gravity, increased serum osmolarity, and dehydration. There's no evidence that the client is experiencing renal failure. Providing emollients to prevent skin breakdown is important but doesn't need to be performed immediately. A physician's order is necessary to slow the I.V. rate, and lowering the rate would contribute to dehydration when polyuria is present.
CN: Physiological integrity; CNS: Physiological adaptation; CL: Analysis

Knowing why you do something can help prevent errors.

16. Stool softeners would be given to a client after a repair of a cerebral aneurysm for which reason?
  1. To stimulate the bowel because of loss of nerve innervation
  2. To prevent straining, which increases intracranial pressure (ICP)
  3. To prevent the Valsalva maneuver, which may lead to bradycardia
  4. To prevent constipation when osmotic diuretics are used

16. 2. Straining when having a bowel movement, sneezing, coughing, or suctioning may lead to increased ICP and should be avoided when potential increased ICP exists. Although the Valsalva maneuver may lead to bradycardia and reflex tachycardia, this rationale doesn't apply to this client. Osmotic diuretics may lead to diarrhea, not constipation.
CN: Physiological integrity; CNS: Reduction of risk potential; CL: Application

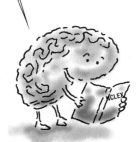

17. A client with a subdural hematoma becomes restless and confused, with dilation of the ipsilateral pupil. The physician orders mannitol for which reason?
  1. To reduce intraocular pressure
  2. To prevent acute tubular necrosis
  3. To promote osmotic diuresis to decrease intracranial pressure (ICP)
  4. To draw water into the vascular system to increase blood pressure

17. 3. Mannitol promotes osmotic diuresis by increasing the pressure gradient, drawing fluid from intracellular to intravascular spaces. Although mannitol is used for all the reasons described, the reduction of ICP in this client is a concern.
CN: Physiological integrity; CNS: Pharmacological therapies; CL: Application

CN: Client needs category   CNS: Client needs subcategory   CL: Cognitive level

18. A client with a subdural hematoma was given mannitol to decrease intracranial pressure (ICP). Which result would <u>best</u> show the mannitol was effective?
1. Urine output increases.
2. Pupils are 8 mm and nonreactive.
3. Systolic blood pressure remains at 150 mm Hg.
4. Blood urea nitrogen (BUN) and creatinine levels return to normal.

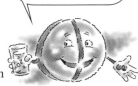

My name is mannitol and I can help your client "go with the flow," if you catch my drift.

19. When evaluating an arterial blood gas from a client with a subdural hematoma, the nurse notes the $Paco_2$ is 30 mm Hg. Which response best describes this result?
1. Appropriate; lowering carbon dioxide (CO_2) reduces intracranial pressure (ICP)
2. Emergent; the client is poorly oxygenated
3. Normal
4. Significant; the client has alveolar hypoventilation

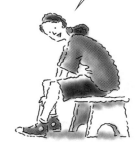

Hmmm, does health insurance cover high-top sneakers?

20. Which nursing intervention should be used to prevent footdrop and contractures in a client recovering from a subdural hematoma?
1. High-top sneakers
2. Low-dose heparin therapy
3. Physical therapy consultation
4. Sequential compression device

21. A client who's diagnosed with a right subarachnoid hemorrhage should be placed in which position?
1. With the head of the bed elevated
2. On his right side
3. On his left side
4. Flat in bed

22. Why is vasopressin given I.M. after a hypophysectomy?
1. To prevent GI bleeding
2. To prevent the syndrome of inappropriate antidiuretic hormone (SIADH)
3. To reduce cerebral edema and lower intracranial pressure
4. To replace antidiuretic hormone (ADH) normally secreted from the pituitary

18. 1. Mannitol promotes osmotic diuresis by increasing the pressure gradient in the renal tubules. No information is given about abnormal BUN and creatinine levels or that mannitol is being given for renal dysfunction or blood pressure maintenance. Fixed and dilated pupils are symptoms of increased ICP or cranial nerve damage.
CN: Physiological integrity; CNS: Physiological adaptation; CL: Application

19. 1. A normal $Paco_2$ value is 35 to 45 mm Hg. CO_2 has vasodilating properties; therefore, lowering $Paco_2$ through hyperventilation will lower ICP caused by dilated cerebral vessels. Alveolar hypoventilation would be reflected in an increased $Paco_2$. Oxygenation is evaluated through Pao_2 and oxygen saturation.
CN: Physiological integrity; CNS: Physiological adaptation; CL: Analysis

20. 1. High-top sneakers are used to prevent footdrop and contractures in neurologic clients. Low-dose heparin therapy and sequential compression boots will prevent deep vein thrombosis. Although a consultation with physical therapy is important to prevent footdrop, a nurse may use high-top sneakers independently.
CN: Physiological integrity; CNS: Reduction of risk potential; CL: Application

21. 1. Elevating the head of the bed enhances cerebral venous return and thereby decreases intracranial pressure (ICP). The other positions wouldn't decrease ICP.
CN: Safe, effective care environment; CNS: Safety and infection control; CL: Application

22. 4. After hypophysectomy, or removal of the pituitary gland, the body can't synthesize ADH. Although vasopressin tannate may be used I.V. to decrease portal pressure, it isn't correct in this instance. SIADH results from excessive ADH secretion. Mannitol or corticosteroids are used to decrease cerebral edema.
CN: Physiological integrity; CNS: Pharmacological therapies; CL: Application

CN: Client needs category   CNS: Client needs subcategory   CL: Cognitive level

23. Which value is considered normal for intracranial pressure (ICP)?
1. 0 to 15 mm Hg
2. 25 mm Hg
3. 35 to 45 mm Hg
4. 120/80 mm Hg

24. A 33-year-old client undergoes an L4-L5 laminectomy. Which method would best prevent skin breakdown??
1. Apply an alternating air mattress to the bed.
2. Use a foam wedge when propping the client on his side.
3. Logroll the client with assistance, if necessary, to keep his back in alignment.
4. Teach the client to reach for the side rail with his dominant hand to pull himself onto his side.

25. Voiding small, frequent amounts of urine after a lumbar laminectomy may indicate which condition?
1. Diabetes insipidus
2. Diabetic ketoacidosis
3. Urine retention
4. Urinary tract infection (UTI)

26. A client with lower back pain and a herniated nucleus pulposus should be taught that strengthening which muscle after laminectomy will prevent lower back pain?
1. Rectus abdominis
2. Diaphragm
3. Gluteus
4. Rectus femoris

27. When preparing a client with suspected herniated nucleus pulposus (HNP) for myelography, which nursing intervention should be done before the test?
1. Question the client about allergy to iodine.
2. Mark distal pulses on the foot in ink.
3. Assess and document pain along the sciatic nerve.
4. Tell the client he may be asked to cough or pant to clear the dye.

We all know the value of a good education. Becoming familiar with normal laboratory values can be indispensable to your nursing career.

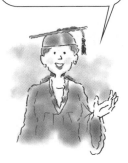

There's nothing "ab"-normal about client teaching. In fact, it's the nurse's responsibility.

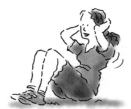

23. 1. Normal ICP is 0 to 15 mm Hg.
CN: Physiological integrity; CNS: Physiological adaptation; CL: Comprehension

24. 3. Turning the client as a unit by logrolling is necessary to relieve pressure on the sacral area and prevent stress on the intradiskal area. An air mattress will help prevent skin breakdown, but the postlaminectomy client needs a firm mattress to support the spine. A foam wedge will maintain the client's position but won't prevent breakdown. Having the client reach out will cause lordosis of the spine.
CN: Physiological integrity; CNS: Reduction of risk potential; CL: Application

25. 3. Swelling or pressure on the peripheral nerves controlling micturition, anesthesia, or use of an indwelling urinary catheter may lead to urine retention with overflow of small, frequent amounts of urine. UTI may be shown by dysuria and small, frequent amounts of voided urine, but would be less likely in this situation. Diabetes insipidus and diabetic ketoacidosis are shown by polyuria.
CN: Physiological integrity; CNS: Basic care and comfort; CL: Analysis

26. 1. Strengthening the rectus abdominis and all of the abdominal muscles will support the back, preventing lower back pain.
CN: Physiological integrity; CNS: Reduction of risk potential; CL: Application

27. 1. A radiopaque dye, commonly iodine-based, is instilled into the spinal canal to outline structures during myelography, so asking about iodine allergy is needed. Pain may be expected along the sciatic nerve with HNP. During cardiac catheterization, a client coughs or pants to clear the dye; before cardiac catheterization or arteriogram, the nurse marks pedal pulses in ink.
CN: Physiological integrity; CNS: Reduction of risk potential; CL: Application

CN: Client needs category   CNS: Client needs subcategory   CL: Cognitive level

28. A client recovering from a stroke has residual dysphagia. When assisting the client to eat, which teaching points should the nurse provide? Select all that apply.
1. "Look up at the ceiling when you swallow."
2. "Tuck your chin in when you swallow."
3. "Turn your head toward your weaker side when you swallow."
4. "After you swallow food, wait a few seconds and then swallow again."
5. "Swallow softly between each bite of food."

29. When prioritizing care, which client should the nurse assess <u>first</u>?
1. A 17-year-old client 24 hours postappendectomy
2. A 33-year-old client with a recent diagnosis of Guillain-Barré syndrome
3. A 50-year-old client 3 days post–myocardial infarction (MI)
4. A 50-year-old client with diverticulitis

30. A client is newly diagnosed with myasthenia gravis. Client teaching would include which condition as the cause of this disease?
1. A postviral illness characterized by ascending paralysis
2. Loss of the myelin sheath surrounding peripheral nerves
3. Inability of basal ganglia to produce sufficient dopamine
4. Destruction of acetylcholine receptors, causing muscle weakness

31. Which condition is an early symptom commonly seen in myasthenia gravis?
1. Dysphagia
2. Fatigue improving at the end of the day
3. Ptosis
4. Respiratory distress

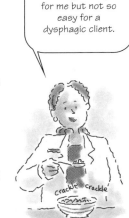

Eating is easy for me but not so easy for a dysphagic client.

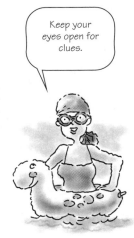

Keep your eyes open for clues.

28. 2, 3, 4. Tucking the chin in reduces the size of the airway opening, which helps prevent aspiration, and a double swallow helps clear the pharynx between bites of food. Having the client turn his head toward his weaker side makes swallowing easier. Swallowing forcefully reduces the amount of residual food in his pharynx.
CN: Physiological integrity; CNS: Basic Care and Comfort; CL: Application

29. 2. Guillain-Barré syndrome is characterized by ascending paralysis and potential respiratory failure. The order of client assessment should follow client priorities, with disorders of airway, breathing, and then circulation. There's no information to suggest the post-MI client has an arrhythmia or other complication. There's no evidence to suggest hemorrhage or perforation for the remaining clients as a priority of care.
CN: Safe, effective care environment; CNS: Coordinated care; CL: Analysis

30. 4. Myasthenia gravis, an autoimmune disorder, is caused by the destruction of acetylcholine receptors. Multiple sclerosis is caused by loss of the myelin sheath. Guillain-Barré syndrome is a postviral illness characterized by ascending paralysis, and Parkinson's disease is caused by the inability of basal ganglia to produce sufficient dopamine.
CN: Health promotion and maintenance; CNS: None; CL: Comprehension

31. 3. Ptosis and diplopia are early signs of myasthenia gravis; respiratory distress and dysphagia occur later. Symptoms are typically milder in the morning and may be exacerbated by stress or lack of rest.
CN: Health promotion and maintenance; CNS: Prevention and early detection of disease; CL: Application

32. One hour after receiving pyridostigmine (Mestinon), a client reports difficulty swallowing and excessive respiratory secretions. The nurse notifies the physician and prepares to administer which medication?
1. Additional pyridostigmine
2. Atropine
3. Edrophonium (Tensilon)
4. Neostigmine (Prostigmin)

32. 2. These symptoms suggest cholinergic crisis or excessive acetylcholinesterase medication, typically appearing 45 to 60 minutes after the last dose of acetylcholinesterase inhibitor. Atropine, an anticholinergic drug, is used to antagonize acetylcholinesterase inhibitors. The other drugs are acetylcholinesterase inhibitors. Tensilon is used to diagnose myasthenia gravis, and Mestinon and Prostigmin are used to treat the condition and would worsen the symptoms.
CN: Physiological integrity; CNS: Pharmacological therapies; CL: Analysis

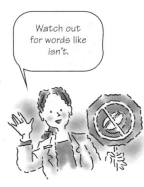

Watch out for words like *isn't.*

33. A client with suspected myasthenia gravis is to undergo a Tensilon test. Tensilon is used to diagnose—but not treat—myasthenia gravis. Why <u>isn't</u> it used for treatment?
1. It isn't available in an oral form.
2. With repeated use, immunosuppression may occur.
3. Dry mouth and abdominal cramps may be intolerable adverse effects.
4. The short half-life of Tensilon makes it impractical for long-term use.

33. 4. The duration of action of Tensilon is 1 to 2 minutes, making it impractical for the long-term management of myasthenia gravis. Immunosuppression with repeated use is an adverse effect of steroid administration, a medication used to treat myasthenia gravis. Dry mouth and abdominal cramps are adverse effects of increased acetylcholine in the parasympathetic nervous system.
CN: Physiological integrity; CNS: Pharmacological therapies; CL: Application

34. A 20-year-old client with myasthenia gravis will undergo plasmapheresis. Which of the following describes the purpose of this procedure?
1. To prevent exacerbations during pregnancy
2. To remove T and B lymphocytes that attack acetylcholine receptors
3. To deliver acetylcholinesterase inhibitor directly into the bloodstream
4. To separate and remove acetylcholine receptor antibodies from the blood

34. 4. The purpose of plasmapheresis in myasthenia gravis is to separate and remove circulating acetylcholine receptor antibodies from the blood of clients refractory to the usual therapies or clients in crisis. Although stress, including pregnancy, may precipitate crisis, this isn't the purpose of the procedure. Plasmapheresis doesn't remove T and B lymphocytes, nor does it deliver acetylcholinesterase inhibitor directly into the bloodstream.
CN: Physiological integrity; CNS: Pharmacological therapies; CL: Application

You've completed more than 25% of the questions. Good for you!

35. When assessing a client with glaucoma, the nurse expects which finding?
1. Complaints of double vision
2. Complaints of halos around lights
3. Intraocular pressure of 15 mm Hg
4. Soft globe on palpation

35. 2. Glaucoma is largely asymptomatic. Symptoms that occur can include loss of peripheral vision or blind spots, reddened sclera, firm globe, decreased accommodation, halos around lights, and occasional eye pain. Normal intraocular pressure is 10 to 21 mm Hg.
CN: Physiological integrity; CNS: Physiological adaptation; CL: Application

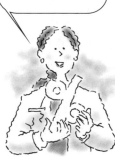

36. A client at the eye clinic is newly diagnosed with glaucoma. Client teaching includes the need to take his medication because noncompliance may lead to which condition?
1. Diplopia
2. Permanent vision loss
3. Progressive loss of peripheral vision
4. Pupillary constriction

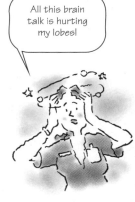

All this brain talk is hurting my lobes!

37. The nurse is caring for a client with a cerebral injury that has impaired his speech and hearing. The client has most likely experienced damage to the:
1. frontal lobe.
2. parietal lobe.
3. occipital lobe.
4. temporal lobe.

38. When evaluating the extent of Parkinson's disease, a nurse observes for which condition?
1. Bulging eyeballs
2. Diminished distal sensation
3. Increased dopamine levels
4. Muscle rigidity

39. Which statement best describes the cause of Parkinson's disease?
1. Loss of the myelin sheath surrounding peripheral nerves
2. Degeneration of the substantia nigra, depleting dopamine
3. Bleeding into the brain stem, resulting in motor dysfunction
4. An autoimmune disorder that destroys acetylcholine receptors

Don't be nervous…I'm sure the answer will come to you if you think about it!

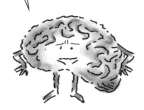

36. 2. Without treatment, glaucoma may progress to irreversible blindness. Treatment won't restore visual damage but will halt disease progression. Miotics, which constrict the pupil, are used in the treatment of glaucoma to permit outflow of the aqueous humor. Central vision loss and blurred or foggy vision (not diplopia) are typical in glaucoma.
CN: Physiological integrity; CNS: Pharmacological therapies; CL: Application

37. 4. The portion of the cerebrum that controls speech and hearing is the temporal lobe. Injury to the frontal lobe causes personality changes, difficulty speaking, and disturbances in memory, reasoning, and concentration. Injury to the parietal lobe causes sensory alterations and problems with spatial relationships. Damage to the occipital lobe causes vision disturbances.
CN: Physiological integrity; CNS: Physiological adaptation; CL: Comprehension

38. 4. Parkinson's disease is characterized by the slowing of voluntary muscle movement, muscular rigidity, and resting tremor. Dopamine is deficient in this disorder. Diminished distal sensation doesn't occur in Parkinson's disease. Bulging eyeballs (exophthalmos) occur in Graves disease.
CN: Physiological integrity; CNS: Physiological adaptation; CL: Application

39. 2. Parkinson's disease is caused by degeneration of the substantia nigra in the basal ganglia of the brain, where dopamine is produced and stored. This results in motor dysfunction. Loss of the myelin sheath around the peripheral nerves describes multiple sclerosis. Myasthenia gravis is an autoimmune disorder that destroys acetylcholine receptors, and bleeding into the brain stem resulting in motor dysfunction describes a hemorrhagic stroke.
CN: Physiological integrity; CNS: Physiological adaptation; CL: Comprehension

CN: Client needs category CNS: Client needs subcategory CL: Cognitive level

40. Which client would be <u>most</u> at risk for secondary Parkinson's disease caused by pharmacotherapy?
1. A 30-year-old client with schizophrenia taking chlorpromazine (Thorazine)
2. A 50-year-old client taking nitroglycerin tablets for angina
3. A 60-year-old client taking prednisone for chronic obstructive pulmonary disease
4. A 75-year-old client using naproxen for rheumatoid arthritis

41. Which symptom occurs <u>initially</u> in Parkinson's disease?
1. Akinesia
2. Aspiration of food
3. Dementia
4. Pill-rolling movements of the hand

42. To evaluate the effectiveness of levodopa-carbidopa, a nurse would watch for which result?
1. Improved visual acuity
2. Increased dyskinesia
3. Reduction in short-term memory
4. Lessened rigidity and tremor

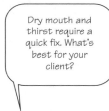

Dry mouth and thirst require a quick fix. What's best for your client?

43. Two days after starting therapy with trihexyphenidyl (Artane), a client complains of a dry mouth. Which nursing intervention would best relieve the client's dry mouth?
1. Offering the client ice chips and frequent sips of water
2. Withholding the drug and notifying the physician
3. Changing the client's diet to clear liquid until the symptoms subside
4. Encouraging the use of supplemental puddings and shakes to maintain weight

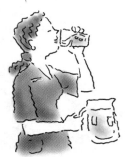

44. Which anti-Parkinson drug can cause drug tolerance or toxicity if taken for too long at one time?
1. Amantadine (Symmetrel)
2. Levodopa-carbidopa (Sinemet)
3. Pergolide (Permax)
4. Selegiline (Eldepryl)

40. 1. Phenothiazines, such as Thorazine, deplete dopamine, which may lead to tremor and rigidity (extrapyramidal effects). The other clients aren't at a greater risk for developing Parkinson's disease.
CN: Physiological integrity; CNS: Pharmacological therapies; CL: Application

41. 4. Early symptoms of Parkinson's disease include coarse resting tremors of the fingers and thumb. Akinesia and aspiration are late signs of Parkinson's disease. Dementia occurs in only 20% of the clients with Parkinson's disease.
CN: Health promotion and maintenance; CNS: None; CL: Application

42. 4. Levodopa-carbidopa increases the amount of dopamine in the central nervous system, allowing for more smooth, purposeful movements. The drug doesn't affect visual acuity and should improve dyskinesia and short-term memory.
CN: Physiological integrity; CNS: Pharmacological therapies; CL: Application

43. 1. Trihexyphenidyl is an anticholinergic agent that causes blurred vision, dry mouth, constipation, and urine retention. There's no need to withhold the drug unless hypotension or tachyarrhythmia occurs. Weight loss may occur with Parkinson's disease; however, the question relates to effects of trihexyphenidyl. A clear liquid diet doesn't provide adequate nutrition and may be more difficult to swallow than thickened liquids if dysphagia is present; it isn't indicated at this time.
CN: Physiological integrity; CNS: Pharmacological therapies; CL: Analysis

44. 2. Long-term therapy with levodopa can result in drug tolerance or toxicity, shown by confusion, hallucinations, or decreased drug effectiveness. The other drugs don't require that the client stop using them for a short period.
CN: Physiological integrity; CNS: Pharmacological therapies; CL: Application

45. Which client would be <u>most likely</u> to develop multiple sclerosis (MS)?
1. A 20-year-old Asian soccer player
2. A 35-year-old White female teacher
3. A 45-year-old type A male smoker
4. A 50-year-old Black female with hypertension

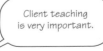

Sometimes your client's age can be a clue.

45. 2. MS is more common in White females ages 20 to 40, with a secondary onset between ages 40 and 60.
CN: Physiological integrity; CNS: Physiological adaptation; CL: Comprehension

46. Which pathophysiologic process is involved in multiple sclerosis (MS)?
1. Destruction of the brain stem and basal ganglia in the brain
2. Degeneration of the nucleus pulposus, causing pressure on the spinal cord
3. Chronic inflammation of rhizomes just outside the central nervous system
4. Development of demyelinization of the myelin sheath, interfering with nerve transmission

46. 4. MS results from chronic progressive demyelination of the myelin sheath, interfering with nerve impulse transmission. The other processes don't describe MS.
CN: Physiological integrity; CNS: Physiological adaptation; CL: Comprehension

47. Which symptom frequently occurs <u>early</u> in multiple sclerosis (MS)?
1. Diplopia
2. Grief
3. Hemiparesis
4. Recent memory loss

47. 1. Early symptoms of MS include slurred speech and diplopia. Paralysis is a late symptom. Although depression and a short attention span may occur, dementia is rarely associated with MS.
CN: Physiological integrity; CNS: Physiological adaptation; CL: Application

48. Which measure would be included in teaching for the client with multiple sclerosis (MS) to avoid <u>exacerbation</u> of the disease?
1. Patch the affected eye.
2. Sleep 8 hours each night.
3. Take hot baths for relaxation.
4. Drink 1,500 to 2,000 ml of fluid daily.

48. 2. MS is exacerbated by exposure to stress, fatigue, and heat. Clients should balance activity with rest. Patching the affected eye may result in improvement in vision and balance but won't prevent exacerbation of the disease. Adequate hydration will help prevent urinary tract infections secondary to a neurogenic bladder.
CN: Physiological integrity; CNS: Reduction of risk potential; CL: Application

49. Which condition or activity may exacerbate multiple sclerosis (MS)?
1. Pregnancy
2. Range-of-motion (ROM) exercises
3. Swimming
4. Urine retention

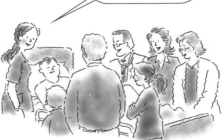

Client teaching is very important.

49. 1. Pregnancy, stress, fatigue, and heat may exacerbate MS. Urine retention is common as a result of neurogenic bladder but doesn't lead to the exacerbation of symptoms. Exercise to maintain ROM is encouraged; swimming is particularly effective because of weightlessness and the cooling of nerves.
CN: Physiological integrity; CNS: Reduction of risk potential; CL: Application

CN: Client needs category   CNS: Client needs subcategory   CL: Cognitive level

50. A client with suspected multiple sclerosis (MS) undergoes a lumbar puncture. Which abnormality is typically found in the cerebrospinal fluid (CSF) of clients with MS?
1. Blood or increased red blood cells
2. Elevated white blood cells (WBCs) or pus
3. Increased glucose concentrations
4. Increased protein levels

51. Which term describes involuntary, jerking, rhythmic movements of the eyes?
1. Diplopia
2. Exophthalmos
3. Nystagmus
4. Oculogyric crisis

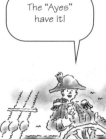

The "Ayes" have it!

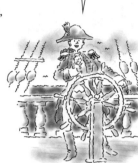

52. Which nursing intervention takes <u>priority</u> for the client having a tonic-clonic seizure?
1. Maintaining a patent airway
2. Timing the duration of the seizure
3. Noting the origin of seizure activity
4. Inserting a padded tongue blade to prevent the client from biting his tongue

53. A client recalls smelling an unpleasant odor before his seizure. Which term describes this?
1. Atonic seizure
2. Aura
3. Icterus
4. Postictal experience

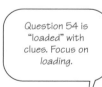

Question 54 is "loaded" with clues. Focus on loading.

54. A client with new-onset seizures of unknown cause is started on phenytoin (Dilantin), 750 mg I.V. now and 100 mg P.O. t.i.d. Which statement best describes the purpose of the <u>loading</u> dose?
1. To ensure that the drug reaches the cerebrospinal fluid
2. To prevent the need for surgical excision of the epileptic focus
3. To reduce secretions in case another seizure occurs
4. To more quickly attain therapeutic levels

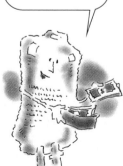

50. 4. Elevated gamma globulin fraction in CSF without an elevated level in the blood occurs in MS. Blood may be found with trauma or subarachnoid hemorrhage. Increased glucose concentration is a nonspecific finding indicating infection or subarachnoid hemorrhage. WBCs or pus indicates infection.
CN: Physiological integrity; CNS: Physiological adaptation; CL: Analysis

51. 3. Nystagmus refers to jerking movements of the eye. Oculogyric crisis involves deviation of the eyes. Exophthalmos refers to bulging eyeballs, seen in Graves disease. Diplopia means double vision.
CN: Health promotion and maintenance; CNS: None; CL: Application

52. 1. The priority during and after a seizure is to maintain a patent airway. Nothing should be placed in the client's mouth during a seizure because teeth may be dislodged or the tongue pushed back, further obstructing the airway. Noting the origin of motor dysfunction and timing the seizure activity are done, but not first.
CN: Physiological integrity; CNS: Reduction of risk potential; CL: Application

53. 2. An aura occurs in some clients as a warning before a seizure. The client may experience a certain smell, a vision such as flashing lights, or a sensation. Postictal experience occurs after a seizure, during which the client may be confused and somnolent or may need to sleep. Atonic seizure or drop attack refers to an abrupt loss of muscle tone. Icterus refers to jaundice.
CN: Physiological integrity; CNS: Physiological adaptation; CL: Application

54. 4. A loading dose of phenytoin and other drugs is given to reach therapeutic levels more quickly; maintenance dosing follows. A loading dose of phenytoin can be oral or parenteral. Surgical excision of an epileptic focus is considered when seizures aren't controlled with anticonvulsant therapy. Phenytoin doesn't reduce secretions.
CN: Physiological integrity; CNS: Pharmacological therapies; CL: Application

55. Which adverse effect may occur during phenytoin (Dilantin) therapy?
1. Dry mouth
2. Furry tongue
3. Somnolence
4. Tachycardia

56. Which symptoms may occur with a phenytoin level of 32 mg/dl?
1. Ataxia and confusion
2. Sodium depletion
3. Tonic-clonic seizure
4. Urinary incontinence

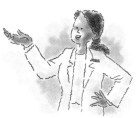

Caution! Can you find the clues here?

57. Which precaution must be taken when giving phenytoin (Dilantin) to a client with a nasogastric (NG) tube for feeding?
1. Check the phenytoin level after giving the drug to check for toxicity.
2. Elevate the head of the bed before giving phenytoin through the NG tube.
3. Give phenytoin 1 hour before or 2 hours after NG tube feedings to ensure absorption.
4. Verify proper placement of the NG tube by placing the end of the tube in a glass of water and observing for bubbles.

58. Why should clients taking phenytoin avoid drinking alcohol?
1. Alcohol increases phenytoin activity.
2. Alcohol raises the seizure threshold.
3. Alcohol impairs judgment and coordination.
4. Alcohol decreases the effectiveness of phenytoin.

Alcohol and phenytoin don't mix!

59. When obtaining vital signs in a client with a seizure disorder, which measure is used?
1. Check for a pulse deficit.
2. Check for pulsus paradoxus.
3. Take an axillary temperature instead of an oral temperature.
4. Check the blood pressure for an auscultatory gap.

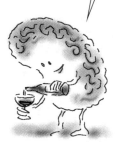

55. 3. Adverse effects of phenytoin include sedation, drowsiness, gingival hyperplasia, blood dyscrasia, and toxicity. The other symptoms aren't adverse effects of phenytoin.
CN: Physiological integrity; CNS: Pharmacological therapies; CL: Application

56. 1. A therapeutic phenytoin level is 10 to 20 mg/dl. A level of 32 mg/dl indicates phenytoin toxicity. Symptoms of toxicity include confusion and ataxia. Phenytoin doesn't cause hyponatremia, seizure, or urinary incontinence. Incontinence may occur during or after a seizure.
CN: Physiological integrity CNS: Pharmacological therapies; CL: Analysis

57. 3. Nutritional supplements and milk interfere with the absorption of phenytoin, decreasing its effectiveness. The nurse verifies NG tube placement by checking for stomach contents before giving drugs and feedings. The head of the bed is elevated when giving all drugs or solutions and isn't specific to phenytoin administration. Phenytoin levels are checked before giving the drug, and the drug is withheld for elevated levels to avoid compounding toxicity.
CN: Physiological integrity; CNS: Pharmacological therapies; CL: Application

58. 4. Although alcohol impairs judgment and coordination, the larger concern is a lowered phenytoin level and lower threshold for seizures.
CN: Physiological integrity; CNS: Pharmacological therapies; CL: Application

59. 3. To reduce the risk of injury, the nurse should take an axillary temperature or use a metal thermometer when taking an oral temperature to prevent injury if a seizure occurs. An auscultatory gap occurs in hypertension. Pulse deficit occurs in an arrhythmia. Pulsus paradoxus may occur with cardiac tamponade.
CN: Physiological integrity; CNS: Reduction of risk potential; CL: Application

CN: Client needs category   CNS: Client needs subcategory   CL: Cognitive level

60. A client in status epilepticus arrives at the emergency department. The family is interviewed to determine the cause of this problem. Which event may have predisposed the client to this condition?
1. Abruptly stopping anticonvulsant therapy
2. Airplane travel
3. Exposure to sunlight
4. Recent upper respiratory infection

61. A client comes to the emergency department after hitting his head in a motor vehicle collision. He's alert and oriented. Which nursing intervention should be done <u>first</u>?
1. Collect data about his full range of motion (ROM) to determine the extent of injuries.
2. Call for an immediate chest X-ray.
3. Immobilize the client's head and neck.
4. Open the airway with the head-tilt chin-lift maneuver.

62. A client with a C6 spinal injury would most likely have which symptom?
1. Aphasia
2. Hemiparesis
3. Paraplegia
4. Tetraplegia

63. A 22-year-old client has a spinal cord transection at the T4 level. The nurse can expect the client to have which symptom?
1. Paraplegia
2. Quadriplegia
3. Autonomic dysreflexia
4. No deficits

The hint hunt is on! See it?

Let's see, what do these spinal cord areas have in common?

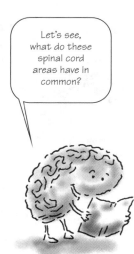

60. 1. Status epilepticus (seizures not responsive to usual therapies) occurs with the abrupt cessation of anticonvulsant drugs or ethanol intake. The other options don't cause status epilepticus.
CN: Physiological integrity; CNS: Physiological adaptation; CL: Analysis

61. 3. All clients with a head injury are treated as if a cervical spine injury is present until X-rays confirm their absence. Determining ROM would be contraindicated at this time. There's no indication the client needs a chest X-ray. The airway doesn't need to be opened because the client appears alert and not in respiratory distress. In addition, the head-tilt chin-lift maneuver wouldn't be used until cervical spine injury is ruled out.
CN: Physiological integrity; CNS: Reduction of risk potential; CL: Application

62. 4. Tetraplegia (quadriplegia) occurs as a result of cervical spine injuries. Paraplegia occurs as a result of injury to the thoracic cord and below. Hemiparesis describes weakness of one side of the body. Aphasia refers to difficulty expressing or understanding spoken words.
CN: Physiological integrity; CNS: Physiological adaptation; CL: Application

63. 1. Spinal cord injuries at the T4 level affect all motor and sensory nerves below the level of injury and result in dysfunction of legs, bowel, and bladder. Paraplegic injuries involve the thoracic, lumbar, or sacral region of the spinal cord. Quadraplegia injuries result from damage to the cervical region of the spine. Autonomic dysreflexia occurs because of a massive sympathetic discharge of stimuli from the autonomic nervous system.
CN: Physiological integrity; CNS: Physiological adaptation; CL: Application

CN: Client needs category CNS: Client needs subcategory CL: Cognitive level

64. A 30-year-old client is admitted to the progressive care unit with a C5 fracture from a motorcycle collision. Which assessment would take priority?
1. Bladder distention
2. Neurologic deficit
3. Pulse oximetry readings
4. The client's feelings about the injury

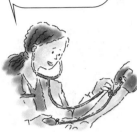

Understanding the significance of vital signs is—well—vital.

65. While in the emergency department, a client with C8 quadriplegia develops a blood pressure of 80/44 mm Hg, pulse of 48 beats/minute, and respiratory rate of 18 breaths/minute. The nurse suspects which condition?
1. Autonomic dysreflexia
2. Hemorrhagic shock
3. Neurogenic shock
4. Pulmonary embolism

66. A client is admitted with a spinal cord injury at the level of T12. He has no movement of his lower extremities. Which medication would be used to control edema of the spinal cord?
1. Acetazolamide (Diamox)
2. Furosemide (Lasix)
3. Methylprednisolone (Solu-Medrol)
4. Sodium bicarbonate

67. A 22-year-old client with quadriplegia is apprehensive and flushed, with a blood pressure of 210/100 mm Hg and heart rate of 50 beats/minute. Which nursing intervention should be done first?
1. Place the client flat in bed.
2. Assess patency of the indwelling urinary catheter.
3. Give one sublingual nitroglycerin tablet.
4. Raise the head of the bed immediately to 90 degrees.

64. 3. After a spinal cord injury, ascending cord edema may cause a higher level of injury. The diaphragm is innervated at the level of C4, so assessment of adequate oxygenation and ventilation through pulse oximetry readings is necessary. Although the other options would be necessary at a later time, observation for respiratory failure is the priority.
CN: Safe, effective care environment; CNS: Coordinated care; CL: Application

65. 3. Symptoms of neurogenic shock include hypotension, bradycardia, and warm, dry skin due to loss of adrenergic stimulation below the level of the lesion. Hypertension, bradycardia, flushing, and sweating of the skin are seen with autonomic dysreflexia. Hemorrhagic shock presents with anxiety, tachycardia, and hypotension; this wouldn't be suspected without an injury. Pulmonary embolism presents with chest pain, hypotension, hypoxemia, tachycardia, and hemoptysis; this may be a later complication of spinal cord injury due to immobility.
CN: Health promotion and maintenance; CNS: None; CL: Analysis

66. 3. High doses of methylprednisolone are used within 24 hours of spinal cord injury to reduce cord swelling and limit neurologic deficits. The other drugs aren't indicated in this circumstance.
CN: Physiological integrity; CNS: Pharmacological therapies; CL: Application

67. 4. Anxiety, flushing above the level of the lesion, piloerection, hypertension, and bradycardia are symptoms of autonomic dysreflexia, typically caused by such noxious stimuli as a full bladder, fecal impaction, or pressure ulcer. Putting the client flat will cause the blood pressure to increase more. Nitroglycerin is given to relieve chest pain and reduce preload; it isn't used for hypertension or dysreflexia. The indwelling urinary catheter should be assessed immediately after the head of the bed is raised.
CN: Physiological integrity; CNS: Physiological adaptation; CL: Analysis

68. A client with paraplegia from a T10 injury is getting ready to transfer to a rehabilitation hospital. When a nurse offers to assist him, the client throws his suitcase on the floor and says, "You don't want to help me." Which response would be the most appropriate for the nurse to give?
1. "You know I want to help you; I offered."
2. "I'll pick these things up for you and come back later."
3. "You seem angry today. How do you feel about your transfer to rehab?"
4. "When you get to rehab, they won't let you behave like a spoiled brat."

69. A client with a cervical spine injury has cervical tongs inserted for which reason?
1. To hasten wound healing
2. To immobilize the surgical spine
3. To prevent autonomic dysreflexia
4. To hold bony fragments of the skull together

70. When a client with a halo vest is discharged from the hospital, which instruction should the nurse give the client and family?
1. Don't use the wheelchair while the halo vest is in place.
2. Clean the pin sites weekly.
3. Keep the wrench that opens the vest attached to the client at all times.
4. Perform range-of-motion (ROM) exercises to the neck and shoulders four times daily.

71. A 20-year-old with structural scoliosis has spinal fusion surgery. Which position would be best during the postoperative period?
1. Supine in bed
2. Side-lying
3. Semi-Fowler's
4. High Fowler's

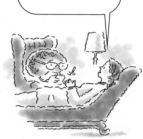

I know I must choose the most therapeutic response.

Teaching involves the whole nursing team.

68. 3. The nurse should always focus on the feelings underlying a particular action. The nurse saying that she offered to help or calling the client a spoiled brat is confrontational. Offering to pick up the client's belongings doesn't deal with the situation and assumes he can't do it alone.
CN: Psychosocial integrity; CNS: None; CL: Application

69. 2. Cervical tongs immobilize the spine until surgical stabilization is accomplished. Tongs don't hasten wound healing, prevent autonomic dysreflexia, or hold bony fragments of the skull together.
CN: Physiological integrity; CNS: Physiological adaptation; CL: Comprehension

70. 3. The wrench must be attached at all times to remove the vest in case the client needs cardiopulmonary resuscitation. The vest is designed to improve mobility; the client may use a wheelchair. The pins are cleaned daily. The purpose of the vest is to immobilize the neck; ROM exercises to the neck are prohibited but should be performed to other areas.
CN: Physiological integrity; CNS: Reduction of risk potential; CL: Application

71. 1. After spinal fusion surgery, the client must remain flat in bed. The latch on a manual bed should be taped and electric beds should be unplugged to prevent the client from raising the head or foot of the bed. Other positions, such as side-lying, semi-Fowler, and high Fowler positions, could prove damaging because the spine must be maintained in a straight position.
CN: Physiological integrity; CNS: Reduction of risk potential; CL: Application

72. Which early intervention describes an appropriate bladder program for a client in rehabilitation for spinal cord injury?
1. Insert an indwelling urinary catheter.
2. Schedule intermittent catheterization every 2 to 4 hours.
3. Perform a straight catheterization every 8 hours while awake.
4. Perform Credé's maneuver to the lower abdomen before the client voids.

73. A 46-year-old client with breast cancer complains of back pain and difficulty moving her legs. Which nursing intervention is <u>most</u> appropriate?
1. Notify the physician.
2. Position the client on her side, and prop her with a foam wedge.
3. Ask the physician for a physical therapy consultation.
4. Give acetaminophen, and reassure the client the pain will resolve soon.

74. A client was admitted to the hospital because of a transient ischemic attack secondary to atrial fibrillation. He would be given which medication to prevent further neurologic deficit?
1. Digoxin (Lanoxin)
2. Diltiazem (Cardizem)
3. Heparin
4. Quinidine gluconate

75. A client is diagnosed with Ménière's disease. Which nursing diagnosis would take priority for this client?
1. *Ineffective tissue perfusion (cerebral)*
2. *Imbalanced nutrition: More than body requirements*
3. *Impaired social interaction*
4. *Risk for injury*

76. Which position would be the most appropriate for a client who has undergone stapedectomy?
1. On the affected side
2. On the unaffected side
3. Prone
4. Sims'

72. 2. Intermittent catheterization should begin every 2 to 4 hours early in treatment. When residual volume is less than 400 ml, the schedule may advance to every 4 to 6 hours. Indwelling catheters may predispose the client to infection and are removed as soon as possible. Credé's maneuver is applied after voiding to enhance bladder emptying.
CN: Physiological integrity; CNS: Basic care and comfort; CL: Application

73. 1. Symptoms of back pain and neurologic deficits may indicate metastasis; therefore, the physician should be notified. Repositioning the client, physical therapy, or acetaminophen may help the pain but may delay evaluation and treatment.
CN: Health promotion and maintenance; CNS: None; CL: Analysis

74. 3. Atrial fibrillation may lead to the formation of mural thrombi, which may embolize to the brain. Heparin will prevent further clot formation and clot enlargement. The other drugs are used in the treatment and control of atrial fibrillation but won't affect clot formation.
CN: Physiological integrity; CNS: Pharmacological therapies; CL: Application

75. 4. Ménière's disease results in dizziness, so the client should be protected from falling. Although hearing loss may occur, causing impaired social interaction, this isn't a priority. Ménière's disease doesn't alter cerebral tissue perfusion or directly affect nutrition.
CN: Safe, effective care environment; CNS: Safety and infection control; CL: Application

76. 2. The client should be positioned with the operative ear up, on the unaffected side. Although Sims' position is a side-lying position, the option doesn't consider which side is best for after-ear surgery.
CN: Physiological integrity; CNS: Basic care and comfort; CL: Application

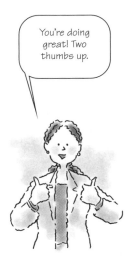

You're doing great! Two thumbs up.

CN: Client needs category   CNS: Client needs subcategory   CL: Cognitive level

77. Which symptom would the nurse expect to find when collecting data from a client with Ménière's disease?
1. Epistaxis
2. Facial pain
3. Ptosis
4. Tinnitus

78. Which nursing intervention has <u>priority</u> for an occupational nurse treating a client with a foreign body protruding from the eye?
1. Irrigating the eye with sterile saline
2. Assessing visual acuity with a Snellen chart
3. Removing the foreign body with sterile forceps
4. Patching both eyes until seen by the ophthalmologist

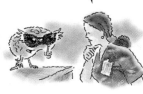

This might give you a clue about the correct response.

79. A client with severe eye pain requests a prescription for the topical anesthetic the ophthalmologist instilled. A nurse explains that these drugs shouldn't be used on an ongoing basis for which reason?
1. They're a way for pathogens to enter the eye.
2. They cause dependence and rebound pain.
3. Damage could occur to the cornea because of lack of sensation.
4. The resulting blurred vision from mydriasis makes activity hazardous.

80. An 86-year-old client admitted to the hospital with chest pain is hard of hearing. Which method should be used when collecting data from this client?
1. Obtain an ear wick.
2. Shout into his better ear.
3. Lower your voice pitch while facing the client.
4. Ask the family to go home and get the client's hearing aid.

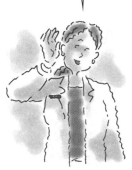

Talk so they can hear ya!

77. 4. Tinnitus, dizziness, and vertigo occur in Ménière's disease. Facial pain may occur with trigeminal neuralgia. Ptosis occurs with a variety of conditions, including myasthenia gravis. Epistaxis may occur with a variety of blood dyscrasias or local lesions.
CN: Physiological integrity; CNS: Physiological adaptation; CL: Application

78. 4. One or both eyes may be patched to prevent pain with extraocular movement or accommodation. Assessment of visual acuity isn't a priority, although it may be done after treatment. Chemicals or small foreign bodies may be irrigated. Protruding objects aren't removed by the nurse because the vitreous body may rupture.
CN: Safe, effective care environment; CNS: Safety and infection control; CL: Application

79. 3. Corneal damage may occur with the prolonged use of topical anesthetics. Dependence and rebound pain don't occur from topical anesthetics. Anesthetics don't cause mydriasis. If the bottle isn't touched to the eye or lashes, the entry of pathogens should be limited.
CN: Physiological integrity; CNS: Reduction of risk potential; CL: Application

80. 3. Hearing loss in the elderly typically involves the upper ranges; lowering the pitch of the voice and facing the client is essential for the client to use other means of understanding, such as lip reading, mood, and so on. Shouting is typically in the upper ranges and could increase anxiety in an already anxious client. An ear wick is used to allow medications to enter the ear canal. Alternate means of communication, such as writing, may also be used to assess chest pain while waiting for the family to bring the hearing aid from home.
CN: Physiological integrity; CNS: Basic care and comfort; CL: Application

81. A client is scheduled for magnetic resonance imaging (MRI) of the head. Which area is essential to assess before the procedure?
1. Food or drink intake within the past 8 hours
2. Metal fillings, prostheses, or a pacemaker
3. The presence of carotid artery disease
4. Voiding before the procedure

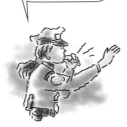

Sorry, you can't proceed any further until we check out a few things.

81. 2. Strong magnetic waves may dislodge metal in the client's body, causing tissue injury. Although the client may be told to restrict food for 8 hours, particularly if contrast is used, metal is an absolute contraindication for this procedure. Voiding beforehand would make the client more comfortable and better able to remain still during the procedure, but it isn't essential for the test. Having carotid artery disease isn't a contraindication to having an MRI.
CN: Safe, effective care environment; CNS: Safety and infection control; CL: Application

82. When giving hydrocortisone, 1 gtt each ear t.i.d., which method would the nurse use?
1. One drop into each ear three times daily
2. One drop into each ear two times daily
3. One mg into each ear three times daily
4. Three drops into the right ear once daily

82. 1. gtt is the abbreviation for drop. tid is the abbreviation for three times per day.
CN: Physiological integrity; CNS: Pharmacological therapies; CL: Comprehension

83. Which is the correct method to properly instill eardrops in a 28-year-old client with otitis externa?
1. Pull the pinna down and back.
2. Pull the pinna up and back.
3. Pull the tragus up and back.
4. Separate the palpebral fissures with a clean gauze pad.

83. 2. To straighten the ear canal of an adult, the pinna is pulled up and back. The palpebral fissures are in the eye. The other options aren't appropriate methods for preparing the ear to receive eardrops.
CN: Physiological integrity; CNS: Pharmacological therapies; CL: Application

84. A female client who has had cataract surgery on her right eye is being discharged. Which discharge instructions should the nurse give the client? Select all that apply.
1. Avoid bending over at the waist.
2. Reduce your sodium intake to reduce intraocular pressure.
3. When you sleep, lie on the same side as your surgery.
4. You can apply eye makeup tomorrow.
5. Call your physician if you have vision loss or see flashing lights.
6. When you sleep, lie on the side opposite to your surgery.

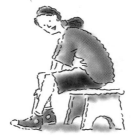

This action is a no-no after cataract surgery—and I don't mean tying my shoes!

84. 1, 5, 6. Bending over may increase intraocular pressure and strain the sutures. Vision loss or seeing flashing lights may signal complications, such as retinal detachment or increased intraocular pressure, and should be reported. Intraocular pressure is reduced when sleeping on the nonsurgical side. Reducing sodium intake doesn't decrease intraocular pressure. Applying eye makeup may introduce infection and cause irritation.
CN: Physiological integrity; CNS: Reduction of risk potential; CL: Application

85. Which symptom of increased intracranial pressure (ICP) after head trauma would appear first?
1. Bradycardia
2. Large amounts of very dilute urine
3. Restlessness and confusion
4. Widened pulse pressure

85. 3. The earliest symptom of increased ICP is a change in mental status. Bradycardia, widened pulse pressure, and bradypnea occur later. The client may void large amounts of very dilute urine if there's damage to the posterior pituitary.
CN: Physiological integrity; CNS: Physiological adaptation; CL: Application

CN: Client needs category   CNS: Client needs subcategory   CL: Cognitive level

86. A client admitted to the emergency department for head trauma is diagnosed with an epidural hematoma. The underlying cause of epidural hematoma is <u>usually</u> related to which condition?
1. Laceration of the middle meningeal artery
2. Rupture of the carotid artery
3. Thromboembolism from a carotid artery
4. Venous bleeding from the arachnoid space

87. A 23-year-old client has been hit on the head with a baseball bat. The nurse notes clear fluid draining from his ears and nose. Which nursing intervention is appropriate?
1. Positioning the client flat in bed
2. Checking the fluid for dextrose with a dipstick
3. Suctioning the nose to maintain airway patency
4. Inserting nasal and ear packing with sterile gauze

88. When observing a client in the emergency department after a head trauma, the nurse knows to monitor the client for a lucid interval. Which statement best describes a lucid interval?
1. An interval when the client's speech is garbled
2. An interval when the client is alert but can't recall recent events
3. An interval when the client is oriented but then becomes somnolent
4. An interval when the client has a "warning" symptom, such as an odor or visual disturbance

89. When teaching the family of a client with C4 quadriplegia how to suction his tracheostomy, the nurse includes which instruction?
1. Suction for 10 to 15 seconds at a time.
2. Regulate the suction machine to 300 cm suction.
3. Apply suction to the catheter during insertion only.
4. Pass the suction catheter into the opening of the tracheostomy tube 2 to 3 cm.

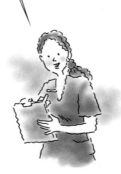

Hint: How do you determine whether the fluid is mucus or cerebral spinal fluid?

86. 1. Epidural hematoma or extradural hematoma is usually caused by laceration of the middle meningeal artery. An embolic stroke is a thromboembolism from a carotid artery that ruptures. Venous bleeding from the arachnoid space is usually observed with subdural hematoma.

CN: Physiological integrity; CNS: Physiological adaptation; CL: Comprehension

87. 2. Clear liquid from the nose (rhinorrhea) or ear (otorrhea) can be determined to be cerebral spinal fluid or mucus by the presence of dextrose. Placing the client flat in bed may increase intracranial pressure and promote pulmonary aspiration. Nothing is inserted into the ears or nose of a client with a skull fracture because of the risk of infection. The nose wouldn't be suctioned because of the risk of suctioning brain tissue through the sinuses.

CN: Physiological integrity; CNS: Physiological adaptation; CL: Analysis

88. 3. A lucid interval is described as a brief period of unconsciousness at the time of the trauma followed by alertness; after several hours, the client deteriorates neurologically. Garbled speech is known as *dysarthria*. An interval in which the client is alert but can't recall recent events is known as *amnesia*. Warning symptoms or auras typically occur before seizures.

CN: Health promotion and maintenance; CNS: None; CL: Comprehension

89. 1. Suction should be applied for 10 to 15 seconds at a time. When suctioning the trachea, the catheter is inserted 4 to 6 inches or until resistance is felt. Suction should be applied only during withdrawal of the catheter. Suction is regulated to 80 to 120 cm.

CN: Physiological integrity; CNS: Reduction of risk potential; CL: Application

CN: Client needs category   CNS: Client needs subcategory   CL: Cognitive level

90. Which condition is a risk factor for hemorrhagic stroke?
1. Coronary artery disease
2. Diabetes
3. Hypertension
4. Recent viral infection

91. An 86-year-old client with a stroke in evolution and a history of coronary artery disease is brought to the medical-surgical floor. His medications include heparin, isosorbide, and verapamil. Which condition should be avoided in a client with a stroke?
1. Dehydration
2. Hypocarbia
3. Hypotension
4. Tube feeding

92. Which client on the rehabilitation unit is most likely to develop autonomic dysreflexia?
1. A client with brain injury
2. A client with herniated nucleus pulposus
3. A client with a high cervical spine injury
4. A client with a stroke

93. Which condition indicates that spinal shock is <u>resolving</u> in a client with C7 quadriplegia?
1. Absence of pain sensation in chest
2. Spasticity
3. Spontaneous respirations
4. Urinary continence

94. When discharging a client from the hospital after a laminectomy, the nurse recognizes that the client needs further teaching when he makes which statement?
1. "I'll sleep on a firm mattress."
2. "I won't drive for 2 to 4 weeks."
3. "When I pick things up, I'll bend my knees."
4. "I can't wait to toss my granddaughter up in the air."

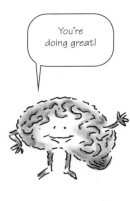

You're doing great!

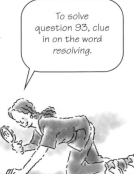

To solve question 93, clue in on the word resolving.

90. 3. Uncontrolled hypertension is the major cause of hemorrhagic stroke. The other options aren't directly linked to this problem.
CN: Physiological integrity; CNS: Reduction of risk potential; CL: Application

91. 3. Isosorbide and verapamil can cause hypotension, which reduces brain perfusion, and should be avoided in a client with a stroke. A hypocarbic state helps reduce intracranial pressure through cerebral vasoconstriction. Nutrition may be delivered by tube when dysphagia exists. Dehydration is unrelated to the client's condition.
CN: Physiological integrity; CNS: Physiological adaptation; CL: Application

92. 3. Autonomic dysreflexia refers to uninhibited sympathetic outflow in clients with spinal cord injuries above the level of T10. The other clients aren't prone to dysreflexia.
CN: Physiological integrity; CNS: Physiological adaptation; CL: Application

93. 2. Spasticity, the return of reflexes, is a sign of resolving shock. Spinal or neurogenic shock is characterized by hypotension, bradycardia, dry skin, flaccid paralysis, or the absence of reflexes below the level of injury. Slight muscle contraction at the bulbocavernosus reflex occurs, but not enough for urinary continence. Spinal shock descends from the injury, and respiratory difficulties occur at C4 and above. The absence of pain sensation in the chest doesn't apply to spinal shock.
CN: Physiological integrity; CNS: Physiological adaptation; CL: Application

94. 4. Lifting more than 10 lb (4.5 kg) for several weeks after surgery is contraindicated. The other responses are appropriate.
CN: Physiological integrity; CNS: Reduction of risk potential; CL: Analysis

CN: Client needs category   CNS: Client needs subcategory   CL: Cognitive level

95. When assessing a client with herniated nucleus pulposus (HNP) of L4-L5, the nurse would expect to find which symptom that's specific to spinal cord compression?

1. Low back pain
2. Pain radiating across the buttocks
3. Positive Kernig's sign
4. Urinary incontinence

96. A nurse assesses a client who has episodes of autonomic dysreflexia. Which condition can cause autonomic dysreflexia?

1. Headache
2. Lumbar spinal cord injury
3. Neurogenic shock
4. Noxious stimuli

97. The nurse is teaching a client and his family about dietary practices related to Parkinson's disease. Which signs and symptoms would be most important for the nurse to address?

1. Fluid overload and drooling
2. Aspiration and anorexia
3. Choking and diarrhea
4. Dysphagia and constipation

98. A client recovering from a spinal cord injury has a great deal of spasticity. Which medication may be used to control spasticity?

1. Hydralazine (Apresoline)
2. Baclofen (Lioresal)
3. Lidocaine (Xylocaine)
4. Methylprednisolone (Medrol)

99. In some clients with multiple sclerosis (MS), plasmapheresis diminishes symptoms. Plasmapheresis achieves this effect by removing which blood component?

1. Catecholamines
2. Antibodies
3. Plasma proteins
4. Lymphocytes

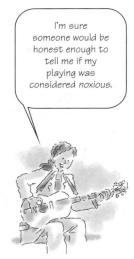

I'm sure someone would be honest enough to tell me if my playing was considered noxious.

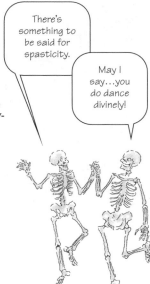

There's something to be said for spasticity.

May I say...you do dance divinely!

95. 4. Progressive neurologic deficits at L4-L5, including worsening muscle weakness, paresthesia, and loss of bowel and bladder control, are symptoms of spinal cord compression. The other symptoms are indicative of HNP.
CN: Physiological integrity; CNS: Reduction of risk potential; CL: Analysis

96. 4. Noxious stimuli, such as a full bladder, fecal impaction, or a pressure ulcer, may cause autonomic dysreflexia. Neurogenic shock isn't a cause of dysreflexia. Autonomic dysreflexia is most commonly seen with injuries at T10 or above. A headache is a symptom, not a cause, of autonomic dysreflexia.
CN: Physiological integrity; CNS: Physiological adaptation; CL: Application

97. 4. The eating problems associated with Parkinson's disease include dysphagia, risk of choking, aspiration, and constipation. Fluid overload, anorexia, and diarrhea aren't problems specifically related to Parkinson's disease.
CN: Physiological integrity; CNS: Reduction of risk potential; CL: Analysis

98. 2. Baclofen is a skeletal muscle relaxant used to decrease spasms. Methylprednisolone, an anti-inflammatory drug, is used to decrease spinal cord edema. Hydralazine is an antihypertensive and afterload reducing agent. Lidocaine is an antiarrhythmic and a local anesthetic agent.
CN: Physiological integrity; CNS: Pharmacological therapies; CL: Application

99. 2. In plasmapheresis, antibodies are removed from the client's plasma. Antibodies attack the myelin sheath of the neuron, causing the manifestations of MS. The treatment of MS with plasmapheresis isn't for the purpose of removing catecholamines, plasma proteins, or lymphocytes.
CN: Physiological integrity; CNS: Physiological adaptation; CL: Comprehension

CN: Client needs category   CNS: Client needs subcategory   CL: Cognitive level

100. A client with a T1 spinal cord injury arrives at the emergency department with a blood pressure of 82/40 mm Hg, pulse rate of 34 beats/minute, dry skin, and flaccid paralysis of the lower extremities. Which condition would most likely be suspected?
1. Autonomic dysreflexia
2. Hypertension
3. Neurogenic shock
4. Sepsis

101. A client has a cervical spinal cord injury at the level of C5. Which condition would the nurse anticipate during the <u>acute</u> phase?
1. Absent corneal reflex
2. Decerebrate posturing
3. Movement of only the right or left half of the body
4. The need for mechanical ventilation

102. When caring for a client with quadriplegia, which nursing intervention takes priority?
1. Forcing fluids to prevent renal calculi
2. Maintaining skin integrity
3. Obtaining adaptive devices for more independence
4. Preventing atelectasis

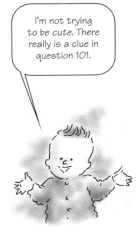

I'm not trying to be cute. There really is a clue in question 101.

103. A client with C7 quadriplegia is flushed and anxious and complains of a pounding headache. Which symptom would also be anticipated?
1. Decreased urine output or oliguria
2. Hypertension and bradycardia
3. Respiratory depression
4. Symptoms of shock

104. A client has a diagnosis of stroke versus transient ischemic attack (TIA). Which statement shows the difference between a TIA and a stroke?
1. TIAs typically resolve in 24 hours.
2. TIAs may be hemorrhagic in origin.
3. TIAs may cause a permanent motor deficit.
4. TIAs may predispose the client to a myocardial infarction (MI).

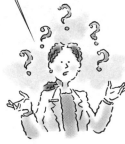

TIA or stroke? Make sure you know the difference in symptoms.

100. 3. Loss of sympathetic control and unopposed vagal stimulation below the level of the injury typically cause hypotension, bradycardia, pallor, flaccid paralysis, and warm, dry skin in the client in neurogenic shock. Autonomic dysreflexia occurs after neurogenic shock abates. Signs of sepsis would include elevated temperature, increased heart rate, and increased respiratory rate.
CN: Physiological integrity; CNS: Physiological adaptation; CL: Analysis

101. 4. The diaphragm is stimulated by nerves at the level of C4. Initially, this client may need mechanical ventilation because of cord edema. This may resolve in time. Decerebrate posturing, hemiplegia, and absent corneal reflexes occur with brain injuries, not spinal cord injuries.
CN: Physiological integrity; CNS: Physiological adaptation; CL: Application

102. 4. Clients with quadriplegia have paralysis or weakness of the diaphragm, abdominal, or intercostal muscles. Maintenance of airway and breathing take top priority. Although forcing fluids, maintaining skin integrity, and obtaining adaptive devices for more independence are all important interventions, preventing atelectasis has more priority.
CN: Physiological integrity; CNS: Reduction of risk potential; CL: Application

103. 2. Hypertension, bradycardia, anxiety, blurred vision, and flushing above the lesion occur with autonomic dysreflexia due to uninhibited sympathetic nervous system discharge. The other options are incorrect.
CN: Physiological integrity; CNS: Physiological adaptation; CL: Analysis

104. 1. Symptoms of TIA result from a transient lack of oxygen to the brain and usually resolve within 24 hours. Hemorrhage into the brain has the worst neurologic outcome and isn't associated with a TIA. Permanent motor deficits don't result from TIA. Unstable angina, not a TIA, may predispose the client to a future MI.
CN: Physiological integrity; CNS: Physiological adaptation; CL: Comprehension

CN: Client needs category   CNS: Client needs subcategory   CL: Cognitive level

105. A client with a right stroke has a flaccid left side. Which intervention would best prevent shoulder subluxation?
1. Splinting the wrist
2. Using an air splint
3. Putting the affected arm in a sling
4. Performing range-of-motion exercises on the affected side

105. 3. Because of the weight of the flaccid extremity, the shoulder may disarticulate. A sling will support the extremity. The other options won't support the shoulder.
CN: Physiological integrity; CNS: Basic care and comfort; CL: Application

106. A 40-year-old paraplegic must perform intermittent catheterization of the bladder. Which instruction should be given?
1. Clean the meatus from back to front.
2. Measure the quantity of urine.
3. Gently rotate the catheter during removal.
4. Clean the meatus with soap and water.

106. 4. Intermittent catheterization may be performed chronically with clean technique, using soap and water to clean the urinary meatus. The meatus is always cleaned from front to back in a woman, or in expanding circles working outward from the meatus in a man. The catheter doesn't need to be rotated during removal. It isn't necessary to measure the urine.
CN: Physiological integrity; CNS: Basic care and comfort; CL: Application

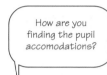

How are you finding the pupil accomodations?

107. Which method should be used to assess pupil accommodation?
1. Assess for peripheral vision.
2. Touch the cornea lightly with a wisp of cotton.
3. Have the client follow an object upward, downward, obliquely, and horizontally.
4. Observe for pupil constriction and convergence while focusing on an object coming toward the client.

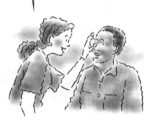

107. 4. Accommodation refers to convergence and constriction of the pupil while focusing on a nearing object. Touching the cornea lightly with a wisp of cotton describes assessment of the corneal reflex. Having the client follow an object upward, downward, obliquely, and horizontally refers to cardinal fields of gaze. Assessing for peripheral vision refers to visual fields.
CN: Physiological integrity; CNS: Physiological adaptation; CL: Application

108. A client at the eye clinic reports difficulty seeing at night. This may result from which nutritional deficiency?
1. Vitamin A
2. Vitamin B₆
3. Vitamin C
4. Vitamin K

108. 1. Night blindness (nyctalopia) may be caused from a vitamin A deficiency or dysfunctional rod receptors. None of the other deficiencies leads to nyctalopia.
CN: Physiological integrity; CNS: Physiological adaptation; CL: Application

See if you can determine which one of us is deficient.

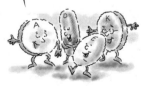

109. A client with a spinal cord injury has a neurogenic bladder. When planning for discharge, the nurse anticipates that the client will need which procedure or program?
1. Intermittent catheterization program
2. Kock pouch
3. Transurethral prostatectomy
4. Ureterostomy

109. 1. Intermittent catheterization, starting with 2-hour intervals and increasing to 4- to 6-hour intervals, is used to manage neurogenic bladder. A Kock pouch is a continent ileostomy. An ileostomy or ureterostomy isn't necessary. Transurethral prostatectomy is indicated for obstruction to urinary outflow by benign prostatic hyperplasia or for the treatment of cancer.
CN: Physiological integrity; CNS: Basic care and comfort; CL: Application

110. When using a Snellen alphabet chart, the nurse records the client's vision as 20/40. Which statement best describes 20/40 vision?
1. The client has alterations in near vision and is legally blind.
2. The client can see at 20 feet what the person with normal vision sees at 40 feet.
3. The client can see at 40 feet what the person with normal vision sees at 20 feet.
4. The client has a 20% decrease in acuity in one eye and a 40% decrease in the other eye.

111. Which instrument is used to record intraocular pressure?
1. Goniometer
2. Ophthalmoscope
3. Slit lamp
4. Tonometer

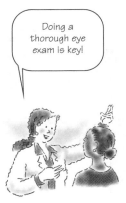

Doing a thorough eye exam is key!

112. After a nurse instills atropine drops into both eyes for a client undergoing an ophthalmic examination, which instruction would be given to the client?
1. Be careful because the blink reflex is paralyzed.
2. Avoid wearing your regular glasses when driving.
3. Be aware that the pupils may be unusually small.
4. Wear dark glasses in bright light because the pupils are dilated.

113. Which procedure or assessment must the nurse perform when preparing a client for eye surgery?
1. Clip the client's eyelashes.
2. Verify the affected eye has been patched for 24 hours before surgery.
3. Verify the client has had nothing by mouth since midnight or at least 8 hours before surgery.
4. Obtain informed consent with the client's signature, and place the forms in the chart.

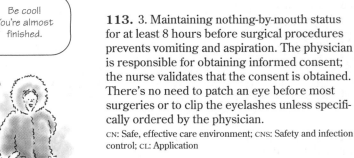

Be cool! You're almost finished.

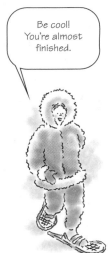

110. 2. The numerator refers to the client's vision while comparing the normal vision in the denominator. Legal blindness refers to 20/150 or less. Alterations in near vision may be due to loss of accommodation caused by the aging process (presbyopia) or farsightedness.
CN: Physiological integrity; CNS: Physiological adaptation; CL: Analysis

111. 4. A tonometer is a device used in glaucoma screening to record intraocular pressure. A goniometer measures joint movement and angles. An ophthalmoscope examines the interior of the eye, especially the retina. A slit lamp evaluates structures in the anterior chamber of the eye.
CN: Physiological integrity; CNS: Reduction of risk potential; CL: Comprehension

112. 4. Atropine, an anticholinergic drug, has mydriatic effects causing pupil dilation. This allows more light onto the retina and causes photophobia and blurred vision. Atropine doesn't paralyze the blink reflex or cause miosis (pupil constriction). Driving may be contraindicated because of blurred vision.
CN: Physiological integrity; CNS: Reduction of risk potential; CL: Application

113. 3. Maintaining nothing-by-mouth status for at least 8 hours before surgical procedures prevents vomiting and aspiration. The physician is responsible for obtaining informed consent; the nurse validates that the consent is obtained. There's no need to patch an eye before most surgeries or to clip the eyelashes unless specifically ordered by the physician.
CN: Safe, effective care environment; CNS: Safety and infection control; CL: Application

CN: Client needs category   CNS: Client needs subcategory   CL: Cognitive level

114. Which statement indicates that a client needs additional teaching after cataract surgery?

 1. "I'll avoid eating until the nausea subsides."
 2. "I can't wait to pick up my granddaughter."
 3. "I'll avoid bending over to tie my shoelaces."
 4. "I'll avoid touching the dropper to my eye when using my eyedrops."

115. Cataract surgery results in aphakia. Which statement best describes this term?

 1. Absence of the crystalline lens
 2. A "keyhole" pupil
 3. Loss of accommodation
 4. Retinal detachment

116. When developing a teaching session on glaucoma for the community, which statement would the nurse stress?

 1. Glaucoma is easily corrected with eyeglasses.
 2. White and Asian individuals are at the highest risk for glaucoma.
 3. Yearly screening for people ages 20 to 40 is recommended.
 4. Glaucoma can be painless, and vision may be lost before the person is aware of a problem.

117. For a client having an episode of acute narrow-angle glaucoma, the nurse expects to give which medication?

 1. Acetazolamide (Diamox)
 2. Atropine
 3. Furosemide (Lasix)
 4. Streptokinase (Streptase)

118. Which symptom would occur in a client with a detached retina?

 1. Flashing lights and floaters
 2. Homonymous hemianopia
 3. Loss of central vision
 4. Ptosis

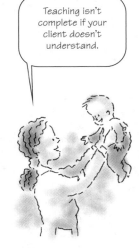

Teaching isn't complete if your client doesn't understand.

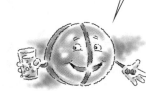

Knowing who I am should take away some of the pressure.

114. 2. Lifting, often involving the Valsalva maneuver, increases intraocular pressure and strain on the surgical site. Preventing nausea and subsequent vomiting will prevent increased intraocular pressure, as will avoiding bending or placing the head in a dependent position. Touching the eye dropper to the eye will contaminate the dropper and thus the entire bottle of medication.
CN: Physiological integrity; CNS: Reduction of risk potential; CL: Analysis

115. 1. Aphakia means "without lens." A keyhole pupil results from iridectomy. Loss of accommodation is a normal response to aging. A retinal detachment is usually associated with retinal holes created by vitreous traction.
CN: Physiological integrity; CNS: Physiological adaptation; CL: Comprehension

116. 4. Open-angle glaucoma causes a painless increase in intraocular pressure with loss of peripheral vision. Individuals older than age 40 should be screened. Blacks have a threefold greater chance of developing glaucoma with an increased chance of blindness than other groups. A variety of miotics and agents to decrease intraocular pressure and occasionally surgery are used to treat glaucoma.
CN: Health promotion and maintenance; CNS: None; CL: Application

117. 1. Acetazolamide, a carbonic anhydrase inhibitor, decreases intraocular pressure by decreasing the secretion of aqueous humor. Streptokinase is a thrombolytic agent, and furosemide is a loop diuretic; these aren't used in the treatment of glaucoma. Atropine dilates the pupil and decreases outflow of aqueous humor, causing a further increase in intraocular pressure.
CN: Physiological integrity; CNS: Pharmacological therapies; CL: Application

118. 1. Signs and symptoms of retinal detachment include abrupt flashing lights, floaters, loss of peripheral vision, or a sudden shadow or curtain in the vision. Occasionally, vision loss is gradual.
CN: Physiological integrity; CNS: Physiological adaptation; CL: Application

CN: Client needs category   CNS: Client needs subcategory   CL: Cognitive level

119. A client underwent an enucleation of the right eye for a malignancy. Which intervention will the nurse perform?
1. Instill miotics, as ordered, to the affected eye.
2. Teach the client to clean the prosthesis in soap and water.
3. Assess reactivity of the pupils to light and accommodation.
4. Teach the client to avoid straining at stool to prevent intraocular pressure.

120. A nurse would question an order to irrigate the ear canal in which circumstance?
1. Ear pain
2. Hearing loss
3. Otitis externa
4. Perforated tympanic membrane

121. Which intervention is essential when instilling Cortisporin suspension, 2 gtt in the right ear?
1. Verify the proper client and route.
2. Warm the solution to prevent dizziness.
3. Hold an emesis basin under the client's ear.
4. Place the client in the semi-Fowler's position.

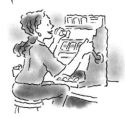

Giving drugs isn't a game of chance. Know the right way to do it.

122. When teaching the client with Ménière's disease, which instruction would a nurse give about vertigo?
1. Report dizziness at once.
2. Drive in daylight hours only.
3. Get up slowly, turning the entire body.
4. Change your position using the logroll technique.

123. Which response by a client <u>best</u> indicates an understanding of the adverse effects of phenytoin (Dilantin)?
1. "I should take the medication with food to prevent nausea."
2. "I need to take this medication until my seizures stop."
3. "I need to see the dentist every 6 months."
4. "I need to report any drowsiness to the physician immediately."

119. 2. Enucleation of the eye refers to surgical removal of the entire eye; therefore, the client needs instructions about the prosthesis. There are no activity restrictions or need for eyedrops; however, prophylactic antibiotics may be used in the immediate postoperative period.
CN: Physiological integrity; CNS: Physiological adaptation; CL: Application

120. 4. Irrigation of the ear canal is contraindicated with perforation of the tympanic membrane because solution entering the inner ear may cause dizziness, nausea, vomiting, and infection. The other conditions aren't contraindications to irrigation of the ear canal.
CN: Physiological integrity; CNS: Reduction of risk potential; CL: Application

121. 1. When giving medications, a nurse follows the five "R's" of medication administration: right client, right drug, right dose, right route, and right time. Put the client in the lateral position, not semi-Fowler's position, for 5 minutes to prevent the drops from draining out. The drops may be warmed to prevent pain or dizziness, but this action isn't essential. An emesis basin would be used for irrigation of the ear.
CN: Physiological integrity; CNS: Pharmacological therapies; CL: Application

122. 3. Turning the entire body, not the head, will prevent vertigo. Turning the client in bed slowly and smoothly will be helpful; logrolling isn't needed. The client shouldn't drive because he may reflexively turn the wheel to correct for vertigo. Dizziness is expected with Ménière's disease but can be prevented.
CN: Physiological integrity; CNS: Reduction of risk potential; CL: Application

123. 3. Phenytoin can cause hypertrophy of the gums and gingivitis; therefore, regular dental checkups are essential. Phenytoin doesn't need to be taken with food and should never be discontinued unless ordered by a physician. Some drowsiness is expected initially; however, this usually decreases with continued use.
CN: Physiological therapy; CNS: Pharmacological therapies; CL: Analysis

CN: Client needs category   CNS: Client needs subcategory   CL: Cognitive level

124. An 18-year-old client was hit in the head with a baseball during practice. When discharging him to the care of his mother, the nurse gives which instruction?
1. Watch him for keyhole pupil for the next 24 hours.
2. Expect profuse vomiting for 24 hours after the injury.
3. Wake him every hour, and assess orientation to person, time, and place.
4. Notify the physician immediately if he has a headache.

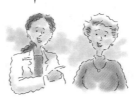

Instruct the client's mother about the care for her son's injury.

125. A client taking carbamazepine (Tegretol) should be monitored for which potential complication?
1. Acute respiratory distress syndrome (ARDS)
2. Diplopia
3. Elevated levels of phenytoin (Dilantin)
4. Leukocytosis

126. When assessing the pupil's ability to constrict, which cranial nerve (CN) is being tested?
1. II
2. III
3. IV
4. V

127. Nursing care of a client with damage to the thalamus, hypothalamus, and pineal gland would be based on knowing the client has problems in which area?
1. Seizure control
2. Identifying foreign agents
3. Difficulty regulating emotions
4. Initiating movements and maintaining temperature control and the sleep-awake cycle

Different areas of the brain (Hey, that's me!) regulate different functions.

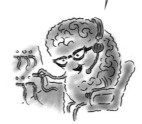

124. 3. Changes in level of consciousness (LOC) may indicate expanding lesions such as subdural hematoma; orientation and LOC are assessed frequently for 24 hours. Profuse or projectile vomiting is a symptom of increased intracranial pressure and should be reported immediately. A slight headache may last for several days after concussion; severe or worsening headaches should be reported. A keyhole pupil is found after iridectomy.
CN: Physiological integrity; CNS: Physiological adaptation; CL: Application

125. 2. Carbamazepine is more likely to cause diplopia, dizziness, ataxia, and a rash. Carbamazepine causes agranulocytosis because of the reduction in leukocytes. ARDS isn't a complication of carbamazepine. Carbamazepine decreases blood levels of phenytoin and oral contraceptives.
CN: Physiological integrity; CNS: Pharmacological therapies; CL: Comprehension

126. 2. CN III, the oculomotor nerve, controls pupil constriction. CN II is the optic nerve, which controls vision. CN IV is the trochlear nerve, which coordinates eye movement. CN V is the trigeminal nerve, which innervates the muscles of chewing.
CN: Physiological integrity; CNS: Physiological adaptation; CL: Application

127. 4. The thalamus is the relay center of communication of sensory and motor information between the higher and lower regions of the brain. The hypothalamus regulates temperature control, and the pineal gland is important to the sleep-awake cycle. Seizure control is more related to neurotransmitter dysfunction. Identifying foreign agents is a function of the immune system. Regulating emotions is a function of the limbic system.
CN: Physiological integrity; CNS: Physiological adaptation; CL: Knowledge

128. Problems with memory and learning would relate to which lobe?
1. Frontal
2. Occipital
3. Parietal
4. Temporal

129. While cooking, your client couldn't feel the temperature of a hot oven. Which lobe could be dysfunctional?
1. Frontal
2. Occipital
3. Parietal
4. Temporal

130. Which neurotransmitter is responsible for many of the functions of the frontal lobe?
1. Dopamine
2. Gamma-aminobutyric acid (GABA)
3. Histamine
4. Norepinephrine

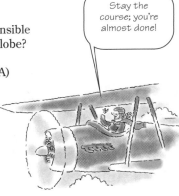

Stay the course; you're almost done!

131. The nurse is discussing the purpose of an EEG with the family of a client with massive cerebral hemorrhage and loss of consciousness. It would be most accurate for the nurse to tell family members that the test measures which of the following?
1. Extent of intracranial bleeding
2. Sites of brain injury
3. Activity of the brain
4. Percent of functional brain tissue

132. The nurse is observing a client with cerebral edema for evidence of increasing intracranial pressure. She monitors his blood pressure for signs of widening pulse pressure. His current blood pressure is 170/80 mm Hg. What's the client's pulse pressure?

128. 4. The temporal lobe functions to regulate memory and learning problems because of the integration of the hippocampus. The parietal lobe primarily functions with sensory function. The occipital lobe functions to regulate vision. The frontal lobe primarily functions to regulate thinking, planning, and judgment.
CN: Physiological integrity; CNS: Physiological adaptation; CL: Knowledge

129. 3. The parietal lobe regulates sensory function, which would include the ability to sense hot or cold objects. The occipital lobe is primarily responsible for vision function. The temporal lobe regulates memory, and the frontal lobe regulates thinking, planning, and judgment.
CN: Safe, effective care environment; CNS: Safety and infection control; CL: Knowledge

130. 1. The frontal lobe primarily functions to regulate thinking, planning, and affect. Dopamine is known to circulate widely throughout this lobe, which is why it's such an important neurotransmitter in schizophrenia. GABA is widely circulated in the hippocampus and hypothalamus. Histamine is primarily found in the hypothalamus. Norepinephrine primarily functions with the hippocampal region not located in the frontal lobe.
CN: Physiological integrity; CNS: Physiological adaptation; CL: Knowledge

131. 3. An EEG measures the electrical activity of the brain. Extent of intracranial bleeding and location of the injury site would be determined by computerized tomography or magnetic resonance imaging. Percent of functional brain tissue would be determined by a series of tests.
CN: Physiological integrity; CNS: Physiological adaptation; CL: Comprehension

132. 90. Pulse pressure is the difference between the systolic blood pressure and the diastolic blood pressure. For this client, pulse pressure = 170 − 80 = 90.
CN: Physiological integrity; CNS: Reduction of risk potential; CL: Application

133. The nurse is caring for a client with multiple sclerosis (MS). Which problems should the nurse expect the client to experience? Select all that apply:
  1. Vision disturbances
  2. Coagulation abnormalities
  3. Balance problems
  4. Immunity compromise
  5. Mood disorders

134. The nurse is teaching a client with trigeminal neuralgia how to minimize pain episodes. Which comments by the client indicate that he understands the instructions? Select all that apply:
  1. "I'll eat food that's very hot."
  2. "I'll try to chew my food on the unaffected side."
  3. "I can wash my face with cold water."
  4. "Drinking fluids at room temperature should reduce pain."
  5. "If tooth brushing is too painful, I'll try to rinse my mouth instead."

135. A client is experiencing problems with balance and fine gross motor function. Identify the area of the client's brain that's malfunctioning.

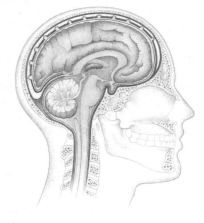

133. 1, 3, 5. MS, a neuromuscular disorder, may cause vision disturbances, balance problems, and mood disorders. MS doesn't cause coagulation abnormalities or immunity problems.
CN: Physiological integrity; CNS: Reduction of risk potential; CL: Application

134. 2, 4, 5. The facial pain of trigeminal neuralgia is triggered by mechanical or thermal stimuli. Chewing food on the unaffected side and rinsing the mouth rather than brushing teeth reduce mechanical stimulation. Drinking fluids at room temperature reduces thermal stimulation. Eating hot food and washing the face with cold water are likely to trigger pain.
CN: Health promotion and maintenance; CNS: None; CL: Comprehension

135.

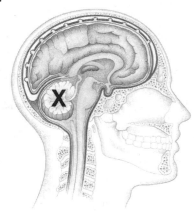

The cerebellum is the portion of the brain that controls balance and fine and gross motor function.
CN: Physiological integrity; CNS: Reduction of risk potential; CL: Comprehension

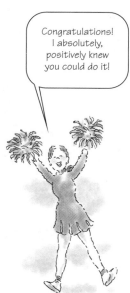

Congratulations! I absolutely, positively knew you could do it!

CN: Client needs category   CNS: Client needs subcategory   CL: Cognitive level

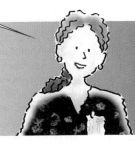

Here's a test that covers nursing care for clients with a disorder of the musculoskeletal system. So get moving and break a leg. Oh—I mean good luck!

Chapter 7
Musculoskeletal disorders

1. Osteoblast activity is needed for which function?

1. Bone formation
2. Estrogen production
3. Hematopoiesis
4. Muscle formation

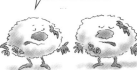

Your hint here is in the Latin root of the word osteoblast.

1. 1. Osteoblast activity is necessary for bone formation. Osteoblasts are bone-forming cells; they don't have a role in muscle formation. Estrogen is linked to calcium reuptake and building of bone tissue. Hematopoiesis is the production of red blood cells in the bone marrow.

CN: Physiological integrity; CNS: Physiological adaptation; CL: Knowledge

2. A 70-year-old female client complains of pain in her lower back. She has a markedly aged appearance and says she doesn't eat well. She's diagnosed with osteoporosis. The nurse teaches the client about injury prevention because she's concerned about preventing which condition that's the primary complication of osteoporosis?

1. Pain
2. Fractures
3. Hardening of the bones
4. Increased bone matrix and remineralization

2. 2. The primary complication of osteoporosis is fractures. Bones soften, and there's a decrease in bone matrix and remineralization. Pain may occur, but fractures can be life-threatening.

CN: Physiological integrity; CNS: Physiological adaptation; CL: Application

3. Which condition is the cause of <u>primary</u> osteoporosis?

1. Alcoholism
2. Hormonal imbalance
3. Malnutrition
4. Osteogenesis imperfecta

3. 2. Hormonal imbalance, faulty metabolism, and poor dietary intake of calcium cause primary osteoporosis. Malnutrition, alcoholism, osteogenesis imperfecta, rheumatoid arthritis, liver disease, scurvy, lactose intolerance, hyperthyroidism, and trauma cause secondary osteoporosis.

CN: Physiological integrity; CNS: Physiological adaptation; CL: Knowledge

4. A 42-year-old client recently had a total hysterectomy. Which response by the client indicates that teaching has been effective?

1. "My risk for osteoporosis is low because I still have my thyroid gland."
2. "Osteoporosis affects only women over 65 years old."
3. "I'm still producing hormones, so I don't have to worry about osteoporosis."
4. "I need to take precautions to protect myself from osteoporosis because I've had surgically induced menopause."

Is this woman at risk for osteoporosis?

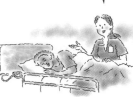

4. 4. Menopause at any age puts women at risk for osteoporosis because of the associated hormonal imbalance. This client's thyroid gland won't protect her from menopause. With her ovaries removed, she's no longer producing the necessary hormones.

CN: Physiological integrity; CNS: Physiological adaptation; CL: Analysis

CN: Client needs category   CNS: Client needs subcategory   CL: Cognitive level

5. Primary prevention of osteoporosis includes which measure?
1. Placing items within reach of the client
2. Installing bars in the bathroom to prevent falls
3. Maintaining optimal calcium and vitamin D intake
4. Using a professional alert system in the home in case a fall occurs when the client is alone

In question 5, primary refers to a level of prevention.

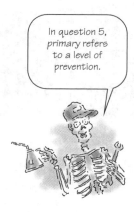

5. 3. Primary prevention of osteoporosis includes maintaining optimal calcium and vitamin D intake. Using a professional alert system in the home, installing bars in bathrooms to prevent falls, and placing items within reach of the client are all secondary and tertiary prevention methods.
CN: Health promotion and maintenance; CNS: None; CL: Application

6. A client asks the nurse why she has applied a cold pack to a sprained ankle. Which response by the nurse would be most appropriate?
1. "It decreases pain and increases circulation."
2. "It numbs the nerves and dilates the blood vessels."
3. "It promotes circulation and reduces muscle spasm."
4. "It constricts local blood vessels and decreases swelling."

6. 4. Application of a cold pack causes the blood vessels to constrict, which reduces the leakage of fluid into the tissues and prevents swelling. It may have an effect on muscle spasms. Cold therapy may reduce pain by numbing the nerves and tissues. Cold therapy doesn't promote circulation or dilate the blood vessels.
CN: Physiological integrity; CNS: Basic care and comfort; CL: Application

7. A client complains of joint pain in his great toe. He states that the joint becomes inflamed and painful but then subsides and recurs at irregular intervals. Which mechanism is believed to cause this?
1. Overproduction of calcium
2. Underproduction of calcium
3. Overproduction of uric acid
4. Underproduction of uric acid

7. 3. This patient is experiencing classic symptoms of gout. Although the exact cause of primary gout remains unknown, it seems linked to a genetic defect in purine metabolism that causes overproduction of uric acid, retention of uric acid, or both. Gout isn't related to calcium production.
CN: Physiological integrity; CNS: Physiological adaptation; CL: Analysis

Dietary restrictions can be an important component of disease management.

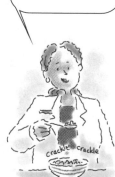

8. A 52-year-old client complains of severe pain in his left great toe. He states that the pain lasts from 1 to 2 weeks and then improves. He has had these symptoms intermittently for the last several years and is pain-free between the attacks. The nurse recognizes that the symptoms described by the client are associated with which disorder?
1. Chronic gout
2. Acute gout
3. Osteoporosis
4. Rheumatoid arthritis

8. 2. The usual pattern of acute gout involves painful episodes with pain-free periods. Chronic gout is marked by frequent painful periods with persistently painful joints. Osteoporosis causes thinning bones and leads to fractures. Rheumatoid arthritis is a systemic disease that affects joints symmetrically.
CN: Physiological integrity; CNS: Physiological adaptation; CL: Application

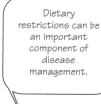

CN: Client needs category   CNS: Client needs subcategory   CL: Cognitive level

9. A client has been prescribed a diet that limits purine-rich foods. Which food would the nurse teach her to avoid eating?

1. Bananas and dried fruits
2. Milk, ice cream, and yogurt
3. Wine, cheese, preserved fruits, meats, and vegetables
4. Anchovies, sardines, kidneys, sweetbreads, and lentils

10. A 61-year-old male client has had gout for a long time and has developed nodules. While teaching the client, the nurse explains that these nodules are referred to by which term?

1. Cysts
2. Stones
3. Tophi
4. Calculi

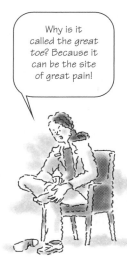

Why is it called the great toe? Because it can be the site of great pain!

11. The nurse is collecting a health history from a 63-year-old man who may have gout. What joint is most commonly affected in the client with gout?

1. Great toe
2. Wrist
3. Ankle
4. Knee

12. A client who has been recently diagnosed with gout asks the nurse to explain why he needs to take colchicine. The nurse plans her response based on the understanding that colchicine:

1. increases estrogen levels in the bloodstream.
2. decreases the risk of infection.
3. decreases inflammation.
4. decreases bone demineralization.

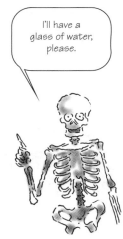

I'll have a glass of water, please.

13. Which statement by a client diagnosed with gout indicates that he understands his discharge instructions?

1. "I'll increase my fluids so that the inflammation will be reduced."
2. "Increasing fluid intake will increase the calcium my body absorbs."
3. "Increasing fluid intake will cause my body to excrete more uric acid."
4. "Increasing fluids will help provide a cushion for my bones."

9. 4. Anchovies, sardines, kidneys, sweetbreads, and lentils are high in purines. Bananas and dried fruits are high in potassium. Milk, ice cream, and yogurt are rich in calcium. Wine, cheese, preserved fruits, meats, and vegetables contain tyramine.

CN: Health promotion and maintenance; CNS: None; CL: Application

10. 3. Tophi are nodular deposits of sodium urate crystals. They can occur as a result of chronic gout. A cyst is a closed sac or pouch with a definite wall that contains fluid, semifluid, or solid material. Stones are abnormal concretions usually composed of mineral salts. Calculi is another name for stones formed by mineral salts.

CN: Physiological integrity; CNS: Reduction of risk potential; CL: Comprehension

11. 1. The great toe is most commonly affected in clients with gout. Gout can affect any joint but most commonly affects the great toe.

CN: Physiological integrity; CNS: Reduction of risk potential; CL: Knowledge

12. 3. The action of colchicine is to decrease inflammation by reducing the migration of leukocytes to synovial fluid. Colchicine doesn't decrease the risk of infection, increase estrogen levels, or decrease bone demineralization.

CN: Physiological integrity; CNS: Pharmacological therapies; CL: Application

13. 3. Fluids promote the excretion of uric acid. Fluids don't decrease inflammation, increase calcium absorption, or provide a cushion for bones.

CN: Physiological integrity; CNS: Physiological adaptation; CL: Application

CN: Client needs category   CNS: Client needs subcategory   CL: Cognitive level

14. The physician has ordered tests for a client to diagnose a suspected case of gout. The nurse should expect to see which result?
1. Presence of urate crystals in the synovial fluid of the affected area
2. Presence of urate crystals in the bloodstream
3. Elevated blood calcium levels
4. Decreased red blood cell (RBC) count

15. A client with gout is receiving indomethacin (Indocin) for pain. Which instruction should the nurse give to a client taking nonsteroidal antiinflammatory drugs (NSAIDs)?
1. Bleeding isn't a problem with NSAIDs.
2. Take NSAIDs with food to avoid an upset stomach.
3. Take NSAIDs on an empty stomach to increase absorption.
4. Don't take NSAIDs at bedtime because they may cause excitement.

16. A client asks for information about osteoarthritis. Which statement should you include in teaching the client about this condition?
1. "Osteoarthritis is rarely debilitating."
2. "Osteoarthritis is a rare form of arthritis."
3. "Osteoarthritis is the most common form of arthritis."
4. "Osteoarthritis afflicts people older than age 60."

17. A 60-year-old female client has received teaching by her nurse about the causes of osteoarthritis. Which statement by the client indicates that further teaching is needed?
1. "My weight has played a role in my developing osteoarthritis."
2. "The broken bones I've had over the years have resulted in osteoarthritis."
3. "I'm getting older, which is associated with osteoarthritis."
4. "I have osteoarthritis because I haven't had enough calcium in my diet."

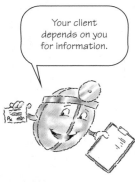

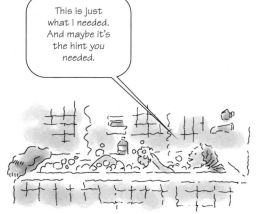

14. 1. Gout causes urate crystals to be deposited in the synovial fluid of affected joints. High levels of uric acid, not urate cyrstals, are found in the bloodstream. Gout doesn't affect calcium or RBC levels. The pain of gout is usually found in joints.
CN: Physiological integrity; CNS: Physiological adaptation; CL: Application

15. 2. Indomethacin, like other NSAIDs, should be taken with food because it can be irritating to the GI mucosa and lead to GI bleeding. It can cause drowsiness and complications from bleeding.
CN: Physiological integrity; CNS: Pharmacological therapies; CL: Application

16. 3. Osteoarthritis is the most common form of arthritis. It can afflict people of any age, although most are elderly, and it can be extremely debilitating.
CN: Physiological integrity; CNS: Physiological adaptation; CL: Application

17. 4. Osteoarthritis may be caused by trauma, aging, or obesity. Calcium doesn't affect osteoarthritis.
CN: Physiological integrity; CNS: Physiological adaptation; CL: Application

18. The nurse knows that a client with osteoarthritis of the knee understands the discharge instructions when the client makes which statement?

1. "I'll take my ibuprofen (Motrin) on an empty stomach."
2. "I'll try taking a warm shower in the morning."
3. "I'll wear my knee splint every night."
4. "I'll jog at least a mile every evening."

19. A client is taking salicyates for osteoarthritis. The presence of which of the following indicates that further assessment is needed?

1. Hearing loss
2. Increased pain in joints
3. Decreased calcium absorption
4. Increased bone demineralization

20. Clients with osteoarthritis may be on bed rest for prolonged periods. Which nursing intervention would be appropriate for these clients?

1. Encouraging coughing and deep breathing, and limiting fluid intake
2. Providing only passive range of motion (ROM), and decreasing stimulation
3. Having the client lie as still as possible, and giving adequate pain medicine
4. Turning the client every 2 hours, and encouraging coughing and deep breathing

21. A client asks the nurse, "What's the difference between rheumatoid arthritis and osteoarthritis?" Which statement is the correct response?

1. "Osteoarthritis is gender-specific; rheumatoid arthritis isn't."
2. "Osteoarthritis is a localized disease; rheumatoid arthritis is systemic."
3. "Osteoarthritis is a systemic disease; rheumatoid arthritis is localized."
4. "Osteoarthritis has dislocations and subluxations; rheumatoid arthritis doesn't."

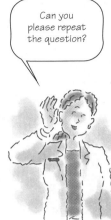

Can you please repeat the question?

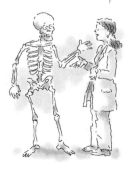

I'd say it's important to know the difference between these two common diseases. Wouldn't you agree?

18. 2. A client with osteoarthritis has joint stiffness that may be partially relieved with a warm shower on arising in the morning. Ibuprofen should be taken with food, as should all nonsteroidal anti-inflammatory medications. Splints are usually used by clients with rheumatoid arthritis. Because the problem is one of continued stress on the joint, the client may want to try to an exercise that puts less strain on the joint, such as swimming.
CN: Physiological integrity; CNS: Basic care and comfort; CL: Application

19. 1. Many elderly people already have diminished hearing, and salicylate use can lead to further or total hearing loss. Salicylates don't increase bone demineralization, decrease calcium absorption, or increase pain in joints.
CN: Physiological integrity; CNS: Pharmacological therapies; CL: Application

20. 4. A bedridden client needs to be turned every 2 hours, have adequate nutrition, and cough and deep-breathe. Adequate pain medication, active and passive ROM, and hydration are also appropriate nursing measures. The client shouldn't lie as still as possible, to prevent contractures, or limit his fluid intake.
CN: Physiological integrity; CNS: Basic care and comfort; CL: Application

21. 2. Osteoarthritis is a localized disease; rheumatoid arthritis is systemic. Osteoarthritis isn't gender-specific, but rheumatoid arthritis is. Clients have dislocations and subluxations in both disorders.
CN: Physiological integrity; CNS: Physiological adaptation; CL: Application

22. A 67-year-old male is seen in the clinic with complaints of right hip pain that worsens after activity, decreased range of motion (ROM) of the right hip, and difficulty getting up after sitting for long periods. The nurse observes crepitus in the right hip upon movement. The nurse recognizes that these symptoms are associated with which condition?
1. Gout
2. Osteoarthritis
3. Rheumatoid arthritis
4. Hip fracture

23. Which instruction would be considered <u>primary</u> prevention of injury from osteoarthritis?
1. Stay on bed rest.
2. Avoid physical activity.
3. Perform only repetitive tasks.
4. Warm up before exercise, and avoid repetitive tasks.

24. Which statement by the client indicates that client teaching regarding osteoarthritis has been effective?
1. "It's a systemic inflammatory disease of the joints."
2. "It involves fusing of the joints in the hand."
3. "It's an inflammatory joint disease that causes loss of articular cartilage in the synovial joint."
4. "It's a noninflammatory joint disease that causes degeneration of the joints."

25. Use of which types of clothing would help a client with osteoarthritis perform activities of daily living at home?
1. Zippered clothing
2. Tied shoes
3. Velcro clothing, slip-on shoes, and rubber grippers
4. Buttoned clothing, slip-on shoes, and rubber grippers

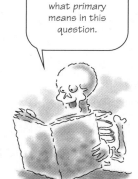

Read carefully to understand what *primary* means in this question.

22. 2. Osteoarthritis of the hip is associated with joint pain that worsens with activity, diminished ROM, joint crepitus, and difficulty arising after long periods of rest. Gout is associated with intermittent periods of joint pain that resolve. Rheumatoid arthritis is a systemic disease that affects multiple joints. Clients with hip fractures have severe pain in the hip or groin and are unable to bear weight, and the leg may be externally rotated.
CN: Physiological integrity; CNS: Physiological adaptation; CL: Analysis

23. 4. Primary prevention of injury from osteoarthritis includes warming up and avoiding repetitive tasks. Physical activity is important to remain fit and healthy and to maintain joint function. Bed rest would contribute to many other systemic complications.
CN: Health promotion and maintenance; CNS: None; CL: Application

24. 4. Osteoarthritis is a noninflammatory joint disease, with degeneration and loss of articular cartilage in synovial joints. Rheumatoid arthritis is a systemic inflammatory joint disease. Arthrodesis is fusion of the joints.
CN: Physiological integrity; CNS: Physiological adaptation; CL: Application

25. 3. Velcro clothing, slip-on shoes, and rubber grippers make it easier for the client to dress and grip objects. Zippers, ties, and buttons may be difficult for the client to use.
CN: Physiological integrity; CNS: Basic care and comfort; CL: Application

CN: Client needs category   CNS: Client needs subcategory   CL: Cognitive level

26. A client with osteoarthritis is refusing to perform her own daily care. Which approach would be <u>most appropriate</u> to use with this client?
1. Perform the care for the client.
2. Explain that she needs to maintain complete independence.
3. Encourage her to perform as much care as her pain will allow.
4. Tell her that after she has completed her care, she'll receive her pain medication.

27. Clients in the late stages of osteoarthritis commonly use which term to describe joint pain?
1. Grating
2. Dull ache
3. Deep aching pain
4. Deep aching, relieved with rest

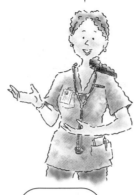

What would be the best way to help the client?

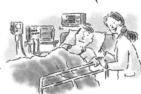

Ask your client about the pain.

28. A client uses a cane for assistance in walking. Which statement is true about a cane or other assistive devices?
1. "A walker is a better choice than a cane."
2. "The cane should be used on the affected side."
3. "The cane should be used on the unaffected side."
4. "A client with osteoarthritis should be encouraged to ambulate without the cane."

29. Which discharge instruction about home activity should be given to a client with osteoarthritis?
1. Learn to pace activity.
2. Remain as sedentary as possible.
3. Return to a normal level of activity.
4. Include vigorous exercise in your daily routine.

26. 3. A client with osteoarthritis should be encouraged to perform as much of her care as possible. The nurse's goal should be to allow her to maintain her self-care abilities with help as needed. It's never appropriate to use pain medication as a bargaining tool.
CN: Psychosocial integrity; CNS: None; CL: Application

27. 1. In the late stages of osteoarthritis, the client typically describes joint pain as grating. As the disease progresses, the cartilage covering the ends of bones is destroyed and bones rub against each other. Osteophytes, or bone spurs, may also form on the ends of bones. A dull ache and deep aching pain that's relieved with or without rest is usually seen in the earlier stages of osteoarthritis.
CN: Physiological integrity; CNS: Physiological adaptation; CL: Analysis

28. 3. A cane should be used on the unaffected side. A client with osteoarthritis should be encouraged to ambulate with a cane, walker, or other assistive device as needed; such use takes weight and stress off joints.
CN: Physiological integrity; CNS: Physiological adaptation; CL: Application

29. 1. A client with osteoarthritis should pace his activities and avoid overexertion. Overexertion can increase degeneration and cause pain. The client shouldn't become sedentary because he'll have a high risk of pneumonia and contractures.
CN: Physiological integrity; CNS: Physiological adaptation; CL: Application

30. A client has been prescribed an anti-inflammatory for osteoarthritis, and the nurse has instructed the client about taking the medication. Which statement by the client indicates that the nurse's teaching has been effective?

1. "If I'm not free from pain in a week, I'll come back to the clinic."
2. "It can take up to 2 to 3 weeks for me to feel the full effects from the medication."
3. "I'll increase my dose if I'm not better in a few days."
4. "If I don't experience pain relief in a few days, I need to stop taking the medication."

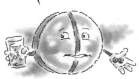

Make sure your client understands how long he may have to wait before feeling the benefits of his medication.

30. 2. Anti-inflammatory drugs may take up to 2 to 3 weeks for full benefits to be appreciated. If the client can tolerate the pain, he should continue on the present dose and offer other pain reduction measures, such as rest, massage, heat, or cold. Clients should never adjust their dosage or discontinue a medication without consulting the physician.
CN: Physiological integrity; CNS: Pharmacological therapies; CL: Application

31. A client is diagnosed with a herniated nucleus pulposus (HNP), or herniated disk. Given her knowledge of HNP, how would the nurse most accurately explain the cause of pain in this condition?

1. The disk slips out of alignment.
2. The disk shatters, and fragments place pressure on nerve roots.
3. The nucleus tissue itself remains centralized, and the surrounding tissue is displaced.
4. The nucleus of the disk puts pressure on the anulus, causing pressure on the nerve root.

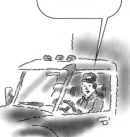

More than one-third down! Keep on truckin'!

31. 4. With an HNP, or herniated disk, the nucleus of the disk puts pressure on the anulus, causing pressure on the nerve root. The disk itself doesn't slip, rupture, or shatter. The nucleus tissue usually moves from the center of the disk.
CN: Physiological integrity; CNS: Physiological adaptation; CL: Application

32. A client complains of low back pain that radiates down the right leg, with numbness and weakness of the right leg. The nurse recognizes these complaints as related to which disorder?

1. Herniated nucleus pulposus (HNP)
2. Muscular dystrophy
3. Parkinson's disease
4. Osteoarthritis

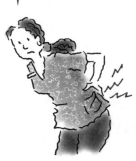

Sometimes I just need some TLC, what you would call a conservative approach.

32. 1. Compression of nerves by the HNP causes back pain that radiates into the leg, with numbness and weakness of the leg. Muscular dystrophy causes wasting of skeletal muscles. Parkinson's disease is characterized by progressive muscle rigidity and tremors. Osteoarthritis causes deep, aching joint pain.
CN: Physiological integrity; CNS: Physiological adaptation; CL: Analysis

33. Conservative treatment of a herniated nucleus pulposus (HNP) would include which measure?

1. Surgery
2. Bone fusion
3. Bed rest, pain medication, and physiotherapy
4. Strenuous exercise, pain medication, and physiotherapy

33. 3. Conservative treatment of an HNP may include bed rest, pain medication, and physiotherapy. Aggressive treatment may include surgery such as a bone fusion.
CN: Physiological integrity; CNS: Reduction of risk potential; CL: Application

CN: Client needs category   CNS: Client needs subcategory   CL: Cognitive level

34. A client is admitted for closed spine surgery to repair a herniated disk. The nurse is discussing the surgery with the client. Which statement should she include in the discussion?
1. "It's riskier than open spine surgery."
2. "Intense physical therapy is needed."
3. "An endoscope is used to perform the surgery."
4. "Recovery time is longer than with open spine surgery."

35. Which description best identifies the position of an intervertebral disk?
1. Encloses the anulus fibrosus
2. Surrounds the nucleus pulposus
3. Located between the vertebrae and the spinal column
4. Located between spinal nerves in the vertebral column

36. Which areas of vertebral herniation are the most common?
1. L1-L2, L4-L5
2. L1-L2, L5-S1
3. L4-L5, L5-S1
4. L5-S1, S2-S3

37. A 50-year-old client is admitted to the emergency department with severe lower back pain, weakness, and atrophy of her leg muscles. Suspecting a herniated disk, which diagnostic test would the nurse expect a physician to order?
1. Chest X-ray, magnetic resonance imaging (MRI), computed tomography (CT) scan
2. Lumbar puncture, chest X-ray, MRI, CT scan
3. Lumbar puncture, chest X-ray, myelography
4. Myelography, MRI, CT scan

38. Which response by the client indicates that the nurse's teaching regarding back safety has been effective?
1. "I'll start carrying objects at arm's length from my body."
2. "I'll sleep on my back at night."
3. "I'll carry objects close to my body."
4. "I'll lift items by bending over at my waist."

Now this is my idea of the ultimate back protection!

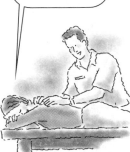

34. 3. Closed spine surgery uses endoscopy to fix a herniated disk. It's less risky than open surgery and has a shorter recovery time; it's commonly done as a same-day surgical procedure. Physical therapy may be less intensive or not needed at all.
CN: Physiological integrity; CNS: Physiological adaptation; CL: Analysis

35. 3. Intervertebral disks are between the vertebrae and the spinal column. The other answers are incorrect descriptions of vertebral disks.
CN: Physiological integrity; CNS: Physiological adaptation; CL: Knowledge

36. 3. The most common areas of herniation are L4-L5, L5-S1.
CN: Physiological integrity; CNS: Physiological adaptation; CL: Knowledge

37. 4. Tests used to diagnose a herniated nucleus pulposus include myelography, MRI, and CT scan. Chest X-ray and lumbar puncture aren't conclusive for a herniated disk.
CN: Physiological integrity; CNS: Physiological adaptation; CL: Application

38. 3. Keeping objects close to the body's center of gravity by carrying them close to the body lessens strain on the back. Carrying objects away from the body, sleeping on the back, and bending over at the waist to lift objects all increase back strain.
CN: Health promotion and maintenance; CNS: None; CL: Application

CN: Client needs category   CNS: Client needs subcategory   CL: Cognitive level

39. A client has been prescribed a skeletal muscle relaxant to treat a herniated nucleus pulposus. After the nurse has instructed the client about taking the medication, which client statement indicates that further teaching is needed?
1. "I'll stand up slowly to avoid dizziness."
2. "If I miss a dose of the medicine, I'll take an extra pill at the next dose."
3. "I'll call my doctor before taking over-the-counter medications."
4. "I'll avoid activities that require alertness while taking the medication."

40. A client with a recent fracture is suspected of having compartment syndrome. Data findings may include which symptoms?
1. Bodywide decrease in bone mass
2. A growth in and around the bone tissue
3. Inability to perform active movement, pain with passive movement
4. Inability to perform passive movement, pain with active movement

41. Compartment syndrome occurs under which condition?
1. Increase in scar tissue
2. Increase in bone mass
3. Decrease in bone mass
4. Hemorrhage into the muscle

42. A client who was casted for a recent fracture of the right ulna complains of severe pain, numbness, and tingling of the right arm. What would be the nurse's <u>most</u> appropriate response?
1. Administer acetaminophen (Tylenol) as prescribed.
2. Lower the arm below the level of the heart.
3. Immediately report the client's symptoms.
4. Apply a heating pad to the area.

43. In compartment syndrome, how long would it take for tissue death to occur?
1. 2 to 4 hours
2. 6 to 8 hours
3. 24 hours
4. 72 hours

CN: Client needs category CNS: Client needs subcategory CL: Cognitive level

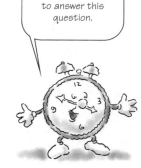

Data collection is like finding all the pieces to a puzzle.

You won't need to take long to answer this question.

39. 2. It isn't appropriate to take more than the prescribed dosage, as serious adverse effects can occur. Changing position slowly will help avoid dizziness. Over-the-counter medications may intensify adverse effects. Skeletal muscle relaxants can cause drowsiness.
CN: Physiological integrity; CNS: Pharmacological therapies; CL: Application

40. 3. With compartment syndrome, the client is unable to perform active movement and pain occurs with passive movement. A bone tumor shows growth in and around the bone tissue. Osteoporosis has a bodywide decrease in bone mass.
CN: Physiological integrity; CNS: Physiological adaptation; CL: Application

41. 4. Compartment syndrome occurs when pressure within the muscle compartment, resulting from edema or bleeding, increases to the point of interfering with circulation. Crush injuries, burns, bites, and fractures requiring casts or dressings may cause this syndrome. It isn't a result of scar tissue or an increase or decrease in bone mass.
NP: Data collection; CN: Physiological integrity; CNS: Physiological adaptation; CL: Knowledge

42. 3. Severe pain, numbness, and tingling are symptoms of impaired circulation due to compartment syndrome, which is a medical emergency. Don't give analgesics until the client has been assessed and treated. Lowering the arm below the level of the heart and applying heat will decrease venous outflow and impair the circulation even more.
CN: Physiological integrity; CNS: Physiological adaptation; CL: Application

43. 1. Tissue death can occur in 2 to 4 hours in compartment syndrome.
CN: Physiological integrity; CNS: Physiological adaptation; CL: Knowledge

44. Treatment of compartment syndrome includes which measure?
1. Amputation
2. Casting
3. Fasciotomy
4. Observation; no treatment is necessary

45. A client is admitted to the emergency department with a foot fracture. Which reason explains why the foot is placed in a brace?
1. To act as a splint
2. To prevent infection
3. To allow for movement
4. To encourage direct contact

46. After treatment of compartment syndrome, a client reports experiencing paresthesia. Which symptoms would be seen with paresthesia?
1. Fever and chills
2. Change in range of motion (ROM)
3. Pain and blanching
4. Numbness and tingling

47. Which characteristic of the fascia can cause it to develop compartment syndrome?
1. It's highly flexible.
2. It's fragile and weak.
3. It's unable to expand.
4. It's the only tissue within the compartment.

48. Which of the following best describes how compartment syndrome can occur?
1. From internal pressure
2. From external pressure
3. From increased blood pressure
4. From internal and external pressure

49. A nurse is instructing a client with a recent leg fracture and cast. Which statements by the client indicate that further teaching is needed? Select all that apply.
1. "I need to report any numbness or tingling in my leg at once."
2. "It's normal to have some numbness or tingling following a fracture."
3. "It's normal to have severe pain even after the cast is on."
4. "I need to keep my leg elevated as much as possible."
5. "The color and temperature of my toes will be checked frequently."
6. "It's normal to have swelling and for the cast to feel really tight."

CN: Client needs category   CNS: Client needs subcategory   CL: Cognitive level

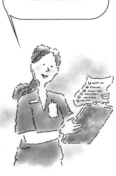

Here's a question your client with a similar problem is bound to ask.

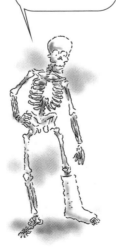

Believe it or not, I get goosebumps just thinking about how you'll answer this one!

44. 3. Treatment of compartment syndrome includes fasciotomy. A fasciotomy involves cutting the fascia over the affected area to permit muscle expansion. Casting, observation, and amputation aren't treatments for compartment syndrome.
CN: Physiological integrity; CNS: Physiological adaptation; CL: Comprehension

45. 1. The purpose of the brace is to act as a splint, prevent direct contact, and maintain immobility. A brace doesn't prevent infection.
CN: Physiological integrity; CNS: Reduction of risk potential; CL: Comprehension

46. 4. Paresthesia is described as numbness and tingling. It doesn't include pain or blanching and isn't associated with fever and chills or change in ROM.
CN: Physiological integrity; CNS: Physiological adaptation; CL: Comprehension

47. 3. Compartment syndrome occurs because the fascia can't expand. It isn't flexible or weak. The compartment contains blood vessels and nerves.
CN: Physiological integrity; CNS: Physiological adaptation; CL: Comprehension

48. 4. Compartment syndrome can occur from internal (bleeding) and external pressure (cast or dressing). Blood pressure doesn't affect compartment syndrome.
CN: Physiological integrity; CNS: Physiological adaptation; CL: Knowledge

49. 2, 3, 6. Paresthesia (numbness or tingling) is the earliest sign; severe pain is a later sign of compartment syndrome and should be reported at once. Elevating the leg will help prevent venous stasis, edema, and impaired circulation. Circulation and limb sensation need to be monitored frequently.
CN: Physiological integrity; CNS: Physiological adaptation; CL: Analysis

50. Which symptoms are considered signs of a fracture?
1. Tingling, coolness, loss of pulses
2. Loss of sensation, redness, warmth
3. Coolness, redness, pain at the site of injury
4. Redness, warmth, pain at the site of injury

51. Which areas would be included in a neurovascular assessment?
1. Orientation, movement, pulses, warmth
2. Capillary refill, movement, pulses, warmth
3. Orientation, pupillary response, temperature, pulses
4. Respiratory pattern, orientation, pulses, temperature

52. A nurse has instructed a client to accurately measure the circumference of both calves each morning and to report any increase in circumference. Which client statement indicates that the teaching has been effective?
1. "I'll use a measuring tape to check circumference."
2. "I only have to call if one leg is significantly larger than the other."
3. "I can measure my calves either near the knee or closer to the ankle."
4. "I'll use the standardized chart for limb circumference."

53. If pulses aren't palpable, which intervention should be performed <u>first</u>?
1. Check again in 1 hour.
2. Alert the nurse in charge immediately.
3. Verify the findings with a handheld Doppler.
4. Alert the physician immediately.

54. A client describes a foul odor from his cast. Which response or intervention would be most appropriate?
1. Assessing further because this may be a sign of infection
2. Teaching him proper cast care, including hygiene measures
3. Doing nothing (This is normal, especially when a cast is in place for a few weeks.)
4. Assessing further because this may be a sign of neurovascular compromise

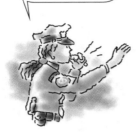

Stop! Don't take a wrong turn in your data collection. Know the signs to watch out for.

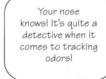

Your nose knows! It's quite a detective when it comes to tracking odors!

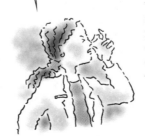

50. 4. Signs of a fracture may include redness, warmth, and intense pain at the fracture site. Coolness, tingling, and loss of pulses are signs of arterial insufficiency.
CN: Physiological integrity; CNS: Physiological adaptation; CL: Application

51. 2. A thorough neurovascular assessment should include checking capillary refill, movement, pulses, and warmth. Neurovascular assessment involves nerve and blood supply to an area. Respiratory pattern, orientation, temperature, and pupillary response aren't part of a neurovascular examination.
CN: Physiological integrity; CNS: Physiological adaptation; CL: Application

52. 1. The correct method for measuring calf circumference is to use a measuring tape, place the tape at the level where the calf circumference is largest, and measure at this same place each time. The client was instructed to report any increase in circumference. A significant increase in calf circumference size might be unilateral or bilateral. There's no standardized chart for limb circumference.
CN: Health promotion and maintenance; CNS: None; CL: Application

53. 3. If pulses aren't palpable, verify the observation with Doppler ultrasonography. If pulses can't be found with a handheld Doppler, immediately notify the physician.
CN: Physiological integrity; CNS: Physiological adaptation; CL: Application

54. 1. A foul odor from a cast may be a sign of infection. The nurse needs to monitor the client for fever, malaise, and possibly an elevation in white blood cells. Odor from a cast is never normal, and it isn't a sign of neurovascular compromise, which would include decreased pulses, coolness, and paresthesia.
CN: Health promotion and maintenance; CNS: None; CL: Analysis

CN: Client needs category   CNS: Client needs subcategory   CL: Cognitive level

55. To reduce the roughness of a cast, which measure should be used?
1. Petal the edges.
2. Elevate the limb.
3. Break off the rough area.
4. Distribute pressure evenly.

56. Elevating a limb with a cast will prevent swelling. Which action best describes how this is done?
1. Place the limb with the cast close to the body.
2. Place the limb with the cast at the level of the heart.
3. Place the limb with the cast below the level of the heart.
4. Place the limb with the cast above the level of the heart.

57. A client who's being discharged with an arm cast wants to shower at home. The nurse teaches her how to shower without getting the cast wet. For which reason is this important?
1. A wet cast can cause a foul odor.
2. A wet cast will weaken or decompose.
3. A wet cast is heavy and difficult to maneuver.
4. It's all right to get the cast wet; just use a hair dryer to dry it off.

58. A male client with a fractured femur is in Russell's traction. He asks the nurse to help him with back care. Which nursing action is most appropriate?
1. Telling the client that he can't have back care while he's in traction
2. Removing the weight to give the client more slack to move
3. Supporting the weight to give the client more slack to move
4. Telling the client to use the trapeze to lift his back off the bed

59. A client is involved in an automobile accident and is being sent to a trauma center. Which classic fractures that typically occur from trauma should the staff be prepared to assess for?
1. Brachial and clavicle
2. Brachial and humerus
3. Humerus and clavicle
4. Occipital and humerus

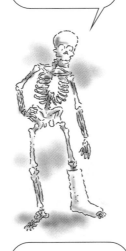

Being in a cast can be especially rough.

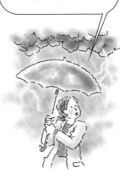

This is tricky...just how *do* you shower without getting wet?

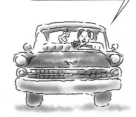

The word *classic* clues you in to a commonly occurring sign, symptom, or event.

55. 1. To reduce the roughness of the cast, petal the edges. Elevating the limb will prevent swelling. Distributing pressure evenly will prevent pressure ulcers. Never break a rough area off the cast.
CN: Physiological integrity; CNS: Basic care and comfort; CL: Application

56. 4. To reduce swelling, place the limb with the cast above the level of the heart. Placing it below or at the level of the heart won't reduce swelling. To elevate a cast, the limb may need to be extended from the body.
CN: Physiological integrity; CNS: Physiological adaptation; CL: Application

57. 2. A wet cast will weaken or decompose. A foul odor is a sign of infection. It's never appropriate to get a cast wet.
CN: Physiological integrity; CNS: Physiological adaptation; CL: Application

58. 4. The traction must not be disturbed, to maintain correct alignment. Therefore, the client should use the trapeze to lift his back off of the bed. The client can have back care as long as he uses the trapeze and doesn't disturb the alignment. The weight shouldn't be moved without a physician's order; it should hang freely without touching anything.
CN: Physiological integrity; CNS: Reduction of risk potential; CL: Application

59. 3. Classic fractures that occur with trauma are those of the humerus and clavicle. There are no brachial bones, and occipital bones aren't usually involved in a traumatic injury.
CN: Physiological integrity; CNS: Physiological adaptation; CL: Analysis

CN: Client needs category   CNS: Client needs subcategory   CL: Cognitive level

60. Which characteristic applies to a closed fracture?
1. Extensive tissue damage
2. Increased risk of infection
3. Same as for a compound fracture
4. Intact skin over the fracture site

61. A client asks why he's being placed in traction prior to surgery. Which response by the nurse is <u>most</u> appropriate?
1. Traction will help prevent skin breakdown.
2. Traction helps with repositioning while in bed.
3. Traction allows for more activity.
4. Traction helps to prevent trauma and overcome muscle spasms.

62. A fracture line that's straight across the bone represents what type of fracture?
1. Linear
2. Longitudinal
3. Oblique
4. Transverse

63. A 75-year-old client with Paget's disease is undergoing tests for a suspected fracture. The nurse should expect to see which type of fracture?
1. Linear
2. Longitudinal
3. Oblique
4. Transverse

64. A 20-year-old female is complaining of severe pain in her right upper arm. Which X-ray finding would indicate the need for further investigation?
1. Longitudinal fracture
2. Oblique fracture
3. Spiral fracture
4. Transverse fracture

65. Which mechanism or condition causes healing of a fracture?
1. Scar tissue
2. Displacement
3. Necrotic tissue formation
4. Formation of new bone tissue

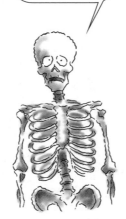

60. 4. A closed fracture maintains intact skin over the fracture site. An open fracture has extensive tissue damage and an increased risk of infection; it's also known as a *compound fracture*.
CN: Physiological integrity; CNS: Physiological adaptation; CL: Knowledge

61. 4. Traction prevents trauma and overcomes muscle spasms. Traction doesn't help in preventing skin breakdown, repositioning the client, or allowing the client to become active.
CN: Physiological integrity; CNS: Basic care and comfort; CL: Application

62. 4. A fracture line straight across the bone is called a transverse fracture. A linear fracture has an intact fracture line. A fracture line at a 45-degree angle to the shaft of the bone is an oblique fracture. A longitudinal fracture has a fracture line that runs lengthwise down the bone.
CN: Physiological integrity; CNS: Physiological adaptation; CL: Knowledge

63. 4. A transverse fracture commonly occurs with Paget's disease. Linear, longitudinal, and oblique fracturs generally occur with trauma.
CN: Physiological integrity; CNS: Physiological adaptation; CL: Application

64. 3. Spiral fractures are commonly seen in the upper extremities and are related to physical abuse. Oblique and longitudinal fractures generally occur with trauma. A transverse fracture commonly occurs with such bone diseases as osteomalacia and Paget's disease.
CN: Physiological integrity; CNS: Physiological adaptation; CL: Application

65. 4. Healing of a fracture occurs by the formation of new bone tissue. Bone doesn't heal by forming scar tissue or necrotic tissue or by displacement.
CN: Physiological integrity; CNS: Physiological adaptation; CL: Knowledge

CN: Client needs category   CNS: Client needs subcategory   CL: Cognitive level

66. A 20-year-old male client has just had a plaster cast applied to his right forearm following reduction of a closed radius fracture due to an in-line skating accident. It's <u>most important</u> for the nurse to check which of the following?
1. Whether the cast is completely dry
2. Sensation and movement of the fingers
3. Whether the client is having any pain
4. Whether the cast needs petaling

67. A 45-year-old client is diagnosed with a long bone fracture. A nurse who's aware of the most serious complications of long bone fracture should monitor the client closely for which potential complication?
1. Bone emboli
2. Fat emboli
3. Platelet emboli
4. Serous emboli

68. A client is diagnosed with a fat emboli. Which signs and symptoms would the nurse expect to find when assessing this client?
1. Tachypnea, tachycardia, shortness of breath, paresthesia
2. Paresthesia, bradypnea, bradycardia, petechial rash on chest and neck
3. Bradypnea, bradycardia, shortness of breath, petechial rash on chest and neck
4. Tachypnea, tachycardia, shortness of breath, petechial rash on chest and neck

69. The community health nurse found an elderly female client lying in the snow, unable to move her right leg because of a fracture. What's the nurse's <u>first priority</u>?
1. Realign the fracture ends.
2. Reduce the fracture.
3. Immobilize the fracture in its present position.
4. Elevate the leg on whatever is available.

70. A high-protein diet is ordered for a client recovering from a fracture. High protein is ordered for which reason?
1. Protein promotes gluconeogenesis.
2. Protein has anti-inflammatory properties.
3. Protein promotes cell growth and bone union.
4. Protein decreases pain medication requirements.

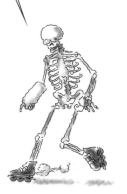

Don't fall down on this question. It's *most important* that you select the correct answer.

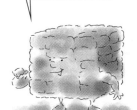

I'm important... you need me! Hey, sometimes you need to promote yourself to get ahead.

66. 2. Neurovascular checks are most important because they're used to determine if any impairment exists after cast application and reduction of the fracture. Checking to see if the cast is completely dry isn't the nurse's highest priority. Checking to see if the client has pain is important but not the highest priority. Petaling to smooth the cast edge is done when the cast is completely dry.
CN: Physiological integrity; CNS: Reduction of risk potential; CL: Application

67. 2. A serious complication of long bone fractures is the development of fat emboli. Platelet or bone emboli are rare occurrences. There aren't emboli known as *serous emboli*.
CN: Physiological integrity; CNS: Physiological adaptation; CL: Application

68. 4. Signs and symptoms of fat emboli include tachypnea, tachycardia, shortness of breath, and a petechial rash on the chest and neck. The fat molecules enter the venous circulation and travel to the lung, obstructing pulmonary circulation. Bradycardia, bradypnea, and paresthesia aren't usual symptoms.
CN: Health promotion and maintenance; CNS: None; CL: Analysis

69. 3. Initial treatment of obvious and suspected fractures includes immobilizing and splinting the limb. Any attempt to realign or rest the fracture at the site may cause further injury and complications. The leg may be elevated only after immobilization.
CN: Physiological integrity CNS: Physiological adaptation; CL: Application

70. 3. High-protein intake promotes cell growth and bone union. Protein doesn't decrease pain medication requirements, exert anti-inflammatory properties, or promote gluconeogenesis.
CN: Physiological integrity; CNS: Basic care and comfort; CL: Application

CN: Client needs category   CNS: Client needs subcategory   CL: Cognitive level

71. The nurse is instructing a nursing assistant on the proper care of a client in Buck's extension traction following a fracture of his left fibula. Which observation indicates that the teaching was effective?
 1. The weights are allowed to hang freely over the end of the bed.
 2. The nursing assistant lifts the weights when assisting the client to move up in bed.
 3. The leg in traction is kept externally rotated.
 4. The nursing assistant instructs the client to perform ankle rotation exercises.

72. Which type of traction is used to treat lower back pain?
 1. Bryant's traction
 2. Buck's traction
 3. Pelvic traction belt
 4. Russell traction

73. The nurse is instructing a nursing assistant on how to properly position a 45-year-old male client who underwent total hip replacement. The nurse explains that the client's hip needs to be in which position?
 1. Straight with the knee flexed
 2. In an abducted position
 3. In an adducted position
 4. Externally rotated

74. A 51-year-old client has undergone a total hip replacement on her right side. After surgery, how often should the nurse turn the client?
 1. Every 1 to 2 hours, from the unaffected side to the back
 2. Every 1 to 2 hours, from the affected side to the back
 3. Every 4 to 6 hours, from the unaffected side to the back
 4. Every 4 to 6 hours, from the affected side to the back

71. 1. In Buck's extension traction, the weights should hang freely without touching the bed or floor. Lifting the weights would break the traction. The client should be moved up in bed, allowing the weights to move freely along with the client. The leg should be kept in straight alignment. Performing ankle rotation exercises could cause the leg to go out of alignment.
CN: Physiological integrity; CNS: Basic care and comfort; CL: Knowledge

72. 3. A pelvic traction belt is conservative treatment for lower back pain. Bryant's traction is used to reduce developmental hip dislocations for children who weigh less than 35 lb (15.9 kg). Russell traction is used for leg traction. Buck's traction is used for leg or arm traction.
CN: Physiological integrity; CNS: Physiological adaptation; CL: Knowledge

73. 2. An abducted position keeps the new joint from becoming displaced out of the socket. The client can keep his hip straight with the knee flexed as long as an abductor pillow is kept in place. Keeping the hip adducted or externally rotated can dislocate the hip joint.
CN: Physiological integrity; CNS: Basic care and comfort; CL: Application

74. 1. The client should be turned at least every 2 hours and always from the unaffected side to the back. The client should never be placed on the affected side. Turning the client every 4 to 6 hours places her at greater risk for skin breakdown.
CN: Physiological integrity; CNS: Reduction of risk potential; CL: Application

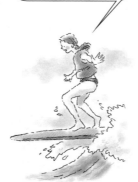

They say location is everything in real estate. Well, position can be everything when caring for a client with a fracture. Speaking of position…I'd better shift!

CN: Client needs category   CNS: Client needs subcategory   CL: Cognitive level

75. Which intervention would help prevent deep vein thrombosis (DVT) after hip surgery?
1. Immobility
2. Convoluted foam mattress
3. Vigorous pulmonary care
4. Subcutaneous heparin and pneumatic compression boots

76. The nurse is caring for a client who's on complete bed rest following complete hip replacement. In an effort to reduce sensory deprivation, the nursing assistant should be instructed to do which of the following?
1. Provide mouth care before meals.
2. Monitor the client's urine output every 2 hours.
3. Check bilateral hand grasps every 4 hours.
4. Orient the client to date and time frequently.

77. A client who had a recent total hip replacement is being seen by the home care nurse. When the nurse arrives, she notes a large number of small carpets scattered throughout the client's home. Which action should the nurse take as a result of this finding?
1. Ask the client why there are so many scattered carpets throughout the home.
2. Collect the small carpets, and place them together near the main door of the home.
3. Review with the client the hazard small carpets play, especially for a person with musculoskeletal impairment.
4. Nothing; there's nothing wrong with having small carpets scattered throughout the home.

78. Which nursing intervention is appropriate for a client in traction?
1. Assessing the pin sites every shift and as needed
2. Adding and removing weights as the client desires
3. Making sure the knots in the rope catch on the pulley
4. Giving range of motion (ROM) to all joints, including those immediately proximal and distal to the fracture, every shift

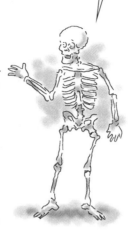

Wow! You've finished 76 questions! Outstanding!

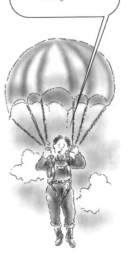

Don't jump to conclusions! Read question 77 carefully, and you won't make the wrong move.

75. 4. To prevent DVT after hip surgery, subcutaneous heparin and pneumatic compression boots are used. Convoluted foam mattresses and pulmonary care don't prevent DVT. Immobility can cause DVT.
CN: Health promotion and maintenance; CNS: None; CL: Application

76. 1. Cleaning the mouth before meals enhances sensual stimuli and taste bud function. Checking urine output doesn't affect sensory input. Checking hand grasps and orienting the client would help to assess neurologic deficits and stimulate the nervous system.
CN: Safe, effective care environment; CNS: Coordinated care; CL: Application

77. 3. Questioning the client about the small scattered carpets would be just the beginning of helping the client understand the role they play in causing home injuries, especially for a person with an alteration in her musculoskeletal status. Collecting the small carpets and doing nothing aren't appropriate actions for the nurse. The nurse should review the hazards of having small carpets on the floors so that the client can take the appropriate action and reduce her likelihood of injury by removing the carpets.
CN: Safe, effective care environment; CNS: Safety and infection control; CL: Application

78. 1. Nursing care for a client in traction may include assessing pin sites every shift and as needed and making sure the knots in the rope don't catch on the pulley. The nurse should add and remove weights only as the physician orders, and give ROM to all joints except those immediately proximal and distal to the fracture every shift.
CN: Physiological integrity; CNS: Basic care and comfort; CL: Application

CN: Client needs category   CNS: Client needs subcategory   CL: Cognitive level

79. A nurse reads this progress notes entry on a client who has had surgical repair of a right hip fracture. The nurse knows these findings are consistent with which condition?

Progress notes	
10/04/08	Client reports new left calf pain (4/5) on pain scale,
1400	that worsens to touch and with dorsiflexion of left
	foot. +4 nonpitting edema left foot to knee noted.
	Prominent superficial veins noted on left leg. Dr.
	Smith notified.————————Ann Jones, R.N.

1. Deep vein thrombosis (DVT)
2. Fat embolus
3. Infection
4. Pulmonary embolism

79. 1. Unilateral leg pain and edema with a positive Homans' sign (calf pain with dorsiflexion of the foot and that isn't always present) might be symptoms of DVT. Tachycardia, chest pain, and shortness of breath may be symptoms of a pulmonary embolism. It's unlikely an infection would occur on the opposite side of the fracture without cause. Symptoms of fat emboli include restlessness, tachypnea, and tachycardia; they're more common in long-bone injuries.
CN: Physiological integrity; CNS: Reduction of risk potential; CL: Application

80. A female client who fell while washing her outside windows has a fractured right ankle and is being fitted with a cast. After assisting with the cast application, what instructions should the nurse give the client?
1. Go home and stay in bed for about 5 days.
2. Keep the cast covered with plastic until it feels dry.
3. Move the right toes for several minutes every hour.
4. Expect some swelling and blueness of the toes.

80. 3. Moving the toes is encouraged to facilitate circulation and prevent swelling. By moving the toes, the client will be aware of any numbness or swelling and can take appropriate action, such as elevating the extremity and reporting the findings to her physician. Usually, clients are instructed to remain in bed for 24 hours while the cast dries. Prolonged immobility creates problems for the client. While the cast is still damp, the ankle should be elevated on a pillow that's protected with plastic; the cast itself should be left open to the air. Swelling and a bluish color of the toes aren't expected; they indicate compromised circulation and should be reported immediately.
CN: Physiological integrity CNS: Reduction of risk potential; CL: Application

81. Synthetic casts take approximately how long to set?
1. Immediately
2. 20 minutes
3. 45 minutes
4. 2 hours

81. 2. Synthetic casts take about 20 minutes to set.
CN: Physiological integrity; CNS: Reduction of risk potential; CL: Knowledge

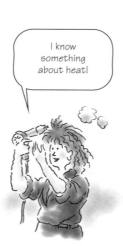

I know something about heat!

82. Which statement by a client who recently had a cast applied indicates that the nurse's teaching has been effective?
1. "The cast will need to be removed if I feel any heat."
2. "Heat is a normal sensation as a cast dries."
3. "The heat I feel is most likely caused by an infection."
4. "I'll call my physician if I feel any heat."

82. 2. Normally, as the cast dries, a client may complain of heat from the cast. Offer reassurance. The cast won't need to be removed and the physician doesn't need to be notified. Heat from the cast isn't a sign of infection.
CN: Physiological integrity; CNS: Reduction of risk potential; CL: Application

CN: Client needs category   CNS: Client needs subcategory   CL: Cognitive level

83. A nurse is providing care for a client with a leg cast. To help prevent footdrop, which action by the nurse is the <u>most</u> appropriate?
1. Encouraging bed rest
2. Supporting the foot with 45 degrees of flexion
3. Supporting the foot with 90 degrees of flexion
4. Placing a stocking on the foot to provide warmth

83. 3. To prevent footdrop in a leg with a cast, the foot should be supported with 90 degrees of flexion. Bed rest can cause footdrop. Keeping the extremity warm won't prevent footdrop.

CN: Health promotion and maintenance; CNS: None; CL: Application

84. The physician has just removed the cast from a 20-year-old male client's lower leg. During the removal, a small superficial abrasion occurred over the ankle. Which statement by the client indicates the need for additional client teaching?
1. "I must use a moisturizing lotion on the dry areas."
2. "The dry, peeling skin will go away by itself."
3. "I can wash the abrasion on my ankle with soap and water."
4. "I'll wait until the abrasion is healed before I go swimming."

84. 1. The dry, peeling skin will heal in a few days with normal cleaning; therefore, lotions are unnecessary. Vigorous scrubbing isn't necessary. Washing the abrasion and delaying swimming until healing are correct procedures to follow after removal of a cast.

CN: Physiological integrity; CNS: Reduction of risk potential; CL: Application

85. Which information is critical to include in the discharge plan for a client leaving the hospital in a leg cast?
1. Cast care procedures and devices to relieve itching
2. Skin care, mouth care, and cast removal procedures
3. Cast care, neurovascular checks, and hygiene measures
4. Cast removal procedures, neurovascular checks, and devices to relieve itching

85. 3. Proper cast care procedures include observing the skin nearest the cast edges for signs of pressure ulcers, keeping the cast dry and intact, and avoiding the use of insertable devices (such as wire hangers or sticks) to relieve itching. Frequent neurovascular checks can reveal evidence of pressure or impaired circulation to the leg under the cast. This includes checking the toes frequently for discoloration, swelling, or lack of movement or sensation. Hygiene measures should focus on the client's normal elimination patterns and the importance of cleanliness after elimination as well as on the need to maintain skin integrity by taking sponge baths and caring for dry skin. Devices should never be inserted between the cast and the skin. Although mouth care and cast removal are important issues, they aren't priority discharge instructions in this case.

CN: Physiological integrity; CNS: Physiological adaptation; CL: Application

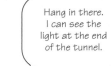

Hang in there. I can see the light at the end of the tunnel.

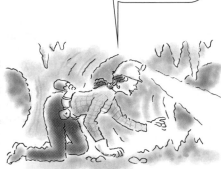

CN: Client needs category   CNS: Client needs subcategory   CL: Cognitive level

86. The nurse is caring for a client with a cast on his left arm. Which assessment finding is most significant for this client?
1. Normal capillary refill in the great toe
2. Presence of a normal popliteal pulse
3. Intact skin around the cast edges
4. Ability to move all toes

86. 3. Because a cast can irritate the skin, the nurse should inspect for this complication. Usually, the skin remains intact around the cast edges. Normally, capillary refill in the left thumb and fingers is more significant than in the great toe because an arm cast can impair circulation in the affected arm. Similarly, the presence of a normal radial pulse is more noteworthy than popliteal pulse because a cast on the left arm could affect circulation in that limb. Movement of this client's fingers is more critical than movement of the toes because a left arm cast could compress a nerve, preventing movement of fingers in the left arm.
CN: Physiological integrity; CNS: Physiological adaptation; CL: Application

87. A client has just returned from the post-anesthesia care unit after undergoing internal fixation of a left femoral neck fracture. The nurse should place the client in which position?
1. On his left side with his right knee bent
2. On his back with two pillows between his legs
3. On his right side with his left knee bent
4. Sitting at a 90-degree angle

87. 2. The operative leg must be kept abducted to prevent dislocation of the hip. Placing the client on the left or right side with knee bent doesn't promote abduction. Acute flexion of the operated hip may cause dislocation. The head of the bed may be raised 35 to 40 degrees.
CN: Physiological integrity; CNS: Reduction of risk potential; CL: Application

88. A 20-year-old client developed osteomyelitis 2 weeks after a fishhook was removed from his foot. Which rationale best explains the expected long-term antibiotic therapy?
1. Bone has poor circulation.
2. Tissue trauma requires antibiotics.
3. Feet are normally difficult to treat.
4. Fishhook injuries are highly contaminated.

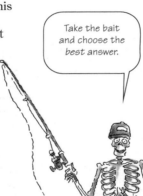

Take the bait and choose the best answer.

88. 1. Bone has poor circulation, making it difficult to treat an infection in the bone. This requires long-term use of I.V. antibiotics to make sure the infection is cleared. Tissue trauma doesn't always require antibiotics, at least not long term. Fishhooks may not be any more contaminated than another instrument that caused an injury. Feet aren't more difficult to treat than other parts of the body unless the client has a circulatory problem or diabetes mellitus.
CN: Physiological integrity; CNS: Pharmacological therapies; CL: Application

89. Client education about gout includes which information?
1. Good foot care will reduce complications.
2. Increased dietary intake of purine is needed.
3. Production of uric acid in the kidney affects joints.
4. Uric acid crystals cause inflammatory destruction of the joint.

89. 4. The client needs to know that uric acid crystals collect in the joint of the great toe and cause inflammation. The kidney excretes uric acid, an end product of metabolism. A diet low in purines would be indicated. Good foot care doesn't affect the development of complications, but increasing water intake may help prevent urinary calculi formation.
CN: Physiological integrity; CNS: Reduction of risk potential; CL: Application

CN: Client needs category   CNS: Client needs subcategory   CL: Cognitive level

90. If I.V. antibiotics don't eliminate osteomyelitis, which treatment is <u>most commonly</u> used next?
1. Bone grafts
2. Hyperbaric oxygen therapy
3. Amputation of the extremity
4. Debridement of necrotic tissue

90. 4. The tissues may need to be debrided to eliminate necrotic tissue and allow new tissue to form. Amputation isn't indicated in the treatment of acute osteomyelitis. A bone graft would be done after debridement. Hyperbaric oxygen therapy has been used in the successful treatment of osteomyelitis, but it isn't always readily available or as common as debridement.
CN: Physiological integrity; CNS: Physiological adaptation; CL: Comprehension

91. A 64-year-old client has just had total hip replacement surgery. The physician orders heparin 8,000 units to be administered subcutaneously. The label on the heparin vial reads: heparin 10,000 units/ml. How many milliliters of heparin should the nurse draw up in the syringe to administer the correct dose? Record your answer using one decimal place.

_____ ml

91. 0.8. This formula is used to calculate drug dosages:
Dose on hand/Quantity on hand = Dose desired/X
In this example, the equation is as follows:
10,000 units/ml = 8,000 units/X; X = 0.8 ml.
CN: Physiological integrity; CNS: Pharmacological therapies; CL: Application

92. A client is diagnosed with gout. Which foods should the nurse instruct the client to <u>avoid</u>? Select all that apply:
1. Green leafy vegetables
2. Liver
3. Cod
4. Chocolate
5. Sardines
6. Eggs
7. Whole milk

92. 2, 3, 5. The client with gout should avoid foods that are high in purines, such as liver, cod, and sardines. Other foods that should be avoided include anchovies, kidneys, sweetbreads, lentils, and alcoholic beverages, especially beer and wine. Green leafy vegetables, chocolate, eggs, and whole milk aren't high in purines and, therefore, aren't restricted in the diet of a client with gout.
CN: Physiological integrity; CNS: Basic care and comfort; CL: Application

CN: Client needs category   CNS: Client needs subcategory   CL: Cognitive level

93. A client is about to undergo total hip replacement surgery. Before the surgery, the nurse conducts a preoperative teaching session with him. The nurse can tell that her teaching has been effective when the client verbalizes the importance of <u>avoiding</u> which actions? Select all that apply:

1. Keeping the legs apart while lying in bed
2. Periodically tightening the leg muscles
3. Internally rotating the feet
4. Bending to pick items up from the floor
5. Sleeping in a side-lying position

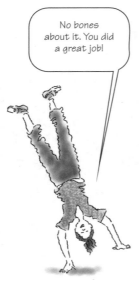

93. 3, 4. After hip replacement surgery, the client should avoid internally rotating his feet and bending more than 90 degrees. These activities can compromise the hip joint. The client should lie with his legs abducted. Leg-strengthening exercises, such as periodically tightening the leg muscles, are recommended to maintain muscle strength and reduce the risk of thrombus formation. A side-lying position is acceptable; however, some physicians restrict lying on the operative side.

CN: Physiological integrity; CNS: Reduction of risk potential; CL: Analysis

---

CN: Client needs category   CNS: Client needs subcategory   CL: Cognitive level

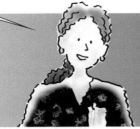

From hiatal hernia to diverticulitis to pancreatitis, this chapter covers all the GI disorders you could ask for, in one handy package. Gotta love it!

Chapter 8
Gastrointestinal disorders

1. Which condition can <u>cause</u> a hiatal hernia?
1. Increased intrathoracic pressure
2. Weakness of the esophageal muscle
3. Increased esophageal muscle pressure
4. Weakness of the diaphragmatic muscle

Read #1 carefully. This question is looking for a cause.

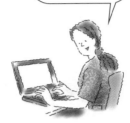

2. Which statement by a client with a sliding hiatal hernia indicates that the client has understood instructions to promote his comfort?
1. "I'll drink carbonated cola beverages with my meals."
2. "I'll be sure to lie down immediately after eating."
3. "I should eat three large, high-carbohydrate meals each day."
4. "I'll sleep with my head elevated about 3 to 4 inches."

3. A 38-year-old client is complaining of reflux in his esophagus 1 to 2 hours after eating or when lying down for the last 2 weeks. The nurse recognizes that this symptom is related to which disorder?
1. Myocardial infarction (MI)
2. Lumbar strain
3. Hiatal hernia
4. Intestinal infection

Which test allows the radiologist to see the stomach in relation to the diaphragm?

4. A nurse would expect to prepare a client for which test to aid in diagnosing a hiatal hernia?
1. Colonoscopy
2. Lower GI series
3. Barium swallow
4. Abdominal X-ray series

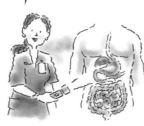

1. 4. A hiatal hernia is caused by weakness of the diaphragmatic muscle and increased intra-abdominal—not intrathoracic—pressure. This weakness allows the stomach to slide into the esophagus. The esophageal supports weaken, but esophageal muscle weakness or increased esophageal muscle pressure isn't a factor in hiatal hernia.
CN: Physiological integrity; CNS: Physiological adaptation; CL: Knowledge

2. 4. With a hiatal hernia, sleeping with the head of the bed elevated 30 degrees (about 3″ to 4″ [7.5 to 10 cm]) prevents stomach acids from refluxing into the esophagus. Carbonated beverages would create gas and possibly irritate the herniated area as the client begins to tolerate bland foods. Lying down immediately after eating would facilitate the reflux of stomach acids, causing irritation and possible aspiration. Small meals are recommended for clients with hiatal hernia.
CN: Physiological integrity; CNS: Physiological adaptation; CL: Analysis

3. 3. Esophageal reflux is a common symptom of hiatal hernia. This condition seems to be associated with chronic exposure of the lower esophageal sphincter to the lower pressure of the thorax, making it less effective. MI may present with indigestion but not reflux. This symptom isn't associated with the other conditions.
CN: Physiological integrity; CNS: Physiological adaptation; CL: Analysis

4. 3. A barium swallow with fluoroscopy shows the position of the stomach in relation to the diaphragm. A colonoscopy and a lower GI series show disorders of the intestine. An abdominal X-ray series will show structural defects but not necessarily a hiatal hernia, unless it's sliding or rolling at the time of the X-ray.
CN: Health promotion and maintenance; CNS: None; CL: Application

CN: Client needs category CNS: Client needs subcategory CL: Cognitive level

5. When is the best time for a nurse to teach a client scheduled for an appendectomy about incision splinting and leg exercises?
1. On the client's admission to the postanesthesia care unit (PACU)
2. Before the surgical procedure
3. During the intraoperative period
4. When the client returns from the PACU

6. Which term best describes the pain associated with appendicitis?
1. Aching
2. Fleeting
3. Intermittent
4. Steady

> The last two items are similar. Know the difference before answering this one.

7. A nurse would place a client with appendicitis in which position to help relieve pain?
1. Prone
2. Sitting
3. Supine, stretched out
4. Lying with legs drawn up

8. Which nursing intervention should be the priority when caring for a client with appendicitis?
1. Monitoring for pain relief
2. Encouraging oral intake of clear fluids
3. Providing discharge teaching
4. Monitoring for symptoms of peritonitis

5. 2. Teaching is most effective when done before the surgical procedure. During this time, the nurse should tell the client what to expect in the immediate postoperative period. On admission to the PACU, the client is usually very drowsy, making this an inopportune time for teaching. During the intraoperative period, anesthesia alters the client's mental status, rendering teaching ineffective. On the client's return from the PACU, the client may remain drowsy.
CN: Physiological integrity; CNS: Reduction of risk potential; CL: Application

6. 4. The pain begins in the epigastrium or periumbilical region, then shifts to the right lower quadrant and becomes steady. The pain may be moderate to severe. Sudden cessation of pain may indicate rupture of the appendix.
CN: Physiological integrity; CNS: Physiological adaptation; CL: Knowledge

7. 4. Lying still with the legs drawn up toward the chest helps relieve tension on the abdominal muscles, which helps to reduce the amount of discomfort felt. Lying flat or sitting may increase the amount of pain experienced.
CN: Physiological integrity; CNS: Physiological adaptation; CL: Application

8. 4. The focus of care is to monitor for peritonitis, or inflammation of the peritoneal cavity. Peritonitis is most commonly caused by appendix rupture and invasion of bacteria, which could be lethal. The client with appendicitis will have pain. However, pain medications are given only after the diagnosis of appendicitis has been confirmed to prevent masking of symptoms. The nurse should prevent oral intake in preparation for surgery. Discharge teaching is important; however, in the acute phase, management should focus on minimizing preoperative complications and recognizing when they may be occurring.
CN: Physiological integrity; CNS: Reduction of risk potential; CL: Application

CN: Client needs category   CNS: Client needs subcategory   CL: Cognitive level

9. Which definition best describes gastritis?
1. Erosion of the gastric mucosa
2. Inflammation of a diverticulum
3. Inflammation of the gastric mucosa
4. Reflux of stomach acid into the esophagus

9. 3. Gastritis is an inflammation of the gastric mucosa that may be acute (commonly resulting from exposure to local irritants) or chronic (associated with autoimmune infections or atrophic disorders of the stomach). Erosion of the mucosa results in ulceration. Inflammation of a diverticulum is called *diverticulitis;* reflux of stomach acid is known as *gastroesophageal reflux disease.*

CN: Physiological integrity; CNS: Physiological adaptation; CL: Knowledge

10. A 27-year-old, Spanish-speaking woman comes to the clinic complaining of abdominal cramping, nausea, and diarrhea for the past 3 days. She has brought her 5-year-old son to interpret. He's worried about his mother. What should be the nurse's next course of action?
1. Reassure the boy and allow him to remain with her. Have an interpreter translate medication and follow-up care with the mother.
2. Have the boy ask his mother whether she has taken medication or had blood in her stools.
3. Give medication instructions to the boy; have him schedule a follow-up appointment.
4. Take the boy into the waiting room to play. Offer the mother follow-up instructions and handouts written in Spanish.

Congratulations! You've finished the first 10 questions!

10. 1. It's inappropriate for a 5-year-old child to assume adult responsibilities and the burden of being a translator for his parent. By obtaining the services of an adult interpreter, you can more accurately provide medication and follow-up instructions and better assess the client's level of comprehension. Allowing the boy to remain in the exam room could provide needed reassurance and potentially benefit mother and child.

CN: Psychosocial integrity; CNS: None; CL: Application

11. Which task would be the priority in the immediate postoperative care of a client who has undergone gastric resection?
1. Monitoring gastric pH to detect complications
2. Monitoring bowel sounds
3. Providing nutritional support
4. Monitoring for symptoms of hemorrhage

Know what signs to look for in your client with a gastric resection.

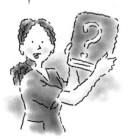

11. 4. The client should be monitored closely for signs and symptoms of hemorrhage, such as bright red blood in the nasogastric tube suction, tachycardia, or a drop in blood pressure. Gastric pH may be monitored to evaluate the need for histamine-2 receptor antagonists. Bowel sounds may not return for up to 72 hours postoperatively. Nutritional needs should be addressed soon after surgery.

CN: Physiological integrity; CNS: Reduction of risk potential; CL: Application

CN: Client needs category   CNS: Client needs subcategory   CL: Cognitive level

12. Which treatment should be included in the immediate care of a client with acute gastritis?
1. Reducing work stress
2. Completing gastric resection
3. Treating the underlying cause
4. Administering enteral tube feedings

13. When reviewing the medical record of a client, which factor would lead the nurse to suspect that the client is at risk for chronic gastritis?
1. Young age
2. Antibiotic usage
3. Gallbladder disease
4. *Helicobacter pylori* infection

14. Which factor associates chronic gastritis with pernicious anemia?
1. Increased absorption of vitamin B_{12}
2. Inability to absorb vitamin B_{12}
3. Overproduction of stomach acid
4. Overproduction of vitamin B_{12}

15. A client diagnosed with diverticulosis asks the nurse to describe this condition. Which concept would the nurse incorporate into the description?
1. An inflamed outpouching of the intestine
2. A noninflamed outpouching of the intestine
3. The partial impairment of the forward flow of intestinal contents
4. An abnormal protrusion of an organ through the structure that usually holds it

16. Which statement by a client indicates that he understands the nurse's teaching regarding the relationship between diet and the development of diverticulosis?
1. "A low-fiber diet may cause diverticulosis."
2. "A high-fiber diet may cause diverticulosis."
3. "A high-protein diet may cause diverticulosis."
4. "A low-carbohydrate diet may cause diverticulosis."

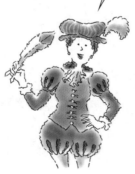

Inflamed or noninflamed? That is the question!

12. 3. Discovering and treating the cause of gastritis is the most beneficial approach. Reducing or eliminating oral intake until the symptoms are gone and reducing the amount of stress are important in the recovery phase. A gastric resection is an option only when serious erosion has occurred.
CN: Safe, effective care environment; CNS: Coordinated care; CL: Comprehension

13. 4. *H. pylori* infection can lead to chronic atrophic gastritis. Chronic gastritis can occur at any age but is more common in older adults. It may be caused by conditions that allow reflux of bile acids into the stomach. Drugs such as nonsteroidal anti-inflammatory agents, not antibiotics, may cause gastritis. Chronic gastritis isn't related to gallbladder disease.
CN: Physiological integrity; CNS: Physiological adaptation; CL: Application

14. 2. With gastritis, the stomach lining becomes thin and atrophic, decreasing stomach acid secretion (the source of intrinsic factor). This decrease causes a reduction in the absorption of vitamin B_{12}, leading to pernicious anemia.
CN: Physiological integrity; CNS: Physiological adaptation; CL: Comprehension

15. 2. Diverticulosis involves a noninflamed outpouching of the intestine. Diverticulitis involves an inflamed outpouching. Partial impairment of the forward flow of the intestine is an obstruction; abnormal protrusion of an organ is a hernia.
CN: Physiological integrity; CNS: Physiological adaptation; CL: Application

16. 1. A low-fiber diet has been implicated in the development of diverticula because this diet decreases the bulk in the stools and predisposes the person to the development of constipation. A high-fiber diet is recommended to help prevent diverticulosis. A high-protein or low-carbohydrate diet has no effect on the development of diverticulosis.
CN: Physiological integrity; CNS: Basic care and comfort; CL: Analysis

CN: Client needs category CNS: Client needs subcategory CL: Cognitive level

17. Which foods should be avoided by a client with diverticulosis to reduce the risk of complications?
1. Bran cereal and lettuce
2. Dried apricots and raisins
3. Cucumbers and tomatoes
4. Brown rice and fresh peeled apples

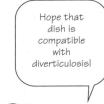
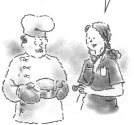

Hope that dish is compatible with diverticulosis!

18. When collecting data from a client with suspected diverticulosis, which symptom would the nurse expect the client to report?
1. Absence of symptoms
2. Change in bowel habits
3. Anorexia and low-grade fever
4. Episodic, dull, or steady midabdominal pain

19. Which test should be administered to a client suspected of having diverticulosis?
1. Abdominal ultrasound
2. Barium enema
3. Barium swallow
4. Gastroscopy

20. A client was hospitalized and treated for acute diverticulitis. The nurse has provided discharge teaching. Which statement by the client indicates that he understands his discharge instructions?
1. "I'll reduce my fluid intake."
2. "I'll decrease the fiber in my diet."
3. "I'll take all of my antibiotics."
4. "I'll exercise to increase my intra-abdominal pressure."

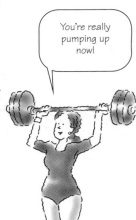

You're really pumping up now!

17. 3. A client with diverticulosis should avoid cucumbers and fresh tomatoes because their seeds can irritate the bowel and contribute to diverticular obstruction. To promote regular bowel movements, the client should consume foods that are high in undigestible fiber, such as bran cereal, lettuce, apricots, raisins, brown rice, and fresh peeled apples.
CN: Health promotion and maintenance; CNS: None; CL: Knowledge

18. 1. Diverticulosis is an asymptomatic condition. The other choices are signs and symptoms of diverticulitis.
CN: Physiological integrity; CNS: Physiological adaptation; CL: Application

19. 2. A barium enema will cause diverticula to fill with barium and be easily seen on an X-ray. An abdominal ultrasound can tell more about such structures as the gallbladder, liver, and spleen than the intestine. A barium swallow and gastroscopy view upper GI structures.
CN: Health promotion and maintenance; CNS: None; CL: Comprehension

20. 3. Antibiotics are used to reduce inflammation. The client with acute diverticulitis typically isn't allowed anything orally until the acute episode subsides. Parenteral fluids are given until the client feels better; then it's recommended that the client drink eight 8-oz (237-ml) glasses of water per day and gradually increase fiber in the diet to improve intestinal motility. During the acute phase, activities that increase intra-abdominal pressure should be avoided to decrease pain and the chance of intestinal obstruction.
CN: Safe, effective care environment; CNS: Safety and infection control; CL: Analysis

CN: Client needs category   CNS: Client needs subcategory   CL: Cognitive level

21. The nurse has taught a teenage client and his parents about Crohn's disease and the dietary changes needed to manage it. Which statement by the parents indicates an accurate understanding of their child's dietary needs?
   1. "We'll need to include plenty of calories in the diet."
   2. "We'll need to make certain that all food is gluten-free."
   3. "We'll be sure to use only low-sodium foods."
   4. "We'll provide high-fiber foods."

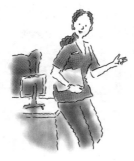

It's important to include the client's family in the teaching process.

22. Which area of the alimentary canal is the <u>most common</u> location of Crohn's disease?
   1. Ascending colon
   2. Descending colon
   3. Sigmoid colon
   4. Terminal ileum

23. When reviewing the history of a client with Crohn's disease, which factor would the nurse associate with this disorder?
   1. Constipation
   2. Diet
   3. Heredity
   4. Lack of exercise

24. Which factor is believed to cause ulcerative colitis?
   1. Acidic diet
   2. Altered immunity
   3. Chronic constipation
   4. Emotional stress

21. 1. Crohn's disease is an inflammatory bowel disease that causes diarrhea with subsequent weight loss and malnutrition. A high-calorie, nutritious diet helps replenish nutrients that are lost through the affected bowel. A gluten-free diet is appropriate for a client with celiac disease, not Crohn's disease. A client with Crohn's disease doesn't need to restrict dietary sodium but should avoid high-fiber foods during a flare-up of the disease because they can contribute to bowel irritation.
CN: Physiological integrity; CNS: Basic care and comfort; CL: Application

22. 4. Studies have shown that the terminal ileum is the most common site for recurrence in clients with Crohn's disease. The other areas may be involved but aren't as common.
CN: Physiological integrity; CNS: Physiological adaptation; CL: Knowledge

23. 3. Although the definitive cause of Crohn's disease is unknown, it's thought to be associated with infectious or immune factors. Because it has a higher incidence in siblings, it may have a genetic cause. Constipation isn't linked to Crohn's disease. On the contrary, Crohn's disease causes bouts of diarrhea. Diet may contribute to exacerbations of Crohn's disease but isn't considered a cause. A lack of exercise isn't considered a cause of Crohn's disease.
CN: Health promotion and maintenance; CNS: None; CL: Application

24. 2. Several theories exist regarding the cause of ulcerative colitis. One suggests altered immunity as the cause based on the extraintestinal characteristics of the disease, such as peripheral arthritis and cholangitis. Diet and constipation have no effect on the development of ulcerative colitis. Emotional stress may exacerbate the attacks but isn't believed to be the primary cause.
CN: Health promotion and maintenance; CNS: None; CL: Comprehension

CN: Client needs category   CNS: Client needs subcategory   CL: Cognitive level

25. The nurse would consider a client with which condition as most at risk for developing a fistula?
1. Crohn's disease
2. Diverticulitis
3. Diverticulosis
4. Ulcerative colitis

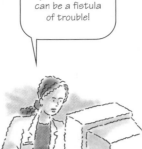

Exam questions sure can be a fistula of trouble!

26. Which area is the <u>most common</u> site of fistulas in clients with Crohn's disease?
1. Anorectal
2. Ileum
3. Rectovaginal
4. Transverse colon

27. A client who reports a number of GI-related symptoms is diagnosed with ulcerative colitis. The nurse explains that ulcerative colitis is:
1. an inflammatory disease of the colon and rectum.
2. an inflammatory disease of the GI tract from the mouth to the anus.
3. a disease that forms outpouches in the large colon.
4. an opening between two or more body structures or spaces.

Many GI disorders have similar symptoms. Pay attention to which one the question is asking about.

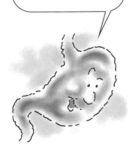

28. A 28-year-old client has been diagnosed with Crohn's disease. The nurse knows that the client may develop which associated disorder?
1. Ankylosing spondylitis
2. Colon cancer
3. Malabsorption syndrome
4. Pernicious anemia

29. Which symptom, if reported by a client, should lead the nurse to suspect Crohn's disease?
1. Bloody diarrhea
2. Weight gain
3. Nausea and vomiting
4. Excessive amounts of fats in the feces

25. 1. The lesions of Crohn's disease are *transmural;* that is, they involve all thicknesses of the bowel. These lesions may perforate the bowel wall, forming fistulas in adjacent structures. Fistulas don't develop in diverticulitis or diverticulosis. The ulcers that occur in the submucosal and mucosal layers of the intestine in ulcerative colitis usually don't progress to fistula formation as in Crohn's disease.
CN: Physiological integrity; CNS: Physiological adaptation; CL: Application

26. 1. Fistulas occur in all these areas, but the anorectal area is most common because of the relative thinness of the intestinal wall in this area.
CN: Physiological integrity; CNS: Physiological adaptation; CL: Comprehension

27. 1. Ulcerative colitis is an inflammatory disease that affects the mucosal lining of the colon and rectum. Crohn's disease commonly affects the entire GI tract, from the mouth to the anus. Diverticulitis causes outpouching in the large colon. A fistula is an opening between two or more body structures.
CN: Physiological integrity; CNS: Physiological adaptation; CL: Application

28. 3. Because of the transmural nature of Crohn's disease lesions, malabsorption may occur. Ankylosing spondylitis and colon cancer are more commonly associated with ulcerative colitis. Pernicious anemia is associated with vitamin B_{12} deficiency.
CN: Physiological integrity; CNS: Physiological adaptation; CL: Application

29. 4. Excessive amounts of fats in the feces due to malabsorption can occur with Crohn's disease. Weight loss (not weight gain) is common. Nausea, vomiting, and bloody diarrhea are symptoms of ulcerative colitis.
CN: Health promotion and maintenance; CNS: None; CL: Application

CN: Client needs category   CNS: Client needs subcategory   CL: Cognitive level

30. Which statement by a client indicates that the nurse's teaching regarding ulcerative colitis has been effective?
1. "I'll have a nutritional deficit."
2. "I might have rectal bleeding."
3. "I'll have soft stools."
4. "I'll have weight loss."

31. If a client had irritable bowel syndrome, which diagnostic test would determine whether the diagnosis is Crohn's disease or ulcerative colitis?
1. Abdominal computed tomography (CT) scan
2. Abdominal X-ray
3. Barium swallow
4. Colonoscopy with biopsy

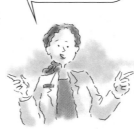

One of these tests can help you distinguish between two GI disorders.

32. Which intervention should be included in the medical management of Crohn's disease?
1. Increasing oral intake of fiber
2. Administering laxatives
3. Using long-term steroid therapy
4. Increasing physical activity

Be sure to consider what the question is asking about. Is it the disease or the treatment?

33. Which effect should a nurse judge as <u>most</u> likely to be caused by antibiotic therapy for a client with Crohn's disease?
1. Decrease in bleeding
2. Increase in body temperature
3. Decrease in body weight
4. Increase in number of stools

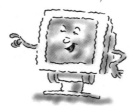

34. A nurse would expect to prepare a client with ulcerative colitis for surgery if the client develops which complication?
1. Gastritis
2. Bowel herniation
3. Bowel outpouching
4. Bowel perforation

30. 2. In ulcerative colitis, rectal bleeding is the predominant symptom. Nutritional deficit, soft stools, and weight loss are more commonly associated with Crohn's disease, in which malabsorption is more of a problem.
CN: Health promotion and maintenance; CNS: None; CL: Application

31. 4. A colonoscopy with biopsy can be performed to determine the state of the colon's mucosal layers, presence of ulcerations, and level of cytologic involvement. An abdominal X-ray or CT scan wouldn't provide the cytologic information necessary to diagnose which disease it is. A barium swallow doesn't involve the intestine.
CN: Physiological integrity; CNS: Physiological adaptation; CL: Application

32. 3. Management of Crohn's disease may include long-term steroid therapy to reduce the extensive inflammation associated with the deeper layers of the bowel wall. Other management focuses on bowel rest (not increasing oral intake) and reducing diarrhea with medications (not giving laxatives). The pain associated with Crohn's disease may require bed rest (not an increase in physical activity).
CN: Physiological integrity; CNS: Basic care and comfort; CL: Application

33. 1. A decrease in bleeding, body temperature, and number of stools indicates the effectiveness of antibiotic therapy. A decrease in body weight may occur during therapy because of inadequate dietary intake but it isn't related to antibiotic therapy.
CN: Physiological integrity; CNS: Pharmacological therapies; CL: Analysis

34. 4. Perforation, obstruction, hemorrhage, and toxic megacolon are common complications of ulcerative colitis that may require surgery. Herniation and gastritis aren't associated with irritable bowel diseases, and outpouching of the bowel wall is diverticulosis.
CN: Safe, effective care environment; CNS: Safety and infection control; CL: Application

CN: Client needs category   CNS: Client needs subcategory   CL: Cognitive level

35. A 35-year-old client with irritable bowel syndome (IBS) is complaining of pain. The nurse should expect which medication to be administered to help alleviate the underlying cause of his pain?
1. Acetaminophen
2. Opiates
3. Steroids
4. Stool softeners

36. During the first few days of recovery from ostomy surgery for ulcerative colitis, which aspect should be the <u>first priority</u> of client care?
1. Body image
2. Ostomy care
3. Sexual concerns
4. Skin care

37. During discharge teaching for a client with ulcerative colitis, the nurse emphasizes the importance of regular physical examinations. The nurse is aware that ulcerative colitis increases the client's risk of developing which disorder?
1. Appendicitis
2. Hemorrhoids
3. Hiatal hernia
4. Colon cancer

38. Which diet is <u>most commonly</u> associated with colon cancer?
1. Low fiber, high fat
2. Low fat, high fiber
3. Low protein, high carbohydrate
4. Low carbohydrate, high protein

39. A nurse is teaching a 52-year-old client about cancer screening. The nurse emphasizes that which diagnostic test should be performed annually after age 50 for a client with average risk to screen for colon cancer?
1. Abdominal computed tomography (CT) scan
2. Abdominal X-ray
3. Colonoscopy
4. Multiple sample fecal occult blood test

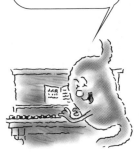

What's a key step in treating a patient who has had ostomy surgery?

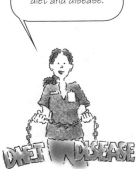

The exam will test your understanding of the links between diet and disease.

35. 3. The pain of IBS is caused by inflammation, which steroids can reduce. Acetaminophen has little effect on the pain, and opiates won't treat its underlying cause. Stool softeners aren't necessary.
CN: Physiological integrity; CNS: Pharmacological therapies; CL: Application

36. 2. Although all of these are concerns the nurse should address, being able to safely manage the ostomy is crucial for the client before discharge.
CN: Physiological integrity; CNS: Basic care and comfort; CL: Application

37. 4. Clients with chronic ulcerative colitis, granulomas, and familial polyposis have an increased risk of developing colon cancer. Clients with ulcerative colitis don't have an increased risk of developing the other disorders.
CN: Health promotion and maintenance; CNS: None; CL: Application

38. 1. A low-fiber, high-fat diet reduces motility and increases the chance of constipation. The metabolic end products of this type of diet are carcinogenic. A low-fat, high-fiber diet is recommended to help avoid colon cancer. Carbohydrates and protein aren't necessarily associated with colon cancer.
CN: Health promotion and maintenance; CNS: None; CL: Knowledge

39. 4. The American Cancer Society guidelines include annual screenings for colon cancer using multiple sample fecal occult blood tests beginning at age 50 for clients at average risk. CT scan and abdominal X-ray can help establish tumor size and metastasis. A colonoscopy can help locate a tumor as well as polyps and can be used for screening every 10 years.
CN: Health promotion and maintenance; CNS: None; CL: Application

40. A client with colon cancer asks the nurse why he's getting radiation therapy before surgery. Which response would be most appropriate?
   1. "It helps reduce the size of the tumor."
   2. "It eliminates the malignant cells."
   3. "The chances of curing the cancer are improved."
   4. "The therapy helps to heal the bowel after surgery."

41. Which symptom is a client with colon cancer most likely to exhibit?
   1. Change in appetite
   2. Change in bowel habits
   3. Increase in body weight
   4. Increase in body temperature

42. A client has just had surgery for colon cancer. The nurse should observe this client for symptoms that might indicate the development of which complication?
   1. Peritonitis
   2. Diverticulosis
   3. Partial bowel obstruction
   4. Complete bowel obstruction

43. Which symptom, if reported by a client, would lead the nurse to suspect possible gastric cancer?
   1. Abdominal cramping
   2. Constant hunger
   3. Feeling of fullness
   4. Weight gain

44. A 56-year-old client is suspected of having gastric cancer. The nurse expects which diagnostic test to aid in confirming the diagnosis of gastric cancer?
   1. Barium enema
   2. Colonoscopy
   3. Gastroscopy
   4. Serum chemistry levels

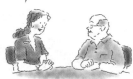

I'll answer your questions to help put you at ease.

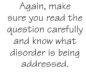

Again, make sure you read the question carefully and know what disorder is being addressed.

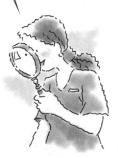

40. 1. Radiation therapy is used to treat colon cancer before surgery to reduce the size of the tumor, making it easier to resect. Radiation therapy can't eliminate the malignant cells (though it helps to define tumor margins), isn't curative, and could slow postoperative healing. CN: Physiological integrity; CNS: Reduction of risk potential; CL: Application

41. 2. The most common complaint of the client with colon cancer is a change in bowel habits. The client may have anorexia, secondary abdominal distention, or weight loss. Fever isn't related to colon cancer. CN: Physiological integrity; CNS: Basic care and comfort; CL: Application

42. 1. Bowel spillage could occur during surgery, resulting in peritonitis. Diverticulosis doesn't result from surgery for colon cancer. Complete or partial intestinal obstruction may occur *before* bowel resection. CN: Physiological integrity; CNS: Physiological adaptation; CL: Application

43. 3. The client with gastric cancer may report a feeling of fullness in the stomach, but not enough to cause him to seek medical care. Abdominal cramping isn't associated with gastric cancer. Anorexia and weight loss (not increased hunger or weight gain) are common symptoms of gastric cancer. CN: Physiological integrity; CNS: Physiological adaptation; CL: Application

44. 3. A gastroscopy will allow direct visualization of the tumor. A barium enema or colonoscopy would help to diagnose *colon* cancer. Serum chemistry levels don't contribute data useful to the assessment of gastric cancer. CN: Health promotion and maintenance; CNS: None; CL: Application

CN: Client needs category   CNS: Client needs subcategory   CL: Cognitive level

45. A client with gastric cancer can expect to have surgery for resection. Which should be the nursing care <u>priority</u> for the preoperative client with gastric cancer?
   1. Discharge planning
   2. Correction of nutritional deficits
   3. Prevention of deep vein thrombosis
   4. Instruction regarding radiation treatment

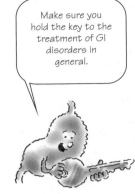

Make sure you hold the key to the treatment of GI disorders in general.

45. 2. Clients with gastric cancer commonly have nutritional deficits and may be cachectic. Discharge planning before surgery is important, but correcting the nutritional deficit is a higher priority. Prevention of deep vein thrombosis also isn't a high priority before surgery, though it assumes greater importance after surgery. At present, radiation therapy hasn't been proven effective for gastric cancer, and teaching about it preoperatively wouldn't be appropriate.
CN: Physiological integrity; CNS: Basic care and comfort; CL: Application

46. When assisting with development of a postoperative care plan for a client after gastric resection, which of the following would be the priority?
   1. Body image
   2. Nutritional needs
   3. Skin care
   4. Spiritual needs

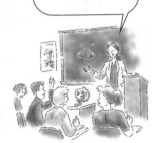

Knowing what to teach your client can help avoid problems down the road.

46. 2. After gastric resection, a client may require total parenteral nutrition or jejunostomy tube feedings to maintain adequate nutritional status. Body image isn't much of a problem for this client because clothing can cover the incision site. Wound care of the incision site is necessary to prevent infection; otherwise, the skin shouldn't be affected. Spiritual needs may be a concern, depending on the client, and should be addressed as the client demonstrates readiness to share concerns.
CN: Physiological integrity; CNS: Basic care and comfort; CL: Application

47. A nurse should teach the client to watch for which complication of gastric resection?
   1. Constipation
   2. Dumping syndrome
   3. Gastric spasm
   4. Intestinal spasms

47. 2. Dumping syndrome is a problem that occurs postprandially after gastric resection because ingested food rapidly enters the jejunum without proper mixing and without the normal duodenal digestive processing. Diarrhea, not constipation, may also be a symptom. Gastric or intestinal spasms don't occur, but antispasmodics may be given to slow gastric emptying.
CN: Health promotion and maintenance; CNS: None; CL: Application

48. A client reports having several episodes of rectal bleeding, ribbon-shaped stools, and abdominal cramping. The nurse recognizes these signs and symptoms as related to which disorder?
   1. Hemorrhoids
   2. Irritable bowel syndrome (IBS)
   3. Colorectal cancer
   4. Liver cancer

48. 3. Rectal bleeding, ribbon-shaped stools, and abdominal cramping are all associated with colorectal cancer but these signs and symptoms aren't all associated with the other conditions. IBS can produce abdominal cramping but not rectal bleeding. Hemorrhoids can cause rectal bleeding. Liver cancer isn't related to these symptoms.
CN: Physiological integrity; CNS: Physiological adaptation; CL: Analysis

CN: Client needs category   CNS: Client needs subcategory   CL: Cognitive level

49. A client with which condition may be <u>likely</u> to develop rectal cancer?
1. Adenomatous polyps
2. Diverticulitis
3. Hemorrhoids
4. Peptic ulcer disease

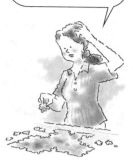

Note the word *likely.* It's an important piece to this puzzle.

49. 1. A client with adenomatous polyps has a higher risk of developing rectal cancer than others do. Clients with diverticulitis are more likely to develop colon cancer. Hemorrhoids don't increase the chance of any type of cancer. Clients with peptic ulcer disease have a higher incidence of gastric cancer.
CN: Health promotion and maintenance; CNS: None; CL: Analysis

50. A nurse is preparing to reinforce the teaching plan for a client with peptic ulcer disease who's scheduled to have a vagotomy. Which teaching point about the vagotomy procedure is correct?
1. Vagotomy is removal of the antrum of the stomach.
2. Vagotomy is removal of 60% to 80% of the stomach.
3. Vagotomy is the severing of the vagus nerve.
4. Vagotomy is the enlargement of the pyloric sphincter.

50. 3. The vagus nerve receives impulses from the brain to secrete hydrochloric acid. A vagotomy severs the vagus nerve, which decreases gastric acid by diminishing cholinergic stimulation to the parietal cells, making them less responsive to gastrin. Removal of the antrum is an antrectomy. Removal of 60% to 80% of the stomach is a gastrectomy. Surgically enlarging the pyloric sphincter is a pyloroplasty.
CN: Physiological integrity; CNS: Physiological adaptation; CL: Application

51. Which condition may cause hemorrhoids?
1. Diarrhea
2. Diverticulosis
3. Portal hypertension
4. Rectal bleeding

This question is looking for the most important assessment for diagnosis.

51. 3. Portal hypertension and other conditions associated with persistently high intra-abdominal pressure, such as pregnancy, can aggravate hemorrhoids. The passing of hard stools, not diarrhea, can lead to hemorrhoids. Diverticulosis has no relationship to hemorrhoids. Rectal bleeding can be a symptom of hemorrhoids.
CN: Physiological integrity; CNS: Physiological adaptation; CL: Analysis

52. A nurse is reviewing data to determine confirmation of a diagnosis of hemorrhoids. Which data would actually confirm hemorrhoids?
1. Palpation of the abdomen
2. Diet history
3. Results of digital rectal examination
4. Sexual history

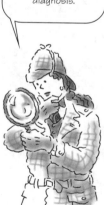

52. 3. Digital rectal examination is important to assess for internal hemorrhoids and determine whether other causes of the pain and bleeding are present. Palpation of the abdomen isn't necessary for hemorrhoids. Diet history is relevant because constipation can worsen hemorrhoids but isn't as important to diagnosis as a digital rectal examination. Sexual history may also be relevant but, again, it isn't as important as a digital rectal examination.
CN: Physiological integrity; CNS: Physiological adaptation; CL: Application

53. Which response by a client with hemorrhoids indicates that the nurse's teaching regarding his medical management has been effective?

1. "I'll eat a high-fiber diet."
2. "I'll apply a cold pack to reduce swelling."
3. "I'll use an astringent lotion to reduce swelling."
4. "I should elevate my buttocks to reduce engorgement."

54. Which response should a nurse offer to a client who asks why he's having a vagotomy to treat his ulcer?

1. To repair a hole in the stomach
2. To reduce the ability of the stomach to produce acid
3. To prevent the stomach from sliding into the chest
4. To remove a potentially malignant lesion in the stomach

55. What's the <u>best</u> postoperative position for a client who had a ruptured appendix and who now has peritonitis?

1. Dorsal decubitus
2. Lateral decubitus
3. Flat
4. Semi-Fowler's

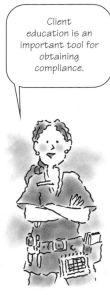

Client education is an important tool for obtaining compliance.

56. A client is admitted with absent bowel sounds, abdominal distention, rebound tenderness, and muscle rigidity. Which diagnosis would the nurse expect to receive?

1. Peritonitis
2. Diverticulitis
3. Dumping syndrome
4. Normal symptoms of diverticulosis

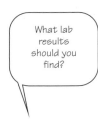

What lab results should you find?

57. Which laboratory result would be expected in a client with peritonitis?

1. Partial thromboplastin time (PTT) longer than 100 seconds
2. Hemoglobin (Hb) level below 10 mg/dl
3. Potassium level above 5.5 mEq/L
4. White blood cell (WBC) count above 15,000/µl

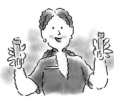

53. 1. A high-fiber diet will add bulk to the stools and ease their passage through the rectum. Application of cold isn't recommended because it can cause injury to the tissue. Astringent lotions can be used to reduce pain. The buttocks should be elevated only when prolapsed hemorrhoids are present.
CN: Physiological integrity; CNS: Physiological adaptation; CL: Application

54. 2. A vagotomy is performed to eliminate the acid-secreting stimulus to gastric cells. A perforation would be repaired with a gastric resection. Repair of hiatal hernia (fundoplication) prevents the stomach from sliding through the diaphragm. Removal of a potentially malignant tumor wouldn't reduce the entire acid-producing mechanism.
CN: Physiological integrity; CNS: Reduction of risk potential; CL: Application

55. 4. Clients with peritonitis are maintained in semi-Fowler's position to keep abdominal contents below the diaphragm to promote lung expansion. The other positions would be inappropriate because the client's head should be elevated to maintain comfort and prevent complications.
CN: Physiological integrity; CNS: Physiological adaptation; CL: Application

56. 1. Absent bowel sounds, abdominal distention, rebound tenderness, and muscle rigidity are symptoms of peritonitis. Diverticulitis is multiple diverticula of the colon. The major signs and symptoms of diverticulitis are intervals of diarrhea, abrupt onset of cramping pain in the lower left quadrant of the abdomen, and a low-grade fever. Dumping syndrome is rapid emptying of the stomach contents into the small intestine. It produces sweating and weakness after eating. Diverticulosis is an asymptomatic condition.
CN: Health promotion and maintenance; CNS: None; CL: Comprehension

57. 4. Because of infection, the client's WBC count will be elevated. A PTT longer than 100 seconds may suggest disseminated intravascular coagulation, a serious complication of septic shock. A hemoglobin level below 10 mg/dl may occur from hemorrhage. A potassium level above 5.5 mEq/L may suggest renal failure.
CN: Physiological integrity; CNS: Physiological adaptation; CL: Application

CN: Client needs category   CNS: Client needs subcategory   CL: Cognitive level

58. A recently admitted client is suspected of having peritonitis. He's requesting a glass of water to drink. The nurse's best response to the client would be which statement?

1. "I can give you small amounts of water frequently."
2. "You're getting your fluids intravenously."
3. "I'll check with the physician."
4. "Until your diagnosis is confirmed and bowel function returns, it wouldn't be safe to give you anything to drink."

59. A client had a gastroscopy while under local anesthesia. Before resuming the client's oral fluid intake, what should the nurse do first?

1. Listen for bowel sounds.
2. Determine whether the client can talk.
3. Check for a gag reflex.
4. Determine the client's mental status.

60. Which factor is most commonly associated with the development of pancreatitis?

1. Alcohol abuse
2. Hypercalcemia
3. Hyperlipidemia
4. Pancreatic duct obstruction

61. A client with pancreatitis asks the nurse how pancreatic enzymes can damage the pancreas. Which explanation by the nurse is <u>most</u> accurate?

1. "The enzymes are utilized by the intestines."
2. "The enzymes autodigest the pancreas."
3. "The enzymes lead to reflux into the gallbladder."
4. "The enzymes block the pancreatic duct."

62. Which laboratory test is used to diagnose pancreatitis?

1. Lipase level
2. Hemoglobin (Hb) level
3. Blood glucose level
4. White blood cell (WBC) count

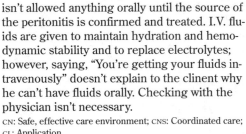

Read question 61 carefully before you answer. Make sure you know what it's asking.

58. 4. The client with peritonitis commonly isn't allowed anything orally until the source of the peritonitis is confirmed and treated. I.V. fluids are given to maintain hydration and hemodynamic stability and to replace electrolytes; however, saying, "You're getting your fluids intravenously" doesn't explain to the clinent why he can't have fluids orally. Checking with the physician isn't necessary.
CN: Safe, effective care environment; CNS: Coordinated care; CL: Application

59. 3. After a gastroscopy, the nurse should check for the presence of a gag reflex before giving oral fluids. This step is essential to prevent aspiration. The presence of bowel sounds, the ability to speak, and mental status within normal limits wouldn't ensure the presence of a gag reflex.
CN: Physiological integrity; CNS: Reduction of risk potential; CL: Application

60. 1. Alcohol abuse is the major cause of acute pancreatitis in males, although gallbladder disease is more commonly implicated in women. Hypercalcemia, hyperlipidemia, and pancreatic duct obstruction are also causes of pancreatitis, but they're less common.
CN: Physiological integrity; CNS: Reduction of risk potential; CL: Comprehension

61. 2. In pancreatitis, pancreatic enzymes become activated and begin to autodigest the pancreas instead of being excreted into the duodenum. The enzymes are activated but aren't used properly by the intestine. Reflux of bile, not enzymes, into the pancreatic duct and clogging of the pancreatic duct may occur before autodigestion of the pancreas occurs.
CN: Physiological integrity; CNS: Physiological adaptation; CL: Application

62. 1. Lipase is an enzyme secreted by the pancreas; when elevated, it's useful in diagnosing pancreatitis. Hb level can be low in pancreatitis, but there are other causes for this. The blood glucose level may be elevated with pancreatitis, but this factor isn't diagnostic. The WBC count may also be elevated in pancreatitis, but this symptom can be caused by infection.
CN: Health promotion and maintenance; CNS: None; CL: Analysis

CN: Client needs category   CNS: Client needs subcategory   CL: Cognitive level

63. A nurse is caring for a client with acute pancreatitis. The nurse knows that it's most important to monitor the client closely for which sign or symptom?
1. Increased appetite
2. Vomiting
3. Hypoglycemia
4. Pain

63. 2. Acute pancreatitis is commonly associated with fluid isolation and accumulation in the bowel secondary to ileus or peripancreatic edema. Fluid and electrolyte loss from vomiting is the primary concern. A client with acute pancreatitis may have increased pain on eating and is unlikely to demonstrate an increased appetite. A client with acute pancreatitis is at risk for hyperglycemia, not hypoglycemia. Although pain is an important concern, it's less significant than vomiting.
CN: Physiological integrity; CNS: Physiological adaptation; CL: Application

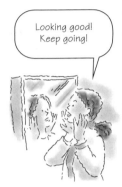

Looking good! Keep going!

64. A nurse is caring for a client with suspected upper GI bleeding. The nurse should monitor this client for:
1. hemoptysis.
2. hematuria.
3. passage of bright red blood in the stools.
4. black, tarry stools.

64. 4. As blood from the GI tract passes through the intestines, bacterial action causes it to become black. Hemoptysis involves coughing up blood from the lungs. Hematuria is blood in the urine. Bright red blood in the stools indicates bleeding from the lower GI tract.
CN: Physiological integrity; CNS: Physiological adaptation; CL: Application

65. What's the <u>most important</u> nursing goal for a client who has had a barium enema?
1. To prevent fecal incontinence
2. To monitor for bleeding
3. To prevent constipation
4. To limit fluid intake

65. 3. Barium should be promptly eliminated from the client's system after it has been introduced into the colon to prevent mass formation and possible bowel obstruction. Therefore, laxatives or enemas are commonly given after a barium enema to prevent the client from becoming constipated. Fecal incontinence isn't an issue because the passage of stools is desired. Bleeding isn't commonly anticipated after a barium enema. The client should be encouraged to increase, not decrease, fluid intake.
CN: Physiological integrity; CNS: Reduction of risk potential; CL: Application

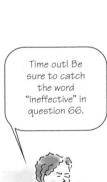

Time out! Be sure to catch the word "ineffective" in question 66.

66. Which action would be <u>ineffective</u> in the immediate management of a client with a perforated gastric ulcer?
1. Blood replacement
2. Antacid administration
3. Nasogastric (NG) tube suction
4. Fluid and electrolyte replacement

66. 2. Antacids aren't helpful in perforation. The client should be treated with antibiotics as well as blood, fluid, and electrolyte replacement. NG tube suction should also be performed to prevent further spillage of stomach contents into the peritoneal cavity.
CN: Physiological integrity; CNS: Physiological adaptation; CL: Application

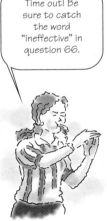

CN: Client needs category   CNS: Client needs subcategory   CL: Cognitive level

67. A nurse is caring for a client with chronic pancreatitis. Which response by the client indicates that discharge teaching has been effective?
1. "I'll eat a low-carbohydrate diet."
2. "I can have an occasional glass of wine."
3. "I'll take pancreatic enzymes with each meal."
4. "I'll take pancreatic enzymes before breakfast and at bedtime."

67. 3. Oral pancreatic enzymes are taken with each meal to aid digestion and control steatorrhea. The client should adhere to a low-fat, not low-carbohydrate, diet. The client should eliminate alcohol from his diet completely as it will continue to cause pancreatic damage.
CN: Physiological integrity; CNS: Physiological adaptation; CL: Analysis

68. In alcohol-related acute pancreatitis, which intervention is the best way to reduce the exacerbation of pain?
1. Lying supine
2. Taking aspirin
3. Eating a low-fat diet
4. Abstaining from alcohol

68. 4. Abstaining from alcohol is imperative to reduce injury to the pancreas; in fact, it may be enough to completely control pain. Lying supine usually aggravates the pain because it stretches the abdominal muscles. Taking aspirin can cause bleeding in hemorrhagic pancreatitis. During an attack of acute pancreatitis, the client usually isn't allowed to ingest anything orally.
CN: Physiological integrity; CNS: Reduction of risk potential; CL: Application

69. A nurse is completing the intake record for a client with chronic pancreatitis. The client has had the following intake during the previous 8 hours. How many milliliters should the nurse record as the client's intake? Record the answer using a whole number.
Intake:
4 oz apple juice
½ cup fruit-flavored gelatin
6 oz water
500 ml 0.45% sodium chloride I.V.
_____ ml

69. 920. Fluid intake for this client includes 4 oz (120 ml) apple juice, ½ cup (120 ml) fruit-flavored gelatin, 6 oz (180 ml) water, and 500 ml 0.45% sodium chloride I.V. for a total of 920 ml.
CN: Physiological integrity; CNS: Basic care and comfort; CL: Application

70. A client with biliary cirrhosis asks the nurse what the cause of this disorder is. What's the most appropriate response by the nurse?
1. "It's caused by an acute viral infection of the liver."
2. "It's caused by alcohol hepatotoxicity."
3. "It's caused by chronic biliary inflammation or obstruction."
4. "It's caused by right-sided heart failure that leads to venous hepatic congestion."

70. 3. Chronic biliary inflammation or obstruction causes biliary cirrhosis. Acute viral hepatitis can cause postnecrotic cirrhosis. Alcohol hepatotoxicity is Laënnec's cirrhosis. Heart failure with prolonged venous hepatic congestion will cause cardiac cirrhosis.
CN: Physiological integrity; CNS: Physiological adaptation; CL: Application

71. A 65-year-old client is admitted with upper GI bleeding from esophageal varices. Which condition can lead to the development of esophageal varices?
1. Cirrhosis of the liver
2. Pancreatitis
3. Ileus
4. Cholecystitis

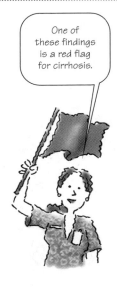

One of these findings is a red flag for cirrhosis.

72. Which diagnostic test helps determine a definitive diagnosis for cirrhosis?
1. Albumin level
2. Bromsulphalein dye excretion
3. Liver biopsy
4. Liver enzyme levels

73. While caring for a client with cirrhosis, the nurse reviews the laboratory data in the client's chart. Which data should the nurse expect to find?
1. Decreased carbon dioxide level
2. Elevated pH level
3. Prolonged prothrombin time (PT)
4. Decreased white blood cell (WBC) count

74. Which measure should a nurse focus on for the client with esophageal varices?
1. Recognizing hemorrhage
2. Controlling blood pressure
3. Encouraging nutritional intake
4. Teaching the client about varices

71. 1. Cirrhosis is marked by scarring of the liver with obstruction of blood flow and development of portal vein hypertension. High portal venous pressures cause enlarged, fragile veins to develop in the stomach and esophagus. Severe pancreatitis can cause bleeding into the abdominal cavity. Ileus is a bowel obstruction. Cholecystitis can lead to perforation and peritonitis but not to portal hypertension.
CN: Physiological integrity; CNS: Physiological adaptation; CL: Application

72. 3. A liver biopsy can reveal the exact cause of the hepatomegaly and this is the test used to determine a definitive diagnosis of cirrhosis. The albumin level will be low, but that can be caused by poor nutritional status. Bromsulphalein dye excretion may be reduced, but other hepatocirculatory disorders could also cause this. Liver enzymes may be elevated, but other liver conditions may cause these elevations.
CN: Physiological integrity; CNS: Physiological adaptation; CL: Comprehension

73. 3. Clotting factors may not be produced normally when a client has cirrhosis, increasing the potential for bleeding. PT measures the time required for a fibrin clot to form. There's no associated change in carbon dioxide level or pH unless the client is developing other comorbidities such as metabolic alkalosis. The WBC count can be elevated in acute cirrhosis but isn't always altered.
CN: Physiological integrity; CNS: Physiological adaptation; CL: Application

74. 1. Recognizing the rupture of esophageal varices, or hemorrhage, is the focus of nursing care because the client could succumb to this quickly. Controlling blood pressure is also important because it helps reduce the risk of variceal rupture. It's also important to teach the client what varices are and what foods he should avoid, such as spicy foods.
CN: Physiological integrity; CNS: Physiological adaptation; CL: Application

75. Which condition is most likely to cause hepatitis?
1. Bacterial infection
2. Biliary dysfunction
3. Metastasis
4. Viral infection

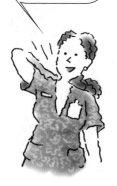

Give yourself a pat on the back! You've completed 75 questions!

75. 4. The most common types of hepatitis are those caused by viruses—hepatitis A, B, C, D, and E. Other types of hepatitis are alcoholic, toxic, and chronic. Bacterial infections rarely cause hepatitis, and biliary dysfunction isn't a cause. Liver metastasis from colon cancer causes liver cancer, not hepatitis.

CN: Health promotion and maintenance; CNS: None; CL: Knowledge

76. Which factor can cause hepatitis A?
1. Blood contact
2. Blood transfusion
3. Contaminated shellfish
4. Sexual contact

76. 3. Hepatitis A can be caused by infected water, milk, or food. Hepatitis B is caused by blood contact and sexual contact. Hepatitis C is usually caused by contact with infected blood, including blood transfusions.

CN: Health promotion and maintenance; CNS: None; CL: Knowledge

77. A nurse is preparing the teaching plan for a client recently diagnosed with hepatitis A. Which teaching statement is correct?
1. The main route of transmission is sputum.
2. The main route of transmission is feces.
3. The main route of transmission is blood.
4. The main route of transmission is urine.

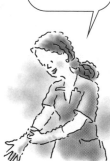

Remember, hepatitis A is highly contagious.

77. 2. The hepatitis A virus is transmitted by the fecal-oral route, primarily through ingestion of contaminated food or liquids. It isn't transmitted via sputum, blood, or urine.

CN: Safe, effective care environment; CNS: Safety and infection control; CL: Application

78. A 25-year-old client reports flulike symptoms, nausea, vomiting, joint pain, and lethargy. The nurse recognizes that these symptoms are most consistent with which condition?
1. Viral hepatitis
2. Nonviral hepatitis
3. Gastric ulcer
4. Cholecystitis

78. 1. Joint pain is very common in clients with viral hepatitis. Other symptoms of viral hepatitis include lethargy, flulike symptoms, anorexia, nausea and vomiting, abdominal pain, diarrhea, constipation, and fever. Nonviral hepatitis doesn't cause joint pain. Gastric ulcer and cholecystitis don't cause joint pain or flulike symptoms.

CN: Physiological integrity; CNS: Physiological adaptation; CL: Application

79. Which client statement indicates that the nurse's teaching about hepatitis A has been effective?
1. "I'll wear a mask all the time."
2. "I should keep my door closed."
3. "I should wash my hands frequently."
4. "I'm allowed to save part of my sandwich to give to my wife."

79. 3. Hepatitis A is transmitted through the fecal-oral route, so frequent hand washing, especially after elimination, will help prevent transmission. It isn't necessary to wear a mask or keep the door closed. Sharing food allows for viral transmission.

CN: Safe, effective care environment; CNS: Safety and infection control; CL: Application

CN: Client needs category   CNS: Client needs subcategory   CL: Cognitive level

80. A nurse is caring for a client with toxic hepatitis. Following the removal of the causative agent, which nursing intervention is a priority?
1. Withholding food and drink
2. Treating adverse effects such as itching
3. Encouraging increased activity
4. Instructing the client about taking corticosteroid medication

81. Which test would be the most accurate for diagnosing liver cancer?
1. Abdominal ultrasound
2. Abdominal flat plate X-ray
3. Cholangiogram
4. Computed tomography (CT) scan

82. Immediately after a liver biopsy, the nurse should closely monitor the client for which complication?
1. Abdominal cramping
2. Hemorrhage
3. Nausea and vomiting
4. Potential infection

83. When a client who has a liver disorder is having an invasive procedure, the nurse helps ensure safety by assessing the results of which test?
1. Coagulation studies
2. Liver enzyme levels
3. Serum chemistries
4. White blood cell count

84. A nurse is giving preoperative and postoperative instructions to a client who will undergo a liver biopsy the next morning. In this situation, patient-teaching information for which problem is most critical?
1. Paralytic ileus
2. Hemorrhage
3. Renal shutdown
4. Constipation

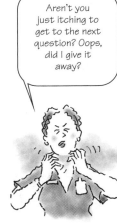

Aren't you just itching to get to the next question? Oops, did I give it away?

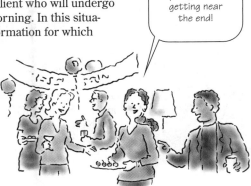

Start the party. You're getting near the end!

80. 2. Along with removal of the causative agent, alleviation of symptoms is the priority. Other interventions include providing a high-calorie diet and promoting rest. Alleviating symptoms and providing comfort will help the client retain the nurse's instructions. The use of corticosteroids is rare; corticosteroids are mainly used to treat autoimmune hepatitis.
CN: Safe, effective care environment; CNS: Coordinated care; CL: Application

81. 4. A client with suspected liver cancer will likely undergo CT imaging to identify tumors. The results of a CT scan are much more definitive than the findings of an ultrasound or X-ray. A cholangiogram evaluates the gallbladder, not the liver.
CN: Health promotion and maintenance; CNS: None; CL: Knowledge

82. 2. The liver is so vascular that taking a biopsy could cause the client to hemorrhage. The client may experience some discomfort but typically not cramping. Nausea and vomiting may be present and infection may occur, but not immediately after the procedure.
CN: Physiological integrity; CNS: Reduction of risk potential; CL: Application

83. 1. The liver produces coagulation factors. If the liver is affected negatively, production of these factors may be altered, placing the client at risk for hemorrhage. The other laboratory tests should be monitored as well, but the results may not necessarily relate to the safety of the procedure.
CN: Physiological integrity; CNS: Reduction of risk potential; CL: Analysis

84. 2. Because the most common adverse effect of a liver biopsy is bleeding, the nurse should provide relevant information regarding the potential for hemorrhage. There's no reason to provide the client with information about a paralytic ileus. Renal shutdown isn't an expected complication after a liver biopsy. The nurse would have no reason to suspect that the client will have a problem with constipation after a liver biopsy.
CN: Physiological integrity; CNS: Reduction of risk potential; CL: Application

CN: Client needs category   CNS: Client needs subcategory   CL: Cognitive level

85. A 53-year-old client was admitted 2 days ago with cirrhosis of the liver. He now appears anxious and irritable, has hand tremors and clammy skin, and wants to leave the hospital. The nurse recognizes these signs and symptoms as indications of which condition?

1. Chronic hepatitis B infection
2. Acute hepatitis C infection
3. Early signs of alcohol withdrawal
4. Late signs of alcohol withdrawal

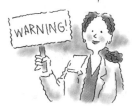

Careful, this question is asking you to identify symptoms.

WARNING!

85. 3. Early signs of alcohol withdrawal include hand tremor, irritability, anxiety, nausea, slight sweating, and alcohol craving. Later signs may include hypertension, hallucinations, seizures, vomiting, tachycardia, and marked confusion. Client's with hepatitis B infection may have nausea, jaundice, and abdominal pain. Client's with acute hepatitis C infection are generally asymptomatic.
CN: Physiological integrity; CNS: Reduction of risk potential; CL: Application

86. When counseling a client in the ways to prevent cholecystitis, which guideline is most important?

1. Eat a low-protein diet.
2. Eat a high-fat, high-cholesterol diet.
3. Limit exercise to 10 minutes per day.
4. Keep weight proportional to height.

86. 4. Obesity is a known cause of gallstones, and maintaining a recommended weight will help to protect against cholecystitis. Excessive dietary intake of cholesterol is associated with the development of gallstones in many people. Dietary protein isn't implicated in cholecystitis. Liquid protein and low-calorie diets (with rapid weight loss of more than 5 lb [2.3 kg] per week) *are* implicated as the cause of some cases of cholecystitis. Regular exercise (30 minutes/three times per week) may help to reduce weight and improve fat metabolism.
CN: Health promotion and maintenance; CNS: None; CL: Application

87. A 45-year-old client is scheduled to undergo a cholecystectomy. He asks the nurse why he is being given atropine sulfate before surgery. The nurse's <u>best</u> response would be which statement?

1. "Atropine is used to relieve pain and anxiety."
2. "Atropine helps ease the induction of anesthesia."
3. "Atropine reduces respiratory secretions."
4. "Atropine prevents infection."

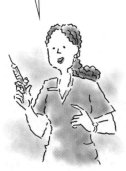

Atropine is ordered preoperatively.

87. 3. Atropine, an anticholinergic agent, is commonly prescribed preoperatively to reduce respiratory tract secretions and prevent the reflex slowing of the heart that occurs during anesthesia. Atropine doesn't relieve pain or anxiety or help ease the induction of anesthesia. Antibiotics may be administered to help prevent infection.
CN: Physiological integrity; CNS: Pharmacological therapies; CL: Application

88. A nurse is reviewing data in a client's chart to determine confirmation of the diagnosis of cholecystitis. Which data would help confirm cholecystitis?

1. Results of a colonoscopy
2. Results of an abdominal ultrasound
3. Results of barium swallow
4. Results of endoscopy

88. 2. An abdominal ultrasound can show if the gallbladder is enlarged, if gallstones are present, if the gallbladder wall is thickened, or if distention of the gallbladder lumen is present. A colonoscopy looks at the inner surface of the colon. A barium swallow looks at the stomach and the duodenum. Endoscopy looks at the esophagus, stomach, and duodenum.
CN: Health promotion and maintenance; CNS: None; CL: Application

89. A nurse has given discharge instructions to a client with chronic cholecystitis. Which response by the client indicates the teaching has been effective?
1. "I need to rest more."
2. "I should avoid taking antacids."
3. "I should increase the fat in my diet."
4. "I will take my anticholinergic medications as prescribed."

90. While a client is being prepared for discharge, the nasogastric (NG) feeding tube becomes clogged. To remedy this problem and teach the client's family how to deal with it at home, what should the nurse do?
1. Irrigate the tube with cola.
2. Advance the tube into the colon.
3. Apply intermittent suction to the tube.
4. Withdraw the clog with a 30-ml syringe.

91. A client with a duodenal ulcer may exhibit which signs and symptoms?
1. Hematemesis
2. Malnourishment
3. Melena
4. Pain with eating

92. Which characteristic is associated with most stress ulcers?
1. A single, well-defined lesion
2. Increased gastric acid production
3. Decreased gastric mucosal blood flow
4. Increased blood flow to gastric mucosa

93. A large group of people has been infected with botulism as a biological weapon. To avoid the need for mechanical ventilation, in which position should each client be placed?
1. Side-lying with a linen roll behind the back to prevent back-lying position
2. Full sitting with suction equipment readily available
3. Flat with the head of the rigid mattress tilted at a 20-degree angle
4. Head of mattress elevated 45 degrees with legs slightly raised above heart level

Control stress, or ulcers may get the best of you!

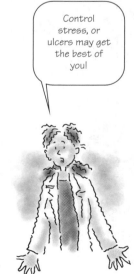

89. 4. Conservative therapy for chronic cholecystitis includes weight reduction by increasing physical activity, a low-fat diet, antacid use to treat dyspepsia, and anticholinergic use to relax smooth muscles and reduce ductal tone and spasm, thereby reducing pain.
CN: Physiological integrity; CNS: Pharmacological therapies; CL: Application

90. 1. The nurse should irrigate the tube with cola because its effervescence and acidity are suited to the purpose, it's inexpensive, and it's readily available in most homes. Advancing the NG tube is inappropriate because the tube is designed to stay in the stomach and isn't long enough to reach the intestines. Applying intermittent suction or using a syringe for aspiration is unlikely to dislodge the clog and may create excess pressure. Intermittent suction may even collapse the tube.
CN: Physiological integrity; CNS: Basic care and comfort; CL: Application

91. 3. The client with a duodenal ulcer may have bleeding at the ulcer site, which shows up as melena. The other findings are consistent with a gastric ulcer.
CN: Physiological integrity; CNS: Physiological adaptation; CL: Comprehension

92. 3. Contrary to popular belief, overproduction of gastric acid is rarely the cause of stress ulcers. Rather, stress states decrease gastric mucosal blood flow, resulting in mucosal breakdown. Stress ulcers are usually more shallow and diffuse than peptic ulcers, which tend to be singular and well-defined.
CN: Physiological integrity; CNS: Physiological adaptation; CL: Comprehension

93. 3. To postpone or avoid the need for mechanical ventilation, the client should be placed on his back, on a rigid mattress, with the head of the mattress elevated 20 degrees. Side-lying and sitting positions aren't indicated.
CN: Safe and effective care environment; CNS: Safety and infection control; CL: Application

CN: Client needs category   CNS: Client needs subcategory   CL: Cognitive level

94. After laparoscopic cholecystectomy, a 43-year-old client complains of pain and nausea. The nurse is preparing meperidine hydrochloride (Demerol) 75 mg and promethazine hydrochloride (Phenergan) 12.5 mg to be administered I.M. in the same syringe. If the label on the Demerol reads 50 mg/ml and the label on the Phenergan reads 25 mg/ml, how many milliliters should the nurse have in the syringe after the correct doses are drawn up? Record your answer using a whole number.

_____ ml

95. A 58-year-old client with osteoarthritis is admitted to the hospital with peptic ulcer disease. Which findings are commonly associated with peptic ulcer disease? Select all that apply:
1. Localized, colicky periumbilical pain
2. History of nonsteroidal anti-inflammatory drug (NSAID) use
3. Epigastric pain that's relieved by antacids
4. Tachycardia
5. Nausea and weight loss
6. Low-grade fever

96. A client undergoes a barium swallow fluoroscopy that confirms gastroesophageal reflux disease (GERD). Based on this diagnosis, the client should be instructed to take which action? Select all that apply:
1. Follow a high-fat, low-fiber diet.
2. Avoid caffeine and carbonated beverages.
3. Sleep with the head of the bed flat.
4. Stop smoking.
5. Take antacids 1 hour and 3 hours after meals.
6. Limit alcohol consumption to one drink per day.

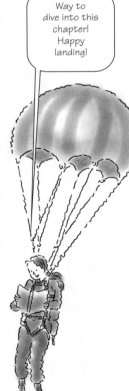

Way to dive into this chapter! Happy landing!

94. 2. This formula is used to calculate drug dosages:

Dose on hand ÷ Quantity on hand = Dose desired ÷ X.

In this example, the formula for calculating the amount of Demerol is as follows:

$50 \text{ mg} \div \text{ml} = 75 \text{ mg} \div X$

$X = 1.5 \text{ ml}.$

The formula for calculating the amount of Phenergan is as follows:

$25 \text{ mg} \div \text{ml} = 12.5 \text{ mg} \div X$

$X = 0.5 \text{ ml}.$

To calculate the total milliliters that should be drawn up in the syringe, the nurse adds the quantity of Demerol and the quantity of Phenergan, as follows:

$1.5 \text{ ml} + 0.5 \text{ ml} = 2 \text{ ml}$ total drawn up in the syringe.

CN: Physiological integrity; CNS: Pharmacological therapies; CL: Application

95. 2, 3, 5. Peptic ulcer disease is characterized by nausea, hematemesis, melena, weight loss, and left-sided epigastric pain—occurring 1 to 2 hours after eating—that's relieved with antacids. NSAID use is also associated with peptic ulcer disease. Appendicitis begins with generalized or localized colicky periumbilical or epigastric pain, followed by anorexia, nausea, a few episodes of vomiting, low-grade fever, and tachycardia.

CN: Physiological integrity; CNS: Physiological adaptation; CL: Analysis

96. 2, 4, 5. The nurse should instruct the client with GERD to follow a low-fat, high-fiber diet. Caffeine, carbonated beverages, alcohol, and smoking should be avoided because they aggravate GERD. In addition, the client should take antacids as prescribed (typically 1 hour and 3 hours after meals and at bedtime). Lying down with the head of the bed elevated, not flat, reduces intra-abdominal pressure, thereby reducing the symptoms of GERD.

CN: Health promotion and maintenance; CNS: None; CL: Application

CN: Client needs category   CNS: Client needs subcategory   CL: Cognitive level

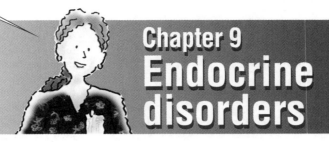

This chapter covers diabetes mellitus and other endocrine disorders, typically a difficult area for nursing students. Don't worry, though, I'll help you through all the tough spots.

Chapter 9
Endocrine disorders

1. After reviewing a client's history and physical examination, which symptoms would lead the nurse to suspect hyperglycemia?
   1. Polydipsia, polyuria, and polyphagia
   2. Weight gain, tiredness, and bradycardia
   3. Irritability, diaphoresis, and tachycardia
   4. Diarrhea, abdominal pain, and weight loss

2. A client presents with diaphoresis, palpitations, jitters, and tachycardia approximately 1½ hours after taking his usual morning insulin. Which treatment is appropriate for this client?
   1. Check blood glucose level, and administer carbohydrates.
   2. Give nitroglycerin, and perform an electrocardiogram (ECG).
   3. Check pulse oximetry, and administer oxygen therapy.
   4. Restrict salt, administer diuretics, and perform paracentesis.

3. Which medication order would be appropriate on the morning of surgery for a client with type 1 diabetes mellitus?
   1. The client should take half of his usual daily insulin.
   2. The client should receive an oral antidiabetic agent.
   3. The client should receive an I.V. insulin infusion.
   4. The client should take his full daily insulin dose with no dextrose infusion.

1. 1. Symptoms of hyperglycemia include polydipsia, polyuria, and polyphagia. Weight gain, tiredness, and bradycardia are symptoms of hypothyroidism. Irritability, diaphoresis, and tachycardia are symptoms of hypoglycemia. Symptoms of Crohn's disease include diarrhea, abdominal pain, and weight loss.
CN: Physiological integrity; CNS: Reduction of risk potential; CL: Analysis

2. 1. The client is experiencing symptoms of hypoglycemia. Checking the blood glucose level and administering carbohydrates will elevate blood glucose. ECG and nitroglycerin are treatments for myocardial infarction. Administering oxygen won't help correct the low blood glucose level. Restricting salt, administering diuretics, and performing paracentesis are treatments for ascites.
CN: Physiological integrity; CNS: Physiological adaptation; CL: Comprehension

3. 1. If the client takes his full daily dose of insulin when he isn't allowed anything orally before surgery, he'll become hypoglycemic. Half the insulin dose will provide all that's needed. Clients with type 1 diabetes don't take oral antidiabetic agents. I.V. insulin infusions aren't standard for routine surgery; they're used in the management of clients undergoing stressful procedures, such as transplants or coronary artery bypass surgery.
CN: Physiological integrity; CNS: Physiological adaptation; CL: Comprehension

What's the appropriate medication order?

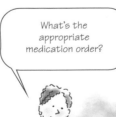

CN: Client needs category   CNS: Client needs subcategory   CL: Cognitive level

4. A physician orders diet, exercise, and oral antidiabetic agents for a client with diabetes. The nurse determines that the client has which diagnosis?
1. Diabetes insipidus
2. Diabetic ketoacidosis
3. Type 1 diabetes mellitus
4. Type 2 diabetes mellitus

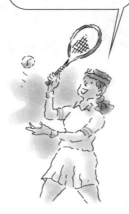

Exercise is just what the doctor ordered!

4. 4. Type 2 diabetes mellitus is controlled primarily through diet, exercise, and oral antidiabetic agents. Desmopressin acetate, a long-acting vasopressin given intranasally, is the treatment of choice for diabetes insipidus. Treatment for diabetic ketoacidosis includes restoration of fluid volume, electrolyte management, reversal of acidosis, and control of blood glucose. Diet and exercise are important in type 1 diabetes mellitus, but blood glucose levels are controlled by insulin injections in that disorder.
CN: Physiological integrity; CNS: Reduction of risk potential; CL: Application

5. Which nursing intervention should be taken for a client who vomits 1 hour after taking his morning glyburide (DiaBeta)?
1. Give glyburide again.
2. Give subcutaneous insulin and monitor blood glucose.
3. Monitor blood glucose closely and look for signs of hypoglycemia.
4. Monitor blood glucose and assess for symptoms of hyperglycemia.

5. 3. When a client who has taken an oral antidiabetic agent vomits, the nurse should monitor glucose and assess him frequently for signs of hypoglycemia. Most of the medication has probably been absorbed. Therefore, repeating the dose would further lower glucose levels later in the day. Giving insulin will also lower glucose levels, causing hypoglycemia. The client wouldn't have hyperglycemia if the glyburide had been absorbed.
CN: Physiological integrity; CNS: Pharmacological therapies; CL: Analysis

6. Which statement by a client indicates that he requires additional teaching regarding the relationship between diabetes mellitus and exercise?
1. "I need to carry candy or juice when I go jogging."
2. "I should wait to eat after I have finished exercising."
3. "I should give my insulin in my abdomen."
4. "I should warm up before my aerobic exercise."

6. 2. The client should eat before exercising to prevent hypoglycemia. Carbohydrate snacking may be necessary with prolonged exercise. Insulin should be given in the abdomen before exercise because it's more rapidly absorbed. Warming up is effective in any exercise plan.
CN: Health promotion and maintenance; CNS: None; CL: Application

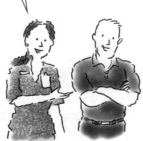

Teaching is very important for a client with diabetes.

7. A client with diabetes mellitus is being taught about possible complications. The nurse should include which conditions in the discussion with the client?
1. Dizziness, dyspnea on exertion, and angina
2. Retinopathy, neuropathy, and coronary artery disease
3. Leg ulcers, cerebral ischemic events, and pulmonary infarcts
4. Fatigue, nausea, vomiting, muscle weakness, and cardiac arrhythmias

7. 2. Retinopathy, neuropathy, and coronary artery disease are all chronic complications of diabetes mellitus. Dizziness, dyspnea on exertion, and angina are symptoms of aortic valve stenosis. Leg ulcers, cerebral ischemic events, and pulmonary infarcts are complications of sickle cell anemia. Hyperparathyroidism causes fatigue, nausea, vomiting, muscle weakness, and cardiac arrhythmias.
CN: Physiological integrity; CNS: Reduction of risk potential; CL: Application

CN: Client needs category CNS: Client needs subcategory CL: Cognitive level

8. Rotating injection sites when administering insulin prevents which complication?
1. Insulin edema
2. Insulin lipodystrophy
3. Insulin resistance
4. Systemic allergic reactions

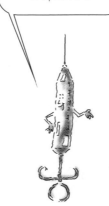

Rotating injection sites is important for preventing complications.

8. 2. Insulin lipodystrophy produces fatty masses at the injection sites, causing unpredictable absorption of insulin injected into these sites. Insulin edema is generalized retention of fluid, sometimes seen after normal blood glucose levels are established in a client with prolonged hyperglycemia. Insulin resistance occurs mostly in overweight clients and is due to insulin binding with antibodies, decreasing the amount of absorption. Systemic allergic reactions range from hives to anaphylaxis; rotating injection sites won't prevent these.
CN: Health promotion and maintenance; CNS: None; CL: Comprehension

9. Which test allows a <u>rapid</u> measurement of glucose in whole blood?
1. Capillary blood glucose test
2. Serum ketone test
3. Serum thyroxine (T_4) test
4. Urine glucose test

9. 1. A capillary blood glucose test is a rapid test used to show blood glucose levels. A serum T_4 test is used to diagnosis thyroid disorders. A serum ketone test is used to document diabetic ketoacidosis by titration and may allow determination of serum ketone concentration. Most of the time, however, neither serum ketone levels nor T_4 levels are useful in determining blood glucose levels. A urine glucose test monitors glucose levels in urine and is influenced by glucose and water excretion. Therefore, results correlate poorly with blood glucose levels.
CN: Physiological integrity; CNS: Reduction of risk potential; CL: Comprehension

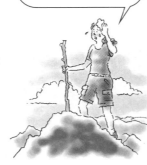

How long does it take to achieve the peak effect?

10. A client is receiving Novolin NPH insulin every morning. When would the nurse expect the client to possibly develop hypoglycemia?
1. 15 minutes to 1 hour
2. 2 to 6 hours
3. 4 to 12 hours
4. 14 to 26 hours

10. 3. Novolin NPH has a peak effect of 4 to 12 hours. The onset of rapid-acting insulin is 15 minutes to 1 hour. The peak effect of rapid-acting insulin is 2 to 6 hours. Long-acting insulin has a peak effect of 14 to 26 hours.
CN: Physiological integrity; CNS: Pharmacological therapies; CL: Application

11. A 52-year-old client reports weight gain and tiredness. On assessment, her vital signs are blood pressure 120/74 mm Hg, pulse rate 52 beats/minute, respiratory rate 20 breaths/minute, and temperature 98° F. Laboratory results show low thyroxine (T_4) and triiodothyronine (T_3) levels. The nurse knows these symptoms are associated with which condition?
1. Tetany
2. Hypothyroidism
3. Hyperthyroidism
4. Hypokalemia

11. 2. Weight gain, lethargy, and slow pulse rate along with decreased T_3 and T_4 levels indicate hypothyroidism. T_3 and T_4 are thyroid hormones that affect growth and development as well as metabolic rate. Tetany is related to low calcium levels. Hypokalemia is a low potassium level.
CN: Physiological integrity; CNS: Physiological adaptation; CL: Analysis

CN: Client needs category   CNS: Client needs subcategory   CL: Cognitive level

12. Which medication would a nurse expect the physician to order for a client with hypothyroidism?
1. Dexamethasone (Decadron)
2. Lactulose (Enulose)
3. Levothyroxine (Synthroid)
4. Lidocaine (Xylocaine)

13. The nurse and a client have just discussed the client's recent diagnosis of hypothyroidism and its causes and effects. Which statement indicates that the client needs further instruction?
1. "Now I see. My clumsiness is caused by a hormone problem."
2. "I just eat too much. That's why I'm depressed and overweight."
3. "No wonder I'm constipated. I'm predisposed to it no matter what I eat."
4. "I'm not cold all the time because I'm getting older. I'm cold because of a metabolic problem."

14. A client with hypothyroidism who experiences trauma, emergency surgery, or severe infection is at risk for developing which condition?
1. Hepatitis B
2. Malignant hyperthermia
3. Myxedema coma
4. Thyroid storm

15. Which potentially serious complication may occur when a client is treated for hypothyroidism?
1. Acute hemolytic reaction
2. Angina or cardiac arrhythmia
3. Retinopathy
4. Thrombocytopenia

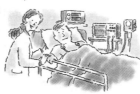

Client-teaching skills are important for all nurses!

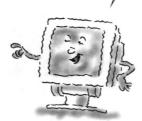

Don't get myxed up on this one! (That's not a typo; it's a hint!)

12. 3. Levothyroxine, a synthetic form of the thyroid hormone thyroxine, is the medication of choice for treating hypothyroidism. Dexamethasone is a steroid and an antithyroid medication. Lactulose is a laxative used to treat constipation. Lidocaine is used to treat ventricular arrhythmias.
CN: Physiological integrity; CNS: Pharmacological therapies; CL: Application

13. 2. Hypothyroidism results from an inadequate secretion of thyroid hormones, which slows metabolic processes and can cause depression and weight gain. A client with hypothyroidism who insists that overeating has caused depression and obesity needs further instruction about the effects of the disease. The other statements reflect an accurate understanding that hypothyroidism can cause clumsiness, constipation, and a feeling of coldness.
CN: Physiological integrity; CNS: Reduction of risk potential; CL: Analysis

14. 3. Myxedema coma represents the most severe form of hypothyroidism. The client develops severe hypothermia and hypoglycemia and becomes comatose. Myxedema coma can be precipitated by opioids, stress (such as surgery), trauma, and infections. Hepatitis B is a virus and isn't caused by thyroid disorders. The client would be hypothermic, not hyperthermic. Thyroid storm is a complication of hyperthyroidism.
CN: Physiological integrity; CNS: Pharmacological therapies; CL: Application

15. 2. Precipitation of angina or cardiac arrhythmia is a potentially serious complication of hypothyroidism treatment, especially for elderly clients or those with underlying heart disease. Acute hemolytic reaction is a complication of blood transfusions. Retinopathy is usually a complication of diabetes mellitus. Thrombocytopenia is defined as a platelet count of less than 150,000/µl and doesn't result from treating hypothyroidism.
CN: Physiological integrity; CNS: Reduction of risk potential; CL: Comprehension

CN: Client needs category   CNS: Client needs subcategory   CL: Cognitive level

16. A client is suspected of having hypothyroidism. Which diagnostic test would be the most appropriate for the nurse to monitor?
1. Liver function studies
2. Hemoglobin A1c
3. Thyroxine (T_4) and thyroid-stimulating hormone (TSH)
4. 24-hour urine for cortisol

17. A nurse can expect to see which symptoms in a client who has hypothyroidism?
1. Polyuria, polydipsia, and weight loss
2. Heat intolerance, nervousness, weight loss, and hair loss
3. Coarsening of facial features and extremity enlargement
4. Tiredness, cold intolerance, weight gain, and constipation

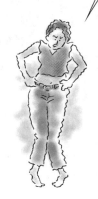

These jeans must have shrunk. Or maybe I should have my thyroid checked.

18. After a client is admitted with an adrenal malfunction, the nurse demonstrates an understanding of the function of the adrenal gland by identifying which hormones as being released by the adrenal medulla?
1. Epinephrine and norepinephrine
2. Glucocorticoids, mineralocorticoids, and androgens
3. Thyroxine (T_4), triiodothyronine (T_3), and calcitonin
4. Insulin, glucagon, and somatostatin

19. When preparing a client scheduled for a thyroid function test, the nurse questions the client about medications. Which medications contain iodine and could alter the results?
1. Acetaminophen and aspirin
2. Estrogen and amphetamines
3. Insulin and oral antidiabetic agents
4. Topical antiseptics and multivitamins

20. While monitoring a client with hypothyroidism, the nurse would expect to observe:
1. hypoactive bowel sounds.
2. hypertension.
3. photophobia.
4. flushed skin.

16. 3. T_4 and TSH are diagnostic tests for hypothyroidism. Liver function studies are indicated in many disorders to check for liver damage. Hemoglobin A1c measurement is used to assess hyperglycemia. Cortisol levels would be checked if adrenal insufficiency is suspected.
CN: Physiological integrity; CNS: Physiological adaptation; CL: Analysis

17. 4. Tiredness, cold intolerance, weight gain, and constipation are symptoms of hypothyroidism, secondary to a decrease in cellular metabolism. Polyuria, polydipsia, and weight loss are symptoms of type 1 diabetes mellitus. Hyperthyroidism has symptoms of heat intolerance, nervousness, weight loss, and hair loss. Coarsening of facial features and extremity enlargement are symptoms of acromegaly.
CN: Physiological integrity; CNS: Physiological adaptation; CL: Application

18. 1. The medulla of the adrenal gland causes the release of epinephrine and norepinephrine. Glucocorticoids, mineralocorticoids, and androgens are released from the adrenal cortex. T_4, T_3, and calcitonin are secreted by the thyroid gland. The islet cells of the pancreas secrete insulin, glucagon, and somatostatin.
CN: Physiological integrity; CNS: Physiological adaptation; CL: Analysis

19. 4. Topical antiseptics and multivitamins contain iodine and can alter thyroid function test results. Estrogen and amphetamines don't contain iodine but may alter thyroid function test results. Insulin, oral antidiabetic agents, acetaminophen, and aspirin won't affect a thyroid test.
CN: Physiological integrity; CNS: Pharmacological therapies; CL: Analysis

20. 1. Hypothyroidism is associated with a general slowing of the body systems, as indicated by hypoactive bowel sounds. The nurse would expect to find the client hypotensive, not hypertensive. Photophobia and flushed skin are symptoms associated with hyperthyroidism.
CN: Physiological integrity; CNS: Physiological adaptation; CL: Application

CN: Client needs category   CNS: Client needs subcategory   CL: Cognitive level

21. A client with Cushing's syndrome is admitted to the medical-surgical unit. During the admission assessment, the nurse notes that the client is agitated and irritable, has poor memory, reports loss of appetite, and appears disheveled. The nurse recognizes that these signs and symptoms are associated with which condition?
  1. Depression
  2. Neuropathy
  3. Hypoglycemia
  4. Hyperthyroidism

22. After teaching a client how to correctly self-administer his daily maintenance dose of 3 units of regular insulin and 4 units of NPH insulin, which client statement demonstrates that the teaching has been successful?
  1. "I'll check my blood sugar after breakfast and give myself shots in my stomach."
  2. "After taking my insulin out of the refrigerator, I'll draw up the clear insulin first to the line for 3 units and then cloudy insulin until there's a total of 7 units in the syringe."
  3. "First, I'll check my blood sugar; then I'll get the insulin from the refrigerator and withdraw 7 units."
  4. "I should inject the insulin into a different site each time and then put it back in the pantry for safekeeping."

23. A 37-year-old client complains of muscle weakness, anorexia, and darkening of his skin. The nurse reviews his laboratory data and notes findings of low serum sodium and high serum potassium levels. The nurse recognizes these signs and symptoms as associated with which condition?
  1. Addison's disease
  2. Cushing's syndrome
  3. Diabetes insipidus
  4. Thyrotoxic crisis

24. Head trauma, brain tumor, or surgical ablation of the pituitary gland can lead to which condition?
  1. Addison's disease
  2. Cushing's syndrome
  3. Diabetes insipidus
  4. Hypothyroidism

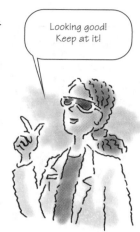

Looking good! Keep at it!

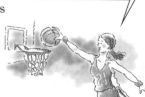

Add another point to your score if you sink this one!

21. 1. Agitation, irritability, poor memory, loss of appetite, and neglect of one's appearance may signal depression, which is common in clients with Cushing's syndrome. Neuropathy affects clients with diabetes mellitus, not Cushing's syndrome. Although hypoglycemia can cause irritability, it also produces increased appetite, rather than loss of appetite. Hyperthyroidism typically causes such signs as goiter, nervousness, heat intolerance, and weight loss despite increased appetite.
CN: Psychosocial integrity; CNS: None; CL: Analysis

22. 2. By indicating the proper dosage and order in which the insulin should be drawn, the client reveals a higher level of knowledge and demonstrates greater readiness to manage his care alone. The next step would be to ask him to demonstrate how an actual injection would be given. Blood sugar should be checked before meals, and insulin should be kept refrigerated. In the third option, the client doesn't demonstrate an understanding of how the insulin is drawn into the syringe.
CN: Health promotion and maintenance; CNS: None; CL: Analysis

23. 1. The clinical picture of Addison's disease includes muscle weakness, anorexia, darkening of the skin's pigmentation, low sodium level, and high potassium level. Cushing's syndrome involves obesity, "buffalo hump," "moonface," and thin extremities. Symptoms of diabetes insipidus include excretion of large volumes of dilute urine. Thyrotoxic crisis can occur with severe hyperthyroidism.
CN: Physiological integrity; CNS: Physiological adaptation; CL: Analysis

24. 3. The cause of diabetes insipidus is unknown, but it may be secondary to head trauma, brain tumors, or surgical ablation of the pituitary gland. Addison's disease is caused by a deficiency of cortical hormones, whereas Cushing's syndrome is an excess of cortical hormones. Hypothyroidism occurs when the thyroid gland secretes low levels of thyroid hormone.
CN: Physiological integrity; CNS: Physiological adaptation; CL: Comprehension

CN: Client needs category   CNS: Client needs subcategory   CL: Cognitive level

25. If fluid intake is limited in a client with diabetes insipidus, which complications will he be at risk for developing?
1. Hypertension and bradycardia
2. Glucosuria and weight gain
3. Peripheral edema and hyperglycemia
4. Severe dehydration and hypernatremia

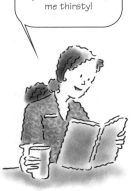

Hmmm. This question is making me thirsty!

26. When caring for a client with a diagnosis of diabetes insipidus, which nursing intervention should be the nurse's priority?
1. Watch for signs of septic shock.
2. Maintain adequate fluid intake.
3. Check weight every 3 days.
4. Monitor urine for specific gravity greater than 1.030.

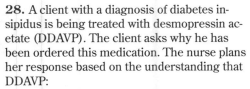

Don't yell at me if you think it's mellitus; it's really an insipid question!

27. Which disorder is suggested by polydipsia and large amounts of waterlike urine with a specific gravity of 1.003?
1. Diabetes mellitus
2. Diabetes insipidus
3. Diabetic ketoacidosis
4. Syndrome of inappropriate antidiuretic hormone (SIADH) secretion

28. A client with a diagnosis of diabetes insipidus is being treated with desmopressin acetate (DDAVP). The client asks why he has been ordered this medication. The nurse plans her response based on the understanding that DDAVP:
1. is a synthetic vasopressin.
2. is a hormone secreted by the adrenal gland.
3. is an antidiabetic agent.
4. is a type of insulin.

25. 4. A client with diabetes insipidus has high volumes of urine, even without fluid replacement. Therefore, limiting fluid intake will cause severe dehydration and hypernatremia. A client undergoing a fluid deprivation test may experience tachycardia and hypotension. A client with diabetes insipidus will usually experience weight loss, and his urine won't contain glucose. Diabetes insipidus has no effect on blood glucose; therefore, the client wouldn't suffer from hyperglycemia. Peripheral edema isn't a symptom of diabetes insipidus.
CN: Physiological integrity; CNS: Physiological adaptation; CL: Comprehension

26. 2. In a client with diabetes insipidus, maintaining fluid intake is essential to prevent severe dehydration. The client is at risk for developing hypovolemic shock because of increased urine output. Weight should be measured on a daily basis to check for adequate fluid balance. Urine specific gravity should be monitored for low osmolality, generally less than 1.005, due to the body's inability to concentrate urine.
CN: Physiological integrity; CNS: Physiological adaptation; CL: Application

27. 2. Diabetes insipidus is characterized by a great thirst (polydipsia) and large amounts of waterlike urine, which has a specific gravity of 1.001 to 1.005. Diabetes mellitus involves polydipsia, polyuria, and polyphagia, but the client also has hyperglycemia. Diabetic ketoacidosis involves weight loss, polyuria, and polydipsia, and the client has severe acidosis. A client with SIADH secretion can't excrete a dilute urine; he retains fluid and develops a sodium deficiency.
CN: Physiological integrity; CNS: Physiological adaptation; CL: Analysis

28. 1. Diabetes insipidus results from a deficiency of circulating antidiuretic hormone (vasopressin). Desmopressin acetate, a synthetic vasopressin, is the medication of choice for treating diabetes insipidus. Glucocorticoids are hormones secreted by the adrenal gland, which isn't involved with diabetes insipidus. Insulin and oral antidiabetic agents are used to treat diabetes mellitus, a disorder of glucose metabolism.
CN: Physiological integrity; CNS: Pharmacological therapies; CL: Application

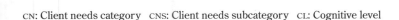
CN: Client needs category   CNS: Client needs subcategory   CL: Cognitive level

29. Diabetes insipidus is a disorder of which gland?

    1. Adrenal gland
    2. Parathyroid gland
    3. Pituitary gland
    4. Thyroid gland

30. A client is diagnosed with diabetes insipidus. The nurse develops a care plan based on the understanding that which hormone is deficient?

    1. Androgen
    2. Epinephrine
    3. Norepinephrine
    4. Vasopressin

31. Which test would a nurse expect to see ordered for a client suspected of having diabetes insipidus?

    1. Capillary blood glucose test
    2. Fluid deprivation test
    3. Serum ketone test
    4. Urine glucose test

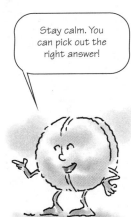

Stay calm. You can pick out the right answer!

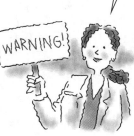

This question calls for crisis intervention.

WARNING!

32. A nurse is reviewing data in the progress notes entry of a client with Addison's disease. Based on the data, the nurse suspects which condition?

Progress notes	
10/04/08 1930	Client reports "headache and nausea, and I'm very weak." Vomited small amount of bile-colored emesis. Vital signs: blood pressure 90/54, heart rate 112, respiratory rate 28, temp 102.4° F. Client is shivering and confused as to time and place but is able to be reoriented. Laboratory results reveal serum cortisol 3 mcg/dl (normal 6 to 23 mcg/dl), fasting blood glucose 62 mg/dl; potassium 5.5 mEq/L; and sodium 128 mEq/L. Dr. Smith notified 1945. ——————Barbara Smith, R.N.

    1. Adrenal crisis
    2. Diabetic ketoacidosis
    3. Myxedema
    4. Thyrotoxic crisis

29. 3. Diabetes insipidus is a disorder of the posterior pituitary gland. The adrenal, thyroid, and parathyroid glands aren't involved.
CN: Physiological integrity; CNS: Reduction of risk potential; CL: Knowledge

30. 4. Clients with diabetes insipidus have a deficiency of vasopressin, the antidiuretic hormone. Androgens, epinephrine, and norepinephrine are hormones secreted by the adrenal gland and aren't related to diabetes insipidus.
CN: Physiological integrity; CNS: Physiological adaptation; CL: Application

31. 2. The fluid deprivation test involves withholding water for 4 to 18 hours and checking urine osmolarity periodically. Plasma osmolarity is also checked. A client with diabetes insipidus will have an increased serum osmolarity (of less than 300 mOsm/kg). Urine osmolarity won't increase. The capillary blood glucose test allows a rapid measurement of glucose in whole blood. The serum ketone test documents diabetic ketoacidosis. The urine glucose test monitors glucose levels in urine, but diabetes insipidus doesn't affect urine glucose levels.
CN: Physiological integrity; CNS: Reduction of risk potential; CL: Analysis

32. 1. As Addison's disease progresses, the client may develop a life-threatening emergency—adrenal crisis, which is related to insufficient levels of cortisol, a hormone produced by the adrenal glands. The crisis occurs as a result of deterioration of the adrenal gland or inadequate treatment of adrenal insufficiency. Diabetic ketoacidosis is a form of hypoglycemia. Myxedema is a form of severe hypothyroidism. Thyrotoxic crisis is a form of severe hyperthyroidism.
CN: Physiological integrity; CNS: Physiological adaptation; CL: Analysis

33. Which disease is caused by a deficiency of cortical hormones?
1. Addison's disease
2. Cushing's syndrome
3. Diabetes mellitus
4. Diabetic ketoacidosis

34. Laboratory findings indicating excessive levels of adrenocortical hormones would correlate with which disease?
1. Addison's disease
2. Cushing's syndrome
3. Diabetes mellitus
4. Hypothyroidism

35. A nurse reviews the laboratory data of a 60-year-old client. The data reveals increased blood and urine levels of triiodothyronine (T_3) and thyroxine (T_4). The nurse knows these values are associated with which condition?
1. Addison's disease
2. Cushing's syndrome
3. Hyperthyroidism
4. Hypopituitarism

36. A physician prescribes an oral antidiabetic medication and weekly glucose monitoring for a 42-year-old male client recently diagnosed with type 2 diabetes. The client is moderately overweight and has a poor diet and a stressful job. He asks how his diagnosis will affect his life. Which response is most appropriate?
1. "The medication will help maintain a steady glucose level, but you need to cut back on snacking."
2. "Type 2 diabetes is common and easily treated. You don't have to make changes."
3. "I'll refer you to a diabetes nurse specialist. She'll help you develop a plan."
4. "You may want to change careers because your job takes so much of your energy."

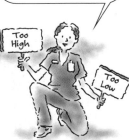

Read question 35 carefully. It states "increased levels."

33. 1. Addison's disease is caused by a deficiency of cortical hormones. Cushing's syndrome is the opposite of Addison's disease and includes excessive adrenocortical activity. Diabetes mellitus is an insulin deficiency. Diabetic ketoacidosis is severe hyperglycemia, causing acidosis.
CN: Physiological integrity; CNS: Physiological adaptation; CL: Knowledge

34. 2. Cushing's syndrome is indicated by excessive levels of adrenocortical hormones. Low levels of glucose and sodium, along with high levels of potassium and white blood cells, are diagnostic of Addison's disease. Diabetes mellitus would have increased blood glucose levels. Hypothyroidism would have low levels of thyroid hormone.
CN: Physiological integrity; CNS: Physiological adaptation; CL: Comprehension

35. 3. Hyperthyroidism has high levels of T_3 and T_4. A definitive diagnosis of Addison's disease must reflect low levels of adrenocortical hormones. Cushing's syndrome would have excessive amounts of adrenocortical hormones. Lower pituitary hormone secretion levels are consistent with hypopituitarism.
CN: Physiological integrity; CNS: Physiological adaptation; CL: Analysis

36. 3. A referral to a nurse specialist who can develop an ongoing relationship and spend more time assessing the client's personal needs and developing a workable plan with him would be most appropriate. Although the medication does help to maintain steady glucose levels, this response ignores the other factors contributing to the client's poor health habits. Telling the client that he won't have to make any lifestyle changes is inappropriate, as is suggesting he change careers.
CN: Health promotion and maintenance; CNS: None; CL: Application

37. An appropriate nursing diagnosis for a client with Addison's disease would include which assessment?
1. *Activity intolerance*
2. *Excess fluid volume*
3. *Ineffective thermoregulation*
4. *Impaired gas exchange*

37. 1. Clients with Addison's disease have inadequate production of adrenal hormones. They commonly experience anorexia, fatigue, and weakness. Hypotension and abdominal and muscle pain also are noted. Therefore, the client commonly experiences activity intolerance. Clients with Addison's disease experience deficient fluid volume, secondary to decreased mineralocorticoid secretion. Heat intolerance is a symptom of hyperthyroidism. The respiratory system isn't directly affected, and gas exchange shouldn't be affected.
CN: Health promotion and maintenance; CNS: None; CL: Analysis

38. A 35-year-old client is admitted with a diagnosis of Addison's disease. Which nursing intervention is most appropriate?
1. Provide frequent rest periods.
2. Administer diuretics.
3. Encourage a high-potassium diet.
4. Maintain fluid restrictions.

I just need to rest, and rest, and rest...

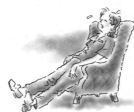

38. 1. A client with Addison's disease is dehydrated, hypotensive, and very weak. Frequent rest periods are needed to prevent exhausting the client. Diuretics would cause further dehydration and are contraindicated in a client with Addison's disease. Potassium levels are usually elevated in Addison's disease because aldosterone secretion is decreased, resulting in decreased sodium and increased potassium. Fluid intake would be encouraged, not restricted, in a dehydrated client.
CN: Physiological integrity; CNS: Physiological adaptation; CL: Analysis

39. A client had a subtotal thyroidectomy in the early morning. During evening rounds, the nurse assesses the client, who now has nausea, a temperature of 105° F (40.6° C), tachycardia, and extreme restlessness. What's the most likely cause of these signs and symptoms?
1. Diabetic ketoacidosis
2. Thyroid crisis
3. Hypoglycemia
4. Tetany

39. 2. Thyroid crisis usually occurs in the first 12 hours after thyroidectomy and causes exaggerated signs of hyperthyroidism, such as high fever, tachycardia, and extreme restlessness. Diabetic ketoacidosis is more likely to produce polyuria, polydipsia, and polyphagia. Hypoglycemia typically produces weakness, tremors, profuse perspiration, and hunger. Tetany typically causes uncontrollable muscle spasms, stridor, cyanosis and, possibly, asphyxia.
CN: Physiological integrity; CNS: Basic care and comfort; CL: Application

Wow! You've finished 40 questions just like that. Now "snap to it" and finish the rest.

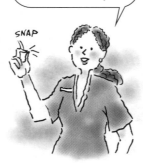

SNAP

40. A nurse can expect to see which signs and symptoms when a client overproduces adrenocortical hormone?
1. Arrested growth and obesity
2. Weight loss and heat intolerance
3. Changes in skin texture and low body temperature
4. Polyuria and dehydration

40. 1. Overproduction of adrenocortical hormone results in growth arrest and obesity. Weight loss and heat intolerance indicate thyroid hormone overproduction. Changes in skin texture and low body temperature indicate thyroid hormone underproduction. Polyuria and dehydration indicate diabetic ketoacidosis.
CN: Physiological integrity; CNS: Physiological adaptation; CL: Application

CN: Client needs category   CNS: Client needs subcategory   CL: Cognitive level

41. Assessment of a client reveals thin extremities but an obese truncal area and a "buffalo hump" at the shoulder area. The client also complains of weakness and disturbed sleep. The nurse interprets this data as indicating which disorder?
   1. Addison's disease
   2. Cushing's syndrome
   3. Graves' disease
   4. Hyperparathyroidism

42. Sodium and water retention in a client with Cushing's syndrome contributes to which commonly seen disorders?
   1. Hypoglycemia and dehydration
   2. Hypotension and hyperglycemia
   3. Pulmonary edema and dehydration
   4. Hypertension and heart failure

43. Which roommate is most appropriate for a client with Cushing's syndrome who has a nursing diagnosis of *Risk for infection?*
   1. Client with uncontrolled hypertension
   2. Client with a tracheostomy
   3. Client with a pressure ulcer
   4. Client with diarrhea

44. A nurse would expect a client with Cushing's syndrome to undergo which test to confirm the diagnosis?
   1. Fluid deprivation test
   2. Glucose tolerance test
   3. Low-dose dexamethasone suppression test
   4. Thallium stress test

> Only one of these tests is used to diagnose Cushing's syndrome. Which one would you choose?

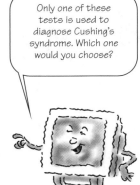

41. 2. Clients with Cushing's syndrome have truncal obesity with thin extremities and a fatty "buffalo hump" at the back of the neck. Clients with Addison's disease show signs of weakness, anorexia, and dark pigmentation of the skin. Clients with Graves' disease (hyperthyroidism) have symptoms of heat intolerance, irritability, and bulging eyes. Hyperparathyroidism is characterized by osteopenia and renal calculi.
CN: Physiological integrity; CNS: Physiological adaptation; CL: Analysis

42. 4. Increased mineralocorticoid activity in a client with Cushing's syndrome commonly contributes to hypertension and heart failure. Hypoglycemia and dehydration are uncommon in a client with Cushing's syndrome. Diabetes mellitus may develop, but hypotension isn't part of the disease process. Pulmonary edema and dehydration also aren't complications of Cushing's syndrome.
CN: Physiological integrity; CNS: Physiological adaptation; CL: Analysis

43. 1. The client with uncontrolled hypertension has the least chance of having an infection that could be transferred to the client with Cushing's syndrome. The clients in the other options are all at higher risk for infection.
CN: Safe, effective care environment; CNS: Safety and infection control; CL: Application

44. 3. A low-dose dexamethasone suppression test is used to detect changes in plasma cortisol levels. A fluid deprivation test is used to diagnosis diabetes insipidus. The glucose tolerance test is used to determine gestational diabetes in pregnant women. A thallium stress test is used to monitor heart function under stress.
CN: Physiological integrity; CNS: Physiological adaptation; CL: Application

CN: Client needs category   CNS: Client needs subcategory   CL: Cognitive level

45. Which nursing intervention should be performed for a client with Cushing's syndrome after adrenalectomy?
1. Monitor laboratory values for hyperglycemia.
2. Monitor blood pressure for hypertension.
3. Monitor laboratory values for hyperkalemia.
4. Monitor laboratory values for hyponatremia.

46. Which nursing diagnosis is appropriate for a client with Addison's disease?
1. *Risk for injury*
2. *Deficient fluid volume*
3. *Acute pain with movement*
4. *Functional urinary incontinence*

47. Which nursing intervention should be performed for a client with Cushing's syndrome?
1. Suggest clothing or bedding that's cool and comfortable.
2. Suggest consumption of high-carbohydrate and low-protein foods.
3. Explain that physical changes are a result of excessive corticosteroids.
4. Explain the rationale for increasing salt and fluid intake in times of illness, increased stress, and very hot weather.

48. A client was recently admitted with a diagnosis of diabetes mellitus. The nurse notices that the client has acetone breath, a weak and rapid pulse, and Kussmaul's respirations. The nurse recognizes these as signs and symptoms of which condition?
1. Hypoglycemia
2. Diabetes insipidus
3. Diabetic ketoacidosis
4. Hyperosmolar hyperglycemic nonketotic syndrome (HHNS)

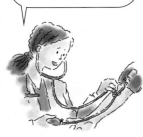

Do you think I'm making the answer to question 45 a little too easy?

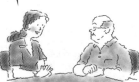

Maybe if I explain the physical changes that may result from corticosteroid use, it will help ease your mind.

45. 2. Removing an adrenal gland may result in postoperative hypertension because handling of the adrenal glands stimulates catecholamine release. A client with Cushing's syndrome would have low potassium and high sodium levels. Hypoglycemia may develop following the removal of the adrenal cortex, which is the source of cortisol.
CN: Physiological integrity; CNS: Physiological adaptation; CL: Application

46. 2. Deficient fluid volume related to inadequate adrenal hormones is common in clients with Addison's disease. Clients with Cushing's syndrome have an increased susceptibility to injury or infection, secondary to the immunosuppression caused by excessive cortisol. Pain and functional incontinence aren't common in Addison's disease.
CN: Physiological integrity; CNS: Reduction of risk potential; CL: Application

47. 3. Clients with Cushing's syndrome have physical changes related to excessive corticosteroids. Clients with hyperthyroidism are heat intolerant and must have comfortable, cool clothing and bedding. Clients with Cushing's syndrome should have a high-protein, not a low-protein, diet. Clients with Addison's disease must increase sodium intake and fluid intake in times of stress to prevent hypotension.
CN: Physiological integrity; CNS: Physiological adaptation; CL: Application

48. 3. Diabetic ketoacidosis is caused by inadequate amounts of insulin or absence of insulin and leads to a series of biochemical disorders. Dizziness, slow cerebration, and tachycardia are signs and symptoms of hypoglycemia; extreme polyuria and dehydration indicate diabetes insipidus; and polyuria, thirst, neurologic abnormalities, and stupor are signs and symptoms of HHNS.
CN: Physiological integrity; CNS: Physiological adaptation; CL: Application

49. An insulin-dependent client who fails to take insulin regularly is at risk for which complication?
  1. Diabetic ketoacidosis
  2. Hypoglycemia
  3. Pancreatitis
  4. Respiratory failure

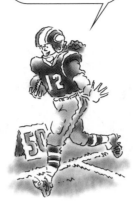

You just crossed the halfway mark. I know you're going to score!

50. A diabetic client has polyphagia, polydipsia, and oliguria; he also complains of headache, malaise, and some vision changes. Assessment shows signs of dehydration. Which diagnosis could be made?
  1. Diabetes insipidus
  2. Diabetic ketoacidosis
  3. Hypoglycemia
  4. Syndrome of inappropriate antidiuretic hormone (SIADH) secretion

51. The thyroid gland is located in which area of the body?
  1. Upper abdomen
  2. Inferior aspect of the brain
  3. Upper portion of the kidney
  4. Lower neck, anterior to the trachea

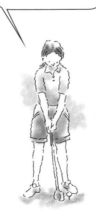

If you studied hard, you'll know this answer to a "T."

52. A client has elevated levels of triiodothyronine (T_3), thyroxine (T_4), and calcitonin. The nurse is aware that these hormones are produced by which gland?
  1. Adrenal gland
  2. Thyroid gland
  3. Pituitary gland
  4. Pancreas

49. 1. A client who fails to regularly take his insulin is at risk for hyperglycemia, which could lead to diabetic ketoacidosis. Hypoglycemia wouldn't occur because the lack of insulin would lead to increased levels of sugar in the blood. A client with chronic pancreatitis may develop diabetes (secondary to the pancreatitis), but insulin-dependent diabetes mellitus doesn't lead to pancreatitis. Respiratory failure isn't related to insulin levels.
CN: Physiological integrity; CNS: Physiological adaptation; CL: Application

50. 2. Early manifestations of diabetic ketoacidosis include polydipsia, polyphagia, and polyuria. As the client dehydrates and loses electrolytes, this condition commonly leads to oliguria, malaise, and vision changes. Diabetes insipidus may result in dehydration but not in polyphagia and polydipsia. Symptoms of hypoglycemia include diaphoresis, tachycardia, and nervousness. A client with SIADH secretion can't excrete a dilute urine, causing hypernatremia.
CN: Physiological integrity; CNS: Physiological adaptation; CL: Application

51. 4. The thyroid gland is in the lower neck, anterior to the trachea. The pancreas is in the upper abdomen. The pituitary gland is located in the inferior aspect of the brain. The adrenal glands are attached to the upper portion of the kidneys.
CN: Health promotion and maintenance; CNS: None; CL: Knowledge

52. 2. The hormones T_3, T_4, and calcitonin are all secreted by the thyroid gland. Glucocorticoids, mineralocorticoids, and androgens are produced by the adrenal gland. The pituitary gland secretes vasopressin, oxytocin, and thyroid-stimulating hormone. Amylase, lipase, and trypsin are enzymes produced by the pancreas that aid in digestion.
CN: Health promotion and maintenance; CNS: None; CL: Application

CN: Client needs category   CNS: Client needs subcategory   CL: Cognitive level

53. Secretion of thyroid-stimulating hormone (TSH) by which gland controls the rate at which thyroid hormone is released?
1. Adrenal gland
2. Parathyroid gland
3. Pituitary gland
4. Thyroid gland

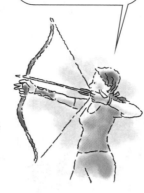

TSH is a hormone with a target gland.

53. 3. By secreting TSH, the pituitary gland controls the rate of thyroid hormone released. The adrenal gland isn't involved in the release of thyroid hormone. The parathyroid gland secretes parathyroid hormones, depending on the levels of calcium and phosphorus in the blood. The thyroid gland secretes thyroid hormone but doesn't control how much is released.
CN: Physiological integrity; CNS: Physiological adaptation; CL: Knowledge

54. When assisting with the development of a care plan for a client with hyperthyroidism, the nurse would anticipate which treatment?
1. Cholelithotomy
2. Irradiation of the thyroid
3. Administration of oral thyroid hormones
4. Whipple procedure

54. 2. Irradiation, involving the administration of ^{131}I, destroys the thyroid gland, thereby treating hyperthyroidism. Cholelithotomy is used to treat gallstones. Oral thyroid hormones are the treatment for hypothyroidism. The Whipple procedure is a surgical treatment for pancreatic cancer.
CN: Physiological integrity; CNS: Pharmacological therapies; CL: Application

55. Which group of symptoms of hyperthyroidism is <u>most commonly</u> found in elderly clients?
1. Depression, apathy, and weight loss
2. Palpitations, irritability, and heat intolerance
3. Cold intolerance, weight gain, and thinning hair
4. Numbness, tingling, and cramping of extremities

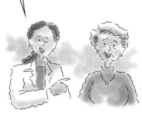

Elderly clients are different from other clients. Be aware of age-related symptoms.

55. 1. Most elderly clients demonstrate depression, apathy, and weight loss, which are typical signs and symptoms of hyperthyroidism. Palpitations, irritability, and heat intolerance can be present with hyperthyroidism, but these aren't typical symptoms in elderly clients. Cold intolerance, weight gain, and thinning hair are some of the signs of hypothyroidism. Numbness, tingling, and cramping of extremities are symptoms of hypocalcemia, which may be a symptom of hypoparathyroidism.
CN: Physiological integrity; CNS: Physiological adaptation; CL: Application

56. A client with hyperthyroidism develops high fever, extreme tachycardia, and altered mental status. The nurse suspects which of the following?
1. Hepatic coma
2. Thyroid storm
3. Myxedema coma
4. Hyperosmolar hyperglycemic nonketotic syndrome (HHNS)

56. 2. Thyroid storm is a form of severe hyperthyroidism that can be precipitated by stress, injury, or infection. Hepatic coma occurs in clients with profound liver failure. Myxedema coma is a rare disorder characterized by hypoventilation, hypotension, hypoglycemia, and hypothyroidism. HHNS occurs in clients with type 2 diabetes mellitus who are dehydrated and have severe hyperglycemia.
CN: Physiological integrity; CNS: Physiological adaptation; CL: Analysis

57. Hyperthyroidism is <u>commonly known</u> as which disorder?
1. Addison's disease
2. Buerger's disease
3. Cushing's syndrome
4. Graves' disease

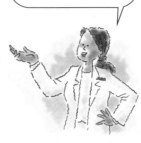

This disorder is also associated with an autoimmune response. But I bet you knew that.

58. Excessive output of thyroid hormone from abnormal stimulation of the thyroid gland is the etiology of which condition?
1. Hyperparathyroidism
2. Hypoparathyroidism
3. Hyperthyroidism
4. Hypothyroidism

59. A client has flushed skin, bulging eyes, and perspiration, and states that he has been "irritable" and having palpitations. The nurse interprets these findings as suggesting:
1. hyperthyroidism.
2. myocardial infarction (MI).
3. pancreatitis.
4. type 1 diabetes mellitus.

60. What can a nurse do to prevent lipodystrophy when administering insulin to a diabetic client?
1. Grasp the skin tightly.
2. Rotate injection sites.
3. Massage the site vigorously.
4. Inject into the deltoid muscle.

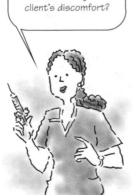

What can you do to minimize your client's discomfort?

57. 4. Hyperthyroidism is known as *Graves' disease*. Addison's disease is a deficiency of cortical hormones. Buerger's disease is a recurring inflammation of arteries in the upper and lower extremities. Cushing's syndrome is an excess of cortical hormones.
CN: Physiological integrity; CNS: Physiological adaptation; CL: Knowledge

58. 3. Excessive output of thyroid hormone is the etiology of hyperthyroidism. Hyperparathyroidism is overproduction of parathyroid hormone, characterized by bone calcification or kidney stones. Hypoparathyroidism is inadequate secretion of parathyroid hormone that occurs after interruption of the blood supply or surgical removal of the parathyroid. Hypothyroidism is slow production of thyroid hormone.
CN: Physiological integrity; CNS: Physiological adaptation; CL: Knowledge

59. 1. Signs and symptoms of hyperthyroidism include nervousness, palpitations, irritability, bulging eyes, heat intolerance, weight loss, and weakness. MI usually involves chest pain that may radiate to the arms, back, or neck and shortness of breath. Pancreatitis involves severe abdominal pain and back tenderness. Type 1 diabetes mellitus involves polyuria, polydipsia, and weight loss.
CN: Physiological integrity; CNS: Physiological adaptation; CL: Analysis

60. 2. The nurse should rotate insulin injection sites systematically to minimize tissue damage, promote absorption, avoid discomfort, and prevent lipodystrophy. Grasping the skin tightly can traumatize the skin; therefore, the nurse should hold it gently but firmly when giving an injection. Massaging the site vigorously is contraindicated because it hastens insulin absorption, which isn't recommended. Usually, insulin is administered subcutaneously, rather than into a muscle, because muscular activity increases insulin absorption.
CN: Physiological integrity; CNS: Pharmacological therapies; CL: Application

61. A client is brought into the emergency department with a brain stem contusion. Two days after admission, the client has a large amount of urine and a serum sodium level of 155 mEq/dl. Which condition may be developing?

1. Myxedema coma
2. Diabetes insipidus
3. Type 1 diabetes mellitus
4. Syndrome of inappropriate antidiuretic hormone (SIADH) secretion

62. A client with a history of diabetes has serum ketones and a serum glucose level above 300 mg/dl. The nurse suspects which of the following?

1. Diabetes insipidus
2. Diabetic ketoacidosis
3. Hypoglycemia
4. Somogyi phenomenon

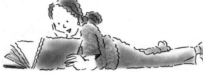

Before you answer, make sure you know which disorder the question is asking you to treat.

63. Objectives for treating <u>diabetic ketoacidosis</u> include administration of which treatment?

1. Glucagon
2. Blood products
3. Glucocorticoids
4. Insulin and I.V. fluids

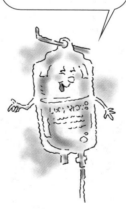

Isn't life a bolus of cherries? (They told me to say that!)

64. Which method of insulin administration would a nurse expect to be used in the initial treatment of hyperglycemia in a client with diabetic ketoacidosis?

1. Subcutaneous
2. I.M.
3. I.V. bolus only
4. I.V. bolus, followed by continuous infusion

61. 2. Two leading causes of diabetes insipidus are hypothalamic or pituitary tumors and closed head injuries. Myxedema coma is a form of hypothyroidism. Type 1 diabetes mellitus isn't caused by a brain injury. A client with SIADH secretion would have hyponatremia; this client's sodium level was 155 mEq/dl, which is above the normal levels of 135 to 145 mEq/dl.

CN: Physiological integrity; CNS: Physiological adaptation; CL: Application

62. 2. Clients with serum ketones and serum glucose levels above 300 mg/dl could be diagnosed with diabetic ketoacidosis. Diabetes insipidus is an overproduction of antidiuretic hormone and doesn't create ketones in the blood. Hypoglycemia causes low blood glucose levels. The Somogyi phenomenon is rebound hyperglycemia following an episode of hypoglycemia.

CN: Physiological integrity; CNS: Physiological adaptation; CL: Analysis

63. 4. A client with diabetic ketoacidosis would receive insulin to lower glucose and would receive I.V. fluids to correct hypotension. Glucagon is given to treat hypoglycemia; diabetic ketoacidosis involves hyperglycemia. Blood products aren't needed to correct diabetic ketoacidosis. Glucocorticoids aren't needed because the adrenal glands aren't involved.

CN: Physiological integrity; CNS: Pharmacological therapies; CL: Application

64. 4. An I.V. bolus of insulin is given initially to control the hyperglycemia, followed by a continuous infusion, titrated to control blood glucose. After the client is stabilized, subcutaneous insulin is given. Insulin is never given I.M.

CN: Physiological integrity; CNS: Pharmacological therapies; CL: Application

65. A physician has ordered a check of glycosylated hemoglobin (HbA_{1c}) levels for a client with diabetes. Which statement by the client regarding this test indicates that teaching has been effective?

1. "It's used to monitor the control of my disease."
2. "It's used to diagnose diabetes."
3. "It's useful in determining if I have anemia."
4. "It reflects the average blood glucose level for the previous 3 weeks."

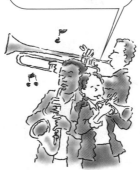

The correct answers may appear in more than one response. Make sure you choose the right combo!

66. Which combination of adverse effects must be carefully monitored when administering I.V. insulin to a client diagnosed with diabetic ketoacidosis?

1. Hypokalemia and hypoglycemia
2. Hypocalcemia and hyperkalemia
3. Hyperkalemia and hyperglycemia
4. Hypernatremia and hypercalcemia

67. A diabetic client suddenly develops hypoglycemia. What should the nurse do first?

1. Give the client a glass of orange juice to drink.
2. Administer 5 more units of regular insulin.
3. Check the client's blood glucose level.
4. Call the client's physician.

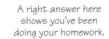

A right answer here shows you've been doing your homework.

68. Which statement by a client demonstrates that he understands foot care teaching instructions related to his diabetes?

1. "I should cut my toenails once a week."
2. "I should wash with very hot water and dry my feet well."
3. "I should inspect the skin on my feet every week for open areas."
4. "I should wear cotton socks."

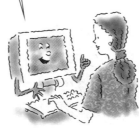

65. 1. The HbA_{1c} is used to gather data and to monitor progress of diabetes control. It isn't used to diagnose diabetes or anemia. Red blood cells live in the body for about 3 months. When the glucose that's attached to the hemoglobin is measured, it reflects the average blood glucose level for the previous 2 to 3 months.

CN: Physiological integrity; CNS: Physiological adaptation; CL: Application

66. 1. Blood glucose must be monitored because there's a chance for hypokalemia or hypoglycemia. Hypokalemia might occur because I.V. insulin forces potassium into cells, thereby lowering the plasma levels of potassium. Hypoglycemia might occur if too much insulin is administered. The client wouldn't have hyperkalemia. Calcium and sodium levels aren't affected.

CN: Physiological integrity; CNS: Pharmacological therapies; CL: Application

67. 1. Drinking a glass of orange juice should raise the client's blood glucose level, thus correcting hypoglycemia. Receiving additional insulin would lower the client's blood glucose level even further, causing hypoglycemia to worsen. The nurse shouldn't take the time to check the client's blood glucose level or call the physician at this time because the client needs immediate attention to prevent loss of consciousness.

CN: Physiological integrity; CNS: Physiological adaptation; CL: Application

68. 4. The client with diabetes is prone to the development of foot problems, such as ulcers and infection, due to the combination of vascular disease and neuropathy. Cotton socks worn with leather shoes keep the feet dry and protected from injury. A podiatrist should routinely examine the feet, and cut the nails as needed. Washing with hot water can result in burns; using lukewarm water is recommended. Visual inspection of the feet should be performed daily.

CN: Physiological integrity; CNS: Reduction of risk potential; CL: Application

CN: Client needs category   CNS: Client needs subcategory   CL: Cognitive level

69. A diabetic client who had a stroke has right-sided paralysis and incontinence and is in the rehabilitation center. Which action should be the nurse's priority in caring for the client?
1. Apply body powder every 4 hours to keep the client dry.
2. To conserve energy, maintain bed rest when the client isn't in therapy.
3. Insert an indwelling urinary catheter to keep the client continent.
4. Wash the client's skin with soap and water, gently patting it dry.

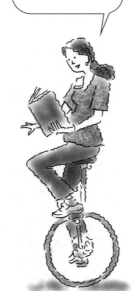

Don't stop now! You're on a roll!

70. An 86-year-old female client who has been on long-term steroid therapy now has drug-induced Cushing's syndrome. She's residing in an extended-care facility because of her multiple chronic health problems. Which condition is closely related to chronic use of steroids?
1. Periods of hypoglycemia
2. Periods of euphoria
3. Thin, easily damaged skin
4. Weight loss

71. A nurse is assessing a client with possible hyperaldosteronism. Which nursing intervention is the <u>priority</u>?
1. Monitoring blood glucose levels
2. Auscultating for breath sounds
3. Monitoring arterial blood gas (ABG) levels
4. Weighing the client weekly

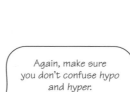

Again, make sure you don't confuse hypo and hyper.

72. Which condition is characterized by osteopenia and renal calculi?
1. Hyperparathyroidism
2. Hypoparathyroidism
3. Hypopituitarism
4. Hypothyroidism

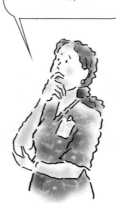

69. 4. The skin of a diabetic client should be kept dry to prevent breakdown and infection. The nurse should avoid excessive use of powders, which can cake with perspiration and cause irritation. Clients undergoing rehabilitation should be upright in a chair, except for short rest periods during the day, to promote optimal recovery. Diabetic clients are especially prone to infections. Urinary tract infections are commonly caused by the use of indwelling catheters. Other methods should be used to encourage continence.
CN: Physiological integrity; CNS: Basic care and comfort; CL: Application

70. 3. Clients taking steroids on a long-term basis lose subcutaneous fat under the skin and are especially vulnerable to skin breakdown and bruising. Such clients should take great care when performing tasks that may injure the skin and should anticipate delayed healing when injuries occur. Clients taking long-term steroids are likely to have hyperglycemia. Prolonged steroid use can cause depression. Clients who experience weight loss should be monitored for weight gain and edema.
CN: Physiological integrity; CNS: Pharmacological therapies; CL: Application

71. 2. Aldosterone is secreted by the adrenal cortex. One of its major functions is causing the kidneys to retain saline in the body. A client with hyperaldosteronism should be observed for signs of respiratory distress, crackles, and the use of accessory muscles. Blood glucose and ABG levels aren't immediate priorities when assessing a client with hyperaldosteronism. Rapid weight gain can indicate fluid volume excess, but the client should be weighed daily, not weekly.
CN: Physiological integrity; CNS: Physiological adaptation; CL: Application

72. 1. Hyperparathyroidism is characterized by osteopenia and renal calculi, secondary to overproduction of parathyroid hormone. Hypoparathyroidism's main symptoms include tetany from hypocalcemia. Hypopituitarism involves extreme weight loss and atrophy of all endocrine glands. Symptoms of hypothyroidism include hair loss, weight gain, and cold intolerance.
CN: Physiological integrity; CNS: Physiological adaptation; CL: Comprehension

CN: Client needs category   CNS: Client needs subcategory   CL: Cognitive level

73. A client with hyperparathyroidism develops renal calculi. The nurse should expect to see which electrolyte levels?
1. Decreased calcium levels
2. Increased calcium levels
3. Increased potassium levels
4. Increased magnesium levels

74. Which laboratory results support a diagnosis of primary hyperparathyroidism?
1. High parathyroid hormone and high calcium levels
2. High magnesium and high thyroid hormone levels
3. Low parathyroid hormone and low potassium levels
4. Low thyroid-stimulating hormone (TSH) and high phosphorus levels

75. Which type of medication is contraindicated in the treatment of clients with hyperparathyroidism?
1. Acetaminophen
2. Aspirin
3. Potassium-wasting diuretics
4. Thiazide diuretics

76. In clients with hyperparathyroidism, which calcium level would be considered an acute hypercalcemic crisis?
1. 2 mg/dl
2. 4 mg/dl
3. 10.5 mg/dl
4. 15 mg/dl

77. A nurse is reviewing the laboratory results on a client's chart, and notes findings of increased serum phosphate levels and decreased serum calcium levels. The nurse is aware that these findings indicate which condition?
1. Cushing's syndrome
2. Graves' disease
3. Hypoparathyroidism
4. Hypothyroidism

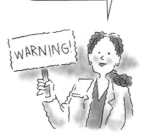

The word contraindicated makes this a tricky question.

WARNING!

73. 2. Renal calculi usually consist of calcium and phosphorus. In hyperparathyroidism, serum calcium levels are high, leading to renal calculi formation. Potassium and magnesium don't form renal calculi, and levels of these aren't high in clients with hyperparathyroidism.
CN: Physiological integrity; CNS: Physiological adaptation; CL: Application

74. 1. A diagnosis of primary hyperparathyroidism is established based on increased serum calcium levels and elevated parathyroid hormone levels. Potassium, magnesium, TSH, and thyroid hormone levels aren't used to diagnose hyperparathyroidism.
CN: Physiological integrity; CNS: Physiological adaptation; CL: Application

75. 4. Thiazide diuretics shouldn't be used because they decrease renal excretion of calcium, thereby raising serum calcium levels even higher. There are no contraindications to aspirin or acetaminophen for clients with hyperparathyroidism. Potassium loss isn't an issue for clients with hyperparathyroidism.
CN: Physiological integrity; CNS: Pharmacological therapies; CL: Application

76. 4. Normal calcium levels are 8.5 to 10.5 mg/dl, so a level of 15 mg/dl is dangerously high.
CN: Physiological integrity; CNS: Physiological adaptation; CL: Knowledge

77. 3. Symptoms of hypoparathyroidism include hyperphosphatemia and hypocalcemia. Excessive adrenocortical activity indicates Cushing's syndrome. Excessive thyroid hormone levels indicate Graves' disease (hyperthyroidism). Low thyroid hormone levels indicate hypothyroidism.
CN: Physiological integrity; CNS: Physiological adaptation; CL: Analysis

78. A 55-year-old client is admitted with hypoparathyroidism. When assessing the client, the nurse should expect to see which sign or symptom?
1. Chest pain
2. Exophthalmos
3. Shortness of breath
4. Hand twitching

79. A client is receiving oral calcium supplements. Which additional vitamin would the nurse encourage the client to consume to enhance absorption of calcium from the GI tract?
1. Vitamin A
2. Vitamin C
3. Vitamin D
4. Vitamin E

80. A nurse is caring for a 30-year-old female client who had a subtotal thyroidectomy to treat hyperthyroidism. Which sign or symptom could indicate bleeding at the incision site?
1. Hoarseness
2. Severe stridor
3. Complaints of a tight dressing
4. Difficulty swallowing

81. Hypersecretion of which hormone would cause pituitary gigantism?
1. Follicle-stimulating hormone (FSH)
2. Growth hormone
3. Parathyroid hormone
4. Thyroid-stimulating hormone (TSH)

82. A 43-year-old client has been diagnosed with hyperthyroidism. Which nursing intervention should be the priority to decrease the client's anxiety?
1. Keeping the client warm
2. Encouraging the client to increase activity
3. Providing a calm, restful environment
4. Placing the client in semi-Fowler's position

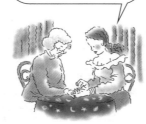

Choose carefully. Identifying the symptom is in your future.

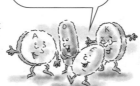

Hey, whose job is it to enhance the absorption of calcium?

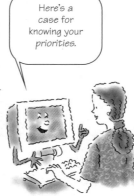

Here's a case for knowing your priorities.

78. 4. Tetany, which is manifested by muscle twitching or spasms, is the chief symptom of hypoparathyroidism. Chest pain and shortness of breath aren't usually symptoms of hypoparathyroidism. Exophthalmos, or bulging eyes, is a common symptom of hyperthyroidism.
CN: Physiological integrity; CNS: Physiological adaptation; CL: Application

79. 3. Variable doses of vitamin D preparations enhance the absorption of calcium from the GI tract. Vitamins A, C, and E aren't involved with this process.
CN: Physiological integrity; CNS: Pharmacological therapies; CL: Application

80. 3. Complaints of a tight dressing indicate postoperative bleeding. Hoarseness or severe stridor indicates damage to the laryngeal nerve. Difficulty swallowing doesn't indicate postoperative bleeding.
CN: Physiological integrity; CNS: Physiological adaptation; CL: Application

81. 2. Hypersecretion of growth hormone causes pituitary gigantism. FSH is involved in the development of ovaries and sperm. Hypersecretion of parathyroid hormone would cause hyperparathyroidism. Hypersecretion of TSH would cause hyperthyroidism.
CN: Physiological integrity; CNS: Physiological adaptation; CL: Knowledge

82. 3. Clients with hyperthyroidism are typically anxious, diaphoretic, nervous, and fatigued; they need a calm, restful environment in which to relax and get adequate rest. Clients with hyperthyroidism are usually warm and diaphoretic and need a cool environment. Activity shouldn't be increased. If a client is exhibiting dyspnea, he would benefit from high Fowler's position.
CN: Physiological integrity; CNS: Basic care and comfort; CL: Application

CN: Client needs category   CNS: Client needs subcategory   CL: Cognitive level

83. A nurse is teaching a client about insulin. The physician has ordered "Regular insulin 6 units U100." Which statement by the client indicates that teaching has been effective?
1. "The insulin is cloudy."
2. "The insulin vial should be shaken vigorously before drawing it into the syringe."
3. "'U100' means that there are 100 units in each milliliter of the insulin and that 6 units are to be administered."
4. "The insulin should be drawn up in a tuberculin syringe."

84. After undergoing a thyroidectomy, a client develops hypocalcemia and tetany. Which medication should the nurse anticipate administering?
1. Calcium gluconate
2. Potassium chloride
3. Sodium bicarbonate
4. Sodium phosphorus

85. Which disorder may cause acute pancreatitis?
1. Gallstones
2. Crohn's disease
3. High gastric acid levels
4. Low thyroid hormone level

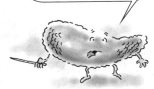

I can't believe we had the gall to ask you this question! (Oooh, that one hurt.)

86. Severe abdominal pain in the midepigastric region, back tenderness, nausea, and vomiting are symptoms of which condition?
1. Acute pancreatitis
2. Crohn's disease
3. Hypophysectomy
4. Pheochromocytoma

83. 3. There are 100 units of insulin in each milliliter of U100 insulin, and it should be drawn up in a U100 syringe (orange needle cap). Regular insulin is clear. Cloudy insulin has a zinc precipitate that must be evenly distributed in the solution. Insulin syringes are the only type of syringe used for drawing up insulin.
CN: Safe, effective care environment; CNS: Safety and infection control; CL: Application

84. 1. Immediate treatment for a client who develops hypocalcemia and tetany after thyroidectomy is calcium gluconate. Potassium chloride and sodium bicarbonate aren't indicated. Sodium phosphorus wouldn't be given because phosphorus levels are already elevated.
CN: Physiological integrity; CNS: Pharmacological therapies; CL: Application

85. 1. Gallstones may cause obstruction and swelling at the ampulla of Vater, preventing flow of pancreatic juices into the duodenum and leading to pancreatitis. Gallbladder obstruction and alcoholism are the major causes of acute pancreatitis. Crohn's disease usually involves the terminal ileum and wouldn't affect the pancreas. Low thyroid hormone levels and high gastric acid levels aren't related to an acute pancreatitis attack.
CN: Physiological integrity; CNS: Physiological adaptation; CL: Comprehension

86. 1. Severe abdominal pain in the midepigastric region, back tenderness, nausea, and vomiting are caused by irritation of the pancreas. A client with Crohn's disease would have abdominal pain, but the pain would be in the lower quadrant; the client would also have diarrhea. Hypophysectomy is removal of the pituitary gland. Pheochromocytoma is a benign tumor of the adrenal medulla.
CN: Physiological integrity; CNS: Physiological adaptation; CL: Analysis

CN: Client needs category   CNS: Client needs subcategory   CL: Cognitive level

87. A 48-year-old client has been admitted with complaints of acute abdominal pain in the midepigastric region, back tenderness, nausea, and vomiting. The nurse recognizes these findings to be associated with which condition?
1. Acute pancreatitis
2. Crohn's disease
3. Hypophysectomy
4. Pheochromocytoma

87. 1. Signs and symptoms of acute pancreatitis include midepigastric abdominal pain, back pain, nausea, and vomiting. Crohn's disease is associated with right lower quadrant abdominal pain (in acute disease) and cramping abdominal pain (in chronic disease). Hypophysectomy is the surgical removal of the pituitary gland. Pheochromocytoma is a tumor of the adrenal gland and doesn't cause abdominal or back symptoms.
CN: Physiological integrity; CNS: Physiological adaptation; CL: Application

88. A physician has ordered famotidine (Pepcid) for a client with acute pancreatitis. The client asks the nurse why this has been ordered. The nurse plans her response based on the understanding that famotidine acts to:
1. inhibit gastric acid secretion.
2. decrease nausea and vomiting.
3. decrease itching.
4. reduce diarrhea.

88. 1. Famotidine is classified as a histamine antagonist and inhibits gastric acid secretions. Antiemetics act to reduce nausea and vomiting. Antihistamines reduce itching and antidiarrheals reduce diarrhea.
CN: Physiological integrity; CNS: Pharmacological therapies; CL: Application

89. If a pancreatitis attack has been brought on by gallstones or gallbladder disease, a client may require reinforcement about the need to follow which type of diet?
1. High-calorie, high-protein diet
2. High-fiber diet, encouraging fluid intake
3. Low-fat diet, avoiding heavy meals
4. Diet high in protein, calcium, and vitamin D

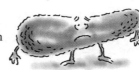

Oh, my. I think my eyes are bigger than my stomach!

89. 3. A client who survives an acute pancreatitis attack caused by gallstones or gallbladder disease requires reinforcement to maintain a low-fat diet and to avoid heavy meals. A high-calorie, high-protein diet is appropriate for clients with hyperthyroidism. A diet high in fiber, encouraging fluid intake, is recommended for constipation. A client with Cushing's syndrome should follow a diet high in protein, calcium, and vitamin D.
CN: Physiological integrity; CNS: Reduction of risk potential; CL: Application

90. Which disorder is an inflammatory disease characterized by progressive anatomic and functional destruction of the pancreas?
1. Acute pancreatitis
2. Addison's disease
3. Chronic pancreatitis
4. Graves' disease

90. 3. Chronic pancreatitis is an inflammatory disease characterized by progressive anatomic and functional destruction of the pancreas. Acute pancreatitis is a digestion of the pancreas by the enzymes it produces. Addison's disease is a deficiency of adrenocortical hormones. Graves' disease is another name for hyperthyroidism.
CN: Physiological integrity; CNS: Physiological adaptation; CL: Knowledge

CN: Client needs category   CNS: Client needs subcategory   CL: Cognitive level

91. A client has diabetic ketoacidosis secondary to infection. As the condition progresses, which signs and symptoms might the nurse see?
  1. Kussmaul's respirations and a fruity odor on the breath
  2. Shallow respirations and severe abdominal pain
  3. Decreased respirations and increased urine output
  4. Cheyne-Stokes respirations and foul-smelling urine

92. A client with diabetes mellitus and a hearing impairment is admitted to the medical-surgical unit. For this client, the nursing team is developing a care plan that includes daily self-administration of insulin. Which intervention should the team include in this plan?
  1. Use facial expressions as needed.
  2. Chew gum while giving instructions.
  3. Shine a light on the client's face.
  4. Raise an arm or hand to get attention.

> The most effective client teaching depends on making sure the client can understand the instructions.

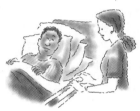

93. Clients with insulin-dependent diabetes mellitus may require which change to their daily routine during periods of infection?
  1. No changes
  2. Less insulin
  3. More insulin
  4. Oral antidiabetic agents

94. A nurse is preparing to administer regular insulin 4 units to a client with type 1 diabetes mellitus. Which equipment does the nurse need to perform the injection? Select all that apply:
  1. Medication administration record
  2. Nursing assessment sheet
  3. 27-gauge, ½″ needle
  4. 22-gauge, ½″ needle
  5. 27-gauge, 1″ needle
  6. 22-gauge, 1″ needle

91. 1. Coma and severe acidosis are ushered in with Kussmaul's respirations (very deep but not labored respirations) and a fruity odor on the breath (acidemia). Shallow respirations and severe abdominal pain may be symptoms of pancreatitis. Decreased respirations and increased urine output aren't symptoms related to diabetic ketoacidosis. Cheyne-Stokes respirations and foul-smelling urine don't result from diabetic ketoacidosis.
CN: Physiological integrity; CNS: Physiological adaptation; CL: Application

92. 4. To get the client's attention, the nurse should raise an arm or hand before presenting instructions. The nurse should avoid relying on facial expressions because they may be misinterpreted as signs of annoyance or other feelings by a client who depends on visual cue. The nurse shouldn't chew gum when teaching a client with limited hearing because it can distort the sounds that the client can hear. If needed, a light may be shone on the nurse's face—not the client's face—to help the client lip-read.
CN: Safe, effective care environment; CNS: Coordinated care; CL: Application

93. 3. During periods of infection or illness, insulin-dependent clients may need even more insulin, rather than reducing the levels or not making any changes in their daily insulin routines, to compensate for increased blood glucose levels. Clients usually aren't switched from injectable insulin to oral antidiabetic agents during periods of infection.
CN: Physiological integrity; CNS: Pharmacological therapies; CL: Application

94. 1, 3. To administer medication, the nurse needs the medication administration record to verify the correct client, medication, dose, time, and route. A subcutaneous injection, such as insulin, is administered with a 25-gauge to 27-gauge, ⅝″ to ½″ needle. The nursing assessment sheet isn't necessary for administering insulin. A 22-gauge needle is too large for a subcutaneous injection. A 1″ needle will deliver the medication into muscle rather than subcutaneous tissue.
CN: Physiological integrity; CNS: Pharmacological therapies; CL: Application

CN: Client needs category   CNS: Client needs subcategory   CL: Cognitive level

95. After falling off a ladder and suffering a brain injury, a client develops syndrome of inappropriate antidiuretic hormone (SIADH). Which findings indicate the effectiveness of the treatment he's receiving? Select all that apply:
1. Decrease in body weight
2. Rise in blood pressure and drop in heart rate
3. Absence of wheezes in the lungs
4. Increased urine output
5. Decreased urine osmolarity

96. A client is admitted to the hospital with diabetes mellitus. Which findings is the nurse most likely to observe in this client? Select all that apply:
1. Excessive thirst
2. Weight gain
3. Constipation
4. Excessive hunger
5. Urine retention
6. Frequent, high-volume urination

97. A client is seen in the clinic with suspected parathyroid hormone (PTH) deficiency. Part of the diagnosis of this condition includes the analysis of serum electrolyte levels. Which electrolyte levels would the nurse expect to be abnormal in a client with PTH deficiency? Select all that apply:
1. Sodium
2. Potassium
3. Calcium
4. Chloride
5. Phosphorus

Congratulations! You finished! Take a bow before you dive in to the next chapter.

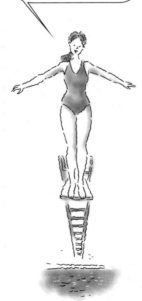

95. 1, 4, 5. SIADH is an abnormality in which there's an abundance of antidiuretic hormone. The predominant feature is water retention, accompanied by oliguria, edema, and weight gain. Evidence of successful treatment includes a reduction in weight, an increase in urine output, and a decrease in the urine's concentration (urine osmolarity). SIADH doesn't manifest as symptoms associated with blood pressure, heart rate, or abnormal breath sounds.
CN: Physiological integrity; CNS: Physiological adaptation; CL: Analysis

96. 1, 4, 6. Classic signs of diabetes mellitus include polydipsia (excessive thirst), polyphagia (excessive hunger), and polyuria (excessive urination). Because the body is starving from the lack of glucose the cells are using for energy, the client has weight loss, not weight gain. Clients with diabetes mellitus usually don't have constipation.
CN: Health promotion and maintenance; CNS: None; CL: Analysis

97. 3, 5. A client with PTH deficiency has abnormal serum calcium and phosphorus levels because PTH regulates these two electrolytes. PTH deficiency doesn't affect sodium, potassium, or chloride.
CN: Physiological integrity; CNS: Physiological adaptation; CL: Analysis

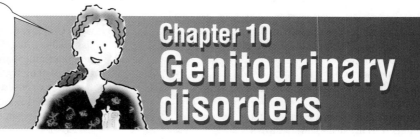

For more information about genitourinary system disorders, visit the Web site of the National Institute of Diabetes and Digestive and Kidney Diseases at *www.niddk.nih.gov/*.

Chapter 10
Genitourinary disorders

1. To treat cervical cancer, a client has had an applicator of radioactive material placed in her vagina. Which observation by the nurse indicates a radiation hazard?
1. The client is on strict bed rest.
2. The head of the bed is set at a 30-degree angle.
3. The client receives a complete bed bath each morning.
4. The nurse checks the applicator's position every 4 hours.

2. A physician tells a client to return 1 week after treatment to have a repeat culture done to verify the cure. This order would be appropriate for a woman with which condition?
1. Genital warts
2. Genital herpes
3. Gonorrhea
4. Syphilis

3. A nurse is caring for a client in the clinic. Which sign or symptom may indicate that the client has gonorrhea?
1. Burning on urination
2. Dry, hacking cough
3. Diffuse skin rash
4. Painless chancre

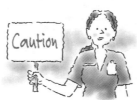

Ask yourself: Which observation indicates a radiation hazard?

1. 3. The client shouldn't receive a complete bed bath while the applicator is in place. In fact, she shouldn't be bathed below the waist because of the risk of radiation exposure to the nurse. During this treatment, the client should remain on strict bed rest. The nurse should check the applicator's position every 4 hours to ensure that it remains in the proper place.
CN: Safe, effective care environment; CNS: Safety and infection control; CL: Application

2. 3. Gonococcal infections can be completely eliminated by drug therapy. This cure is documented by a negative culture 4 to 7 days after therapy is finished. Genital warts aren't curable and are identified by appearance, not culture. Genital herpes isn't curable and is identified by the appearance of the lesions or cytologic studies. The diagnosis of syphilis is done using dark-field microscopy or serologic tests.
CN: Physiological integrity; CNS: Physiological adaptation; CL: Application

3. 1. Burning on urination may be a symptom of gonorrhea or urinary tract infection. A dry, hacking cough is a sign of a respiratory infection, not gonorrhea. A diffuse rash may indicate secondary stage syphilis. A painless chancre is the hallmark of primary syphilis. It appears wherever the organisms enter the body, such as on the genitalia, anus, or lips.
CN: Physiological integrity; CNS: Physiological adaptation; CL: Analysis

CN: Client needs category   CNS: Client needs subcategory   CL: Cognitive level

4. Which statement made by a client with a chlamydial infection indicates understanding of the potential complications?

1. "I'm glad I'm not pregnant; I'd hate to have a malformed baby from this disease."
2. "I hope this medicine works before this disease gets into my urine and destroys my kidneys."
3. "If I had known a diaphragm would put me at risk for this, I would have taken birth control pills."
4. "I need to treat this infection so it doesn't spread into my pelvis because I want to have children some day."

5. A nurse is teaching personal hygiene care techniques to a client with genital herpes. Which statement by the client indicates the teaching has been effective?

1. "I will wear loose cotton underwear."
2. "I will apply a water-based lubricant to my lesions."
3. "I should rub rather than scratch in response to itching."
4. "I can pour hydrogen peroxide and water over my lesions."

6. A client with nephritis is taking the diuretic furosemide (Lasix) as prescribed. To avoid potassium depletion, the nurse teaches the client prevention techniques. Which client statement indicates an accurate understanding of these techniques?

1. "I'll avoid consuming magnesium-rich foods."
2. "I'll watch for and report signs of hypercalcemia."
3. "I'll eat such foods as apricots, dates, and citrus fruits."
4. "I'll take furosemide with the usual dose of my antihypertensive drug."

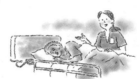

Teaching good hygiene techniques contributes to your client's overall well-being.

4. 4. Chlamydia is a common cause of pelvic inflammatory disease and infertility. It doesn't affect the kidneys or cause birth defects. It can cause conjunctivitis and respiratory infection in neonates exposed to infected cervicovaginal secretions during delivery. Use of a diaphragm isn't a risk factor.
CN: Physiological integrity; CNS: Reduction of risk potential; CL: Application

5. 1. Wearing loose cotton underwear promotes drying and helps avoid irritation of the lesions. The use of lubricants is contraindicated because they can prolong healing time and increase the risk of secondary infection. Lesions shouldn't be rubbed or scratched because of the risk of tissue damage and additional infection. Cool, wet compresses can be used to soothe the itch. The use of hydrogen peroxide and water on lesions isn't recommended.
CN: Physiological integrity; CNS: Basic care and comfort; CL: Analysis

6. 3. Because furosemide is a potassium-wasting diuretic, the client should eat potassium-rich foods, such as apricots, dates, and citrus fruits, to prevent potassium depletion. The other client statements have no relationship to potassium balance. The client may consume magnesium-rich foods as desired. The client should watch for signs of adverse reactions to furosemide such as hypocalcemia—not hypercalcemia. The client should take furosemide with an antihypertensive drug only if prescribed; the combination may produce hypotension but doesn't cause potassium depletion.
CN: Health promotion and maintenance; CNS: None; CL: Application

7. A nurse is examining the following laboratory values in the chart of a male client with chronic renal failure. Which value indicates that hemodialysis is an effective treatment for this client?

1. RBCs
2. WBCs
3. Calcium
4. BUN

Laboratory slip

Dialysis laboratory results

Laboratory values	Before dialysis	After dialysis
Red blood cells (RBCs)	5 million/mm³	4 million/mm³
White blood cells (WBCs)	11 million/mm³	4.8 million/mm³
Calcium	8.5 mg/dl	8.5 mg/dl
Blood urea nitrogren (BUN)	30 mg/dl	15 mg/dl

7. 4. The BUN level reflects the amount of urea and nitrogenous waste products in the blood. Dialysis removes excess amounts of these elements from the blood, which is reflected in a lower BUN level. Hemodialysis doesn't affect the RBC or WBC count. Calcium levels are usually low in clients with chronic renal failure. These levels are corrected by giving calcium supplements, not through hemodialysis.
CN: Physiological integrity; CNS: Physiological adaptation; CL: Analysis

You know what they say...an ounce of prevention...

8. A nurse has performed disease prevention teaching with a female client who has genital herpes. Which client behavior indicates that the teaching has been successful?

1. The client keeps the affected area moist.
2. The client keeps her fingernails long.
3. The client wears tight-fitting jeans.
4. The client washes her hands before and after touching lesions.

8. 4. Because hand-to-body contact is a common method of transmitting the herpes simplex virus, the client should wash her hands before and after touching the lesions to prevent the spread of the disease. To promote lesion drying and client comfort, the client should keep the affected area dry. To prevent scratching of the lesions, the client should keep her fingernails short, instead of long. Because tight-fitting clothes help retain heat and moisture, which can delay healing and cause discomfort, the client should wear loose-fitting garments.
CN: Safe, effective care environment; CNS: Safety and infection control; CL: Application

9. In which group is it <u>most important</u> for the client to understand the importance of an annual Papanicolaou test?

1. Clients with a history of recurrent candidiasis
2. Clients with a pregnancy before age 20
3. Clients infected with the human papillomavirus (HPV)
4. Clients with a long history of hormonal contraceptive use

9. 3. HPV causes genital warts, which are associated with an increased incidence of cervical cancer. Recurrent candidiasis, pregnancy before age 20, and use of hormonal contraceptives don't increase the risk of cervical cancer.
CN: Health promotion and maintenance; CNS: None; CL: Application

CN: Client needs category CNS: Client needs subcategory CL: Cognitive level

10. Which factor in a client's history indicates she's at risk for candidiasis?
 1. Nulliparity
 2. Menopause
 3. Use of corticosteroids
 4. Use of spermicidal jelly

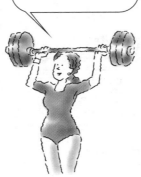

You've already finished 10 questions. Get pumped!

11. Copious amounts of frothy, greenish vaginal discharge would be a symptom of which infection?
 1. Candidiasis
 2. *Gardnerella vaginalis* vaginitis
 3. Gonorrhea
 4. Trichomoniasis

12. A 19-year-old woman reports an intermittent milky vaginal discharge. She isn't sexually active and doesn't report itching or burning. Which factor is the most likely cause of the milky discharge?
 1. Inadequate cleaning of the perineal area
 2. Sensitivity to a feminine hygiene product
 3. Normal fluctuation in estrogen and progesterone levels
 4. Reaction to heat and moisture from wearing tight clothing

Any of these factors might be the cause, but this item is asking you to choose the most likely cause, right?

13. A 59-year-old female client underwent a left mastectomy yesterday. The client has a saline lock for intermittent I.V. access in her lower right arm. Which technique for obtaining a blood pressure reading would be most appropriate for this client?
 1. Using the right arm, and placing the cuff above the saline lock insertion site
 2. Using the left arm, and pumping the cuff only as necessary
 3. Using the leg, and placing the cuff on the client's thigh
 4. Using the right arm, and placing the cuff below the saline lock insertion site

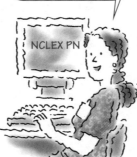

NCLEX PN

10. 3. Small numbers of the fungus *Candida albicans* are commonly in the vagina. Because corticosteroids decrease host defense, they increase the risk of candidiasis. Pregnancy, not nulliparity, increases the risk of candidiasis. Candidiasis is rare before menarche and after menopause. The use of hormonal contraceptives, not spermicidal jelly, increases the risk of candidiasis.
CN: Health promotion and maintenance; CNS: None; CL: Application

11. 4. The discharge associated with infection caused by *Trichomonas* organisms is homogenous, greenish gray, watery, and frothy or purulent. The discharge associated with candidiasis is thick, white, and resembles cottage cheese in appearance while that associated with infection due to *G. vaginalis* is thin and grayish white, with a marked fishy odor. With gonorrhea, vaginal discharge is purulent when present but, in many women, gonorrhea produces no symptoms.
CN: Physiological integrity; CNS: Physiological adaptation; CL: Application

12. 3. Vaginal fluid is clear, milky, or cloudy, depending on the fluctuating levels of estrogen and progesterone. A milky vaginal discharge is normal and isn't associated with sensitivity, reaction to heat or moisture, or inadequate cleaning.
CN: Health promotion and maintenance; CNS: None; CL: Application

13. 1. To obtain a blood pressure reading, the nurse should always use the arm opposite the side of the mastectomy. Never take a blood pressure reading in the arm on the affected side without a physician's order. Blood pressure readings may be taken in the leg in some cases, but doing so isn't necessary in this case. It isn't necessary to place the cuff below the saline lock to obtain a blood pressure reading.
CN: Health promotion and maintenance; CNS: None; CL: Application

14. A nurse must administer a douche to a client scheduled for a vaginal hysterectomy. How should she perform the procedure?

1. Separate the labia, clean the vaginal orifice, insert the douche nozzle 2″ (5.1 cm), and administer room temperature solution well above the client's hip level.
2. Separate the labia, clean the vaginal orifice, insert the douche nozzle 2″, and administer cool solution well above the client's hip level.
3. Separate the labia, clean the vaginal orifice, insert the douche nozzle 2″, and administer 100° F (37.8° C) solution 2′ (61 cm) above the client's hip level.
4. Separate the labia, clean the vaginal orifice, insert the douche nozzle 2″, and administer 100° F solution 3′ (91.4 cm) above the client's hip level.

14. 3. The correct procedure for administering a douche is to separate the labia, clean the vaginal orifice, insert the douche nozzle 2″, and administer 100° F solution 2′ above the client's hip level.

CN: Safe, effective care environment; CNS: Safety and infection control; CL: Application

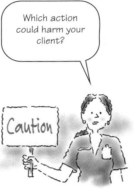

Which action could harm your client?

Caution

15. A nurse enters the room of a client who had a left modified mastectomy 8 hours earlier. Which observation indicates that the nursing assistant assigned to the client needs <u>further instruction</u> and guidance?

1. The client is squeezing a ball in her left hand.
2. The client is wearing a robe with elastic cuffs.
3. The client's affected arm is elevated on a pillow.
4. A blood pressure cuff is on the client's right arm.

15. 2. Elastic cuffs can contribute to the development of lymphedema and should be avoided. Simple exercises such as squeezing a ball help promote circulation and should be started as soon as possible after surgery. Elevation of the affected arm promotes venous and lymphatic return from the extremity. Blood pressure measurements in the affected arm should also be avoided.

CN: Safe, effective care environment; CNS: Coordinated care; CL: Analysis

16. For which signs and symptoms should a client at risk for evisceration be monitored after an abdominal hysterectomy?

1. Tachycardia accompanied by a weak, thready pulse
2. Hypotension with a decreased level of consciousness (LOC)
3. Shallow, rapid respirations and increasing vaginal drainage
4. Low-grade fever with increasing serosanguineous incisional drainage

16. 4. Signs of impending evisceration are low-grade fever and increasing serosanguineous drainage. Tachycardia; weak, thready pulse; shallow, rapid respirations; hypotension; decreased LOC; and vaginal drainage after abdominal hysterectomy are all unrelated to impeding evisceration, although they may be associated with other serious problems such as shock.

CN: Physiological integrity; CNS: Reduction of risk potential; CL: Comprehension

CN: Client needs category   CNS: Client needs subcategory   CL: Cognitive level

17. Which finding indicates that oxycodone (Percodan) given to a client with breast cancer metastasized to the bone is exerting the desired effect?

1. Bone density is increased.
2. Pain is 0 to 2 on a 10-point scale.
3. Alpha-fetoprotein level is decreased.
4. Serum calcium level is within normal range.

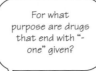

For what purpose are drugs that end with "-one" given?

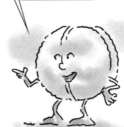

18. Which instruction should be given to a client with prostatitis who's receiving co-trimoxazole double strength (Bactrim DS)?

1. Don't expect improvement of symptoms for 7 to 10 days.
2. Drink six to eight glasses of fluid daily while taking this medication.
3. If a sore mouth or throat develops, take the medication with milk or an antacid.
4. Use a sunscreen of at least SPF-15 with PABA to protect against drug-induced photosensitivity.

19. Which factor should be checked when evaluating the effectiveness of an alpha-adrenergic blocker given to a client with benign prostatic hyperplasia (BPH)?

1. Voiding pattern
2. Size of the prostate
3. Creatinine clearance
4. Serum testosterone level

20. A nursing diagnosis of *Risk for impaired tissue integrity* would be most appropriate for which client?

1. Client with endometriosis
2. Client taking hormonal contraceptives
3. Client with a vaginal packing in place
4. Client having reconstructive breast surgery

The appropriate nursing diagnosis helps everyone work toward the same goal.

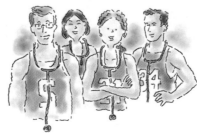

17. 2. Oxycodone is an opioid analgesic used for alleviating severe pain, especially in terminal illness. If a client's pain has decreased to 0 to 2 on a 10-point scale (where 0 is no pain and 10 is the worst pain), the medication is working as desired. The drug doesn't directly affect bone density, alpha-fetoprotein level, or serum calcium level.

CN: Physiological integrity; CNS: Pharmacological therapies; CL: Analysis

18. 2. Six to eight glasses of fluid daily are needed to prevent renal problems, such as crystalluria and calculi formation. The symptoms should improve in a few days if the drug is effective. Sore throat and sore mouth are adverse effects that should be reported right away. The drug causes photosensitivity, but a PABA-free sunscreen should be used because PABA can interfere with the drug's action.

CN: Physiological integrity; CNS: Pharmacological therapies; CL: Application

19. 1. The prostate gland has alpha-adrenergic receptors. Thus, alpha-adrenergic blockers relax the smooth muscle of the bladder neck and prostate, so the urinary symptoms of BPH (frequency, urgency, hesitancy) are reduced in many clients. These drugs don't affect the size of the prostate, renal function, or production or metabolism of testosterone.

CN: Physiological integrity; CNS: Pharmacological therapies; CL: Application

20. 4. Reconstructive breast surgery places the client at risk for insufficient blood supply to the muscle graft and skin, which can lead to tissue necrosis. Endometriosis or hormonal contraceptives aren't generally associated with altered tissue perfusion. Pressure from vaginal packing can sometimes put pressure on the bladder neck and interfere with voiding, not tissue perfusion.

CN: Physiological integrity; CNS: Reduction of risk potential; CL: Analysis

21. A physician has ordered a condom catheter for a client. The nurse cleans the client's perineal area before application of the condom catheter and sees irritation, excoriation, and swelling of the penis. Which nursing intervention should be the nurse's <u>priority</u>?
1. Twisting the condom after application
2. Applying the condom with adhesive tape
3. Informing the charge nurse of the findings
4. Rolling the condom down securely over the tip of the penis

22. Which instruction is the <u>most important</u> to give women to decrease the risk of toxic shock syndrome?
1. Avoid douching.
2. Wear loose cotton underwear.
3. Use pads, not tampons, overnight.
4. Avoid sexual intercourse during menses.

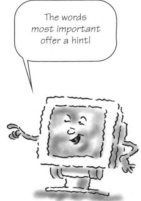

The words most important offer a hint!

23. Which response is the most appropriate when a client asks what activity limitations are necessary after a dilatation and curettage procedure?
1. Tampons may be used during exercise.
2. Avoid strenuous work and sexual intercourse for at least 2 weeks.
3. Stay on bed rest for 3 days; then gradually resume normal activity.
4. Engage in activity as tolerated, and take a soaking tub bath each day to promote relaxation.

24. Which assessment finding is <u>abnormal</u> in a 72-year-old man?
1. Decreased sperm count
2. Small firm testes on palpation
3. History of slowed sexual response
4. Decreased plasma testosterone level

Abnormal or normal? Always consider your client's age.

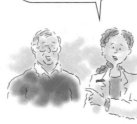

21. 3. The nurse should inform the charge nurse of the baseline data because a condom catheter shouldn't be used on a client with penile irritation, excoriation, swelling, or discoloration. Further inflammation and ulceration may occur. A condom catheter shouldn't be twisted because twisting can obstruct urine flow. It should be secured with elastic tape or Velcro rather than adhesive tape, which is inflexible and can stop blood flow. It should have a 1″ (2.5-cm) gap between the tip of the penis and the connecting tube to prevent penile irritation and allow complete urine drainage.
CN: Safe, effective care environment; CNS: Coordinated care; CL: Application

22. 3. The cause of toxic shock syndrome is a toxin produced by *Staphylococcus aureus* bacteria. It is most common in menstruating women using tampons. Tampons, particularly when left in place for more than 8 hours (such as overnight), are believed to provide a good environment for growth of the bacteria, which then enter the bloodstream through breaks in the vaginal mucosa. Douching, use of loose cotton underwear, and sexual intercourse during menstruation have no direct association with toxic shock syndrome.
CN: Health promotion and maintenance; CNS: None; CL: Comprehension

23. 2. Strenuous work, which can result in increased bleeding, should be avoided for 2 weeks to allow time for healing. Sexual intercourse should also be avoided for 2 weeks to allow healing and decrease the risk of infection. Overall activity should be gradually resumed, reaching preoperative levels in the 2-week period, but bed rest isn't necessary. Tampons and tub baths should be avoided for 1 week. No other restrictions are routinely necessary.
CN: Physiological integrity; CNS: Reduction of risk potential; CL: Application

24. 1. Normal sperm production continues despite the age-related degenerative changes that occur in the male reproductive system. Among the normal age-related changes are decreased size and increased firmness of the testes, a decrease in sexual potency, and decreased production of testosterone and progesterone.
CN: Physiological integrity; CNS: Physiological adaptation; CL: Application

CN: Client needs category   CNS: Client needs subcategory   CL: Cognitive level

25. After having transurethral resection of the prostate (TURP), a client returns to the unit with a three-way indwelling urinary catheter and continuous closed bladder irrigation. Which finding suggests that the client's catheter is occluded?
1. The urine in the drainage bag appears red to pink.
2. The client reports bladder spasms and the urge to void.
3. The normal saline irrigation is infusing at the rate of 50 gtt/minute.
4. About 1,000 ml of irrigant have been instilled, and 1,200 ml of drainage have been returned.

26. Which comment made by a client being treated for chronic prostatitis indicates that self-care instructions should be clarified?
1. "I miss not being able to have sex."
2. "I enjoy frequent soaking in a hot tub of water."
3. "Cutting down on coffee hasn't been as hard as I expected."
4. "I'm used to getting up and moving."

27. Perineal pain in the absence of an observable cause suggests which condition?
1. Endometriosis
2. Internal hemorrhoids
3. Prostatitis
4. Renal calculi

28. Which finding observed in a client taking finasteride (Proscar) would be a cause for alarm?
1. Azotemia
2. Breast enlargement
3. Decreased prostate size
4. Flushing

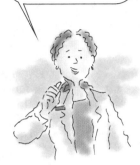

Client teaching includes making sure your client understands your instructions.

I think I detect an alarming situation!

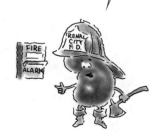

25. 2. Reports of bladder spasms and the urge to void suggest that a blood clot may be occluding the catheter. After TURP, urine normally appears red to pink, and normal saline irrigant is usually infused at a rate of 40 to 60 gtt/minute or according to facility protocol. The amount of returned fluid (1,200 ml) should correspond to the amount of instilled fluid, plus the client's urine output (1,000 ml + 200 ml), which reflects catheter patency.
CN: Physiological integrity; CNS: Basic care and comfort; CL: Application

26. 1. Ejaculation can aid in the treatment of chronic prostatitis by decreasing the retention of prostatic fluid. Coffee should be eliminated from the diet because it can increase prostate secretion. Warm sitz baths and not sitting for too long at a time promote comfort.
CN: Physiological integrity; CNS: Physiological adaptation; CL: Application

27. 3. Prostatitis can cause prostate pain, which is felt as perineal discomfort. Endometriosis can cause pain low in the abdomen, deep in the pelvis, or in the rectal or sacrococcygeal area, depending on the location of the ectopic tissue. Hemorrhoids cause rectal pain and pressure. Renal calculi typically produce flank pain.
CN: Health promotion and maintenance; CNS: None; CL: Comprehension

28. 1. Azotemia, a buildup of nitrogenous waste products in the blood, indicates impaired renal function. Finasteride is prescribed for chronic urine retention with large residual volumes secondary to benign prostatic hyperplasia (BPH). Azotemia in a client on finasteride therapy can indicate the drug isn't effective in relieving the urinary symptoms associated with BPH or that an unrelated renal problem has occurred. Breast enlargement, decrease in prostate size, and flushing are expected effects of finasteride, an antiandrogenic agent.
CN: Physiological integrity; CNS: Pharmacological therapies; CL: Application

CN: Client needs category   CNS: Client needs subcategory   CL: Cognitive level

29. Which treatment is appropriate for a client with cervical polyps who has been treated with cryosurgery?
1. Daily douche
2. Oral antibiotics
3. Intravaginal antibiotic cream
4. Use of tampons for 72 hours

30. Which intervention would be <u>contraindicated</u> for a woman having intracavitary radiation for cancer of the cervix?
1. Low-residue diet
2. Fowler's position when in bed
3. Indwelling urinary catheter to gravity drainage
4. Diphenoxylate hydrochloride with atropine (Lomotil) 2 mg four times daily

31. Which condition of the female reproductive system generally requires the identification and treatment of sexual partners?
1. Bartholinitis
2. Candidiasis
3. *Chlamydia trachomatis* infection
4. Endometriosis

32. Which piece of information should be given to a client taking metronidazole (Flagyl)?
1. Breathlessness and cough are common adverse effects.
2. Urine may develop a greenish tinge while the client is taking this drug.
3. Mixing this drug with alcohol causes severe nausea and vomiting.
4. Heart palpitations may occur and should be immediately reported.

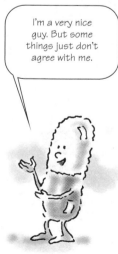

I'm a very nice guy. But some things just don't agree with me.

29. 3. Intravaginal antibiotic cream is commonly used to aid healing and prevent infection. Oral antibiotics are used for clients with acute cervicitis or perimetritis. Douching is generally avoided for 2 weeks, as is the use of tampons.
CN: Physiological integrity; CNS: Reduction of risk potential; CL: Application

30. 2. Clients having intracavitary radiation therapy are on strict bed rest to avoid displacing the radiation source. An order for Fowler's position when in bed is incorrect. An indwelling urinary catheter is used to prevent urine from distending the bladder and changing the position of tissues relative to the radiation source. A low-residue diet and diphenoxylate hydrochloride with atropine are used to prevent diarrhea during treatment.
CN: Physiological integrity; CNS: Reduction of risk potential; CL: Analysis

31. 3. Chlamydia is a common sexually transmitted disease (STD) requiring the treatment of all current sexual partners to prevent reinfection. Bartholinitis results from obstruction of a duct. Candidiasis is a yeast infection that commonly occurs as a result of antibiotic use. Sexual partners may become infected, although men can usually be treated with over-the-counter products. Endometriosis occurs when endometrial cells are seeded throughout the pelvis and isn't an STD.
CN: Health promotion and maintenance; CNS: None; CL: Application

32. 3. When mixed with alcohol, metronidazole causes a disulfiram-like effect involving nausea, vomiting, and other unpleasant symptoms. Urine may turn reddish brown, not greenish, from the drug. Cardiovascular or respiratory effects aren't associated with use of this drug.
CN: Physiological integrity; CNS: Pharmacological therapies; CL: Application

CN: Client needs category   CNS: Client needs subcategory   CL: Cognitive level

33. Which symptom is an <u>adverse effect</u> of hydrocodone with acetaminophen (Percocet) that a client with metastatic prostate cancer should report to the physician?
1. Blurred vision
2. Diarrhea
3. Unusual dreams
4. Vomiting

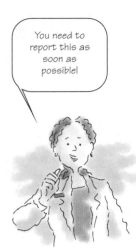

You need to report this as soon as possible!

34. Which intervention is appropriate for a client having hysterosalpingography?
1. Give the client a perineal pad to wear after the procedure.
2. Give the client nothing by mouth after midnight the night before the procedure.
3. Position the client in the knee-chest position during the procedure.
4. Keep the client in a dorsal recumbent position for 4 hours after the procedure.

35. Which instruction applies to a vaginal irrigation?
1. Insert the nozzle about 3″ (7.6 cm) into the vagina.
2. Direct the tip of the nozzle toward the sacrum.
3. Instill the solution in a constant flow over 5 to 10 minutes.
4. Raise the solution at least 24″ (61 cm) above the client's hip level.

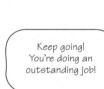

Keep going! You're doing an outstanding job!

36. A 36-year-old man who has never had mumps reports that he was just notified that an 8-year-old child of a family with whom he stayed recently has been diagnosed with mumps. Which treatment should the man receive?
1. I.V. antibiotics
2. Ice packs to the scrotum
3. Application of a scrotal support
4. Administration of gamma globulin

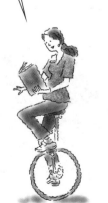

33. 4. Vomiting is an adverse effect of the drug that should be reported because it impairs the client's quality of life and places the client at risk for dehydration. Taking the medication with food may prevent vomiting. If not, other opiate analgesics may be better tolerated. Blurred vision and diarrhea aren't associated with the use of hydrocodone with acetaminophen. Unusual dreams are a common adverse effect but don't need to be reported unless bothersome to the client.
CN: Physiological integrity; CNS: Pharmacological therapies; CL: Application

34. 1. A perineal pad is needed after hysterosalpingography because the contrast medium may leak from the vagina for several hours and stain the clothing. The bowel must be cleaned before the procedure, but the client doesn't have to refrain from having anything by mouth after midnight. The procedure is performed with the client in the lithotomy position, and no special positioning is required after the procedure.
CN: Physiological integrity; CNS: Basic care and comfort; CL: Application

35. 2. The normal position of the vagina slants up and back toward the sacrum. Directing the tip of the nozzle toward the sacrum allows it to follow the normal slant of the vagina and minimizes tissue trauma. The nozzle should be inserted about 2″ (5.1 cm). The fluid can be instilled intermittently and, for best therapeutic results, over 20 to 30 minutes. The container should be no higher than 24″ above the client's hip level to avoid forcing fluid and bacteria through the cervical os into the uterus.
CN: Safe, effective care environment; CNS: Safety and infection control; CL: Comprehension

36. 4. Gamma globulin provides passive immunity to mumps. Antibiotic therapy is used in the treatment of bacterial orchitis. Ice and the use of a scrotal support are used as comfort measures in the treatment of orchitis.
CN: Health promotion and maintenance; CNS: None; CL: Application

CN: Client needs category   CNS: Client needs subcategory   CL: Cognitive level

37. Which statement by a man scheduled for a vasectomy indicates he needs further teaching about the procedure?
  1. "If I decide I want a child, I'll just get a reversal."
  2. "Amazing! I can make sperm but classify as sterile."
  3. "I'm sure glad I made some deposits in the sperm bank."
  4. "I can't believe I still have to worry about contraception after this surgery."

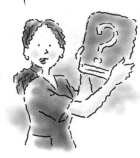

Look for signs that your client doesn't understand the information.

38. Which area of client teaching should be stressed when the goal is to prevent the development of phimosis in a 20-year-old uncircumcised man?
  1. Proper cleaning of the prepuce
  2. Importance of regular ejaculation
  3. Technique of testicular self-examination
  4. Proper hand washing before touching the genitals

39. Which statement should be included when teaching a client newly diagnosed with testicular cancer?
  1. Testicular cancer isn't responsive to chemotherapy, but it's highly curative with surgery.
  2. Radiation therapy is never used, so the unaffected testicle remains healthy.
  3. Testicular self-examination is still important because there's an increased risk of a second tumor.
  4. Taking testosterone after orchiectomy prevents changes in appearance and sexual function.

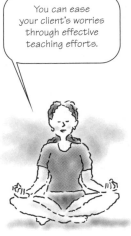

You can ease your client's worries through effective teaching efforts.

40. Which statement shows the significance of a persistent elevation in alpha-fetoprotein (AFP) level after orchiectomy for testicular cancer?
  1. Fertility is maintained.
  2. The cancer has recurred.
  3. There's metastatic disease.
  4. Testosterone levels are low.

37. 1. Vasectomy procedures can be reversed but with varying degrees of success. Because of the variable success, a client can't be sure of reversibility and needs to consider vasectomy a permanent sterilization procedure when deciding to have it done. After vasectomy, the client remains fertile until sperm stored distal to the severed vas are evacuated. Once this occurs, sperm are still produced, but they don't enter the ejaculate and are absorbed by the body.
CN: Physiological integrity; CNS: Physiological adaptation; CL: Application

38. 1. Proper cleaning of the preputial area to remove secretions is critical to the prevention of noncongenital phimosis. Regular ejaculation can decrease the symptoms of chronic prostatitis, but it has no effect on the development of phimosis. Testicular self-examination is important in the early detection and treatment of testicular cancer. Hand washing is important in preventing the spread of infection.
CN: Health promotion and maintenance; CNS: None; CL: Application

39. 3. A history of a testicular malignancy puts the client at increased risk for a second tumor. Testicular self-examination enables early detection and treatment and is critical. Chemotherapy is added for clients who have evidence of metastasis after irradiation. Radiation therapy is used on the retroperitoneal lymph nodes. Testosterone isn't usually needed because the unaffected testis usually produces sufficient hormone.
CN: Physiological integrity; CNS: Reduction of risk potential; CL: Application

40. 3. AFP is a tumor marker elevated in nonseminomatous malignancies of the testicle. After the tumor is removed, the level should decrease. A persistent elevation after orchiectomy indicates tumor is present someplace outside the testicle that was removed. A recurrence of the cancer is indicated by a postsurgical decrease in AFP level followed by an elevation as a new tumor starts to grow. The level of AFP isn't related to fertility or testosterone level.
CN: Physiological integrity; CNS: Physiological adaptation; CL: Analysis

41. Which discharge instruction should be given to a client after a prostatectomy?
1. Avoid straining at stool.
2. Report clots in the urine right away.
3. Soak in a warm tub daily for comfort.
4. Return to your usual activities in 3 weeks.

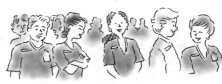

Good client teaching is an important responsibility for any nurse.

42. After a biopsy of the prostate, which symptom should be reported?
1. Pain on ejaculation
2. Blood in the semen
3. Difficulty urinating
4. Temperature of more than 99°F (37.2° C)

43. Two days after a transrectal biopsy of the prostate, a client calls the clinic to report his stools are streaked with blood. Which response is appropriate?
1. Tell the client to take a laxative.
2. Tell the client to come in for examination.
3. Reassure the client that this is an expected occurrence.
4. Ask the client to collect a stool specimen for testing.

44. A nurse is caring for the following clients who have a history of genital herpes infection. Which client is <u>most</u> at risk for an outbreak of genital herpes?
1. A client who complains of a headache and fever
2. A client who complains of vaginal and urethral discharge
3. A client who complains of dysuria and lymphadenopathy
4. A client who complains of genital pruritus and paresthesia

41. 1. Straining at stool after prostatectomy can cause bleeding. Small blood clots or pieces of tissue commonly are passed in the urine for up to 2 weeks postoperatively. Tub baths are prohibited because they cause dilation of pelvic blood vessels. Other activities are resumed based on the guidance of the physician. Sexual intercourse and driving are usually prohibited for about 3 weeks. Exercising and returning to work are usually prohibited for about 6 weeks.
CN: Physiological integrity; CNS: Reduction of risk potential; CL: Comprehension

42. 3. Difficulty urinating suggests urethral obstruction. Blood in the semen is an expected finding for months, and discomfort on ejaculation is expected for weeks. Temperature of more than 101°F (38.3° C) should be reported because it suggests infection.
CN: Physiological integrity; CNS: Reduction of risk potential; CL: Comprehension

43. 3. After a transrectal prostatic biopsy, blood in the stools is expected for a number of days. Stool softeners are prescribed if the client complains of constipation; straining at stool can precipitate bleeding, but laxatives generally aren't necessary. Because blood in the stools is expected, testing the stools or examining the client isn't necessary.
CN: Physiological integrity; CNS: Reduction of risk potential; CL: Application

44. 4. Pruritus and paresthesia as well as redness of the genital area are prodromal symptoms of recurrent herpes infection. These symptoms occur 30 minutes to 48 hours before the lesions appear. Headache and fever are symptoms of viremia associated with the primary infection. Vaginal and urethral discharge is also a local sign of primary infection. Dysuria and lymphadenopathy are local symptoms of primary infection that may also occur with recurrent infection.
CN: Physiological integrity; CNS: Physiological adaptation; CL: Analysis

CN: Client needs category   CNS: Client needs subcategory   CL: Cognitive level

45. Which instruction should be given to a woman newly diagnosed with genital herpes?
1. Obtain a Papanicolaou (Pap) test every 3 years.
2. Have your partner use a condom when lesions are present.
3. Use a water-soluble lubricant for relief of pruritus.
4. Limit stress and emotional upset as much as possible.

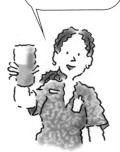

Your glass is half full of the right answers! Keep going!

46. A client has been admitted with primary syphilis. Which signs or symptoms should the nurse expect to see with this diagnosis?
1. A painless genital ulcer that appeared about 3 weeks after unprotected sex
2. Copper-colored macules on the palms and soles that appeared after a brief fever
3. Patchy hair loss and red, broken skin involving the scalp, eyebrows, and beard areas
4. One or more flat, wartlike papules in the genital area that are sensitive to touch

47. During a routine physical examination, a firm mass is palpated in the right breast of a 35-year-old woman. Which finding or client history would suggest cancer of the breast as opposed to fibrocystic disease?
1. History of early menarche
2. Cyclic change in mass size
3. History of anovulatory cycles
4. Increased vascularity of the breast

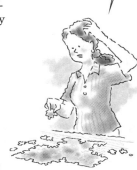

The client's history can provide the missing piece of the puzzle.

48. After which procedure is the use of sterile technique in the provision of client hygiene most critical?
1. Radical prostatectomy
2. Perineal prostatectomy
3. Suprapubic prostatectomy
4. Transurethral prostatectomy (TURP)

45. 4. Stress, anxiety, and emotional upset seem to predispose a client to recurrent outbreaks of genital herpes. Sexual intercourse should be avoided during outbreaks, and a condom should be used between outbreaks; it isn't known whether the virus can be transmitted at this time. During an outbreak, creams and lubricants should be avoided because they may prolong healing. Because a relationship has been found between genital herpes and cervical cancer, a Pap test is recommended every year.
CN: Physiological integrity; CNS: Physiological adaptation; CL: Application

46. 1. A painless genital ulcer is a symptom of primary syphilis. Macules on the palms and soles after fever are indicative of secondary syphilis, as is patchy hair loss. Wartlike papules are indicative of genital warts.
CN: Physiological integrity; CNS: Physiological adaptation; CL: Analysis

47. 4. Increase in breast size or vascularity is consistent with breast cancer. Early menarche as well as late menopause or a history of anovulatory cycles is associated with fibrocystic disease. Masses associated with fibrocystic disease of the breast are firm, are most commonly located in the upper outer quadrant of the breast, and increase in size before menstruation. They may be bilateral in a mirror image and are typically well demarcated and freely moveable.
CN: Health promotion and maintenance; CNS: None; CL: Application

48. 2. The incision in a perineal prostatectomy is close to the rectum, which normally contains gram-negative organisms that can cause infection if introduced into other areas of the body. The use of proper sterile technique, including washing front to back, in providing hygiene is more critical to these clients than those with either no external incision, as with TURP, or abdominal incisions, as with radical or suprapubic prostatectomy.
CN: Physiological integrity; CNS: Reduction of risk potential; CL: Application

CN: Client needs category   CNS: Client needs subcategory   CL: Cognitive level

49. Which condition is a <u>common</u> cause of prerenal acute renal failure?
1. Atherosclerosis
2. Decreased cardiac output
3. Prostatic hypertrophy
4. Rhabdomyolysis

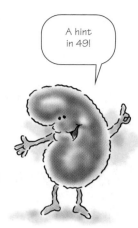

A hint in 49!

49. 2. Prerenal acute renal failure refers to renal failure due to an interference with renal perfusion. Decreased cardiac output causes a decrease in renal perfusion, which leads to a lower glomerular filtration rate. Atherosclerosis and rhabdomyolysis are renal causes of acute renal failure. Prostatic hypertrophy would be an example of a postrenal cause of acute renal failure.

CN: Physiological integrity; CNS: Physiological adaptation; CL: Knowledge

50. A client admitted for acute pyelonephritis is about to start antibiotic therapy. Which symptom would be expected in this client?
1. Hypertension
2. Flank pain on the affected side
3. Pain that radiates toward the unaffected side
4. No tenderness with deep palpation over the costovertebral angle

50. 2. The client may complain of pain on the affected side because the kidney is enlarged and might have formed an abscess. Hypertension is associated with chronic pyelonephritis. The client would have tenderness with deep palpation over the costovertebral angle. Pain may radiate down the ureters or to the epigastrium.

CN: Physiological integrity; CNS: Physiological adaptation; CL: Knowledge

51. Discharge instructions for a client treated for acute pyelonephritis should include which statement?
1. Avoid taking any dairy products.
2. Return for follow-up urine cultures.
3. Stop taking the prescribed antibiotics when the symptoms subside.
4. Recurrence is unlikely because you've been treated with antibiotics.

51. 2. The client needs to return for follow-up urine cultures because bacteriuria may be present but may not produce symptoms. Intake of dairy products won't contribute to pyelonephritis. Antibiotics must be taken for the full course of therapy regardless of symptoms. Pyelonephritis commonly recurs as a relapse or new infection and usually recurs within 2 weeks of completing therapy.

CN: Health promotion and maintenance; CNS: None; CL: Comprehension

52. A client is complaining of severe flank and abdominal pain. A flat plate of the abdomen shows urolithiasis. Which intervention is important?
1. Strain all urine.
2. Limit fluid intake.
3. Enforce strict bed rest.
4. Encourage a high-calcium diet.

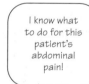

I know what to do for this patient's abdominal pain!

52. 1. Urine should be strained for calculi and sent to the laboratory for analysis. Fluid intake of 3 to 4 L/day is encouraged to flush the urinary tract and prevent further calculi formation. Ambulation is encouraged to help pass the calculi through gravity. A low-calcium diet is recommended to help prevent the formation of calcium calculi.

CN: Physiological integrity; CNS: Reduction of risk potential; CL: Application

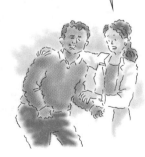

CN: Client needs category   CNS: Client needs subcategory   CL: Cognitive level

53. A client is receiving a radiation implant for the treatment of bladder cancer. Which intervention is appropriate?
   1. Flush all urine down the toilet.
   2. Restrict the client's fluid intake.
   3. Place the client in a semiprivate room.
   4. Monitor the client for signs and symptoms of cystitis.

54. A client has undergone a radical cystectomy and has an ileal conduit for the treatment of bladder cancer. Which postoperative assessment finding must be reported to the physician immediately?
   1. A red, moist stoma
   2. A dusky-colored stoma
   3. Urine output more than 30 ml/hour
   4. Slight bleeding from the stoma when changing the appliance

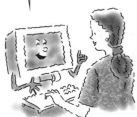

Question 54 asks you to prioritize responses according to which is most urgent.

55. Which statement by a client with an ileal conduit indicates the need for further teaching?
   1. "I'll change my appliance at bedtime."
   2. "I'll cover the stoma with gauze while changing the appliance."
   3. "I'll clean the skin around the stoma with mild soap and water, and dry it thoroughly."
   4. "I'll cut the hole in the appliance wafer no more than 3 mm larger than the stoma."

56. A client is diagnosed with cystitis. Client teaching aimed at preventing a recurrence should include which instruction?
   1. Bathe in a tub.
   2. Wear cotton underpants.
   3. Use a feminine hygiene spray.
   4. Limit your intake of cranberry juice.

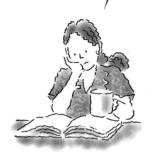

Stay awake now. You're closer to home!

53. 4. Cystitis is the most common adverse reaction of clients undergoing radiation therapy; symptoms include dysuria, frequency, urgency, and nocturia. Urine of clients with radiation implants for bladder cancer should be sent to the radioisotopes laboratory for monitoring. It's recommended that fluid intake be increased. Clients with radiation implants require a private room.
CN: Physiological integrity; CNS: Reduction of risk potential; CL: Knowledge

54. 2. The stoma should be red and moist, indicating adequate blood flow. A dusky or cyanotic stoma indicates insufficient blood supply and is an emergency needing prompt intervention. Urine output less than 30 ml/hour or no urine output for more than 15 minutes should be reported. Slight bleeding from the stoma when changing the appliance may occur because the intestinal mucosa is very fragile.
CN: Physiological integrity; CNS: Reduction of risk potential; CL: Comprehension

55. 1. The client should change the appliance in the morning, when urine output is lowest, to decrease the amount of urine that might come in contact with the skin, causing irritation. Covering the stoma with gauze while changing the appliance helps prevent urine seepage onto the skin. Cleaning the skin around the stoma with soap and water and drying it thoroughly help prevent irritation from urine. The faceplate or wafer of the appliance shouldn't be more than 3 mm larger than the stoma to reduce the skin area in contact with urine.
CN: Physiological integrity; CNS: Basic care and comfort; CL: Analysis

56. 2. Cotton underpants prevent infection because they allow air to flow to the perineum. Women should shower instead of taking a tub bath to prevent infection. Feminine hygiene spray can act as an irritant. Cranberry juice helps prevent cystitis because it increases urine acidity; alkaline urine supports bacterial growth.
CN: Health promotion and maintenance; CNS: None; CL: Application

CN: Client needs category   CNS: Client needs subcategory   CL: Cognitive level

57. Care for an indwelling urinary catheter should include which intervention?
1. Insert the catheter using clean technique.
2. Keep the drainage bag on the bed with the client.
3. Clean around the catheter at the meatus with soap and water.
4. Lay the drainage bag on the floor to enable maximum drainage through gravity.

58. A nurse is preparing to obtain a urine culture from a male client. Which urine-collection technique is appropriate for this client?
1. Have the client void in a clean container, being careful not to touch the rim.
2. Clean the foreskin of the uncircumcised male before specimen collection.
3. Have the client void into a urinal and then pour the urine into the specimen container.
4. Have the client begin to void and then catch some urine in a sterile container midstream.

59. A client with chronic renal failure is admitted with pulmonary edema following a missed dialysis treatment yesterday. The nurse should monitor the client closely for which condition?
1. Alkalemia
2. Hyperkalemia
3. Hypernatremia
4. Hypokalemia

60. Dialysis allows for the exchange of particles across a semipermeable membrane by which action?
1. Osmosis and diffusion
2. Passage of fluid toward a solution with a lower solute concentration
3. Allowing the passage of blood cells and protein molecules through it
4. Passage of solute particles toward a solution with a higher concentration

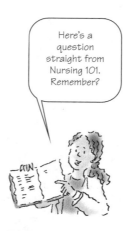

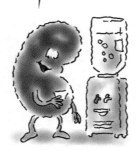

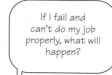

57. 3. It's important to clean the catheter at the meatus to decrease the chance of infection. The catheter should be inserted using sterile technique. Keeping the drainage bag in the bed with the client causes backflow of urine into the urethra, increasing the chance of infection. The drainage bag shouldn't be placed on the floor because of the increased risk of infection due to microorganisms. It should hang on the bed in a dependent position.
CN: Physiological integrity; CNS: Reduction of risk potential; CL: Comprehension

58. 4. Catching urine midstream reduces the amount of contamination by microorganisms at the meatus. Voiding in a clean container is done for a random specimen, not a clean-catch specimen for urine culture. When cleaning an uncircumcised male, the foreskin should be retracted, and the glans penis should be cleaned to prevent specimen contamination. Voiding in a urinal doesn't allow for an uncontaminated specimen because the urinal isn't sterile.
CN: Physiological integrity; CNS: Reduction of risk potential; CL: Analysis

59. 2. The kidneys are responsible for excreting potassium. In renal failure, the kidneys can no longer excrete potassium, resulting in hyperkalemia. The kidneys are responsible for regulating the acid-base balance; in renal failure, acidemia, not alkalemia, would be seen. Generally, hyponatremia, not hypernatremia, would be seen because of the dilutional effect of water retention. Hypokalemia is generally seen in clients undergoing diuresis.
CN: Physiological integrity; CNS: Physiological adaptation; CL: Application

60. 1. Osmosis allows for the removal of fluid from the blood by allowing it to pass through the semipermeable membrane to an area of high concentration (dialysate), and diffusion allows for passage of particles (electrolytes, urea, and creatinine) from an area of higher concentration to an area of lower concentration. Fluid passes to an area with a higher solute concentration. The pores of the semipermeable membrane are small, thus preventing the flow of blood cells and protein molecules through it.
CN: Physiological integrity; CNS: Physiological adaptation; CL: Knowledge

CN: Client needs category   CNS: Client needs subcategory   CL: Cognitive level

61. A client has just received a renal transplant and has started cyclosporine (Sandimmune) therapy to prevent graft rejection. Which condition indicates to the nurse that the client is experiencing a major adverse effect related to the medication?
1. Depression
2. Hemorrhage
3. Infection
4. Peptic ulcer disease

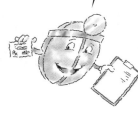

Remember, cyclosporine is an immune system suppressant.

62. A client received a kidney transplant 2 months ago. He's admitted to the hospital with the diagnosis of acute rejection. Which assessment finding would be expected?
1. Hypotension
2. Normal body temperature
3. Decreased white blood cell (WBC) counts
4. Elevated blood urea nitrogen (BUN) and creatinine levels

63. A client is undergoing peritoneal dialysis. The dialysate dwell time is completed, and the clamp is opened to allow the dialysate to drain. The nurse notes that drainage has stopped and that only 500 ml has drained; the amount of dialysate instilled was 1,500 ml. Which intervention would be done <u>first</u>?
1. Change the client's position.
2. Call the physician.
3. Check the catheter for kinks or obstruction.
4. Clamp the catheter, and instill more dialysate at the next exchange time.

There's a lot of information given here. Look closely for the common patterns.

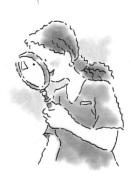

64. A client receiving hemodialysis treatment arrives at the hospital with a blood pressure of 200/100 mm Hg, a heart rate of 110 beats/minute, and a respiratory rate of 36 breaths/minute. Oxygen saturation on room air is 89%. He complains of shortness of breath, and +2 pedal edema is noted. His last hemodialysis treatment was yesterday. Which intervention should be done first?
1. Administer oxygen.
2. Elevate the foot of the bed.
3. Restrict the client's fluids.
4. Prepare the client for hemodialysis.

61. 3. Infection is the major complication to watch for in clients on cyclosporine therapy because cyclosporine is an immunosuppressive drug. Depression may occur posttransplantation, but not because of cyclosporine. Hemorrhage is a complication associated with anticoagulant therapy. Peptic ulcer disease is a complication of steroid therapy.
CN: Physiological integrity; CNS: Pharmacological therapies; CL: Analysis

62. 4. In a client with acute renal graft rejection, evidence of deteriorating renal function, including elevated BUN and creatinine levels, is expected. The client would most likely have acute hypertension. The nurse would see elevated, not decreased, WBC counts as well as fever because the body is recognizing the graft as foreign and is attempting to fight it.
CN: Physiological integrity; CNS: Reduction of risk potential; CL: Analysis

63. 3. The first intervention should be to check for kinks and obstructions because they could be preventing drainage. After checking for kinks, have the client change position to promote drainage. If unable to get more output despite checking for kinks and changing the client's position, the nurse should then call the physician to determine the proper intervention. Don't give the next scheduled exchange until the dialysate is drained because abdominal distention will occur, unless the output is within the parameters set by the physician.
CN: Physiological integrity; CNS: Reduction of risk potential; CL: Analysis

64. 1. Airway and oxygenation are always the first priority. Because the client is complaining of shortness of breath and his oxygen saturation is only 89%, the nurse must try to increase the partial pressure of arterial oxygen by administering oxygen. The foot of the bed may be elevated to reduce edema, but this isn't a priority. The client is experiencing pulmonary edema from fluid overload and will need to be dialyzed and have his fluids restricted, but the first intervention should be aimed at the immediate treatment of hypoxia.
CN: Physiological integrity; CNS: Physiological adaptation; CL: Analysis

CN: Client needs category   CNS: Client needs subcategory   CL: Cognitive level

65. A client with renal insufficiency is admitted with a diagnosis of pneumonia. He's being treated with I.V. antibiotics and has had episodes of hypotension. Which laboratory value would be monitored closely?
1. Blood urea nitrogen (BUN) and creatinine levels
2. Arterial blood gas (ABG) levels
3. Platelet count
4. Potassium level

66. A client had transurethral prostatectomy for benign prostatic hypertrophy. He's currently being treated with a continuous bladder irrigation and is complaining of an increase in severity of bladder spasms. What should the nurse do first for this client?
1. Administer an oral analgesic.
2. Stop the irrigation and call the physician.
3. Administer a belladonna and opium suppository as ordered by the physician.
4. Check for the presence of clots, and make sure the catheter is draining properly.

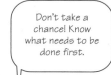

Don't take a chance! Know what needs to be done first.

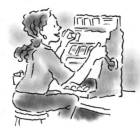

67. A client with bladder cancer has had his bladder removed and an ileal conduit created for urine diversion. While changing this client's pouch, the nurse observes that the area around the stoma is red, weeping, and painful. What should the nurse conclude?
1. The skin wasn't lubricated before the pouch was applied.
2. The pouch faceplate doesn't fit the stoma.
3. A skin barrier was applied properly.
4. Stoma dilation wasn't performed.

68. A client has an indwelling urinary catheter, and urine is leaking from a hole in the collection bag. Which nursing intervention would be most appropriate?
1. Cover the hole with tape.
2. Remove the catheter, and insert a new one using sterile technique.
3. Disconnect the drainage bag from the catheter, and replace it with a new bag.
4. Place a towel under the bag to prevent spillage of urine on the floor, which could cause the client to slip and fall.

Here are those words most appropriate again. Don't you just love 'em?

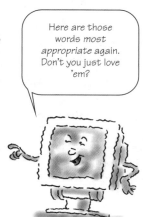

65. 1. BUN and creatinine levels are used to monitor renal function. Because the client is receiving I.V. antibiotics, which can be nephrotoxic, these tests would be used to closely monitor renal function. The client is also hypotensive, which is a prerenal cause of acute renal failure. ABG determinations are inappropriate for this situation. Platelets and potassium levels should be monitored according to routine.
CN: Physiological integrity; CNS: Reduction of risk potential; CL: Analysis

66. 4. Blood clots and blocked outflow of the urine can increase spasms. The irrigation shouldn't be stopped as long as the catheter is draining because clots will form. A belladonna and opium suppository should be given to relieve spasms but only *after* assessment of the drainage. Oral analgesics should be given if the spasms are unrelieved by the belladonna and opium suppository.
CN: Physiological integrity; CNS: Physiological adaptation; CL: Analysis

67. 2. If the pouch faceplate doesn't fit the stoma properly, the skin around the stoma will be exposed to continuous urine flow from the stoma, causing excoriation and red, weeping, painful skin. A lubricant shouldn't be used because it would prevent the pouch from adhering to the skin. When properly applied, a skin barrier prevents skin excoriation. Stoma dilation isn't performed with an ileal conduit, although it may be done with a colostomy, if ordered.
CN: Physiological integrity; CNS: Basic care and comfort; CL: Analysis

68. 2. The system is no longer a closed system, and bacteria might have been introduced into the system, so a new sterile catheter should be inserted. Placing a towel under the bag and taping up the hole leave the system open, which increases the risk of infection. Replacing the drainage bag by disconnecting the old one from the catheter opens up the entire system and isn't recommended because of the increased risk of infection.
CN: Safe, effective care environment; CNS: Safety and infection control; CL: Analysis

CN: Client needs category   CNS: Client needs subcategory   CL: Cognitive level

69. During a health history, which statement by a client indicates a risk of renal calculi?
1. "I've been drinking a lot of cola soft drinks lately."
2. "I've been jogging more than usual."
3. "I've had more stress since we adopted a child last year."
4. "I'm a vegetarian and eat cheese two or three times each day."

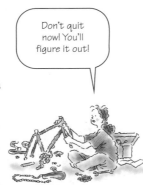

Don't quit now! You'll figure it out!

70. A client is admitted with severe nausea, vomiting, and diarrhea and is hypotensive. She's noted to have severe oliguria with elevated blood urea nitrogen (BUN) and creatinine levels. The physician will most likely write an order for which treatment?
1. Encourage oral fluids.
2. Give furosemide (Lasix) 20 mg I.V.
3. Start hemodialysis after temporary access is obtained.
4. Start I.V. fluid of normal saline solution bolus followed by a maintenance dose.

71. A woman who reports painful urination during or after voiding might have a problem in which location?
1. Bladder
2. Kidneys
3. Ureters
4. Urethra

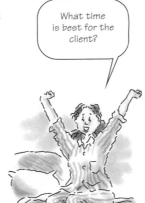

What time is best for the client?

72. What's the best time of day to give diuretics?
1. Anytime
2. Bedtime
3. Morning
4. Noon

73. Which intervention would be <u>inappropriate</u> to help a client with postoperative urine retention?
1. Give a diuretic.
2. Pour warm water over the perineum.
3. Consider inserting a bladder catheter.
4. Place the client in a sitting or semi-Fowler position.

69. 4. Renal calculi are commonly composed of calcium. Diets high in calcium may predispose a person to renal calculi. Milk and milk products are high in calcium. Cola soft drinks don't contain ingredients that would increase the risk of renal calculi. Jogging and increased stress aren't considered risk factors for renal calculi formation.
CN: Health promotion and maintenance; CNS: None; CL: Analysis

70. 4. The client is experiencing prerenal failure secondary to hypovolemia. I.V. fluids should be given to rehydrate the client, urine output should increase, and the BUN and creatinine levels will normalize. The client wouldn't be able to tolerate oral fluids because of the nausea, vomiting, and diarrhea. The client isn't fluid overloaded, and her urine output won't increase with furosemide. The client won't need dialysis because the oliguria and increased BUN and creatinine levels are due to dehydration.
CN: Physiological integrity; CNS: Physiological adaptation; CL: Analysis

71. 1. Pain during or after voiding indicates a bladder problem, usually infection. Kidney and ureter pain would be in the flank area, and problems of the urethra would cause pain at the external orifice commonly felt at the start of voiding.
CN: Health promotion and maintenance; CNS: None; CL: Knowledge

72. 3. A diuretic given in the morning has time to work throughout the day. Diuretics given at nighttime will cause the client to get up to go to the bathroom frequently, interrupting sleep.
CN: Physiological integrity; CNS: Pharmacological therapies; CL: Application

73. 1. Urine retention reflects bladder distention from urine. A diuretic isn't necessary. Sitting upright and pouring water over the perineum may help the client void. If these measures aren't successful, the nurse should consider inserting a bladder catheter to drain the bladder, which requires an order from the physician.
CN: Physiological integrity; CNS: Basic care and comfort; CL: Application

CN: Client needs category   CNS: Client needs subcategory   CL: Cognitive level

74. Which factor may place a surgical client at risk for urine retention?
1. Dehydration
2. History of smoking
3. Duration of surgery
4. Anticholinergic medication before surgery

75. Which type of catheter is generally used for the client with urine retention?
1. Coudé
2. Indwelling urinary
3. Straight
4. Three-way

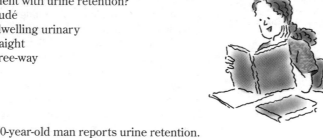

All these catheters aren't the same.

76. An 80-year-old man reports urine retention. Which factor may contribute to this client's problem?
1. Benign prostatic hyperplasia
2. Diabetes
3. Diet
4. Hypertension

77. A client with chronic renal failure (CRF) is admitted to the urology unit. Which diagnostic test results are consistent with CRF?
1. Increased pH with decreased hydrogen ions
2. Increased serum levels of calcium
3. Blood urea nitrogen (BUN) level of 100 mg/dl and serum creatinine level of 6.5 mg/dl
4. Uric acid level of 3.5 mg/dl and phenol-sulfonphthalein (PSP) excretion of 75%

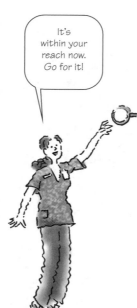

It's within your reach now. Go for it!

74. 4. Anticholinergic medications, such as atropine and scopolamine (Scopace), may cause urine retention, particularly for the client who has surgery in the pelvic area (inguinal hernia, hysterectomy). Dehydration, smoking, and duration of surgery aren't risk factors for urine retention.
CN: Physiological integrity; CNS: Reduction of risk potential; CL: Comprehension

75. 3. Urine retention is usually a temporary problem. The three-way catheter is used for clients who need bladder irrigation such as after a prostate resection. A catheter coudé is used only when it's difficult to insert a standard catheter, usually because of an enlarged prostate. The other catheters are used for longer-term bladder problems.
CN: Physiological integrity; CNS: Basic care and comfort; CL: Comprehension

76. 1. An enlarged prostate gland is common among elderly men and commonly results in urine retention, frequency, dribbling, and difficulty starting the urine stream. Diabetes, diet, and hypertension usually don't affect urine retention. Diabetes can cause renal failure.
CN: Physiological integrity; CNS: Reduction of risk potential; CL: Application

77. 3. The normal BUN level ranges from 8 to 23 mg/dl, and the normal serum creatinine level ranges from 0.7 to 1.5 mg/dl. A BUN level of 100 mg/dl and a serum creatinine level of 6.5 mg/dl are abnormally elevated, reflecting CRF and the kidneys' decreased ability to remove nonprotein nitrogen waste from the blood. CRF causes decreased pH and increased hydrogen ions, not vice versa. CRF also increases serum levels of potassium, magnesium, and phosphatase and decreases serum levels of calcium. A uric acid level of 3.5 mg/dl falls within the normal range of 2.7 to 7.7 mg/dl; PSP excretion of 75% also falls within the normal range of 60% to 75%.
CN: Physiological integrity; CNS: Physiological adaptation; CL: Knowledge

CN: Client needs category CNS: Client needs subcategory CL: Cognitive level

78. Which steps should a nurse follow to insert a straight urinary catheter?
1. Create a sterile field, drape the client, clean the meatus, and insert the catheter only 6″ (15.2 cm).
2. Put on gloves, prepare the equipment, create a sterile field, expose the urinary meatus, and insert the catheter 6″.
3. Prepare the client and equipment, create a sterile field, put on gloves, clean the urinary meatus, and insert the catheter until the urine flows.
4. Prepare the client, prepare the equipment, create a sterile field, test the catheter balloon, clean the meatus, and insert the catheter until urine flows.

79. A client is injected with radiographic contrast medium and immediately shows signs of dyspnea, flushing, and pruritus. Which intervention should take priority?
1. Check vital signs.
2. Make sure the airway is patent.
3. Apply a cold pack to the I.V. site.
4. Call the physician.

80. An 80-year-old man is admitted for a cystoscopy with biopsy of the bladder. After the physician obtains a history, the surgery is postponed. What would be an inappropriate reason to postpone this client's surgery?
1. The client is taking an anticoagulant.
2. The client has a urinary tract infection (UTI).
3. The client might have carcinoma of the bladder.
4. The client reports chest pain at rest for the past 3 days.

78. 3. Preparing the client and equipment, creating a sterile field, putting on gloves, cleaning the urinary meatus, and inserting the catheter until the urine flows are the vital steps for inserting a straight catheter. The nurse must prepare the client and equipment *before* creating a sterile field. The nurse shouldn't put on gloves before creating a sterile field or performing the other tasks. The nurse would test a catheter balloon when inserting a retention catheter, not a straight catheter.
CN: Safe, effective care environment; CNS: Safety and infection control; CL: Knowledge

This word—priority—is your biggest hint.

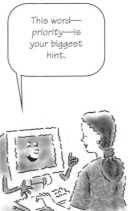

79. 2. The client is showing symptoms of an allergy to the iodine in the contrast medium. The first action is to make sure the client's airway is patent. If compromised, call a cardiac arrest code. Checking vital signs and calling for the physician are important nursing actions but should follow making sure the airway is patent. A cold pack isn't indicated.
CN: Physiological integrity; CNS: Physiological adaptation; CL: Application

80. 3. Suspected bladder carcinoma is probably the reason for the planned biopsy. Anticoagulants should be discontinued for 3 to 5 days before the procedure. Bladder biopsies shouldn't be done when an active UTI is present because sepsis may result. Chest pain at rest may indicate myocardial ischemia and would be an indication to postpone the biopsy until it can be further investigated.
CN: Physiological integrity; CNS: Reduction of risk potential; CL: Analysis

CN: Client needs category   CNS: Client needs subcategory   CL: Cognitive level

81. Unless there are postoperative complications, a cystoscopy client is typically discharged to home within 24 hours. Which instruction is given at discharge?
  1. Expect bloody urine for about a week.
  2. Drink 8 to 10 glasses of water every 8 hours.
  3. Try to urinate frequently, and measure your output.
  4. Check the color, consistency, and amount of urine in the indwelling urinary catheter bag every 4 to 8 hours.

82. Before a renal biopsy, which piece of information is most important to tell a physician?
  1. The client signed a consent.
  2. The client understands the procedure.
  3. The client has normal urinary elimination.
  4. The client regularly takes aspirin or non-steroidal anti-inflammatory drugs (NSAIDs).

83. Kegel exercises are used to gain control of bladder function in women with stress incontinence, and in some men after prostate surgery. Which instruction would help a client perform these exercises?
  1. Completely empty the bladder.
  2. Do the exercise 200 times per day.
  3. Sit or stand with your legs together.
  4. Drink small amounts of fluid frequently.

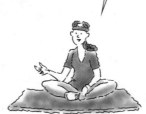

Kegel exercises can improve muscle tone and help you gain bladder control.

84. Which instruction is given to clients with chronic pyelonephritis?
  1. Stay on bed rest for up to 2 weeks.
  2. Use analgesia on a regular basis for up to 6 months.
  3. Have a urine culture every 2 weeks for up to 6 months.
  4. You may need antibiotic treatment for several weeks or months.

81. 3. The bladder must be emptied frequently, and output should be measured to make sure the bladder is emptying. Blood in the urine isn't normal except for small amounts during the first 24 hours after the procedure. Large amounts of fluids help flush microorganisms out of the body, but 8 to 10 glasses every 8 hours may not be reasonable. Also, families don't tend to think in time periods, so instructions should be given per day. The client may not have an indwelling urinary catheter.
CN: Physiological integrity; CNS: Reduction of risk potential; CL: Application

82. 4. Aspirin and NSAIDs cause increased bleeding times and commonly result in hemorrhaging when biopsies are performed. It's the physician's responsibility to make sure the client understands the procedure, which is needed for informed consent. It isn't necessary to report that the client has normal urinary elimination.
CN: Physiological integrity; CNS: Reduction of risk potential; CL: Application

83. 2. Exercises begin with tightening and relaxing the vagina, rectum, and urethra four or five times during each session and gradually increasing to 25 times for each session. The client stops the flow of urine during urination to practice holding the flow. Standing or sitting with the legs apart facilitates the exercise. Clients should drink plenty of fluids to prevent urinary problems.
CN: Physiological integrity; CNS: Physiological adaptation; CL: Application

84. 4. Chronic pyelonephritis can be a long-term condition and requires close monitoring to prevent permanent damage to the kidneys. Analgesia and bed rest may be used during the acute stage but usually aren't required for the long term. A urine culture is done 2 weeks after stopping antibiotics to make sure the infection has been eradicated.
CN: Physiological integrity; CNS: Reduction of risk potential; CL: Application

CN: Client needs category   CNS: Client needs subcategory   CL: Cognitive level

85. A nurse is caring for a client with renal failure who's complaining of nausea. Which factor best explains how nausea is related to renal failure?

1. Oliguria
2. Gastric ulcer
3. Electrolyte imbalance
4. Accumulation of metabolic wastes

86. Which client is at greatest risk for developing acute renal failure?

1. A dialysis client who gets influenza
2. A teenager who has an appendectomy
3. A pregnant woman who has a fractured femur
4. A client with diabetes who has a heart catheterization

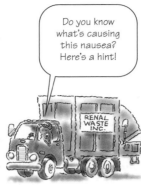

Do you know what's causing this nausea? Here's a hint!

87. Which intervention would be done for a client with urinary calculus?

1. Save any stone larger than 0.25 cm.
2. Strain the urine, limit oral fluids, and give pain medications.
3. Encourage fluid intake, strain the urine, and give pain medications.
4. Insert an indwelling urinary catheter, check intake and output, and give pain medications.

88. A nurse is assessing a client who has a urinary tract infection (UTI). Which statement should the nurse expect the client to make? Select all that apply:

1. "I urinate large amounts."
2. "I need to urinate frequently."
3. "It burns when I urinate."
4. "My urine smells sweet."
5. "I need to urinate urgently."

85. 4. Although a client with renal failure can develop stress ulcers, nausea is usually related to the poisons of metabolic wastes that accumulate when the kidneys can't eliminate them. Although a client may have electrolyte imbalances and oliguria, these conditions don't directly cause nausea.

CN: Physiological integrity; CNS: Physiological adaptation; CL: Analysis

86. 4. Diabetes can damage the smaller arteries of the kidneys, and clients with diabetes are prone to renal insufficiency and renal failure. The contrast used for heart catheterization must be eliminated by the kidneys, which further stresses them and may produce acute renal failure. A dialysis client already has end-stage renal disease and wouldn't develop acute renal failure. A teenager who has an appendectomy and a pregnant woman who fractures a femur aren't at increased risk for renal failure.

CN: Health promotion and maintenance; CNS: None; CL: Analysis

87. 3. Encourage fluids and strain all urine, saving all calculi, including "flecks." Give pain medications because renal calculi are extremely painful. Indwelling urinary catheters usually aren't needed.

CN: Physiological integrity; CNS: Basic care and comfort; CL: Application

88. 2, 3, 5. Typical assessment findings for a client with a UTI include urinary frequency, burning on urination, and urinary urgency. The client with a UTI typically reports that he voids frequently in small amounts, not large amounts. The client with a UTI complains of foul-smelling, not sweet-smelling, urine.

CN: Physiological integrity; CNS: Physiological adaptation; CL: Application

89. A nurse is collecting a sterile urine specimen for culture and sensitivity from an indwelling urinary catheter. Identify the area on the indwelling urinary catheter where the nurse should insert the sterile syringe to obtain the urine specimen.

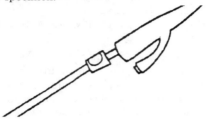

90. A nurse is completing an intake and output record for a client who's receiving continuous bladder irrigation after transurethral resection of the prostate. How many milliliters of urine should the nurse record as output for her shift if the client received 1,800 ml of normal saline irrigating solution and the output in the urine drainage bag is 2,400 ml? Record your answer as a whole number.

_____ml

91. A 26-year-old client with chronic renal failure plans to receive a kidney transplant. Recently, the physician told the client that he's a poor candidate for transplant because of chronic uncontrolled hypertension and diabetes mellitus. Now, the client tells the nurse, "I want to go off dialysis. I'd rather not live than be on this treatment for the rest of my life." Which response is appropriate? Select all that apply:
1. Take a seat next to the client and sit quietly.
2. Say to the client, "We all have days when we don't feel like going on."
3. Leave the room to allow the client to collect his thoughts.
4. Say to the client, "You're feeling upset about the news you got about the transplant."
5. Say to the client, "The treatments are only 3 days a week. You can live with that."

89.

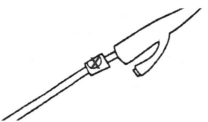

A sterile urine specimen is obtained from an indwelling urinary catheter by clamping the catheter briefly, cleaning the rubber port with an alcohol wipe, and using a sterile syringe to withdraw the urine.
CN: Physiological integrity; CNS: Reduction of risk potential; CL: Application

90. 600. To calculate urine output, subtract the amount of irrigation solution infused into the bladder from the total amount of fluid in the drainage bag (2,400 ml − 1,800 ml = 600 ml).
CN: Physiological integrity; CNS: Reduction of risk potential; CL: Application

91. 1, 4. Silence is a therapeutic communication technique that allows the nurse and client to reflect on what has been said or taken place. By waiting quietly and attentively, the nurse encourages the client to initiate and maintain conversation. By reflecting the client's implied feelings, the nurse promotes communication. Using such platitudes as "We all have days when we don't feel like going on" fails to address the client's needs. The nurse shouldn't leave the client alone because he may harm himself. Reminding the client of the treatment frequency doesn't address his feelings.
CN: Psychosocial integrity; CNS: None; CL: Analysis

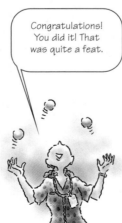

Congratulations! You did it! That was quite a feat.

CN: Client needs category   CNS: Client needs subcategory   CL: Cognitive level

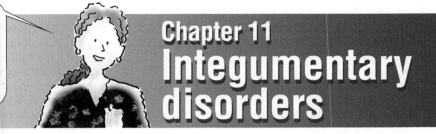

Chapter 11
Integumentary disorders

1. A nurse is caring for a 50-year-old client with a burn injury. Which statement best describes the client's nutritional needs?
  1. The client needs 100 cal/kg throughout hospitalization.
  2. The hypermetabolic state after a burn injury leads to poor healing.
  3. Controlling the temperature of the environment decreases caloric demands.
  4. Maintaining a hypermetabolic rate decreases the client's risk of infection.

2. A 30-year-old client is admitted to the emergency department with a deep partial-thickness burn on his arm after a fire in his workplace. Which signs and symptoms should the nurse expect to see?
  1. Pain and redness
  2. Minimal damage to the epidermis
  3. Necrotic tissue through all layers of skin
  4. Necrotic tissue through most of the dermis

3. A client is seen in the physician's office with a suspected brown recluse spider bite. Which sign would best indicate this type of spider bite?
  1. Bull's-eye rash
  2. Painful rash around a necrotic lesion
  3. Herald patch of oval lesions
  4. Line of papules and vesicles that appear 1 to 3 days after exposure

I think my chances of being bitten by a spider today are pretty low.

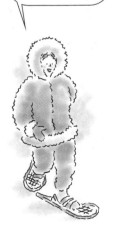

1. 2. A burn injury causes a hypermetabolic state resulting in protein and lipid catabolism that affects wound healing. Caloric intake must be 1½ to 2 times the basal metabolic rate, with at least 1.5 to 2 g/kg of body weight of protein daily. An environmental temperature within normal range lets the body function efficiently and devote caloric expenditure to healing and normal physiologic processes. If the temperature is too warm or too cold, the body gives energy to warming or cooling, which takes away from energy used for tissue repair. High metabolic rates increase the risk of infection.
CN: Physiological integrity; CNS: Basic care and comfort; CL: Application

2. 4. A deep partial-thickness burn causes necrosis of the epidermal and dermal layers. Redness and pain are characteristics of a superficial injury. Superficial burns cause slight epidermal damage. With deep burns, the nerve fibers are destroyed and the client doesn't feel pain in the affected area. Necrosis through all skin layers is seen with full-thickness injuries.
CN: Physiological integrity; CNS: Physiological adaptation; CL: Application

3. 2. Necrotic, painful rashes are associated with the bite of a brown recluse spider. A bull's-eye rash located primarily at the site of the bite is a classic sign of Lyme disease. A herald patch—a slightly raised, oval lesion about 2 to 6 cm in diameter and appearing anywhere on the body—is indicative of pityriasis rosea. A linear, papular, vesicular rash is characteristic of exposure to poison ivy.
CN: Physiological integrity; CNS: Physiological adaptation; CL: Analysis

CN: Client needs category   CNS: Client needs subcategory   CL: Cognitive level

4. A nurse is about to administer a Mantoux test. Which instruction should be followed when administering this test?
1. Use the deltoid muscle.
2. Rub the site to help absorption.
3. Read the results within 72 hours.
4. Read the results by checking for a rash.

5. A female client is worried she might have lice. Which finding should the nurse look for?
1. Diffuse, pruritic wheals
2. Oval, white dots stuck to the hair shafts
3. Pain, redness, and edema with an embedded stinger
4. Pruritic nodules and linear burrows of the finger and toe webs

6. A client is brought to the emergency department with second- and third-degree burns on his left arm, left anterior leg, and anterior trunk. Using the Rule of Nines, what percentage of the total body surface area has been burned?
1. 18%
2. 27%
3. 30%
4. 36%

7. A 19-year-old female client comes to the clinic with dark red lesions on her hands, wrist, and waistline. She has scratched several of the lesions so they're open and bleeding. The nurse instructs the client to try pressing on the itchy lesions. What's the rationale for this intervention?
1. Pressing the skin spreads beneficial microorganisms.
2. Pressing is suggested before scratching.
3. Pressing the skin promotes breaks in the skin.
4. Pressing the skin stimulates nerve endings.

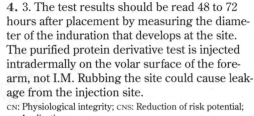

Follow the Rule of Nines when caring for clients with burns.

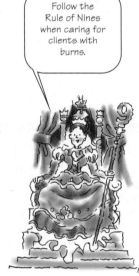

4. 3. The test results should be read 48 to 72 hours after placement by measuring the diameter of the induration that develops at the site. The purified protein derivative test is injected intradermally on the volar surface of the forearm, not I.M. Rubbing the site could cause leakage from the injection site.
CN: Physiological integrity; CNS: Reduction of risk potential; CL: Application

5. 2. Nits, the eggs of lice, are seen as white, oval dots. Diffuse, itchy wheals are associated with an allergic reaction. Bites from honeybees are associated with a stinger, pain, and redness. Pruritic nodules and linear burrows are diagnostic for scabies.
CN: Physiological integrity; CNS: Physiological adaptation; CL: Application

6. 4. The Rule of Nines divides body surface into percentages that, when totaled, equal 100%. According to the Rule of Nines, the arms account for 9% each, the anterior legs account for 9% each, and the anterior trunk accounts for 18%. Therefore, this client's burns cover 36% of his body surface area.
CN: Physiological integrity; CNS: Physiological adaptation; CL: Comprehension

7. 4. Pressing the skin stimulates nerve endings and can reduce the sensation of itching. Scratching (not pressing) the skin spreads microorganisms and opens portals of entry for bacteria. Scratching isn't recommended at all. Pressing the skin doesn't promote breaks in the skin.
CN: Physiological integrity; CNS: Physiological adaptation; CL: Application

8. A client arrives at the office of his physician complaining of several palpable elevated masses. Which term accurately describes these masses?
1. Erosions
2. Macules
3. Papules
4. Vesicles

9. A nurse is teaching a client about isotretinoin (Accutane). Which statement by the client indicates a need for further teaching?
1. "My husband and I are trying to have a baby."
2. "Some acne medications can lead to diarrhea."
3. "My friend has had folliculitis since taking another acne medicine, Cleocin."
4. "Sometimes drugs used for skin problems can cause yeast infections."

10. A nurse is caring for a 12-year-old child with a diagnosis of eczema. Which nursing interventions are appropriate for a child with eczema?
1. Administer antibiotics as prescribed.
2. Administer antifungals as ordered.
3. Administer tepid baths, and use moisturizers immediately after the bath.
4. Administer hot baths, and pat dry or air-dry the affected areas.

11. Which of the following instructions is given to a client taking nystatin oral solution?
1. Take the drug right after meals.
2. Take the drug right before meals.
3. Mix the drug with small amounts of food.
4. Take half the dose before and half after meals.

12. A client is examined and found to have pinpoint, pink-to-purple, nonblanching macular lesions 1 to 3 mm in diameter. Which term best describes these lesions?
1. Ecchymosis
2. Hematoma
3. Petechiae
4. Purpura

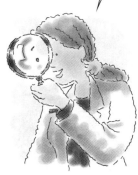

Masses, smasses. I know a papule when I see one!

You're doing petechiae-ly well so far. Keep going!

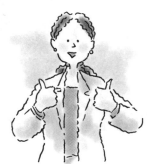

8. 3. Papules are elevated up to 0.5 cm, and nodules and tumors are masses elevated more than 0.5 cm. Erosions are characterized by loss of the epidermal layer. Macules and patches are nonpalpable, flat changes in skin color. Fluid-filled lesions are vesicles and pustules.
CN: Health promotion and maintenance; CNS: None; CL: Knowledge

9. 1. Even small amounts of Accutane are associated with severe birth defects. Most female clients are also prescribed hormonal contraceptives. Tetracycline, which can be used to treat acne, is associated with yeast infections. Clindamycin phosphate (Cleocin T Gel), another medicine used in the treatment of acne, can cause diarrhea and gram-negative folliculitis.
CN: Health promotion and maintenance; CNS: None; CL: Application

10. 3. Tepid baths and moisturizers are indicated to keep the infected areas clean and minimize itching. Antibiotics are given only when superimposed infection occurs. Antifungals aren't usually administered in the treatment of eczema. Hot baths can exacerbate the condition and increase itching.
CN: Physiological integrity; CNS: Physiological adaptation; CL: Application

11. 1. Nystatin oral solution should be swished around the mouth after eating for the best contact with mucous membranes. Taking the drug before or with meals doesn't allow for the best contact with the mucous membranes.
CN: Physiological integrity; CNS: Pharmacological therapies; CL: Application

12. 3. Petechiae are small macular lesions 1 to 3 mm in diameter. Ecchymosis is a purple-to-brown bruise, macular or papular, and varied in size. A hematoma is a collection of blood from ruptured blood vessels that's more than 1 cm in diameter. Purpura are purple macular lesions larger than 1 cm.
CN: Physiological integrity; CNS: Physiological adaptation; CL: Knowledge

CN: Client needs category CNS: Client needs subcategory CL: Cognitive level

13. A client has a rash consisting of scattered lesions on various parts of the body. Which type of rash is this?
1. Annular
2. Confluent
3. Diffuse
4. Linear

14. During a clinic visit for an active flare-up of psoriasis, a physician sees several bruises on the female client's arms. The client explains they were caused by her "bumping into things." She later privately confides in the nurse that her husband has been physically abusive. What's the most appropriate nursing intervention?
1. Immediately inform the physician about the physical violence.
2. Tell the client you'll talk to the physician and obtain referrals for personal counseling.
3. Tell the client that you'll need to call the local police.
4. Make sure the client has a safe place to go if needed.

15. A nurse is developing a care plan to maintain skin integrity in an adult client. Which nursing intervention would <u>best</u> meet the client's needs?
1. Applying a pleasantly scented dusting powder to the axillae and groin, beneath the breasts, and between the toes
2. Remembering to apply a deodorant or antiperspirant immediately after shaving under the arms
3. Trying to keep skin intact because healthy skin is the body's first line of defense
4. Always using alcohol for back rubs instead of lotion

16. A client has rough papules on the soles of his feet that are sometimes painful when he walks. Which term best describes this condition?
1. Filiform wart
2. Flat wart
3. Plantar wart
4. Venereal wart

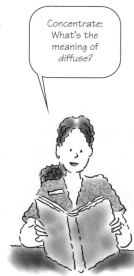

Concentrate: What's the meaning of diffuse?

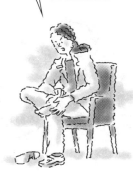

You'll get this question right because you have a lot of—ouch!—sole!

13. 3. A diffuse rash usually has widely distributed scattered lesions. An annular rash is ring-shaped. Confluent lesions are touching or adjacent to each other. Linear rashes are lesions arranged in a line.
CN: Physiological integrity; CNS: Physiological adaptation; CL: Knowledge

14. 4. Because there are physical indicators of violence, ensuring the client's safety is a priority. Therefore, the nurse should make sure the client has a safe place to go if needed. Options 1, 2, and 3 are inappropriate because they undermine the trust the client has placed in the nurse and could be damaging if her secret is revealed to the physician or legal authorities without her permission.
CN: Physiological integrity; CNS: Reduction of risk potential; CL: Analysis

15. 3. Because healthy skin is the body's first line of defense, a key nursing goal is to keep the skin intact. To reduce moisture, the nurse can apply a nonirritating dusting powder, such as cornstarch, to the client's axillae and groin, beneath the breasts, and between the toes after those areas are dry. However, scented powder shouldn't be used because it can irritate the skin. Deodorants and antiperspirants shouldn't be applied to the skin immediately after shaving because they may cause irritation. The nurse should use lotion for back rubs because alcohol dries the skin and can irritate it.
CN: Physiological integrity; CNS: Basic care and comfort; CL: Application

16. 3. Plantar warts are rough papules commonly found on the soles of the feet. Filiform warts are long spiny projections from the skin surface. Flat warts are flat-topped, smooth-surfaced lesions. Venereal warts appear on the genital mucosa and are confluent papules with rough surfaces.
CN: Physiological integrity; CNS: Physiological adaptation; CL: Knowledge

CN: Client needs category   CNS: Client needs subcategory   CL: Cognitive level

17. A nurse receives a report on a client who has circular lesions on his neck. Which condition is the client most likely to have?
   1. Candidiasis
   2. Molluscum contagiosum
   3. Tinea corporis
   4. Tinea pedis

Build your knowledge of the identifying shapes and sizes of various skin lesions.

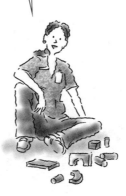

18. A client has thick, discolored nails with splintered hemorrhages, easily separated from the nail bed. There are also "ice pick" pits and ridges. Which term best describes these symptoms?
   1. Paronychia
   2. Psoriasis
   3. Seborrhea
   4. Scabies

19. A nurse is reviewing a newly admitted client's chart. Based on this progress notes entry, the nurse knows the data are consistent with which condition?

Color can be a classic sign of some conditions.

Progress note	
10/04/08 1830	Client admitted from ED after having been found unconscious at home. Client is unresponsive to painful stimuli. Blood pressure 90/60 mm Hg; heart rate 110 in sinus rhythm; respiratory rate 14 breaths/minute. Nail beds and all mucous membranes appear cherry red. ————Barbara Smith, R.N.

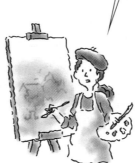

   1. Spider bite
   2. Aspirin ingestion
   3. Hydrocarbon ingestion
   4. Carbon monoxide poisoning

20. Which term describes a fungal infection of the scalp?
   1. Tinea capitis
   2. Tinea corporis
   3. Tinea cruris
   4. Tinea pedis

17. 3. Tinea corporis, or *ringworm,* is a flat, scaling, papular lesion with raised borders. Candidiasis is a fungal infection of the skin or mucous membranes commonly found in the oral, vaginal, and intestinal mucosal tissue. Molluscum contagiosum is a viral skin infection with small, red, papular lesions. Tinea pedis is a superficial fungal infection on the feet, commonly called *athlete's foot,* that causes itching, sweating, and a foul odor.
CN: Physiological integrity; CNS: Physiological adaptation; CL: Analysis

18. 2. Psoriasis, a chronic skin disorder with an unknown cause, shows these characteristic skin changes. A paronychia is a bacterial infection of the nail bed. Seborrhea is a chronic inflammatory dermatitis known as cradle cap. Scabies are mites that burrow under the skin, generally between the webbing of the fingers and toes.
CN: Physiological integrity; CNS: Physiological adaptation; CL: Knowledge

19. 4. Cherry-red skin indicates exposure to high levels of carbon monoxide. Spider bite reactions are usually localized to the area of the bite. Nausea and vomiting and pale skin are symptoms of aspirin ingestion. Hydrocarbon or petroleum ingestion usually causes respiratory symptoms and tachycardia.
CN: Physiological integrity; CNS: Physiological adaptation; CL: Analysis

20. 1. Tinea capitis is a fungal infection of the scalp. Tinea corporis describes fungal infections of the body. Tinea cruris describes fungal infections of the inner thigh and inguinal creases, and tinea pedis is the term for fungal infections of the foot.
CN: Physiological integrity; CNS: Physiological adaptation; CL: Application

CN: Client needs category   CNS: Client needs subcategory   CL: Cognitive level

21. In a client with burns on his legs, which nursing intervention helps prevent contractures?
1. Applying knee splints
2. Elevating the foot of the bed
3. Hyperextending the client's palms
4. Performing shoulder range-of-motion (ROM) exercises

21. 1. Applying knee splints prevents leg contractures by holding the joints in a position of function. Elevating the foot of the bed can't prevent contractures because this action doesn't hold the joints in a position of function. Hyperextending a body part for an extended time is inappropriate because it can cause contractures. Performing shoulder ROM exercises can prevent contractures in the shoulders, but not in the legs.
CN: Physiological integrity; CNS: Reduction of risk potential; CL: Application

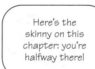

Prioritize!

22. A nurse is planning care for a client with burns on the upper torso. Which nursing diagnosis should take the <u>highest</u> priority?
1. *Ineffective airway clearance related to edema of the respiratory passages*
2. *Impaired physical mobility related to the disease process*
3. *Disturbed sleep pattern related to facility environment*
4. *Risk for infection related to breaks in the skin*

22. 1. When caring for a client with upper torso burns, the nurse's primary goal is to maintain respiratory integrity. Therefore, a diagnosis of *Ineffective airway clearance related to edema of the respiratory passages* should take the highest priority. The second diagnosis isn't appropriate because burns aren't a disease. Although the third and fourth diagnoses may be appropriate, they don't command a higher priority than the first because they don't reflect immediate life-threatening problems.
CN: Physiological integrity; CNS: Physiological adaptation; CL: Application

23. A client has just arrived at the emergency department after sustaining a major burn injury. Which metabolic alterations are expected during the first 8 hours postburn?
1. Hyponatremia and hypokalemia
2. Hyponatremia and hyperkalemia
3. Hypernatremia and hypokalemia
4. Hypernatremia and hyperkalemia

23. 2. During the first 48 hours after a burn, capillary permeability increases, allowing fluids to shift from the plasma to the interstitial spaces. This fluid is high in sodium, causing a decrease in serum sodium levels. Potassium also leaks from the cells into the plasma, causing hyperkalemia.
CN: Physiological integrity; CNS: Physiological adaptation; CL: Analysis

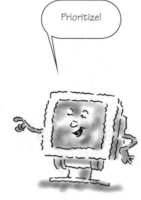

Here's the skinny on this chapter: you're halfway there!

24. In a client who has been burned, which medication should the nurse expect to use to prevent infection?
1. Malathion (Ovide)
2. Diazepam (Valium)
3. Mafenide (Sulfamylon)
4. Meperidine (Demerol)

24. 3. The topical antibiotic mafenide is prescribed to prevent infection in clients with second- and third-degree burns. Malathion is a pediculicide used to treat lice infestation. Diazepam is an antianxiety agent that may be administered to clients with burns, but not to prevent infection. The opioid analgesic meperidine is used to help control pain in clients with burns.
CN: Physiological integrity; CNS: Pharmacological therapies; CL: Comprehension

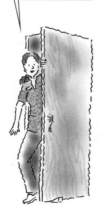

CN: Client needs category   CNS: Client needs subcategory   CL: Cognitive level

25. Which method is best for making sure a client receives an ordered dressing change each shift?
    1. Write the order in the client's care Kardex.
    2. Put a sign above the head of the client's bed.
    3. Tell the nurse about the treatment in the report.
    4. Document the dressing change in the narrative note.

26. Which nursing diagnosis is correct for a client with a reddened sacrum unrelieved by position change?
    1. *Risk for pressure ulcer*
    2. *Risk for impaired skin integrity*
    3. *Impaired skin integrity* related to infrequent turning and positioning
    4. *Impaired skin integrity* related to the effects of pressure and shearing force

27. A surgical client has just been admitted to a unit from the postanesthesia care unit. When should the nurse change the dressing for the first time?
    1. 2 hours after admission
    2. When it becomes saturated
    3. Based on written orders for dressing changes
    4. The surgeon changes the first dressing; then follow written orders

28. An alert, 96-year-old hemiplegic client slips on the floor after climbing out of bed to get to the bathroom. You observe slight ecchymosis and edema on the right hip, notify the physician, and fill out an incident report. What would be the most appropriate nursing action to prevent this client from falling in the future?
    1. Make sure he's adequately medicated at bedtime.
    2. Have him wear elbow and knee pads at night.
    3. Lower the bed and place pads near the bathroom door.
    4. Ask him about his elimination patterns to better anticipate his needs.

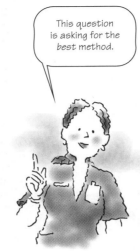

This question is asking for the best method.

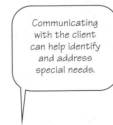

Communicating with the client can help identify and address special needs.

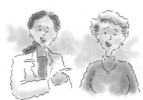

25. 1. Writing the order in the client's care Kardex notifies everyone of the treatment. Posting a sign above the head of the bed is a good reminder but doesn't ensure that the treatment will be performed. Verbally reporting to the nurse on the upcoming shift doesn't ensure the dressing change will be done. Although the intervention should be documented in the narrative note, this doesn't guarantee that the next nurse will do the treatment.
CN: Safe, effective care environment; CNS: Coordinated care; CL: Application

26. 4. The client's impaired skin integrity is the result of pressure and shearing forces. The first option isn't an approved nursing diagnosis. This client has an actual—not potential—skin impairment. The third option is an improperly written nursing diagnosis. The use of infrequent turning and positioning noted in the statement implies the nurse hasn't done the required nursing care.
CN: Physiological integrity; CNS: Basic care and comfort; CL: Application

27. 4. The surgeon should always perform the first postoperative dressing change. Generally, the surgeon will change the dressing and assess the wound the next morning during rounds. The dressing shouldn't need to be changed 2 hours after the procedure. If the first dressing becomes saturated, it may be secured with additional tape or bandages. If the nurse notes hemorrhage or excessive amount of drainage, the surgeon should be notified.
CN: Physiological integrity; CNS: Basic care and comfort; CL: Application

28. 4. Asking the client about his elimination patterns indicates that the nurse is aware that the client can give her information to help her better meet his needs. By talking with the client, the nurse is recognizing his worth and engaging participation in his own care. Options 1 and 2 are inappropriate. Lowering the bed would be helpful; however, the cushioning pads must be placed by the sides of the bed, not by the bathroom.
CN: Health promotion and maintenance; CNS: None; CL: Analysis

CN: Client needs category   CNS: Client needs subcategory   CL: Cognitive level

29. A client has a possible postoperative wound infection. Which technique should the nurse use to obtain a wound culture from a surgical site?
1. Thoroughly irrigate the wound before collecting the culture.
2. Use a sterile swab, and wipe the crusty area around the outside of the wound.
3. Gently roll a sterile swab from the center of the wound outward to collect drainage.
4. Use one sterile swab to collect drainage from several possible infected sites along the incision.

30. Which characteristic of an abdominal incision would indicate a potential for <u>delayed</u> wound healing?
1. Sutures dry and intact
2. Wound edges in close approximation
3. Purulent drainage on a soiled wound dressing
4. Sanguineous drainage in a wound collection drainage bag

31. A nursing assistant will be changing the soiled bed linens of a client with a draining pressure ulcer. Which protective equipment should the nursing assistant wear?
1. Mask
2. Clean gloves
3. Sterile gloves
4. Shoe protectors

32. Which intervention is most appropriate for preventing pressure ulcers in a bedridden elderly client?
1. Slide instead of lift the client when turning.
2. Turn and reposition the client at least every 8 hours.
3. Apply lotion after bathing the client, and vigorously massage the skin.
4. Post a turning schedule at the client's bedside, and adapt position changes to the client's situation.

Preventive care is a focus of many NCLEX questions.

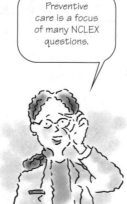

29. 3. Rolling a swab from the center outward is the right way to culture a wound. Irrigating the wound washes away drainage, debris, and many of the microorganisms colonizing or infecting the wound. The outside of the wound may be colonized with microorganisms from this wound or another wound or normal microorganisms on the client's skin. These microorganisms may grow in culture and confuse the interpretation of results. All sources of drainage in an incision or surgical wound may not be infected or may be infected with different microorganisms, so each swab should be used on only one site.

CN: Safe, effective care environment; CNS: Safety and infection control; CL: Application

30. 3. Purulent drainage contains white blood cells, which fight infection. The sutures from a wound draining purulent secretions would pull away with an infection. Wound edges can't approximate with an infection in the wound. Sanguineous drainage indicates bleeding, not infection.

CN: Physiological integrity; CNS: Physiological adaptation; CL: Comprehension

31. 2. Clean gloves protect the nursing assistant's hands and wrists from microorganisms in the linens. A mask protects the wearer from droplet nuclei and large particle aerosols. Sterile gloves would allow her to touch a sterile object or area without contaminating it. Shoe protectors prevent static and microorganism transmission from the floor of one room to another.

CN: Safe, effective care environment; CNS: Safety and infection control; CL: Analysis

32. 4. A turning schedule with a signing sheet will ensure that the client gets turned. When moving a client, lift, rather than slide, the client to avoid shearing. A client in bed for prolonged periods should be turned every 1 to 2 hours. Apply lotion to keep the skin moist, but refrain from vigorous massage to avoid damaging capillaries.

CN: Safe, effective care environment; CNS: Safety and infection control; CL: Analysis

CN: Client needs category CNS: Client needs subcategory CL: Cognitive level

33. Which instruction is the <u>most important</u> to give a client who has recently had a skin graft?
1. Continue physical therapy.
2. Protect the graft from direct sunlight.
3. Use cosmetic camouflage techniques.
4. Apply lubricating lotion to the graft site.

34. A client is diagnosed with basal cell epithelioma. Given her knowledge of basal cell epithelioma and its most common cause, which condition would the nurse expect to find in this client's medical history?
1. Burns
2. Exposure to sun
3. Immunosuppression
4. Exposure to radiation

35. Which statement is correct regarding skin turgor?
1. Overhydration causes the skin to tent.
2. Normal skin turgor is moist and boggy.
3. Inelastic skin turgor is a normal part of aging.
4. Dehydration causes the skin to appear edematous and spongy.

36. A nurse is caring for a geriatric client with a pressure ulcer on the sacrum. When teaching the client about dietary intake, which foods should the nurse plan to emphasize?
1. Legumes and cheese
2. Whole-grain products
3. Fruits and vegetables
4. Lean meats and low-fat milk

37. Which water temperature is correct for a bed bath?
1. 97° to 100° F (36.1° to 37.8° C)
2. 100° to 110° F (37.8° to 43.3° C)
3. 110° to 115° F (43.3° to 46.1° C)
4. 115° to 120° F (46.1° to 48.9° C)

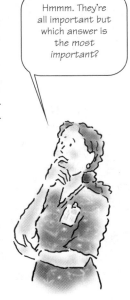

Hmmm. They're all important but which answer is the most important?

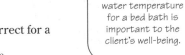

The correct water temperature for a bed bath is important to the client's well-being.

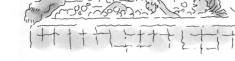

33. 2. To avoid burning and sloughing, the client must protect the graft from direct sunlight. The other three interventions are all helpful to the client and his recovery but aren't as important.
CN: Physiological integrity; CNS: Physiological adaptation; CL: Analysis

34. 2. The sun is the best known and most common cause of basal cell epithelioma. Burns, immunosuppression, and radiation are less common causes.
CN: Physiological integrity; CNS: Reduction of risk potential; CL: Analysis

35. 3. Inelastic skin turgor is a normal part of aging. Overhydration causes the skin to appear edematous and spongy. Normal skin turgor is dry and firm. Dehydration causes inelastic skin with tenting.
CN: Physiological integrity; CNS: Basic care and comfort; CL: Knowledge

36. 4. Although the client should eat a balanced diet with foods from all food groups, the diet should emphasize foods that supply complete protein, such as lean meats and low-fat milk. Protein helps build and repair body tissue, which promotes healing. Legumes provide incomplete protein. Cheese contains complete protein but also fat, which should be limited to 30% or less of caloric intake. Whole-grain products supply incomplete proteins and carbohydrates. Fruits and vegetables provide mainly carbohydrates.
CN: Physiological integrity; CNS: Basic care and comfort; CL: Application

37. 3. The client should be protected from becoming chilled. The water temperature should be 110° to 115° F to compensate for evaporative body cooling during and after the bath. Water temperature the same as body temperature, slightly cooler, or slightly warmer will eventually cool, which could cause discomfort and increase evaporative body cooling. Water of 115° to 120° F would be too hot and put the client at risk for burns or discomfort. Always test water with a bath thermometer.
CN: Physiological integrity; CNS: Basic care and comfort; CL: Knowledge

CN: Client needs category   CNS: Client needs subcategory   CL: Cognitive level

38. A client received burns to his entire back and left arm. Using the Rule of Nines, the nurse calculates that he has sustained burns to which percentage of his body?
  1. 9%
  2. 18%
  3. 27%
  4. 36%

39. Which technique will maintain surgical asepsis?
  1. Change the sterile field after sterile water is spilled on it.
  2. Put on sterile gloves; then open a container of sterile saline.
  3. Place a sterile dressing ½″ (1.3 cm) from the edge of the sterile field.
  4. Clean the wound with a circular motion, moving from outer circles toward the center.

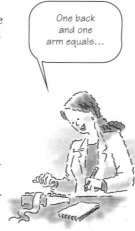

One back and one arm equals...

40. A nurse is performing a skin assessment on a recently admitted client. Which factor is most important in planning care for the client?
  1. Family history of pressure ulcers
  2. Presence of existing pressure ulcers
  3. Overall risk of developing pressure ulcers
  4. Potential areas of pressure ulcer development

41. Which piece of equipment for the wheelchair- or bed-bound client impedes circulation to the area it's meant to protect?
  1. Waterbed
  2. Ring or donut
  3. Gel flotation pad
  4. Polyurethane foam mattress

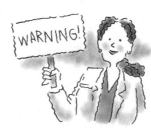

WARNING!

38. 3. According to the Rule of Nines, the posterior trunk, anterior trunk, and legs are each 18% of the total body surface. The head, neck, and arms are each 9% of total body surface, and the perineum is 1%. In this case, the client received burns to his back (18%) and one arm (9%), totaling 27% of his body.
CN: Physiological integrity; CNS: Reduction of risk potential; CL: Application

39. 1. A sterile field is considered contaminated when it becomes wet. Moisture can act as a wick, allowing microorganisms to contaminate the field. The outside of containers such as sterile saline bottles aren't sterile. The containers should be opened before sterile gloves are put on, and the solution poured over the sterile dressings placed in a sterile basin. Wounds should be cleaned from the most contaminated area to the least contaminated area, for example, from the center outward. The outer inch of a sterile field isn't considered sterile.
CN: Safe, effective care environment; CNS: Safety and infection control; CL: Application

40. 2. Areas of existing pressure ulcers need immediate treatment, and therefore are most important. Family history of pressure ulcers isn't a risk factor for development of pressure ulcers. Overall risk and potential areas of pressure development are important in planning care but don't take priority.
CN: Physiological integrity; CNS: Reduction of risk potential; CL: Application

41. 2. Rings or donuts shouldn't be used because they restrict circulation. The waterbed distributes pressure over the entire surface. Gel pads give with weight. Foam mattresses evenly distribute pressure.
CN: Physiological integrity; CNS: Reduction of risk potential; CL: Application

CN: Client needs category   CNS: Client needs subcategory   CL: Cognitive level

42. A client develops wound evisceration following abdominal surgery. Which intervention should be the nurse's <u>priority</u> for this client?
1. Giving prophylactic antibiotics as ordered
2. Having the client drink as much fluid as possible
3. Explaining to the client what's happening and giving support
4. Covering the protruding internal organs with sterile gauze moistened with sterile saline

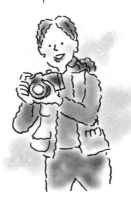

Priority is the key word to focus on here.

42. 4. Evisceration requires emergency surgical repair. Covering the wound with sterile gauze moistened with sterile saline is essential to prevent the organs from drying. The gauze and saline must be sterile to reduce the risk of infection. Antibiotics will usually be ordered and started as soon as possible but aren't the priority. The nurse should place the client on nothing-by-mouth status immediately, but covering the wound takes priority. While the nurse works quickly to get the client treated, providing emotional support will help reduce the client's anxiety but isn't the priority for this client.
CN: Physiological integrity; CNS: Physiological adaptation; CL: Application

43. Which intervention is performed <u>first</u> when changing a dressing or giving wound care?
1. Put on gloves.
2. Wash hands thoroughly.
3. Slowly remove the soiled dressing.
4. Observe the dressing for the amount, type, and odor of drainage.

43. 2. The first thing the nurse must do is wash her hands. Putting on gloves, removing the dressing, and observing the drainage are all parts of the dressing change procedure that come after hand washing.
CN: Physiological integrity; CNS: Basic care and comfort; CL: Application

44. When caring for a client who spends all or most of his time in bed, a turning schedule prevents the development of complications. Which schedule is best for most clients?
1. Turn every 30 minutes.
2. Turn every 1 to 2 hours.
3. Turn once every 8 hours.
4. Keep the client on his back as much as possible.

44. 2. Turning the client every 1 to 2 hours will prevent pressure areas from developing and help prevent atelectasis and other pulmonary complications. Turning every half-hour is too frequent, and every 8 hours would make the client vulnerable to the development of complications. The client should spend time on his back according to the turning schedule. During that period, the head of the bed should be raised to prevent the client from aspirating.
CN: Physiological integrity; CNS: Basic care and comfort; CL: Application

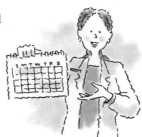

Timing is everything when reading skin test results.

45. Which instruction is <u>most important</u> when teaching a client about hypersensitivity skin test results?
1. Wash the sites daily with a mild soap.
2. Have the sites read on the correct date.
3. Keep the skin test areas moist with a mild lotion.
4. Stay out of direct sunlight until the tests are read.

45. 2. An important facet of evaluating skin tests is to read the skin test results at the proper time. Evaluating the skin test too late or too early will give inaccurate, unreliable results. There's no need to wash the sites with soap. The sites should be kept dry. Direct sunlight isn't prohibited.
CN: Health promotion and maintenance; CNS: None; CL: Application

CN: Client needs category   CNS: Client needs subcategory   CL: Cognitive level

46. Despite conventional treatment, a client's psoriasis has worsened. His physician prescribes methotrexate (Trexall) 25 mg by mouth as a single weekly dose. The pharmacy dispenses 2.5-mg scored tablets. How many tablets should the nurse instruct the client to consume to achieve the prescribed dose? Record your answer using a whole number.

_____ tablets

We need to know the correct formula to calculate the correct dose.

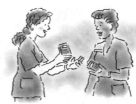

47. A 35-year-old client is brought to the emergency department with second- and third-degree burns over 15% of his body. His admission vital signs are as follows: blood pressure 100/50 mm Hg, heart rate 130 beats/minute, and respiratory rate 26 breaths/minute. Which nursing interventions are appropriate for this client? Select all that apply:
1. Clean the burns with hydrogen peroxide.
2. Cover the burns with saline-soaked towels.
3. Begin an I.V. infusion of lactated Ringer's solution.
4. Place ice directly on the burn areas.
5. Administer 6 mg of morphine I.V.
6. Administer tetanus prophylaxis, as ordered.

48. An elderly client who's 5'4" and weighs 145 lb is admitted to the long-term care facility. The admitting nurse takes this report: "The client sits for long periods in his wheelchair and has bowel and bladder incontinence. He can feed himself and has a fair appetite, eating best at breakfast and poorly thereafter. He doesn't have family members living nearby and is often noted to be crying and depressed. He also frequently requires large doses of sedatives." Which factors place the client at risk for developing a pressure ulcer? Select all that apply:
1. Weight
2. Incontinence
3. Sitting for long periods
4. Sedation
5. Crying and depression
6. Eating poorly at lunch and dinner

You did it! Now take a break, have a nutritious snack, and then forge ahead. Nothing can stop you now!

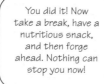

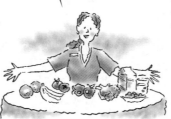

46. 10. The correct formula to calculate a drug dose is:
    Dose on hand/Quantity on hand = Dose desired/X.
    The physician prescribes 25 mg, which is the dose desired. The pharmacy dispenses 2.5-mg tablets, which is the dose on hand. So:
    2.5 mg/1 tablet = 25 mg/X;
    X = 10 tablets.
CN: Physiological integrity; CNS: Pharmacological therapies; CL: Application

47. 3, 5, 6. Immediate interventions for this client should aim to stop the burning and relieve the pain. The nurse should begin I.V. therapy with a crystalloid, such as lactated Ringer's solution, to prevent hypovolemic shock and to maintain cardiac output. Typically, 2 to 25 mg of morphine (Duramorph) or 5 to 15 mg of meperidine (Demerol) are administered I.V. in small increments to treat pain. Tetanus prophylaxis should also be administered, as ordered. Hydrogen peroxide and povidone-iodine solution could further damage tissue, and saline-soaked towels could lead to hypothermia. Ice placed directly on burn wounds could cause further thermal damage.
CN: Physiological integrity; CNS: Physiological adaptation; CL: Application

48. 2, 3, 4. Inactivity, immobility, incontinence, and sedation are all risk factors for developing pressure ulcers. The client's weight and poor eating habits at lunch and dinner aren't directly related to the risk of developing pressure ulcers, but a calorie count should be taken to see if the client is getting adequate calories and fluids because poor nutrition can contribute to pressure ulcers. The fact that the client cries and is depressed has no direct bearing on this client's risk for developing a pressure ulcer. However, clients with depression are commonly not as active, so his activity levels should be monitored closely.
CN: Physiological integrity; CNS: Reduction of risk potential; CL: Analysis

CN: Client needs category   CNS: Client needs subcategory   CL: Cognitive level

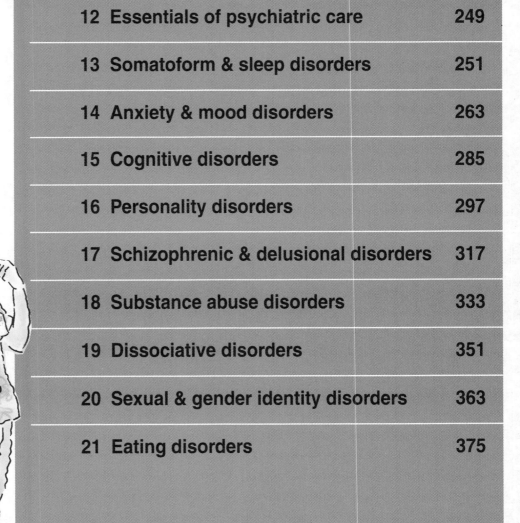

Part III Care of the psychiatric client

Before you take the tests related to psychiatric care, try these practice questions. They may help clear your head!

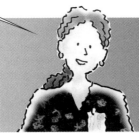

Chapter 12
Essentials of psychiatric care

1. The nurse is explaining the Bill of Rights for psychiatric patients to a client who has voluntarily sought admission to an inpatient psychiatric facility. Which rights should the nurse include in the discussion? Select all that apply:
   1. Right to select health care team members
   2. Right to refuse treatment
   3. Right to a written treatment plan
   4. Right to obtain disability
   5. Right to confidentiality
   6. Right to personal mail

2. A client with bipolar disorder becomes verbally aggressive in a group therapy session. Which response by the nurse would be best?
   1. "You're behaving in an unacceptable manner and you need to control yourself."
   2. "If you continue to talk like that, no one will want to be around you."
   3. "You're frightening everyone in the group. Leave the room immediately."
   4. "Other people are disturbed by your profanity. I'll walk with you down the hall to help release some of that energy."

3. The nurse is caring for a female client who had been extremely suicidal but now appears very serene. She says she has finally gotten things worked out. What would be the best way to respond to this client?
   1. "I'm glad things are working out for you."
   2. "How have you managed to work things out so quickly?"
   3. "I'm not clear about what has changed for you; tell me more."
   4. "You look so much better; you must be feeling relieved."

All of these options might be acceptable, but only one is the best option.

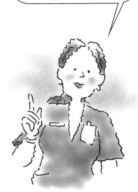

1. 2, 3, 5, 6. An inpatient client usually receives a copy of the Bill of Rights for psychiatric patients, which includes options 2, 3, 5, and 6. However, a client in an inpatient setting can't select health care team members. A client may apply for disability as a result of a chronic, incapacitating illness; however, disability isn't a patient right, and members of a psychiatric institution don't decide who should receive it.
CN: Psychosocial integrity; CNS: None; CL: Application

2. 4. This response informs the client that, although the behavior is unacceptable, the client is still worthy of help. The other responses indicate that the client is in control of the behavior.
CN: Safe, effective care environment; CNS: Coordinated care; CL: Application

3. 3. Asking the client to tell her more allows the nurse to seek further clarification without placing words in the client's mouth. Options 1 and 4 block further exploration and indicate the nurse's lack of insight. Option 2 allows the client to give an answer that hides underlying intent (for example, the client may respond, "I prayed about it and believe that God is now in charge of my life").
CN: Psychosocial integrity; CNS: None; CL: Application

CN: Client needs category   CNS: Client needs subcategory   CL: Cognitive level

4. While reviewing the hospital progress record, a nurse notes the chart entry below on a client with a diagnosis of depression. Which response by the nurse is <u>most</u> appropriate?

Progress notes	
9/4/08	Client observed sitting in a chair looking
0900	out the window or down at her hands;
	doesn't make eye contact. Client
	encouraged to visit the dayroom. Client
	states, "I don't want to go to the
	dayroom today. I don't like going down
	there. I'm just going to stay in my
	room." ————————Barbara Smith, L.P.N.

1. Allow the client to remain in her room.
2. Insist that the client interact with others throughout the day.
3. Sit with the client in her room for brief intervals to establish a trusting relationship.
4. Have other clients go to the client's room to keep her company.

5. Two 16-year-old clients are being treated in an adolescent unit. During a recreational activity, they begin a physical fight. How should the nurse intervene?
1. Remove the teenagers to separate areas and set limits.
2. Remind the teenagers of the unit rules.
3. Obtain an order to place the teenagers in seclusion.
4. Obtain an order to place the teenagers in restraints.

6. Which statement best describes the key advantage of using groups in psychotherapy?
1. Decreases the focus on the individual
2. Fosters the physician-client relationship
3. Confronts individuals with their shortcomings
4. Fosters a new learning environment

4. 3. Depressed people shouldn't be allowed to isolate themselves, as isolation only further lowers their self-esteem. Brief periods of interaction would accomplish two goals: to prevent the client's withdrawal, and to begin establishing trust and demonstrating genuine interest in the client. Allowing her to remain alone in her room wouldn't be therapeutic. Insisting that she interact with others or having other clients go to her room would be too threatening to the client at this time.
CN: Psychosocial integrity; CNS: None; CL: Application

5. 1. Setting limits and removing the clients from the situation is the best way to handle aggression. Reminders of appropriate behaviors aren't likely to be effective at this time, and seclusion and restraints are reserved for more serious situations.
CN: Physiological integrity; CNS: Physiological adaptation; CL: Application

6. 4. In a group, the individual has the opportunity to learn that others have the same problems and needs. The group can also provide an arena where new methods of relating to others can be tried. Decreasing focus on the individual isn't a key advantage (and sometimes isn't an advantage at all). Groups don't, by themselves, foster the physician-client relationship, and they aren't always used to confront individuals.
CN: Psychosocial integrity; CNS: None; CL: Application

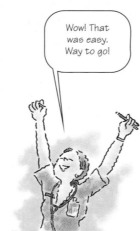

Wow! That was easy. Way to go!

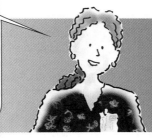
Can't remember much about a particular somatoform disorder? Type this address into your Internet browser: www.emedicine.com. Then search for the disorder. Cool!

1. Which statement is correct about clients who have somatoform disorders?
1. They usually seek medical attention.
2. They have organic pathologic disorders.
3. They regularly attend psychotherapy sessions without encouragement.
4. They're eager to discover the true reasons for their physical symptoms.

2. Which statement is correct about the diagnosis of somatoform disorders?
1. The somatic complaints are limited to one organ system.
2. The event preceding the physical illness occurred recently.
3. They're physical conditions with organic pathologic causes.
4. They're disorders that occur in the absence of organic findings.

3. Which action best accounts for the physical symptoms in a client with a somatoform disorder?
1. To cope with delusional thinking
2. To provide attention for the individual
3. To prevent or relieve symptoms of anxiety
4. To protect the client from family conflict

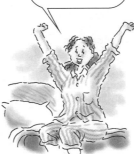

A good night's sleep is important before taking an exam.

1. 1. A client with a somatoform disorder usually seeks medical attention. These clients have a history of multiple physiological complaints without associated demonstrable organic pathologic causes. The expected behavior for this type of disorder is to seek treatment from several medical physicians for somatic complaints, not psychiatric evaluation.
CN: Health promotion and maintenance; CNS: None; CL: Knowledge

2. 4. The essential feature of somatoform disorders is a physical or somatic complaint without any demonstrable organic findings to account for the complaint. There are no known physiological mechanisms to explain the findings. Somatic complaints aren't limited to one organ system. The diagnostic criteria for somatoform disorders state that the client has a history of many physical complaints beginning before age 30 that occur over several years.
CN: Psychosocial integrity; CNS: None; CL: Analysis

3. 3. Anxiety and depression commonly occur in somatoform disorders. The client prevents or relieves symptoms of anxiety by focusing on physical symptoms. Somatic delusions occur in schizophrenia. The symptoms allow the client to avoid unpleasant activity, not to seek individual attention. Somatization in dysfunctional families shifts the open conflict to the client's illness, thus providing some stability for the family, not the client.
CN: Psychosocial integrity; CNS: None; CL: Analysis

CN: Client needs category   CNS: Client needs subcategory   CL: Cognitive level

4. Which ego <u>defense mechanism</u> describes the underlying dynamics of somatization disorder?
1. Repression of anger
2. Suppression of grief
3. Denial of depression
4. Preoccupation with pain

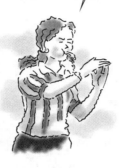

Time out! Remember you're looking for a defense mechanism.

5. For the past 6 months, an 86-year-old client in an extended care facility has been complaining about breast pain and is convinced she has cancer despite medical diagnostic tests indicating that she doesn't. The symptoms—feelings of pain and a belief that she has a serious disease—may indicate which disorder?
1. Conversion disorder
2. Hypochondriasis
3. Severe anxiety
4. Sublimation

6. A client reports severe pain in the back and joints. On reviewing the client's history, the nurse notes a diagnosis of depression and frequent hospitalizations for psychosomatic illness. What should the nurse encourage this client to do?
1. Tell the physician about the pain so that its cause can be determined.
2. Remember all the previous health problems that weren't real.
3. Try to get more rest and use relaxation techniques.
4. Ignore the pain and focus on happy things.

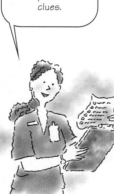

The client's history can provide important clues.

4. 1. One psychodynamic theory states that somatization is the transformation of aggressive and hostile wishes toward others into physical complaints. Repressed anger originating from past disappointments and unfilled needs for nurturing and caring are expressed by soliciting other people's concern and rejecting them as ineffective. Suppression, denial, and preoccupation aren't the defense mechanisms underlying the dynamics of somatization disorder.
CN: Psychosocial integrity; CNS: None; CL: Knowledge

5. 2. Hypochondriasis is defined as a morbid fear or belief that one has a serious disease, though none exists. No neurologic symptoms are apparent as with conversion disorders. There are no apparent symptoms related to severe anxiety. There's no evidence of channeling maladaptive feelings or impulses into socially acceptable behavior that would be evident in a client experiencing sublimation.
CN: Physiological integrity; CN: Physiological adaptation; CL: Analysis

6. 1. Initially, the nurse should treat all symptoms as indicators of possible pathology because a history of psychosomatic illness doesn't rule out a physical illness as a cause of the client's current symptoms. The other options assume that the client has a psychosomatic illness, which could lead to ignoring a physical illness or condition. A client with a psychosomatic illness experiences real physical symptoms that are triggered or exacerbated by psychological issues. The physical symptoms aren't imagined or fabricated by the client.
CN: Physiological integrity; CNS: Reduction of risk potential; CL: Application

CN: Client needs category   CNS: Client needs subcategory   CL: Cognitive level

7. A college student frequently visited the health center before course examinations. Physical causes for these visits have been eliminated. Based on the following progress note entry in the client's chart, the nurse suspects which disorder?

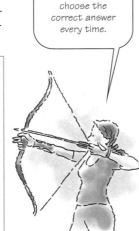

Aim to choose the correct answer every time.

Progress notes	
9/4/08 2130	19-year-old client states, "I'm having abdominal discomfort. It happens on and off, especially the last week while I'm trying to study for mid-term exams. I know that there's something really wrong." Client denies that these symptoms are related to eating. Normal bowel sounds auscultated. Abdomen soft and nontender to palpation. Vital signs: Temp, 98.2° F; BP, 114/72 mm Hg; heart rate, 76 beats/minute; respiratory rate, 20 breaths/minute. Denies nausea, vomiting, diarrhea, or loss of appetite.— ————————————————N. Jones, L.P.N.

1. Conversion disorder
2. Depersonalization
3. Hypochondriasis
4. Somatoform disorder

8. A nursing goal for a client diagnosed with hypochondriasis should focus on which area?
   1. Determining the cause of a sleep disturbance
   2. Relieving the fear of serious illness
   3. Recovering the lost or altered function
   4. Giving positive reinforcement for accomplishments related to physical appearance

9. Which nursing intervention is <u>appropriate</u> for a client diagnosed with hypochondriasis?
   1. Teach the client adaptive coping strategies.
   2. Help the client eliminate the stress in her life.
   3. Confront the client with the statement, "It's all in your head."
   4. Encourage the client to focus on identification of physical symptoms.

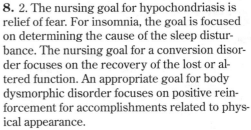

Pay close attention to the word *appropriate*.

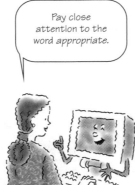

7. 3. Hypochondriasis in this case is shown by the client's belief she has a serious illness, although pathologic causes have been eliminated. The disturbance usually lasts at least 6 months, and the GI system is commonly affected. Exacerbations are usually associated with identifiable life stressors that, in this case, can be related to the client's examinations. Conversion disorders are characterized by one or more neurologic symptoms. Depersonalization refers to persistent, recurrent episodes of feeling detached from one's self or body. Somatoform disorders generally have a chronic course with few remissions.
CN: Psychosocial integrity; CNS: None; CL: Analysis

8. 2. The nursing goal for hypochondriasis is relief of fear. For insomnia, the goal is focused on determining the cause of the sleep disturbance. The nursing goal for a conversion disorder focuses on the recovery of the lost or altered function. An appropriate goal for body dysmorphic disorder focuses on positive reinforcement for accomplishments related to physical appearance.
CN: Psychosocial integrity; CNS: None; CL: Application

9. 1. Because of weak ego strength, a client with hypochondriasis is unable to use coping mechanisms effectively. The nursing focus is to teach adaptive coping mechanisms. It isn't realistic to eliminate all stress. A client should never be confronted with the statement, "It's all in your head," because this wouldn't facilitate a long-term therapeutic relationship, which is necessary to offer reassurance that no physical disease is present. The client is already aware of his physical symptoms and encouraging him to focus on them wouldn't be therapeutic.
CN: Psychosocial integrity; CNS: None; CL: Application

10. A client is exhibiting anxiety, which is evidenced by muscle tension, distractibility, and increased heart rate and blood pressure. Which nursing intervention has <u>top priority</u>?

1. Remain with the client and use a soft voice and reassuring approach.
2. Assist the client to identify factors that contribute to anxiety.
3. Teach relaxation techniques, such as deep breathing and muscle relaxation.
4. Administer antianxiety medications as appropriate.

11. Which therapeutic strategy can a nurse use to reduce anxiety in a client diagnosed with hypochondriasis?

1. Suicide precautions
2. Relaxation exercises
3. Electroconvulsive therapy
4. Pharmacologic intervention

12. A client is given triazolam (Halcion) for a sleep disorder. The nurse is reinforcing some teaching precautions concerning the medication. The nurse determines that the client understands the precautions when the client states:

1. "I take the medication with citrus juice."
2. "I shouldn't confuse this medication with Haldol."
3. "It's okay to take a short drive after taking the medication."
4. "It's okay to smoke while I take this medication."

13. Which measure should be included when teaching a client strategies to help promote sleep?

1. Keep the room warm.
2. Eat a large meal before bedtime.
3. Schedule bedtime when you feel tired.
4. Avoid caffeine, excessive fluid intake, alcohol, and stimulating drugs before bedtime.

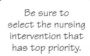

Be sure to select the nursing intervention that has top priority.

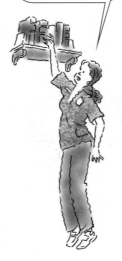

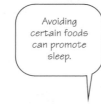

Avoiding certain foods can promote sleep.

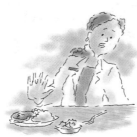

10. 1. The priority nursing intervention is to remain with the client and use a soft voice and reassuring approach. Remaining with the client provides for his safety and a soft voice is calming and reassuring, which will add to his feelings of safety and protection. Interventions, such as identifying factors that contribute to anxiety, teaching relaxation techniques, and administering antianxiety medications, are included in the client's care plan but should be addressed later.
CN: Psychosocial integrity; CNS: None; CL: Application

11. 2. A nurse can initiate relaxation exercises to decrease anxiety without an order from the physician. In a hypochondriasis disorder, no threat of suicide exists. Medical intervention would include electroconvulsive therapy and pharmacologic intervention.
CN: Physiological integrity; CNS: Physiological adaptation; CL: Application

12. 2. Haldol is an antipsychotic that has a spelling similar to Halcion and is used for clients with psychoses, Tourette's syndrome, severe behavioral problems in children, and emergency sedation of severely agitated psychotic clients. Halcion is one of a group of sedative-hypnotic medications that can be used only for a limited time because of the risk of dependence. Grapefruit and grapefruit juices can alter the absorption of Halcion. The client should avoid driving and tasks that require alertness or motor skills because the medication may cause drowsiness. Smoking reduces drug effectiveness.
CN: Physiological integrity; CNS: Pharmacological therapies; CL: Analysis

13. 4. Caffeine, excessive fluid intake, alcohol, and stimulating drugs act as stimulants; avoiding them should promote sleep. Maintaining a cool temperature in the room will better facilitate sleeping. Excessive fullness or hunger may interfere with sleep. Setting a regular bedtime and wake-up time facilitates physiological patterns.
CN: Health promotion and maintenance; CNS: None; CL: Application

CN: Client needs category   CNS: Client needs subcategory   CL: Cognitive level

14. Which sleep disorder indicates that an individual can't prevent falling asleep, even in the middle of a task or sentence?
  1. Hypersomnia
  2. Insomnia
  3. Narcolepsy
  4. Parasomnia

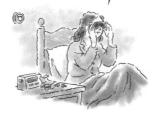

14. 3. Narcolepsy is also known as *sleep attacks.* Hypersomnia, or *somnolence,* refers to excessive sleepiness or seeking excessive amounts of sleep. Insomnia is a sleep disorder in which an individual has difficulty initiating or maintaining sleep. Parasomnia refers to unusual or undesired behavior that occurs during sleep, such as nightmares and sleepwalking.
CN: Physiological integrity; CNS: Physiological adaptation; CL: Knowledge

15. Treatments for sleep disorders include which method?
  1. Behavior therapy
  2. Biofeedback
  3. Group therapy
  4. Insight-oriented psychotherapy

15. 2. Biofeedback, relaxation therapy, and psychopharmacology are appropriate treatments for sleep disorders. Behavior therapy, group therapy, and insight-oriented psychotherapy are treatments related to somatoform disorders.
CN: Physiological integrity; CNS: Basic care and comfort; CL: Application

16. Which nursing intervention would be <u>most appropriate</u> for a depressed client with a nursing diagnosis of *Disturbed sleep pattern related to external factors?*
  1. Consult the physician about prescribing a bedtime sleep medication.
  2. Allow the client to sit at the nurses' station for comfort.
  3. Allow the client to watch television until he's sleepy.
  4. Encourage the client to take a warm bath before retiring.

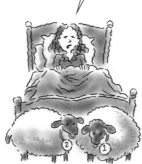

16. 4. Sleep-inducing activities, such as a warm bath, help promote relaxation and sleep. Although consulting a physician about prescribing a bedtime sleep medication is possible, it wouldn't be the best nursing intervention for this client. Encouraging the client to watch television or sit at the nurses' station wouldn't necessarily promote sleep. In fact, these activities may provide too much stimulation, further preventing sleep.
CN: Physiological integrity; CNS: Basic care and comfort; CL: Application

17. The nurse is reviewing a nursing care plan for a 45-year-old male client with a psychophysiological disorder. Her interventions should address which of the following?
  1. Only the physical symptoms that are life-threatening
  2. Only the physical symptoms that are distressing the client
  3. Physical symptoms as well as psychosocial and spiritual problems
  4. Only psychosocial symptoms

17. 3. Physical, psychosocial, and spiritual problems are thoroughly and continuously assessed with each client. The nurse must include all symptoms, even those that aren't life-threatening, and consider all physical symptoms, even those the client doesn't find distressing. Psychosocial symptoms should be considered but all three areas must be assessed to provide a thorough care plan.
CN: Psychosocial integrity; CNS: None; CL: Comprehension

18. A nurse is instructing a 38-year-old male client undergoing treatment for anxiety and insomnia. The practitioner has prescribed lorazepam (Ativan) 1 mg by mouth three times per day. The nurse determines that the teaching regarding the client's diagnosis and medication has been effective when the client gives which response?
1. "I'll avoid caffeine."
2. "I'll avoid aged cheese."
3. "I'll avoid sunlight."
4. "I'll maintain adequate salt intake."

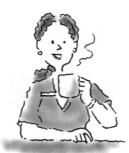

I don't know why I'm so anxious about this question.

19. A home health nurse is caring for a client diagnosed with a conversion disorder manifested by paralysis in the left arm. An organic cause for the deficit has been ruled out. Which nursing intervention is <u>most appropriate</u> for this client?
1. Perform all physical tasks for the client to foster dependence.
2. Allot an hour each day to discuss the paralysis and its cause.
3. Identify primary or secondary gains that the physical symptom provides.
4. Allow the client to withdraw from all physical activities.

20. A 35-year-old female client is diagnosed with conversion disorder with paralysis of the legs. What's the <u>best</u> nursing intervention for the nurse to use?
1. Discuss with the client ways to live with the paralysis.
2. Focus interactions on results of medical tests.
3. Encourage the client to move her legs as much as possible.
4. Avoid focusing on the client's physical limitations.

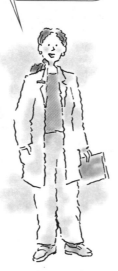

Don't lose sleep over question 21—focus on the most appropriate answer.

21. Which outcome criteria is <u>most appropriate</u> for a teenager who's irritable, hasn't slept well in 6 months, and has dropped out of social activities?
1. The client will sleep well at night.
2. The parents will stop worrying about the client.
3. The client will obtain appropriate mental health services.
4. The parents will impose strict behavior guidelines for the client to follow.

CN: Client needs category   CNS: Client needs subcategory   CL: Cognitive level

18. 1. Lorazepam is a benzodiazepine used to treat various forms of anxiety and insomnia. Caffeine is contraindicated because it's a stimulant and increases anxiety. A client on a monoamine oxidase inhibitor should avoid aged cheeses. Clients taking certain antipsychotic medications should avoid sunlight. Salt intake has no effect on lorazepam.
CN: Physiological integrity; CNS: Pharmacological therapies; CL: Analysis

19. 3. Primary or secondary gains should be identified because they're etiological factors that can be used in problem resolution. The nurse should encourage the client to be as independent as possible and intervene only when the client requires assistance. The nurse shouldn't focus on the disability. The nurse should encourage the client to perform physical activities to the greatest extent possible.
CN: Psychosocial integrity; CNS: None; CL: Application

20. 4. The paralysis is used as an unhealthy way of expressing unmet psychological needs. The nurse should avoid speaking about the paralysis to shift the client's attention to the mental aspect of the disorder. The other options focus too much on the paralysis, which doesn't allow recognition of the underlying psychological motivations.
CN: Psychosocial integrity; CNS: None; CL: Application

21. 3. Mental health services can protect the client and offer the best means of regaining mental health. The client could reestablish a healthy sleeping pattern without addressing underlying issues. The parents' worrying is unrelated to the child's immediate need for help. The child's behavior suggests the need for professional service, not disciplinary measures.
CN: Psychosocial integrity; CNS: None; CL: Application

22. The mother of a client approaches the nurses' station in tears. She says that she's upset about her daughter's diagnosis of conversion disorder. Which response is best?
   1. "What is it that upsets you the most?"
   2. "Are you afraid your daughter will never get well?"
   3. "Her behavior is typical of someone with conversion disorder."
   4. "Let me give you some information about her illness."

23. Which intervention would most likely be found in a teaching plan for an anxious client who reports difficulty settling down for sleep?
   1. Teaching time management skills
   2. Teaching conflict resolution skills
   3. Teaching progressive muscle relaxation
   4. Teaching adverse effects of antipsychotic medication

24. Which statement is correct about conversion disorders?
   1. The symptoms can be controlled.
   2. The psychological conflict is repressed.
   3. The client is aware of the psychological conflict.
   4. The client shouldn't be made aware of the conflicts underlying the symptoms.

25. A client is admitted for abrupt onset of paralysis in her left arm. Although no physiological cause has been found, the symptoms are exacerbated when she speaks of losing custody of her children in a recent divorce. These findings are characteristic of which disorder?
   1. Body dysmorphic disorder
   2. Conversion disorder
   3. Delusional disorder
   4. Malingering

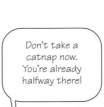

Don't take a catnap now. You're already halfway there!

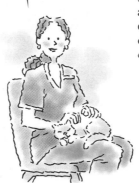

22. 1. Asking the mother an open-ended question permits the nurse to collect data reported in the mother's own words. The other options narrow the data collection process prematurely. Also, it's important to hear what the mother has to say without planting suggestions about her daughter's condition.
CN: Psychosocial integrity; CNS: None; CL: Application

23. 3. Progressive muscle relaxation is a systematic tensing and relaxing of separate muscle groups. As the technique is mastered, relaxation results. Time management skills and conflict resolution skills are helpful in an overall effort to reduce stress and anxiety but don't provide immediate relief in an effort to sleep. Antipsychotic medications aren't usually used to treat anxiety or difficulty with sleep.
CN: Psychosocial integrity; CNS: None; CL: Application

24. 2. In conversion disorders, the client isn't conscious of intentionally producing symptoms that can't be self-controlled. The symptoms are characterized by one or more neurologic symptoms. Understanding the principles and conflicts behind the symptoms can prove helpful during a client's therapy.
CN: Psychosocial integrity; CNS: None; CL: Comprehension

25. 2. Conversion disorders are characterized by one or more neurologic symptoms associated with psychological conflict. Body dysmorphic disorder is an imagined belief that there's a defect in the appearance of all or part of the body. The client isn't experiencing a delusion, which would be the criteria for a delusional disorder. Malingering is the intentional production of symptoms to avoid obligations or obtain rewards.
CN: Psychosocial integrity; CNS: None; CL: Analysis

CN: Client needs category   CNS: Client needs subcategory   CL: Cognitive level

26. A client has been diagnosed with conversion-disorder blindness. The client shows "la belle indifference." Which statement <u>best</u> describes this term?
1. The client is suppressing her true feelings.
2. The client's anxiety has been relieved through her physical symptoms.
3. The client is acting indifferent because she doesn't want to show her actual fear.
4. The client's needs are being met, so she doesn't need to be anxious.

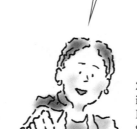

Don't be indifferent to question 26. Just select the best response.

26. 2. Conversion accomplishes anxiety reduction through the production of a physical symptom symbolically linked to an underlying conflict. The client isn't aware of the internal conflict. Hospitalization doesn't remove the source of the conflict.
CN: Psychosocial integrity; CNS: None; CL: Analysis

27. A client with hypochondriasis complains of pain in her right side that she hasn't had before. Which response is the <u>most appropriate</u>?
1. "It's time for group therapy now."
2. "Tell me about this new pain you're having. You'll miss group therapy today."
3. "I'll report this pain to your physician. In the meantime, group therapy starts in 5 minutes. You must leave now to be on time."
4. "I'll call your physician and see if he'll order a new pain medication. Why don't you get some rest for now?"

27. 3. The amount of time focused on discussing physical symptoms should be decreased. Lack of positive reinforcement may help stop the maladaptive behavior. All physical complaints need to be evaluated for physiological causes by the physician. Avoiding the statement demeans the client and doesn't address the underlying problem. Allowing verbalization of the new onset of pain emphasizes physical symptoms and prevents the client from attending group therapy.
CN: Psychosocial integrity; CNS: None; CL: Application

28. Which intervention would help a client with conversion-disorder blindness to eat?
1. Direct the client to independently locate items on the tray and feed himself.
2. See to the needs of the other clients in the dining room, then feed this client last.
3. Establish a "buddy" system with other clients who can feed the client at each meal.
4. Expect the client to feed himself after explaining the location of food on the tray.

28. 4. The client is expected to maintain some level of independence by feeding himself. At the same time, the nurse should be supportive in a matter-of-fact way. Feeding the client leads to dependence.
CN: Psychosocial integrity; CNS: None; CL: Application

29. A client diagnosed with conversion disorder who's experiencing left-sided paralysis tells the nurse she has received a lot of attention in the hospital and it's unfortunate that others outside the hospital don't find her interesting. Which nursing diagnosis is appropriate for this client?
1. *Interrupted family processes*
2. *Ineffective health maintenance*
3. *Ineffective coping*
4. *Social isolation*

29. 3. The client can't express her internal conflicts in appropriate ways. There are no defining characteristics to support the other nursing diagnoses.
CN: Psychosocial integrity; CNS: None; CL: Application

CN: Client needs category   CNS: Client needs subcategory   CL: Cognitive level

30. To help a client with conversion disorder increase self-esteem, which nursing intervention is appropriate?
  1. Set large goals so the client can see positive gains.
  2. Focus attention on the client as a person rather than on the symptom.
  3. Discuss the client's childhood to link present behaviors with past traumas.
  4. Encourage the client to use avoidant-interactional patterns rather than assertive patterns.

31. According to diagnostic criteria, which condition occurs with conversion disorders?
  1. Delusions
  2. Feelings of depression or euphoria
  3. A feeling of dread accompanied by somatic signs
  4. One or more neurologic symptoms associated with psychological conflict or need

32. A client diagnosed with conversion disorder has a nursing diagnosis of *Interrupted family processes related to the client's disability.* Which goal is appropriate for this client?
  1. The client will resume former roles and tasks.
  2. The client will take over roles of other family members.
  3. The client will rely on family members to meet all client needs.
  4. The client will focus energy on problems occurring in the family.

33. Which nursing diagnosis is appropriate for a client with conversion disorder who has little energy to expend on activities or interactions with friends?
  1. *Powerlessness*
  2. *Hopelessness*
  3. *Impaired social interaction*
  4. *Compromised family coping*

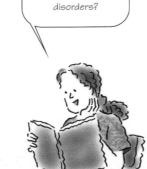

Let's see. What do I need to know about conversion disorders?

Social interaction is important for the client with conversion disorder.

30. 2. Focusing on the client directs attention away from the symptom. This approach eventually reduces the client's need to gain attention through physical symptoms. Small goals ensure success and reinforce self-esteem. Discussion of childhood has no correlation with self-esteem. Avoiding interactional situations doesn't foster self-esteem.
CN: Psychosocial integrity; CNS: None; CL: Application

31. 4. Symptoms of conversion disorders are neurologic in nature (paralysis, blindness). Delusional disorders are characterized by delusions. Mood disorders are characterized by abnormal feelings of depression or euphoria. Anxiety is characterized by a feeling of dread.
CN: Health promotion and maintenance; CNS: None; CL: Knowledge

32. 1. The client who uses somatization has typically adopted a sick role in the family, characterized by dependence. Increasing independence and resumption of former roles are necessary to change this pattern. The client shouldn't be expected to take on the roles or responsibilities of other family members.
CN: Psychosocial integrity; CNS: None; CL: Application

33. 3. When clients focus their mental and physical energy on somatic symptoms, they have little energy to expend on social or diversional activities. Such a client needs nursing assistance to become involved in social interactions. Although the other diagnoses are common for a client with conversion disorder, the information given doesn't support them.
CN: Psychosocial integrity; CNS: None; CL: Application

CN: Client needs category   CNS: Client needs subcategory   CL: Cognitive level

34. A new client admitted to a psychiatric unit is diagnosed with conversion disorder. The client shows a lack of concern for her sudden paralysis, though her athletic abilities have always been a source of pride to her. This manifestation is known as which condition?
1. Acute dystonia
2. La belle indifference
3. Malingering
4. Secondary gain

35. Which nursing intervention is the <u>most appropriate</u> for a client who had pseudoseizures and is diagnosed with conversion disorder?
1. Explain that the pseudoseizures are imaginary.
2. Promote dependence so that unfilled dependency needs are met.
3. Encourage the client to discuss his feelings about the pseudoseizures.
4. Promote independence and withdraw attention from the pseudoseizures.

36. Which therapeutic approach would enable a client to cope effectively with life stress without using conversion?
1. Focus on the symptoms.
2. Ask for clarification of the symptoms.
3. Listen to the client's symptoms in a matter-of-fact manner.
4. Point out that the client's symptoms are an escape from dealing with conflict.

37. Which statement made by a client shows the nurse that the goal of stress management was attained?
1. "My arm hurts."
2. "I enjoy being dependent on others."
3. "I don't really understand why I'm here."
4. "My muscles feel relaxed after that progressive relaxation exercise."

38. Pain disorders, such as headaches and musculoskeletal pain, are most commonly associated with which group?
1. Men
2. Women
3. Less educated population
4. Low socioeconomic population

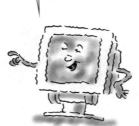

The phrase most appropriate is a hint! Don't miss it!

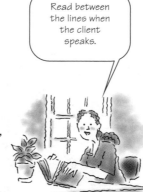

Read between the lines when the client speaks.

34. 2. La belle indifference is a lack of concern about the present illness in some clients. Acute dystonia refers to muscle spasms. Malingering is voluntary production of symptoms. Secondary gain refers to the benefits of illness.
CN: Psychosocial integrity; CNS: None; CL: Knowledge

35. 4. Successful performance of independent activities enhances self-esteem. Confronting the client with a statement that the symptoms are imaginary may jeopardize a long-term relationship with the client. Positive reinforcement encourages the continual use of the maladaptive responses. Focus shouldn't be on the disability because it may provide positive gains for the client.
CN: Physiological integrity; CNS: Physiological adaptation; CL: Application

36. 3. Listening in a matter-of-fact manner doesn't focus on the client's symptoms. All other interventions focus on the client's symptoms, which draw attention to the physical symptoms, not the underlying cause.
CN: Health promotion and maintenance; CNS: None; CL: Application

37. 4. The client is experiencing positive results from the relaxation exercise. All other responses alert the nurse that the client needs further interventions.
CN: Physiological integrity; CNS: Physiological adaptation; CL: Analysis

38. 2. Pain disorders are more common in women than men. Pain disorders can occur at any age, especially from ages 30 to 49. There isn't a high correlation of pain disorders with less educated individuals or those from a low socioeconomic population.
CN: Physiological integrity; CNS: Physiological adaptation; CL: Knowledge

39. Which description <u>best</u> defines a somatoform pain disorder?
1. A preoccupation with pain in the absence of physical disease
2. A physical or somatic complaint without any demonstrable organic findings
3. A morbid fear or belief that one has a serious disease where none exists
4. One or more neurologic symptoms associated with psychological conflict or need

40. Which feature is least likely to be associated with malingering?
1. A collection of symptoms inconsistent with any one medical profile
2. An exaggeration of symptoms
3. A medical condition confirmed by diagnostic testing
4. A group of symptoms not believable

41. A 45-year-old client has been diagnosed with malingering. The nursing assistant caring for the client asks the nurse what this diagnosis is. Which response by the nurse would be most appropriate?
1. "It's a preoccupation with pain in the absence of physical disease."
2. "It's a voluntary production of a physical symptom for a secondary gain."
3. "It's a morbid fear or belief that one has a serious disease where none exists."
4. "It's associated with a psychological need or conflict in which the client shows one or more neurologic symptoms."

42. Based on a nursing diagnosis of *Ineffective coping* for a client with somatoform pain disorder, which nursing goal is most realistic?
1. The client will be free from injury.
2. The client will recognize sensory impairment.
3. The client will discuss beliefs about spiritual issues.
4. The client will verbalize absence or significant reduction of physical symptoms.

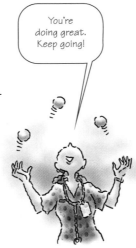

You're doing great. Keep going!

Remember, diagnostic criteria for psychological problems come from the latest edition of the *Diagnostic & Statistical Manual of Mental Disorders*, currently known as *DSM-IV-TR*.

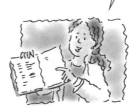

39. 1. Somatoform pain disorder is a preoccupation with pain in the absence of physical disease. A physical or somatic complaint refers to somatoform disorders in general. A morbid fear of serious illness is hypochondriasis. Neurologic symptoms are associated with conversion disorders.
CN: Psychosocial integrity; CNS: None; CL: Knowledge

40. 3. Although there's no specific method to determine whether an individual is a malingerer, all of the above features except confirmation of a medical condition are seen in this condition. Psychological tests may also help to detect this condition.
CN: Psychosocial integrity; CNS: None; CL: Knowledge

41. 2. Malingering is defined as a voluntary production of physical or psychological symptoms to accomplish a specific goal or secondary gain (avoidance of a specific situation, such as a jail term or to obtain money). The other statements are associated with conversion, hypochondriasis, and pain disorders.
CN: Health promotion and maintenance; CNS: None; CL: Application

42. 4. Expression of feelings enables the client to ventilate emotions, which decreases anxiety and draws attention away from the physical symptoms. The client isn't experiencing a safety issue. Spiritual issues are related to spiritual distress, and no evidence exists to support that the client is having spiritual distress. There's also no apparent correlation with any sensory-perceptual alterations.
CN: Physiological integrity; CNS: Basic care and comfort; CL: Analysis

CN: Client needs category CNS: Client needs subcategory CL: Cognitive level

43. Which nursing diagnosis is appropriate for a client with a somatoform disorder?
1. *Interrupted family processes*
2. *Disturbed thought processes*
3. *Ineffective denial*
4. *Ineffective coping*

44. Which statement made by a client best meets the diagnostic criteria for pain disorder?
1. "I can't move my right leg."
2. "I'm having severe stomach and leg pain."
3. "I'm so afraid I might have human immunodeficiency virus."
4. "I'm having chest pain and pain radiating down my left arm that began more than 1 hour ago."

45. Which conditions or situations are most likely to result in difficulty sleeping? Select all that apply:
1. Shift work
2. Sleep apnea
3. Reduction of external stimuli
4. Caffeine intake in the evening
5. Consistent bedtime routine
6. Excessive worry or anxiety

46. A client has primary insomnia and requires pharmaceutical assistance to sleep. The physician orders secobarbital sodium (Seconal) 75 mg by mouth at bedtime. The nurse has secobarbital sodium 25-mg tablets on hand. How many tablets should she administer to the client? Record you answer using a whole number.

_____ tablets

43. 4. A somatoform pain disorder is closely associated with the client's inability to handle stress and conflict. Disturbed thought processes aren't directly correlated with this disorder. While interrupted family processes and ineffective denial may be present, they aren't the primary focus.
CN: Psychosocial integrity; CNS: None; CL: Application

44. 2. Pain in one or more anatomic sites is the predominant focus of the clinical presentation and is of sufficient severity to warrant clinical attention. A client with a conversion disorder can experience a motor neurologic symptom such as paralysis. Hypochondriasis is a morbid fear or belief that one has a serious disease where none exists. Unremitting chest pain with radiation of pain down the left arm is symptomatic of a myocardial infarction.
CN: Psychosocial integrity; CNS: None; CL: Application

45. 1, 2, 4, 6. Shift work can disrupt the circadian rhythm. Sleep apnea can cause a reduction in oxygen to the brain, which can reduce the quality of rest. Caffeine is a stimulant and, if taken too close to bedtime, it can interfere with falling asleep. Excessive worry or anxiety causes an increase in adrenaline, which enhances alertness and reduces sleepiness. A consistent bedtime routine and reduction of external stimuli promote good sleep.
CN: Health promotion and maintenance; CNS: None; CL: Analysis

46. 3. Each tablet contains 25 mg of the medication. The correct formula to calculate this drug dose is:
Dose of each tablet × X = Prescribed dose
25 mg × X (# of tablets) = 75 mg;
25X = 75;
X = 75/25;
X = 3.
CN: Physiological integrity; CNS: Pharmacological therapies; CL: Analysis

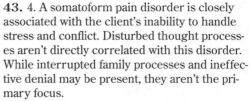

Good for you! Now take a nap and don't be anxious about chapter 14.

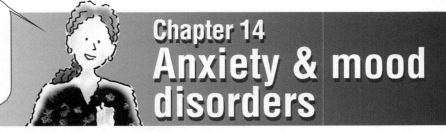

Chapter 14
Anxiety & mood disorders

Want more information on anxiety and mood disorders to help you prepare for the NCLEX? Check out the Web site of the National Alliance for the Mentally III at *www.nami.org/.*

1. Which condition(s) should the nurse expect to find in a client with a history of panic attacks?
1. Restlessness and fragmented sleep
2. Difficulty falling asleep
3. Wild and vivid dreams
4. Abrupt awakening and feelings of fear

2. During the admission assessment, a client with a panic disorder begins to hyperventilate and says, "I'm going to die if I don't get out of here right now!" What's the nurse's best response?
1. "Just calm down. You're getting overly anxious."
2. "What do you think is causing your panic attack?"
3. "You can rest alone in your room until you feel better."
4. "You're having a panic attack. I'll stay here with you."

3. A client with a history of panic attacks who says, "I felt so trapped," right after an attack <u>most likely</u> has which fear?
1. Loss of control
2. Loss of identity
3. Loss of memory
4. Loss of maturity

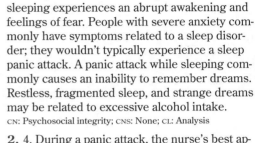

Which answer to question 3 is *most likely* to get you off to a good start?

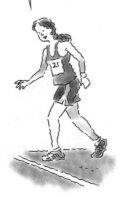

1. 4. A person who suffers a panic attack while sleeping experiences an abrupt awakening and feelings of fear. People with severe anxiety commonly have symptoms related to a sleep disorder; they wouldn't typically experience a sleep panic attack. A panic attack while sleeping commonly causes an inability to remember dreams. Restless, fragmented sleep, and strange dreams may be related to excessive alcohol intake.
CN: Psychosocial integrity; CNS: None; CL: Analysis

2. 4. During a panic attack, the nurse's best approach is to orient the client to what's happening and provide reassurance that the client won't be left alone. The client's anxiety level is likely to increase—and the panic attack is likely to continue—if the client is told to calm down, asked the reasons for the attack, or is left alone.
CN: Psychosocial integrity; CNS: None; CL: Application

3. 1. People who fear loss of control during a panic attack commonly make statements about feeling trapped, getting hurt, or having little to no personal control over their situations. People who experience panic attacks don't tend to have memory impairment or loss of identity. People who have panic attacks also don't regress or become immature.
CN: Psychosocial integrity; CNS: None; CL: Application

CN: Client needs category   CNS: Client needs subcategory   CL: Cognitive level

4. Which factor should the nurse be most concerned about when caring for a client taking an antianxiety medication?
1. Physical and psychological dependence
2. Transient hypertension
3. Abrupt withdrawal
4. Constipation

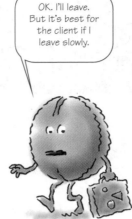

OK. I'll leave. But it's best for the client if I leave slowly.

5. A nurse is caring for a patient experiencing a panic attack. Which intervention by the nurse would be most appropriate?
1. Tell the client to take deep breaths.
2. Have the client talk about the anxiety.
3. Encourage the client to verbalize feelings.
4. Ask the client about the cause of the attack.

6. Which instruction should the nurse include in a teaching session about panic disorder for clients and their families?
1. Identifying when anxiety is escalating
2. Determining how to stop a panic attack
3. Addressing strategies to reduce physical pain
4. Preventing the client from depending on others

For the NCLEX, you should know the definitions of common fears such as agoraphobia.

7. Which finding would the nurse expect to see in a client with agoraphobia who's experiencing a panic attack?
1. Family history of panic attacks
2. Inability to set realistic goals
3. Inability to be alone in public places
4. Poor impulse control

4. 3. Abrupt discontinuation of an antianxiety drug can lead to withdrawal symptoms. Antianxiety medications are usually prescribed for short periods. However, if used over a prolonged period, such drugs may produce psychological or physical dependence. Transient hypertension and constipation aren't associated with antianxiety drugs.
CN: Physiological integrity; CNS: Pharmacological therapies; CL: Application

5. 1. During a panic attack, the nurse should remain with the client and direct what's said toward changing the physiological response, such as taking deep breaths. During an attack, the client is unable to talk about anxious situations and isn't able to address feelings, especially uncomfortable feelings and frustrations. While having a panic attack, the client is also unable to focus on anything other than the symptoms, so the client won't be able to discuss the cause of the attack.
CN: Psychosocial integrity; CNS: None; CL: Analysis

6. 1. By identifying the presence of anxiety, it's possible to take steps to prevent its escalation. A panic attack can't be stopped. The nurse can take steps to assist the client safely through the attack. Later, the nurse can assist the client to alleviate the precipitating stressors. Clients who experience panic disorder don't tend to be in physical pain. The client experiencing a panic disorder may need to periodically depend on other people when having a panic attack.
CN: Psychosocial integrity; CNS: None; CL: Comprehension

7. 3. The client with agoraphobia commonly restricts himself to home and is unable to carry out normal socializing and life-sustaining activities. Clients with panic disorders as evidenced by agoraphobia are able to set realistic goals and tend to be cautious and reclusive rather than impulsive. Although there's a familial tendency toward panic disorder, information about client needs must be obtained to determine how agoraphobia affects the client's life.
CN: Psychosocial integrity; CNS: None; CL: Analysis

CN: Client needs category   CNS: Client needs subcategory   CL: Cognitive level

8. Which explanation about the relationship between consumed substances and panic attacks should the nurse reinforce as part of a behavior modification program?
1. Cigarettes can trigger panic episodes.
2. Fermented foods can cause panic attacks.
3. Hormonal therapy can induce panic attacks.
4. Tryptophan can predispose a person to panic attacks.

9. The nurse is caring for a 27-year-old male client who's in the panic level of anxiety. Which action is the nurse's <u>highest</u> priority?
1. Encourage the client to discuss his feelings.
2. Provide for the client's safety needs.
3. Decrease environmental stimuli.
4. Respect the client's personal space.

10. Which short-term client outcome is appropriate for a client with panic disorder?
1. Identify childhood trauma.
2. Monitor nutritional intake.
3. Institute suicide precautions.
4. Decrease episodes of disorientation.

11. A client diagnosed with panic disorder with agoraphobia is talking with the nurse about the progress made in treatment. Which statement indicates a positive client response?
1. "I went to the mall with my friend last Saturday."
2. "I'm hyperventilating only when I have a panic attack."
3. "Today I decided that I can stop taking my medication."
4. "Last night I decided to eat more than a bowl of cereal."

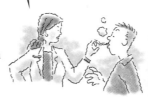

You need to understand the relationship between consumed substances and panic attacks.

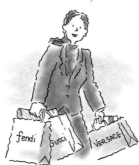

I've always said that shopping is good therapy.

8. 1. Cigarettes are considered stimulants and can trigger panic attacks. Fermented foods, hormonal therapy, and tryptophan don't cause panic attacks.
CN: Psychosocial integrity; CNS: None; CL: Analysis

9. 2. A client in the panic level of anxiety doesn't comprehend and can't follow instructions or care for his own basic needs. The client is unable to express feelings due to the level of anxiety. Decreased environmental stimulus is needed but only after the client's safety needs and other basic needs are met. The nurse must enter the client's personal space to provide personal care because a client in panic can't do so for himself.
CN: Psychosocial integrity; CNS: None; CL: Knowledge

10. 3. Clients with panic disorder are at risk for suicide. Childhood trauma is associated with posttraumatic stress disorder, *not* panic disorder. Nutritional problems don't typically accompany panic disorder. Clients with panic disorder aren't typically disoriented; they may have a temporarily altered sense of reality, but that lasts only for the duration of the attack.
CN: Psychosocial integrity; CNS: None; CL: Comprehension

11. 1. Clients with panic disorder tend to be socially withdrawn. Going to the mall is a sign of working on avoidance behaviors. Hyperventilation is a key symptom of panic disorder. Teaching breathing control is a major intervention for clients with panic disorder. The client taking medications for panic disorder, such as tricyclic antidepressants and benzodiazepines, must be weaned off these drugs. Most clients with panic disorder with agoraphobia don't have nutritional problems.
CN: Psychosocial integrity; CNS: None; CL: Analysis

CN: Client needs category   CNS: Client needs subcategory   CL: Cognitive level

12. Which group therapy intervention would be of <u>primary</u> importance to a client with panic disorder?
  1. Explore how secondary gains are derived from the disorder.
  2. Discuss new ways of thinking and feeling about panic attacks.
  3. Work to eliminate manipulative behavior used for meeting needs.
  4. Learn the risk factors and other demographics associated with panic disorder.

13. A nurse is caring for a client with social phobia. Which statement is <u>most</u> accurate regarding clients with social phobia?
  1. They avoid social situations.
  2. They are at risk for self-harm.
  3. They exhibit compulsive behavior.
  4. They have poor self-esteem.

14. Which statement is typical of a client with social phobia?
  1. "Without people around, I just feel so lost."
  2. "There's nothing wrong with my behavior."
  3. "I always feel like I'm the center of attention."
  4. "I know I can't accept that award for my brother."

15. Clients with a social phobia would <u>most</u> <u>likely</u> fear which situation?
  1. Dental procedures
  2. Meeting strangers
  3. Being bitten by a dog
  4. Having a car accident

16. Which intervention by the nurse would be <u>most</u> appropriate when caring for a client newly diagnosed with insulin-dependent diabetes who also has blood-injection-injury phobia?
  1. Teach the client to avoid fainting by tensing the muscles of the legs and abdomen.
  2. Quickly expose the client to feared situations.
  3. Have the client avoid as much medical care as possible.
  4. Focus on treating the symptoms with antianxiety medication.

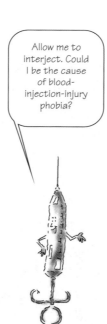

Allow me to interject. Could I be the cause of blood-injection-injury phobia?

12. 2. Discussion of new ways of thinking and feeling about panic attacks can enable others to learn and benefit from a variety of intervention strategies. There are usually no secondary gains obtained from having a panic disorder. People with panic disorder aren't using the disorder as a way to manipulate others. Learning the risk factors could be accomplished in another format such as a psychoeducational program.
CN: Psychosocial integrity; CNS: None; CL: Analysis

13. 1. Clients with social phobia avoid social situations for fear of being humiliated or embarrassed. They generally don't tend to be at risk for self-harm and usually don't demonstrate compulsive behavior. Not all individuals with social anxiety have low self-esteem.
CN: Psychosocial integrity; CNS: None; CL: Analysis

14. 4. People who have a social phobia usually undervalue themselves and their talents. They fear social gatherings and dislike being the center of attention. They tend to stay away from situations in which they may feel humiliated and embarrassed. They don't like to be in feared social situations or around many people. They're very critical of themselves and believe that others will also be critical.
CN: Psychosocial integrity; CNS: None; CL: Application

15. 2. Fear of meeting strangers is a common example of social phobia. Fears of having a dental procedure, being bitten by a dog, or having an accident *aren't* social phobias.
CN: Psychosocial integrity; CNS: None; CL: Knowledge

16. 1. The client may be able to avoid fainting and relieve hypotension by tensing the large muscle groups. Desensitization by slowly, not quickly, exposing the client to blood injection is indicated to reduce fear. Clients with blood-injection-injury phobia may avoid all medical care, which is dangerous to their health. Antianxiety medications may help on a short-term basis only.
CN: Psychosocial integrity; CNS: None; CL: Application

CN: Client needs category   CNS: Client needs subcategory   CL: Cognitive level

17. A client on the sixth floor of a psychiatric unit has a morbid fear of elevators. She's scheduled to attend occupational therapy, which is located on the ground floor of the hospital. The client refuses to take the elevator, insisting that the stairs are safer. Which nursing action would be <u>best</u> given the client's refusal to use the elevator?
1. Insist that she take the elevator.
2. Offer a special reward if she rides the elevator.
3. Withhold her occupational therapy privileges until she's able to ride the elevator.
4. Allow her to use the stairs.

18. Which behavior modification technique is useful in the treatment of phobias?
1. Aversion therapy
2. Imitation or modeling
3. Positive reinforcement
4. Systematic desensitization

19. Which statement would be useful when teaching the client and family about phobias and the need for a strong support system?
1. The use of a family support system is only temporary.
2. The need to be assertive can be reinforced by the family.
3. The family must set limits on inappropriate behaviors.
4. The family plays a role in promoting client independence.

20. Which nursing diagnosis would the nurse expect to find on the care plan of a client with a phobia about elevators?
1. *Social isolation related to a lack of social skills*
2. *Disturbed thought processes related to a fear of elevators*
3. *Ineffective coping related to poor coping skills*
4. *Anxiety related to fear of elevators*

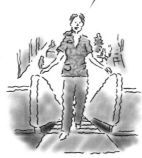

It's important to know the ups and downs of phobias.

17. 4. This client has a phobia and must not be forced to ride the elevator because of the risk of panic-level anxiety, which can occur if she's forced to contact the phobic object. This client can't control her fear; therefore, stating that she must take the elevator or promising a reward won't work. Occupational therapy is a treatment the client needs, not a reward.
CN: Psychosocial integrity; CNS: None; CL: Application

18. 4. Systematic desensitization is a common behavior modification technique successfully used to help treat phobias. Aversion therapy and positive reinforcement *aren't* behavior modification techniques used with treatment of phobias. The techniques of imitation or modeling are social learning techniques, not behavior modification techniques.
CN: Psychosocial integrity; CNS: None; CL: Application

19. 4. The family plays a vital role in supporting the client in treatment and preventing the client from using the phobia to obtain secondary gains. Family support must be ongoing, not temporary. The family can be more helpful by focusing on effective handling of anxiety, rather than focusing energy on developing assertiveness skills. People with phobias are already restrictive in their behavior; more restrictions aren't necessary.
CN: Psychosocial integrity; CNS: None; CL: Analysis

20. 3. Poor coping skills can cause ineffective coping. Such a client isn't relegated to social isolation, and lack of social skills has nothing to do with phobia. Fear of elevators is a manifestation, not the cause, of altered thoughts and anxiety.
CN: Psychosocial integrity; CNS: None; CL: Analysis

CN: Client needs category   CNS: Client needs subcategory   CL: Cognitive level

21. A nurse is caring for a client suspected of having posttraumatic stress disorder (PTSD). The nurse is aware that the client is also <u>commonly</u> at high risk for developing which condition?
1. Self-harm and violent behavior
2. Eating disorder
3. Schizophrenia
4. "Sundown" syndrome

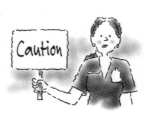

22. Which action explains why tricyclic antidepressant medication is given to a client who has severe posttraumatic stress disorder?
1. It prevents hyperactivity and purposeless movements.
2. It increases the client's ability to concentrate.
3. It helps prevent experiencing the trauma again.
4. It facilitates the grieving process.

23. Which nursing action would be included in a care plan for a client with posttraumatic stress disorder who states that the experience was "bad luck"?
1. Encourage the client to verbalize the experience.
2. Assist the client in defining the experience as a trauma.
3. Work with the client to take steps to move on with life.
4. Help the client accept positive and negative feelings.

> A client describing a trauma as "bad luck" may be in denial.

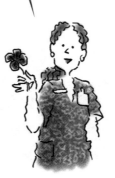

24. A client was in a plane crash a year ago and several people were killed. The client is now experiencing nightmares, insomnia, headaches, loss of appetite, and fatigue. Which disorder is the client <u>most likely</u> experiencing?
1. Panic disorder
2. Posttraumatic stress disorder
3. Bipolar disorder
4. Conversion disorder

21. 1. Clients who experience PTSD are at high risk for suicide and other forms of violent behavior. Eating disorders are possible, but not a common complication of PTSD. Clients with PTSD don't usually have their extreme anxiety manifest itself as schizophrenia. "Sundown" syndrome is an increase in agitation accompanied by confusion. It's commonly seen in clients with dementia, not those with PTSD.
CN: Psychosocial integrity; CNS: None; CL: Analysis

22. 3. Tricyclic antidepressant medication will decrease the frequency of reenactment of the trauma for the client. It will help memory problems and sleeping difficulties and will decrease numbing. The medication won't prevent hyperactivity and purposeless movements nor increase the client's concentration. No medication will facilitate the grieving process.
CN: Physiological integrity; CNS: Pharmacological therapies; CL: Application

23. 2. The client must define the experience as traumatic to realize the situation wasn't under personal control. Encouraging the client to verbalize the experience without first addressing the denial isn't a useful strategy. The client can move on with life only after acknowledging the trauma and processing the experience. Acknowledgment of the actual trauma and verbalization of the event should come *before* the acceptance of feelings.
CN: Psychosocial integrity; CNS: None; CL: Analysis

24. 2. The client is reliving the crash because it's close to the first anniversary of the accident. Panic disorder isn't correct because the client is still able to function. Bipolar disorder isn't appropriate because the client isn't exhibiting mania and depression. Conversion disorder isn't correct because the client isn't exhibiting any physical symptoms, such as paralysis, that aren't supported by a medical diagnosis.
CN: Psychosocial integrity; CNS: None; CL: Application

25. Which statement by a family member most closely reflects accurate understanding of the <u>most common</u> symptoms of posttraumatic stress disorder (PTSD)?
1. "My son started having bad dreams 6 months after returning from war."
2. "My son washes his hands several dozen times a day."
3. "My son is afraid to leave the house."
4. "My son is withdrawn and cries a lot."

26. While caring for a client with posttraumatic stress disorder, the family notices that loud noises cause a serious anxiety response. Which explanation would help the family understand the client's response?
1. Environmental triggers can cause the client to react emotionally.
2. Clients commonly experience extreme fear of normal environmental stimuli.
3. After a trauma, the client can't respond to stimuli in an appropriate manner.
4. The response indicates another emotional problem needs investigation.

27. A client was the lone survivor of a train wreck 6 months ago. Which statement by the client would indicate a maladaptive response to the trauma?
1. "I don't want to talk about it."
2. "I'm able to concentrate on reading a book."
3. "I've started to sleep through the night."
4. "I jump when I hear a train whistle because it reminds me of the wreck."

28. If a client suffering from posttraumatic stress disorder (PTSD) says, "I've decided to just avoid everything and everyone," the nurse might suspect the client is at <u>greatest</u> risk for which behavior?
1. Becoming homeless
2. Exhausting finances
3. Terminating employment
4. Using substances

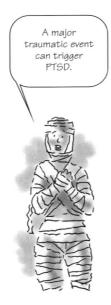

A major traumatic event can trigger PTSD.

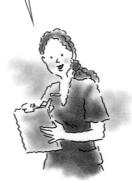

All of the answers may be possible risks, but you've got to choose the greatest risk.

25. 1. PTSD occurs following a major traumatic event and can be manifested by recurrent dreams and intense psychological distress. Excessive hand washing would indicate an obsessive-compulsive disorder. Agoraphobia is characterized by fear of leaving the house. Withdrawal and crying may be present in PTSD, but are more indicative of depression.
CN: Psychosocial integrity; CNS: None; CL: Analysis

26. 1. Repeated exposure to environmental triggers can cause the client to experience a hyperarousal state because there's a loss of physiological control of incoming stimuli. After experiencing a trauma, the client may have strong reactions to stimuli similar to those that occurred during the traumatic event. However, not *all* stimuli will cause an anxiety response. The client's anxiety response is typically seen after a traumatic experience and doesn't indicate the presence of another problem.
CN: Psychosocial integrity; CNS: None; CL: Application

27. 1. Denial is used as a protective response to posttraumatic stress. Concentration and sleeping through the night indicate resolution of conflicts. Startling sounds can provoke anxiety in a client with posttraumatic stress disorder, but the client expresses understanding of why this happens to him.
CN: Psychosocial integrity; CNS: None; CL: Application

28. 4. The use of substances is a way for the client to deny problems and self-medicate distress. There are few homeless people with PTSD as the cause of their homelessness. Most clients with PTSD can manage money and maintain employment.
CN: Psychosocial integrity; CNS: None; CL: Application

CN: Client needs category   CNS: Client needs subcategory   CL: Cognitive level

29. Which action would be most appropriate when speaking to a client with posttraumatic stress disorder (PTSD) about the trauma?
    1. Obtain validation of what the client says from another party.
    2. Request that the client write down what's being said.
    3. Ask questions to convey an interest in the details.
    4. Listen attentively.

30. Which client statement indicates an understanding of survivor guilt?
    1. "I think I can see the purpose of my survival."
    2. "I can't help but feel that everything is their fault."
    3. "I now understand why I'm not able to forgive myself."
    4. "I wish I could stop sabotaging my family relationships."

31. Which nursing intervention would best help the client with posttraumatic stress disorder and his family handle interpersonal conflict at home?
    1. Have the family teach the client to identify defensive behaviors.
    2. Have the family discuss how to change dysfunctional family patterns.
    3. Have the family agree not to tell the client what to do about problems.
    4. Have the family arrange for the client to participate in social activities.

32. The effectiveness of monoamine oxidase (MAO) inhibitor drug therapy in a client with posttraumatic stress disorder (PTSD) can be demonstrated by which client self-report?
    1. "I'm sleeping better and don't have nightmares."
    2. "I'm not losing my temper as much."
    3. "I've lost my craving for alcohol."
    4. "I've lost my phobia of water."

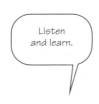

Listen and learn.

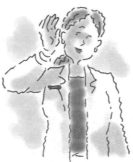

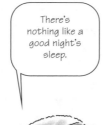

There's nothing like a good night's sleep.

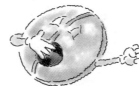

29. 4. An effective communication strategy for a nurse to use with a PTSD client is listening attentively and staying with the client. There's no need to obtain validation about what the client says by asking for information from another party, asking them to write what's being said, or distracting them by asking questions.
CN: Psychosocial integrity; CNS: None; CL: Application

30. 3. Survivor guilt occurs when the person has almost constant thoughts about the other people who perished in the event. They don't understand why they survived when their friend or loved one didn't. Blaming self, rather than blaming others, is a component of survivor guilt. Survivor guilt and impaired interpersonal relationships are two different categories of responses to trauma and don't indicate that the person understands survivor guilt.
CN: Psychosocial integrity; CNS: None; CL: Analysis

31. 2. Discussion of dysfunctional family patterns allows the family to determine why and how these patterns are maintained. Having family members point out the defensive behaviors of the client may inadvertently produce more defensive behavior. Families can be a source of support and assistance. Therefore, inflexible rules, such as not telling the client what to do about his problems, aren't useful to the client or the family. The family shouldn't be encouraged to arrange social activities for the client. Social activities outside of the home don't assist the family handling conflict within the home.
CN: Psychosocial integrity; CNS: None; CL: Application

32. 1. MAO inhibitors are used to treat sleep problems, nightmares, and intrusive daytime thoughts in individuals with PTSD. MAO inhibitors aren't used to help control temper or phobias or to decrease the craving for alcohol.
CN: Physiological integrity; CNS: Pharmacological therapies; CL: Analysis

33. The nurse is caring for a Vietnam veteran with a history of explosive anger, unemployment, and depression since being discharged from the service. The client reports feeling ashamed of being "weak" and of letting past experiences control his present thoughts and actions. What's the nurse's <u>best</u> response?
1. "Many people who have been in your situation experience similar emotions and behaviors."
2. "No one can predict how he'll react in a traumatic situation."
3. "It's not too late for you to make changes in your life."
4. "Weak people don't want to make changes in their lives."

34. Which result is the <u>major purpose</u> for providing group therapy to a group of adolescents who witnessed the violent death of a peer?
1. To learn violence prevention strategies
2. To talk about appropriate expression of anger
3. To discuss the effect of the trauma on their lives
4. To develop trusting relationships among their peers

35. The nurse is caring for a 53-year-old male client with posttraumatic stress disorder who's experiencing a frightening flashback. The nurse can <u>best</u> offer reassurance of safety and security through which nursing action?
1. Encouraging the client to talk about the traumatic event
2. Assessing for maladaptive and coping strategies
3. Staying with the client
4. Acknowledging feelings of guilt or self-blame

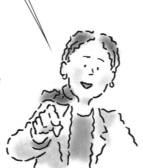

The term *major purpose* indicates that there may be more than one right answer. You need to choose the best answer.

33. 1. By saying that extreme anger and other reactions are normal responses to trauma, the nurse assists the client in dealing with his shame over a perceived lack of control of feelings. It also helps him gain confidence in his ability to alter behaviors. The other responses are clichés and don't address the client's feelings.
CN: Psychosocial integrity; CNS: None; CL: Application

34. 3. By discussing the effect of the trauma on their lives, the adolescents can grieve and develop effective coping strategies. Learning violence prevention strategies isn't the most immediate concern after a trauma occurs nor is working on developing healthy relationships. It's appropriate to talk about how to express anger appropriately after the trauma is addressed.
CN: Psychosocial integrity; CNS: None; CL: Application

35. 3. The nurse should stay with the client during periods of flashbacks and nightmares, offer reassurance of safety and security, and assure the client that these symptoms aren't uncommon following a severe trauma. Encouraging him to talk about the traumatic event, observing for maladaptive and coping strategies, and acknowledging feelings of guilt or self-blame may be carried out in the future. The nurse's top priority during the flashback is to stay with the client.
CN: Psychosocial integrity; CNS: None; CL: Application

CN: Client needs category   CNS: Client needs subcategory   CL: Cognitive level

36. Which nursing behavior would demonstrate caring to clients with a diagnosis of anxiety disorder?
1. Verbalize concern about the client.
2. Arrange group activities for clients.
3. Have the client sign the treatment plan.
4. Hold psychoeducational groups on medications.

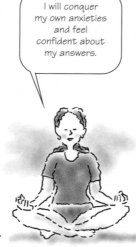

> I will conquer my own anxieties and feel confident about my answers.

36. 1. The nurse who verbally expresses concern about a client's well-being is acting in a caring and supportive manner. Arranging for group activities may be an action where the nurse has no direct client contact and is therefore unable to demonstrate caring to clients. Having a client sign the treatment plan may not be viewed as a sign of caring. Having a psychoeducational group on medications may be viewed by clients as a teaching experience and not caring because the nurse may have limited interaction with them.
CN: Health promotion and maintenance; CNS: None; CL: Application

37. Which finding should the nurse expect when talking about school to a child diagnosed with a generalized anxiety disorder?
1. The child has been fighting with peers for the past month.
2. The child can't stop lying to parents and teachers.
3. The child has gained 15 lb (6.8 kg) in the past month.
4. The child expresses concerns about grades.

37. 4. Children with generalized anxiety disorder will worry about how well they're performing in school. Children with generalized anxiety disorder don't tend to be involved in conflict. They're more oriented toward good behavior. Children with generalized anxiety disorder don't tend to lie to others. They would want to do their best and try to please others. A weight gain of 15 lb isn't a typical characteristic of a child with anxiety disorder.
CN: Psychosocial integrity; CNS: None; CL: Analysis

38. A client with a generalized anxiety disorder may also have which concurrent diagnosis?
1. Bipolar disorder
2. Gender identity disorder
3. Panic disorder
4. Schizoaffective disorder

38. 3. Approximately 75% of clients with generalized anxiety disorder may also have a diagnosis of phobia, panic disorder, or substance abuse. Clients with generalized anxiety disorder don't tend to have a coexisting diagnosis of bipolar disorder, gender identity disorder, or schizoaffective disorder.
CN: Psychosocial integrity; CNS: None; CL: Application

39. Which statement indicates a positive response from a generalized anxiety disorder client to a nurse's teaching about nutrition?
1. "I've stopped drinking so much diet cola."
2. "I've reduced my intake of carbohydrates."
3. "I now eat less at dinner and before bedtime."
4. "I've cut back on my use of dairy products."

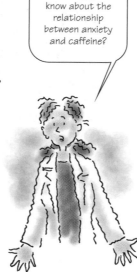

> What do you know about the relationship between anxiety and caffeine?

39. 1. Clients with generalized anxiety disorder can decrease anxiety by eliminating caffeine from their diets. It isn't necessary for clients with generalized anxiety to decrease their carbohydrate intake, eat less at dinner or before bedtime (unless there are other compelling health reasons), or cut back on their use of dairy products.
CN: Health promotion and maintenance; CNS: None; CL: Application

CN: Client needs category   CNS: Client needs subcategory   CL: Cognitive level

40. A client with generalized anxiety disorder is prescribed a benzodiazepine, but the client doesn't want to take the medication. Which explanation for this behavior would most likely be correct?

1. "I don't think the psychiatrist likes me."
2. "I want to solve my problems on my own."
3. "I'll wait several weeks to see if I need to take it."
4. "I think my family gains by keeping me medicated."

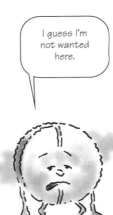

I guess I'm not wanted here.

40. 2. Many clients don't want to take medications because they believe that using a medication is a sign of personal weakness and that they can't solve their problems by themselves. Thinking that the psychiatrist dislikes them reflects paranoid thinking that isn't usually seen in clients with generalized anxiety disorder. By waiting several weeks to take the medication, the client could be denying that the medication is necessary or beneficial. By focusing on the negative motives of family members, the client could be avoiding talking about himself.
CN: Psychosocial integrity; CNS: None; CL: Analysis

41. A female client describes her unpredictable episodes of acute anxiety as "just awful." She says that she feels like she's about to die and can hardly breathe. The nurse recognizes that the symptoms described by the client are associated with which condition?

1. Agoraphobia
2. Dissociative disorder
3. Posttraumatic stress disorder (PTSD)
4. Panic disorder

41. 4. This client is describing the characteristics of someone with panic disorder. Agoraphobia is characterized by fear of public places; dissociative disorder, by lost periods of time; and PTSD, by hypervigilance and sleep disturbance.
CN: Psychosocial integrity; CNS: None; CL: Application

42. Which statement by a 44-year-old client with a diagnosis of generalized anxiety disorder would convince the nurse that anxiety has been a long-standing problem?

1. "I was, and still am, an impulsive person."
2. "I've always been hyperactive, but not in useful ways."
3. "When I was in college, I never thought I would finish."
4. "All my life I've had intrusive dreams and scary nightmares."

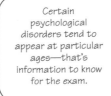

Certain psychological disorders tend to appear at particular ages—that's information to know for the exam.

42. 3. For many people who have a generalized anxiety disorder, the age of onset is during young adulthood. The symptoms of impulsiveness and hyperactivity aren't commonly associated with a diagnosis of generalized anxiety disorder. The symptom of intrusive dreams and nightmares is associated with posttraumatic stress disorder rather than generalized anxiety disorder.
CN: Psychosocial integrity; CNS: None; CL: Comprehension

43. Which symptom would the client with generalized anxiety disorder <u>most likely</u> display when assessed for muscle tension?

1. Difficulty sleeping
2. Restlessness
3. Strong startle response
4. Tachycardia

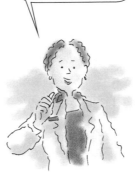

43. 2. Restlessness is a symptom associated with muscle tension. Difficulty sleeping and a strong startle response are considered symptoms of vigilance and scanning of the environment, not muscle tension. Tachycardia is classified as a symptom of autonomic hyperactivity, not muscle tension.
CN: Physiological integrity; CNS: Physiological adaptation; CL: Knowledge

CN: Client needs category   CNS: Client needs subcategory   CL: Cognitive level

44. When planning the care of a client with general anxiety disorder, which intervention is <u>most important</u> to include?
1. Encourage the client to engage in activities that increase feelings of power and self-esteem.
2. Promote the client's interaction and socialization with others.
3. Assist the client to make plans for regular periods of leisure time.
4. Encourage the client to use a diary to record when anxiety occurred, its cause, and which interventions may have helped.

45. Which intervention helps the nurse deal with escalating client anxiety?
1. Explore feelings about current life stressors.
2. Discuss the need to flee from painful situations.
3. Have the client develop a realistic view of self.
4. Provide appropriate phone numbers for hotlines and clinics.

46. The nurse is teaching a 53-year-old male client with the nursing diagnosis *Anxiety related to lack of knowledge about an impending surgical procedure.* Which of the following is an appropriate nursing intervention?
1. Reassure the client that there are many treatments for the problem.
2. Calmly ask the client to describe the procedure that is to be done.
3. Tell the client that the nursing staff will help in any way they can.
4. Tell the client that he shouldn't keep his feelings to himself.

47. A client with a diagnosis of generalized anxiety disorder wants to stop taking his lorazepam (Ativan). Which important fact should the nurse discuss with the client about discontinuing the medication?
1. Stopping the drug may cause depression.
2. Stopping the drug increases cognitive abilities.
3. Stopping the drug decreases sleeping difficulties.
4. Stopping the drug can cause withdrawal symptoms.

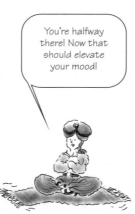

You're halfway there! Now that should elevate your mood!

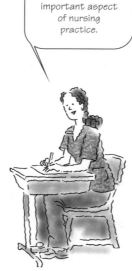

Teaching is an important aspect of nursing practice.

44. 4. One of the nurse's goals is to help the client associate symptoms with an event, thereby beginning to learn appropriate ways to eliminate or reduce distress. A diary can be a beneficial tool for this purpose. Although encouraging the client to engage in activities that increase feelings of power and self-esteem, promoting interaction and socialization with others, and assisting the client to make plans for regular periods of leisure time may be appropriate, they aren't the priority.
CN: Psychosocial integrity; CNS: None; CL: Application

45. 4. By having information on hotlines and clinics, the client can pursue help and support when the anxiety is escalating. Discussion about current life stressors isn't useful when focusing on how best to handle the client's escalating anxiety. Fleeing from painful situations and discussing views of oneself aren't the best strategies; neither allows for problem solving.
CN: Psychosocial integrity; CNS: None; CL: Application

46. 2. An appropriate short-term goal in this case is, "The client will repeat to the nurse the major points of the procedure." By asking the client to describe the procedure, the nurse can assess his level of understanding and address his anxiety by providing necessary teaching. Reassuring him that there are many treatments, instructing him that the nursing staff will help, and telling him that he shouldn't keep his feelings to himself don't address the client's anxiety or lack of knowledge about the procedure.
CN: Psychosocial integrity; CNS: None; CL: Comprehension

47. 4. Stopping antianxiety drugs such as benzodiazepines can cause the client to have withdrawal symptoms. Stopping a benzodiazepine doesn't tend to cause depression, increase cognitive abilities, or decrease sleeping difficulties.
CN: Physiological integrity; CNS: Pharmacological therapies; CL: Application

CN: Client needs category   CNS: Client needs subcategory   CL: Cognitive level

48. Five days after running out of medication, a client taking clonazepam (Klonopin) says to the nurse, "I know I shouldn't have just stopped the drug like that, but I'm okay." Which response would be best?
1. "Let's monitor you for problems, in case something else happens."
2. "You could go through withdrawal symptoms for up to 2 weeks."
3. "You've handled your anxiety and you now know how to cope with stress."
4. "If you're fine now, chances are you won't experience withdrawal symptoms."

49. A client taking alprazolam (Xanax) reports light-headedness and nausea every day while getting out of bed. Which action should the nurse take to objectively validate this client's problem?
1. Take the client's blood pressure.
2. Monitor body temperature.
3. Teach Valsalva's maneuver.
4. Obtain a blood chemical profile.

50. A client with chronic anxiety disorder complains of chest pain. Which nursing intervention is most appropriate?
1. Reassure the client that the episode will pass.
2. Stay with the patient.
3. Obtain vital signs.
4. Administer prescribed antianxiety medication.

51. Which communication guideline should the nurse use when talking with a client experiencing mania?
1. Address the client in a light and joking manner.
2. Focus and redirect the conversation as necessary.
3. Allow the client to talk about several different topics.
4. Ask only open-ended questions to facilitate conversation.

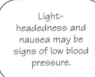

Light-headedness and nausea may be signs of low blood pressure.

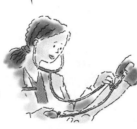

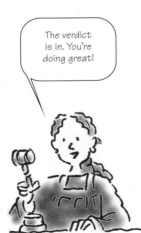

The verdict is in. You're doing great!

48. 2. Withdrawal symptoms can appear after 1 or 2 weeks because the benzodiazepine has a long half-life. Looking for another problem unrelated to withdrawal isn't the nurse's best strategy. The act of discontinuing an antianxiety medication doesn't indicate that a client has learned to cope with stress. Every client taking medication needs to be monitored for withdrawal symptoms when the medication is stopped abruptly.
CN: Physiological integrity; CNS: Pharmacological therapies; CL: Analysis

49. 1. The nurse should take a blood pressure reading to monitor for orthostatic hypotension. A body temperature reading or chemistry profile won't yield useful information about hypotension. Valsalva's maneuver is performed to lower the heart rate and isn't an appropriate intervention.
CN: Physiological integrity; CNS: Reduction of risk potential; CL: Knowledge

50. 3. Although the client with chronic anxiety disorder may have somatic symptoms, physiologic causes for chest pain must be thoroughly assessed. Reassuring the client would be acceptable only after ruling out a physiologic cause for the symptoms. Staying with the client may be therapeutic, but obtaining vital signs would take precedence. Administering antianxiety agents might mask signs of cardiac problems.
CN: Psychosocial integrity; CNS: None; CL: Analysis

51. 2. To decrease stimulation, the nurse should attempt to redirect and focus the conversation, not allow the client to talk about different topics. By addressing the client in a light and joking manner, the conversation may contribute to the client feeling out of control. For a manic client, it's best to ask closed questions because open-ended questions may enable the client to talk endlessly, again possibly contributing to the client feeling out of control.
CN: Psychosocial integrity; CNS: None; CL: Comprehension

52. Which adverse effect would the nurse explain to the client with bipolar disorder and the client's family before administering electroconvulsive therapy (ECT)?
1. Cholestatic jaundice
2. Hypertensive crisis
3. Mouth ulcers
4. Respiratory arrest

53. A client who has just had electroconvulsive therapy (ECT) asks for a drink of water. Which intervention would be the nurse's <u>priority</u>?
1. Check the client's blood pressure.
2. Assess the gag reflex.
3. Obtain a body temperature.
4. Determine level of consciousness.

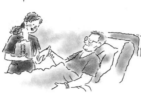

You can probably have a drink, but I need to check something first.

54. A client who's in the manic phase of bipolar disorder constantly belittles other clients and demands special favors from the nurses. Which nursing intervention would be <u>most appropriate</u> for this client?
1. Ask other clients and staff members to ignore the client's behavior.
2. Set limits with consequences for belittling or demanding behavior.
3. Offer the client an antianxiety agent when this behavior occurs.
4. Offer the client a variety of stimulating activities.

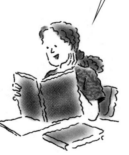

The client is most likely experiencing which problem?

55. A client with bipolar disorder who complains of headache, agitation, and indigestion is <u>most likely</u> experiencing which problem?
1. Depression
2. Cyclothymia
3. Hypomania
4. Mania

56. A client with bipolar disorder has abruptly stopped taking his prescribed medication. Which behavior would indicate the client has experienced a manic episode?
1. Binge eating
2. Relationship avoidance
3. Sudden relocation
4. Thoughtless spending

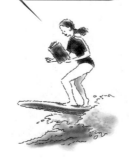

Know the specific behaviors associated with each disorder.

52. 4. Respiratory arrest may occur as a complication of the anesthesia used with ECT. Cholestatic jaundice, hypertensive crisis, and mouth ulcers don't occur during or as a result of ECT.
CN: Physiological integrity; CNS: Physiological adaptation; CL: Knowledge

53. 2. The nurse must check the client's gag reflex before allowing the client to have a drink after an ECT procedure. Blood pressure and body temperature don't influence whether the client may have a drink after the procedure. The client would obviously be conscious if he's requesting a glass of water.
CN: Safe, effective care environment; CNS: Safety and infection control; CL: Application

54. 2. By setting limits with consequences for noncompliance, the nurse can protect others from a client who exhibits belittling and demanding behaviors. Asking others to ignore the client is likely to increase those behaviors. Offering the client an antianxiety agent or stimulating activities provides no motivation for the client to change the problematic behaviors.
CN: Psychosocial integrity; CNS: None; CL: Application

55. 4. Headache, agitation, and indigestion are symptoms that suggest mania in a client with a history of bipolar disorder. These symptoms *aren't* suggestive of depression, cyclothymia, or hypomania.
CN: Physiological integrity; CNS: Physiological adaptation; CL: Knowledge

56. 4. Thoughtless or reckless spending is a common symptom of a manic episode. Binge eating isn't a behavior that's characteristic of a client during a manic episode. Relationship avoidance doesn't occur in a client experiencing a manic episode. During episodes of mania, a client may, in fact, interact with many people and participate in unsafe sexual behavior. Sudden relocation isn't a characteristic of impulsive behavior demonstrated by a client with bipolar disorder.
CN: Psychosocial integrity; CNS: None; CL: Application

CN: Client needs category   CNS: Client needs subcategory   CL: Cognitive level

57. Which intervention would help the client with bipolar disorder to maintain adequate nutrition?
1. Determine the client's metabolic rate.
2. Make the client sit down for each meal and snack.
3. Give the client foods to be eaten while he's active.
4. Have the client interact with a dietitian twice a week.

58. Which adverse reaction does the client with bipolar disorder taking lithium need to report?
1. Black tongue
2. Increased lacrimation
3. Periods of disorientation
4. Persistent GI upset

59. When providing discharge instructions for a client with bipolar disorder who's receiving lithium carbonate, the nurse should stress which of the following?
1. The client should take the medication with food.
2. The client should have blood serum levels checked regularly.
3. The client should take the medication on an empty stomach.
4. The client should avoid operating heavy machinery.

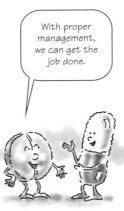

With proper management, we can get the job done.

60. Which activity is appropriate for a client with a diagnosis of bipolar disorder in the manic phase?
1. Playing a card game
2. Playing a vigorous basketball game
3. Playing a board game
4. Painting

61. A client with bipolar disorder is having difficulty sleeping. Which behavior modification technique should the nurse reinforce with the client?
1. Use a sleep medication.
2. Work on solving a problem.
3. Exercise before bedtime.
4. Develop a sleep ritual.

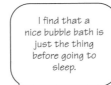

I find that a nice bubble bath is just the thing before going to sleep.

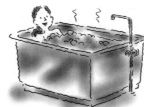

57. 3. By giving the client high-calorie foods that can be eaten while he's active, the nurse facilitates the client's nutritional intake. Determining the client's metabolic rate isn't useful information when the client is experiencing mania. During a manic episode, the client can't be still or focused long enough to interact with a dietitian or sit still long enough to eat.
CN: Psychosocial integrity; CNS: None; CL: Knowledge

58. 4. Persistent GI upset indicates a mild-to-moderate toxic reaction. Black tongue is an adverse reaction of mirtazapine (Remeron), not lithium. Increased lacrimation isn't an adverse effect of lithium. Periods of disorientation don't tend to occur with the use of lithium.
CN: Physiological integrity; CNS: Pharmacological therapies; CL: Knowledge

59. 2. Regularly checking serum lithium levels is a critical part of medication management. The client is at high risk for toxicity with this drug, so regular monitoring is key to the success of treatment. Taking lithium carbonate with food or on an empty stomach and avoiding operating heavy machinery aren't necessary when taking this medication.
CN: Physiological integrity; CNS: Reduction of risk potential; CL: Application

60. 4. An activity, such as painting, that promotes minimal stimulation is the best choice. Activities, such as playing cards, basketball, or a board game, may escalate hyperactivity and should be avoided.
CN: Psychosocial integrity; CNS: None; CL: Application

61. 4. A sleep ritual or nighttime routine helps the client to relax and prepare for sleep. Obtaining sleep medication is a temporary solution. Working on problem solving may excite the client rather than tire him. Exercise before retiring is inappropriate.
CN: Physiological integrity; CNS: Reduction of risk potential; CL: Application

CN: Client needs category CNS: Client needs subcategory CL: Cognitive level

62. Which topic should the nurse discuss with the family of a client with bipolar disorder if the family is distressed about the client's episodes of manic behavior?

1. Ways to protect themselves from the client's behavior
2. How to proceed with an involuntary commitment
3. Where to confront the client about the reckless behavior
4. When to safely increase medication during manic periods

63. Which explanation should the nurse give to a client newly diagnosed with bipolar disorder who doesn't understand why <u>frequent blood work</u> is necessary while he's taking lithium?

1. Frequent measurement of lithium levels will help the primary care provider spot liver and renal damage early.
2. Frequent measurement of lithium levels will demonstrate whether the client is taking a high enough dosage.
3. Frequent measurement of lithium levels will indicate whether the drug passes through the blood-brain barrier.
4. Frequent measurement of lithium levels are unnecessary if the client takes the drug as ordered.

64. A client with a diagnosis of bipolar disorder in the manic phase is at risk for exhaustion and inadequate food intake. How can the nurse best meet the client's nutritional needs?

1. Establish a set time to eat meals.
2. Order high-protein milk shakes between meals.
3. Allow family members to bring the client's favorite foods to the hospital.
4. Provide finger foods that can be eaten on the go.

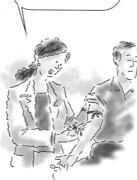

Monitoring blood levels helps ensure that adequate doses of lithium are being administered.

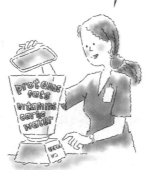

Anxiety and mood disorders can affect the nutritional status of your client.

62. 1. Family members need to assess their needs and develop ways to protect themselves. Clients who have symptoms of impulsive or reckless behavior might not be candidates for hospitalization. Confronting the client during a manic episode may escalate the behavior. The family must never increase the dosage of prescribed medication without first consulting the primary health care provider.

CN: Safe, effective care environment; CNS: Safety and infection control; CL: Application

63. 2. Measurement of lithium levels in the blood determines whether an effective dose of lithium is being given to maintain a therapeutic level of the drug. The drug is contraindicated for clients with renal, cardiac, or liver disease. Lithium levels aren't measured to determine if the drug passes through the blood-brain barrier. Taking the drug as ordered doesn't eliminate the need for blood work.

CN: Physiological integrity; CNS: Pharmacological therapies; CL: Comprehension

64. 4. Finger foods that can be eaten quickly while the client is in a highly energetic state are best. This client can't sit still long enough to eat. Favorite foods and high-protein shakes may help with the client's intake but don't necessarily provide balanced nutrition.

CN: Physiological integrity; CNS: Basic care and comfort; CL: Application

65. Which statement made by a client with bipolar disorder indicates that the nurse's teaching on coping strategies was effective?
1. "I can decide what to do to prevent family conflict."
2. "I can handle problems without asking for any help."
3. "I can stay away from my friends when I feel distressed."
4. "I can ignore things that go wrong instead of getting upset."

66. A client with depression is admitted to the hospital following a suicide attempt. Which nursing diagnosis would be <u>most</u> appropriate at this time?
1. *Disturbed body image related to depression*
2. *Imbalanced nutrition: Less than body requirements related to depression*
3. *Hygiene self-care deficit related to depression*
4. *Risk for self-directed violence related to depression*

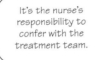

It's the nurse's responsibility to confer with the treatment team.

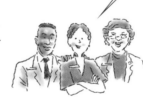

67. A nurse is caring for a client who reports that he thinks about suicide every day. In conferring with the treatment team, which recommendation by the nurse would be <u>most</u> appropriate for this client?
1. A no-suicide contract
2. Weekly outpatient therapy
3. A second psychiatric opinion
4. Intensive inpatient treatment

Hmmm. Question 68 asks about short-term goals.

68. Which short-term goal should the nurse focus on for a client who makes statements about not deserving things?
1. Identify distorted thoughts.
2. Describe self-care patterns.
3. Discuss family relationships.
4. Explore communications skills.

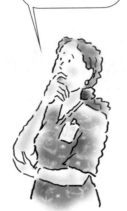

65. 1. The client should be focusing on his strengths and abilities to prevent family conflict. Not being able to ask for help is problematic and not a good coping strategy. Avoiding problems also isn't a good coping strategy. It's better to identify and handle problems as they arise. Ignoring situations that cause discomfort won't facilitate solutions or allow the client to demonstrate effective coping skills.
CN: Psychosocial integrity; CNS: None; CL: Analysis

66. 4. A client who has attempted suicide must be considered a safety risk. Although clients with depression may have disturbed body image or a self-care deficit, safety insurance takes a higher priority, especially when the client is newly admitted. Imbalanced nutritional status may or may not be present in clients with depression.
CN: Safe, effective care environment; CNS: Safety and infection control; CL: Analysis

67. 4. For a client thinking about suicide on a daily basis, inpatient care would be the best intervention. Although a no-suicide contract is an important strategy, this client needs additional care. The client needs a more intensive level of care than weekly outpatient therapy. Immediate intervention is paramount, not a second psychiatric opinion.
CN: Safe, effective care environment; CNS: Safety and infection control; CL: Application

68. 1. It's important to identify distorted thinking such as self-deprecating thoughts because they can lead to depression. Self-care patterns don't necessarily reflect distorted thinking. Family relationships might not influence distorted thinking patterns. A form of communication called *negative self-talk* would be explored only after distorted thinking patterns were identified.
CN: Psychosocial integrity; CNS: None; CL: Application

CN: Client needs category   CNS: Client needs subcategory   CL: Cognitive level

69. Which intervention should be of primary importance to the nurse working with a client to modify the client's negative expectations?

1. Encourage the client to discuss spiritual matters.
2. Help the client learn how to problem solve.
3. Help the client explore issues related to loss.
4. Have the client identify positive aspects of self.

70. A nurse is caring for a client how has been diagnosed with depression and is suspected of being suicidal. When reviewing the progress note in the client's chart, the nurse notes the entry below. Which nursing intervention would be the <u>most</u> appropriate?

Progress notes	
9/4/08 1230	Client found sitting in a chair in her room with curtains drawn. Client states, "Leave me alone. I don't want to be here anymore."——————Barbara Smith, L.P.N.

1. Speak to family members to ascertain if the client is suicidal.
2. Talk to the client to determine if the client is an attention-seeker.
3. Arrange for the client to be placed on immediate suicide precautions.
4. Ask a direct question such as, "Do you ever think about killing yourself?"

71. Which instruction should the nurse include when teaching the family of a client with major depression?

1. Address how depression is a lifelong illness.
2. Explain that depression is an illness and can be treated.
3. Describe how depression masks a person's true feelings.
4. Teach how depression causes frequent disorganized thinking.

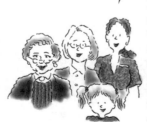

You may have misconceptions about depression.

69. 4. An important intervention used to counter negative expectations is to focus on the positive and have the client explore positive aspects of himself. Discussion of spiritual matters doesn't address the need to change negative expectations. Learning how to problem solve won't modify the client's negative expectations. If the client dwells on the negative and focuses on loss, it will be natural to have negative expectations.

CN: Psychosocial integrity; CNS: None; CL: Application

70. 4. The best approach to determining if a client is suicidal is to ask about thoughts of suicide in a direct and caring manner. The client should be assessed directly, not through family members. Assessing for attention-seeking behaviors doesn't deal directly with the problem. Assessment must be performed before determining if suicide precautions are necessary.

CN: Psychosocial integrity; CNS: None; CL: Application

71. 2. The nurse must help the family understand depression, its effect on the family, and recommended treatments. Depression doesn't need to be a lifelong illness. It's important to help families understand that depression can be successfully treated and that, in some situations, depression can reoccur during the life cycle. The feelings expressed by the client are genuine; they reflect cognitive distortions and disillusionment. Disorganized thinking is more commonly associated with schizophrenia rather than depression.

CN: Psychosocial integrity; CNS: None; CL: Application

72. A client with major depression asks why he is taking mirtazapine (Remeron), a serotonin reuptake inhibitor, instead of imipramine (Tofranil), a tricyclic antidepressant. Which explanation is <u>most accurate</u>?

1. The newer serotonin reuptake inhibitor drugs are better-tested drugs.
2. The serotonin reuptake inhibitors have few adverse effects.
3. The serotonin reuptake inhibitors require a low dose of an antidepressant drug.
4. The serotonin reuptake inhibitors are as good as other antidepressant drugs.

73. Which intervention is most likely to promote a positive sense of self in a client with depression whose goal is enhancing self-esteem?

1. Playing cards
2. Praying daily
3. Taking medication
4. Writing poetry

74. An adolescent who's depressed and reported by his parents as having difficulty in school is brought to the community mental health center to be evaluated. Which other health problem would the nurse suspect?

1. Anxiety disorder
2. Behavioral difficulties
3. Cognitive impairment
4. Labile moods

75. Which nursing intervention is <u>most effective</u> in lowering a client's risk of suicide?

1. Using a caring approach
2. Developing a strong relationship with the client
3. Establishing a suicide contract to ensure his safety
4. Encouraging avoidance of overstimulating activities

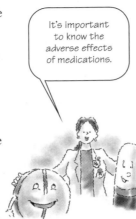

It's important to know the adverse effects of medications.

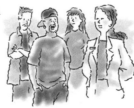

These teens may not be subtle or quiet.

72. 2. The serotonin reuptake inhibitors are drugs with few adverse effects and are unlikely to be toxic in an overdose. All drugs must be tested through a government-specified protocol. The dosage strength of the drug shouldn't be relevent to the client. Comparison of two different types of antidepressant medications isn't useful. The final statement doesn't give the client helpful information.
CN: Physiological integrity; CNS: Pharmacological therapies; CL: Analysis

73. 4. Writing poetry or engaging in some other creative outlet will enhance self-esteem. Playing cards and praying don't necessarily promote self-esteem. Taking medication will decrease symptoms of depression after a therapeutic blood level is established but it won't, by itself, promote self-esteem.
CN: Psychosocial integrity; CNS: None; CL: Comprehension

74. 2. Adolescents tend to demonstrate severe irritability and behavioral problems rather than simply a depressed mood. Anxiety disorder is more commonly associated with small children rather than adolescents. Cognitive impairment is typically associated with delirium or dementia. Labile mood is more characteristic of a client with cognitive impairment or bipolar disorder.
CN: Psychosocial integrity; CNS: None; CL: Analysis

75. 3. Establishing a suicide contract with the client demonstrates that the nurse's concern for his safety is a priority and that his life is of value. When a client agrees to a suicide contract, it decreases his risk for a successful attempt. Caring alone ignores the underlying mechanism of the client's wish to commit suicide. Merely developing a strong relationship with the client isn't addressing the potential the client has for harming himself. Encouraging the client to stay away from activities could cause isolation, which would be detrimental to the client's well-being.
CN: Safe, effective care environment; CNS: Safety and infection control; CL: Application

CN: Client needs category   CNS: Client needs subcategory   CL: Cognitive level

76. The nurse is instructing a 53-year-old female client about using the antianxiety medication lorazepam (Ativan). Which statement by the client indicates a need for further teaching?
1. "I should get up slowly from a sitting or lying position."
2. "I shouldn't stop taking this medicine abruptly."
3. "I usually drink a beer every night to help me sleep."
4. "If I have a sore throat, I should report it to the physician."

77. Which of the following is typically the etiology for posttraumatic stress disorder (PTSD)?
1. Ineffective coping
2. A life-threatening or catastrophic event
3. Posttraumatic phobia and uncontrolled anxiety
4. Altered role performance

78. A client has been receiving treatment for depression for 3 weeks. Which behavior suggests that the client is less depressed?
1. Talking about the difficulties of returning to college after discharge
2. Spending most of the day sitting alone in the corner of the room
3. Wearing a hospital gown instead of street clothes
4. Showing no emotion when visitors leave

79. A lack of dietary salt intake can have which effect on lithium levels?
1. Decrease
2. Increase
3. Increase then decrease
4. No effect at all

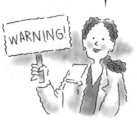

Your client shouldn't drink alcoholic beverages while taking this drug.

WARNING!

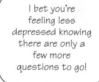

I bet you're feeling less depressed knowing there are only a few more questions to go!

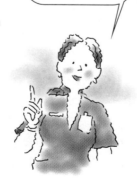

76. 3. The client shouldn't consume alcohol or any other central nervous system depressant while taking this drug. All of the other statements indicate that the client understands the nurse's instructions.
CN: Physiological integrity; CNS: Pharmacological therapies; CL: Application

77. 2. PTSD is usually caused by some life-threatening or catastrophic event, such as a war, rape, and natural disaster. Ineffective coping, posttraumatic phobia and uncontrolled anxiety, and altered role performance are all manifestations, not causes, of this disorder.
CN: Psychosocial integrity; CNS: None; CL: Knowledge

78. 1. By talking about returning to college, the client is demonstrating an interest in making plans for the future, which is a sign of beginning recovery from depression. Decreased socialization, lack of interest in personal appearance, and lack of emotion are all symptoms of depression.
CN: Physiological integrity; CN: Reduction of risk potential; CL: Application

79. 2. There's a direct relationship between the amount of salt and the plasma levels of lithium. Lithium plasma levels increase when there's a decrease in dietary salt. An increase in dietary salt causes the opposite effect of decreasing lithium plasma levels. It's important that the nurse monitors adequate dietary sodium.
CN: Physiological integrity; CNS: Pharmacological therapies; CL: Knowledge

CN: Client needs category   CNS: Client needs subcategory   CL: Cognitive level

80. A client with bipolar disorder has been taking lithium (Lithotabs), as prescribed, for the past 3 years. Today, family members brought this client to the hospital because the client hadn't slept, bathed, or changed clothes for 4 days; had lost 10 lb (4.5 kg) in the past month; and woke the entire family at 4 a.m. with plans to fly them to Hawaii for a vacation. Based on this information, what may the nurse assume?

1. The family isn't supportive of the client.
2. The client had stopped taking the prescribed medication.
3. The client hasn't accepted the diagnosis of bipolar disorder.
4. The lithium level should be measured before the client receives the next lithium dose.

81. A client taking antidepressants for major depression for about 3 weeks is expressing that he's feeling better. Which complication should he now be assessed for?

1. Manic depression
2. Potential for violence
3. Substance abuse
4. Suicidal ideation

82. A 40-year-old client has been brought to the hospital by her husband because she has refused to get out of bed for 2 days. She won't eat, she has been neglecting household responsibilities, and she's tired all the time. Her diagnosis on admission is major depression. Which question is most appropriate for the admitting nurse to ask <u>at this point</u>?

1. "What has been troubling you?"
2. "Why do you dislike yourself?"
3. "How do you feel about your life?"
4. "What can we do to help?"

83. A client on the psychiatric unit is receiving lithium therapy and has a lithium level of 1 mEq/L. The nurse notes that the client has fine tremors of the hands. What should the nurse do?

1. Hold the client's next lithium dose.
2. Notify the physician immediately.
3. Have the lithium level measurement repeated.
4. Realize that a fine tremor is expected.

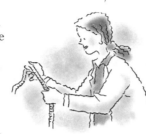

Something just doesn't measure up!

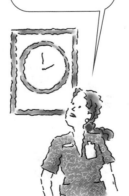

Timing is critical here. Read the question again if you have any doubts about what is being asked.

80. 4. Measuring the lithium level is the best way to evaluate the effectiveness of lithium therapy and begin to assess the client's current status. The client's unsupportive family, stopping of the medication, and not accepting the diagnosis may contribute to his manic episode, but the nurse can't assume these to be true until after assessing the client and family more fully.
CN: Psychosocial integrity; CNS: Reduction of risk potential; CL: Application

81. 4. After a client has been on antidepressants and is feeling better, he commonly then has the energy to harm himself. Manic depression isn't treated with antidepressants. Nothing in the client's history suggests a potential for violence. There are no signs or symptoms suggesting substance abuse.
CN: Safe, effective care environment; CNS: Safety and infection control; CL: Analysis

82. 3. The nurse must develop nursing interventions based on the client's perceived problems and feelings. Asking the client to draw a conclusion may be difficult for her at this time. *Why* questions can place the client in a defensive position. Requiring the client to find possible solutions is beyond the scope of her present abilities.
CN: Psychosocial integrity; CNS: None; CL: Analysis

83. 4. Fine tremors of the hands are considered normal with lithium therapy. The lithium level is within normal limits so there's no need to hold a dose, notify the physician, or repeat the blood work.
CN: Psychosocial integrity; CNS: None; CL: Application

CN: Client needs category   CNS: Client needs subcategory   CL: Cognitive level

84. Following an examination by the forensic nurse in the emergency department, a rape victim is being prepared for discharge. The nurse is aware that the client is at risk for posttraumatic stress disorder (PTSD) and instructs the client that it's important that she report which symptoms associated with PTSD? Select all that apply.
  1. Recurrent, intrusive recollections or nightmares
  2. Gingival and dental problems
  3. Sleep disturbances
  4. Flight of ideas
  5. Unusual talkativeness
  6. Difficulty concentrating

85. The nurse is caring for a client who talks freely about feeling depressed. The nurse hears the client state, "Things will never change." What other indications of hopelessness would the nurse look for? Select all that apply:
  1. Bouts of anger
  2. Periods of irritability
  3. Preoccupation with delusions
  4. Feelings of worthlessness
  5. Self-destructive statements
  6. Intense interpersonal relationship

86. The nurse interviews the family of a client who's hospitalized with severe depression and suicidal ideation. Which family assessment information is essential to formulating an effective care plan? Select all that apply:
  1. Physical pain
  2. Personal responsibilities
  3. Employment skills
  4. Communication patterns
  5. Role expectations
  6. Current family stressors

87. A nurse is preparing discharge instructions for a client prescribed sertraline (Zoloft), a selective serotonin reuptake inhibitor. The nurse should monitor the client for which adverse drug effects? Select all that apply.
  1. Agitation
  2. Agranulocytosis
  3. Sleep disturbance
  4. Intermittent tachycardia
  5. Dry mouth
  6. Seizure

84. 1, 3, 6. Clients diagnosed with PTSD typically experience recurrent, intrusive recollections or nightmares, sleep disturbances, difficulty concentrating, chronic anxiety or panic attacks, memory impairment, and feelings of detachment or estrangement that destroy interpersonal relationships. Gingival and dental problems are associated with bulimia. Flight of ideas and unusual talkativeness are characteristic of the acute manic phase of bipolar affective disorder.
CN: Psychosocial integrity; CNS: None; CL: Application

85. 1, 2, 4. Clients who are depressed and express hopelessness also tend to manifest inappropriate expressions of anger, periods of irritability, and feelings of worthlessness. Options 3 and 6 are usually seen in clients with schizophrenia; they aren't typically seen in those who express hopelessness. Not all self-destructive behavior is suicidal in intent but may be a way for the client to feel alive.
CN: Psychosocial integrity; CNS: None; CL: Analysis

86. 4, 5, 6. When working with the family of a depressed client, it's helpful for the nurse to be aware of the family's communication style, the role expectations for its members, and current family stressors. This information can help identify family difficulties and teaching points that could benefit the client and the family. Information concerning physical pain, personal responsibilities, and employment skills wouldn't be helpful because these areas aren't directly related to their experience of having a depressed family member.
CN: Psychosocial integrity; CNS: None; CL: Analysis

87. 1, 3, 5. Common adverse effects of Zoloft include agitation, sleep disturbance, and dry mouth. Agranulocytosis, intermittent tachycardia, and seizures are adverse effects of clozapine (Clozaril).
CN: Physiological integrity; CNS: Pharmacological therapies; CL: Application

Congratulations! You did it! Good job!

CN: Client needs category   CNS: Client needs subcategory   CL: Cognitive level

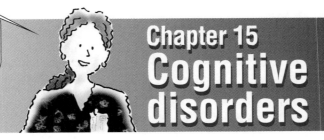

This chapter covers a host of cognitive disorders. Are your own cognitive powers ready? Ok, let's go!

Chapter 15
Cognitive disorders

1. Dementia is related to which disorder?
1. Alcohol withdrawal
2. Alzheimer's disease
3. Obsessive-compulsive disorder (OCD)
4. Postpartum depression

1. 2. Dementia occurs in Alzheimer's disease and is generally progressive and deteriorating. The symptoms related to alcohol withdrawal result from alcohol intoxication. Effects of alcohol on the central nervous system include loss of memory, concentration, insight, and motor control. OCDs are recurrent ideas, impulses, thoughts, or patterns of behavior that produce anxiety if resisted. Postpartum depression doesn't lead to dementia.
CN: Physiological integrity; CNS: Physiological adaptation; CL: Comprehension

2. A physician diagnoses a client with dementia of the Alzheimer's type. Which statement about possible causes of this disorder is <u>most</u> accurate?
1. Alzheimer's disease is most commonly caused by cerebral abscess.
2. Chronic alcohol abuse plays a significant role in Alzheimer's disease.
3. Multiple small brain infarctions typically lead to Alzheimer's disease.
4. The cause of Alzheimer's disease is currently unknown.

Researchers continue to explore the cause of Alzheimer's disease.

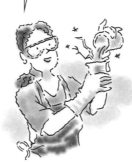

2. 4. Several hypotheses suggest genetic factors, trauma, accumulation of aluminum, alterations in the immune system, or alterations in acetylcholine as contributing to the development of Alzheimer's disease, but the exact cause of Alzheimer's disease is unknown. Chronic alcohol abuse hasn't been associated with the development of Alzheimer's disease, nor have the presence of cerebral abscesses or small brain infarctions.
CN: Health promotion and maintenance; CNS: None; CL: Application

3. Of the following conditions that can cause a dementia similar to Alzheimer's disease, which is <u>reversible</u>?
1. Multiple sclerosis
2. Electrolyte imbalance
3. Multiple small brain infarctions
4. Human immunodeficiency virus infection

3. 2. Electrolyte imbalance is a correctable metabolic abnormality. The other conditions are irreversible.
CN: Physiological integrity; CNS: Physiological adaptation; CL: Application

4. In the <u>early</u> stages of Alzheimer's disease, which symptom is expected?
1. Dilated pupils
2. Rambling speech
3. Elevated blood pressure
4. Significant recent memory impairment

4. 4. Significant recent memory impairment, indicated by the inability to verbalize remembrances after several minutes to an hour, can be assessed in the early stages of Alzheimer's disease. Dilated pupils, elevated blood pressure, and rambling speech are expected symptoms of delirium.
CN: Physiological integrity; CNS: Physiological adaptation; CL: Application

CN: Client needs category   CNS: Client needs subcategory   CL: Cognitive level

5. Which pathophysiological change in the brain causes the symptoms of Alzheimer's disease?

1. Glucose inadequacy
2. Atrophy of the frontal lobe
3. Degeneration of the cholinergic system
4. Intracranial bleeding in the limbic system

6. Which data collection finding shows impairment in abstract thinking and reasoning?

1. The client can't repeat a sentence.
2. The client has problems calculating simple problems.
3. The client doesn't know the name of the president of the United States.
4. The client can't find similarities and differences between related words or objects.

7. In addition to disturbances in cognition and orientation, a client with Alzheimer's disease may also show changes in which area?

1. Appetite
2. Energy levels
3. Hearing
4. Personality

8. Which intervention would help a client diagnosed with Alzheimer's disease perform activities of daily living?

1. Have the client perform all basic care without help.
2. Tell the client that morning care must be done by 9 a.m.
3. Give the client a written list of activities he's expected to do.
4. Encourage the client, and give ample time to complete basic tasks.

9. Which medication for Alzheimer's disease, approved by the Food and Drug Administration, is a moderately long-acting inhibitor of cholinesterase?

1. Bupropion (Wellbutrin)
2. Haloperidol (Haldol)
3. Donepezil (Aricept)
4. Triazolam (Halcion)

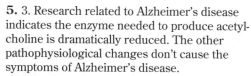

Data collection is a skill of critical importance!

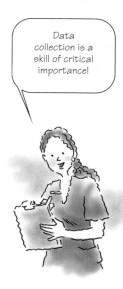

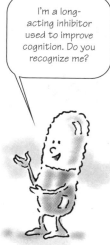

I'm a long-acting inhibitor used to improve cognition. Do you recognize me?

5. 3. Research related to Alzheimer's disease indicates the enzyme needed to produce acetylcholine is dramatically reduced. The other pathophysiological changes don't cause the symptoms of Alzheimer's disease.
CN: Physiological integrity; CNS: Physiological adaptation; CL: Analysis

6. 4. Abstract thinking is assessed by noting similarities and differences between related words or objects. Not being able to do a simple calculation or repeat a sentence shows a client's inability to concentrate and focus on thoughts. Not knowing the name of the president of the United States is a deficiency in general knowledge.
CN: Physiological integrity; CNS: Physiological adaptation; CL: Analysis

7. 4. Personality change is common in dementia. It's less common to see changes in appetite, energy, or hearing.
CN: Physiological integrity; CNS: Physiological adaptation; CL: Application

8. 4. Clients with Alzheimer's disease respond to the affect of those around them. A gentle, calm approach is comforting and nonthreatening, and a tense, hurried approach may agitate the client. The client has problems performing independently; expecting him to perform self-care independently may lead to frustration.
CN: Safe, effective care environment; CNS: Coordinated care; CL: Application

9. 3. Donepezil is used to improve cognition and functional autonomy in mild to moderate dementia of the Alzheimer's type. Bupropion is used for depression. Haloperidol is used for agitation, aggression, hallucinations, thought disturbances, and wandering. Triazolam is used for sleep disturbances.
CN: Physiological integrity; CNS: Pharmacological therapies; CL: Knowledge

CN: Client needs category   CNS: Client needs subcategory   CL: Cognitive level

10. A nurse places an object in the hand of a client with Alzheimer's disease and asks the client to identify the object. Which term represents the client's inability to name the object?
1. Agnosia
2. Aphasia
3. Apraxia
4. Perseveration

11. Which nursing intervention will help a client with progressive memory deficit function in his environment?
1. Help the client do simple tasks by giving step-by-step directions.
2. Avoid frustrating the client by performing basic care routines for the client.
3. Stimulate the client's intellectual functioning by bringing new topics to the client's attention.
4. Promote the use of the client's sense of humor by telling jokes or riddles and discussing cartoons.

12. Which intervention is an important part of providing care to a client diagnosed with Alzheimer's disease?
1. Avoid physical contact.
2. Apply wrist and ankle restraints.
3. Provide a high level of sensory stimulation.
4. Monitor the client carefully.

13. Which nursing intervention is the <u>most important</u> in caring for a client diagnosed with Alzheimer's disease?
1. Make sure the environment is safe to prevent injury.
2. Make sure the client receives food she likes to prevent hunger.
3. Make sure the client meets other clients to prevent social isolation.
4. Make sure the client takes care of her daily physical care to prevent dependence.

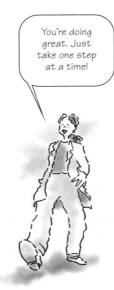

You're doing great. Just take one step at a time!

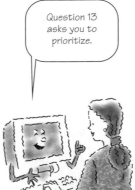

Question 13 asks you to prioritize.

10. 1. Agnosia is the inability to recognize familiar objects. Aphasia is characterized by an impaired ability to speak. Apraxia refers to the client's inability to use objects properly. All three impairments usually occur in stage 3 of Alzheimer's disease. Perseveration is continued repetition of a meaningless word or phrase that occurs in stage 2 of Alzheimer's disease.
CN: Health promotion and maintenance; CNS: None; CL: Application

11. 1. Clients with cognitive impairment should do all the tasks they can. By giving simple directions in a step-by-step fashion, the client can better process information and perform tasks. Clients with cognitive impairment may not be able to understand the joke or riddle, and cartoons may add to their confusion. Stimulation of intellect can be accomplished by discussing familiar topics with them; changes in topics may add to their confusion.
CN: Psychosocial integrity; CNS: None; CL: Application

12. 4. Whenever client safety is at risk, careful observation and supervision are of ultimate importance in avoiding injury. Physical contact is implemented during basic care. Applying restraints may cause agitation and combativeness. A high level of sensory stimulation may be too stimulating and distracting.
CN: Safe, effective care environment; CNS: Coordinated care; CL: Application

13. 1. Providing for client safety is the number one priority when caring for any client but particularly when a client is already compromised and at greater risk for injury. Promoting adequate nutrition, socialization, and self-care are important, but not the priority nursing intervention.
CN: Safe, effective care environment; CNS: Safety and infection control; CL: Application

CN: Client needs category   CNS: Client needs subcategory   CL: Cognitive level

14. Which medication is used to decrease the agitation, violence, and bizarre thoughts associated with dementia?
　1. Diazepam (Valium)
　2. Ergoloid (Hydergine)
　3. Haloperidol (Haldol)
　4. Donepezil (Aricept)

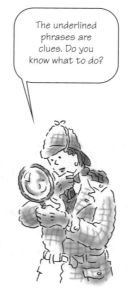

The underlined phrases are clues. Do you know what to do?

14. 3. Haloperidol is an antipsychotic that decreases the symptoms of agitation, violence, and bizarre thoughts. Diazepam is used for anxiety and muscle relaxation. Ergoloid is an adrenergic blocker used to block vascular headaches. Donepezil is used for improvement of cognition.

CN: Physiological integrity; CNS: Reduction of risk potential; CL: Application

15. A client diagnosed with Alzheimer's disease tells the nurse that today she has a luncheon date with her daughter, who isn't visiting that day. Which response by the nurse would be most appropriate for this situation?
　1. "Where are you planning to have your lunch?"
　2. "You're confused and don't know what you're saying."
　3. "I think you need some more medication, and I'll bring it to you."
　4. "Today is Monday, March 8, and we'll be eating lunch in the dining room."

15. 4. The best nursing response is to reorient the client to the date and environment. Confrontation can provoke an outburst. Medication won't provide immediate relief for memory impairment.

CN: Psychosocial integrity; CNS: None; CL: Application

16. Which feature is characteristic of cognitive disorders?
　1. Catatonia
　2. Depression
　3. Feeling of dread
　4. Deficit in cognition or memory

16. 4. Cognitive disorders represent a significant change in cognition or memory from a previous level of functioning. Catatonia is a type of schizophrenia characterized by periods of physical rigidity, negativism, excitement, and stupor. Depression is a feeling of sadness and apathy and is part of major depressive and other mood disorders. A feeling of dread is characteristic of an anxiety disorder.

CN: Physiological integrity; CNS: Physiological adaptation; CL: Application

17. Which disorder is a degenerative disorder of cognition primarily associated with age or metabolic deterioration?
　1. Delirium
　2. Dementia
　3. Neurosis
　4. Psychosis

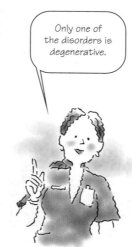

Only one of the disorders is degenerative.

17. 2. Dementia is progressive and commonly associated with aging or underlying metabolic or organic deterioration. Delirium is characterized by abrupt, spontaneous cognitive dysfunction with an underling organic mental disorder. Neurosis and psychosis are psychological diagnoses.

CN: Physiological integrity; CNS: Physiological adaptation; CL: Knowledge

CN: Client needs category　CNS: Client needs subcategory　CL: Cognitive level

18. Which characteristic best defines dementia?
1. Personal neglect in self-care
2. Poor judgment, especially in social situations
3. Memory loss occurring as a natural consequence of aging
4. Loss of intellectual abilities that impair the ability to perform basic care

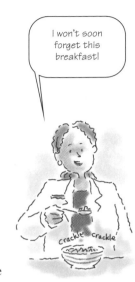

I won't soon forget this breakfast!

18. 4. The ability to perform self-care is an important measure of the progression of dementia. Personal neglect and poor judgment typically occur in dementia but aren't considered defining characteristics. Memory loss reflects underlying physical, metabolic, and pathologic processes.
CN: Physiological integrity; CNS: Physiological adaptation; CL: Knowledge

19. Asking a client with a suspected dementia disorder to recall what she ate for breakfast would assess which area?
1. Food preferences
2. Recent memory
3. Remote memory
4. Speech capacity

19. 2. Persons with dementia have difficulty in recent memory or learning, which may be a key to early detection. Assessing food preferences may be helpful in determining what the client likes to eat, but this assessment has no direct correlation in assessing dementia. Speech difficulties, such as rambling, irrelevance, and incoherence, may be related to delirium.
CN: Health promotion and maintenance; CNS: None; CL: Application

20. It's important to collect data for a definitive diagnosis of a dementia disorder to determine which factor?
1. Prognosis
2. Genetic information
3. Degree of impairment
4. Implications for treatment

20. 4. The reversibility of dementia is a function of the underlying pathologic states, so it's important to collect data and treat the underlying cause. Prognosis isn't the most important factor when making a diagnosis. Genetic information isn't relevant. The degree of impairment is necessary information for developing a care plan.
CN: Health promotion and maintenance; CNS: None; CL: Comprehension

21. Which factor is considered a cause of vascular dementia?
1. Head trauma
2. Genetic factors
3. Acetylcholine alteration
4. Interruption of blood flow to the brain

This question asks you to select the most significant cause.

21. 4. The cause of vascular dementia is directly related to an interruption of blood flow to the brain. Head trauma, genetic factors, and acetylcholine alteration are causative factors related to dementia of the Alzheimer's type.
CN: Physiological integrity; CNS: Physiological adaptation; CL: Comprehension

22. Which factor is considered the most significant cause of vascular dementia?
1. Arterial hypertension
2. Hypoxia
3. Infection
4. Toxins

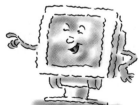

22. 1. Arterial hypertension, cerebral emboli, and cerebral thrombosis are causes of vascular dementia. Hypoxia, infection, and toxins are causes of delirium.
CN: Physiological integrity; CNS: Reduction of risk potential; CL: Knowledge

CN: Client needs category   CNS: Client needs subcategory   CL: Cognitive level

23. Which assessment finding is expected for a client with vascular dementia?
1. Hypersomnolence
2. Insomnia
3. Restlessness
4. Small-stepped gait

24. In which way is vascular dementia different from Alzheimer's disease?
1. Vascular dementia has a more abrupt onset.
2. The duration of vascular dementia is usually brief.
3. Personality change is common in vascular dementia.
4. The inability to perform motor activities is common in vascular dementia.

25. A progression of symptoms that occurs in steps rather than a gradual deterioration indicates which type of dementia?
1. Alzheimer's dementia
2. Parkinson's dementia
3. Substance-induced dementia
4. Vascular dementia

26. Which disorder is characterized by a general impairment in intellectual functioning?
1. Alzheimer's disease
2. Amnesia
3. Delirium
4. Dementia

23. 4. Focal neurologic signs commonly seen with vascular dementia include weakness of the limbs, small-stepped gait, and difficulty with speech. Hypersomnolence, insomnia, and restlessness are symptoms related to delirium.
CN: Physiological integrity; CNS: Physiological adaptation; CL: Application

24. 1. Vascular dementia differs from Alzheimer's disease in that it has a more abrupt onset and runs a highly variable course. The duration of delirium is usually brief. Personality change is common in vascular dementia. The inability to carry out motor activities is common in vascular dementia.
CN: Health promotion and maintenance; CNS: None; CL: Analysis

25. 4. Vascular dementia has a more abrupt onset and progresses in steps. At times, the dementia seems to clear up, and the individual shows fairly lucid thinking. Dementia of the Alzheimer's type has a slow onset with a progressive, deteriorating course. Parkinson's dementia sometimes resembles the dementia of Alzheimer's disease. Substance-induced dementia is related to the persisting effects of substance use.
CN: Physiological integrity; CNS: Physiological adaptation; CL: Analysis

26. 4. Dementia is characterized by general impairment in intellectual functioning and occurs in a progressive, irreversible course. Alzheimer's disease is a progressive dementia in which all known reversible causes are eliminated. Amnesia refers to recent short-term and long-term memory loss. One of the distinguishing characteristics of delirium is the development of symptoms over a short time, usually hours to days.
CN: Physiological integrity; CNS: Physiological adaptation; CL: Knowledge

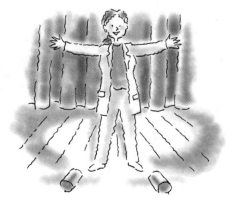

You've reached the halfway mark. Take a bow!

CN: Client needs category   CNS: Client needs subcategory   CL: Cognitive level

27. An elderly client has experienced memory and attention deficits that developed over a 3-day period. These symptoms are characteristic of which disorder?
1. Alzheimer's disease
2. Amnesia
3. Delirium
4. Dementia

27. 3. Delirium is characterized by an abrupt onset of fluctuating levels of awareness, clouded consciousness, perceptual disturbances, and disturbed memory and orientation. Alzheimer's disease is a progressive dementia in which all known reversible causes are eliminated. Amnesia refers to recent short-term and long-term memory loss. Dementia is characterized by general impairment in intellectual functioning and occurs in a progressive, irreversible course.
CN: Physiological integrity; CNS: Physiological adaptation; CL: Application

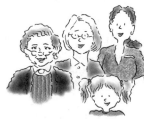

Age can be a determining factor in certain cognitive disorders.

28. Which age-group is at <u>high risk</u> for developing a state of delirium?
1. Adolescent
2. Elderly
3. Middle-aged
4. School-aged

28. 2. Because of normal physiological changes, the elderly population is highly susceptible to delirium. Adolescent, middle-aged, and school-aged groups are less likely to experience the multiple etiologies that can be associated with delirium.
CN: Health promotion and maintenance; CNS: None; CL: Application

29. Which nursing diagnosis is <u>best</u> for an elderly client experiencing visual and auditory hallucinations?
1. *Interrupted family processes*
2. *Ineffective role performance*
3. *Impaired verbal communication*
4. *Disturbed sensory perception*

29. 4. The client is experiencing visual and auditory hallucinations related to a sensory alteration. *Interrupted family processes, Ineffective role performance,* and *Impaired verbal communication* don't address the hallucinations the client is experiencing.
CN: Health promotion and maintenance; CNS: None; CL: Application

30. Which intervention is the <u>most appropriate</u> for clients with cognitive disorders?
1. Promote socialization.
2. Maintain optimal physical health.
3. Provide frequent changes in personnel.
4. Provide an overstimulating environment.

30. 2. A client's cognitive impairment may hinder self-care abilities. More socialization, frequent changes in staff members, and an overstimulating environment would only increase anxiety and confusion.
CN: Health promotion and maintenance; CNS: None; CL: Application

Sometimes my friends and I can be quite intoxicating.

31. A newly admitted client diagnosed with delirium has a history of hypertension and anxiety. The client had been taking digoxin, furosemide (Lasix), and diazepam (Valium) for anxiety. This client's impairment may be related to which condition?
1. Infection
2. Metabolic acidosis
3. Drug intoxication
4. Hepatic encephalopathy

31. 3. This client has been taking several medications that have a propensity for producing delirium: digoxin (a cardiac glycoside), furosemide (a thiazide diuretic), and diazepam (a benzodiazepine). Sufficient supporting data don't exist to suspect infection, metabolic acidosis, or hepatic encephalopathy as causes.
CN: Physiological integrity; CNS: Physiological adaptation; CL: Analysis

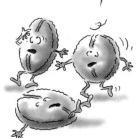

CN: Client needs category   CNS: Client needs subcategory   CL: Cognitive level

32. Which environment is the <u>most appropriate</u> for a client experiencing sensory-perceptual alterations?
1. A room with continuous soft lighting
2. A room with continuous bright lighting
3. Sitting by the nurses' desk while out of bed
4. A quiet, well-lit room without glare during the day and a darkened room for sleeping

33. As a nurse enters a client's room, the client says, "They're crawling on my sheets! Get them off my bed!" Which assessment is the most accurate?
1. The client is experiencing aphasia.
2. The client is experiencing dysarthria.
3. The client is experiencing a flight of ideas.
4. The client is experiencing visual hallucinations.

34. A delirious client is shouting for someone to get the bugs off her. Which response is the most appropriate?
1. "Don't worry, I'll stay here and brush away the bugs for you."
2. "Try to relax. The crawling sensation will go away sooner if you can relax."
3. "There are no bugs on your legs. It's just your imagination playing tricks on you."
4. "I know you're frightened. I don't see bugs crawling on your legs, but I'll stay here with you."

35. Which description of a client's experience and behavior can be assessed as an illusion?
1. The client tries to hit the nurse when vital signs must be taken.
2. The client says, "I keep hearing a voice telling me to run away."
3. The client becomes anxious whenever the nurse leaves the bedside.
4. The client looks at the shadows on a wall and tells the nurse she sees frightening faces.

Don't be bugged by this question. The answer is easy to see.

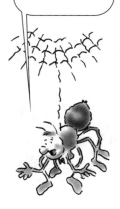

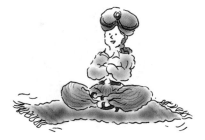

It isn't an illusion. You're doing great!

32. 4. A quiet, shadow-free environment produces the fewest sensory-perceptual distortions for a client with cognitive impairment associated with delirium.
CN: Safe, effective care environment; CNS: Safety and infection control; CL: Application

33. 4. The presence of a sensory stimulus correlates with the definition of a hallucination, which is a false sensory perception. Aphasia refers to a communication problem. Dysarthria is difficulty in speech production. Flight of ideas is rapid shifting from one topic to another.
CN: Health promotion and maintenance; CNS: None; CL: Application

34. 4. Never argue about hallucinations with a client. Instead, promote an environment of trust and safety by acknowledging the client's perceptions.
CN: Physiological integrity; CNS: Basic care and comfort; CL: Application

35. 4. An illusion is an inaccurate perception or false response to a sensory stimulus. Auditory hallucinations are associated with sound and are more common in schizophrenia. Anxiety and agitation can be secondary to illusions.
CN: Physiological integrity; CNS: Physiological adaptation; CL: Analysis

CN: Client needs category   CNS: Client needs subcategory   CL: Cognitive level

36. Which neurologic change is an <u>expected</u> characteristic of aging?
1. Widening of the sulci
2. Depletion of neurotransmitters
3. Neurofibrillary tangles and plaques
4. Degeneration of the frontal and temporal lobes

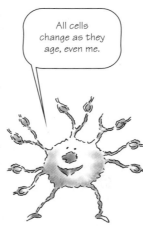

All cells change as they age, even me.

37. A major consideration in assessing memory impairment in an elderly individual includes which factor?
1. Allergies
2. Past surgery
3. Age at onset of symptoms
4. Social and occupational lifestyle

38. The nurse is caring for an 88-year-old female client in a nursing home. The client is confused and thinks she's in a train station. Which response to this behavior is the nurse's <u>top priority</u>?
1. Correct errors in the client's perception of reality in a matter-of-fact manner.
2. Have a conversation with the client when this behavior occurs.
3. Observe the client and know her whereabouts at all times.
4. Refer to the date, time, and place during interactions with the client.

39. A nursing assistant tells a nurse, "The client with amnesia looks fine but responds to questions in a vague, distant manner. What should I be doing for her?" Which response is the <u>most appropriate</u>?
1. "Give her lots of space to test her independence."
2. "Keep her busy and make sure she doesn't take naps during the day."
3. "Whenever you think she needs direction, use short, simple sentences."
4. "Spend as much time with her as you can, and ask questions about her recent life."

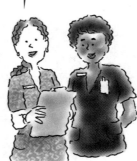

Teaching nursing assistants helps improve the quality of care they provide.

36. 4. Aging isn't necessarily associated with significant decline, but degeneration of the frontal and temporal lobes is an expected change. Widening of the sulci, depletion of neurotransmitters, and neurofibrillary tangles and plaques are changes characteristic of Alzheimer's disease.
CN: Physiological integrity; CNS: Physiological adaptation; CL: Analysis

37. 4. Minor memory problems are distinguished from dementia by their minor severity and their lack of significant interference with the client's social or occupational lifestyle. Allergies, past surgery, or age at onset of symptoms would be included in the history data but don't directly correlate with the client's memory impairment.
CN: Psychosocial integrity; CNS: None; CL: Analysis

38. 3. The nurse's top priority is to maintain safety and security for the client by observing her and knowing her whereabouts at all times; otherwise, the client may wander off and endanger herself. Correcting errors in the client's perception, conversing with her, and orienting her to the date, time, and place are important but aren't the highest priority in this case.
CN: Psychosocial integrity; CNS: None; CL: Application

39. 3. Disruptions in the ability to perform basic care, confusion, and anxiety are commonly apparent in clients with amnesia. Offering simple directions to promote daily functions and reduce confusion helps increase feelings of safety and security. Giving this client lots of space may make her feel insecure. There's no significant rationale for keeping her busy all day with no rest periods; the client may become more tired and less functional at other basic tasks. Asking her many questions that she won't be able to answer just intensifies her anxiety level.
CN: Safe, effective care environment; CNS: Coordinated care; CL: Application

CN: Client needs category   CNS: Client needs subcategory   CL: Cognitive level

40. With amnesic disorders, in which cognitive area is a change expected?
1. Speech
2. Concentration
3. Intellectual function
4. Recent short-term and long-term memory

41. Which nursing action is the <u>best</u> way to help a client with mild Alzheimer's disease remain functional?
1. Obtain a physician's order for a mild anxiolytic to control behavior.
2. Call attention to all mistakes so they can be quickly corrected.
3. Advise the client to move into a retirement center.
4. Maintain a stable, predictable environment and daily routine.

42. The nurse is providing nursing care to a client with Alzheimer-type dementia. Which nursing intervention takes <u>top priority</u>?
1. Establish a routine that supports former habits.
2. Maintain physical surroundings that are cheerful and pleasant.
3. Maintain an exact routine from day to day.
4. Control the environment by providing structure, boundaries, and safety.

43. The nurse finds a 78-year-old client with Alzheimer's type dementia wandering in the hall at 3 a.m. The client has removed his clothing and says to the nurse, "I'm just taking a stroll through the park." What's the <u>best</u> approach to this behavior?
1. Immediately help the client back to his room and into some clothing.
2. Tell the client that such behavior won't be tolerated.
3. Tell the client it's too early in the morning to be taking a stroll.
4. Ask the client if he would like to go back to his room.

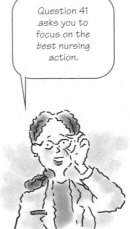

Question 41 asks you to focus on the best nursing action.

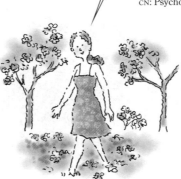

You're almost there. The remaining questions should be a walk in the park!

40. 4. The primary area affected in amnesia is memory; all other areas of cognition are normal.
CN: Physiological integrity; CNS: Physiological adaptation; CL: Application

41. 4. Clients in the early stages of Alzheimer's disease remain fairly functional with familiar surroundings and a predictable routine. They become easily disoriented with surprises and social overstimulation. Anxiolytics can impair memory and worsen the problem. Calling attention to all the client's mistakes is nonproductive and serves to lower the client's self-esteem. Moving to an unfamiliar environment will heighten the client's agitation and confusion.
CN: Psychosocial integrity; CNS: None; CL: Application

42. 4. By controlling the environment and providing structure and boundaries, the nurse is helping to keep the client safe and secure, which is a top-priority nursing measure. Establishing a routine that supports former habits and maintaining cheerful, pleasant surroundings and an exact routine foster a supportive environment; however, keeping the client safe and secure takes priority.
CN: Psychosocial integrity; CNS: None; CL: Application

43. 1. The nurse shouldn't allow the client to embarrass himself in front of others. Intervene as soon as the behavior is observed. Scolding the client isn't helpful because it isn't something the client can understand. Don't engage in social chatter. The interaction with this client should be concrete and specific. Don't ask the client to choose unnecessarily. The client may not be able to make appropriate choices.
CN: Psychosocial integrity; CNS: None; CL: Application

CN: Client needs category   CNS: Client needs subcategory   CL: Cognitive level

44. Which nursing diagnosis is appropriate for a client diagnosed with an amnesic disorder?
1. *Anticipatory grieving related to loss of functional ability*
2. *Ineffective denial*
3. *Ineffective coping*
4. *Risk for injury related to impaired cognition*

45. The nurse is planning care for a client who was admitted with dementia due to Alzheimer's disease. The family reports that the client has to be watched closely for wandering behavior at night. Which nursing diagnosis is the nurse's top priority for this client?
1. *Disturbed sleep pattern*
2. *Activity intolerance*
3. *Disturbed sensory perception*
4. *Risk for injury*

46. Which medical condition may be associated with an amnesic disorder?
1. Drug overdose
2. Cerebral anoxia
3. Medications (anticonvulsants)
4. Lead, mercury, and carbon dioxide toxins

47. Which laboratory evaluation is an expected part of the initial workup for an amnesic disorder?
1. Angiography
2. Cardiac catheterization
3. Electrocardiography
4. Metabolic and endocrine tests

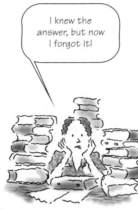

I knew the answer, but now I forgot it!

44. 4. Changes in cognitive ability place a client at high risk for injury. The client isn't aware of a loss and therefore doesn't grieve for it or experience ineffective denial. The client isn't aware of a need to cope.
CN: Safe, effective care environment; CNS: Safety and infection control; CL: Analysis

45. 4. Providing a safe, effective care environment takes priority in this case. *Disturbed sleep pattern, Activity intolerance,* and *Disturbed sensory perception* fall under physical integrity and, although important, they aren't as important as providing a safe, effective care environment.
CN: Safe, effective care environment; CNS: Safety and infection control; CL: Application

46. 2. A variety of medical conditions are related to amnesic disorders, such as head trauma, stroke, cerebral neoplastic disease, herpes simplex, encephalitis, poorly controlled insulin-dependent diabetes, and cerebral anoxia. Drug overdose, medications, and toxins cause substance-induced amnesia and aren't medical conditions.
CN: Physiological integrity; CNS: Physiological adaptation; CL: Application

47. 4. An amnesic disorder is characterized by impairment in memory from direct physiological effects of a medical condition or effects of a substance, medication, or toxin. Metabolic and endocrine tests will identify such causes. Angiography, cardiac catheterization, and electrocardiography are diagnostic tests related to the cardiovascular system.
CN: Health promotion and maintenance; CNS: None; CL: Application

48. A nurse is working with the family of a client who has Alzheimer's disease. The nurse notes that the client's spouse is too exhausted to continue providing care all alone. The adult children live too far away to provide relief on a weekly basis. Which nursing intervention would be most helpful? Select all that apply:
1. Telling the absent children that they must participate in helping the client
2. Suggesting the spouse seek counseling to help cope with exhaustion
3. Recommending community resources for adult day care and respite care
4. Encouraging the spouse to talk about the difficulties involved in caring for a loved one with Alzheimer's disease
5. Asking whether friends or church members can help with errands or provide short periods of relief
6. Recommending that the client be placed in a long-term care facility

49. The nurse is assigned to care for a client with early stage Alzheimer's disease. Which nursing intervention should be included in the client's care plan? Select all that apply:
1. Change the client's routine often.
2. Engage the client in complex discussions to improve memory.
3. Furnish the client's environment with familiar possessions.
4. Assist the client with activities of daily living (ADLs) as necessary.
5. Assign tasks in simple steps.

50. The nurse is assessing a client to determine whether he's suffering from dementia or depression. Which information helps the nurse suspect a diagnosis of dementia rather than depression? Select all that apply:
1 The progression of symptoms is slow.
2. The client answers questions with, "I don't know."
3. The client acts apathetic and pessimistic.
4. The family can't identify when the symptoms first appeared.
5. The client's personality has changed.
6. The client has great difficulty paying attention to others.

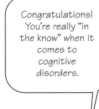

Congratulations! You're really "in the know" when it comes to cognitive disorders.

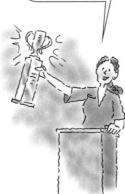

48. 3, 4, 5. Many community services exist for Alzheimer's clients and their families. Encouraging use of these resources may make it possible for the client to stay at home and alleviate the spouse's exhaustion. The nurse can also support the caregiver by urging her to talk about the difficulties she's facing in caring for a spouse. Friends and church members may be able to help provide care to the client, allowing the caregiver time for rest, exercise, or an enjoyable activity. Telling the children to participate more would probably be ineffective and may evoke anger or guilt. Counseling may be helpful, but it wouldn't alleviate the caregiver's physical exhaustion and wouldn't address the client's immediate needs. A long-term care facility isn't an option until the family is ready to make that decision.
CN: Psychosocial integrity; CNS: None; CL: Analysis

49. 3, 4, 5. A client with Alzheimer's disease experiences progressive deterioration in cognitive functioning. Familiar possessions may help to orient the client. The client should be encouraged to perform ADLs but may need assistance with certain activities. Using a step-by-step approach helps the client complete tasks independently. A client with Alzheimer's disease functions best with consistent routines. Complex discussions don't improve the memory of a client with Alzheimer's disease.
CN: Psychosocial integrity; CNS: None; CL: Application

50. 1, 4, 5, 6. Common characteristics of dementia include a slow onset of symptoms, difficulty identifying when the symptoms first occurred, noticeable changes in the client's personality, and impaired ability to pay attention to other people. Options 2 and 3 are symptoms of depression, not dementia.
CN: Psychosocial integrity; CNS: None; CL: Analysis

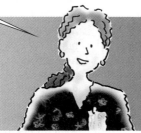

No, this chapter doesn't cover quirks of the rich and famous. It's all about mental disorders affecting the personality. Have a blast!

Chapter 16
Personality disorders

1. A client tells the nurse that her coworkers are sabotaging her computer. When the nurse asks questions, the client becomes argumentative. This behavior shows personality traits associated with which personality disorder?
  1. Antisocial
  2. Histrionic
  3. Paranoid
  4. Schizotypal

2. A nurse notices a client is mistrustful and shows hostile behavior. Which type of personality disorder is associated with these characteristics?
  1. Antisocial
  2. Avoidant
  3. Borderline
  4. Paranoid

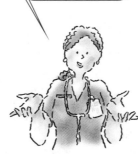

Don't be paranoid. The questions are straightforward and not intended to trick you.

3. The nurse is caring for a client with paranoid personality disorder. Which behavior is a common characteristic of this disorder?
  1. The client can't follow limits set on his behavior.
  2. The client is afraid another person will inflict harm.
  3. The client avoids responsibility for his health care.
  4. The client depends on others to make important decisions.

1. 3. Because of their suspiciousness, paranoid personalities ascribe malevolent activities to others and tend to be defensive, becoming quarrelsome and argumentative. Clients with antisocial personality disorder can also be antagonistic and argumentative, but are less suspicious than paranoid personalities. Clients with a histrionic personality disorder are dramatic, not suspicious and argumentative. Clients with schizotypal personality disorder are usually detached from others and tend to have eccentric behavior.
CN: Psychosocial integrity; CNS: None; CL: Comprehension

2. 4. Paranoid individuals have a need to constantly scan the environment for signs of betrayal, deception, and ridicule, appearing mistrustful and hostile. They expect to be tricked or deceived by others. The extreme suspiciousness is lacking in antisocial personalities, who tend to be more arrogant and self-assured despite their vigilance and mistrust. Individuals with avoidant personality disorders are guarded, fearing interpersonal rejection and humiliation. Clients with borderline personality disorders behave impulsively and tend to manipulate others.
CN: Psychosocial integrity; CNS: None; CL: Knowledge

3. 2. A client with paranoid personality disorder is afraid others will inflict harm. An individual with antisocial personality disorder won't be able to follow the limits set on behavior. An individual with an avoidant personality might avoid responsibility for health care because he tends to scan the environment for threatening things. A client with dependent personality disorder is likely to want others to make important decisions for him.
CN: Psychosocial integrity; CNS: None; CL: Analysis

4. Which statement is typical of a client diagnosed with paranoid personality disorder?

    1. "I understand you're to blame."

    2. "I must be seen first; it's not negotiable."

    3. "I see nothing humorous in this situation."

    4. "I wish someone would select the outfit for me."

5. The nurse is caring for a 33-year-old male client diagnosed with borderline personality disorder. The nurse tells the client that they'll be meeting for 1 hour every week on Monday at 1 p.m. Which statement best describes the rationale for setting limits for a client with borderline personality disorder?

    1. It helps the client clarify limits.

    2. It encourages the client to be manipulative.

    3. It provides the nurse with leverage against unacceptable behavior.

    4. It provides an opportunity for the client to assess the situation.

6. A nurse suspects a client has paranoid personality disorder. Which finding confirms the nurse's suspicion?

    1. Exhibitionism

    2. Impulsiveness

    3. Secretiveness

    4. Self-destructiveness

7. Which type of behavior is expected from a client diagnosed with paranoid personality disorder?

    1. Eccentric

    2. Exploitative

    3. Hypersensitive

    4. Seductive

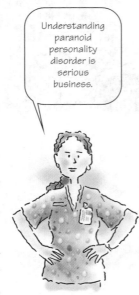

Understanding paranoid personality disorder is serious business.

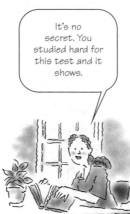

It's no secret. You studied hard for this test and it shows.

4. 3. Clients with paranoid personality disorder tend to be extremely serious and lack a sense of humor. Clients with borderline personality disorder tend to blame others for their problems. Clients with narcissistic personality disorders have a sense of self-importance and entitlement. Clients with dependent personality disorder want others to make their decisions.
CN: Psychosocial integrity; CNS: None; CL: Analysis

5. 1. Clarifying limits and making clear what may be unclear to the client helps the client establish boundaries himself, which fosters a therapeutic, trusting relationship between the nurse and the client. The nurse should never encourage manipulation or attempt to gather leverage against the client, which would be unprofessional. The client must understand his behavior patterns before he can start assessing the situation.
CN: Psychosocial integrity; CNS: None; CL: Application

6. 3. Clients with paranoid personality disorder tend to be secretive. Clients with histrionic personality disorder tend to be exhibitionists, and those with borderline personality disorder tend to be impulsive and self-destructive.
CN: Psychosocial integrity; CNS: None; CL: Comprehension

7. 3. People with paranoid personality disorders are hypersensitive to perceived threats. Schizotypal personalities appear eccentric and engage in activities others find perplexing. Clients with narcissistic personality disorder are interpersonally exploitative to enhance themselves or indulge their own desires. A client with histrionic personality disorder can be extremely seductive when in search of stimulation and approval.
CN: Psychosocial integrity; CNS: None; CL: Analysis

CN: Client needs category   CNS: Client needs subcategory   CL: Cognitive level

8. A client with paranoid personality disorder is discussing current problems with a nurse. Which nursing intervention has <u>priority</u> in the care plan?
1. Have the client look at sources of frustration.
2. Have the client focus on ways to interact with others.
3. Have the client discuss the use of defense mechanisms.
4. Have the client clarify thoughts and beliefs about an event.

9. A client with a paranoid personality disorder makes an inappropriate and unreasonable report to a nurse. Which principle of good communication skills is important to use?
1. Use logic to address the client's concern.
2. Confront the client about the stated misperception.
3. Use nonverbal communication to address the issue.
4. Tell the client matter-of-factly that you don't share his interpretation.

10. Which short-term goal is <u>most appropriate</u> for the client with paranoid personality disorder who has impaired social skills?
1. Obtain feedback from other people.
2. Discuss anxiety-provoking situations.
3. Address positive and negative feelings about self.
4. Identify personal feelings that hinder social interaction.

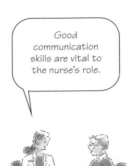

Good communication skills are vital to the nurse's role.

8. 4. Clarifying thoughts and beliefs helps the client avoid misinterpretations. Clients with a paranoid personality disorder tend to be aggressive and argumentative rather than frustrated. They tend to mistrust people and don't see interacting with others as a way to handle problems. The client's priority must be to interpret his thoughts and beliefs realistically, rather than discuss defense mechanisms. A paranoid client will focus on defending himself rather than acknowledging the use of defense mechanisms.
CN: Psychosocial integrity; CNS: None; CL: Analysis

9. 4. Telling the client you don't share his interpretation helps the client differentiate between realistic and emotional thoughts and conclusions. When the nurse uses logic to respond to a client's inappropriate statement, the nurse risks creating a power struggle with the client. It's unwise to confront a client with a paranoid personality disorder because the client will immediately become defensive. The use of nonverbal communication will probably be misinterpreted and arouse the client's suspicion.
CN: Psychosocial integrity; CNS: None; CL: Analysis

10. 4. The client must address the feelings that impede social interactions before developing ways to address impaired social skills. Feedback can be obtained only after action is taken to improve or change the situation. Discussion of anxiety-provoking situations is important but doesn't help the client with impaired social skills. Addressing the client's positive and negative feelings about himself won't directly influence impaired social skills.
CN: Psychosocial integrity; CNS: None; CL: Application

CN: Client needs category   CNS: Client needs subcategory   CL: Cognitive level

11. The nurse is caring for a client diagnosed with histrionic personality disorder. The client is observed tearing pages out of the books in the unit library and putting them into the ventilation system. Which of the following is the best initial nursing intervention?
   1. Place the client in a safe, secluded environment.
   2. Help the client develop more acceptable methods of seeking attention.
   3. Withdraw attention from the client at this time.
   4. Identify inappropriate behaviors to the client in a matter-of-fact manner.

12. Which approach should be used with a client with paranoid personality disorder who misinterprets many things the health care team says?
   1. Limit interaction to activities of daily living.
   2. Address only problems and causes of distress.
   3. Explore anxious situations and offer reassurance.
   4. Speak in simple messages without details.

13. A client with paranoid personality disorder responds aggressively during a psychoeducational group to something another client said about him. Which explanation is the most likely?
   1. The client doesn't want to participate in the group.
   2. The client took the statement as a personal criticism.
   3. The client is impulsive and was acting out frustrations.
   4. The client was attempting to handle emotional distress.

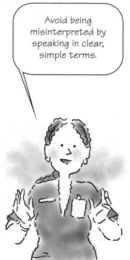

Avoid being misinterpreted by speaking in clear, simple terms.

11. 1. If the client begins destroying property or presenting potential harm to himself or others, it may be necessary to immediately place him in a safe, secluded environment. When the client regains control and ceases the behavior, then attempt to talk to him to explore more acceptable ways of handling frustration and expressing feelings. Lack of attention from the nurse wouldn't reduce the client's attention-seeking behaviors. When the client regains control and ceases the behavior, the nurse must make it clear which behaviors are inappropriate.
CN: Psychosocial integrity; CNS: None; CL: Analysis

12. 4. If the nurse speaks to the client using clear, simple messages, there's less chance that information will be misinterpreted. Interaction can't be limited because it will interfere with working on identified treatment goals. Discussing complex topics creates a situation in which the client will have additional information to misinterpret. If the nurse addresses only problems and specific stressors, it will be difficult to establish a trusting relationship.
CN: Psychosocial integrity; CNS: None; CL: Application

13. 2. Clients with paranoid personality disorder tend to be hypersensitive and take what other people say as a personal attack on their character. The client is driven by the suspicion that others will inflict harm. The client's participation in group therapy would be minimal because the client is directing energy toward emotional self-protection. Clients with a paranoid personality disorder tend to be rigid and guarded rather than impulsive and acting out. The client with a paranoid personality disorder is acting to defend himself, not handle emotional distress.
CN: Psychosocial integrity; CNS: None; CL: Analysis

CN: Client needs category   CNS: Client needs subcategory   CL: Cognitive level

14. A client with a paranoid personality disorder tells a nurse of his decision to stop talking to his wife. Which area should be assessed?
 1. The client's doubts about the partner's loyalty
 2. The client's need to be alone and have time for self
 3. The client's decision to separate from the marital partner
 4. The client's fears about becoming too much like the partner

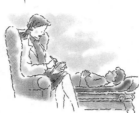

Try to establish a therapeutic relationship with the client.

15. Which characteristic of a client with a paranoid personality disorder makes it <u>difficult</u> for a nurse to establish an interpersonal relationship?
 1. Dysphoria
 2. Hypervigilance
 3. Indifference
 4. Promiscuity

16. The wife of a client diagnosed with paranoid personality disorder tells the client she wants a divorce. When discussing this situation with the couple, which factor would help the nurse form a care plan for this couple?
 1. Denied grief
 2. Intense jealousy
 3. Exploitation of others
 4. Self-destructive tendencies

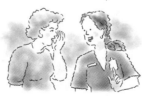

Avoid behaviors that may cause the client distress.

17. A client with a paranoid personality disorder tells a nurse that another nurse is out to get him. Which action by the nurse may cause distress for this paranoid client?
 1. Giving as-needed medication to another client
 2. Taking the clients outside the unit for exercise
 3. Checking vital signs of each person on the unit
 4. Talking to another client in the corner of the lounge

14. 1. Clients with paranoid personality disorder are preoccupied with the loyalty or trustworthiness of people, especially family and friends. People commonly withdraw from a client with paranoid personality disorder due to the difficulty in maintaining a healthy relationship. The client's need to be alone and have time for self isn't related to the decision to stop talking to a partner. These clients focus on the belief that others will harm them, not that they may become like a marital partner.
CN: Psychosocial integrity; CNS: None; CL: Application

15. 2. Clients with paranoid personality disorder think others will harm, deceive, or exploit them in some way, and they're commonly guarded and ready to defend themselves from actual or perceived attacks. They don't tend to be dysphoric, indifferent, or promiscuous.
CN: Psychosocial integrity; CNS: None; CL: Knowledge

16. 2. Clients with paranoid personality disorder are commonly extremely suspicious and jealous and make frequent accusations of partners and family members. Clients with paranoid personality disorder don't tend to struggle with the denial of grief. Clients with narcissistic personality disorder tend to exploit other people. Clients with borderline personality disorder have self-destructive tendencies.
CN: Psychosocial integrity; CNS: None; CL: Comprehension

17. 4. Clients with paranoid personality disorder tend to interpret any discussion that doesn't include them as evidence of a plot against them. Giving medication to another client wouldn't alarm the client. Checking vital signs on each client on the unit or taking the clients outside for exercise probably wouldn't be seen as a threat to the client's well-being.
CN: Psychosocial integrity; CNS: None; CL: Application

CN: Client needs category   CNS: Client needs subcategory   CL: Cognitive level

18. Which statement made by a client with paranoid personality disorder shows teaching about social relationships is effective?

    1. "As long as I live, I won't abide by social rules."

    2. "Sometimes I can see what causes relationship problems."

    3. "I'll find out what problems others have so I won't repeat them."

    4. "I don't have problems in social relationships; I never really did."

19. Which <u>long-term</u> goal is appropriate for a client with paranoid personality disorder who's trying to improve peer relationships?

    1. The client will verbalize a realistic view of self.

    2. The client will take steps to address disorganized thinking.

    3. The client will become appropriately interdependent on others.

    4. The client will become involved in activities that foster social relationships.

20. A family of a client with paranoid personality disorder is trying to understand the client's behavior. Which intervention would help the family?

    1. Help the family find ways to handle stress.

    2. Explore the possibility of finding respite care.

    3. Help the family manage the client's eccentric actions.

    4. Encourage the family to focus on the client's strengths.

21. A client with antisocial personality disorder is trying to convince a nurse that he deserves special privileges and that an exception to the rules should be made for him. Which response is the most <u>appropriate</u>?

    1. "I believe we need to sit down and talk about this."

    2. "Don't you know better than to try to bend the rules?'

    3. "What you're asking me to do for you is unacceptable."

    4. "Why don't you bring this request to the community meeting?"

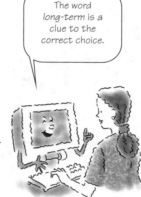

The word long-term is a clue to the correct choice.

18. 2. Progress is shown when the client addresses behaviors that negatively affect relationships. Clients with paranoid personality disorder struggle to understand and express their feelings about social rules. Knowing other people's problems isn't useful; the client must focus on his own issues. Clients with paranoid personality disorder tend to have impaired social relationships and are very uncomfortable in social settings. Not recognizing the problem indicates the client is in denial.
CN: Psychosocial integrity; CNS: None; CL: Application

19. 4. An appropriate long-term goal is for the client to increase interactions, social skills, and make the commitment to become involved with others on a long-term basis. To verbalize a realistic view of self is a short-term goal. The client with a paranoid personality disorder doesn't tend to have disorganized thinking. A client with paranoid personality disorder won't allow himself to be interdependent on others.
CN: Psychosocial integrity; CNS: None; CL: Analysis

20. 3. The family needs to know how to handle the client's symptoms and eccentric behaviors. All people need to learn strategies for handling stress, but the focus must be on helping the family learn how to handle symptoms. There's no need to find respite care for a client with a paranoid personality disorder. Focusing on the client's strengths is a positive action, but the family in this situation must learn how to manage the client's behavior.
CN: Psychosocial integrity; CNS: None; CL: Application

21. 3. These clients commonly try to manipulate the nurse to get special privileges or make exceptions to the rules on their behalf. By informing the client directly when actions are inappropriate, the nurse helps the client learn to control unacceptable behaviors by setting limits. By sitting down to talk about the request, the nurse is telling the client there's room for negotiation when there isn't. By implying that the client wants to bend the rules humiliates him. The client's behavior is unacceptable and shouldn't be brought to a community meeting.
CN: Psychosocial integrity; CNS: None; CL: Application

22. A client with antisocial personality disorder tells a nurse, "Life has been full of problems since childhood." Which situation or condition would the nurse explore in the assessment?

 1. Birth defects
 2. Distracted easily
 3. Hypoactive behavior
 4. Substance abuse

23. Which behavior by a client with antisocial personality disorder alerts a nurse to the need for teaching related to interaction skills?

 1. Frequently crying
 2. Having panic attacks
 3. Avoiding social activities
 4. Failing to follow social norms

24. When reviewing a client's chart, the nurse notes the progress note below. Which statement about the client's condition is <u>most</u> accurate?

Progress notes
9/4/08 / 1130 — Client, age 28, admitted to unit with diagnosis of antisocial personality disorder and suicide attempt after cutting his right wrist. Right wrist dressing appears dry and intact. Client states, "I don't want to be here and I'm not following your treatment plan or any of your rules. I'm going to tell everyone here not to follow your rules."———Barbara Jones, L.P.N.

> To answer this question, you should know the characteristics of antisocial personality disorder.

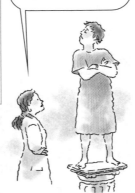

 1. The client requires psychotropic drugs to treat his condition, which he refuses.
 2. The client manipulates other clients but not his family.
 3. The client may not be motivated to change his behavior or his lifestyle.
 4. The client could quickly make behavior changes if motivated.

22. 4. Clients with antisocial personality disorder commonly engage in substance abuse during childhood. They don't have a higher incidence of birth defects than other people. Clients with antisocial personality disorder are commonly manipulative and are no more distracted from issues than others. They tend to be hyperactive, not hypoactive.
CN: Psychosocial integrity; CNS: None; CL: Comprehension

23. 4. Failure to abide by social norms influences the client's ability to interact in a healthy manner with peers. Clients with antisocial personality disorders don't have frequent crying episodes or panic attacks. Avoiding social activities is more likely observed in an avoidance personality style.
CN: Psychosocial integrity; CNS: None; CL: Analysis

24. 3. Clients with antisocial personality disorder feel nothing is wrong with their behavior and have no desire to change. These clients don't benefit from psychotropic drug therapy. They attempt to manipulate all people with whom they come in contact. A quick behavior change isn't a realistic expectation for clients with this disorder.
CN: Psychosocial integrity; CNS: None; CL: Application

25. Which intervention should be done <u>first</u> for a client who has an antisocial personality disorder and a history of polysubstance abuse?
1. Human immunodeficiency virus (HIV) testing
2. Electrolyte profile
3. Anxiety screening
4. Psychological testing

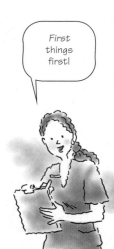

First things first!

25. 1. A client who engages in high-risk behaviors such as polysubstance abuse should undergo HIV testing. This client would benefit from an entire chemistry profile as part of a complete medical examination, rather than a single test for electrolytes. An anxiety screen isn't needed for a client with antisocial personality disorder. Information from psychological testing is valuable when developing a treatment plan but isn't an immediate concern.
CN: Physiological integrity; CNS: Reduction of risk potential; CL: Application

26. Which short-term goal is appropriate for a client with an antisocial personality disorder who acts out when distressed?
1. Develop goals for personal improvement.
2. Identify situations that are out of the client's control.
3. Encourage the client to identify traumatic life events.
4. Learn to express feelings in a nondestructive manner.

26. 4. By working on appropriate expression of feelings, the client learns how to talk about what's stressful, rather than hurt himself or others. The most pressing need is to learn to cope and talk about problems rather than act out. Developing goals for personal improvement is a long-term goal, not a short-term one. Although it's important to differentiate what is and isn't under the client's control, the most important goal for handling distress is to talk about feelings appropriately. The identification of traumatic life events will occur only after the client begins to express feelings appropriately.
CN: Safe, effective care environment; CNS: Safety and infection control; CL: Application

27. A nurse notices other clients on the unit avoiding a client diagnosed with antisocial personality disorder. When discussing appropriate behavior in group therapy, which comment is <u>expected</u> about this client by his peers?
1. "He's never honest."
2. "He's superstitious."
3. "He has temper tantrums."
4. "He constantly needs attention."

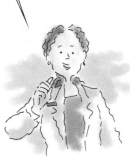

Read this question carefully. It seems to be asking you for a positive response, but it isn't.

27. 1. Clients with antisocial personality disorder tend to engage in acts of dishonesty, shown by lying. Clients with schizotypal personality disorder tend to be superstitious. Clients with histrionic personality disorders tend to overreact to frustrations and disappointments, have temper tantrums, and seek attention.
CN: Psychosocial integrity; CNS: None; CL: Application

28. During a family meeting for a client with an antisocial personality disorder, which statement is expected from an exasperated family member?
1. "Today I'm the enemy, but tomorrow I'll be a saint to him."
2. "When he's wrong, he never apologizes or even acts sorry."
3. "Sometimes I can't believe how he exaggerates about everything."
4. "There are times when his compulsive behavior is too much to handle."

28. 2. The client with antisocial personality disorder has no remorse. The client with a borderline personality disorder shows splitting. The client with an antisocial personality disorder doesn't tend to exaggerate about life events or be compulsive.
CN: Psychosocial integrity; CNS: None; CL: Analysis

CN: Client needs category   CNS: Client needs subcategory   CL: Cognitive level

29. Which goal is <u>most appropriate</u> for a client with antisocial personality disorder with a high risk of violence directed at others?
1. The client will discuss the desire to hurt others rather than act.
2. The client will be given something to destroy to displace the anger.
3. The client will develop a list of resources to use when anger escalates.
4. The client will understand the difference between anger and physical symptoms.

30. A client with antisocial personality disorder says, "I always want to blow things off." Which response is the most appropriate?
1. "Try to focus on what needs to be done and just do it."
2. "Let's work on considering some options and strategies."
3. "Procrastinating is a part of your illness that we'll work on."
4. "The best thing to do is decide on some useful goals to accomplish."

31. Which goal for the family of a client with antisocial disorder should the nurse stress in her teaching?
1. The family must assist the client to decrease ritualistic behavior.
2. The family must learn to live with the client's impulsive behavior.
3. The family must stop reinforcing inappropriate negative behavior.
4. The family must start to use negative reinforcement of the client's behavior.

32. Which nursing intervention has priority in the care plan for a client with antisocial personality disorder who shows defensive behaviors?
1. Help the client accept responsibility for his own decisions and behaviors.
2. Work with the client to feel better about himself by taking care of basic needs.
3. Teach the client to identify the defense mechanisms used to cope with distress.
4. Confront the client about the disregard of social rules and the feelings of others.

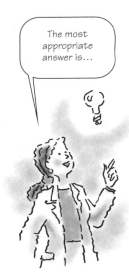

The most appropriate answer is...

Part of the nurse's job is teaching the family.

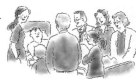

29. 1. By discussing the desire to be violent toward others, the nurse can help the client get in touch with the pain associated with the angry feelings. It isn't helpful to have the client destroy something. The client needs to talk about strong feelings in a nonviolent manner, not refer to a list of crisis references. Helping the client understand the relationship between feelings and physical symptoms can be done after discussing the desire to hurt others.
CN: Psychosocial integrity; CNS: None; CL: Analysis

30. 2. By considering options or strategies, the client gains skills to overcome ineffective behaviors. The client tends to be irresponsible and needs guidance on what specifically to focus on to change behavior. Clients with an antisocial personality disorder don't tend to struggle with procrastination; instead, they show reckless and irresponsible behaviors. It's premature to decide on goals when the client needs to address the mental mindset and work to change the irresponsible behavior.
CN: Psychosocial integrity; CNS: None; CL: Analysis

31. 3. The family needs help learning how to stop reinforcing inappropriate client behavior. Clients with antisocial personality disorder don't show ritualistic behaviors. The family can set limits and reinforce consequences when the client shows shortsightedness and poor planning. Negative reinforcement is an inappropriate strategy for the family to use to support the client.
CN: Psychosocial integrity; CNS: None; CL: Analysis

32. 1. Clients with antisocial personality disorder tend to blame other people for their behaviors and must learn how to take responsibility for their actions. Clients with antisocial personality disorder don't tend to have problems with self-care habits or meeting basic needs. Clients with antisocial personality disorder will deny they're defensive or distressed. Most commonly, these clients feel justified in retaliatory behavior. To confront the client would only cause him to become even more defensive.
CN: Psychosocial integrity; CNS: None; CL: Analysis

CN: Client needs category   CNS: Client needs subcategory   CL: Cognitive level

33. A client with antisocial personality disorder is trying to manipulate the health care team. Which strategy is important for the staff to use?
1. Focus on how to teach the client more effective behaviors for meeting basic needs.
2. Help the client verbalize underlying feelings of hopelessness and learn coping skills.
3. Remain calm and don't respond emotionally to the client's manipulative actions.
4. Help the client eliminate the intense desire to have everything in life turn out perfectly.

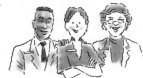

The staff must work together to help the client.

34. A client with dependent personality disorder is working to increase self-esteem. Which statement by the client shows teaching was <u>successful</u>?
1. "I'm not just going to look at the negative things about myself."
2. "I'm most concerned about my level of competence and progress."
3. "I'm not as envious of the things other people have as I used to be."
4. "I find I can't stop myself from taking over things others should be doing."

35. A client is suspected of having antisocial personality disorder. Which finding would <u>most</u> support this diagnosis?
1. The client has delusional thinking.
2. The client has feelings of inferiority.
3. The client has disorganized thinking.
4. The client has multiple criminal charges.

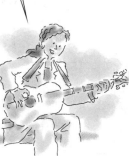

You've got to accentuate the positive and eliminate the negative.

36. A nurse on the psychiatric unit is caring for a client with an antisocial personality disorder. Which behavior is the nurse <u>most likely</u> to observe?
1. Manipulation, shallowness, and the need for immediate gratification
2. Tendency to profit from mistakes or learn from past experiences
3. Expression of guilt and anxiety regarding behavior
4. Acceptance of authority and discipline

33. 3. The best strategy to use with a client trying to manipulate staff is to stay calm and refrain from responding emotionally. Negative reinforcement of inappropriate behavior increases the chance it will be repeated. Later, it may be possible to address how to meet the client's basic needs. Clients with antisocial personality disorder don't tend to experience feelings of hopelessness or the desire for life events to turn out perfectly. In most cases, these clients negate responsibility for their behavior.
CN: Psychosocial integrity; CNS: None; CL: Analysis

34. 1. As the client makes progress on improving self-esteem, self-blame and negative self-evaluations will decrease. A client with dependent personality disorder tends to feel fragile and inadequate and would be extremely unlikely to discuss their level of competence and progress. These clients focus on self and aren't envious or jealous. Individuals with dependent personality disorders don't take over situations because they see themselves as inept and inadequate.
CN: Psychosocial integrity; CNS: None; CL: Application

35. 4. Clients with antisocial personality disorder are commonly sent for treatment by the court after multiple crimes or for the use of illegal substances. Clients with antisocial personality disorder don't tend to have delusional thinking, feelings of inferiority, or disorganized thinking.
CN: Psychosocial integrity; CNS: None; CL: Application

36. 1. Due to the client's lack of scruples and underlying powerlessness, the nurse expects to see manipulation, shallowness, impulsivity, and self-centered behavior. This client doesn't profit from mistakes and learn from past experiences, lacks anxiety and guilt, and is unable to accept authority and discipline.
CN: Psychosocial integrity; CNS: None; CL: Application

CN: Client needs category CNS: Client needs subcategory CL: Cognitive level

37. Which finding is consistent with a diagnosis of antisocial personality disorder?
1. Problematic work history
2. Struggle with severe anxiety
3. Severe physical health conditions
4. Being critical of positive feedback

38. A client with antisocial personality disorder is beginning to practice several socially acceptable behaviors in the group setting. Which outcome will result from this change?
1. Fewer panic attacks
2. Acceptance of reality
3. Improved self-esteem
4. Decreased physical symptoms

39. A client with a diagnosis of borderline personality disorder is admitted to the unit after slashing his wrist. The nurse is preparing a care plan with a nursing diagnosis of *Risk for self-directed violence*. Which goal is <u>most</u> appropriate for a client with this disorder?
1. Establish a therapeutic relationship with the client.
2. Identify if splitting is present in the client's thoughts.
3. Talk about his acting out and self-destructive tendencies.
4. Encourage the client to understand why he blames others.

40. Which nursing intervention is <u>most appropriate</u> in helping a client with a borderline personality disorder identify appropriate behaviors?
1. Schedule a family meeting.
2. Place the client in seclusion.
3. Formulate a behavioral contract.
4. Perform a mental status assessment.

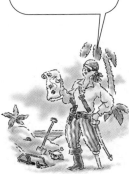

A client's work history may be a clue to antisocial behavior.

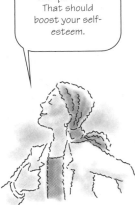

You've answered half of the questions. That should boost your self-esteem.

37. 1. Clients with a diagnosis of antisocial personality disorder tend to have problems in their job roles and poor work histories. They don't have severe anxiety disorders or severe physical health problems and are able to accept positive feedback from others.
CN: Psychosocial integrity; CNS: None; CL: Comprehension

38. 3. When clients with antisocial personality disorder begin to practice socially acceptable behaviors, they also commonly experience a more positive sense of self. Clients with antisocial personality disorder don't tend to have panic attacks, alteration in their perception of reality, or somatic manifestations of their illness.
CN: Psychosocial integrity; CNS: None; CL: Comprehension

39. 1. After promoting client safety, the nurse establishes a rapport with the client to facilitate appropriate expression of feelings. At this time, the client isn't ready to address unhealthy behavior. A therapeutic relationship must be established before the nurse can effectively work with the client on splitting, self-destructive tendencies, and blaming others.
CN: Psychosocial integrity; CNS: None; CL: Application

40. 3. The use of a behavioral contract establishes a framework for healthier functioning and places responsibility for actions back on the client. Seclusion will reinforce the fear of abandonment found in clients with borderline personality. Performing a mental status assessment or scheduling a family meeting won't help the client identify appropriate behaviors.
CN: Psychosocial integrity; CNS: None; CL: Application

CN: Client needs category   CNS: Client needs subcategory   CL: Cognitive level

41. Which statement is <u>typical</u> of a client with borderline personality disorder who has recurrent suicidal thoughts?

  1. "I can't believe how everyone has suddenly stopped believing in me."

  2. "I don't care what other people say, I know how bad I looked to them."

  3. "I might as well check out because my boyfriend doesn't want me anymore."

  4. "I won't stop until I've gotten revenge on all those people who blamed me."

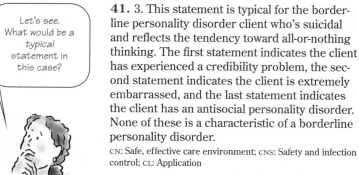

Let's see. What would be a typical statement in this case?

42. Which finding is expected when taking a health history from a client with borderline personality disorder?

  1. A negative sense of self

  2. A tendency to be compulsive

  3. A problem with communication

  4. An inclination to be philosophical

43. Which characteristic or situation is indicated when a client with borderline personality disorder has a crisis?

  1. Antisocial behavior

  2. Suspicious behavior

  3. Relationship problems

  4. Auditory hallucinations

44. Which assessment finding is seen in a client diagnosed with borderline personality disorder?

  1. Abrasions in various healing stages

  2. Intermittent episodes of hypertension

  3. Alternating tachycardia and bradycardia

  4. Mild state of euphoria with disorientation

45. Which <u>short-term</u> goal is appropriate for a client with borderline personality disorder with low self-esteem?

  1. Write in a journal daily.

  2. Express fears and feelings.

  3. Stop obsessive-compulsive behaviors.

  4. Decrease dysfunctional family conflicts.

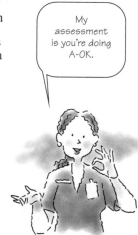

My assessment is you're doing A-OK.

41. 3. This statement is typical for the borderline personality disorder client who's suicidal and reflects the tendency toward all-or-nothing thinking. The first statement indicates the client has experienced a credibility problem, the second statement indicates the client is extremely embarrassed, and the last statement indicates the client has an antisocial personality disorder. None of these is a characteristic of a borderline personality disorder.

CN: Safe, effective care environment; CNS: Safety and infection control; CL: Application

42. 1. Clients with a borderline personality disorder have low self-esteem and a negative sense of self. They have little or no problem expressing themselves and communicating with others. Although they have a tendency to be impulsive, they aren't usually compulsive or philosophical.

CN: Psychosocial integrity; CNS: None; CL: Comprehension

43. 3. Relationship problems can precipitate a crisis because they bring up issues of abandonment. Clients with borderline personality disorder aren't usually suspicious; they're more likely to be depressed or highly anxious. They don't have symptoms of antisocial behavior or auditory hallucinations.

CN: Psychosocial integrity; CNS: None; CL: Analysis

44. 1. Clients with borderline personality disorder tend to self-mutilate and have abrasions in various stages of healing. Intermittent episodes of hypertension, alternating tachycardia and bradycardia, or a mild state of euphoria with disorientation don't tend to occur with this disorder.

CN: Psychosocial integrity; CNS: None; CL: Application

45. 2. Acknowledging fears and feelings can help the client identify parts of himself that make him uncomfortable, and he can begin to work on developing a positive sense of self. Writing in a daily journal isn't a short-term goal to enhance self-esteem. A client with borderline personality disorder doesn't struggle with obsessive-compulsive behaviors. Decreasing dysfunctional family conflicts is a long-term goal.

CN: Psychosocial integrity; CNS: None; CL: Analysis

CN: Client needs category   CNS: Client needs subcategory   CL: Cognitive level

46. Which intervention is important to include in a teaching plan for the family of a client diagnosed with borderline personality disorder?
1. Teach the family methods for handling the client's anxiety.
2. Explore how the family reinforces the sick role with the client.
3. Encourage the family to have the client express intense emotions.
4. Help the family put pressure on the client to improve current behavior.

47. In planning care for a client with borderline personality disorder, a nurse must be aware that this client is prone to developing which condition?
1. Binge eating
2. Memory loss
3. Cult membership
4. Delusional thinking

48. Which statement is expected from a client with borderline personality disorder with a history of dysfunctional relationships?
1. "I won't get involved in another relationship."
2. "I'm determined to look for the perfect partner."
3. "I've decided to learn better communication skills."
4. "I'm going to be an equal partner in a relationship."

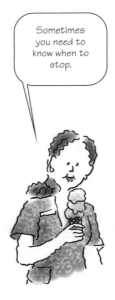

Sometimes you need to know when to stop.

46. 1. The family needs to learn how to handle the client's intense stress and low tolerance for frustration. Family members don't want to reinforce the sick role; they're more concerned with preventing anxiety from escalating. Clients with borderline personality disorder already maintain intense emotions and it's not safe to encourage further expression of them. The family doesn't need to put pressure on the client to change behavior; this approach will only cause inappropriate behavior to escalate.
CN: Health promotion and maintenance; CNS: None; CL: Application

47. 1. Clients with borderline personality disorder are likely to develop dysfunctional coping and act out in self-destructive ways such as binge eating. They aren't prone to develop memory loss or delusional thinking. Becoming involved in cults may be seen in some clients with antisocial personality disorder.
CN: Psychosocial integrity; CNS: None; CL: Analysis

48. 2. Clients with borderline personality disorder would decide to look for a perfect partner. This characteristic is a result of the dichotomous manner in which these clients view the world. They go from relationship to relationship without taking responsibility for their behavior. It's unlikely an unsuccessful relationship will cause clients to make a change. Because they tend to blame others for problems, it's unlikely they would express a desire to learn communication skills. They tend to be demanding and impulsive in relationships. There's no thought given to what one wants or needs from a relationship.
CN: Psychosocial integrity; CNS: None; CL: Analysis

CN: Client needs category   CNS: Client needs subcategory   CL: Cognitive level

49. Which nursing intervention is the <u>most appropriate</u> for a client with borderline personality disorder working on developing healthy relationships?

1. Have the client assess current behaviors.
2. Work with the client to develop outgoing behavior.
3. Limit the client's interactions to family members only.
4. Encourage the client to approach others for interactions.

50. Which defense mechanism is most likely to be seen in a client with borderline personality disorder?

1. Compensation
2. Displacement
3. Identification
4. Projection

51. Which condition is <u>most</u> likely to coexist in clients with a diagnosis of borderline personality disorder?

1. Avoidance
2. Delirium
3. Depression
4. Disorientation

52. Which nursing intervention has <u>priority</u> for a client with borderline personality disorder?

1. Maintain consistent, realistic limits.
2. Give instructions for meeting basic self-care needs.
3. Engage in daytime activities to stimulate wakefulness.
4. Have the client attend group therapy on a daily basis.

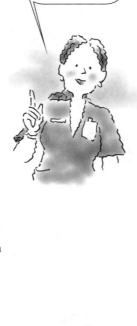

There's only one answer that's most appropriate.

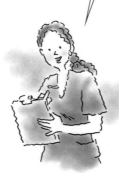

Prioritizing is a crucial part of nursing!

49. 1. Self-assessment of behavior enables the client to look at himself and identify social behaviors that need to be changed. Clients with borderline personality disorder don't tend to have difficulty approaching and interacting with other people. It's unrealistic to have clients with borderline personality disorder limit their interactions to family members only. Clients with borderline personality disorder tend to be demanding and the center of attention. It isn't useful to work on developing outgoing behavior.
CN: Psychosocial integrity; CNS: None; CL: Analysis

50. 4. Clients with borderline personality disorder tend to blame and project their feelings and inadequacies onto others. They don't identify with other people or tend to use compensation to handle distress. Clients with borderline personality disorder are impulsive and tend to react immediately. It's unlikely they would displace their feelings onto others.
CN: Psychosocial integrity; CNS: None; CL: Analysis

51. 3. Chronic feelings of emptiness and sadness predispose a client to depression. About 40% of the clients with borderline personality disorder struggle with depression. Clients with borderline personality disorder tend to disregard boundaries and limits. Avoidance isn't an issue with these clients. Clients with borderline personality disorder don't tend to develop delirium or become disoriented. These conditions are only a possibility if the client becomes intoxicated.
CN: Psychosocial integrity; CNS: None; CL: Comprehension

52. 1. Clients with borderline personality disorder who are needy, dependent, and manipulative will benefit greatly from maintaining consistent, realistic limits. They don't tend to have difficulty meeting their self-care needs and don't tend to have sleeping difficulties. They enjoy attending group therapy because they typically attempt to use the opportunity to become the center of attention.
CN: Psychosocial integrity; CNS: None; CL: Application

53. Which outcome indicates individual therapy has been effective for a client with borderline personality disorder?
1. The client accepts that medication isn't a treatment of choice.
2. The client agrees to undergo hypnosis for suppression of memories.
3. The client understands the organic basis for the problematic behavior.
4. The client verbalizes awareness of the consequences for unacceptable behaviors.

54. Which action by a client with borderline personality disorder indicates adequate learning about personal behavior?
1. The client talks about intense anger.
2. The client smiles while making demands.
3. The client decides never to engage in conflict.
4. The client stops the family from controlling finances.

55. A nurse is planning care for a client with borderline personality disorder who has been agitated. Which instruction is included for the client and family?
1. Encourage the rebuilding of family relationships.
2. Help the client handle anxiety before it escalates.
3. Have the client participate in a weekly support group.
4. Discuss the client's bad habits that must be changed.

56. A client with a borderline personality disorder isn't making progress on the identified goals. Which client factor should be reevaluated?
1. Memory
2. Motivation
3. Orientation
4. Perception

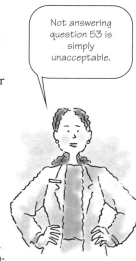

Not answering question 53 is simply unacceptable.

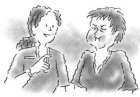

When treatment isn't working, reevaluation may be necessary.

53. 4. An indication of effective individual therapy for this client is his expressed awareness of consequences for unacceptable behaviors. Medications can control symptoms; however, monitoring for reckless use or abuse of drugs must be done for the client with borderline personality disorder. Hypnosis isn't a treatment for a client with borderline personality disorder. There's no organic basis for the development of this disorder.
CN: Psychosocial integrity; CNS: None; CL: Application

54. 1. Learning has occurred when anger is discussed rather than acted out in unhealthy ways. The behavior to change would be the demands placed on others. Smiling while making these demands shows manipulative behavior. Not engaging in conflict is unrealistic. It's important to help this client slowly develop financial responsibility rather than just stopping the family from monitoring the client's overspending.
CN: Psychosocial integrity; CNS: None; CL: Application

55. 2. The client needs help handling anxiety because escalating anxiety can trigger self-destructive behaviors in clients with borderline personality disorder. When a client with borderline personality disorder is agitated, it's difficult to communicate, let alone rebuild family relationships. Participation in a weekly support group won't be enough to help the client handle agitation. When a client is agitated, it isn't appropriate to discuss bad habits that must be changed. This action may further agitate the client.
CN: Psychosocial integrity; CNS: None; CL: Application

56. 2. Clients with borderline personality disorders tend to be poorly motivated regarding treatment. They don't tend to have memory problems, problems in orientation, or perception problems, such as hallucinations and illusions.
CN: Psychosocial integrity; CNS: None; CL: Analysis

57. A nurse is assessing a client diagnosed with dependent personality disorder. Which characteristic is a major component of this disorder?
1. Abrasive to others
2. Indifferent to others
3. Manipulative of others
4. Overreliance on others

58. A client with dependent personality disorder is working on goals for self-care. Which short-term goal is <u>most important</u> to the client's everyday activities of daily living?
1. Do all self-care activities independently.
2. Write a daily schedule for each day of the week.
3. Do self-care activities in a minimal amount of time.
4. Determine activities that can be performed without help.

59. Which information must be included for the family of a person diagnosed with dependent personality disorder?
1. Address coping skills.
2. Explore panic attacks.
3. Promote exercise programs.
4. Decrease aggressive outbursts.

60. Which strategy is appropriate for a client with dependent personality disorder?
1. Orient the client to current surroundings.
2. Reassure the client about personal safety.
3. Ask questions to help the client recall problems.
4. Differentiate between positive and negative feedback.

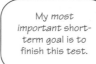
My most important short-term goal is to finish this test.

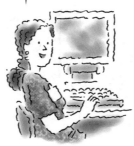

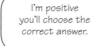
I'm positive you'll choose the correct answer.

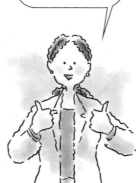

57. 4. Clients with dependent personality disorder are extremely overreliant on other people; they aren't abrasive or assertive. People with dependent personality disorder rely on others and want to be taken care of. They aren't indifferent. They're clinging and demanding of others; they don't manipulate.
CN: Psychosocial integrity; CNS: None; CL: Knowledge

58. 4. By determining activities that can be performed without assistance, the client can then begin to practice them independently. If the nurse only encourages a client to perform self-care activities independently, nothing may change. Writing a daily schedule doesn't help the client focus on what needs to be done to promote self-care. The amount of time needed to perform self-care activities isn't important. If time pressure is put on the client, there may be more reluctance to perform self-care activities.
CN: Psychosocial integrity; CNS: None; CL: Comprehension

59. 1. The family needs information about coping skills to help the client learn to handle stress. Clients with dependent personality disorder don't tend to have panic attacks. Exercise is a health promotion activity for all clients. Clients with dependent personality disorder wouldn't need exercise promoted more than others. These clients don't have aggressive outbursts; they tend to be passive and submit to others.
CN: Safe, effective care environment; CNS: Coordinated care; CL: Comprehension

60. 4. Clients with dependent personality disorder tend to view all feedback as criticism; they commonly misinterpret another's remarks. Clients with dependent personality disorder don't need orientation to their surroundings. Personal safety isn't an issue because a person with dependent personality disorder typically isn't self-destructive. Memory problems aren't associated with this disorder, so asking questions to stimulate one's memory isn't necessary.
CN: Psychosocial integrity; CNS: None; CL: Application

CN: Client needs category   CNS: Client needs subcategory   CL: Cognitive level

61. A client with dependent personality disorder is crying after a family meeting. Which statement by a family member is <u>most likely</u> the cause of upset to this client?
1. "You take advantage of people, especially the people in our family."
2. "You act as if you love me one minute, but hate me the next minute."
3. "You feel as if you deserve everything, whether you work for it or not."
4. "You always agree to everything, but deep down inside you feel differently."

62. A 31-year-old male client with borderline personality is instructed to stay in the game room. He asks the nurse to "bend the rules a little, just this one time." Which response is <u>most appropriate</u>?
1. "No."
2. "OK, but just this once."
3. Ignore the client.
4. "Let me explain the rules to you."

63. A client with borderline personality disorder confides in one nurse that she's disappointed in the other nurses because of their lack of sensitivity to her. What's the <u>best</u> action for the nurse to take?
1. Explain the other nurses' behaviors to the client.
2. Ask for more information about the client's disappointment.
3. Call a team meeting to help others understand the client better.
4. Advise the client to seek out the nurses and tell them directly.

64. In planning care for a client with borderline personality disorder, the nurse must account for which behavioral trait?
1. An inability to make decisions independently
2. A propensity to act out when feeling afraid, alone, or devalued
3. A belief she deserves special privileges not accorded to others
4. A display of inappropriately seductive appearance and behavior

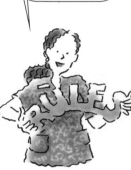

Know the appropriate response to a client who asks you to bend the rules.

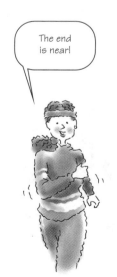

The end is near!

61. 4. Most likely, the client was confronted by a family member about behavior that doesn't represent the client's true feelings. Clients with dependent personality disorder are afraid they won't be taken care of if they disagree. They don't have a sense of entitlement and don't take advantage of other people, but they subordinate their needs to others. They don't show the defense mechanism of splitting, where a person is valued and then devalued.
CN: Psychosocial integrity; CNS: None; CL: Analysis

62. 4. Explaining the rules allows the nurse to be firm but not confrontational with the client. A simple "no" is too harsh by itself. The nurse's response needs more of an explanation. By agreeing to bend the rules, the nurse would allow the client to manipulate the caregiver. Ignoring the client would do nothing but frustrate him.
CN: Psychosocial integrity; CNS: None; CL: Application

63. 4. One communication strategy when working with a client with borderline personality disorder is to never engage in third-party conversations. Explaining the other nurses' behaviors to the client, asking for more information about his disappointment, or calling a team meeting encourage splitting behaviors and are nonproductive.
CN: Psychosocial integrity; CNS: None; CL: Application

64. 2. Clients with borderline personality disorder have an intense fear of abandonment. These clients are able to make decisions independently. Feeling deserving of special privileges is characteristic of a person with narcissistic personality disorder. Inappropriate seductive appearance and behavior is characteristic of someone with histrionic personality disorder.
CN: Psychosocial integrity; CNS: None; CL: Application

CN: Client needs category CNS: Client needs subcategory CL: Cognitive level

65. Which information is expected in a history of a client with dependent personality disorder?
1. Lack of relationships
2. Lack of self-confidence
3. Preoccupation with rules
4. Tendency to overvalue self

66. Which short-term goal is appropriate for a client with dependent personality disorder experiencing excessive dependency needs?
1. Verbalize self-confidence in own abilities.
2. Decide relationships don't take energy to sustain.
3. Discuss feelings related to frequent mood swings.
4. Stop obsessive thinking that impedes daily social functioning.

67. A client with dependent personality disorder is thinking about getting a part-time job. Which nursing intervention will help this client when employment is obtained?
1. Help the client develop strategies to control impulses.
2. Explain there are consequences for inappropriate behaviors.
3. Have the client work to sustain healthy interpersonal relationships.
4. Help the client decrease the use of regression as a defense mechanism.

68. A client with dependent personality disorder has difficulty expressing personal concerns. Which communication technique is best to teach the client?
1. Questioning
2. Reflection
3. Silence
4. Touch

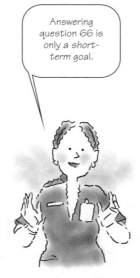

Answering question 66 is only a short-term goal.

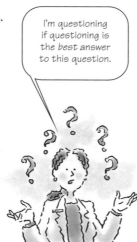

I'm questioning if questioning is the best answer to this question.

65. 2. Clients with a dependent personality disorder lack self-confidence and have low self-esteem. They have unhealthy relationships, allowing others to take over their lives. They aren't preoccupied with rules. They focus on their need to be taken care of by others. They tend to undervalue, not overvalue self.
CN: Psychosocial integrity; CNS: None; CL: Knowledge

66. 1. Individuals with dependent personalities believe they must depend on others to be competent for them. They need to gain more self-confidence in their own abilities. The client must realize relationships take energy to develop and sustain. Clients with dependent personality disorder usually don't have mood swings or obsessive thinking that interferes with their socialization.
CN: Psychosocial integrity; CNS: None; CL: Application

67. 3. Sustaining healthy relationships will help the client be comfortable with peers in the job setting. Clients with dependent personality disorder don't usually have trouble with impulse control or offensive behavior that would lead to negative consequences. They don't usually use regression as a defense mechanism. It's common to see denial and introjection used.
CN: Psychosocial integrity; CNS: None; CL: Analysis

68. 1. Questioning is a way to learn to identify feelings and express self. The use of reflection isn't a communication technique that will help the client express personal feelings and concerns. Using silence won't help the client identify and discuss personal concerns. The use of touch to express feelings and personal concerns must be used very judiciously.
CN: Psychosocial integrity; CNS: None; CL: Application

69. A nurse is evaluating the effectiveness of an assertiveness group that a client with dependent personality disorder attended. Which client statement indicates the group had therapeutic value?
1. "I can't seem to do the things other people do."
2. "I wish I could be more organized like other people."
3. "I want to talk about something that's bothering me."
4. "I just don't want people in my family to fight anymore."

70. After a family visit, a client with dependent personality disorder becomes anxious. Which situation is a possible cause of the anxiety?
1. Sensitivity to criticism
2. Discussion of family rules
3. Being asked personal questions
4. Identification of eccentric behavior

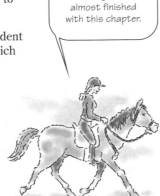

Keep on trotting! You're almost finished with this chapter.

71. A 46-year-old male client undergoing treatment for paranoia refuses to take his fluphenazine (Prolixin) because he says he thinks it's poisoned. Which response is best?
1. Omit the dose and notify the physician.
2. Tell him that he'll receive an injection if he refuses the oral medication.
3. Put the medication in his juice without informing him.
4. Allow him to examine the medication to see that it isn't poisoned.

72. Which emotional health problem may potentially coexist in a client with dependent personality disorder?
1. Psychotic disorder
2. Acute stress disorder
3. Alcohol-related disorder
4. Posttraumatic stress disorder (PTSD)

69. 3. By asking to talk about a bothersome situation, the client has taken the first step toward assertive behavior. The first statement reflects a lack of self-confidence; it isn't an assertive statement. Statements that express the client's wishes aren't assertive statements. To smooth over or minimize troubling events isn't an assertive position.
CN: Psychosocial integrity; CNS: None; CL: Application

70. 1. Clients with dependent personality disorder are extremely sensitive to criticism and can become very anxious when they feel interpersonal conflict or tension. When they have discussions about family rules, they try to become submissive and please others rather than become anxious. When they're asked personal questions, they don't necessarily become anxious. Clients with dependent personality disorder don't tend to show eccentric behavior that causes them anxiety.
CN: Psychosocial integrity; CNS: None; CL: Application

71. 1. The nurse's best response is to omit the dose and notify the physician because insisting that the client take the medication will only increase his paranoia and agitation. Forcing injections and tricking clients into taking medication is illegal. Don't put the medication in his juice without informing him. A rational approach (such as allowing the client to examine the medication) to irrational ideas seldom works.
CN: Psychosocial integrity; CNS: None; CL: Application

72. 2. Because they have placed their own needs in the hands of others, clients with dependent personalities are extremely vulnerable to acute stress disorder. They don't tend to have coexisting problems of psychotic disorder, alcohol-related disorder, or PTSD.
CN: Psychosocial integrity; CNS: None; CL: Analysis

CN: Client needs category   CNS: Client needs subcategory   CL: Cognitive level

73. While collecting data on a client who was diagnosed with impulse control disorder (and who displays violent, aggressive, and assaultive behavior), the nurse can expect to find which assessment? Select all that apply:

1. The client functions well in other areas of his life.
2. The degree of aggressiveness is out of proportion to the stressor.
3. The client typically uses a stressor to justify the violent behavior.
4. The client has a history of parental alcoholism and a chaotic, abusive family life.
5. The client shows no remorse about his inability to control his behavior.

74. A client with paranoid schizophrenia is becoming dangerously agitated. The nurse gives him an as-needed dose of haloperidol (Haldol). How is this medication administered? Select all that apply.

1. Sublingually
2. I.V.
3. Intradermally
4. I.M.
5. Orally

75. A client has borderline personality disorder. Which behaviors would substantiate this diagnosis? Select all that apply:

1. Recurrent suicidal behaviors, gestures, or threats
2. Chronically depressed affect, slowed thinking, and slurred speech
3. Frantic attempts to avoid real or imagined abandonment
4. Chronic feelings of emptiness
5. Eating disorders, such as binging and purging

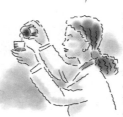

Know the proper methods of administration for various medications.

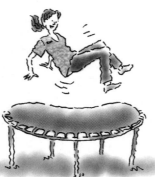

You're finished! So go ahead and jump for joy.

73. 1, 2, 4. A client with an impulse control disorder who displays violent, aggressive, and assaultive behavior generally functions well in other areas of his life. The degree of the client's aggressiveness is disproportionate to the stressor, and the client commonly has a history of parental alcoholism, as well as a chaotic family life. The client usually verbalizes sincere guilt and remorse for the aggressive behavior.
CN: Psychosocial integrity; CNS: None; CL: Application

74. 4, 5. I.M. administration of Haldol is the most effective means of calming psychotic agitation. It can also be given orally two or three times per day. This medication doesn't come in a sublingual form and isn't given I.V. Intradermal administration would be inappropriate because the drug must be absorbed rapidly to obtain the desired effect.
CN: Physiological integrity; CNS: Pharmacological therapies; CL: Analysis

75. 1, 3, 4. Options 1, 3, and 4 are correct because they're typical behaviors seen in borderline personality disorder. Though no etiology is known, it's believed to result from a severely disrupted or disconnected attachment with the primary caregiver at an early developmental age. This disruption of normal emotional development causes a sense of "core emptiness" that persists for life and is generally resistant to treatment. The symptoms in option 2 are more indicative of a mood disorder, and those in option 5 are consistent with an eating disorder.
CN: Psychosocial integrity; CNS: None; CL: Analysis

CN: Client needs category   CNS: Client needs subcategory   CL: Cognitive level

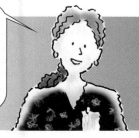

It's no delusion. You'll do great on this chapter if you use your nursing skills—knowledge, experience, compassion, insight...

Chapter 17
Schizophrenic & delusional disorders

1. A schizophrenic client tells his primary nurse that he's scheduled to meet the King of Samoa at a special time, making it impossible for the client to leave his room for dinner. Which response by the nurse is the <u>most appropriate</u>?
1. "It's meal time. Let's go so you can eat."
2. "The King of Samoa told me to take you to dinner."
3. "Your physician expects you to follow the unit's schedule."
4. "People who don't eat on this unit aren't being cooperative."

2. While looking out the window, a client with schizophrenia remarks, "That school across the street has creatures in it that are waiting for me." Which nursing action is the <u>most</u> appropriate for this client?
1. Ask the client why the creatures are waiting for him.
2. Acknowledge the client's fears and insecurities.
3. Explain to the client that there are no creatures in the school.
4. Ignore the remark and redirect the client to group activities.

3. Which nursing intervention is <u>most</u> important for a client with schizophrenia?
1. Teaching the client about the illness
2. Initiating a behavioral contract with the client
3. Requiring the client to attend all unit functions
4. Providing a consistent, predictable environment

Sometimes I can't sort out what's real and what isn't. You'll see what I mean as you work your way through this chapter.

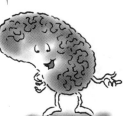

1. 1. A delusional client is so wrapped up in his false beliefs that he tends to disregard activities of daily living, such as nutrition and hydration. He needs clear, concise, firm directions from a caring nurse to meet his needs. The second response belittles and tricks the client, possibly evoking mistrust on the part of the client. The third response evades the issue of meeting his basic needs. The last response is demeaning and doesn't address the delusion.
CN: Health promotion and maintenance; CNS: None; CL: Application

2. 2. Acknowledging the client's fears and insecurities helps to establish a trusting relationship and increase feelings of safety. Asking the client why the creatures are waiting only serves to reinforce the delusional thoughts. Challenging the client's delusion may lead to agitation. Ignoring the remark does nothing to reassure the client. A delusional client isn't able to participate in group activities.
CN: Psychosocial integrity; CNS: None; CL: Application

3. 4. A consistent, predictable environment helps the client remain as functional as possible and prevents sensory overload. Teaching the client about his illness is important but not a priority. A behavioral contract and required attendance at all functions aren't particularly effective with schizophrenia.
CN: Psychosocial integrity; CNS: None; CL: Application

CN: Client needs category   CNS: Client needs subcategory   CL: Cognitive level

4. A 22-year-old schizophrenic client was admitted to the psychiatric unit during the night. The next morning, he begins to misidentify the nurse and call her by his sister's name. Which intervention is best?
1. Assessing the client for potential violence
2. Taking the client to his room, where he'll feel safer
3. Assuming the misidentification makes the client feel more comfortable
4. Correcting the misidentification and orienting the client to the unit and staff

4. 4. Misidentification can contribute to anxiety, fear, aggression, and hostility. Orienting a new client to the hospital unit, staff, and other clients, along with establishing a nurse-client relationship, can decrease these feelings and help the client feel in control. Assessing for potential violence is an important nursing function for any psychiatric client, but a perceived supportive environment reduces the risk of violence. Withdrawing to his room, unless interpersonal relationships have become nontherapeutic for him, encourages the client to remain in his fantasy world.
CN: Psychosocial integrity; CNS: None; CL: Application

5. Which term describes an effect of isolation?
1. Delusions
2. Hallucinations
3. Lack of volition
4. Waxy flexibility

5. 2. Prolonged isolation can produce sensory deprivation, manifested by hallucinations. A delusion is a false perception caused by misinterpretation of a real object. Lack of volition is a symptom associated with type I negative symptoms of schizophrenia. Waxy flexibility is a motor disturbance that's a predominant feature of catatonic schizophrenia.
CN: Psychosocial integrity; CNS: None; CL: Application

6. A client diagnosed with schizophrenia several years ago tells the nurse that he feels "very sad." The nurse observes that he's smiling when he says it. Which term best describes the nurse's observation?
1. Inappropriate affect
2. Extrapyramidal
3. Insight
4. Inappropriate mood

6. 1. Affect refers to behaviors, such as facial expression, that can be observed when a person is expressing and experiencing feelings. If the client's affect doesn't reflect the emotional content of the statement, the affect is considered inappropriate. Extrapyramidal symptoms are adverse effects of some categories of medication. Insight is a component of the mental status examination and is the ability to perceive oneself realistically and understand if a problem exists. Mood is an extensive and sustained feeling.
CN: Psychosocial integrity; CNS: None; CL: Comprehension

This word salad doesn't sound very appetizing. I think I'll go with the Caesar instead.

7. A nurse asks a client diagnosed with schizophrenia to go to the dayroom for activities. He replies, "Look, bread, table, cow." Based on this interaction, the nurse suspects that the client has which type of schizophrenia?
1. Paranoid
2. Catatonic
3. Disorganized
4. Residual

7. 3. The client's reply is an example of word salad and is associated with the disorganized type of schizophrenia. The paranoid schizophrenic is extremely suspicious and may feel persecuted. Catatonic schizophrenia predominantly involves disturbances of movement. Clients with residual schizophrenia, although no longer having hallucinations or delusions, may still experience avolition (lack of motivation) and anhedonia (loss of pleasure in things that are usually pleasurable).
CN: Psychosocial integrity; CNS: None; CL: Application

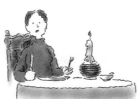

CN: Client needs category   CNS: Client needs subcategory   CL: Cognitive level

8. A client on the psychiatric unit is copying and imitating the movements of his primary nurse. During recovery, he said, "I thought the nurse was my mirror. I felt connected only when I saw my nurse." This behavior is known by which term?
   1. Modeling
   2. Echopraxia
   3. Ego-syntonicity
   4. Ritualism

9. The teenage son of a father with schizophrenia is worried that he might have schizophrenia as well. Which behavior would be an indication that he should be evaluated for signs of the disorder?
   1. Moodiness
   2. Preoccupation with his body
   3. Spending more time away from home
   4. Changes in sleep patterns

10. Which manifestation is usually responsive to <u>traditional</u> antipsychotic drugs?
   1. Apathy
   2. Delusions
   3. Social withdrawal
   4. Attention impairment

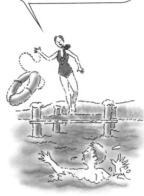

A nurse can be a lifeline to a family member who's dealing with anxiety and guilt. Just check out questions 9 and 11 if you have any doubt.

11. A client was hospitalized after his son filed a petition for involuntary hospitalization for safety reasons. The son seeks out the nurse because his father is angry and refuses to talk with him. He's frustrated and feeling guilty about his decision. Which response to the son is the <u>most</u> empathic?
   1. "Your father is here because he needs help."
   2. "He'll feel differently about you as he gets better."
   3. "It sounds like you're feeling guilty about leaving your father here."
   4. "This is a stressful time for you, but you'll feel better as he gets well."

8. 2. Echopraxia is the involuntary copying of another's behaviors and is the result of the loss of ego boundaries. Modeling is the conscious copying of someone's behaviors. Ego-syntonicity refers to behaviors that correspond with the individual's sense of self. Ritualistic behaviors are repetitive and compulsive.
CN: Psychosocial integrity; CNS: None; CL: Application

9. 4. In conjunction with other signs, changes in sleep patterns are distinctive initial signs of schizophrenia. Other signs include changes in personal care habits and social isolation. Moodiness, preoccupation with the body, and spending more time away from home are normal adolescent behaviors.
CN: Health promotion and maintenance; CNS: None; CL: Application

10. 2. Positive symptoms, such as delusions, hallucinations, thought disorder, and disorganized speech, respond to traditional antipsychotic drugs. Apathy, social withdrawal, and attention impairment are part of the category of negative symptoms, which also include affective flattening, restricted thought and speech, and anhedonia, and are more responsive to the atypical antipsychotics, such as clozapine (Clozaril), risperidone (Risperdal), and olanzapine (Zyprexa).
CN: Physiological integrity CNS: Pharmacological therapies; CL: Comprehension

11. 3. This response focuses on the son and helps him discuss and deal with his feelings. Unresolved feelings of guilt, shame, isolation, and loss of hope impact the family's ability to manage the crisis and be supportive to the client. The other responses offer premature reassurance and cut off the opportunity for the son to discuss his feelings.
CN: Psychosocial integrity; CNS: None; CL: Application

12. A client is about to be discharged with a prescription for the antipsychotic agent haloperidol (Haldol), 10 mg by mouth b.i.d. During a discharge teaching session, the nurse should reinforce which instruction with the patient?

    1. Take the medication 1 hour before a meal.

    2. Decrease the dosage if signs of illness decrease.

    3. Apply a sunscreen before being exposed to the sun.

    4. Increase the dosage up to 50 mg twice per day if signs of illness don't decrease.

13. Which symptom indicates tardive dyskinesia?

    1. Involuntary movements

    2. Blurred vision

    3. Restlessness

    4. Sudden fever

14. A client approaches a nurse and tells her that he hears a voice telling him that he's evil and deserves to die. Which term describes the client's perception?

    1. Delusion

    2. Disorganized speech

    3. Hallucination

    4. Idea of reference

15. A 49-year-old client is admitted to the emergency department frightened and reporting that he's hearing voices telling him to do bad things. Which intervention should be the nurse's <u>priority</u>?

    1. Tell the client he's safe and the voices aren't real.

    2. Tell the client he's safe now and promise the staff will protect him.

    3. Assess the nature of the commands by asking the client what the voices are saying.

    4. Administer a neuroleptic medication.

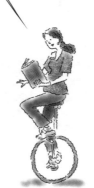

12. 3. Because haloperidol can cause photosensitivity and precipitate severe sunburn, the nurse should instruct the client to apply a sunscreen before exposure to the sun. The nurse should teach the client to take haloperidol with meals to prevent gastric upset or irritation, rather than 1 hour before, and should instruct the patient not to decrease or increase the dosage unless the physician orders it.

CN: Physiological integrity; CNS: Pharmacological therapies; CL: Application

13. 1. Symptoms of tardive dyskinesia include tongue protrusion, lip smacking, chewing, blinking, grimacing, choreiform movements of limbs and trunk, and foot tapping. Blurred vision is a common adverse reaction of antipsychotic drugs and usually disappears after a few weeks of therapy. Restlessness is associated with akathisia. Sudden fever may be a symptom of a malignant neurologic disorder.

CN: Physiological integrity; CNS: Reduction of risk potential; CL: Application

14. 3. Hallucinations are sensory experiences that are misrepresentations of reality or have no basis in reality. Delusions are beliefs not based in reality. Disorganized speech is characterized by jumping from one topic to the next or using unrelated words. An idea of reference is a belief that an unrelated situation holds special meaning for the client.

CN: Psychosocial integrity; CNS: None; CL: Knowledge

15. 3. Safety is the priority. The nurse should directly ask the client about the nature of the auditory commands to adequately assess the safety of the client and the staff. The nurse should never make promises to the client that she may not be able to fulfill. The physician may order a neuroleptic, but the nurse's priority is to address safety.

CN: Psychosocial integrity; CNS: None; CL: Application

CN: Client needs category   CNS: Client needs subcategory   CL: Cognitive level

16. What's the ideal number of members in an inpatient therapy group?
1. 1 to 4
2. 4 to 7
3. 7 to 10
4. 10 to 15

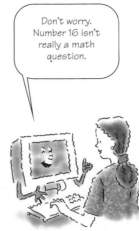

Don't worry. Number 16 isn't really a math question.

17. A client admitted to an inpatient unit approaches a nursing student saying he descended from a long line of people of a "super-race." Which action by the student is correct?
1. Smile and walk into the nurse's station.
2. Challenge the client's false belief.
3. Listen for hidden messages in themes of delusion, indicating unmet needs.
4. Introduce herself, shake hands, and sit down with the client in the day room.

18. The nurse assesses a schizophrenic client for auditory hallucinations. Which behavior is most suggestive of this symptom?
1. Speaking loudly when engaged in conversation
2. Ignoring comments by the nurse
3. Responding only to the same person
4. Tilting the head to one side

19. A nurse is assisting with morning care when a client suddenly throws off the covers and starts shouting, "My body is changing and disintegrating because I'm not of this world!" Which term best describes this behavior?
1. Depersonalization
2. Ideas of reference
3. Looseness of association
4. Paranoid ideation

16. 3. The ideal number of members in an inpatient group is 7 to 10. Having fewer than 7 members provides inadequate interaction and material for successful group process. Having more than 10 members doesn't allow for adequate time for individual participation.
CN: Psychosocial integrity; CNS: None; CL: Application

17. 4. The first goal is to establish a relationship with the client, which includes creating psychological space for the creation of trust. The student should sit and make herself available, reflecting concern and interest. Walking into the nurse's station would indicate disinterest and lack of concern about the client's feelings. Delusions are firmly maintained false beliefs, and attempts to dismiss or challenge them don't work. After establishing a relationship and lessening the client's anxiety, the student can orient the client to reality, listen to his concerns and fears, and try to understand the feelings reflected in the delusions.
CN: Safe, effective care environment; CNS: Coordinated care; CL: Application

18. 4. A client who's having auditory hallucinations may tilt his head to one side, as if listening to someone or something. Speaking loudly, ignoring comments, and responding only to one person are indicative of hearing deficit, anxiety, and paranoid behavior, respectively.
CN: Psychosocial integrity; CNS: None; CL: Analysis

19. 1. Depersonalization is a state in which the client feels unreal or believes parts of the body are being distorted. Ideas of reference are beliefs unrelated to situations and hold special meaning for the individual. The term *looseness of association* refers to sentences that have a vague connection to one another. Paranoid ideations are beliefs that others intend to harm the client in some way.
CN: Psychosocial integrity; CNS: None; CL: Analysis

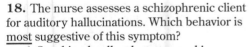

CN: Client needs category   CNS: Client needs subcategory   CL: Cognitive level

20. Many clients with schizophrenia simultaneously have opposing emotions. Which term describes this phenomenon?
1. Double bind
2. Ambivalence
3. Loose associations
4. Inappropriate affect

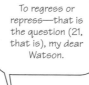

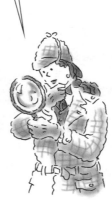

To regress or repress—that is the question (21, that is), my dear Watson.

21. A 16-year-old client with a diagnosis of undifferentiated schizophrenia has become very clingy and begins sucking her thumb while interacting with the nurse. The nurse understands that these behaviors indicate which defense mechanism?
1. Repression
2. Regression
3. Rationalization
4. Projection

22. A nurse on a psychiatric unit observes a client in the corner of the room moving his lips as if he were talking to himself. Which action is the <u>most appropriate</u>?
1. Asking him why he's talking to himself
2. Leaving him alone until he stops talking
3. Telling him it isn't good for him to talk to himself
4. Inviting him to join in a card game with the nurse

23. A client makes vague statements with no logical connections. He asks whether the nurse understands. Which response is <u>best</u>?
1. "Why don't we wait until later to talk about it?"
2. "You're not making sense, so I won't talk about this topic."
3. "Yes, I understand the overall sense of the logical connections from the idea."
4. "I want to understand what you're saying, but I'm having difficulty following you."

Shhh. Don't tell anyone I told you, but the answer to one of these questions is in the cards!

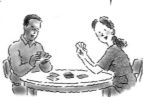

20. 2. Ambivalence, one of the symptoms associated with schizophrenia, immobilizes the person from acting. A double bind presents two conflicting messages—for example, saying that you trust someone but then not allowing the person in your room. Loose association involves rapid shifts of ideas from one subject to another in an unrelated manner. Inappropriate affect refers to an observable expression of emotion incongruent with the emotion felt.
CN: Psychosocial integrity; CNS: None; CL: Comprehension

21. 2. Regression, a return to earlier behavior in order to reduce anxiety, is the basic defense mechanism in schizophrenia. Repression is the blocking of unacceptable thoughts or impulses from the consciousness. Rationalization is a defense mechanism used to justify one's behavior. Projection is a defense mechanism in which one blames others and attempts to justify actions.
CN: Psychosocial integrity; CNS: None; CL: Application

22. 4. Being with the nurse and playing a game provide stimulation that competes with the hallucinations. Being alone keeps the client in his fantasy world. Telling him it isn't good to talk to himself fails to show an understanding of how real his fantasy world and hallucinations are.
CN: Psychosocial integrity; CNS: None; CL: Application

23. 4. The nurse must communicate that she wants to understand without blaming the client for the lack of understanding. Asking the client to wait because he's too confused cuts off an attempt to communicate and asks the client to do what he can't at present. Telling the client that he isn't making sense is judgmental and could impair the therapeutic relationship. Pretending to understand is a violation of trust and can damage the therapeutic relationship.
CN: Psychosocial integrity; CNS: None; CL: Application

CN: Client needs category   CNS: Client needs subcategory   CL: Cognitive level

24. A client asks a nurse if she hears the voice of the nonexistent man speaking to him. Which response is best?
1. "No one is in your room except you."
2. "Yes, I hear him, but I won't listen to him."
3. "What has he told you? Is it helpful advice?"
4. "No, I don't hear him, but I know you do. What's he saying?"

25. Which instruction is correct for a client taking chlorpromazine (Thorazine)?
1. Reduce the dosage if you feel better.
2. Occasional social drinking isn't harmful.
3. Stop taking the drug immediately if adverse reactions develop.
4. Schedule routine medication checks.

26. A 34-year-old woman is referred to a mental health clinic by the court. The client harassed a couple next door to her with charges that the husband was in love with her. She wrote love notes and called him on the telephone throughout the night. The client is employed and has had no problems with her job. Which disorder is suspected?
1. Major depression
2. Paranoid schizophrenia
3. Delusional disorder
4. Bipolar affective disorder

27. A client with a diagnosis of paranoid-type schizophrenia is receiving an antipsychotic medication. His physician has just prescribed benztropine (Cogentin). The nurse realizes that this medication was most likely prescribed in response to which possible adverse reaction?
1. Tardive dyskinesia
2. Hypertensive crisis
3. Acute dystonia
4. Orthostatic hypotension

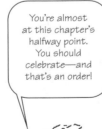

You're almost at this chapter's halfway point. You should celebrate—and that's an order!

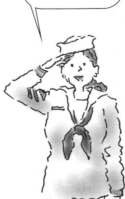

24. 4. This response points out reality and shows concern and support. Attempting to argue the client out of the belief might entrench him more firmly in his belief, making him feel more out of control because of the negative and fearful nature of hallucinations. The other two responses violate the trust of the therapeutic relationship.
CN: Safe, effective care environment; CNS: Coordinated care; CL: Application

25. 4. Ongoing assessment by a practitioner is important to assess for adverse reactions and continued therapeutic effectiveness. The dosage should be cut only after checking with the practitioner. Alcoholic beverages are contraindicated while taking an antipsychotic drug. Adverse reactions should be reported immediately to determine if the drug should be discontinued.
CN: Physiological integrity; CNS: Pharmacological therapies; CL: Application

26. 3. The client has a delusional disorder with erotomanic delusions as her primary symptom, and believes she's loved intensely by a married person showing no interest in her. No symptoms of major depression exist. The client doesn't believe someone is trying to harm her (the hallmark characteristic of paranoia). Bipolar affective disorder is characterized by cycles of extreme emotional highs (mania) and lows (depression).
CN: Psychosocial integrity; CNS: None; CL: Application

27. 3. Benztropine is used as adjunctive therapy in parkinsonism and for all conditions and medications that produce extrapyramidal symptoms except tardive dyskinesia. Its anticholinergic effect reduces the extrapyramidal effects associated with antipsychotic drugs. Hypertensive crisis and orthostatic hypotension aren't associated with extrapyramidal symptoms.
CN: Physiological integrity; CNS: Pharmacological therapies; CL: Analysis

CN: Client needs category   CNS: Client needs subcategory   CL: Cognitive level

28. A 20-year-old client is admitted to the hospital with a diagnosis of schizophrenia. During the initial assessment, he points to the nurse's stethoscope and says it's a snake. Which term describes this phenomenon?
1. Abstraction
2. Delusion
3. Hallucination
4. Illusion

29. A 52-year-old schizophrenic client was admitted to the hospital 2 days ago and began medication treatment with haloperidol (Haldol). When reviewing the progress record, the nurse notes the entry below. Which laboratory result needs to be reported immediately?

Progress notes
9/4/08 1345 — Client is pale and diaphoretic, with warm skin. She has tremors and difficulty speaking. Vital signs: Temp, 102.6° F; BP, 160/98 mm Hg; heart rate, 94 beats/minute; respiratory rate, 20 breaths/minute. Laboratory results received: CK, 500 units/L; WBC, 15,000/l; HCT, 38%; Hb, 14 g/dl.————Barbara Smith, L.P.N.

1. CK and HCT
2. WBC and HCT
3. CK and WBC
4. WBC and Hb

30. A client can't eat because he believes his bowels have turned against him. Which term describes this phenomenon?
1. Conversion hysteria
2. Depersonalization
3. Hypochondriasis
4. Somatic delusion

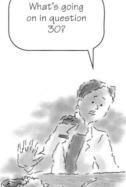

What's going on in question 30?

31. Which action by the nurse is an appropriate therapeutic intervention for a client experiencing hallucinations?
1. Confining him to his room until he feels better
2. Providing a competing stimulus that distracts from the hallucinations
3. Discouraging attempts to understand what precipitates his hallucinations
4. Supporting perceptual distortions until he gives them up of his own accord

28. 4. An illusion is a misinterpretation of an actual sensory stimulation. An abstraction is an idea or concept, such as love or a belief that can't be represented by a concrete object. A delusion is a fixed belief and a hallucination is a false sensory perception without a stimulus.
CN: Psychosocial integrity; CNS: None; CL: Comprehension

29. 3. The client's symptoms and elevated CK level and WBC count indicate she's probably suffering from neuroleptic malignant syndrome (NMS), a potentially fatal reaction to antipsychotic medications. Signs and symptoms of NMS include elevated blood pressure, hyperthermia, muscle rigidity, diaphoresis, and pale skin. HCT and Hb are within normal range.
CN: Psychosocial integrity; CNS: Reduction of risk potential; CL: Analysis

30. 4. A somatic delusion is a fixed false belief pertaining to the body and body parts. Conversion hysteria is a somatoform disorder in which there are symptoms of some physical illness without any underlying organic cause. Depersonalization is a feeling of unreality concerning self and a loss of self-identity, with things around the person seeming different, strange, or unreal. Hypochondriasis is somatic overconcern with a morbid attention to details of body functioning.
CN: Psychosocial integrity; CNS: None; CL: Comprehension

31. 2. Providing a competing stimulus acknowledges the presence of the hallucinations and teaches ways to decrease their frequency. The other nursing actions support and maintain hallucinations or deny their existence.
CN: Psychosocial integrity; CNS: None; CL: Application

CN: Client needs category CNS: Client needs subcategory CL: Cognitive level

32. A client with schizophrenia reports that her hallucinations have decreased in frequency. Which intervention would be appropriate to begin addressing the client's problem with social isolation?
1. Having the client join in a group game
2. Naming the client as the leader of the client support group
3. Having the client play solitaire
4. Asking the client to participate in a group sing-along

33. A single, 24-year-old client is admitted with acute schizophrenic reaction. Which method is appropriate therapy for this type of schizophrenia?
1. Counseling to produce insight into behavior
2. Biofeedback to reduce agitation associated with schizophrenia
3. Drug therapy to reduce symptoms associated with acute schizophrenia
4. Electroconvulsive therapy to treat the mood component of schizophrenia

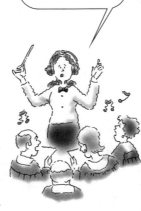

This kind of activity might be therapeutic for a client but, to me, it's painful!

34. A client tells a nurse that voices are telling him to do "terrible things." Which action is part of the initial therapy?
1. Finding out what the voices are telling him
2. Letting him go to his room to decrease his anxiety
3. Beginning to talk to the client about an unrelated topic
4. Telling the client the voices aren't real

35. A newly admitted client is diagnosed with schizophrenia. The client tells the nurse that the police are looking for him and will kill him if they find him. The nurse recognizes this as a delusion of which type?
1. Paranoid
2 Religious
3. Grandiose
4. Somatic

32. 4. Having the client participate in a noncompetitive group activity that doesn't require individual participation won't present a threat to the client. Games can become competitive and can lead to anxiety or hostility. The client probably lacks sufficient social skills to lead a group at this time. Playing solitaire doesn't encourage socialization.
CN: Psychosocial integrity; CNS: None; CL: Application

33. 3. Drug therapy is usually successful in normalizing behavior and reducing or eliminating hallucinations, delusions, thought disorder, affect flattening, apathy, avolition, and asociality. Counseling to produce insight into the client's behavior usually isn't appropriate in an acute schizophrenic reaction. Biofeedback reduces anxiety and modifies behavioral responses but isn't the major component in the treatment of schizophrenia. Electroconvulsive therapy might be considered for schizoaffective disorder (which has a mood component) and is a treatment of choice for clinical depression.
CN: Psychosocial integrity; CNS: None; CL: Comprehension

34. 1. For safety purposes, the nurse must find out whether the voices are directing the client to harm himself or others. Further assessment can help identify appropriate therapeutic interventions. Isolating a person during this intense sensory confusion commonly reinforces the psychosis. Changing the topic indicates that the nurse isn't concerned about the client's fears. Dismissing the voices shuts down communication between the client and the nurse.
CN: Safe, effective care environment; CNS: Safety and infection control; CL: Application

35. 1. This client is exhibiting paranoid delusions, which are excessive or irrational suspicions or distrust of others. A religious delusion is the belief that one is favored by a higher being or is an instrument of a higher being. A grandiose delusion is the belief that one possesses greatness or special powers. A somatic delusion is the belief that one's body or body parts are distorted or diseased.
CN: Psychosocial integrity; CNS: None; CL: Knowledge

36. Which instructions are <u>most appropriate</u> for a client who has started taking haloperidol (Haldol)?
1. "You should report feelings of restlessness or agitation at once."
2. "You can take your herbal supplements safely with this drug."
3. "Be aware that you'll feel increased energy taking this drug."
4. "This drug will indirectly control essential hypertension."

37. The nurse is having an interaction with a 38-year-old male delusional client. Which is the <u>best</u> nursing action?
1. Telling the client the delusions aren't real
2. Explaining the delusion to the client
3. Encouraging the client to remain delusional
4. Beginning to develop a trusting relationship with the client

38. Which cluster of symptoms would indicate schizophrenia?
1. Persistent, intrusive thoughts leading to repetitive, ritualistic behaviors
2. Feelings of helplessness and hopelessness
3. Unstable moods and delusions of grandeur
4. Hallucinations or delusions and decreased ability to function in society

39. The nurse is caring for a 58-year-old male client diagnosed with paranoid schizophrenia. When the client says, "The earth and the roof of the house rule the political structure with particles of rain," the nurse recognizes this as which type of expression?
1. Tangentiality
2. Perseveration
3. Loose association
4. Thought blocking

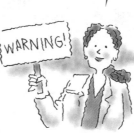

Arguing with a delusional client will set in motion a struggle that just can't be won!

WARNING!

36. 1. Agitation and restlessness are adverse effects of haloperidol and can be treated with anticholinergic drugs. Using herbal supplements while taking haloperidol may interfere with the drug's effectiveness. Although the client may experience increased concentration and activity, these effects are due to a decrease in symptoms, not the drug itself. Haloperidol isn't likely to cause essential hypertension.
CN: Physiological integrity; CNS: Pharmacological therapies; CL: Application

37. 4. Developing a trusting relationship gives the nurse more therapeutic time with the client. Never argue with or try to talk the client out of a delusion. The delusions are very real to him. Explaining the delusions helps the nurse, not the client. Encouraging the client to remain delusional isn't therapeutic.
CN: Psychosocial integrity; CNS: None; CL: Application

38. 4. Schizophrenia is a brain disease characterized by a variety of symptoms, including hallucinations, delusions, and asociality. Clients with obsessive-compulsive disorder experience intrusive thoughts and ritualistic behaviors. Feelings of helplessness and hopelessness are pivotal symptoms of clinical depression. Unstable moods and delusions of grandeur are characteristics of bipolar affective disorder.
CN: Psychosocial integrity; CNS: None; CL: Comprehension

39. 3. Loose association refers to changing ideas from one unrelated theme to another, as exhibited by the client. Tangentiality is the wandering from topic to topic. Perseveration is involuntary repetition of the answer to a question in response to a new question. Thought blocking is having difficulty articulating a response or stopping midsentence.
CN: Psychosocial integrity; CNS: None; CL: Application

40. During the initial interview, a schizophrenic client states to the nurse, "I don't enjoy things anymore. I used to love to read mystery books, but even that isn't enjoyable now." The nurse correctly identifies the client is experiencing which of the following conditions?
1. Avolition
2. Anhedonia
3. Alogia
4. Flat affect

41. A client is admitted after being found on a highway, hitting at cars and yelling at motorists. When approached by the nurse, the client shouts, "You're the one who stole my husband from me." Which condition describes the client's condition?
1. Hallucinatory experience
2. Delusional experience
3. Disorientation to the environment
4. Asking for limit-setting from the staff

42. When teaching the family of a client with schizophrenia, the nurse should provide which information?
1. Relapse can be prevented if the client takes medication.
2. Support is available to help family members meet their own needs.
3. Improvement should occur if the client has a stimulating environment.
4. Stressful situations in the family can precipitate a relapse in the client.

43. A nurse is caring for a client hospitalized on a psychiatric unit. The client repeats the nurse's phrases and shows motor immobility with prominent grimacing. Which medical diagnosis is most likely?
1. Catatonic schizophrenia
2. Disorganized schizophrenia
3. Residual schizophrenia
4. Undifferentiated schizophrenia

40. 2. Anhedonia is the loss of pleasure in things that are usually pleasurable. Avolition is the lack of motivation. Alogia, also called *poverty of speech,* is a decrease in the amount of richness of speech. A flat affect is absence of emotional expression.
CN: Psychosocial integrity; CNS: None; CL: Application

41. 2. A delusion is a false belief manufactured without appropriate or sufficient evidence to support it. The client's statements don't represent hallucinations because they aren't perceptual disorders. No information in the question addresses orientation. Although limit-setting is integral to a safe environment, the client's statement reflects issues about self-esteem.
CN: Psychosocial integrity; CNS: None; CL: Application

42. 2. Because family members of a client with schizophrenia face difficult situations and great stress, the nurse should inform them of support services that can help them cope with such problems. The nurse should also teach them that medication can't prevent relapses and that environmental stimuli may precipitate symptoms. Although stress can trigger symptoms, the nurse shouldn't make the family feel responsible for relapses.
CN: Health promotion and maintenance; CNS: None; CL: Application

43. 1. Motor immobility, parroting phrases, and grimacing are characteristics of catatonic schizophrenia. Symptoms of disorganized schizophrenia are disorganized speech and behaviors with flat or inappropriate affect. Symptoms of residual schizophrenia include odd beliefs, eccentric behavior, and illogical thinking. Undifferentiated schizophrenia is characterized by delusions or hallucinations and other behaviors common to other types of schizophrenia.
CN: Psychosocial integrity; CNS: None; CL: Comprehension

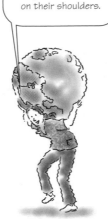

The family members of a client with schizophrenia commonly feel like they have the weight of the world on their shoulders.

44. A nurse on an inpatient unit is having a discussion with a client with schizophrenia about his schedule for the day. The client comments that he was highly active at home, and then explains the volunteer job he held. Which term describes the client's thinking?
1. Circumstantiality
2. Loose associations
3. Referential
4. Tangentiality

45. While talking to a client with schizophrenia, a nurse notes that the client frequently uses unrecognizable words with no common meaning. Which term describes this?
1. Echolalia
2. Clang association
3. Neologisms
4. Word salad

46. While caring for a hospitalized client diagnosed with schizophrenia, a nurse observes the client watching television. The client tells the nurse the television is speaking directly to him. Which term describes this belief?
1. Autistic thinking
2. Concrete thinking
3. Paranoid thinking
4. Referential thinking

47. A nurse is talking with a family of a client diagnosed with schizophrenia. The mother asks, "What causes this disease?" Which explanation for the disorder is the most widely accepted?
1. Prenatal or postpartum central nervous system damage
2. Bacterial infections of the mother during pregnancy or delivery
3. A biological predisposition exacerbated by environmental stressors
4. Lack of bonding and attachment during infancy, which leads to depression in later life

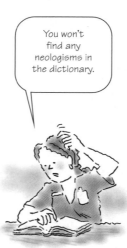

You won't find any neologisms in the dictionary.

44. 4. Tangentiality describes thought patterns loosely connected but not directly related to the topic. In circumstantiality, the person digresses with unnecessary details. Loose associations are rapid shifts in the expression of ideas from one subject to another in an unrelated manner. An individual who demonstrates referential thinking incorrectly interprets neutral incidents and external events as having a particular or special meaning for him.
CN: Psychosocial integrity; CNS: None; CL: Application

45. 3. Neologisms are newly coined words with personal meaning to the client with schizophrenia. Word salads are words strung in sequence that have no connection to one another. Echolalia is parrotlike echoing of spoken words or sounds. Clanging is the association of words by sound rather than meaning.
CN: Psychosocial integrity; CNS: None; CL: Application

46. 4. Referential, or primary process, thinking is a belief that incidents and events in the environment have special meaning for the client. Autistic thinking is a disturbance in thought due to the intrusion of a private fantasy world, internally stimulated, resulting in abnormal responses to people. Concrete thinking is the literal interpretation of words and symbols. A client with paranoid thinking believes that others are trying to harm him.
CN: Psychosocial integrity; CNS: None; CL: Comprehension

47. 3. The holistic theory, currently the most widely accepted theory of its type, states that an interaction between biological predisposition and environmental stressors is the cause of schizophrenia. The biological explanation states that schizophrenia is caused by a brain disease, a bacterial infection in utero, or early brain damage. The psychoanalytic perspective involves the belief that the mother-infant bond is the source of the schizophrenia.
CN: Physiological integrity; CNS: Physiological adaptation; CL: Application

48. A 31-year-old female client with a diagnosis of schizophrenia walks with the nurse to the dayroom but refuses to speak. What's the most therapeutic nursing intervention?
1. Ignoring the refusal to speak and talking about something such as the weather
2. Telling the client that the refusal to speak is making others uncomfortable
3. Spending time with the client, even in silence
4. Making the client attend therapy with others so the other clients can encourage talking

48. 3. Spending time with the client lets her know that the nurse cares. Although sitting in silence can be awkward, it's therapeutic. Ignoring the behavior and using small talk encourages the silence. Telling the client about making others uncomfortable usually has no effect on the behavior. Coercing the client to attend therapy with others would encourage continued silence.

CN: Psychosocial integrity; CNS: None; CL: Application

49. A client is taking chlorpromazine (Thorazine) for the treatment of schizophrenia. This drug blocks the transmission of which substance?
1. Dopamine
2. Epinephrine
3. Norepinephrine
4. Thyroxine

49. 1. Most antipsychotic agents block the transmission of dopamine to the brain. Other transmitters linked to schizophrenia include serotonin, acetylcholine, and norepinephrine. Epinephrine, norepinephrine, and thyroxine aren't blocked by chlorpromazine.

CN: Physiological integrity; CNS: Pharmacological therapies; CL: Knowledge

50. In preparation for discharge, a client diagnosed with schizophrenia was taught self–symptom monitoring as part of a relapse prevention program. Which statement indicates the client understands symptom monitoring?
1. "When I hear voices, I become afraid I'll relapse."
2. "My parents aren't involved enough to be aware if I begin to relapse."
3. "My family is more protected from stress if I keep them out of my illness process."
4. "When I'm feeling stressed, I go to a quiet room of the house by myself and do imagery."

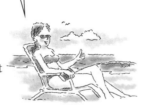

I'm using imagery to picture myself at the beach, in a comfortable chair, and completely stress-free. Wow! This stuff really works.

50. 4. This statement indicates the client has learned a technique for coping with stress with the use of imagery. The other statements don't show an understanding of self–symptom monitoring and may result in symptom intensification and possible relapse.

CN: Psychosocial integrity; CNS: None; CL: Application

51. A client diagnosed with schizophrenia has been taking haloperidol (Haldol) for 1 week when a nurse observes that the client's gaze is fixed on the ceiling. Which <u>specific</u> condition is the client exhibiting?
1. Akathisia
2. Neuroleptic malignant syndrome
3. Oculogyric crisis
4. Tardive dyskinesia

51. 3. An oculogyric crisis involves a fixed positioning of the eyes, typically in an upward gaze. The condition is uncomfortable but not life-threatening. Akathisia is a restlessness that can cause pacing and tapping of the fingers or feet. High fever, sweating, unstable blood pressure, stupor, and muscular rigidity are signs of neuroleptic malignant syndrome. Stereotyped involuntary movements (tongue protrusion, lip smacking, chewing, blinking, and grimacing) characterize tardive dyskinesia.

CN: Physiological integrity; CNS: Pharmacological therapies; CL: Application

CN: Client needs category   CNS: Client needs subcategory   CL: Cognitive level

52. A 50-year-old schizophrenic client becomes agitated and confronts the nurse with clenched fists. Which would be the <u>most</u> appropriate intervention by the nurse?

1. Take the client by the hand and lead him to the activity room for cards.
2. Step up to the client and tell him his behavior is inappropriate.
3. Call for security to take him to a seclusion room.
4. Speak to him in a quiet voice and offer him medication to help him calm down.

53. A client taking antipsychotic medications shows dystonic reactions, including torticollis and oculogyric crisis. Which medication is typically prescribed to treat these adverse reactions?

1. Benztropine (Cogentin)
2. Chlordiazepoxide (Librium)
3. Diazepam (Valium)
4. Fluoxetine (Prozac)

54. A 22-year-old woman was brought to the hospital by her parents because of her bizarre behavior. The parents reported that she stayed in her room, refused to eat meals with the family, and talked to herself almost constantly. She lost interest in her job and had been fired because of her inability to perform. During the intake process, the nurse notes that the client is unkempt, has body odor, exhibits illogical thought patterns, and appears to be listening to someone no one else can see or hear. Which nursing goal is the <u>priority</u> for this client?

1. Maintaining safety
2. Ensuring adequate nutrition
3. Orienting the client
4. Providing hygiene measures

52. 4. Always use the least restrictive means to calm a client. Never touch an agitated client; touch can be misinterpreted as a threat and further escalate the situation. Stepping up to an agitated client can be seen as an aggressive act. Seclusion is a last resort.
CN: Physiological integrity; CNS: Reduction of risk potential; CL: Application

53. 1. Benztropine and trihexyphenidyl (Artane) are anticholinergic drugs used to counteract the dystonic reactions and other adverse reactions of antipsychotic drugs. The antihistamine diphenhydramine (Benadryl) is also effective in treating extrapyramidal symptoms. Fluoxetine is an antidepressant, and diazepam and chlordiazepoxide are minor tranquilizers or antianxiety agents.
CN: Physiological integrity; CNS: Pharmacological therapies; CL: Application

54. 1. Whenever a client is hallucinating or otherwise out of touch with reality, safety is always the primary concern. Although ensuring adequate nutrition, orienting the client, and providing hygiene measures are valid concerns, they're all secondary to ensuring a safe environment.
CN: Safe, effective care environment; CNS: Safety and infection control; CL: Application

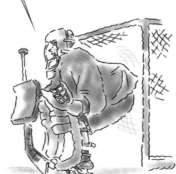

When in danger of being hit in the face with a puck—or when caring for a client who's out of touch with reality—think safety first!

55. As a nurse approaches the nurses' station, a client diagnosed with a delusional disorder raises his voice and says, "You're following me. What do you want?" To prevent escalating fear and anger, the nurse takes a nonthreatening posture and makes which response in a calm voice?
1. "Are you frightened?"
2. "You know I'm not following you."
3. "You'll have to go into seclusion if you continue to threaten me."
4. "I'm sorry if I frightened you. I was returning to the nurses' station after going out for lunch."

56. Which action by a client with stable schizophrenia is <u>most important</u> for preventing relapse?
1. Attending group therapy sessions
2. Participating in family support meetings
3. Attending social skills training sessions
4. Consistently taking prescribed medications

57. A client approaches the nurse and points at the sky, showing her where the men would be coming from to get him. Which response is <u>most therapeutic</u>?
1. "Why do you think the men are coming here?"
2. "You're safe here; we won't let them harm you."
3. "It seems like the world is pretty scary for you, but you're safe here."
4. "There are no bad men in the sky because no one lives that close to earth."

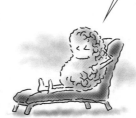

It's easier for me to relax when I know relapse is less likely. Check out question 56 and you'll understand what I mean.

58. A client is brought to the crisis response center by his family. During evaluation, he reports being depressed for the last month and complains about voices constantly whispering to him. Which diagnosis is the <u>most likely</u>?
1. Catatonic schizophrenia
2. Disorganized schizophrenia
3. Paranoid schizophrenia
4. Schizoaffective disorder

55. 4. Being clear in communication, remaining calm, and showing concern increases the chance the client will cooperate, lessening the potential for violence. The first response tries to identify the client's feelings but doesn't convey warmth and concern. The second response isn't empathic and shows no indication of trying to reach the client at a level beyond content of communication. The third response may increase the client's anxiety, fear, and mistrust when the nurse engages in a power struggle and triggers competitiveness within the client.
CN: Psychosocial integrity; CNS: None; CL: Application

56. 4. Although all of the choices are important for preventing relapse, compliance with the medication regimen is central to the treatment of schizophrenia, a brain disease.
CN: Safe, effective care environment; CNS: Coordinated care; CL: Application

57. 3. This response acknowledges the client's fears, listens to his feelings, and offers a sense of security as the nurse tries to understand the concerns behind the symbolism. She reflects these concerns to the client, along with reassurance of safety. The first response validates the delusion, not the feelings and fears, and doesn't orient the client to reality. The second response gives false reassurance. Because the nurse isn't sure of the symbolism, she can't make this promise. The last response rejects the client's feelings and doesn't address his fears.
CN: Safe, effective care environment; CNS: Coordinated care; CL: Application

58. 4. A client with a major depressive episode who begins to hear voices is most likely schizoaffective. The client who repeats phrases and shows waxy flexibility or stupor with prominent grimaces is most likely catatonic. The client with disorganized speech and behavior and a flat or inappropriate affect most likely has disorganized schizophrenia. The client who expresses thoughts of people spying on him, attributes ulterior motives to others, and has a flat affect is most likely paranoid schizophrenic.
CN: Psychosocial integrity; CNS: None; CL: Analysis

CN: Client needs category   CNS: Client needs subcategory   CL: Cognitive level

59. The nurse monitoring a client who appears to be hallucinating notes paranoid content in the client's speech. The client appears agitated, gesturing at a figure on the television. Which nursing intervention is appropriate? Select all that apply:

1. Instruct the client to stop the behavior.
2. Reinforce that the client isn't in danger.
3. Acknowledge the presence of the hallucinations.
4. Instruct other team members to ignore the client's behavior.
5. Immediately apply physical restraints.
6. Use a calm voice and simple commands.

59. 2, 3, 6. Using a calm voice, the nurse should reassure the client that he's safe. She shouldn't challenge the client; rather, she should acknowledge his hallucinatory experience. It isn't appropriate to request that the client stop the behavior or that other team members ignore the client's behavior. Implementing restraints isn't warranted at this time. Although the client is agitated, no evidence exists that he's at risk for harming himself or others.
CN: Psychosocial integrity; CNS: None; CL: Application

60. A client with schizophrenia is taking the atypical antipsychotic medication clozapine (Clozaril). Which signs and symptoms indicate the presence of adverse effects associated with this medication? Select all that apply:

1. Sore throat
2. Pill-rolling movements
3. Polyuria
4. Fever
5. Polydipsia
6. Orthostatic hypotension

60. 1, 4. Sore throat, fever, and sudden onset of other flulike symptoms are signs of agranulocytosis, an adverse effect of clozapine caused by an insufficient number of granulocytes, which causes the individual to be susceptible to infection. The client's white blood cell count should be monitored at least weekly throughout the course of treatment. Pill-rolling movements can occur in those experiencing extrapyramidal adverse effects associated with antipsychotic medication prescribed for much longer than a medication such as clozapine. Polydipsia (excessive thirst) and polyuria (increased urine) are common adverse effects of lithium. Orthostatic hypotension is an adverse effect of tricyclic antidepressants.
CN: Physiological integrity; CNS: Pharmacological therapies; CL: Application

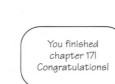

You finished chapter 17! Congratulations!

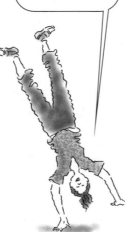

61. A physician starts a client on the antipsychotic medication haloperidol (Haldol). The nurse is aware that this medication has extrapyramidal adverse effects. Which measures should the nurse take when administering this drug? Select all that apply:

1. Review subcutaneous injection technique.
2. Closely monitor vital signs, especially temperature.
3. Provide the client with the opportunity to pace.
4. Monitor blood glucose levels.
5. Provide the client with hard candy.
6. Monitor for signs and symptoms of urticaria.

61. 2, 3, 5. Neuroleptic malignant syndrome is a life-threatening extrapyramidal adverse effect of antipsychotic medications such as haloperidol. It's associated with a rapid increase in temperature. The most common extrapyramidal adverse effect, akathisia, is a form of psychomotor restlessness that can commonly be relieved by pacing. Haloperidol and the anticholinergic medications that are provided to alleviate its extrapyramidal effects can result in dry mouth. Providing the client with hard candy to suck on can help alleviate this problem. Haloperidol isn't given subcutaneously and doesn't affect blood glucose levels. Urticaria isn't usually associated with this drug's administration.
CN: Physiological integrity; CNS: Pharmacological therapies; CL: Analysis

CN: Client needs category   CNS: Client needs subcategory   CL: Cognitive level

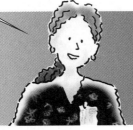

Substance abuse is
serious business—as is
answering these questions
carefully and thoughtfully.

Chapter 18
Substance abuse disorders

1. Family members of a client who abuses alcohol ask a nurse to help them intervene. Which action is essential for a successful intervention?
    1. All family members must tell the client they're powerless.
    2. All family members must describe how the addiction affects them.
    3. All family members must come up with their share of financial support.
    4. All family members must become caregivers during the detoxification period.

2. A client who abuses alcohol tells a nurse, "I'm sure I can become a social drinker." Which response is <u>most appropriate</u>?
    1. "When do you think you can become a social drinker?"
    2. "What makes you think you'll learn to drink normally?"
    3. "What examples of major problems in your life are related to your alcohol use?"
    4. "How many alcoholic beverages can a social drinker consume?"

3. A client asks a nurse not to tell his parents about his alcohol problem. Which response is <u>most appropriate</u>?
    1. "How can you not tell them? Is that being honest?"
    2. "Don't you think you'll need to tell them someday?"
    3. "Do alcohol problems run in either side of your family?"
    4. "What do you think will happen if you tell your parents?"

The fear of being
judged can keep a
client from asking for
the help he so
desperately needs.

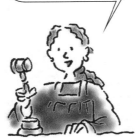

1. 2. After the family is taught about addiction, they must write down examples of how the addiction has affected each of them and use this information during the intervention. It isn't necessary to tell the client the family is powerless. The family is empowered through this intervention experience. In many cases, a third-party payer will help with treatment costs. Doing an intervention doesn't make family members responsible for financial support or providing care and support during the detoxification period.
CN: Psychosocial integrity; CNS: None; CL: Analysis

2. 3. This question may help the client recall the problematic results of using alcohol and the reasons the client began treatment. Asking when he believes he can become a social drinker will only encourage the addicted person to deny the problem and develop an unrealistic, self-defeating goal. Asking how many alcoholic beverages a social drinker can consume, and why the client thinks he can drink normally will encourage the addicted person to defend himself and deny the problem.
CN: Psychosocial integrity; CNS: None; CL: Application

3. 4. Clients who struggle with addiction problems commonly believe people will be judgmental, rejecting, and uncaring if they're told that the client is recovering from alcohol abuse. The first response challenges the client and will put him on the defensive. The second response will make the client defensive and construct rationalizations about why his parents don't need to know. The third response is a good assessment question, but isn't appropriate to ask a client who's afraid to tell others about his addiction.
CN: Psychosocial integrity; CNS: None; CL: Analysis

4. A nurse assesses a client for signs of alcohol withdrawal. During the period of <u>early</u> withdrawal, which finding is expected?
1. Depression
2. Hyperactivity
3. Insomnia
4. Nausea

5. Which condition is <u>most commonly</u> found in a client who chronically abuses alcohol?
1. Enlarged liver
2. Nasal irritation
3. Muscle wasting
4. Limb paresthesia

6. Within 8 hours of her last drink, an alcoholic client experiences tremors, loss of appetite, and disordered thinking. The nurse believes this client is in second-stage withdrawal. What should the nurse do next?
1. Give disulfiram (Antabuse) as prescribed.
2. Obtain a physician's order for lorazepam (Ativan).
3. Help the client engage in progressive muscle-relaxation techniques.
4. Provide the client with constant one-on-one monitoring.

7. A client who abuses alcohol tells a nurse, "Alcohol helps me sleep." Which information about alcohol use affecting sleep is <u>most accurate</u>?
1. Alcohol doesn't help promote sleep.
2. Continued alcohol use causes insomnia.
3. One glass of alcohol at dinnertime can induce sleep.
4. Sometimes alcohol can make one drowsy enough to fall asleep.

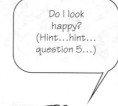

Do I look happy? (Hint...hint... question 5...)

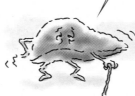

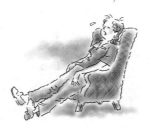

Are sleep and alcohol a good mix? If I told you, I'd be giving away the answer to question 7!

4. 4. Nausea and, later, vomiting are early signs of alcohol withdrawal. Depression, hyperactivity, and insomnia aren't associated with early alcohol withdrawal.
CN: Psychosocial integrity; CNS: None; CL: Knowledge

5. 1. A major effect of alcohol on the body is liver impairment, and an enlarged liver is a common physical finding. Nasal irritation is commonly seen in clients who snort cocaine. Muscle wasting and limb paresthesia don't tend to occur in clients who abuse alcohol.
CN: Psychosocial integrity; CNS: None; CL: Knowledge

6. 2. A client in second-stage withdrawal should be medicated with a benzodiazepine, such as lorazepam, to prevent progression of symptoms to alcohol-withdrawal delirium, a life-threatening withdrawal syndrome. Disulfiram is used during early recovery, not during detoxification. Progressive muscle relaxation isn't particularly effective during withdrawal. Close monitoring during withdrawal is appropriate after the client has been medicated for withdrawal symptoms.
CN: Psychosocial integrity ; CNS: None; CL: Application

7. 2. Alcohol use may initially promote sleep but, with continued use, it causes insomnia. Evidence shows that alcohol doesn't facilitate sleep. One glass of alcohol at dinnertime won't induce sleep. The statement that alcohol can make one drowsy enough to fall asleep doesn't give information about how alcohol affects sleep. It makes the client think alcohol use to induce sleep is an appropriate strategy.
CN: Psychosocial integrity; CNS: None; CL: Analysis

CN: Client needs category   CNS: Client needs subcategory   CL: Cognitive level

8. A family expresses concern when a family member withdrawing from alcohol is given lorazepam (Ativan). What information should be given to the family about the medication?
1. The medication promotes a sense of well-being during the client's difficult withdrawal period.
2. The medication is given for a short time to help the client complete the withdrawal process.
3. The medication will help the client forget about the physical sensations that accompany alcohol withdrawal.
4. The medication helps in the treatment of coexisting diseases, such as cardiac problems and hypertension.

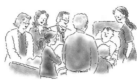

It's important to teach the client's family too.

8. 2. Lorazepam is a short-acting benzodiazepine that may be given for 1 week to help the client in alcohol withdrawal. However, there's some debate over its use due to a potential risk for cross-addiction. The medication isn't given to help forget the experience; it lessens the symptoms of withdrawal. It isn't used to treat coexisting cardiovascular problems or promote a sense of well-being.
CN: Physiological integrity; CNS: Pharmacological therapies; CL: Comprehension

9. A client who abuses alcohol tells a nurse that everyone in his family has an alcohol problem and nothing can be done about it. Which response is the most appropriate?
1. "You're right; it's much harder to become a recovering person."
2. "This is just an excuse for you so you don't have to work on becoming sober."
3. "Sometimes nothing can be done, but you may be the exception in this family."
4. "Alcohol problems can occur in families, but you can decide to take the steps to become and stay sober."

9. 4. This statement challenges the client to become proactive and take the steps necessary to maintain a sober lifestyle. The first response agrees with the client's denial and isn't a useful response. The second response confronts the client and may make him more adamant in defense of this position. The third response agrees with the client's denial and isn't a useful response.
CN: Psychosocial integrity; CNS: None; CL: Application

10. Which major cardiovascular problem may occur in a client with chronic alcoholism?
1. Arteriosclerosis
2. Heart failure
3. Heart valve damage
4. Pericarditis

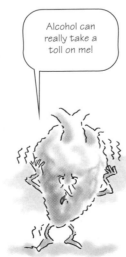

Alcohol can really take a toll on me!

10. 2. Heart failure is a severe cardiac consequence associated with long-term alcohol use. Arteriosclerosis, heart valve damage, and pericarditis aren't medical consequences of alcoholism.
CN: Physiological integrity; CNS: Reduction of risk potential; CL: Knowledge

11. Which finding is commonly associated with abuse of alcohol in a young, depressed adult woman?
1. Defiant responses
2. Infertility
3. Memory loss
4. Sexual abuse

11. 4. Many women diagnosed with substance abuse problems also have a history of physical or sexual abuse. Alcohol abuse isn't a common finding in a young woman showing defiant behavior or experiencing infertility. Memory loss isn't a common finding in a young woman dealing with alcohol abuse.
CN: Psychosocial integrity; CNS: None; CL: Analysis

CN: Client needs category CNS: Client needs subcategory CL: Cognitive level

12. A nurse determines that a client who abused alcohol has nutritional problems. Which strategy is <u>best</u> for addressing the client's nutritional needs?
1. Encouraging the client to eat a diet high in calories
2. Helping the client recognize and follow a balanced diet
3. Having the client drink liquid protein supplements daily
4. Having the client monitor the calories consumed each day

13. A client with a history of alcohol abuse refuses to take vitamins. Which statement is <u>most appropriate</u> for explaining why vitamins are important?
1. "It's important to take vitamins to stop your craving."
2. "Prolonged use of alcohol can cause vitamin depletion."
3. "For every vitamin you take, you'll help your liver heal."
4. "By taking vitamins, you won't need to worry about your diet."

14. Which behavior in a client who abuses alcohol indicates a nutrition-related knowledge <u>deficit</u>?
1. Avoiding foods high in fat
2. Eating only one adequate meal each day
3. Taking vitamin and mineral supplements
4. Eating large amounts of fiber

15. A nurse is caring for a client who typically consumes 15 to 20 beers per week and is extremely defensive about his alcohol intake. He admits to experiencing blackouts and has had three alcohol-related motor vehicle accidents. What's the <u>best</u> action for this client?
1. Monitor his alcohol intake.
2. Switch to low-alcohol beer or wine coolers.
3. Limit his intake to no more than three beers per drinking occasion.
4. Abstain from alcohol altogether.

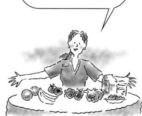

Don't forget the food! Proper nutrition is especially important for people dealing with alcohol abuse.

12. 2. Clients who abuse alcohol are commonly malnourished and need help to follow a balanced diet, which is especially important because episodes of hypoglycemia and hyperglycemia may occur due to the high sugar content of alcohol. Increasing calories may cause the client to eat empty calories. The client must be involved in the decision to supplement daily dietary intake; the nurse can't force him to drink liquid protein supplements. Having the client monitor calorie intake could be done only after the client recognizes the need to maintain a balanced diet. Calorie counts aren't needed in most recovering clients who begin to eat from basic food groups.
CN: Physiological integrity; CNS: Reduction of risk potential; CL: Comprehension

13. 2. Chronic alcoholism interferes with the metabolism of many vitamins. Vitamin supplements can prevent deficiencies. Taking vitamins won't stop the craving for alcohol or help a damaged liver heal. A balanced diet is essential *in addition* to taking multivitamins.
CN: Physiological integrity; CNS: Reduction of risk potential; CL: Application

14. 2. If the client eats only one adequate meal each day, there will be a deficit of essential nutrients. It's appropriate for the client to take vitamin and mineral supplements to prevent deficiency in these nutrients. Avoiding foods high in fat content and consuming large portions of foods containing fiber indicate the client has good knowledge about nutrition.
CN: Physiological integrity; CNS: Reduction of risk potential; CL: Knowledge

15. 4. This client demonstrates behaviors consistent with middle-stage addiction. Once addicted, the only way to control intake is to abstain altogether—monitoring or limiting intake, or switching to low-alcoholic drinks won't work for this client.
CN: Psychosocial integrity; CNS: None; CL: Comprehension

16. A nurse is caring for a client who's undergoing treatment for acute alcohol dependence. The client tells the nurse, "I don't have a problem. My wife made me come here." Which defense mechanism is the client using?
1. Projection and suppression
2. Denial and rationalization
3. Rationalization and repression
4. Suppression and denial

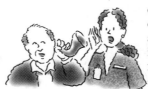

A client with alcohol dependence can sometimes have a hard time hearing the truth.

16. 2. The client is using denial and rationalization. Denial is the unconscious disclaimer of unacceptable thoughts, feelings, needs, or certain external factors. Rationalization is the unconscious effort to justify intolerable feelings, behaviors, and motives. The client isn't using projection, suppression, or repression. Emotions, behavior, and motives, which are consciously intolerable, are denied and then attributed to others in projection. Suppression is a conscious effort to control and conceal unacceptable ideas and impulses into the unconscious. Repression is the unconscious placement of unacceptable feelings into the unconscious mind.
CN: Physiological integrity; CNS: Physiological adaptation; CL: Application

17. Which short-term goal should be a <u>priority</u> for a client with a knowledge deficit about the effects of alcohol on the body?
1. Test blood chemistries daily.
2. Verbalize the results of substance use.
3. Talk to a pharmacist about the substance.
4. Attend a weekly aerobic exercise program.

17. 2. It's important for the client to talk about the health consequences of the continued use of alcohol. Testing blood chemistries daily gives the client minimal knowledge about the effects of alcohol on the body and isn't the most useful information in a teaching plan. A pharmacist isn't the appropriate health care professional to educate the client about the effects of alcohol use on the body. Although exercise is an important goal of self-care, it doesn't address the client's knowledge deficit about the effects of alcohol on the body.
CN: Physiological integrity; CNS: Reduction of risk potential; CL: Application

18. A nurse is assigned to care for a recently admitted client who has attempted suicide. What should the nurse be sure to do?
1. Search the client's belongings and room carefully for items that could be used to attempt suicide.
2. Express trust that the client won't cause self-harm while in the facility.
3. Respect the client's privacy and don't search any belongings.
4. Remind all staff members to check on the client frequently.

18. 1. Because a client who has attempted suicide could try again, the nurse should search the client's belongings and room to remove any items that could be used in another suicide attempt; the need to maintain a safe environment supersedes the client's right to privacy. Expressing trust that the client won't cause self-harm may increase guilt and pain if the client can't live up to that trust. Although frequent checks by staff members are helpful, they aren't enough because the client may attempt suicide between checks.
CN: Safe, effective care environment; CNS: Safety and infection control; CL: Application

CN: Client needs category   CNS: Client needs subcategory   CL: Cognitive level

19. A client experiencing alcohol withdrawal says he's worried about periodic hallucinations. Which intervention is best for this client's problem?
1. Pointing out that the sensation doesn't exist
2. Allowing the client to talk about the experience
3. Encouraging the client to wash his body areas well
4. Determining if the client has a cognitive impairment

20. A client who has been drinking alcohol for 30 years asks a nurse if permanent damage has occurred to his immune system. Which response is the best?
1. "There's usually less resistance to infections."
2. "Sometimes the body's metabolism will increase."
3. "Put your energies into maintaining sobriety for now."
4. "Drinking puts you at high risk for disease later in life."

21. A client experiencing alcohol withdrawal is upset about going through detoxification. Which of these goals is the priority?
1. The client will commit to a drug-free lifestyle.
2. The client will work with the nurse to remain safe.
3. The client will drink plenty of fluids on a daily basis.
4. The client will make a personal inventory of strengths.

22. A client recovering from alcohol abuse needs to develop effective coping skills to handle daily stressors. Which intervention is most useful to the client?
1. Determining the client's verbal skills
2. Helping the client avoid conflict
3. Discussing examples of successful coping behavior
4. Teaching the client to accept uncomfortable situations

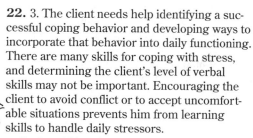

When a client stops drinking, the day-to-day stressors remain. Finding new ways to cope is essential.

19. 2. The client needs to talk about the periodic hallucinations to prevent them from becoming triggers to acting out behaviors and possible self-injury. The client's experience of sensory-perceptual alterations must be acknowledged. Determining if the client has a cognitive impairment and encouraging the client to wash his body areas well don't address the problem of periodic hallucinations.
CN: Psychosocial integrity; CNS: None; CL: Application

20. 1. Chronic alcohol use depresses the immune system and causes increased susceptibility to infections. A nutritionally well-balanced diet that includes foods high in protein and B vitamins will help develop a strong immune system. The potential damage to the immune system doesn't increase the body's metabolism. The third response negates the client's concern and isn't an appropriate or caring response. Drinking alcohol may put the client at risk for immune system problems at any time in life.
CN: Physiological integrity; CNS: Physiological adaptation; CL: Analysis

21. 2. The most important goal is client safety. Although drinking enough fluids, identifying personal strengths, and committing to a drug-free lifestyle are important goals, promoting client safety must be the nurse's first priority.
CN: Psychosocial integrity; CNS: None; CL: Analysis

22. 3. The client needs help identifying a successful coping behavior and developing ways to incorporate that behavior into daily functioning. There are many skills for coping with stress, and determining the client's level of verbal skills may not be important. Encouraging the client to avoid conflict or to accept uncomfortable situations prevents him from learning skills to handle daily stressors.
CN: Psychosocial integrity; CNS: None; CL: Analysis

CN: Client needs category CNS: Client needs subcategory CL: Cognitive level

23. A client is struggling with alcohol dependence. Which <u>communication strategy</u> would be most effective?

1. Speaking briefly and directly
2. Avoiding blaming or preaching to the client
3. Confronting feelings and examples of perfectionism
4. Determining if nonverbal communication will be more effective

24. A 30-year-old woman signed herself into an alcohol treatment program. During the first visit with the nurse, she vehemently maintains that she has no problem with alcohol. She states that she's in this program only because her husband issued an ultimatum. Which response is best?

1. "I wonder why your husband would issue such an ultimatum?"
2. "Because you came voluntarily, you're free to leave anytime you wish."
3. "From your point of view, what is most important for me to know about you?"
4. "You sound pretty definite about not having a problem with alcohol."

25. A client recovering from alcohol addiction has limited coping skills. Which characteristic would indicate relationship problems?

1. The client is prone to panic attacks.
2. The client doesn't pay attention to details.
3. The client has poor problem-solving skills.
4. The client ignores the need to relax and rest.

26. A nurse suggests to a client struggling with alcohol addiction that keeping a journal may be helpful. Which reason <u>best</u> explains this?

1. The client can identify stressors and responses to them.
2. The client will be better able to understand the diagnosis.
3. The client can help others by reading the journal to them.
4. The client will develop an emergency plan for use in a crisis.

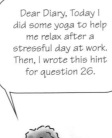

Dear Diary, Today I did some yoga to help me relax after a stressful day at work. Then, I wrote this hint for question 26.

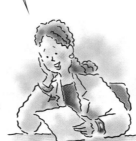

23. 2. Blaming or preaching to the client causes negativity and prevents the client from hearing what the nurse has to say. Speaking briefly to the client may not allow time for adequate communication. Perfectionism doesn't tend to be an issue. Determining if nonverbal communication will be more effective is better suited to a client with a cognitive impairment.
CN: Psychosocial integrity; CNS: None; CL: Analysis

24. 3. The third response allows the nurse to collect more information. The first response focuses on the husband, who isn't the client. The second response is abrasive and blocks communication. The fourth response doesn't allow for further exploration.
CN: Psychosocial integrity; CNS: None; CL: Application

25. 3. To have satisfying relationships, a person must be able to communicate and problem solve. Relationship problems don't predispose people to panic attacks more than other psychosocial stressors. Paying attention to details isn't a major concern when addressing the client's relationship difficulties. Although ignoring the need for rest and relaxation is unhealthy, it shouldn't pose a major relationship problem.
CN: Psychosocial integrity; CNS: None; CL: Analysis

26. 1. Keeping a journal enables the client to identify problems and patterns of coping. From this information, the difficulties the client faces can be addressed. A journal may help to promote better understanding of the client's illness. However, its primary purpose is to help the client gain insight. Journals aren't read to other people unless the client wants to share a particular part. Journals aren't typically used for identifying an emergency plan for use in a crisis.
CN: Psychosocial integrity; CNS: None; CL: Application

CN: Client needs category   CNS: Client needs subcategory   CL: Cognitive level

27. What information is <u>most important</u> to use in a teaching plan for a client who has abused alcohol?
    1. Personal needs
    2. Illness exacerbation
    3. Cognitive distortions
    4. Communication skills

27. 4. Addicted clients commonly have difficulty communicating their needs in an appropriate way. Learning appropriate communication skills is a major goal of treatment. Next, behavior that focuses on the self and meeting personal needs will be addressed. Teaching about illness exacerbation isn't a skill, but is essential for relaying information about relapse. Identifying cognitive distortions would be difficult if the client has poor communication skills.
CN: Psychosocial integrity; CNS: None; CL: Analysis

28. A nurse is preparing for a teaching session with a client who abuses alcohol. What client data would be <u>most</u> important for the nurse to obtain?
    1. Sleep patterns
    2. Decision making
    3. Willingness to learn
    4. Communication skills

28. 3. It's important to know if the client's current situation helps or hinders his potential to learn. Sleep patterns, decision making, and communication skills aren't factors that must be assessed before teaching about addiction.
CN: Psychosocial integrity; CNS: None; CL: Analysis

29. A nurse is developing strategies to prevent relapse with a client who abuses alcohol. Which client intervention is important?
    1. Avoiding taking over-the-counter (OTC) medications
    2. Limiting monthly contact with the family
    3. Refraining from becoming involved in group activities
    4. Avoiding people, places, and activities from the former lifestyle

29. 4. Changing the client's old habits is essential for sustaining a sober lifestyle. Certain OTC medications that don't contain alcohol will probably need to be used by the client at certain times. It's unrealistic to have the client abstain from all such medications. Contact with the client's family may not be a trigger to relapse, so limiting contact wouldn't be useful. Refraining from group activities isn't a good strategy to prevent relapse. Going to Alcoholics Anonymous and other support groups will help prevent relapse.
CN: Psychosocial integrity; CNS: None; CL: Analysis

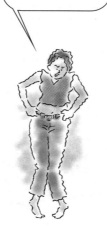

Changing old habits can be difficult. Changing these jeans is downright painful!

30. A client asks a nurse, "Why is it important to talk to my peers in group therapy?" Which response is <u>most appropriate</u>?
    1. "Group therapy lets you see what you're doing wrong in your life."
    2. "Group therapy acts as a defense against your disorganized behavior."
    3. "Group therapy provides a way to ask for support as well as to support others."
    4. "In group therapy, you can vent your frustrations and others will listen."

30. 3. The best response addresses how group therapy provides opportunities to communicate, learn, and give and get support. Group members will give a client feedback, not just point out what a client is doing wrong. Group therapy isn't a defense against disorganized behavior. People can express all kinds of feelings and discuss a variety of topics in group therapy. Interactions are goal-oriented and not just vehicles to vent one's frustrations.
CN: Psychosocial integrity; CNS: None; CL: Application

31. A family meeting is held with a client who abuses alcohol. While listening to the family, which unhealthy communication pattern might be identified?
1. Use of descriptive jargon
2. Disapproval of behaviors
3. Avoidance of issues that cause conflict
4. Unlimited expression of nonverbal communication

32. A client addicted to alcohol begins individual therapy with a nurse. Which intervention should be a <u>priority</u>?
1. Learning to express feelings
2. Establishing new roles in the family
3. Determining new strategies for socializing
4. Decreasing preoccupation with physical health

33. A client recovering from alcohol addiction asks a nurse how to talk to his children about the impact of his addiction on them. Which response by the nurse is most appropriate?
1. "Try to limit references to the addiction and focus on the present."
2. "Talk about all the hardships you've had in working to remain sober."
3. "Tell them you're sorry and emphasize that you're doing so much better now."
4. "Talk to them by acknowledging the difficulties and pain your drinking caused."

34. A client with alcoholism has just completed a residential treatment program. What can this client reasonably expect?
1. Her family will no longer be dysfunctional.
2. She'll need ongoing support to remain abstinent.
3. She doesn't need to be concerned about abusing alcohol in the future.
4. She can learn to consume alcohol without problems.

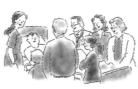

Recovery from alcohol addiction is a family affair.

31. 3. The interaction pattern of a family with a member who abuses alcohol commonly revolves around denying the problem, avoiding conflict, or rationalizing the addiction. Health care providers are more likely to use jargon. The family might have problems setting limits and expressing disapproval of the client's behavior. Nonverbal communication usually gives the nurse insight into family dynamics.
CN: Psychosocial integrity; CNS: None; CL: Analysis

32. 1. The client must address issues, learn ways to cope effectively with life stressors, and express his needs appropriately. Only after the client establishes sobriety can the possibility of taking on new roles become a reality. Determining new strategies for socializing isn't the priority intervention for an addicted client. Usually, these clients need to change former socializing habits. Clients addicted to alcohol don't tend to be preoccupied with physical health problems.
CN: Psychosocial integrity; CNS: None; CL: Comprehension

33. 4. Part of the healing process for the family is to acknowledge the pain, embarrassment, and overall difficulties the client's drinking problem caused family members. The first response facilitates the client's ability to deny the problem. The second prevents the client from acknowledging the difficulties the children endured. The third leads the client to believe only a simple apology is needed. The addiction must be addressed, and the children's pain acknowledged.
CN: Psychosocial integrity; CNS: None; CL: Appication

34. 2. Addiction is a relapsing illness. Support is helpful to most people in maintaining an abstinent lifestyle. The family dynamics probably will change as a result of the client's abstinence; however, there's no way to predict whether these changes will be healthy. An alcoholic client always remains at risk for abusing alcohol. Addicted people can't consume alcohol in moderation.
CN: Psychosocial integrity; CNS: None; CL: Application

CN: Client needs category   CNS: Client needs subcategory   CL: Cognitive level

35. A client who abused alcohol for more than 20 years is diagnosed with cirrhosis of the liver. Which statement by the client shows that teaching has been effective?

1. "If I decide to stop drinking, my health may improve."
2. "If I watch my blood pressure, I should be okay."
3. "If I take vitamins, I can undo some liver damage."
4. "If I use nutritional supplements, I won't have problems."

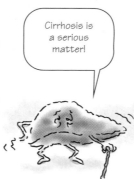

Cirrhosis is a serious matter!

35. 1. This statement reflects the client's perception of the severity of the condition and the life-threatening complications that can result from continued use of alcohol. Aggressive treatment is required, not merely watching one's blood pressure. At this point in the illness, there's little likelihood that liver damage from cirrhosis can be altered. The fourth statement denies the severity of the problem and negates the life-threatening complications common with a diagnosis of cirrhosis.
CN: Physiological integrity; CNS: Reduction of risk potential; CL: Analysis

36. A client tells a nurse, "I'm not going to have health problems from smoking marijuana." Which response by the nurse is <u>most accurate</u>?

1. "Evidence shows it isn't associated with health problems."
2. "Marijuana can cause reproductive and other problems later in life."
3. "Smoking marijuana isn't as dangerous as smoking cigarettes."
4. "Some people have minor or no reactions to smoking marijuana."

36. 2. Marijuana causes cardiac, respiratory, immune, and reproductive health problems. The residues from marijuana are more toxic than those from cigarettes. All people who smoke marijuana have symptoms of intoxication.
CN: Physiological integrity; CNS: Reduction of risk potential; CL: Comprehension

37. During an assessment of a client with a history of polysubstance abuse, which information should be obtained after the names of the drugs?

1. Age at last use
2. Route of administration
3. How the drugs were obtained
4. The places the drugs were used

37. 2. The route of administration gives information about the effects of the drugs and what immediate treatment is necessary. Age at last use, how the drugs were obtained, and places they were used aren't essential information for treatment.
CN: Physiological integrity; CNS: Reduction of risk potential; CL: Knowledge

38. A client says, "I started using cocaine as a recreational drug, but now I can't seem to control the use." The nurse knows that the client's statement is <u>most</u> consistent with which drug behavior?

1. Toxic dose
2. Dual diagnosis
3. Cross-tolerance
4. Compulsive use

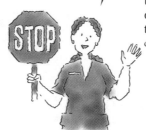

When it comes to substance abuse, stopping is easier said than done.

38. 4. Compulsive drug use involves taking a substance for a period of time significantly longer than intended. A toxic dose is the amount of a drug that causes a poisonous effect. Dual diagnosis is the coexistence of a drug problem and a mental health problem. Cross-tolerance occurs when the effects of a drug are decreased and the client takes larger amounts to achieve the desired drug effect.
CN: Psychosocial integrity; CNS: None; CL: Application

CN: Client needs category   CNS: Client needs subcategory   CL: Cognitive level

39. A client says he used amphetamines to be productive at work. Which symptom <u>commonly</u> occurs when the drugs are abruptly discontinued?

1. Severe anxiety
2. Increased yawning
3. Altered perceptions
4. Amotivational syndrome

40. Using which type of drug since early adolescence could lead to bone marrow depression?

1. Amphetamines
2. Cocaine
3. Inhalants
4. Marijuana

41. Which statement best explains why it's important to monitor behavior in a client who has stopped using phencyclidine (PCP)?

1. Fatigue can cause feelings of being overwhelmed.
2. Agitation and mood swings can occur during withdrawal.
3. Bizarre behavior can be a precursor to a psychotic episode.
4. Memory loss and forgetfulness can cause unsafe conditions.

42. A client is seeking help to stop using amphetamines. In anticipation of withdrawal, the nurse should monitor the client closely for which symptom?

1. Disturbed sleep
2. Increased yawning
3. Psychomotor agitation
4. Inability to concentrate

43. Which condition can occur in a client who has just used cocaine?

1. Increased heart rate
2. Elevated temperature
3. Increased jugular vein distention
4. Decreased respiratory rate

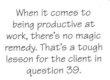

When it comes to being productive at work, there's no magic remedy. That's a tough lesson for the client in question 39.

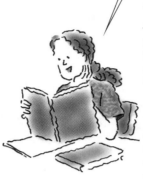

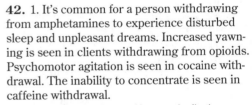

More oxygen!

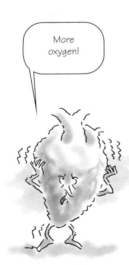

39. 1. When amphetamines are abruptly discontinued, the client may experience severe anxiety or agitation. Increased yawning is a symptom of opioid withdrawal. Altered perceptions occur when a client is withdrawing from hallucinogens. Amotivational syndrome is seen in clients using marijuana.
CN: Psychosocial integrity; CNS: None; CL: Application

40. 3. Inhalants cause severe bone marrow depression. Amphetamines, cocaine, and marijuana don't cause bone marrow depression.
CN: Physiological integrity; CNS: Reduction of risk potential; CL: Knowledge

41. 3. Bizarre behavior and speech are associated with PCP withdrawal and can indicate psychosis. Fatigue isn't necessarily a problem when a client stops using PCP. Agitation, mood swings, memory loss, and forgetfulness don't tend to occur when a client has stopped using PCP.
CN: Psychosocial integrity; CNS: None; CL: Analysis

42. 1. It's common for a person withdrawing from amphetamines to experience disturbed sleep and unpleasant dreams. Increased yawning is seen in clients withdrawing from opioids. Psychomotor agitation is seen in cocaine withdrawal. The inability to concentrate is seen in caffeine withdrawal.
CN: Psychosocial integrity; CNS: None; CL: Application

43. 1. An increase in heart rate is common because cocaine increases the heart's demand for oxygen. Cocaine doesn't increase body temperature, cause increased jugular vein distention, or decrease respiratory rate.
CN: Physiological integrity; CNS: Physiological adaptation; CL: Application

CN: Client needs category   CNS: Client needs subcategory   CL: Cognitive level

44. What information is <u>most important</u> to teach a client who abuses prescription drugs?
1. Herbal substitutes are safer to use.
2. Medication should be used only for the reason prescribed.
3. The client should consult a physician before using a drug.
4. Consider if family members influence the client to use drugs.

44. 2. Drug abusers usually take prescribed drugs for reasons other than those intended primarily to self-medicate or experience a sense of euphoria. The safety and efficacy of most herbal remedies hasn't been established. Sometimes, over-the-counter medications are necessary for minor problems that don't require consulting with a physician. There may be a family history of substance abuse, but it isn't a priority when planning nursing care.
CN: Psychosocial integrity; CNS: None; CL: Application

45. The family of an adolescent who smokes marijuana asks a nurse if the use of marijuana leads to abuse of other drugs. Which response is <u>best</u>?
1. "Use of marijuana is a stage your child will go through."
2. "Many people use marijuana and don't use other street drugs."
3. "Use of marijuana can lead to abuse of more potent substances."
4. "It's difficult to answer that question as I don't know your child."

45. 3. Marijuana is considered a "gateway drug" because it tends to lead to the abuse of more potent drugs. People who use marijuana tend to use or at least experiment with more potent substances. Marijuana isn't part of a developmental stage that adolescents go through. It isn't important that the nurse know the child to address this question.
CN: Psychosocial integrity; CNS: None; CL: Application

46. A pregnant client is thinking about stopping cocaine use. Which statement by the client indicates effective teaching about pregnancy and drug use?
1. "Right after birth I'll give the baby up for adoption."
2. "I'll help the baby get through the withdrawal period."
3. "I don't want the baby to have withdrawal symptoms."
4. "It's scary to think the baby may have Down syndrome."

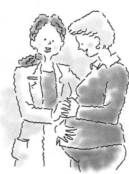

46. 3. Neonates born to mothers addicted to cocaine have withdrawal symptoms at birth. If the client says she'll give the baby up for adoption after birth or help the baby get through the withdrawal period, the teaching was ineffective because the mother doesn't see the impact of her drug use on the child. Use of cocaine during pregnancy doesn't contribute to the possibility of the baby having Down syndrome.
CN: Physiological integrity; CNS: Reduction of risk potential; CL: Analysis

47. After leaving on a pass, a client with a history of cocaine abuse returns to an inpatient drug and alcohol facility showing behavior changes. Which test shows the presence of cocaine in the body?
1. Antibody screen
2. Glucose screen
3. Hepatic screen
4. Urine screen

47. 4. A urine toxicology screen would show the presence of cocaine in the body. Antibody, glucose, or hepatic screening wouldn't show the presence of cocaine in the body.
CN: Psychosocial integrity; CNS: None; CL: Knowledge

CN: Client needs category CNS: Client needs subcategory CL: Cognitive level

48. A nurse is assessing a client admitted to the emergency department with suspected overdose of an antianxiety agent. Which signs and symptoms would be <u>typical findings</u> with this diagnosis?
1. Combativeness, sweating, and confusion
2. Agitation, hyperactivity, and grandiose ideation
3. Emotional lability, euphoria, and impaired memory
4. Suspiciousness, dilated pupils, and increased blood pressure

49. A nurse is developing a care plan for a client recovering from cocaine use. Which intervention should be the nurse's <u>priority</u> for this client?
1. Providing meticulous skin care
2. Initiating suicide precautions
3. Establishing frequent orientation
4. Obtaining nutritional consultation

50. Which clinical condition is commonly seen in substance abuse clients who repeatedly use cocaine?
1. Panic attacks
2. Bipolar cycling
3. Attention deficits
4. Expressive aphasia

51. A client who uses cocaine finally admits other drugs were also abused <u>to equalize the effect</u> of cocaine. Which substance might be included in the client's pattern of polysubstance abuse?
1. Alcohol
2. Amphetamines
3. Caffeine
4. Phencyclidine

52. A mother asks the nurse what she should do about her son's behavior, which has been erratic for 6 months. Which response is best?
1. Telling her how to set daily goals for her son
2. Reassuring her that her child is going through a phase that will pass
3. Discussing the child's specific behaviors, and suggesting possible actions to take
4. Explaining that the child seems fragile and that she needs to be patient with him

When in doubt, think safety first!

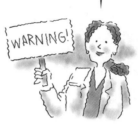

WARNING!

48. 3. Signs of antianxiety agent overdose include emotional lability, euphoria, and impaired memory. Phencyclidine overdose can cause combativeness, sweating, and confusion. Amphetamine overdose can result in agitation, hyperactivity, and grandiose ideation. Hallucinogen overdose can produce suspiciousness, dilated pupils, and increased blood pressure.
CN: Physiological integrity; CNS: Reduction of risk potential; CL: Application

49. 2. Clients recovering from cocaine use are prone to "postcoke depression" and are likely to become suicidal if they can't take the drug. Skin care and frequent orientation are routine nursing interventions but aren't the most immediate considerations for this client. Nutrition consultation isn't the most pressing intervention for this client.
CN: Psychosocial integrity; CNS: None; CL: Analysis

50. 2. Clients who frequently use cocaine will experience the rapid cycling effect of excitement and then severe depression. They don't tend to experience panic attacks, attention deficits, or expressive aphasia.
CN: Psychosocial integrity; CNS: None; CL: Analysis

51. 1. A cocaine addict will usually use alcohol to decrease or equalize the stimulating effects of cocaine. Amphetamines, caffeine, and phencyclidine aren't used to equalize the stimulating effects of cocaine.
CN: Psychosocial integrity; CNS: None; CL: Application

52. 3. This parent requires guidance and direction to consider possible alternatives. The child needs to set his own goals. Erratic behavior isn't typical of a passing phase. More than patience is needed to deal with erratic behavior that persists for 6 months.
CN: Psychosocial integrity; CNS: None; CL: Application

CN: Client needs category   CNS: Client needs subcategory   CL: Cognitive level

53. Which statement by a client indicates teaching about cocaine use has been effective?
1. "I wasn't using cocaine to feel better about myself."
2. "I started using cocaine more and more until I couldn't stop."
3. "I'm not addicted to cocaine because I don't use it every day."
4. "I'm not going to be a chronic user. I only use it on holidays."

53. 2. This statement reflects the trajectory or common pattern of cocaine use and indicates successful teaching. The first statement reflects the client's denial. People gravitate to the drug and continue its use because it gives them a sense of well-being, competency, and power. Cocaine abusers tend to be binge users and can be drug-free for days or weeks between use, but they still have a drug problem. The fourth statement indicates the client is in denial about the drug's potential to become a habit; effective teaching didn't occur.

CN: Psychosocial integrity; CNS: None; CL: Analysis

54. A client is admitted with acute intoxication of lysergic acid diethylamide (LSD). Which signs and symptoms would the nurse <u>commonly</u> expect to find in a client with this diagnosis?
1. Visual distortions
2. Sudden, violent behavior
3. Multiple personalities
4. Generalized anxiety

54. 1. Visual distortions and gross distortion of reality are found in LSD intoxication. LSD intoxication doesn't manifest as sudden, violent behavior; multiple personalities; or generalized anxiety.

CN: Physiological integrity; CNS: Physiological adaptation; CL: Application

55. Which psychiatric or medical emergency is <u>most likely</u> to occur when a client is using phencyclidine (PCP)?
1. Cardiac arrest
2. Seizure disorder
3. Violent behavior
4. Delirium reaction

55. 3. When a client is using PCP, an acute psychotic reaction can occur. The client is capable of sudden, explosive, violent behavior. PCP doesn't tend to cause cardiac arrest or a seizure disorder. Delirium is associated with inhalant intoxication.

CN: Psychosocial integrity; CNS: None; CL: Knowledge

56. A client who smoked marijuana daily for 10 years tells a nurse, "I don't have any goals, and I just don't know what to do." Which communication technique is the <u>most useful</u> when talking to this client?
1. Focusing the interaction
2. Using nonverbal methods
3. Using reflection techniques
4. Using open-ended questions

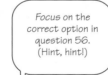

Focus on the correct option in question 56. (Hint, hint!)

56. 1. A client with amotivational syndrome from chronic use of marijuana tends to talk in tangents and needs the nurse to focus the conversation. Nonverbal communication or reflection techniques wouldn't be useful as this client must focus and learn to identify and accomplish goals. Using only open-ended questions won't allow the client to focus and establish specific goals.

CN: Psychosocial integrity; CNS: None; CL: Comprehension

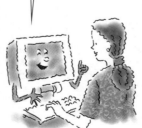

CN: Client needs category   CNS: Client needs subcategory   CL: Cognitive level

57. A nurse is assessing for physical health problems in a client who uses heroin. Which medical consequence of heroin use commonly occurs?
1. Hepatitis
2. Peptic ulcers
3. Hypertension
4. Chronic pharyngitis

58. The family of a client withdrawing from heroin asks a nurse why the client is receiving naltrexone (ReVia). Which response is correct?
1. "It's used to help reverse withdrawal symptoms."
2. "It's used to keep the client sedated during withdrawal."
3. It takes the place of detoxification with methadone."
4. It's given to decrease the client's memory of the withdrawal experience."

59. Which nursing intervention reflects the major component of a cocaine addiction treatment program?
1. Helping the client find ways to be happy and competent
2. Fostering the creative use of self in community activities
3. Teaching the client to handle stresses in the work setting
4. Helping the client acknowledge the current level of dependency

60. A client tells a nurse, "I've been clean from drugs for the past 5 years, but my life really hasn't changed." Which concept should be explored with this client?
1. Further education
2. Conflict resolution
3. Career development
4. Personal development

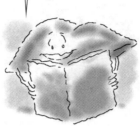

I'm just checking to see if I'm going to make another appearance in this chapter. I think I'm famous.

57. 1. Hepatitis is the most common medical complication of heroin abuse. Peptic ulcers are more likely to be a complication of caffeine use, hypertension is a complication of amphetamine use, and chronic pharyngitis is a complication of marijuana use.
CN: Physiological integrity; CNS: Reduction of risk potential; CL: Application

58. 1. Naltrexone is an opioid antagonist and helps reverse the symptoms of opioid withdrawal. Keeping the client sedated during withdrawal isn't the reason for giving this drug. The drug isn't used in place of detoxification with methadone and doesn't decrease the client's memory of the withdrawal experience.
CN: Physiological integrity; CNS: Reduction of risk potential; CL: Application

59. 1. The major component of a treatment program for a client addicted to cocaine is to help the client discover ways to feel happy and competent without using the drug. Because clients typically credit cocaine for their achievements, helping them discover ways of achieving happiness and success without the drug are paramount. The second intervention may foster use because the client hasn't yet discovered drug-free ways of engaging in challenging activities. The third intervention is appropriate but isn't the major component of treatment. The fourth intervention isn't a major treatment component because the client must first work on remaining drug-free.
CN: Psychosocial integrity; CNS: None; CL: Application

60. 4. True recovery involves changing the client's distorted thinking and working on personal and emotional development. Before the client pursues further education, conflict resolution skills, or career development, it's imperative that the client devote energy to emotional and personal development.
CN: Psychosocial integrity; CNS: None; CL: Analysis

CN: Client needs category   CNS: Client needs subcategory   CL: Cognitive level

61. A client discusses how drug addiction has made life unmanageable. Which information does the client need to <u>start</u> coping with the drug problem?

    1. How peers have committed to sobriety

    2. How to accomplish family of origin work

    3. The addiction process and tools for recovery

    4. How environmental stimuli serve as drug triggers

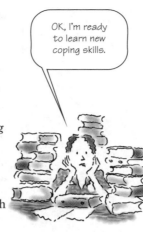

OK, I'm ready to learn new coping skills.

61. 3. When the client admits life has become unmanageable, the best strategy is to teach about the addiction, how to obtain support, and how to develop new coping skills. Information about how peers committed to sobriety would be shared with the client as the treatment process begins. Family of origin work would be a later part of the treatment process. Initially, the client must commit to sobriety and learn skills for recovery. Identifying how environmental stimuli serve as drug triggers would be a later part of the treatment process.

CN: Psychosocial integrity; CNS: None; CL: Analysis

62. A nurse is collecting data from a client with a history of cocaine abuse. Which condition might <u>typically</u> be found with this client?

    1. Glossitis

    2. Pharyngitis

    3. Bilateral ear infections

    4. Perforated nasal septum

62. 4. The client who snorts cocaine frequently commonly develops a perforated nasal septum. Glossitis, bilateral ear infections, and pharyngitis aren't common physical findings for a client with a history of cocaine abuse.

CN: Physiological integrity; CNS: Physiological adaptation; CL: Application

63. A client recovering from cocaine abuse is participating in group therapy. Which statement by the client indicates he has benefited from the group?

    1. "I think the laws about drug possession are too strict in this country."

    2. "I'll be more careful about talking about my drug use to my children."

    3. "I finally realize the short high from cocaine isn't worth the depression."

    4. "I can't understand how I could get all these problems that we talked about in group."

63. 3. This is a realistic appraisal of a client's experience with cocaine and how harmful the experience is. The first statement indicates the client is distracting himself from personal issues and isn't working on goals in the group setting. Talking about drugs to children must be reinforced with nonverbal behavior, and not talking about drugs may give children the wrong message about drug use. The fourth statement indicates the client is in denial about the consequences of cocaine use.

CN: Psychosocial integrity; CNS: None; CL: Analysis

64. A family expresses concern that a member who stopped using amphetamines 3 months ago is acting paranoid. Which explanation is the <u>best</u>?

    1. A person gets symptoms of paranoia with polysubstance abuse.

    2. When a person uses amphetamines, paranoid tendencies may continue for months.

    3. Sometimes family dynamics and a high suspicion of continued drug use make a person paranoid.

    4. Amphetamine abusers may have severe anxiety and paranoid thinking.

64. 2. After a client uses amphetamines, there may be long-term effects that exist for months after use. Two common effects are paranoia and ideas of reference. Even with polysubstance abuse, the paranoia comes from the chronic use of amphetamines. The third explanation blames the family when the paranoia actually comes from the drug use. Severe anxiety isn't typically manifested in paranoid thinking.

CN: Psychosocial integrity; CNS: None; CL: Analysis

65. A nurse is trying to determine if a client who abuses heroin has any drug-related legal problems. Which assessment question is the best to ask the client?
 1. When did your spouse become aware of your use of heroin?
 2. Do you have a probation officer you report to periodically?
 3. Have you received any legal violations related to your drug use?
 4. Do you have a history of frequent visits with the employee assistance program manager?

66. A male client returns to the psychiatric unit after being on a 6-hour pass. The nurse observes that the client is agitated and ataxic and that he exhibits nystagmus and general muscle hypertonicity. The nurse suspects that the client was using drugs while away from the unit. His symptoms are most indicative of intoxication with which drug?
 1. Phencyclidine (PCP)
 2. Crack cocaine
 3. Heroin
 4. Cannabis

67. A client who uses cocaine denies that his drug use is a problem. Which intervention strategy would be best to confront the client's denial?
 1. Stating ways to cope with stress
 2. Repeating the drug facts as needed
 3. Identifying the client's ambivalence
 4. Using open-ended, factual questions

68. A nurse is instructing a client who's to receive disulfiram (Antabuse). Which statement by the client demonstrates that the teaching was effective?
 1. "I can use any aftershave."
 2. "I can use any mouthwash."
 3. "I can use any cough syrups."
 4. "I can use any antacids."

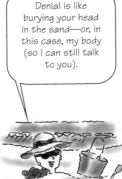

Denial is like burying your head in the sand—or, in this case, my body (so I can still talk to you).

65. 3. This question focuses on obtaining direct information about drug-related legal problems. When a spouse becomes aware of a partner's substance abuse, the first action isn't necessarily to institute legal action. Even if the client reports to a probation officer, the offense isn't necessarily a drug-related problem. Asking if the client has a history of frequent visits with the employee assistance program manager isn't useful; it assumes any such visit is related to drug issues.
CN: Psychosocial integrity; CNS: None; CL: Analysis

66. 1. The client's behavior suggests the use of PCP. Crack cocaine intoxication is characterized by euphoria, grandiosity, aggressiveness, paranoia, and depression. Heroin intoxication is characterized by euphoria followed by sleepiness. Cannabis intoxication is characterized by a panic state and visual hallucinations.
CN: Psychosocial integrity; CNS: None; CL: Application

67. 4. The use of open-ended, factual questions will help the client acknowledge that a drug problem exists. Repeating drug facts won't be effective, as the client will perceive it as preaching or nagging. Stating ways to cope with stress and identifying the client's ambivalence won't be effective for breaking through a client's denial.
CN: Psychosocial integrity; CNS: None; CL: Application

68. 4. Antacids don't interact with disulfiram. The client should avoid anything containing alcohol, including aftershave lotion and some cough medicines and mouthwashes.
CN: Psychosocial integrity; CNS: None; CL: Analysis

CN: Client needs category   CNS: Client needs subcategory   CL: Cognitive level

69. A nurse has developed a relationship with a client who has an addiction problem. What information would indicate that the therapeutic interaction is in the working stage? Select all that apply:

1. The client addresses how the addiction has contributed to family distress.
2. The client reluctantly shares a family history of addiction.
3. The client verbalizes difficulty identifying personal strengths.
4. The client discusses the financial problems related to the addiction.
5. The client expresses uncertainty about meeting with the nurse.
6. The client acknowledges the addiction's effects on the children.

70. A client who's recovering from an appendectomy is alert and ambulatory and complains of pain. The team leader asks the nurse to give him his PRN-ordered oral analgesic. The nurse is aware that this client has had a long history of substance abuse. List in ascending chronological order the steps the nurse would take to administer this particular medication. Use all the options.

| 1. Check the client's two identifiers with the medication administration record. |
| 2. Stay with the client as he takes the medication to ensure the medication hasn't been "pocketed" in his cheeks or under his tongue. |
| 3. Document on the medication sheet that you've given the medication. |
| 4. Administer the medication. |
| 5. Check the physician's orders with the medication administration record to see if it's time for the medication. |
| 6. Place the correct medication and dose in a medication cup. |

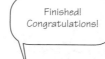

Finished! Congratulations!

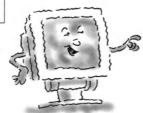

69. 1, 4, 6. Addressing how the addiction has contributed to family distress, discussing financial problems related to addiction, and acknowledging the effects on the children are examples of the nurse-client working phase of an interaction. In the working phase, the client explores, evaluates, and determines solutions to identified problems. Reluctant sharing of family addiction history, difficulty identifying personal strengths, and expressing uncertainty about meeting with the nurse are examples of what happens during the introductory phase of the nurse-client interaction.

CN: Psychosocial integrity; CNS: None; CL: Analysis

70. Ordered response:

| 5. Check the physician's orders with the medication administration record to see if it's time for the medication. |
| 6. Place the correct medication and dose in a medication cup. |
| 1. Check the client's two identifiers with the medication administration record. |
| 4. Administer the medication. |
| 2. Stay with the client as he takes the medication to ensure the medication hasn't been "pocketed" in his cheeks or under his tongue. |
| 3. Document on the medication sheet that you've given the medication. |

The first step is to check the physician's orders to ensure accuracy. The nurse should check for the appropriate time because this is a PRN order. Once the correct medication and dose are obtained and placed in a medication cup, the nurse would go to the client with the medication orders and check the client's two identifiers. Medication is always administered after establishing the correct identity of the client. Because this patient has a history of substance abuse, the nurse should remain with the client as he takes the medication, check his mouth to be sure it has been swallowed, and then document the medication administration.

CN: Safe and effective care environment; CNS: Coordinated care; CL: Analysis

CN: Client needs category CNS: Client needs subcategory CL: Cognitive level

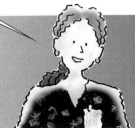

Caring for clients with dissociative disorders can be challenging and rewarding. Doing well in this chapter can be rewarding, too!

Chapter 19
Dissociative disorders

1. Which factor is associated with a client with dissociative identity disorder (DID)?
1. An absent father
2. An inflated sense of self-esteem
3. Vivid memories of childhood trauma
4. A parent who was alternately loving and abusive

2. A nurse is admitting a client with a diagnosis of dissociative identity disorder (DID). The nurse knows that which characteristic might typically be found in a client with this diagnosis?
1. Ritualistic behavior
2. Out-of-body experiences
3. History of severe childhood abuse
4. Ability to give a thorough personal history

3. Which nursing diagnosis would you expect for a client with dissociative identity disorder (DID)?
1. *Disturbed thought processes related to delusional ideations*
2. *Risk for self-directed violence related to suicidal ideations or gestures*
3. *Deficient diversional activity related to lack of environmental stimulation*
4. *Disturbed sensory perception (visual) related to altered sensory reception of visual stimulation*

1. 4. Repeated exposure to a childhood environment that alternates between highly stressful and then loving and supportive can be a factor in the development of DID. Many children grow up in a household without a father but don't develop DID. Because of dissociation from the trauma, a client with DID usually can't recall traumatic childhood events. Clients with DID commonly have low self-esteem.
CN: Psychosocial integrity; CNS: None; CL: Knowledge

2. 3. DID is theorized to develop as a protective response to such traumatic experiences as severe abuse in childhood. Ritualistic behavior is seen with obsessive-compulsive disorders. Out-of-body experiences are more commonly associated with depersonalization disorder. Because of the dissociative response to personal experiences, people with DID are usually unable to give a thorough personal history.
CN: Psychosocial integrity; CNS: None; CL: Application

3. 2. A common reason clients with DID are admitted to a psychiatric facility is because one of the alter personalities is trying to kill another personality. Delusions and hallucinations (as in option 4) are commonly associated with schizophrenic disorders. Because of the assortment of alter personalities controlling the client with DID, diversional activity deficit is rarely a problem.
CN: Safe, effective care environment; CNS: Coordinated care; CL: Application

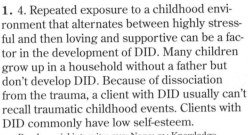

An adult client with DID probably has emotional wounds from a traumatic childhood.

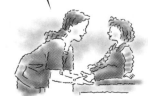

4. Which nursing intervention is important for a client with dissociative identity disorder (DID)?
　1. Giving antipsychotic medications as prescribed
　2. Maintaining consistency when interacting with the client
　3. Confronting the client about the use of alter personalities
　4. Preventing the client from interacting with others when one of the alter personalities is in control

5. A nurse is caring for a 25-year-old woman who's exhibiting signs of low self-esteem. Which client outcome is <u>most</u> desirable?
　1. The client will participate in new activities.
　2. The client will sleep without interruption at night.
　3. The client will be encouraged to confront fear of failure.
　4. The nurse will spend more time with the client.

6. Which goal would be realistic for a client with dissociative identity disorder (DID)?
　1. Confronts the abuser
　2. Attends the unit's milieu meetings
　3. Prevents alter personalities from emerging
　4. Reports no longer having feelings of anger about childhood traumas

7. A nurse is caring for a client with a diagnosis of dissociative identity disorder (DID). Which client behavior should the nurse identify as a safety risk?
　1. The client experiences periods of lost time.
　2. The client expresses a desire to hurt himself.
　3. The client expresses gladness to be in the unit.
　4. The client experiences hearing loud voices.

> Abracadabra! It's no illusion—the difference between client outcomes and nursing interventions is the key to answering question 5.

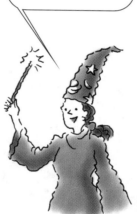

4. 2. Using consistency to establish trust and support is important when interacting with a client with DID. Many of these clients have had few healthy relationships. Medication hasn't proven effective in the treatment of DID. Confronting the client about the alter personalities would be ineffective because the client has little, if any, knowledge of the presence of these other personalities. Isolating the client wouldn't be therapeutic.
CN: Safe, effective care environment; CNS: Coordinated care; CL: Analysis

5. 1. A desired client outcome for a person with low self-esteem is participation in new activities without exhibiting fear of failure. It hasn't been established that this client has difficulty sleeping. Allowing the client to confront fear of failure and spending more time with the client are nursing interventions, not outcomes.
CN: Psychosocial integrity; CNS: None; CL: Application

6. 2. Attending milieu meetings decreases feelings of isolation and shows that the client has begun to trust the nurse. Typically, the abuser was a part of the client's childhood, and confrontation in adulthood may not be possible or therapeutic. The client with DID is commonly unaware of alter personalities and thus can't prevent them from emerging. Clients with DID have dissociated from painful experiences, so the host personality usually doesn't have negative feelings about such experiences.
CN: Psychosocial integrity; CNS: None; CL: Analysis

7. 2. The nurse needs to initiate safety precautions to prevent self-harm. The sensation of lost periods of time isn't a safety issue. Being glad to be in the unit indicates a feeling of security. The client with DID hearing voices doesn't indicate a psychotic episode.
CNS: Safe and effective care environment; CN: Safety and infection control; CL: Application

CN: Client needs category CNS: Client needs subcategory CL: Cognitive level

8. Which finding is expected for a client with dissociative identity disorder (DID)?
1. A close relationship with her mother
2. A history of performing poorly in school
3. Inability to recall certain events or experiences
4. Consistency in the performance of certain tasks or skills

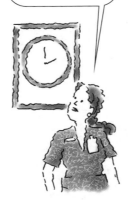

Where does the time go? That's a question that nurses and clients with DID have in common.

9. A hospitalized client with dissociative identity disorder (DID) reports hearing voices. Which nursing intervention is <u>most appropriate</u>?
1. Telling the client to lie down and rest
2. Giving an as-needed dose of haloperidol (Haldol)
3. Encouraging the client to continue with his daily activities
4. Notifying the physician the client is having a psychotic episode

10. Which goal would be <u>most</u> important for a client with dissociative identity disorder (DID)?
1. Learning how to control periods of mania
2. Learning how to integrate all the alternate personalities
3. Developing coping strategies to deal with a traumatic childhood
4. Determining what's causing them to feel they have periods of "lost time"

11. A client with dissociative identity disorder (DID) reports hearing voices and asks the nurse if that means she's "crazy." Which response would be <u>most appropriate</u>?
1. "What do the voices tell you?"
2. "Why would you think you're crazy?"
3. "People with DID commonly report hearing voices."
4. "Hearing voices is typically a symptom of schizophrenia."

8. 3. Clients with DID commonly experience bouts of amnesia when alter personalities are in control. Clients with DID have learned in childhood how to live in two separate worlds: one in the daytime, in which they're able to perform well in school and have friendships, and one at nighttime, when the abuse occurs. The alter personalities may vary in the ability and type of skills and tasks performed. A close relationship with a parent is unlikely because of probable abuse in childhood.
CN: Psychosocial integrity; CNS: None; CL: Comprehension

9. 3. Because many clients with DID hear voices, it's appropriate to have the client continue with daily activities. The voices are probably alter personalities communicating, which doesn't indicate a psychotic episode. Having the client lie down and rest wouldn't be therapeutic. The physician wouldn't be notified to prescribe such antipsychotic medication as haloperidol.
CN: Safe, effective care environment; CNS: Coordinated care; CL: Application

10. 4. The initial symptom many clients with DID experience is the sensation of "lost time." These are times the alter personalities are in control. Depression, not mania, may be another early symptom of clients with DID. Initially, the client with DID isn't aware of the presence of alternate personalities. Before therapeutic interventions, clients with DID may not even be aware of childhood trauma because of dissociation from the event.
CN: Psychosocial integrity; CNS: None; CL: Application

11. 3. The most therapeutic answer is to give correct information. Asking what the voices tell the client would be changing the topic without answering the question. Asking "why" questions can put the client on the defensive. Schizophrenia isn't the only cause of hearing voices, and this response suggests the client may be schizophrenic.
CN: Psychosocial integrity; CNS: None; CL: Analysis

CN: Client needs category   CNS: Client needs subcategory   CL: Cognitive level

12. Which intervention would <u>most likely</u> appear in the care plan of a client with dissociative identity disorder (DID)?
1. Arrange to have staff check on the client every 15 to 30 minutes.
2. Prevent all family from visiting until the third day of hospitalization.
3. Make sure the staff understands the client will be on seizure precautions.
4. Place the client in a quiet room away from the noise of the nurses' station.

13. A client is being treated at a community mental health clinic. A nurse has been instructed to observe for any behaviors indicating dissociative identity disorder (DID). Which behavior would be included?
1. Delusions of grandeur
2. Reports of fatigue
3. Changes in dress, mannerisms, and voice
4. Refusal to make a follow-up appointment

14. Which statement about clients with a dissociative identity disorder (DID) is correct?
1. They rarely marry.
2. They rarely improve with treatment.
3. They can be treated with antianxiety drugs.
4. They commonly improve with long-term therapy.

15. When interacting with a client with a dissociative identity disorder, a nurse observes that one of the alter personalities is in control. Which intervention is the <u>most appropriate</u>?
1. Giving recognition to the alter personality
2. Notifying the physician
3. Immediately stopping interacting with the client
4. Ignoring the alter personality, and asking to speak to the host personality

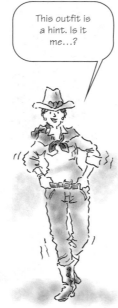

This outfit is a hint. Is it me...?

12. 1. A common reason for hospitalization in clients with DID is suicidal ideations or gestures. For the client's safety, frequent checks should be done. Family interactions might be therapeutic for the client, and the family may be able to provide a more thorough history because of the client's dissociation from traumatic events. Seizure activity isn't an expected symptom of DID. Because of the possibility of suicide, the client's room should be close to the nurses' station.
CN: Safe, effective care environment; CNS: Safety and infection control; CL: Application

13. 3. When alter personalities are in control, the person will have complete personality changes. Delusions of grandeur are more commonly associated with such disorders as manic states and schizophrenia. Complaints of fatigue aren't a main symptom of DID. The refusal to make a follow-up appointment could indicate many problems, including noncompliance.
CN: Psychosocial integrity; CNS: None; CL: Application

14. 4. Most clients with DID can be successfully treated with long-term therapy. Many clients with DID marry. For many dissociative conditions, pharmacologic therapy has little effect.
NP: Data collection; CN: Psychosocial integrity; CNS: None; CL: Knowledge

15. 1. By giving recognition to the alter personality, the nurse conveys to the client that she believes the alter personality exists. Asking to speak to the host personality or immediately stopping interaction with the client won't stop the client from being controlled by alter personalities. The physician doesn't need to be notified because this is an expected occurrence.
CN: Psychosocial integrity; CNS: None; CL: Analysis

16. A nurse on the psychiatric unit is caring for a 51-year-old male client who's suicidal. Which nursing intervention takes <u>priority</u>?
1. Discouraging sleep except at bedtime
2. Making a verbal contract with the client to notify the staff of suicidal thoughts
3. Limiting time spent alone by encouraging the client to participate in group activities
4. Creating a safe physical and interpersonal environment

17. A family member of a client with dissociative identity disorder (DID) asks a nurse if hypnotic therapy might help the client. Which response would be <u>most appropriate</u>?
1. "What would make you think that?"
2. "No, hypnosis is rarely used in the treatment of psychiatric conditions."
3. "Yes, but this treatment is used only after other types of therapy have failed."
4. "Yes, commonly the client doesn't have conscious awareness of alter personalities."

18. Which intervention is appropriate when caring for a client with dissociative identity disorder?
1. Reminding the alter personalities they're part of the host personality
2. Interacting with the client only when the host personality is in control
3. Establishing an empathetic relationship with each emerging personality
4. Providing positive reinforcement to the client when calm, not angry, alter personalities are present

19. While interacting with a client with dissociative identity disorder (DID), a nurse observes characteristics of an alter personality. The client goes from being calm to being angry and shouting. Which response would be most appropriate?
1. "Is one of you upset?"
2. "Why have you become angry?"
3. "Tell me what you're feeling right now."
4. "Let me speak to someone who isn't angry."

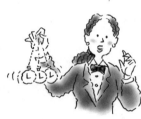

You are getting sleepy...very sleepy...wake up and answer question 17!

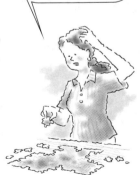

The personalities of a client with DID are like the pieces of a puzzle; each one is a component of the whole.

16. 4. Creating a safe environment, including removing obvious hazards, recognizing nonobvious hazards, maintaining close observation, serving as a client advocate in interpersonal situations, and communicating concern to the client in verbal and nonverbal ways, is the nurse's highest priority. Other interventions, such as discouraging sleep except at bedtime, making a verbal contract, and encouraging participation in group activities, should be included in the client's plan, but these don't have top priority.
CN: Psychosocial integrity; CNS: None; CL: Application

17. 4. Because of dissociation from painful events, hypnosis is usually effective in the treatment of clients with DID. It may be under hypnosis that alter personalities start to emerge. The first response could place the family member on the defensive. Hypnosis is used in a variety of psychiatric conditions. Hypnosis is commonly a first-line treatment for the client with DID.
CN: Psychosocial integrity; CNS: None; CL: Application

18. 3. Establishing an empathetic relationship with each emerging personality (including those that may seem unpleasant) provides a therapeutic environment in which to care for the client. Interacting with the client only when the host personality is in control would be useless because the client has limited, if any, control or awareness when alter personalities are in control.
CN: Psychosocial integrity; CNS: None; CL: Application

19. 3. This response encourages integration and discourages dissociation. When interacting with clients with DID, the nurse always wants to remind the client that the alter personalities are a component of one person. Responses reinforcing interaction with only one alter personality instead of trying to interact with the individual as a single person aren't appropriate. Asking "why" questions can put the client on the defensive and impede further communication.
CN: Psychosocial integrity; CNS: None; CL: Application

CN: Client needs category CNS: Client needs subcategory CL: Cognitive level

20. A client with dissociative identity disorder has been in therapy for 2 years and just learned her father passed away. Her father sexually abused her throughout her childhood. Which intervention would be <u>most appropriate</u>?
  1. Having the client seek inpatient therapy
  2. Encouraging the client's verbalization of feelings of anger and guilt
  3. Encouraging the client's alter personalities to emerge during this stressful time
  4. Stressing to the client that the death of the abuser should be helpful in her healing process

21. A nurse finds a suicidal client trying to hang himself in his room. To preserve the client's self-esteem and safety, what should the nurse do?
  1. Place the client in seclusion with checks every 15 minutes.
  2. Assign a nursing staff member to remain with the client at all times.
  3. Make the client stay with the group at all times.
  4. Refuse to let the client in his room.

22. A nurse observes that an alter personality (a child) of an adult client with dissociative identity disorder is in control. The client is sitting in the dayroom, interacting with others. Which action would be <u>most appropriate</u>?
  1. Allowing the client to continue interacting with clients in the dayroom
  2. Asking to speak to one of the adult alter personalities of the host personality
  3. Removing the client from the dayroom and allowing her to play with toys
  4. Removing the client from the dayroom and reorienting her that she's in a safe place

23. Which feeling or background history is <u>most commonly</u> reported by clients with dissociative identity disorder (DID) who seek help?
  1. Loneliness
  2. Supportive family system
  3. Profound sadness
  4. An almost uncontrollable urge to kill the abuser

20. 2. The death of the abuser may cause the client to experience feelings of anger and guilt. Unless the client becomes suicidal or rapidly deteriorates, inpatient treatment wouldn't be necessary. Encouraging the client's alter personalities to emerge could result in further dissociation. The death of the abuser can be a stressful event and can leave the client with unresolved feelings.
CN: Health promotion and maintenance; CNS: None; CL: Analysis

21. 2. Implementing a one-to-one staff-to-client ratio is the nurse's highest priority. Doing so allows the client to maintain his self-esteem and keeps him safe. Seclusion would damage the client's self-esteem. Forcing the client to stay with the group and refusing to let him in his room don't guarantee his safety.
CN: Psychosocial integrity; CNS: None; CL: Application

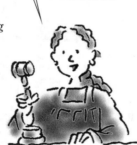

Sometimes, making a judgment call about what's best for a client takes an extra dose of wisdom.

22. 4. Removing the client at this time may protect her from future embarrassment. Reorienting the client discourages dissociation and encourages integration. Asking to speak to an alter personality encourages dissociation. Allowing the client to play with toys also reinforces this behavior and encourages dissociation.
CN: Safe, effective care environment; CNS: Safety and infection control; CL: Analysis

23. 3. Many clients with DID initially experience problems with sadness. Although clients with DID may feel lonely, this is secondary to sadness. Typically, the family is dysfunctional and unlikely to be supportive. Usually, the memories of abuse are repressed; the client may not have a conscious awareness of being angry with the abuser.
CN: Psychosocial integrity; CNS: None; CL: Knowledge

CN: Client needs category   CNS: Client needs subcategory   CL: Cognitive level

24. Which nursing intervention is most appropriate for a client with dissociative identity disorder (DID)?
1. Encouraging the client to confront the abuser
2. Stressing the importance of long-term psychotherapy
3. Suggesting the client name his sub-personalities
4. Teaching the importance of taking prescribed antipsychotic drugs

25. A nurse observes a female client with dissociative identity disorder crying uncontrollably as her parents leave the behavioral unit. Which intervention would be most helpful?
1. Tell the client that you're sorry her family upset her.
2. Leave the client alone to compose herself.
3. Ask the client why she's so upset.
4. Offer to remain quietly beside the client.

26. A client with dissociative identity disorder (DID) is admitted to an inpatient psychiatric unit. A nurse-manager asks all staff to attend a meeting. Which is the most likely reason for the meeting?
1. To review the restraint protocol with the staff
2. To inform the staff that no one should refuse to work with the client
3. To warn the staff that this client may be difficult and challenging to work with
4. To allow staff members to discuss concerns about working with a client with DID

27. A 26-year-old man is reported missing after being the victim of a violent crime. Two months later, a family member finds him working in a city 100 miles from his home. The man doesn't recognize the family member or recall being the victim of a crime. He most likely has which condition?
1. Depersonalization disorder
2. Dissociative amnesia
3. Dissociative fugue
4. Dissociative identity disorder (DID)

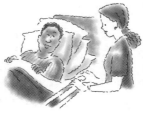

Feelings. Nothing more than feelings. It's all about the feelings.

24. 2. Clients with DID need long-term psychotherapy in order to improve and maintain their mental health. The client with DID has repressed the abuse and would be unable to confront the abuser. Having the client name sub-personalities is nontherapeutic. Antipsychotic drugs aren't prescribed for this disorder.
CN: Psychosocial integrity; CNS: None; CL: Analysis

25. 4. Offering to remain quietly beside the client provides emotional support. Support should be offered to the client before leaving her alone. Telling the client she's sorry her family upset her is an assignment of blame without knowing the facts. The client may not know why she's upset and become defensive.
CN: Psychosocial integrity; CNS: None; CL: Analysis

26. 4. Allowing all staff members to meet together may prevent the staff from splitting into groups of those who believe the validity of this diagnosis and those who don't. Unless this client shows behaviors harmful to himself or others, restraints aren't needed. Telling the staff that no one should refuse to work with the client or that this client will probably be difficult and challenging sets a negative tone as the staff plans and provides care for the client.
CN: Safe, effective care environment; CNS: Coordinated care; CL: Application

27. 3. Dissociative fugue is sudden flight after a traumatic event. During the episode, the person may assume a new identity and may not recognize people from his past. Depersonalization disorder is the sudden loss of the sense of one's own reality. Dissociative amnesia doesn't involve flight from work or home. DID is the coexistence of two or more personalities in one person.
CN: Psychosocial integrity; CNS: None; CL: Knowledge

CN: Client needs category   CNS: Client needs subcategory   CL: Cognitive level

28. Which nursing intervention is most appropriate for a client who has just had an episode of dissociative fugue?
  1. Letting the client verbalize the fear and anxiety he feels
  2. Encouraging the client to share his experiences during the episode
  3. Having the client sign a contract stating he won't leave the premises again
  4. Telling the client he won't resolve his problems by running away from them

29. Which statement best describes the cause of dissociative disorders?
  1. They occur as a result of incest.
  2. They occur as a result of substance abuse.
  3. They occur in more than 40% of all people.
  4. They occur as a result of the brain trying to protect the person from severe stress.

30. Which nursing intervention would be most helpful when working with a client to reduce recurrent episodes of dissociative fugue?
  1. Placing the client on elopement precautions
  2. Helping the client identify resources to deal with stressful situations
  3. Allowing the client to share his experiences about the dissociative fugue episodes
  4. Confronting the client about running away from problems instead of dealing with them

31. A 32-year-old client lost her home in a flood last month. When questioned about her feelings about the loss, she doesn't remember being in a flood or owning a home. This client most likely has which disorder?
  1. Depersonalization disorder
  2. Dissociative amnesia
  3. Dissociative fugue
  4. Dissociative identity disorder (DID)

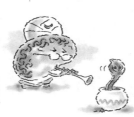

My intentions are good, but sometimes my protective side can have dire consequences.

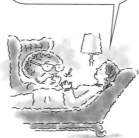

Now I understand! You use dissociative amnesia to protect a person who can't yet handle the pain of remembering a traumatic event.

28. 1. An episode of dissociative fugue can be a frightening experience; encouraging the client to discuss his fears will help establish a plan for coping with them. The client rarely remembers the events during the episode, and asking him to recall them can increase anxiety. Signing a contract would have little effect because a dissociative fugue episode isn't something the client consciously wants. Because he isn't conscious of "running away," the fourth response isn't helpful.
CN: Health promotion and maintenance; CNS: None; CL: Analysis

29. 4. This answer best describes the cause of a dissociative disorder. Incest is only one of many reasons dissociative disorders occur. Typically, substance abuse isn't a cause (but may be an effect) of a dissociative disorder. Dissociative disorders are actually rare.
CN: Psychosocial integrity; CNS: None; CL: Knowledge

30. 2. Dissociative fugue is precipitated by stressful situations. Helping the client identify resources could prevent recurrences. When the dissociative fugue episode is over, the client returns to normal functioning; he wouldn't be an elopement risk. Clients commonly have amnesia about the events during the dissociative fugue episode; therefore, asking them to share or remember their experiences or confronting them about running away from their problems can increase their anxiety.
CN: Psychosocial integrity; CNS: None; CL: Analysis

31. 2. Dissociative amnesia commonly occurs after a person has experienced a traumatic event. Depersonalization disorder is characterized by recurrent sensations of loss of one's own reality. Dissociative fugue is the sudden departure from one's home or work. DID is the coexistence of two or more personalities within the same individual.
CN: Psychosocial integrity; CNS: None; CL: Knowledge

32. Dissociative amnesia is <u>most likely</u> to occur as a result of which circumstance?
1. Binge drinking
2. A hostage situation
3. A closed-head injury
4. A fight with a family member

33. A client was the driver in an automobile accident in which a 3-year-old boy was killed. The client now has dissociative amnesia. He verbalizes an understanding of his treatment plan when he makes which statement?
1. "I won't drive a car again for at least 1 year."
2. "I'll take my Ativan any time I feel upset about this situation."
3. "I'll visit the child's grave as soon as I'm released from the hospital."
4. "I'll attend my hypnotic therapy sessions prescribed by my psychiatrist."

34. A nurse is teaching a client with dissociative identity disorder (DID) about the condition. Which statement by the client indicates that the teaching has been effective?
1. "I'll probably never be able to regain my memories of the fire."
2. "I have problems with my memory due to my abuse of tranquilizers."
3. "If I concentrate hard enough, I'll be able to bring up memories of the car accident."
4. "To protect my mental well-being, my brain has temporarily hidden my memories of the rape from me."

35. Which set of circumstances indicates the <u>highest</u> risk of suicide?
1. Suicide plan, handy means of carrying out plan, and history of previous attempt
2. Preoccupation with morbid thoughts and limited support system
3. Suicidal ideation, active suicide planning, and family history of suicide
4. Threats of suicide, recent job loss, and intact support system

32. 2. Dissociative amnesia typically occurs after the person has experienced a stressful, traumatic situation. Binge drinking doesn't cause dissociative amnesia. A closed-head injury could result in physiologic, but not dissociative, amnesia. Having a fight with a family member typically wouldn't be stressful enough to cause dissociative amnesia.
CN: Psychosocial integrity; CNS: None; CL: Knowledge

33. 4. Hypnosis can be beneficial to this client because it allows repressed feelings and memories to surface. Visiting the child's grave upon release from the hospital may be too traumatic and could encourage continuation of the amnesia. The client needs to learn coping mechanisms other than taking a highly addictive drug such as lorazepam (Ativan). The client may be ready to drive again, and circumstances may dictate that he drives again before 1 year has passed.
CN: Psychosocial integrity; CNS: None; CL: Application

34. 4. One of the cardinal features of DID is that the person has loss of memory of a traumatic event. With this disorder, the loss of memory is a protective function performed by the brain and isn't within the person's conscious control. With therapy and time, the person will probably be able to recall the traumatic events. This type of amnesia isn't related to substance abuse.
CN: Psychosocial integrity; CNS: None; CL: Analysis

When a suicidal client has a detailed plan for attempting suicide, it's time for immediate intervention.

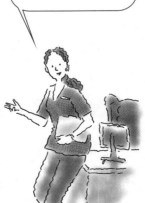

35. 1. A lethal plan with a handy means of carrying it out poses the highest risk and requires immediate intervention. Although all the remaining risk factors can lead to suicide, they aren't considered as high a risk as a formulated, lethal plan and the means at hand. However, a client exhibiting any of these risk factors should be taken seriously and considered at risk for suicide.
CN: Psychosocial integrity; CNS: None; CL: Application

CN: Client needs category   CNS: Client needs subcategory   CL: Cognitive level

36. A client with dissociative amnesia and presently in host personality mode indicates understanding about the use of amobarbital (Amytal) in her treatment when she makes which statement?
1. "This medication helps me sleep."
2. "This medication helps me control my anxiety."
3. "I must take this drug once a day after discharge if the drug is to be therapeutic."
4. "I'm given this medication during therapy sessions to increase my ability to remember forgotten events."

37. A client with dissociative amnesia says, "You must think I'm really stupid because I have no recollection of the accident." Which response would be <u>most appropriate</u>?
1. "Why would I think you're stupid?"
2. "Have I acted like I think you're stupid?'
3. "You'll be fine soon."
4. "As a protective measure, the brain sometimes doesn't let us remember traumatic events."

38. Which nursing intervention is <u>most</u> important in caring for a client with a dissociative disorder?
1. Encouraging the client to participate in unit activities and meetings
2. Questioning the client about the events triggering the dissociative disorder
3. Allowing the client to remain in his room anytime he's experiencing feelings of dissociation
4. Encouraging the client to form friendships with other clients in his therapy groups to decrease his feelings of isolation

39. Which characteristic applies to depersonalization disorder?
1. Disorientation to time, place, and person
2. Sensation of detachment from body or mind
3. Unexpected and sudden travel to another location
4. A feeling that one's environment will never change

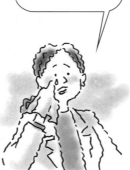

Question 37 cries out for the most appropriate response.

36. 4. This drug is given to the client with dissociative amnesia to help her remember forgotten events. It isn't prescribed as a sleep aid or antianxiety agent. Because the drug is given during therapy to recall forgotten events, there would be no therapeutic benefit to taking this drug at home.
CN: Psychosocial integrity; CNS: None; CL: Analysis

37. 4. This response provides a simple explanation for the client. The use of "why" can put the client on the defensive. The second response takes the focus off the client. The third response gives false reassurance.
CN: Psychosocial integrity; CNS: None; CL: Application

38. 1. Individuals with certain dissociative disorders feel detached from their environment and can experience impaired social functioning. Attending unit activities and meetings helps decrease the client's sense of isolation. Typically, the client can't recall the events that triggered the dissociative disorder. The client would need to be isolated from others only if he couldn't interact appropriately. A client with a dissociative disorder has typically had few healthy relationships. Forming friendships with others in therapy could be setting the client up to continue in unhealthy relationships.
CN: Safe, effective care environment; CNS: Coordinated care; CL: Application

39. 2. In depersonalization disorder, the person feels detached from his body and mental processes. The person is usually oriented to time, place, and person. Unexpected and sudden travel to another location is one of the characteristics of dissociative fugue. Clients with depersonalization disorder commonly feel the outside world has changed.
CN: Psychosocial integrity; CNS: None; CL: Comprehension

40. A client with depersonalization disorder verbalizes understanding of the ways to decrease his symptoms when he makes which statement?
1. "I'll avoid any stressful situation."
2. "Meditation will help control my symptoms."
3. "I'll need to practice relaxation exercises regularly."
4. "I may need to remain on antipsychotic medication for the rest of my life."

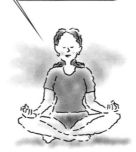

You've made it all the way to question 40! You deserve a hint. Yoga…relaxation… symptom control…

40. 3. Relaxation can lead to a decrease in maladaptive responses. Although stress can be a predisposing factor in depersonalization disorder, it's impossible to avoid all stressful situations. Meditation is the voluntary induction of the sensation of depersonalization. This disorder isn't a psychotic disorder, so antipsychotic medication wouldn't be therapeutic.
CN: Psychosocial integrity; CNS: None; CL: Analysis

41. A client with depersonalization disorder spends much of her day in a dreamlike state, during which she ignores personal care needs. Which nursing diagnosis would you expect to find identified for this client?
1. *Disturbed thought processes related to organic brain damage*
2. *Impaired memory related to frequently being in a dreamlike state*
3. *Dressing or grooming self-care deficit related to perceptual impairment*
4. *Deficient knowledge related to performance of personal care needs due to lack of information*

41. 3. Because of time spent in a dreamlike state, many clients with depersonalization disorder ignore self-care needs. There's no known organic brain damage with this disorder. Memory impairment is more of a problem with other dissociative disorders, such as dissociative identity disorder and dissociative amnesia. The dreamlike state can lead to problems meeting personal care needs, not a knowledge deficit.
CN: Safe, effective care environment; CNS: Safety and infection control; CL: Application

42. A severely depressed client who has made multiple suicide attempts matter-of-factly tells the nurse that her family life was normal and uneventful. Which behaviors would lead the nurse to suspect the diagnosis of a dissociative identity disorder (DID) in this client? Select all that apply:
1. Inability to recall important personal information too severe to be explained by ordinary forgetfulness
2. Absence of any physiological effects of a substance such as alcohol or drugs
3. Ability to selectively and consciously choose to avoid certain painful topics
4. A sense of grandiosity, that she's special and has a particular mission for mankind
5. Posttraumatic symptoms, such as flashbacks, nightmares, and an exaggerated startle response

42. 1, 2, 5. A dissociative disorder is a persistent state of being disconnected from the totality of one's personhood, particularly painful emotions. With dissociative disorder, the inability to recall personal information is far more extensive than ordinary forgetfulness; the symptoms occur apart from any chemical inducement, and the individual doesn't have the ability to consciously make a decision to separate from painful emotions or topics. A sense of grandiosity isn't characteristic of this disorder. Posttraumatic symptoms, such as flashbacks, nightmares, and an exaggerated startle response, are also signs and symptoms of DID.
CN: Psychosocial integrity; CNS: None; CL: Analysis

CN: Client needs category   CNS: Client needs subcategory   CL: Cognitive level

43. The wife of a client reports that her husband often disappears for days at a time, not showing up for work and then returning with no memory of anything out of the ordinary occurring. Which of the following might the nurse suspect? Select all that apply:
1. This client is experiencing sleep terror disorder that's interfering with his activities of daily life.
2. The client is taking drugs, possibly of a hallucinogenic nature.
3. The client is experiencing dissociative fugue.
4. The client has a form of a severe identity disorder.
5. The client may have a serious neurologic disorder and should be further examined by a competent neurologist.

44. A client is awake and sitting quietly in a chair but doesn't respond to verbal or tactile stimuli. He has had repeated episodes of staring into the distance, seemingly oblivious to events or persons in his immediate vicinity. When the client emerges from these episodes, he continues with life as usual. Which statements are accurate based on these assessment findings? Select all that apply:
1. The client has entered a state of self-induced hypnosis.
2. This client may be involved in ritual activity that has led him into a trancelike state.
3. The client is demonstrating signs of a dissociative trance disorder.
4. The client is in a state of malingering to obtain a secondary emotional gain.
5. The client is demonstrating psychotic behavior and decompensation.
6. The client has no control over his behavior.

43. 3, 4. Dissociative fugue is a type of dissociative identity disorder (DID) characterized by sudden, unexpected travel away from home, with the inability to recall what took place during this timeframe. DIDs are considered severe, chronic identity disorders. Sleep terror disorder involves recurrent episodes in which the client awakens abruptly from sleep and experiences feelings of panic. Use of hallucinogenic drugs is unlikely because drugs wouldn't explain the inability to recover lengthy periods of lost time such as this client demonstrates. A serious neurologic disorder is possible but not likely because there are no other physiological symptoms and the predominant complaint is more characteristic of a severe dissociative disorder.
CN: Psychosocial integrity; CNS: None; CL: Analysis

44. 3, 6. The client is demonstrating typical signs of a dissociative trance that isn't consciously induced. There's no basis to make the assumption that the client is in a state of self-induced hypnosis or has any involvement in ritual activities that would account for this behavioral state. There's no evidence to suggest that malingering is a reasonable explanation. The client, though not responsive, does come out of the trances and demonstrates normal behavior, so psychosis with decompensation can be ruled out.
CN: Psychosocial integrity; CNS: None; CL: Analysis

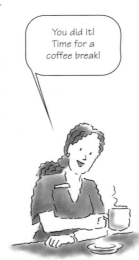

You did it! Time for a coffee break!

This chapter will test your knowledge of disorders of a highly sensitive nature. You'll do great. Good luck!

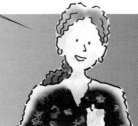

Chapter 20
Sexual & gender identity disorders

1. The wife of a male client who has undergone surgery for the repair of an abdominal aortic aneurysm asks if her husband will be impotent. Which response is <u>most appropriate</u>?
  1. "Don't worry; he'll be okay."
  2. "He has other problems to worry about."
  3. "We'll cross that bridge when we come to it."
  4. "There may be a chance of erectile dysfunction following this type of surgery."

2. Which discharge instruction would be <u>most accurate</u> for a female client who has suffered a spinal cord injury at the C4 level?
  1. "After a spinal cord injury, women usually remain fertile; therefore, you may consider contraception if you don't want to become pregnant."
  2. "After a spinal cord injury, women are usually unable to conceive a child."
  3. "Sexual intercourse shouldn't be different for you."
  4. "After a spinal cord injury, menstruation usually stops."

3. Diagnostic criteria for fetishism include which of the following? Select all that apply:
  1. During a 6-month period, there's recurrent sexual involvement with the use of non-living objects.
  2. Before the diagnostic 6-month period, the individual generally has normal sexual orientation and urges.
  3. These urges, fantasies, or behaviors cause significant impairment in the performance of activities of daily living (ADLs).
  4. The non-living objects involved in this behavior are usually items significant to the individual's childhood.
  5. This disorder generally begins in latency.

1. 4. Erectile dysunction and retrograde ejaculation are sexual dysfunctions commonly experienced after abdominal aortic aneurysm repair. Telling a family member that the client will be all right is offering false assurance. Stating that he has other problems isn't therapeutic and doesn't address the wife's concern. Telling the client's wife to "cross that bridge when we come to it" ignores her concerns and isn't therapeutic.
CN: Psychosocial integrity; CNS: None; CL: Application

2. 1. After a spinal cord injury, women remain fertile and can conceive and deliver a child. If a woman doesn't want to become pregnant, she *must* use contraception. Menstruation isn't affected by a spinal cord injury, but sexual functioning may be different.
CN: Physiological integrity; CNS: Physiological adaptation; CL: Application

3. 1, 3. Diagnostic criteria for fetishism include recurrent sexual involvement with the use of non-living objects during a 6-month period and significant impairment in performing ADLs due to the urges, fantasies, and behaviors. There's no specific indication that the individual has normal sexual orientation and urges prior to the actual development of the behavioral symptoms. The disorder generally begins in adolescence, and doesn't typically involve objects significant to the individual's childhood.
CN: Psychosocial integrity; CNS: None; CL: Comprehension

CN: Client needs category   CNS: Client needs subcategory   CL: Cognitive level

4. A client with chronic obstructive pulmonary disease (COPD) tells the nurse, "I no longer have enough energy to make love to my husband." Which nursing intervention would be <u>most appropriate</u>?

1. Referring the couple to a sex therapist
2. Referring the woman to a gynecologist
3. Suggesting methods and measures that conserve energy
4. Telling the client to discuss it with her husband

5. A client with an ileostomy tells the nurse he can't have an erection. What pertinent information should the nurse know?

1. The client will never regain erectile function.
2. The client needs an abdominal X-ray.
3. The client has no problem with the ability to control sexual functioning.
4. Impotence is uncommon after an ileostomy.

6. A recently divorced 40-year-old male who has undergone radiation therapy for prostate cancer tells the nurse he can't achieve an erection. Which nursing diagnosis would the nurse expect to find on the client's care plan?

1. *Ineffective coping related to cancer diagnosis*
2. *Sexual dysfunction related to the effects of radiation therapy*
3. *Disturbed body image related to the effects of radiation therapy*
4. *Fear related to cancer diagnosis*

7. Which action should the nurse include in the teaching plan of a newly married female client with a cervical spinal cord injury who doesn't wish to become pregnant at this time?

1. Provide the client with brochures on sexual practice.
2. Provide the client's husband with information on vasectomy.
3. Instruct the client on the rhythm method of contraception.
4. Instruct the client's husband on inserting a diaphragm with contraceptive jelly.

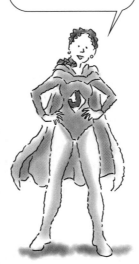

Just call me Super Nurse! I may not be faster than a speeding bullet, but I do deal with sensitive issues with my super-smart, super-compassionate nursing powers!

4. 3. Sexual dysfunction in COPD clients is the direct result of dyspnea and reduced energy levels. Measures to reduce physical exertion, enhance oxygenation, and accommodate decreased energy levels may aid sexual activity. If the problem persists, a consult with a therapist might be necessary. A gynecologic consult isn't necessary. Discussing this with her husband may not resolve the problem.
CN: Physiological integrity; CNS: Reduction of risk potential; CL: Application

5. 4. Sexual dysfunction is uncommon after an ileostomy; psychological causes of impotence should be explored. An abdominal X-ray isn't indicated for sexual dysfunction. An ileostomy can change a person's perception of self-control, making sexual functioning difficult.
CN: Psychosocial integrity; CNS: None; CL: Analysis

6. 2. Radiation or chemotherapy may cause sexual dysfunction. Libido may be only temporarily affected, and the client should be provided with emotional support. The client may experience alopecia or skin changes as well as weight loss, but the client isn't verbalizing concern in this area. The client hasn't verbalized fear or concern related to the cancer.
CN: Psychosocial integrity; CNS: None; CL: Analysis

7. 4. Because the client experienced a cervical spinal cord injury, she can't insert any form of contraception protection; therefore, it's vital to provide her husband with instructions on inserting a diaphragm. Providing the couple with literature on sexual practice doesn't address the client's concerns. During this time of crisis the couple doesn't wish to have children but they may reconsider, so providing information on vasectomy isn't appropriate. The rhythm method isn't the most effective way to prevent pregnancy.
CN: Psychosocial integrity; CNS: None; CL: Application

CN: Client needs category   CNS: Client needs subcategory   CL: Cognitive level

8. A female client tells the nurse she's having her menstrual period every 2 weeks, and it lasts for 1 week. Which term <u>best</u> defines this menstrual pattern?
1. Amenorrhea
2. Dyspareunia
3. Menorrhagia
4. Metrorrhagia

9. A nurse is caring for a 39-year-old male client who recently underwent surgery and is having difficulty accepting changes in his body image. Which nursing intervention is appropriate?
1. Actively listening to the client as he expresses positive and negative feelings about his body image
2. Restricting the client's opportunity to view the incision and dressing because it's upsetting
3. Assisting the client to focus on future plans for recovery
4. Assisting the client to repress anger while discussing the body image alteration

10. A 38-year-old woman must undergo a hysterectomy for uterine cancer. The nurse planning her care should include which action to meet the woman's body image changes?
1. Ask her if she's having pain.
2. Refer her to a psychotherapist.
3. Don't discuss the subject with her.
4. Encourage her to verbalize her feelings.

11. A 50-year-old male who had a myocardial infarction 8 weeks ago tells a nurse, "My wife wants to make love, but I don't think I can. I'm worried that it might kill me." Which response from the nurse would be <u>most appropriate</u>?
1. "Tell me about your feelings."
2. "Let's have you do more rehabilitation."
3. "Let me call the primary health care provider for you."
4. "Tell your wife that, when you're able, you'll make love."

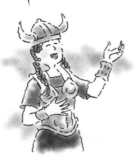

You say menorrhagia, I say metrorrhagia. Let's call the whole thing off!

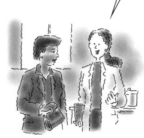

Can we talk? Encouraging a client to verbalize feelings is therapeutic for the client and revealing for the nurse.

8. 3. Menorrhagia is excessive uterine bleeding flow and duration during a menstrual period. Amenorrhea is lack of menstruation. Dyspareunia is painful intercourse. Metrorrhagia is uterine bleeding from a cause other than menstruation.
CN: Physiological integrity; CNS: Reduction of risk potential; CL: Application

9. 1. The nurse must observe for any indication that the client is ready to address his body image change. The client should be allowed to look at the incision and dressing if he wants to do so. It's too soon to focus on the future with this client. The nurse should allow the client to express his feelings and not repress them, because repression prolongs recovery.
CN: Psychosocial integrity; CNS: None; CL: Application

10. 4. The nurse should encourage the client to verbalize her feelings because loss of reproductive organs may bring on feelings of loss related to body image and sexuality. Pain is a concern after surgery, but it has no bearing on body image. Referring her to a psychotherapist may be premature; the client should be given time to work through her feelings. Avoiding the subject isn't a therapeutic nursing intervention.
CN: Psychosocial integrity; CNS: None; CL: Application

11. 1. The nurse should address the client's concerns. Asking the client to verbalize his feelings will permit the nurse to gain insight into the problem. Rehabilitation shouldn't be increased until the nurse assesses the situation and is sure no harm will come to the client. Calling the primary health care provider before a complete assessment is made is inappropriate. Telling the wife that eventually the client will be able to make love may place strain on the marriage.
CN: Psychosocial integrity; CNS: None; CL: Application

CN: Client needs category   CNS: Client needs subcategory   CL: Cognitive level

12. A 55-year-old female client who's in cardiac rehabilitation tells a nurse that she can't make love to her husband because she often feels excessively fatigued and has a sense of doom. Which nursing intervention is <u>most</u> <u>appropriate</u>?
1. Instructing her not to have intercourse until she's ready
2. Instructing her to take a nitroglycerin tablet prior to intercourse
3. Encouraging her to learn additional methods to use for sexual intercourse
4. Collecting data regarding her fatigue and reporting the findings to the physician

13. A 33-year-old female client tells the nurse she has never had an orgasm. She tells the nurse that her partner is upset that he can't meet her needs. Which nursing intervention is <u>most appropriate</u>?
1. Asking the client if she desires intercourse
2. Assessing the couple's perception of the problem
3. Telling the client that most women don't reach orgasm
4. Referring the client to a therapist because she has sexual aversion disorder

14. A 20-year-old female client is in the emergency department after being sexually assaulted by a stranger. Which nursing intervention has the <u>highest priority</u>?
1. Assisting her in identifying which of her behaviors placed her at risk for the attack
2. Making an appointment for her in 6 weeks at a local sexual assault crisis center
3. Encouraging discussion of her early childhood experiences
4. Assisting her in identifying family or friends who could provide immediate support for her

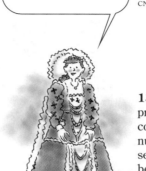

Fortunately, choosing an appropriate nursing intervention is easier than choosing an appropriate outfit. The invitation said "evening casual." What do you think?

12. 4. Because the client has a complaint of fatigue, she should be examined. Instructing her not to have intercourse doesn't address her concerns. She shouldn't take nitroglycerin before intercourse until her fatigue is evaluated. Before recommending alternative methods for intercourse, the nurse should assess the client physically and psychologically.
CN: Psychosocial integrity; CNS: None; CL: Application

13. 2. Assessing the couple's perception of the problem will define the problem and assist the couple and the nurse in understanding it. A nurse can't make a medical diagnosis such as sexual aversion disorder. Most individuals can be taught to reach orgasm if there's no underlying medical condition. When assessing the client, the nurse should be professional and matter-of-fact, and shouldn't make the client feel inadequate or defensive.
CN: Psychosocial integrity; CNS: None; CL: Application

14. 4. The client needs a lot of support to help her through this ordeal. Assisting the client in identifying behaviors that placed her at risk for the attack places the blame on the client. Waiting 6 weeks to make an appointment is incorrect—the local crisis center must be called immediately. Some psychiatric disorders are related to early childhood experiences, but rape isn't.
CN: Psychosocial integrity; CNS: None; CL: Application

CN: Client needs category   CNS: Client needs subcategory   CL: Cognitive level

15. A 50-year-old male client taking antihypertensive medication tells the nurse who's monitoring his blood pressure that he can't have sexual intercourse with his wife anymore because of erectile dysfunction. When teaching the client, which response by the nurse would be <u>most</u> appropriate?
1. "Erectile dysfunction is an inevitable occurrence with advancing age."
2. "Medical treatment for hypertension will improve erectile dysfunction."
3. "Psychological stress is the most common cause of erectile dysfunction."
4. "Erectile dysfunction usually has a physical cause."

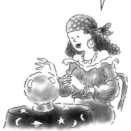

Oh, great powers of nursing. Which option is correct? Actually, hitting the books is probably more reliable than mystical powers!

16. Adult victims of childhood sexual abuse need to be monitored for signs and symptoms of which disorders?
1. Depression and substance abuse disorders
2. Bipolar and somatization disorders
3. Narcissistic disorders and bulimia nervosa
4. Obsessive-compulsive and posttraumatic stress disorders

17. Which condition is <u>most</u> likely to be associated with female infertility?
1. Oral contraceptive use for 2 years
2. Sexually transmitted disease (STD)
3. Anemia
4. Osteoporosis

18. A male client reports to the nurse that he has a strong desire to live and be treated as a woman. He confesses that he's uncomfortable with his assigned sex. What best describes these feelings?
1. Delusions
2. Gender identity issues
3. Homosexuality
4. Hormone imbalances

15. 4. Approximately 70% of cases of erectile dysfunction can be traced to physical causes and about 20% to 30% can be traced to psychological causes. Although the incidence of erectile dysfunction increases with age, the condition isn't an inevitable part of the aging process. Controlling hypertension may help prevent vascular damage, but some antihypertensives may cause erectile dysfunction.
CN: Physiological integrity; CNS: Pharmacological therapies; CL: Application

16. 1. Childhood sexual abuse is closely linked to the development of depression and substance abuse disorders. It's also linked to the development of somatization and posttraumatic stress disorders and bulimia nervosa. Victims of childhood sexual abuse aren't predisposed to developing bipolar, narcissistic, or obsessive-compulsive disorders.
CN: Psychosocial integrity; CNS: None; CL: Analysis

17. 2. If left untreated, some STDs can interfere with fertility. A history of taking oral contraceptives doesn't lead to infertility. Anemia doesn't lead to infertility; however, correcting this condition can make fertility and maintaining a pregnancy more favorable. Osteoporosis is a condition in which bone loss occurs; the risk of developing osteoporosis increases after menopause.
CN: Health promotion and maintenance; CNS: None; CL: Application

18. 2. A persistent cross-gender identification and dissatisfaction with one's assigned gender are major characteristics of gender identity disorders. Delusions are firmly held beliefs not substantiated in reality. Homosexuality is an attraction to members of the same sex. Hormone imbalances aren't relevant to the diagnosis of gender identity issues.
CN: Psychosocial integrity; CNS: None; CL: Knowledge

CN: Client needs category   CNS: Client needs subcategory   CL: Cognitive level

19. Which treatment might be used for a client with gender identity disorder?
1. Group therapy
2. Surgical sexual reassignment
3. Relaxation techniques
4. Antipsychotic agent

20. Which statement by a male client with paraphilia indicates a potential for relapse?
1. "I'll go to outpatient therapy."
2. "I'm going to try to attend all therapy sessions."
3. "I can't imagine why the judge sent me here."
4. "The physician wants me to take leuprolide acetate (Lupron). I think that will help."

21. A 38-year-old woman was returning home from the store late one evening and was sexually assaulted. When she's brought to the emergency department, she's crying. Which intervention for this client should be the nurse's <u>first priority</u>?
1. Filing a police report
2. Calling the client's family
3. Encouraging the client to enroll in a self-defense class
4. Remaining with the client and assisting her through the crisis

22. A 20-year-old single female client in college who has recently been diagnosed with human papillomavirus infection comes to the health clinic. She has researched her condition and appears anxious and tearful. Which nursing intervention would be <u>most</u> appropriate?
1. Asking the client to discuss her concerns
2. Providing her with reliable information about this condition
3. Referring her to her gynecologist
4. Discussing the dangers of multiple sex partners

19. 2. A surgical sexual reassignment operation is the treatment for gender identity disorder. This treatment is undertaken only after careful clinical interviews and evaluations by specialists in this field. Group therapy and relaxation techniques may be helpful to this client, but aren't specific to the treatment of this disorder. Antipsychotic drugs aren't appropriate for this condition.
CN: Psychosocial integrity; CNS: None; CL: Application

20. 3. A lack of insight into his problem may indicate a potential for relapse for this client. Attending all therapy sessions and outpatient therapy demonstrates compliance with the treatment plan. Leuprolide acetate is an antiandrogenic that lowers testosterone levels and decreases the libido.
CN: Psychosocial integrity; CNS: None; CL: Analysis

21. 4. Sexual assault is treated as a medical emergency, and the client requires constant attention and assistance during the crisis. Filing a police report wouldn't take precedence over a medical emergency. Comforting the client by contacting her family should be carried out after her injuries are treated. Encouraging the client to enroll in a self-defense class isn't appropriate during crisis.
CN: Psychosocial integrity; CNS: None; CL: Application

22. 1. Encouraging the client to discuss her concerns establishes a nonjudgmental, therapeutic relationship and would be the best initial response. Other interventions might be appropriate at some point. The nurse should take care to discuss the dangers of multiple sex partners in a nonjudgmental manner.
CN: Psychosocial integrity; CNS: None; CL: Application

23. A client is admitted to the hospital for treatment of pedophilia and tells the nurse that he doesn't want to talk to her about his sexual behaviors. Which response from the nurse is <u>most appropriate</u>?

1. "I need to ask you the questions on the database."
2. "It's your right not to answer my questions."
3. "OK, I'll just write 'no comment.'"
4. "I know this must be difficult for you."

24. A 30-year-old single female client with ulcerative colitis has recently had a colostomy. She appears anxious and says to the nurse, "I don't think I can ever have a sexual relationship now that I have this." Which response by the nurse would be <u>most</u> appropriate?

1. Offer to refer her to a support group.
2. Allow her to express her concerns to the nurse.
3. Offer to research statistics on this topic.
4. Explore the positive aspects of her treatment regimen.

25. A male client is brought to the emergency department after being sexually assaulted by a rival gang member. The nurse observes that the client appears relaxed and is calmly talking to a relative. The nurse determines that the client may be using which defense mechanism?

1. Rationalization
2. Denial
3. Displacement
4. Projection

26. Which goal is appropriate for a client diagnosed with pedophilia?

1. Attending all meetings on the unit
2. Using triggers to initiate sexual behaviors
3. Informing his employer of the reason for his hospitalization
4. Verbalizing appropriate methods to meet sexual needs on discharge

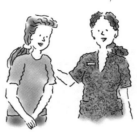

Getting a client to open up and communicate requires a bit more subtlety. Check out question 23 for some better ideas!

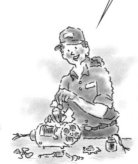

In the toolbox of defense mechanisms, denial is the biggest power tool of all!

23. 4. Stating "I know this must be difficult for you" acknowledges the client's feelings and opens communication. Insisting that the form must be completed doesn't open up communication or acknowledge the client's feelings. Clients have rights, but data collection is necessary so that help with the problem can be offered. Writing "no comment" alone would be inappropriate.

CN: Psychosocial integrity; CNS: None; CL: Application

24. 2. Allowing the client to express her concerns is a therapeutic first step. Referring her to a support group is premature. Offering to research statistics or to explore positive aspects of treatment negate the emotional aspect of this problem, and the client might conclude that it isn't acceptable to discuss her feelings.

CN: Physiological integrity; CNS: Reduction of risk potential; CL: Application

25. 2. The client is demonstrating the defense mechanism of denial, in which a client retreats into himself to reduce the threat of what has happened to his self-concept. Rationalization prevents admitting an inadequacy. Displacement transfers feelings about one person to another. Projection places blame on someone else or on circumstances.

NCN: Psychosocial integrity; CNS: None; CL: Analysis

26. 4. On discharge, the client should be able to verbalize an alternative appropriate method to meet his sexual needs, and effective strategies to prevent relapse. It isn't imperative that the client attend all meetings on the unit, but it's important that the client attend the prescribed group sessions. A client with pedophilia should recognize triggers that initiate inappropriate sexual behavior, and learn ways to direct his impulses. The client may wish to discuss the disorder with his spouse but not necessarily with his employer.

CN: Psychosocial integrity; CNS: None; CL: Analysis

CN: Client needs category   CNS: Client needs subcategory   CL: Cognitive level

27. A client admitted to the hospital with a diagnosis of pedophilia tells his roommate about his problems. His roommate runs down the hall yelling at the nurse, "I don't want to be in here with a child molester." Which response from the nurse is <u>most appropriate</u>?
  1. "Stop acting out."
  2. "Calm down and go back to your room."
  3. "Your roommate isn't a child molester."
  4. "I can see you're upset. Let's sit down and we'll talk."

28. A client states that he has been diagnosed with voyeurism. The nurse knows which action is characteristic of a voyeur?
  1. Observing others while they disrobe
  2. Wearing clothing of the opposite sex
  3. Rubbing against a nonconsenting person
  4. Using rubber sheeting for sexual arousal

29. A female being treated for infertility confides to the nurse that she hasn't told her partner she has been treated for a sexually transmitted disease in the past. What would be the most therapeutic response for the nurse to give?
  1. "Do you think withholding this information is the basis for a trusting relationship?"
  2. "Don't you think your partner deserves to know?"
  3. "What concerns do you have about sharing this information?"
  4. "I can understand why you would want to keep this information from him."

30. After learning that his gay roommate has tested positive for human immunodeficiency virus, a client asks the nurse about moving to another room on the psychiatric unit because the client doesn't feel "safe" now. What should the nurse do <u>first</u>?
  1. Move the client to another room.
  2. Ask the client to describe any fears.
  3. Move the client's roommate to a private room.
  4. Explain that such a move wouldn't be therapeutic for the client or his roommate.

27. 4. Acknowledging that the client is upset and sitting down and talking with him allows the client to verbalize his feelings. Telling the client to stop acting out isn't a therapeutic response. If a client were agitated or anxious over his roommate, it wouldn't be therapeutic or safe to keep those clients together without intervention. Stating that the pedophile isn't a child molester doesn't acknowledge the client's feelings.
CN: Psychosocial integrity; CNS: None; CL: Application

28. 1. Voyeurism is sexual arousal from secretly observing someone who's disrobing. A transvestic fetishism describes the enjoyment of cross-dressing. Rubbing against someone who is nonconsenting is frottage. Using objects for sexual arousal is fetishism.
CN: Psychosocial integrity; CNS: None; CL: Application

29. 3. This response encourages the client to verbalize her concerns in a safe environment and begin to choose a course of action for how to deal with this issue now. Telling the client that she's withholding information that may cause distrust in her relationship, and that her partner deserves to know conveys negative judgments. The fourth response doesn't encourage discussion or problem solving.
CN: Psychosocial integrity; CNS: None; CL: Application

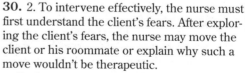

Dealing effectively with clients' conflicting needs and concerns can be a balancing act. Question 30 will help you achieve that delicate balance.

30. 2. To intervene effectively, the nurse must first understand the client's fears. After exploring the client's fears, the nurse may move the client or his roommate or explain why such a move wouldn't be therapeutic.
CN: Psychosocial integrity; CNS: None; CL: Application

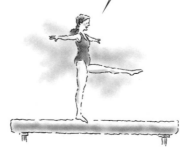

31. A rape victim comes to the emergency department for treatment. Which nursing diagnosis would most likely be identified to address the psychological component of this crisis?
1. *Sexual dysfunction*
2. *Risk for infection*
3. *Acute pain*
4. *Rape-trauma syndrome*

32. A nurse lecturing on paraphilias informs her audience that recidivism is high for paraphilias. Which definition <u>best</u> describes recidivism?
1. Insight into treatment
2. Aggressive sexual assault
3. Behaviors associated with sexual deviation
4. Continued inappropriate behavior after treatment

33. Which aspect of treatment for infertility do couples commonly report as the <u>most</u> stressful?
1. Receiving examinations
2. Giving specimens
3. Scheduling sexual intercourse
4. Finding out which partner is infertile

34. A 42-year-old female client reports that recently she finds intercourse to be painful. Which nursing diagnosis is <u>most</u> useful when planning this client's care?
1. *Ineffective coping*
2. *Disturbed body image*
3. *Ineffective sexuality patterns*
4. *Sexual dysfunction*

35. A nurse knows that <u>gender</u> is part of one's identity. Which event signifies when gender is first ascribed?
1. A neonate is born.
2. A child attends school.
3. A child receives sex-specific toys.
4. A child receives sex-specific clothing.

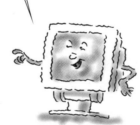

Couples dealing with infertility can experience a range of emotions. If you don't believe me, take a good look at question 33.

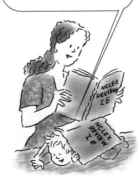

I'm all boy, and I have been since...oops, that would be giving too much away!

31. 4. *Rape-trauma syndrome* is the most likely nursing diagnosis for this client. There's no evidence that this client has a sexual dysfunction. *Risk for infection* and *Acute pain* may be appropriate diagnoses related to the physical aspect of this trauma, but they don't address psychological issues.
CN: Psychosocial integrity; CNS: None; CL: Comprehension

32. 4. Recidivism is defined as continuing in an unacceptable behavior after completing treatment to correct that behavior. High level of insight isn't connected with any specific disorder. Aggressive sexual assault is a type of paraphilia. Sexually deviant behaviors are known as *paraphilias.*
CN: Psychosocial integrity; CNS: None; CL: Analysis

33. 3. The major cause of stress in infertile couples is planning sexual intercourse to correlate with fertility cycles. The inconvenience and discomfort of receiving examinations and producing specimens aren't major stressors. Most couples undergoing fertility treatment understand that one partner is usually infertile.
CN: Health promotion and maintenance; CNS: None; CL: Application

34. 4. *Sexual dysfunction* is the most useful nursing diagnosis for this client because she has identified painful intercourse as a physical problem, which can alter the giving and receiving of pleasure and satisfaction. *Ineffective coping* would apply if the client stated she avoids intercourse or expresses alternative coping mechanisms. *Disturbed body image* isn't appropriate because the client hasn't stated that she's uncomfortable with her body image. *Ineffective sexuality patterns* would apply if the client stated she doesn't engage in intercourse or have the ability to relate to others sexually.
CN: Psychosocial integrity; CNS: None; NP: Application

35. 1. As soon as a neonate is born, gender is ascribed. In the hospital, a neonate is given either a pink or blue name band, card, or blanket. Sexual identity is reaffirmed throughout the school years. Gender identification is perpetuated throughout life with sex-specific clothing and toys.
CN: Psychosocial integrity; CNS: None; CL: Comprehension

CN: Client needs category   CNS: Client needs subcategory   CL: Cognitive level

36. A mother brings her 14-year-old son to the psychiatric crisis room. The client's mother states, "He's always dressing in female clothing. There must be something wrong with him." Which response from the nurse would be <u>most appropriate</u>?

1. "Your son will be evaluated shortly."
2. "I'll tell your son that this isn't appropriate."
3. "You seem to be upset. Would you like to talk?"
4. "I wouldn't want my son to dress in girl's clothing."

37. A female client taking antidepressant medication complains to the nurse that she has a decreased desire for sex, which is causing significant marital stress. Which response by the nurse would be the most appropriate?

1. "Don't stop taking the medication."
2. "What are your thoughts on how you should handle this?"
3. "Doesn't your husband understand the importance of your medication?"
4. "Have you discussed this with your physician?"

38. Which reason explains the rationale for estrogen therapy for a male client who wishes to undergo sexual reassignment surgery?

1. To develop breasts
2. To cause menstruation
3. To assist with cross-dressing
4. To develop body hair and stop menstruation

39. A nurse is assisting in developing a teaching plan on rape prevention. Which guideline would have the <u>highest</u> priority in this plan?

1. Avoid drinking heavily at a party.
2. Avoid walking alone at night.
3. Learn ways to defend yourself.
4. Always take the shortest driving route home.

36. 3. Acknowledging the mother's feelings and offering her an opportunity to verbalize her concerns provides a forum for open communication. Telling the client's mother that he'll be evaluated shortly doesn't address her concerns. Telling the client that this behavior isn't appropriate doesn't assess his feelings, nor does it analyze the behavior. The nurse shouldn't offer an opinion by stating she wouldn't want her son dressing in female clothing.
CN: Psychosocial integrity; CNS: None; CL: Application

37. 2. Encouraging the client to verbalize her thoughts will help the client to problem solve and identify feelings related to different choices. The first response is too directive and doesn't encourage exploration on the part of the client. The third response conveys negative judgment. The fourth response might be appropriate, but it may also give the impression that the nurse doesn't want to discuss this issue with the client.
CN: Psychosocial integrity; CNS: None; CL: Application

38. 1. A male who receives long-term estrogen therapy will develop female secondary sexual characteristics such as breasts. A male on estrogen won't menstruate as he doesn't have a uterus. Estrogen has no bearing on cross-dressing. Androgens would be taken by a female to develop body hair and stop menstruation.
CN: Psychosocial integrity; CNS: None; CL: Analysis

39. 3. Learning self-defense methods helps protect an individual in various situations. Drinking heavily at a party, especially if alone, and walking alone at night would tend to compromise safety. The shortest driving route might take an individual through a high-crime neighborhood; one should learn alternative routes in order to have options if safety seems compromised.
CN: Health promotion and maintenance; CNS: None; CL: Application

Faster isn't always better. Check out question 39 and you'll see what I mean.

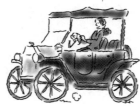

CN: Client needs category   CNS: Client needs subcategory   CL: Cognitive level

40. A nurse is collecting data on a male client with the potential diagnosis of gender identity disorder. The nurse knows that the diagnostic criteria for this disorder in a male must include a persistent identification with femaleness and which other sign or symptom?
1. Significant impairment in social, occupational, or other important area of functioning
2. Co-existing physical intersex condition
3. Simple rejection of sex-role stereotypes without distress
4. Delusional ideas of belonging to the female sex with a secondary diagnosis of schizophrenia

41. A group of female college students was walking back to their dorm at night. Suddenly, a man ran out from the bushes and exposed himself to them. All of the women were initially startled, but all but one began to laugh. This one female went to the health clinic because she was so upset. Which response by the nurse would be <u>most helpful</u> psychologically to this student?
1. "Can you imagine a flasher on campus!"
2. "I'll call security right away."
3. "I can see you're upset. Tell me more about this."
4. "Please describe this person to me."

42. According to Erikson, an adolescent who's suffering from gender identity disorder can't progress through which developmental task?
1. Initiative versus guilt
2. Intimacy versus isolation
3. Industry versus inferiority
4. Identity versus role confusion

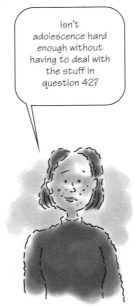

Isn't adolescence hard enough without having to deal with the stuff in question 42?

40. 1. Diagnostic criteria for male gender identity disorder include a pervasive identification with femaleness and feelings of discomfort or inappropriateness with maleness. These feelings cause significant distress and disturbances in functioning and aren't simply a rejection of sex-role stereotypes. Gender identity disorder doesn't usually occur as a result of an intersex condition and rarely occurs along with a diagnosis of schizophrenia.
CN: Psychosocial integrity; CNS: None; CL: Analysis

41. 3. Acknowledging the client's emotions is the best initial step in helping her talk about her concerns. The first response isn't therapeutic. The second and fourth responses are appropriate interventions but don't help the student deal with her emotional reaction.
CN: Psychosocial integrity; CNS: None; CL: Analysis

42. 4. According to developmentalist Erik Erikson, adolescence is a time when role identity is found as a result of independence and sexual maturity; role confusion would result from the inability to integrate all experiences. Initiative versus guilt is when a child begins to conceptualize and interpersonalize relationships. Intimacy versus isolation is a stage in which the adult meets other adults and establishes relationships. Industry versus inferiority is when a child incorporates and acquires social skills.
CN: Health promotion and maintenance; CNS: None; CL: Analysis

CN: Client needs category   CNS: Client needs subcategory   CL: Cognitive level

43. A 35-year-old male who has been married for 10 years arrives at the psychiatric clinic stating, "I can't live this lie any more. I wish I were a woman. I don't want my wife. I need a man." Which nursing intervention would be most appropriate?
1. Calling the primary health care provider
2. Encouraging the client to speak to his wife
3. Having the client admitted
4. Sitting down with the client, and talking about his feelings

44. A 35-year-old male client states he has little or no sexual desire. He states this is causing great distress in his marriage. What further information would be <u>most useful</u> in assessing the situation? Select all that apply:
1. The client's age when he had his first girlfriend
2. When the problem first appeared and potential contributing factors
3. Medications and dosages
4. Report of recent bladder or prostate problems
5. Age of the client's wife

45. Pedophilia is diagnosed by the presence of specifically defined behaviors and characteristics. Which statements regarding pedophilia are true? Select all that apply:
1. A strong sexual attraction to prepubescent children exists.
2. Male children are more commonly the focus of attention than female children.
3. The pedophile is usually very attentive to a child's needs to gain their attention.
4. The disorder generally begins in early adulthood.
5. The pedophile must be age 16 or older or at least 5 years older than the child.

43. 4. Sitting down with the client and exploring his feelings will allow the nurse to assess him. The primary health care provider shouldn't be notified until an assessment is made. The client shouldn't speak to his wife until he has processed his feelings. An assessment of the client should be made *before* admitting him to the unit.
CN: Psychosocial integrity; CNS: None; CL: Application

44. 2, 3. Option 2 is correct and provides opportunity to gather a great deal of useful information in better understanding the client's current condition. Option 3 is correct because certain medications can have a profound effect on sexual desire. The client's age when he started dating has no bearing on the current problem. Reporting previous problems is useful but wouldn't provide a sufficient explanation for the lack of sexual desire. The age of the client's wife is irrelevant and doesn't provide assessment data.
CN: Psychosocial integrity; CNS: None; CL: Analysis

45. 1, 3, 5. Pedophilia is a disorder characterized by a strong sexual attraction to prepubescent children that generally begins to manifest itself in adolescence, not early adulthood. By definition, the pedophile must be age 16 or older or at least 5 years older than the child. The pedophile generally is attentive to the needs of children in order to gain their trust, loyalty, and attention. Female, not male, children are more commonly the focus of attention.
CN: Psychosocial integrity; CNS: None; CL: Comprehension

Congratulations! You're finished! You're at peak performance!

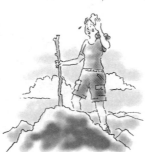

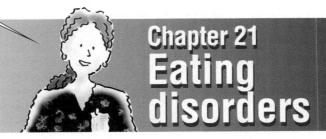

New information about eating disorders is released continuously. Start educating yourself by considering these questions carefully!

Chapter 21
Eating disorders

1. A parent whose daughter is diagnosed with bulimia nervosa asks a nurse, "How can my child have an eating disorder when she isn't underweight?" Which response is best?

1. "A person with bulimia nervosa can maintain a normal weight."
2. "It's hard to face this type of problem in a person you love."
3. "At first there's no weight loss; it comes later in the disease."
4. "This is a serious problem even though there's no weight loss."

2. A nurse is reviewing the chart of an adolescent client who has been admitted to the unit. When reading the progress notes below, the nurse notes a laboratory result that indicates a condition consistent with a diagnosis of bulimia nervosa. Which condition does the nurse suspect?

Progress notes	
9/4/08 1015	Received 15-year-old female admitted with diagnosis of bulimia nervosa. Vital signs: blood pressure, 100/70 mm Hg; heart rate, 82 beats/minute; respiratory rate, 20 breaths/minute; temperature, 98° F (36.7° C). Laboratory results: Na, 136 mEq/L; K, 3.0 mEq/L; Cl, 104 mEq/L; Ca, 9.5 mg/dl; fasting blood glucose, 90 mg/dl. Results called to Dr. L. Smith, M.D. ————Barbara Jones, L.P.N.

1. Hypocalcemia
2. Hypoglycemia
3. Hypokalemia
4. Hyponatremia

1. 1. A person with bulimia nervosa may be of normal weight, overweight, or underweight. Weight loss isn't a clinical criterion for bulimia nervosa. The second and fourth responses don't address the need for information about the relationship between weight change and bulimia nervosa. The third response is incorrect bacause the client may experience little or no weight loss.

CN: Psychosocial integrity; CNS: None; CL: Application

2. 3. Clients who are bulimic will have hypokalemia (decreased potassium levels) due to purging behaviors. Hyponatremia, hypoglycemia, and hypocalcemia don't tend to occur in clients with bulimia nervosa; all of these values are at normal levels for this client.

CN: Physiological integrity; CNS: Physiological adaptation; CL: Analysis

CN: Client needs category   CNS: Client needs subcategory   CL: Cognitive level

3. Which statement about the binge-purge cycle that occurs with bulimia nervosa is correct?
1. There are emotional triggers connected to bingeing.
2. Over time, people usually grow out of bingeing behaviors.
3. Bingeing isn't the problem; purging is the issue to address.
4. When a person gets too hungry, there's a tendency to binge.

4. A client with bulimia and a history of purging by vomiting is hospitalized for further observation because she's at risk for which of the following?
1. Diabetes mellitus
2. Electrolyte imbalances and cardiac arrhythmias
3. GI obstruction
4. Septicemia from a low white blood cell count

5. A client with a diagnosis of bulimia nervosa is working on relationship issues. Which nursing intervention is the <u>most important</u>?
1. Having the client work on developing social skills
2. Focusing on how relationships cause bulimic behavior
3. Helping the client identify feelings about relationships
4. Discussing how to prevent getting overinvolved in relationships

6. A young woman with bulimia nervosa wants to lessen her feelings of powerlessness. Which short-term goal is most important <u>initially</u>?
1. Learning problem-solving skills
2. Decreasing symptoms of anxiety
3. Performing self-care activities daily
4. Verbalizing how to set limits with others

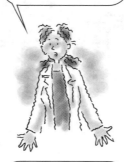

Emotions sure can be powerful. Just ask a client with an eating disorder—or a nurse!

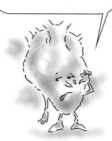

You'll be heart-sick when you learn what purging can do to me.

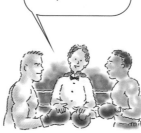

Want to know what can give a client with bulimia nervosa a sense of power? The answer is in question 6.

3. 1. It's important for the client to understand the emotional triggers for bingeing, such as disappointment, depression, and anxiety. People don't outgrow eating disorders. This response leads a person to believe binge-eating is a normal part of growth and development when it definitely isn't. The third statement negates the seriousness of bingeing and leads the client to believe only vomiting is a problem. Physiologic hunger doesn't predispose a client to bingeing behaviors.
CN: Psychosocial integrity; CNS: None; CL: Comprehension

4. 2. People who purge by vomiting are at great risk for electrolyte imbalance and resulting cardiac arrhythmias. Purging doesn't lead to any of the other conditions listed.
CN: Physiological integrity; CNS: Reduction of risk potential; CL: Application

5. 3. The client must address personal feelings, especially uncomfortable ones because they may trigger bingeing behavior. Social skills are important to a client's well-being but they aren't typically a major problem for the client with bulimia nervosa. Relationships *don't cause* bulimic behaviors. It's the inability to handle stress or conflict that arises from interactions that causes the client to be distressed. The client isn't necessarily overinvolved in relationships; the issue may be the lack of satisfying relationships in the person's life.
CN: Psychosocial integrity; CNS: None; CL: Application

6. 1. If the client can learn effective problem-solving skills, she'll gain a sense of control and power over her life. Anxiety is commonly caused by feelings of powerlessness. Performing daily self-care activities won't reduce one's sense of powerlessness. Verbalizing how to set limits and protect herself from the intrusive behavior of others is a necessary life skill, but problem-solving skills take priority in this case.
CN: Psychosocial integrity; CNS: None; CL: Comprehension

7. A client with bulimia nervosa tells a nurse her parents don't know about her eating disorder. Which goal is appropriate for this client and her family?
1. Decreasing the chaos in the family unit
2. Learning effective communication skills
3. Spending time together in social situations
4. Discussing the client's need to be responsible

8. When discussing self-esteem with a client with bulimia nervosa, which area is the <u>most important</u>?
1. Personal fears
2. Family strengths
3. Negative thinking
4. Environmental stimuli

9. Which complication of bulimia nervosa is <u>life-threatening</u>?
1. Amenorrhea
2. Bradycardia
3. Gastric rupture
4. Yellow skin

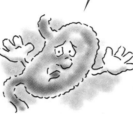

I'm a little queasy. I just read the answer to question 9.

10. A nurse is talking to a client with bulimia nervosa about the complications of laxative abuse. Which statement by the client indicates that she's beginning to understand the risks associated with laxative abuse?
1. "I don't really have much taste for food, so there's no loss in getting it out of my system more quickly."
2. "Laxatives help me get rid of extra calories before they're added to my body. I know I just shouldn't eat the extra calories to begin with."
3. "Laxatives are over-the-counter medications that have no harmful effect."
4. "Using laxatives prevents my body from absorbing essential nutrients, such as protein, fat, and calcium."

7. 2. A major goal for the client and her family is to learn to communicate directly and honestly. To change the chaotic environment, the family must first learn to communicate effectively. Families with a member who has an eating disorder are commonly enmeshed and don't need to spend more time together. Before discussing the client's level of responsibility, the family needs to establish effective ways of communicating with one another.
CN: Psychosocial integrity; CNS: None; CL: Comprehension

8. 3. Clients with bulimia nervosa need to work on identifying and changing their negative thinking and distortion of reality. Personal fears are related to negative thinking. Exploring family strengths isn't a priority; it's more appropriate to explore the client's strengths. Environmental stimuli don't cause bulimic behaviors.
CN: Psychosocial integrity; CNS: None; CL: Application

9. 3. Gastric rupture from purging can be a life-threatening complication of bulimia nervosa. Amenorrhea, bradycardia, and yellow skin are complications of bulimia nervosa that don't tend to be life-threatening.
CN: Physiological integrity; CNS: Reduction of risk potential; CL: Knowledge

10. 4. A serious complication of laxative abuse is malabsorption of nutrients, such as proteins, fats, and calcium. Laxative abuse doesn't tend to affect the client's sense of taste. Clients with bulimia nervosa need to change their negative thinking in regard to calories and the use of laxatives.
CN: Physiological integrity; CNS: Reduction of risk potential; CL: Application

CN: Client needs category   CNS: Client needs subcategory   CL: Cognitive level

11. Which nursing diagnosis should the nurse expect to find in the nursing care plan for a client with bulimia?

1. *Decreased cardiac output related to muscle spasms in the hands and feet*
2. *Risk for infection related to enlargement of salivary and parotid glands*
3. *Disturbed thought processes related to personal identity disturbance*
4. *Ineffective denial related to underlying need for acceptance*

12. A client is talking with a nurse about her binge-purge cycle. Which question should the nurse ask about the cycle?

1. "Do you know how to stop the binge-purge cycle?"
2. "Does the binge-purge cycle help you lose weight?"
3. "Can the binge-purge cycle take away your anxiety?"
4. "How often do you go through the binge-purge cycle?"

13. A nurse is collecting data about possible substance abuse in a client with bulimia nervosa. Which question is best for obtaining information about this possible problem?

1. "Have you ever used diet pills?"
2. "Where would you go to buy drugs?"
3. "At what age did you start drinking?"
4. "Do your peers ever offer you drugs?"

14. A client with bulimia nervosa is discussing her abnormal eating behaviors. Which statement by the client indicates she's beginning to understand this eating disorder?

1. "When my loneliness gets to me, I start to binge."
2. "I know that when my life gets better I'll eat right."
3. "I know I waste food and waste my money on food."
4. "After my parents divorce, I'll talk about bingeing and purging."

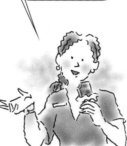

To the person with bulimia nervosa, eating is more about emotions than hunger or nutrition.

11. 4. An unmet need for acceptance can cause denial about self-destructive behaviors and is congruent with the underlying dynamics of eating disorders. Decreased cardiac output isn't caused by muscle spasms in the hands and feet. Enlarged parotid and salivary glands don't cause infection. Disturbed thought processes aren't caused by personal identity disturbance.
CN: Psychosocial integrity; CNS: None; CL: Application

12. 4. This question is important because there's usually a range of frequencies, such as from a once-a-week pattern to multiple times each day. The first question isn't an appropriate question because it will generate feelings of self-blame and shame. It's common for clients with bulimia nervosa to experience daily fluctuations in their weight. Some clients report weight variations of up to 10 lb (4.5 kg). The binge-purge cycle may initially relieve mood symptoms, but it tends to generate overall negative feelings about self.
CN: Psychosocial integrity; CNS: None; CL: Application

13. 1. Some clients with bulimia nervosa have a history of or actively use amphetamines to control weight. The use of alcohol and street drugs is also common. The second and fourth questions could be answered by the client without revealing drug use. The age the client started drinking may not reveal current substance use.
CN: Psychosocial integrity; CNS: None; CL: Application

14. 1. Binge eating is a way to handle the uncomfortable feelings of frustration, loneliness, anger, and fear. The second statement indicates the client is experiencing denial of the eating disorder. The third statement addresses the client's guilt feelings; it doesn't reflect knowledge of her eating disorder. The fourth statement shows the client isn't ready to discuss her eating disorder.
CN: Psychosocial integrity; CNS: None; CL: Analysis

15. A nurse is collecting data on a client to determine the distress experienced after binge eating. Which symptom is <u>typical</u> after bingeing?
1. Loss of taste
2. Headache
3. Pain
4. Sore throat

16. A mother of a client with bulimia nervosa asks a nurse if bulimia nervosa will stop her daughter from menstruating. Which response is best?
1. "All women with anorexia nervosa or bulimia nervosa will have amenorrhea."
2. "When your daughter is bingeing and purging, she won't have normal periods."
3. "The eating disorder must be ongoing for your daughter's menstrual cycle to change."
4. "Your daughter may have a normal or abnormal menstrual cycle, depending on the severity of her problem."

17. Which difficulty is <u>commonly</u> found in families with a member who has bulimia nervosa?
1. Mental illness
2. Multiple losses
3. Chronic anxiety
4. Substance abuse

18. A client with bulimia nervosa tells a nurse her major problem is eating too much food in a short period of time and then vomiting. Which short-term goal is the most <u>important</u>?
1. Helping the client understand every person has a satiety level
2. Encouraging the client to verbalize fears and concerns about food
3. Determining the amount of food the client will eat without purging
4. Obtaining a therapy appointment to look at the emotional causes of bulimia nervosa

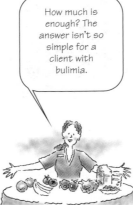

How much is enough? The answer isn't so simple for a client with bulimia.

15. 3. After a binge episode, the client commonly has abdominal distention and stomach pain. Headache and ageusia (loss of taste) aren't associated with binge eating. A sore throat is associated with vomiting.
CN: Physiological integrity; CNS: Physiological adaptation; CL: Knowledge

16. 4. Women with bulimia nervosa may have a normal or abnormal menstrual cycle, depending on the severity of the eating disorder. Not all women with eating disorders have amenorrhea. The eating disorder can disrupt the menstrual cycle at any point in the illness.
CN: Physiological integrity; CNS: Physiological adaptation; CL: Analysis

17. 2. Families with a member who has bulimia nervosa usually struggle with multiple losses. Mental illness, chronic anxiety, and substance abuse don't tend to be themes in the family background of the client with bulimia nervosa.
CN: Psychosocial integrity; CNS: None; CL: Analysis

18. 3. The client must meet her nutritional needs to prevent further complications, so she must identify the amount of food she can eat without purging as her first short-term goal. Obtaining knowledge or verbalizing her fears and feelings about food are *not* priority goals for this client. All clients must first take steps to meet their nutritional needs. Therapy is an important part of dealing with this disorder, but it isn't the first step.
CN: Physiological integrity; CNS: Reduction of risk potential; CL: Application

CN: Client needs category   CNS: Client needs subcategory   CL: Cognitive level

19. Which statement indicates a client with bulimia nervosa is making progress in interrupting the binge-purge cycle?
1. "I called my friend the last two times I got upset."
2. "I know I'll have this problem with eating forever."
3. "I started asking my mother or sister to watch me eat each meal."
4. "I can have my boyfriend bring me home from parties if I want to purge."

20. A client with bulimia nervosa asks a nurse, "How can I ask for help from my family?" Which response is the <u>most appropriate</u>?
1. "When you ask for help, make sure you really need it."
2. "Have you ever asked for help before?"
3. "Ask family members to spend time with you at mealtime."
4. "Think about how you can handle this situation without help."

21. A client with bulimia nervosa tells a nurse that she doesn't eat during the day, but after 5 p.m. she begins to binge and vomit. Which intervention would be the <u>most useful</u> to this client?
1. Helping the client stop eating the foods on which she binges
2. Discussing the effects of fasting on the client's pattern of eating
3. Encouraging the client to become involved in food preparation
4. Teaching the client to eat earlier in the day and decrease intake at night

22. A client with bulimia nervosa tells a nurse she was doing well until last week, when she had a fight with her father. Which nursing intervention would be most helpful?
1. Examining the relationship between feelings and eating
2. Discussing the importance of therapy for the entire family
3. Encouraging the client to avoid certain family members
4. Identifying daily stressors and learning stress management skills

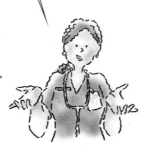

Which statement is a sign of progress? Work through question 19 for the answer.

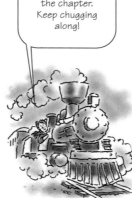

You're almost halfway through the chapter. Keep chugging along!

19. 1. A sign of progress is when the client begins to verbalize feelings and interact with people instead of turning to food for comfort. The second statement indicates the client needs more information on how to handle the disorder. Having another person watch the client eat isn't a helpful strategy as the client will depend on others to help control food intake. The last statement indicates the client is in denial about the severity of the problem.
CN: Psychosocial integrity; CNS: None; CL: Application

20. 2. The nurse should determine whether the client has ever been successful in asking for help because previous experiences affect the client's ability to ask for help now. The client needs to ask for help anytime without analyzing the level of need. Having other people present at mealtime isn't the only way to ask for help. Developing a support system is imperative for this client.
CN: Psychosocial integrity; CNS: None; CL: Analysis

21. 2. It's common for a person who fasts for most of the day to become extremely hungry, overeat by bingeing, and then feel the need to purge. Restricting food intake can actually trigger the binge-purge cycle. In treatment, the client is taught to identify foods that trigger eating, discuss the feelings associated with these foods, and work to eat them in normal amounts. Involvement in food preparation won't promote changes in the client's behaviors. The last intervention doesn't address how fasting can trigger the binge-purge cycle.
CN: Psychosocial integrity; CNS: None; CL: Application

22. 1. The client must understand her feelings and develop healthy coping skills to handle unpleasant situations. Family therapy may be indicated but shouldn't be an immediate intervention. Avoidance isn't a useful coping strategy; eventually the underlying issues must be explored. All clients can benefit from stress management skills but, for this client, care must focus on the relationship between feelings and eating behaviors.
CN: Psychosocial integrity; CNS: None; CL: Application

23. Which statement from a bulimic client shows that she understands the concept of <u>relapse</u>?
1. "If I can't maintain control over things, I'll have problems."
2. "If I have problems, then that says I haven't learned much."
3. "If this illness becomes chronic, I won't be able to handle it."
4. "If I have problems, I can start over again and not feel hopeless."

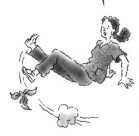

To the client with bulimia nervosa, a relapse is just a slip—not a reason to give up!

24. Which medical condition is commonly found in clients with bulimia nervosa?
1. Allergies
2. Cancer
3. Diabetes
4. Hepatitis A

25. What's the treatment team's <u>priority</u> in planning the care of a client with an eating disorder?
1. Preventing the client from performing any muscle-building exercises
2. Keeping the client on bed rest until she attains a specified weight
3. Meeting daily to discuss manipulation and countertransference
4. Monitoring the client's weight and vital signs daily

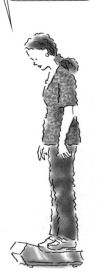

Pound for pound, clients with anorexia nervosa simply don't believe what the scale tells them.

26. A client with anorexia nervosa attended psychoeducational sessions on principles of adequate nutrition. Which statement by the client indicates the teaching was effective?
1. "I should eat while I'm doing things to distract myself."
2. "I should eat all my food at night just before I go to bed."
3. "I should eat small amounts of food slowly at every meal."
4. "I should eat only when I'm with my family and trying to be social."

23. 4. This statement indicates that the client knows a relapse is just a slip, and positive gains made from treatment haven't been lost. Control issues relate to powerlessness, which contribute to relapse. Negative self-statements can lead to relapse.
CN: Psychosocial integrity; CNS: None; CL: Comprehension

24. 3. Diabetes, heart disease, and hypertension are medical complications commonly seen in clients with bulimia nervosa. Allergies, cancer, and hepatitis A are *not* medical complications commonly associated with bulimia nervosa.
CN: Health promotion and maintenance; CNS: None; CL: Knowledge

25. 3. Clients with eating disorders commonly use manipulative ploys and countertransference to resist weight gain (if they restrict food intake) or maintain purging practices (if they're bulimic). They commonly play staff members against one another and hone in on their caretaker's vulnerabilities. Muscle building is acceptable because, compared with aerobic exercise, it burns relatively few calories. Keeping the client on bed rest until she reaches a specified weight can result in unnecessary power struggles and prevent staff from focusing on more pertinent issues and problems. Monitoring the client's weight and vital signs is important but not vital on a daily basis unless the client's physiologic condition warrants such close scrutiny.
CN: Psychosocial integrity; CNS: None; CL: Application

26. 3. Slowly eating small amounts of food facilitates adequate digestion and prevents distention. Healthy eating is best accomplished when a person isn't doing other things while eating. Eating just before bedtime isn't a healthy eating habit. If a client eats only when the family is present or when trying to be social, eating is tied to social or emotional cues rather than nutritional needs.
CN: Physiological integrity; CNS: Reduction of risk potential; CL: Application

CN: Client needs category   CNS: Client needs subcategory   CL: Cognitive level

27. A client with anorexia nervosa tells a nurse, "I'll never have the slender body I want." Which intervention is <u>best</u> to handle this problem?
1. Calling a family meeting to get help from the parents
2. Helping the client work on developing a realistic body image
3. Making an appointment for the client to see the dietitian on a weekly basis
4. Developing an exercise program the client can participate in twice per week

28. For a client with anorexia nervosa, which goal takes the <u>highest</u> priority?
1. The client will establish adequate daily nutritional intake.
2. The client will make a contract with the nurse that sets a target weight.
3. The client will identify self-perceptions about body size as unrealistic.
4. The client will verbalize the possible physiological consequences of self-starvation.

29. Which communication strategy is <u>best</u> to use with a client with anorexia nervosa who's having problems with peer relationships?
1. Use concrete language and maintain a focus on reality.
2. Direct the client to talk about what's causing the anxiety.
3. Teach the client to communicate feelings and express self appropriately.
4. Confront the client about being depressed and self-absorbed.

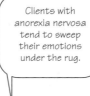

Clients with anorexia nervosa tend to sweep their emotions under the rug.

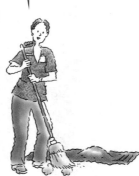

30. A nurse plans to include the parents of a client with anorexia nervosa in therapy sessions along with the client. What fact should the nurse remember about the parents of clients with anorexia?
1. They tend to overprotect their children.
2. They usually have a history of substance abuse.
3. They maintain emotional distance from their children.
4. They alternate between loving and rejecting their children.

27. 2. With anorexia nervosa, the client pursues thinness and has a distorted view of self. A family meeting may not help the client develop a more realistic view of her body. Although meeting with a dietitian might be helpful, it isn't a priority. Clients with anorexia nervosa typically exercise excessively.
CN: Psychosocial integrity; CNS: None; CL: Application

28. 1. According to Maslow's hierarchy of needs, all humans need to meet basic physiological needs first. Because a client with anorexia nervosa eats little or nothing, the nurse must plan to help the client meet this basic, immediate physiological need first. The nurse may give lesser priority to goals that address long-term plans, self-perception, and potential complications.
CN: Physiological integrity; CNS: Basic care and comfort; CL: Application

29. 3. Clients with anorexia nervosa commonly communicate on a superficial level and avoid expressing feelings. Identifying feelings and learning to express them are initial steps in decreasing isolation. Clients with anorexia nervosa are usually able to discuss abstract and concrete issues. Confrontation or directing the client to talk about what's causing the anxiety usually aren't effective communication strategies because they may cause the client to withdraw and become more depressed.
CN: Psychosocial integrity; CNS: None; CL: Application

30. 1. Clients with anorexia nervosa typically come from a family with parents who are controlling and overprotective. These clients use eating to gain control of an aspect of their lives. Having a history of substance abuse, maintaining an emotional distance, and alternating between love and rejection aren't typical characteristics of parents of children with anorexia nervosa.
CN: Psychosocial integrity; CNS: None; CL: Application

31. A nurse is talking to the family of a client with anorexia nervosa. Which family behavior is <u>most likely</u> to be seen during the family's interaction?
1. Sibling rivalry
2. Rage reactions
3. Parental disagreement
4. Excessive independence

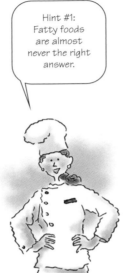

Hint #1: Fatty foods are almost never the right answer.

32. A nurse is working with a client with anorexia nervosa who has dry, flaky skin. Which short-term goal is the <u>most important</u> for the client?
1. Do daily exercises.
2. Eat some fatty foods daily.
3. Check neurologic reflexes.
4. Consume whole grains and fish.

33. A female client with anorexia nervosa is discharged from the hospital after gaining 12 pounds. Which client statement <u>best</u> indicates that the nurse's reinforcement of discharge teaching has been effective?
1. "I plan to eat two small meals a day."
2. "I feel this is scary but I'm not going to write about it in my journal."
3. "I have to cut back on my calorie intake because I've gained 12 pounds."
4. "I'll need to attend therapy for support to stay healthy."

34. A client with anorexia nervosa tells a nurse she always feels fat. Which intervention is <u>best</u> for this client?
1. Talking about how important the client is
2. Encouraging her to look at herself in a mirror
3. Addressing the dynamics of the disorder
4. Talking about how she's different from her peers

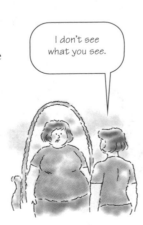

I don't see what you see.

31. 3. In many families with a member with anorexia nervosa, there's marital conflict and parental disagreement. Sibling rivalry is a common occurrence and not specific to a family with a member with anorexia nervosa. In these families, the members tend to be enmeshed and dependent on each other. The family with an anorexic member is usually one that looks good to the outside observer. Emotions are overcontrolled, and there's difficulty appropriately expressing negative feelings.
CN: Psychosocial integrity; CNS: None; CL: Comprehension

32. 4. A lack of essential fatty acids in the diet can cause dry, flaky skin, as well as iron deficiency anemia and estrogen deficiency. Intake of whole grains and fish would be important to supply these fatty acids. Exercise may help prevent contractures and muscle atrophy but it may have only a limited secondary effect in promoting circulation. Intake of fatty foods won't have an impact on the client's skin problems. Checking neurologic reflexes won't necessarily assist with handling skin problems.
CN: Physiological integrity; CNS: Reduction of risk potential; CL: Application

33. 4. The client is planning to attend therapy after discharge and this shows an understanding of the need for continued counseling. Eating only two small meals a day is an unrealistic plan for meeting nutritional needs. Feeling insecure when leaving a controlled environment is a common response to discharge; however, writing about her feelings in a journal would be therapeutic. Gaining 12 pounds indicates that the client's nutritional needs are being met at her present caloric intake levels.
CN: Psychosocial integrity; CNS: None; CL: Analysis

34. 3. The client can benefit from understanding the underlying dynamics of the eating disorder. The client with anorexia nervosa has low self-esteem and won't believe the positive statements. Although the client may look at herself in the mirror, in her mind she'll still see herself as fat. Pointing out differences will only diminish her already low self-esteem.
CN: Psychosocial integrity; CNS: None; CL: Application

CN: Client needs category CNS: Client needs subcategory CL: Cognitive level

35. The grandparents of a client with anorexia nervosa want to support the client but aren't sure what they should do. Which intervention is <u>best</u>?
1. Encouraging positive expressions of affection
2. Encouraging behaviors that promote socialization
3. Discussing how eating disorders create powerlessness
4. Discussing the meaning of hunger and body sensations

36. A 15-year-old adolescent female is brought to the clinic by her parents because of a significant amount of weight loss in the past 4 months. Which accompanying condition would indicate that the client is suffering from anorexia nervosa?
1. Hypertension
2. Amenorrhea
3. Hyperthermia
4. Diarrhea

37. An adolescent client with anorexia nervosa tells a nurse about her outstanding academic achievements and her thoughts about suicide. Which factor must the nurse consider when contributing to the care plan for this client?
1. Self-esteem
2. Physical illnesses
3. Paranoid delusions
4. Relationship avoidance

38. In contributing to the care plan for a family with a member who has anorexia nervosa, what information should be included?
1. Coping mechanisms used in the past
2. Concerns about changes in lifestyle and daily activities
3. Rejection of feedback from family and significant others
4. Appropriate eating habits and social behaviors centering on eating

How do we cope with problems? Asking about the good, the bad, and the ugly will help you plan the best care for me.

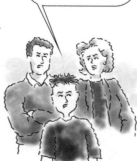

35. 1. Clients with eating disorders need emotional support and expressions of affection from family members. It wouldn't be an appropriate strategy to have the grandparents promote socialization. Although clients with eating disorders feel powerless, it's better to have the grandparents focus on something positive. Talking about hunger and other sensations won't give the grandparents useful strategies.
CN: Psychosocial integrity; CNS: None; CL: Application

36. 2. Anorexia nervosa is characterized by profound weight loss caused by severe restriction of food intake by the client. If severe enough, it causes amenorrhea in females, along with decreased—not increased—body temperature, and hypotension—not hypertension. It usually doesn't produce diarrhea, but it may produce constipation because decreased oral intake leads to decreased GI motility.
CN: Physiological integrity; CNS: Reduction of risk potential; CL: Application

37. 1. The client lacks self-esteem, which contributes to her level of depression and feelings of personal ineffectiveness, which, in turn, may lead to suicidal thoughts. Physical illnesses are common with clients with anorexia nervosa but they don't relate to this situation. Paranoid delusions refer to false ideas that others want to harm you. No evidence exists that this client is socially isolated.
CN: Psychosocial integrity; CNS: None; CL: Analysis

38. 1. Examination of positive and negative coping mechanisms used by the family allows the nurse to build a care plan specific to the family's strengths and weaknesses. The way the family copes with concerns is more important than the concerns themselves. Feedback from the family and significant others is vital when building a care plan. Providing information on appropriate eating habits and social behaviors centered on eating won't assist the family in coping with their family member's illness.
CN: Psychosocial integrity; CNS: None; CL: Application

CN: Client needs category CNS: Client needs subcategory CL: Cognitive level

39. Which goal is best to help a client with anorexia nervosa recognize self-distortions?
1. Identify the client's misperceptions of self.
2. Acknowledge immature and childlike behaviors.
3. Determine the consequences of a faulty support system.
4. Recognize the age-appropriate tasks to be accomplished.

40. The parents of a client with anorexia nervosa ask the nurse about the predisposing risk factors for developing this disorder. After reinforcement of the teaching plan by the nurse, which statement by the parents best indicates that the teaching has been effective?
1. "Risk factors include the inability to be still and emotional lability."
2. "Risk factors include a high level of anxiety and disorganized behavior."
3. "Risk factors include low self-esteem and problems with family relationships."
4. "Risk factors include a lack of life experiences and opportunity to learn life skills."

41. A client with anorexia nervosa has started taking fluoxetine (Prozac). The nurse should closely monitor the client for which adverse reaction?
1. Drowsiness
2. Dry mouth
3. Light-headedness
4. Nausea

42. A client with anorexia nervosa is worried about her rectal bleeding. Which question will help obtain more information about the problem?
1. "How often do you use laxatives?"
2. "How many days ago did you stop vomiting?"
3. "Are you eating anything that causes irritation?"
4. "Do you bleed before or after exercise?"

39. 1. Questioning the client's misperceptions and distortions will create doubt about how the client views herself. Acknowledging immature behaviors or determining the consequences of a faulty support system won't promote recognition of self-distortions. Recognizing the age-appropriate tasks to be accomplished won't help the client recognize distortions.
CN: Psychosocial integrity; CNS: None; CL: Analysis

40. 3. There are several risk factors for eating disorders, including low self-esteem, history of depression, substance abuse, and dysfunctional family relationships. Restlessness and emotional lability are symptoms of manic depressive illness. Anxiety and disorganized behavior could be signs of a psychotic disorder. A lack of life experiences and an absence of opportunities to learn life skills may be a result of anorexia.
CN: Psychosocial integrity; CNS: None; CL: Analysis

41. 4. Nausea is an adverse reaction to the drug that compounds the eating disorder problem, and the client must be closely monitored. Although the adverse reactions of drowsiness, dry mouth, and light-headedness may occur, they aren't likely to interfere with treatment.
CN: Physiological integrity; CNS: Pharmacological therapies; CL: Application

42. 1. Excessive use of laxatives will cause GI irritation and rectal bleeding. If the client stopped vomiting but is still using laxatives, rectal bleeding can occur. Clients who are anorexic eat very little, and what they eat won't cause rectal bleeding. Exercise doesn't cause rectal bleeding.
CN: Health promotion and maintenance; CNS: None; CL: Application

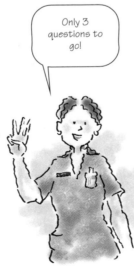

Only 3 questions to go!

43. Which interventions would be supportive for a client with a nursing diagnosis of *Imbalanced nutrition: Less than body requirements due to dysfunctional eating patterns?* Select all that apply:

1. Provide small, frequent feedings.
2. Monitor weight gain.
3. Allow the client to skip meals until the antidepressant levels are therapeutic.
4. Encourage journaling to promote the expression of feelings.
5. Monitor the client at mealtimes and for an hour after meals.
6. Encourage the client to eat three substantial meals per day.

44. Which characteristics are <u>typical</u> findings in a client with anorexia nervosa? Select all that apply:

1. Intense fear of gaining weight
2. Possible amenorrhea
3. Weight 70% or less than her ideal body weight
4. Awareness that she has a problem, but refusal to admit it
5. Self-esteem that's dependent on how she looks
6. Weight loss accomplished through the use of diet pills

45. A nurse should be alert for which findings in a client with bulimia nervosa? Select all that apply:

1. Severe electrolyte imbalances
2. Damaged teeth due to the eroding effects of gastric acids on tooth enamel
3. Pneumonia from aspirated stomach contents
4. Cessation of menses
5. Esophageal tears and gastric rupture
6. Intestinal inflammation

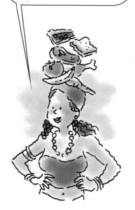

> Some misperceptions—like thinking I look cool in this outfit—are easier to overcome than others. Check out question 43 for the details.

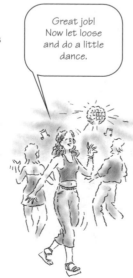

> Great job! Now let loose and do a little dance.

43. 1, 2, 4, 5. Smaller meals may be better tolerated by the client and will gradually increase her daily caloric intake. The nurse should monitor the client's weight because an anorexic will hide weight loss. Anorexics are emotionally restrained and afraid of their feelings, so journaling can be a powerful tool that assists in recovery. Anorexic clients are obsessed with gaining weight and will skip all meals if given the opportunity so encouraging the client to skip meals isn't therapeutic. Because of self-starvation, they seldom can tolerate large meals three times per day.
CN: Psychosocial integrity; CNS: None; CL: Analysis

44. 1, 2, 5. Anorexic individuals are intensely afraid of gaining weight, and females commonly stop menstruating. Self-esteem of anorexic individuals depends on how they look. The diagnostic criteria state that a person is anorexic when her weight is 85% below the expected weight for her height. Individuals with the disorder typically don't believe they have a problem and don't consider their behavior abnormal. Anorexics don't accomplish weight loss through the use of diet pills, but rather through avoidance of food and with excessive exercise.
CN: Psychosocial integrity; CNS: None; CL: Application

45. 1, 2, 4, 5. Constant bingeing and purging behaviors can result in severe electrolyte imbalances, erosion of tooth enamel from constant exposure to gastric acids, menstrual irregularities, esophageal tears and, in severe cases, gastric rupture. Aspiration pneumonia is unlikely because the vomiting is voluntary and controlled. Intestinal inflammation isn't typically associated with bulimia nervosa.
CN: Physiologic integrity; CNS: Physiological adaptation; CL: Application

CN: Client needs category   CNS: Client needs subcategory   CL: Cognitive level

Part IV Maternal-neonatal care

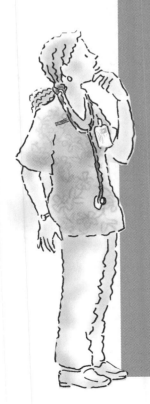

Looking for information about antepartum care before tackling this chapter? Visit *www.obgyn.net/*, an independent Web site dedicated to obstetric and gynecologic health problems.

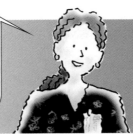

Chapter 22
Antepartum care

1. During an examination, a client who's 32 weeks pregnant becomes dizzy, light-headed, and pale while supine. What should the nurse do <u>first</u>?
    1. Listen to fetal heart tones.
    2. Take the client's blood pressure.
    3. Ask the client to breathe deeply.
    4. Turn the client on her left side.

Think about the development of the fetus at 32 weeks to answer question 1.

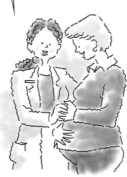

2. A nurse has just taught a client about the signs of true and false labor. Which client statement indicates an accurate understanding of this information?
    1. "False labor contractions are regular."
    2. "False labor contractions intensify with walking."
    3. "False labor contractions usually occur in the abdomen."
    4. "False labor contractions move from the back to the front of the abdomen."

3. In twin-to-twin transfusion syndrome, the arterial circulation of one twin is in communication with the venous circulation of the other twin. One fetus is considered the *donor* twin, and one becomes the *recipient* twin. Observation of the recipient twin would most likely show which condition?
    1. Anemia
    2. Oligohydramnios
    3. Polycythemia
    4. Small fetus

Careful: Be sure to think twice before answering question 3.

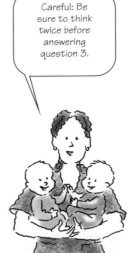

1. 4. As the enlarging uterus increases pressure on the inferior vena cava, it compromises venous return, which can cause dizziness, light-headedness, and pallor when the client is supine. The nurse can relieve these symptoms by turning the client on her left side, which relieves pressure on the vena cava and restores venous return. Although they're valuable assessments, fetal heart tone and maternal blood pressure measurements don't correct the problem. Because deep breathing has no effect on venous return, it can't relieve the client's symptoms.
CN: Physiological integrity; CNS: Reduction of risk potential; CL: Application

2. 3. False labor contractions are usually felt in the abdomen, are irregular, and are typically relieved by walking. True labor contractions move from the back to the front of the abdomen, are regular, and aren't relieved by walking.
CN: Health promotion and maintenance; CNS: None; CL: Comprehension

3. 3. The recipient twin in twin-to-twin transfusion syndrome (also known as *twin-twin transfusion syndrome*) is transfused by the other twin. The recipient twin then becomes polycythemic and commonly has heart failure due to circulatory overload. The donor twin becomes anemic. The recipient twin has polyhydramnios, not oligohydramnios. The recipient twin is usually large, whereas the donor twin is usually small.
CN: Physiological integrity; CNS: Physiological adaptation; CL: Analysis

4. A pregnant client who reports painless vaginal bleeding at 28 weeks' gestation is diagnosed with placenta previa, in which the placental edge reaches the internal os. This type of placenta previa is known as:
1. low-lying placenta previa.
2. marginal placenta previa.
3. partial placenta previa.
4. total placenta previa.

5. A 24-year-old client is diagnosed with placenta previa at 28 weeks' gestation. The physician alerts the nurse that the client will need treatment. Which procedures or treatments should the nurse prepare the client for?
1. Stat culture and sensitivity
2. Antenatal steroids after 34 weeks' gestation
3. Ultrasound examination every 2 to 3 weeks
4. Scheduled delivery of the fetus before fetal maturity in a hemodynamically stable mother

Discussing necessary procedures can help alleviate your stress.

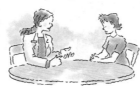

6. A client with painless vaginal bleeding is suspected of having placenta previa. Which procedure would the nurse expect the physician to order to diagnose placenta previa?
1. Amniocentesis
2. Digital or speculum examination
3. External fetal monitoring
4. Ultrasound

Studying will predispose you to doing well on the exam.

7. A client is diagnosed with hyperemesis gravidarum after coming to the antepartum unit with persistent vomiting, weight loss, and hypovolemia. The nurse taking her health history would expect to discover which factor that predisposes the client to developing this condition?
1. Trophoblastic disease
2. Maternal age older than 35 years
3. Malnourished or underweight clients
4. Low levels of human chorionic gonadotropin (HCG)

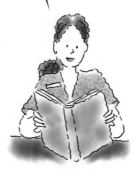

4. 2. A marginal placenta previa is characterized by implantation of the placenta in the margin of the cervical os, not covering the os. A low-lying placenta is implanted in the lower uterine segment but doesn't reach the cervical os. A partial placenta previa is the partial occlusion of the cervical os by the placenta. The internal cervical os is completely covered by the placenta in a total placenta previa.
CN: Physiological integrity; CNS: Physiological adaptation; CL: Analysis

5. 3. Fetal surveillance through ultrasound examination every 2 to 3 weeks is indicated to evaluate fetal growth, amniotic fluid, and placental location in clients with placenta previa being expectantly managed. A stat culture and sensitivity would be done for severe bleeding or maternal or fetal distress and isn't part of expectant management. Antenatal steroids may be given to clients between 26 and 32 weeks' gestation to enhance fetal lung maturity. In a hemodynamically stable mother, delivery of the fetus should be delayed until fetal lung maturity is attained.
CN: Physiological integrity; CNS: Reduction of risk potential; CL: Application

6. 4. When the mother and fetus are stabilized, ultrasound evaluation of the placenta should be done to determine the cause of the bleeding. Amniocentesis is contraindicated in placenta previa. A digital or speculum examination shouldn't be done as this may lead to severe bleeding or hemorrhage. External fetal monitoring won't detect a placenta previa, although it will detect fetal distress, which may result from blood loss or placental separation.
CN: Physiological integrity; CNS: Reduction of risk potential; CL: Application

7. 1. Trophoblastic disease is associated with hyperemesis gravidarum. Obesity and maternal age younger than 20 years are risk factors for developing hyperemesis gravidarum. High levels of estrogen and HCG have been associated with hyperemesis.
CN: Physiological integrity; CNS: Reduction of risk potential; CL: Application

CN: Client needs category CNS: Client needs subcategory CL: Cognitive level

8. A nurse is assisting in developing a teaching plan for a client who's about to enter the third trimester of pregnancy. The teaching plan should include identification of which danger sign that must be reported <u>immediately</u>?
   1. Hemorrhoids
   2. Blurred vision
   3. Dyspnea on exertion
   4. Increased vaginal mucus

9. Which symptom occurs with a hydatidiform mole?
   1. Heavy, bright red bleeding every 21 days
   2. Fetal cardiac motion after 6 weeks' gestation
   3. Benign tumors found in the smooth muscle of the uterus
   4. "Snowstorm" pattern on ultrasound with no fetus or gestational sac

10. A 21-year-old client has just been diagnosed with having a hydatidiform mole. Which trait is considered a risk factor for developing a hydatidiform mole?
   1. Age in 20s or 30s
   2. High socioeconomic status
   3. Primigravida
   4. Prior molar gestation

11. A 21-year-old client arrives at the emergency department with complaints of cramping abdominal pain and mild vaginal bleeding. Pelvic examination shows a left adnexal mass that's tender when palpated. Culdocentesis shows blood in the cul-de-sac. This client probably has which condition?
   1. Abruptio placentae
   2. Ectopic pregnancy
   3. Hydatidiform mole
   4. Pelvic inflammatory disease

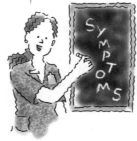

Sometimes it's hard to keep your symptoms straight, isn't it?

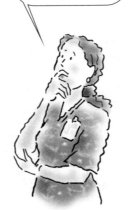

Hmmm. What do these symptoms suggest in a woman of childbearing age?

8. 2. During pregnancy, blurred vision may be a danger sign of preeclampsia or eclampsia, complications that require immediate attention because they can cause severe maternal and fetal consequences. Although hemorrhoids may occur during pregnancy, they don't require immediate attention. Dyspnea on exertion and increased vaginal mucus are common discomforts caused by the physiological changes of pregnancy.
CN: Physiological integrity; CNS: Reduction of risk potential; CL: Application

9. 4. Ultrasound is the technique of choice in diagnosing a hydatidiform mole. The chorionic villi of a molar pregnancy resemble a "snowstorm" pattern on ultrasound. Bleeding with a hydatidiform mole is usually dark brown and may occur erratically for weeks or months. There's no cardiac activity because there's no fetus. Benign tumors found in the smooth muscle of the uterus are leiomyomas or fibroids.
CN: Physiological integrity; CNS: Reduction of risk potential; CL: Analysis

10. 4. A previous molar gestation increases a woman's risk for developing a subsequent molar gestation by 4 to 5 times. Adolescents and women ages 40 years and older are at increased risk for molar pregnancies. Multigravidas, especially women with a prior pregnancy loss, and those with lower socioeconomic status are at an increased risk for this problem.
CN: Physiological integrity; CNS: Physiological adaptation; CL: Analysis

11. 2. Most ectopic pregnancies don't appear as obvious life-threatening medical emergencies. Ectopic pregnancies must be considered in any woman of childbearing age who complains of menstrual irregularity, cramping abdominal pain, and mild vaginal bleeding. Pelvic inflammatory disease, abruptio placentae, and hydatidiform mole won't show blood in the cul-de-sac.
CN: Physiological integrity; CNS: Reduction of risk potential; CL: Analysis

12. A client who's 34 weeks pregnant arrives at the emergency department with severe abdominal pain, uterine tenderness, and increased uterine tone. The client denies vaginal bleeding. The external fetal monitor shows fetal distress with severe, variable decelerations. The client most likely has which condition?
  1. Abruptio placentae
  2. Ectopic pregnancy
  3. Molar pregnancy
  4. Placenta previa

12. 1. A client with severe abruptio placentae will commonly have severe abdominal pain. The uterus will have increased tone with little to no return to resting tone between contractions. The fetus will start to show signs of distress, with decelerations in the heart rate or even fetal death with a large placental separation. An ectopic pregnancy, which usually occurs in the fallopian tubes, would rupture well before 34 weeks. A molar pregnancy generally would be detected before 34 weeks' gestation. Placenta previa usually involves painless vaginal bleeding without uterine contractions.
CN: Physiological integrity; CNS: Reduction of risk potential; CL: Analysis

13. During a routine visit to the clinic, a client tells the nurse that she thinks she may be pregnant. The physician orders a pregnancy test. The nurse should know the purpose of this test is to determine which change in the client's hormone level?
  1. Increase in human chorionic gonadotropin (HCG)
  2. Decrease in HCG
  3. Increase in luteinizing hormone (LH)
  4. Decrease in LH

13. 1. HCG increases in a woman's blood and urine to fairly large concentrations until the 15th week of pregnancy. The other hormone values aren't indicative of pregnancy.
CN: Health promotion and maintenance; CNS: None; CL: Comprehension

14. Which change in respiratory function during pregnancy is considered <u>normal</u>?
  1. Increased tidal volume
  2. Increased expiratory volume
  3. Decreased inspiratory capacity
  4. Decreased oxygen consumption

14. 1. A pregnant client breathes more deeply, which increases the tidal volume of gas moved in and out of the respiratory tract with each breath. The expiratory volume and residual volume decrease as the pregnancy progresses. The inspiratory capacity increases during pregnancy. The increased oxygen consumption in the pregnant client is 15% to 20% greater than in the nonpregnant state.
CN: Health promotion and maintenance; CNS: None; CL: Knowledge

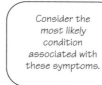

Consider the most likely condition associated with these symptoms.

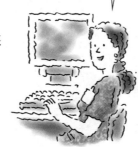

15. A 23-year-old client who's 27 weeks pregnant arrives at her physician's office with complaints of fever, nausea, vomiting, malaise, unilateral flank pain, and costovertebral angle tenderness. Which condition would the nurse <u>most</u> <u>likely</u> suspect?
  1. Asymptomatic bacteriuria
  2. Bacterial vaginosis
  3. Pyelonephritis
  4. Urinary tract infection (UTI)

15. 3. The symptoms indicate acute pyelonephritis, a serious condition in a pregnant client. Asymptomatic bacteriuria doesn't cause symptoms. Bacterial vaginosis causes milky white vaginal discharge but no systemic symptoms. UTI symptoms include dysuria, urgency, frequency, and suprapubic tenderness.
CN: Physiological integrity; CNS: Reduction of risk potential; CL: Analysis

CN: Client needs category   CNS: Client needs subcategory   CL: Cognitive level

16. A pregnant client is visiting the clinic and complains about the tiny, blanched, slightly raised end arterioles on her face, neck, arms, and chest. The nurse should explain that these are normal during pregnancy and referred to as which of the following?
1. Epulis
2. Linea nigra
3. Striae gravidarum
4. Telangiectasias

17. A prenatal client asks the nurse about dizygotic twins. Which statement should the nurse include in her teaching?
1. They occur most commonly in Asian women.
2. There's a decreased risk with increased parity.
3. There's an increased risk with increased maternal age.
4. Use of fertility drugs poses no additional risk.

18. A client in her fifth month of pregnancy is having a routine clinic visit. The nurse should assess the client for which common <u>second</u> trimester condition?
1. Mastitis
2. Metabolic alkalosis
3. Physiological anemia
4. Respiratory acidosis

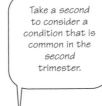

Take a second to consider a condition that is common in the second trimester.

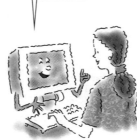

19. A 21-year-old client, 6 weeks' pregnant, is diagnosed with hyperemesis gravidarum. The nurse should be alert for which condition?
1. Bowel perforation
2. Electrolyte imbalance
3. Miscarriage
4. Gestational hypertension

16. 4. The dilated arterioles that occur during pregnancy are due to the elevated level of circulating estrogen and are called *telangiectasias.* An epulis is a red raised nodule on the gums that may develop at the end of the first trimester and continue to grow as the pregnancy progresses. The linea nigra is a pigmented line extending from the symphysis pubis to the top of the fundus during pregnancy. Striae gravidarum, or stretch marks, are slightly depressed streaks that commonly occur over the abdomen, breast, and thighs during the second half of pregnancy.
CN: Health promotion and maintenance; CNS: None; CL: Application

17. 3. Dizygotic twinning is influenced by race (most common in Black women and least common in Asian women), age (increased risk with increased maternal age), parity (increased risk with increased parity), and fertility drugs (increased risk with the use of fertility drugs, especially ovulation-inducing drugs).
CN: Health promotion and maintenance; CNS: None; CL: Application

18. 3. Hemoglobin level and hematocrit decrease during pregnancy as the increase in plasma volume exceeds the increase in red blood cell production. Mastitis is an infection in the breast characterized by a swollen tender breast and flulike symptoms. This condition is most commonly seen in breast-feeding clients. Alterations in acid-base balance during pregnancy result in a state of respiratory alkalosis, compensated by mild metabolic acidosis.
CN: Health promotion and maintenance; CNS: None; CL: Application

19. 2. Excessive vomiting in clients with hyperemesis gravidarum commonly causes weight loss and fluid, electrolyte, and acid-base imbalances. Gestational hypertension and bowel perforation aren't related to hyperemesis. The effects of hyperemesis on the fetus depend on the severity of the disorder. Clients with severe hyperemesis may have a low-birth-weight infant, but the disorder isn't generally life-threatening.
CN: Physiological integrity; CNS: Reduction of risk potential; CL: Analysis

CN: Client needs category   CNS: Client needs subcategory   CL: Cognitive level

20. A 29-year-old client has gestational diabetes. The nurse is teaching her about managing her glucose levels. Which therapy would be most appropriate for this client?

1. Diet
2. Long-acting insulin
3. Oral hypoglycemic drugs
4. Glucagon

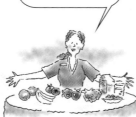

Making proper food choices can usually control gestational diabetes.

20. 1. Clients with gestational diabetes are usually managed by diet alone to control their glucose intolerance. Long-acting insulin usually isn't needed for blood glucose control in the client with gestational diabetes. Oral hypoglycemic drugs are contraindicated in pregnancy. Glucagon raises blood glucose and is used to treat hypoglycemic reactions.

CN: Health promotion and maintenance; CNS: None; CL: Application

21. Magnesium sulfate is given to pregnant clients with preeclampsia to <u>prevent</u> which condition?

1. Hemorrhage
2. Hypertension
3. Hypomagnesemia
4. Seizures

21. 4. The anticonvulsant mechanism of magnesium is believed to depress seizure foci in the brain and peripheral neuromuscular blockade. Magnesium doesn't help prevent hemorrhage in preeclamptic clients. Antihypertensive drugs other than magnesium are preferred for sustained hypertension. Hypomagnesemia isn't a complication of preeclampsia.

CN: Physiological integrity; CNS: Pharmacological therapies; CL: Analysis

22. A pregnant client has a contraction stress test (CST). Which statement describes negative CST results?

1. Persistent late decelerations in fetal heartbeat occurred, with at least three contractions in a 10-minute window.
2. Accelerations of fetal heartbeat occurred, with at least 15 beats/minute, lasting 15 to 30 seconds in a 20-minute period.
3. Accelerations of fetal heartbeat were absent or didn't increase by 15 beats/minute for 15 to 30 seconds in a 20-minute period.
4. There was good fetal heart rate variability and no decelerations from contraction in a 10-minute period in which there were three contractions.

22. 4. A CST measures the fetal response to uterine contractions. A client must have three contractions in a 10-minute period. A negative CST shows good fetal heart rate variability with no decelerations from uterine contractions. Persistent late decelerations with contractions is a positive CST. Reactive nonstress tests (NSTs) have accelerations in the fetal heartbeat of at least 15 beats/minute lasting 15 to 30 seconds in a 20-minute period. No accelerations in the heartbeat of at least 15 beats/minute for 15 to 30 seconds in a 20-minute period indicates a nonreactive NST.

CN: Health promotion and maintenance; CNS: None; CL: Analysis

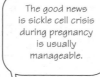

The good news is sickle cell crisis during pregnancy is usually manageable.

23. A pregnant client with sickle cell anemia is at an increased risk for having a sickle cell crisis during pregnancy. Aggressive management for a client experiencing a sickle cell crisis with severe pain includes which measure?

1. Antihypertensive drugs
2. Diuretic drugs
3. I.V. fluids
4. Acetaminophen (Tylenol) for pain

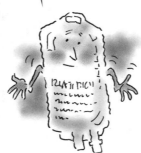

23. 3. A sickle cell crisis during pregnancy is usually managed by exchange transfusion, oxygen, and I.V. fluids. Antihypertensive drugs usually aren't necessary. Diuretics wouldn't be used unless fluid overload resulted. The client usually needs a stronger analgesic than acetaminophen to control the pain of a crisis.

CN: Physiological integrity; CNS: Reduction of risk potential; CL: Analysis

CN: Client needs category   CNS: Client needs subcategory   CL: Cognitive level

24. Which cardiac condition is normal during pregnancy?
   1. Cardiac tamponade
   2. Heart failure
   3. Endocarditis
   4. Systolic murmur

25. While assessing a client in her 24th week of pregnancy, the nurse learns that the client has been experiencing signs and symptoms of pregnancy-induced hypertension, or preeclampsia. Which sign or symptom helps differentiate preeclampsia from eclampsia?
   1. Seizures
   2. Headaches
   3. Blurred vision
   4. Weight gain

26. A client with preeclampsia is diagnosed with pregnancy-induced hypertension (PIH) and is given magnesium sulfate to prevent seizure activity. The nurse can reassure the client that her magnesium levels are therapeutic if they fall within what range?
   1. 4 to 7 mEq/L
   2. 8 to 10 mEq/L
   3. 10 to 12 mEq/L
   4. Greater than 15 mEq/L

27. A client is receiving I.V. magnesium sulfate for severe preeclampsia. Which adverse effect is associated with magnesium sulfate?
   1. Anemia
   2. Decreased urine output
   3. Hyperreflexia
   4. Increased respiratory rate

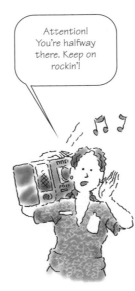

Attention! You're halfway there. Keep on rockin'!

24. 4. Systolic murmurs are heard in up to 90% of pregnant clients, and the murmur disappears soon after the delivery. Cardiac tamponade, which causes effusion of fluid into the pericardial sac, isn't normal during pregnancy. Despite the increases in intravascular volume and work load of the heart associated with pregnancy, heart failure isn't normal in pregnancy. Endocarditis is most commonly associated with I.V. drug use and isn't a normal finding in pregnancy.
CN: Health promotion and maintenance; CNS: None; CL: Knowledge

25. 1. The primary difference between preeclampsia and eclampsia is the occurrence of seizures, which occur when the client becomes eclamptic. Headaches, blurred vision, weight gain, increased blood pressure, and edema of the hands and feet are all indicative of preeclampsia.
CN: Physiological integrity; CNS: Physiological adaptation; CL: Comprehension

26. 1. The therapeutic level of magnesium for clients with PIH is 4 to 7 mEq/L. A serum level of 8 to 10 mEq/L may cause the absence of reflexes in the client. Serum levels of 10 to 12 mEq/L may cause respiratory depression, and a serum level of magnesium greater than 15 mEq/L may result in respiratory paralysis.
CN: Physiological integrity; CNS: Pharmacological therapies; CL: Analysis

27. 2. Decreased urine output may occur in clients receiving I.V. magnesium and should be monitored closely. Urine output should be greater than 30 ml/hour because magnesium is excreted through the kidneys and can easily accumulate to toxic levels. Anemia isn't associated with magnesium therapy. Magnesium infusions may cause depression of deep tendon reflexes. The client should be monitored for respiratory depression and paralysis when serum magnesium levels reach approximately 15 mEq/L.
CN: Physiological integrity; CNS: Pharmacological therapies; CL: Analysis

CN: Client needs category   CNS: Client needs subcategory   CL: Cognitive level

28. The antagonist for magnesium sulfate should be readily available to any client receiving I.V. magnesium. Which drug is the antidote for magnesium toxicity?
1. Calcium gluconate (Kalcinate)
2. Hydralazine (Apresoline)
3. Naloxone (Narcan)
4. Rh$_o$(D) immune globulin (RhoGAM)

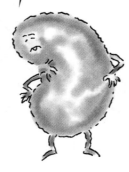

With the right drug, I can get rid of that extra magnesium.

28. 1. Calcium gluconate is the antidote for magnesium toxicity. Ten milliliters of 10% calcium gluconate is given by I.V. push over 3 to 5 minutes. Hydralazine is given for sustained elevated blood pressures in preeclamptic clients. Naloxone is used to correct narcotic toxicity. Rh$_o$(D) immune globulin is given to women with Rh-negative blood to prevent antibody formation from Rh-positive conceptions.
CN: Physiological integrity; CNS: Pharmacological therapies; CL: Analysis

29. A pregnant client is screened for tuberculosis during her first prenatal visit. An intradermal injection of purified protein derivative (PPD) of the tuberculin bacilli is given. Which sign would indicate a positive test result?
1. An indurated wheal under 10 mm in diameter appears in 6 to 12 hours.
2. An indurated wheal over 10 mm in diameter appears in 48 to 72 hours.
3. A flat, circumscribed area under 10 mm in diameter appears in 6 to 12 hours.
4. A flat circumscribed area over 10 mm in diameter appears in 48 to 72 hours.

29. 2. A positive PPD result would be an indurated wheal over 10 mm in diameter that appears in 48 to 72 hours. The area must be a raised wheal, not a flat, circumscribed area.
CN: Health promotion and maintenance; CNS: None; CL: Knowledge

30. A nurse is discussing nutrition with a Chinese-American primigravida. The client states that she knows that calcium is important during pregnancy but that she and her family don't consume many milk or dairy products. What advice should the nurse give?
1. "The prenatal vitamins that are recommended will satisfy all dietary requirements."
2. "You could supplement your diet with 1,800 mg of over-the-counter calcium tablets."
3. "You should consume other non-dairy foods that are high in calcium."
4. "After the first trimester, calcium intake isn't significant because all fetal organ structures are formed."

30. 3. Food is considered the ideal source of nutrients. However, milk and dairy aren't the only food sources of calcium. While prenatal vitamins are generally recommended, they don't satisfy all requirements. The calcium requirement for pregnancy is 1,300 mg/day for females ages 14 to 18 and 1,000 mg/day for females ages 19 to 50. A calcium dose of 1,200 mg/day is recommended for the elderly client. Over-the-counter supplements aren't always safe and should be specifically recommended by the medical practitioner. While it's true that all fetal organs are formed by the end of the first trimester, development continues throughout pregnancy.
CN: Heath promotion and maintenance; CNS: None; CL: Application

31. Rh isoimmunization in a pregnant client develops during which condition?
1. Rh-positive maternal blood crosses into fetal blood, stimulating fetal antibodies.
2. Rh-positive fetal blood crosses into maternal blood, stimulating maternal antibodies.
3. Rh-negative fetal blood crosses into maternal blood, stimulating maternal antibodies.
4. Rh-negative maternal blood crosses into fetal blood, stimulating fetal antibodies.

31. 2. Rh isoimmunization occurs when Rh-positive fetal blood cells cross into the maternal circulation and stimulate maternal antibody production. In subsequent pregnancies with Rh-positive fetuses, maternal antibodies may cross back into the fetal circulation and destroy the fetal blood cells.
CN: Physiological integrity; CNS: Reduction of risk potential; CL: Knowledge

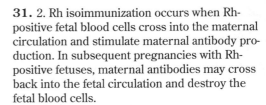
Relax! Things are going quite smoothly.

32. A client who's into week 32 of her pregnancy is having contractions. The physician prescribes terbutaline (Brethine). Which statement by the client indicates that additional teaching about terbutaline is needed?
1. "I understand that taking terbutaline will stabilize my blood pressure."
2. "I will take terbutaline to relax my uterus and stop uterine contractions."
3. "I will continue to take terbutaline until my pregnancy is at term."
4. "I shouldn't have any breathing problems as a side effect of the drug."

32. 1. Terbutaline doesn't stabilize blood pressure. A selective beta$_2$-adrenergic agonist, terbutaline relaxes smooth muscles of the bronchi and uterus. It's commonly used for bronchospasm and premature labor and is given to stop contractions. The client will continue to take terbutaline until the pregnancy is at term (37 weeks).
CN: Physiological integrity; CNS: Pharmacological therapies; CL: Analysis

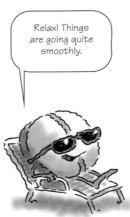

33. A client hospitalized for premature labor tells the nurse she's having occasional contractions. Which nursing intervention would be the <u>most appropriate</u>?
1. Teach the client the possible complications of premature birth.
2. Tell the client to walk around to see if she can get rid of the contractions.
3. Give I.V. fluids and encourage her to empty her bladder and drink plenty of fluids.
4. Notify anesthesia for immediate epidural placement to relieve the pain associated with contractions.

33. 3. An empty bladder and adequate hydration may help decrease or stop labor contractions. Teaching the client potential complications is likely to increase her anxiety rather than help her relax. Walking may encourage contractions to become stronger. It would be inappropriate to call anesthesia and have an epidural placed because further assessment of the contractions is necessary.
CN: Physiological integrity; CNS: Reduction of risk potential; CL: Application

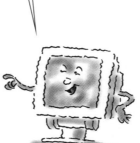
You don't have to be a math whiz to figure this one out.

34. The phrase "gravida 4, para 2" indicates which prenatal history?
1. A client has been pregnant four times and had two miscarriages.
2. A client has been pregnant four times and delivered two live-born children.
3. A client has been pregnant four times and had two cesarean deliveries.
4. A client has been pregnant four times and had two spontaneous abortions.

34. 2. *Gravida* refers to the number of times a client has been pregnant; *para* refers to the number of viable children born. Therefore, the client who's gravida 4, para 2 has been pregnant four times and delivered two live-born children.
CN: Health promotion and maintenance; CNS: None; CL: Knowledge

CN: Client needs category   CNS: Client needs subcategory   CL: Cognitive level

35. Which factor would contribute to a high-risk pregnancy?
1. Blood type O positive
2. First pregnancy at age 33
3. History of allergy to honey bee pollen
4. Type 1 diabetes

36. Which complication can be potentially life-threatening and can occur in a client receiving a tocolytic agent?
1. Diabetic ketoacidosis
2. Hyperemesis gravidarum
3. Pulmonary edema
4. Sickle cell anemia

37. Which hormone would be administered for the stimulation of uterine contractions?
1. Estrogen
2. Fetal cortisol
3. Oxytocin
4. Progesterone

38. Which answer <u>best</u> describes the stage of pregnancy in which maternal and fetal blood are exchanged?
1. Conception
2. 9 weeks' gestation, when the fetal heart is well developed
3. 32 to 34 weeks' gestation (third trimester)
4. Never

39. Which rationale <u>best</u> explains why a pregnant client is urged to lie on her side when resting or sleeping in the later stages of pregnancy?
1. To facilitate digestion
2. To facilitate bladder emptying
3. To prevent compression of the vena cava
4. To avoid the development of fetal anomalies

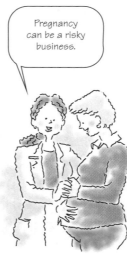

Pregnancy can be a risky business.

35. 4. A woman with a history of diabetes has an increased risk for perinatal complications, including hypertension, preeclampsia, and neonatal hypoglycemia. The age of 33 without other risk factors doesn't increase risk, nor does type O-positive blood or environmental allergens.
CN: Health promotion and maintenance; CNS: None; CL: Comprehension

36. 3. Tocolytics are used to stop labor contractions. The most common adverse effect associated with the use of these drugs is pulmonary edema. Clients who don't have diabetes don't need to be observed for diabetic ketoacidosis. Hyperemesis gravidarum doesn't result from tocolytic use. Sickle cell anemia is an inherited genetic condition and doesn't develop spontaneously.
CN: Physiological integrity; CNS: Pharmacological therapies; CL: Knowledge

37. 3. Oxytocin is the hormone responsible for stimulating uterine contractions. Pitocin, the synthetic form, may be given to clients who are past their due date. Although estrogen has a role in uterine contractions, it isn't given in a synthetic form to help uterine contractility. Fetal cortisol is believed to slow the production of progesterone by the placenta. Progesterone has a relaxing effect on the uterus.
CN: Physiological integrity; CNS: Pharmacological therapies; CL: Knowledge

38. 4. Only nutrients and waste products are transferred across the placenta. Blood exchange never occurs. Complications and some medical procedures can cause an exchange to occur accidentally.
CN: Physiological integrity; CNS: Physiological adaptation; CL: Comprehension

39. 3. The weight of the pregnant uterus is sufficiently heavy to compress the vena cava, which could impair blood flow to the uterus, possibly supplying insufficient oxygen to the fetus. The side-lying position hasn't been shown to prevent fetal anomalies, nor does it facilitate bladder emptying or digestion.
CN: Physiological integrity; CNS: Reduction of risk potential; CL: Analysis

CN: Client needs category   CNS: Client needs subcategory   CL: Cognitive level

40. A pregnant client is concerned about lack of fetal movement. What instructions would the nurse give that might offer reassurance?
1. Start taking an additional prenatal vitamin.
2. Take a warm bath to facilitate fetal movement.
3. Eat foods that contain a high sugar content to enhance fetal movement.
4. Lie down once a day and count the number of fetal movements for 15 to 30 minutes.

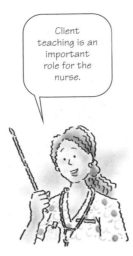

Client teaching is an important role for the nurse.

41. What would be the <u>most appropriate</u> recommendation to a pregnant client who complains of swelling in her feet and ankles?
1. Limit fluid intake.
2. Buy walking shoes.
3. Sit and elevate the feet twice daily.
4. Start taking a diuretic as needed daily.

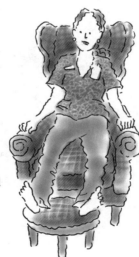

Sometimes you just have to take a break.

42. Which intervention would the nurse recommend to a client having severe heartburn during her pregnancy?
1. Eat several small meals daily.
2. Eat crackers on waking every morning.
3. Drink a preparation of salt and vinegar.
4. Drink orange juice frequently during the day.

43. Which maternal complication is associated with obesity in pregnancy?
1. Mastitis
2. Placenta previa
3. Preeclampsia
4. Rh isoimmunization

40. 4. Having the client lie down once during the day will allow her to concentrate on detecting fetal movement, which can be reassuring. Additionally, when the mother is up and actively walking around, it tends to be soothing to the fetus, resulting in sleep promotion. Lying down will make it easier for the client to detect movement. Instructing her to take an additional prenatal vitamin isn't recommended because vitamins can be toxic. Taking a warm bath is likely to sooth the fetus. There's also a risk for hyperthermia if the water is too warm or the client is immersed too long. Eating additional sugary foods isn't recommended because some pregnant clients are more susceptible to cavities.
CN: Psychosocial integrity; CNS: None; CL: Application

41. 3. Sitting down and putting up her feet at least once daily will promote venous return and, therefore, decrease edema. Limiting fluid intake isn't recommended unless there are additional medical complications such as heart failure. Buying walking shoes won't necessarily decrease edema. Diuretics aren't recommended during pregnancy because it's important to maintain an adequate circulatory volume.
CN: Physiological integrity; CNS: Basic care and comfort; CL: Application

42. 1. Eating small, frequent meals will place less pressure on the esophageal sphincter, reducing the likelihood of the regurgitation of stomach contents into the lower esophagus. None of the other interventions have been shown to decrease heartburn.
CN: Physiological integrity; CNS: Basic care and comfort; CL: Application

43. 3. The incidence of preeclampsia in obese clients is about seven times more than that in a nonobese pregnant client. Placenta previa, mastitis, and Rh isoimmunization aren't associated with increased incidence in obese pregnant clients.
CN: Physiological integrity; CNS: Reduction of risk potential; CL: Analysis

CN: Client needs category   CNS: Client needs subcategory   CL: Cognitive level

44. Because uteroplacental circulation is compromised in clients with preeclampsia, a nonstress test (NST) is performed to detect which condition?
1. Anemia
2. Fetal well-being
3. Intrauterine growth retardation (IUGR)
4. Oligohydramnios

45. A client is 33 weeks pregnant and has had diabetes since age 21. When checking her fasting blood glucose level, which value would indicate the client's disease is controlled?
1. 45 mg/dl
2. 85 mg/dl
3. 120 mg/dl
4. 136 mg/dl

46. A client with diabetes, who is in the late third trimester, has a nonstress test twice weekly. The 20-minute test showed three fetal heart rate accelerations that exceeded the baseline by 15 beats/minute and lasted longer than 15 seconds. The nurse knows these results are consistent with which interpretation of a nonstress test?
1. Reactive test
2. Nonreactive test
3. Positive test
4. Negative test

47. A nurse is reinforcing teaching about the signs of preterm labor to a client who is at 28 weeks' gestation. Which teaching should the nurse reinforce?
1. Irregular contractions that don't dilate the cervix are normal.
2. Regular contractions that dilate the cervix are an indication of labor.
3. Painful contractions without cervical dilation are signs of labor.
4. Irregular contractions with cervical effacement indicate labor.

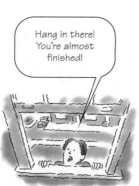

Hang in there! You're almost finished!

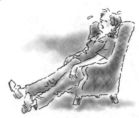

Here's MY reaction to a nonstress test.

44. 2. An NST is based on the theory that a healthy fetus will have transient fetal heart rate accelerations with fetal movement. A fetus with compromised uteroplacental circulation usually won't have these accelerations, which indicate a nonreactive NST. An NST can't detect anemia in a fetus. Serial ultrasounds will detect IUGR and oligohydramnios in a fetus.
CN: Health promotion and maintenance; CNS: None; CL: Analysis

45. 2. Recommended fasting blood glucose levels in pregnant clients with diabetes are 60 to 95 mg/dl. A fasting blood glucose level of 45 g/dl is low and may result in symptoms of hypoglycemia. A blood glucose level below 120 mg/dl is recommended for 2-hour postprandial values. A blood glucose level above 136 mg/dl in a pregnant client indicates hyperglycemia.
CN: Health promotion and maintenance; CNS: None; CL: Analysis

46. 1. The nonstress test is the preferred antepartum heart rate screening test for pregnant clients with diabetes. A reactive nonstress test is two or more fetal heart rate accelerations that exceed baseline by at least 15 beats/minute and last longer than 15 seconds within a 20-minute period. A nonreactive nonstress test lacks accelerations in the fetal heart rate with fetal movement. The terms *positive* and *negative* aren't used to describe the interpretation of nonstress tests.
CN: Physiological integrity; CNS: Reduction of risk potential CL: Analysis

47. 2. Regular uterine contractions before 36 weeks' gestation that occur every 10 minutes or more and are accompanied by cervical dilation changes are considered signs of preterm labor. Uterine contractions without cervical changes aren't considered signs of preterm labor.
CN: Physiological integrity; CNS: Reduction of risk potential; CL: Application

48. Which condition is the <u>most common</u> cause of anemia in pregnancy?
1. Alpha thalassemia
2. Beta thalassemia
3. Iron deficiency anemia
4. Sickle cell anemia

49. Which test should be ordered to <u>confirm</u> a diagnosis of beta thalassemia?
1. Complete blood count (CBC)
2. Hemoglobin A_{1c}
3. Hemoglobin electrophoresis
4. Iron level

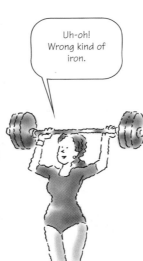

Uh-oh! Wrong kind of iron.

48. 3. Iron deficiency anemia accounts for approximately 95% of anemia in pregnancy. Thalassemias are the most common genetic disorders of the blood. These anemias cause a reduction or absence of the alpha or beta hemoglobin chain. Sickle cell anemia is an inherited chronic disease that results from abnormal hemoglobin synthesis.
CN: Health promotion and maintenance; CNS: None; CL: Knowledge

49. 3. Diagnosis of the specific type of thalassemia is achieved by hemoglobin electrophoresis. This test detects high levels of hemoglobin A_2 or F. The CBC includes white blood cell, hemoglobin, hematocrit, and platelet values. Hemoglobin A_{1c} values show the client's blood glucose levels over the past 120 days. A direct iron level can't be tested. Iron status is indirectly assessed through hemoglobin, hematocrit, mean corpuscular volume, and other such values. A client history and diet record can also help determine iron intake.
CN: Physiological integrity; CNS: Reduction of risk potential; CL: Knowledge

50. Which nursing intervention for a pregnant adolescent client in her first trimester has the <u>highest</u> priority?
1. Schedule the client for a screening glucose tolerance test.
2. Make sure the client receives nutritional counseling and reinforce the teaching.
3. Teach the client she's at increased risk for having a macrosomic neonate.
4. Monitor the client for signs and symptoms of placenta previa.

51. A nurse is teaching a course on the anatomy and physiology of reproduction. In this illustration of the female reproductive organs, identify the area where fertilization occurs.

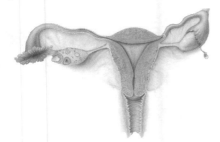

50. 2. Nutritional counseling must be emphasized as part of the prenatal care for adolescent clients. Adolescents aren't at increased risk for developing gestational diabetes or placenta previa. Adolescent clients are at risk for delivering low-birth-weight neonates, not macrosomic neonates.
CN: Health promotion and maintenance; CNS: None; CL: Analysis

51.

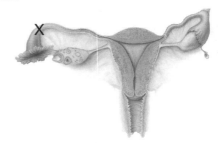

After ejaculation, the sperm travel by flagellar movement through the fluids of the cervical mucus into the fallopian tube to meet the descending ovum in the ampulla, where fertilization occurs.
CN: Health promotion and maintenance; CNS: None; CL: Application

CN: Client needs category   CNS: Client needs subcategory   CL: Cognitive level

52. When teaching an antepartal client about the passage of the fetus through the birth canal during labor, the nurse describes the cardinal mechanisms of labor. Place these events in the proper ascending chronological order. Use all the options.

1. Flexion
2. External rotation
3. Descent
4. Expulsion
5. Internal rotation
6. Extension

52. Ordered response:

3. Descent
1. Flexion
5. Internal rotation
6. Extension
2. External rotation
4. Expulsion

The fetus moving through the birth canal changes position to ensure that the smallest diameter of the fetal head always presents to the smallest diameter of the birth canal. Termed the *cardinal mechanisms of labor,* these position changes occur in this sequence: descent, flexion, internal rotation, extension, external rotation, and expulsion.

CN: Physiological integrity; CNS: Physiological adaptation; CL: Application

53. A client is scheduled for amniocentesis. What should the nurse do to prepare the client for the procedure? Select all that apply:
1. Ask the client to void.
2. Instruct the client to drink 1 L of fluid.
3. Ask the client to lie on her left side.
4. Assess fetal heart rate.
5. Insert an I.V. catheter.
6. Monitor maternal vital signs.

53. 1, 4, 6. To prepare a client for amniocentesis, the nurse should ask her to empty her bladder to reduce the risk of bladder perforation. Before the procedure, the nurse should also assess fetal heart rate and maternal vital signs to establish baselines. The client should be asked to drink 1 L of fluid before transabdominal ultrasound, not amniocentesis. The client should be supine during the procedure; afterward, she should be placed on her left side to avoid supine hypotension, promote venous return, and ensure adequate cardiac output. I.V. access isn't necessary for this procedure.

CN: Physiological integrity; CNS: Reduction of risk potential; CL: Application

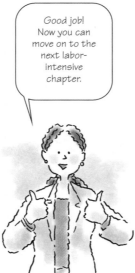

Good job! Now you can move on to the next labor-intensive chapter.

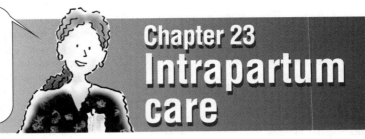

The antepartum and postpartum periods are important to know about. However, the intrapartum period—that's where the action is! This chapter covers the intrapartum period, perhaps the most critical of the three.

Chapter 23
Intrapartum care

1. A client with a full-term, uncomplicated pregnancy comes into the labor-and-delivery unit in early labor saying that she thinks her water has broken. Which action by the nurse would be most appropriate?
1. Prepare the client for delivery.
2. Note the color, amount, and odor of the fluid.
3. Immediately contact the physician.
4. Collect a sample of the fluid for microbial analysis.

2. A client who's 36 weeks pregnant comes into the labor-and-delivery unit with mild contractions. Which complication should the nurse watch for when the client informs her that she has placenta previa?
1. Sudden rupture of membranes
2. Vaginal bleeding
3. Emesis
4. Fever

3. A client's labor doesn't progress. The physician orders I.V. administration of 1,000 ml normal saline solution with oxytocin (Pitocin) 10 units to run at 2 milliunits/minute. Two milliunits/ minute is equivalent to how many ml/minute?
1. 0.002
2. 0.02
3. 0.2
4. 2.0

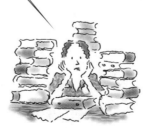

Now I have to be a mathematician, too. Go figure!

1. 2. Noting the color, amount, and odor of the fluid will help guide the nurse in her next action. There's no need to call the client's physician immediately or prepare the client for delivery if the fluid is clear and delivery isn't imminent. Rupture of membranes isn't unusual in the early stages of labor. Fluid collection for microbial analysis isn't routine if there's no concern of infection (maternal fever).

CN: Physiological integrity; CNS: Reduction of risk potential; CL: Application

2. 2. Contractions may disrupt the microvascular network in the placenta of a client with placenta previa and result in bleeding. If the separation of the placenta occurs at the margin of the placenta, the blood will escape vaginally. Sudden rupture of the membranes isn't related to placenta previa. Fever would indicate an infectious process, and emesis isn't related to placenta previa.

CN: Physiological integrity; CNS: Reduction of risk potential; CL: Application

3. 3. The answer is found by setting up a ratio and following through with the calculations shown below. Each unit of oxytocin contains 1,000 milliunits. Therefore, 1,000 ml of I.V. fluid contains 10,000 milliunits (10 units) of Pitocin. Use the following equation:

$$10,000/1,000 = 2/X;$$
$$10,000X = 2,000;$$

Solve for X (equals 0.2 ml).

CN: Physiological integrity; CNS: Pharmacological therapies; CL: Analysis

4. A client in labor has been receiving oxytocin (Pitocin) to aid her progress. The nurse caring for her notes that a contraction has remained strong for 60 seconds. Which action should the nurse take <u>first</u>?

1. Stop the oxytocin infusion.
2. Notify the physician.
3. Monitor fetal heart tones as usual.
4. Turn the client on her left side.

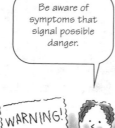

Be aware of symptoms that signal possible danger.

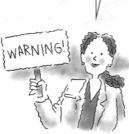

5. A client at term arrives in the labor unit experiencing contractions every 4 minutes. After a brief assessment, she's admitted and an electronic fetal monitor is applied. Which observation would alert the nurse to an increased potential for fetal distress?

1. Total weight gain of 30 lb (13.6 kg)
2. Maternal age of 32 years
3. Blood pressure of 146/90 mm Hg
4. Treatment for syphilis at 15-weeks' gestation

6. Cervical effacement and dilation aren't progressing in a client in labor. The physician orders I.V. administration of oxytocin (Pitocin). During oxytocin administration, why must the nurse monitor the client's fluid intake and output closely?

1. Oxytocin causes water intoxication.
2. Oxytocin causes excessive thirst.
3. Oxytocin is toxic to the kidneys.
4. Oxytocin has a diuretic effect.

7. After an amniotomy, which client goal should take the <u>highest</u> priority?

1. The client will express increased knowledge about amniotomy.
2. The fetus will maintain adequate tissue perfusion.
3. The fetus will display no signs of infection.
4. The client will report relief of pain.

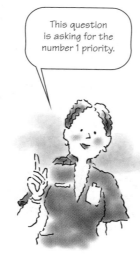

This question is asking for the number 1 priority.

4. 1. A contraction that remains strong for 60 seconds with no sign of letting up signals approaching tetany and could cause rupture of the uterus. Oxytocin stimulates contractions and should be stopped. The nurse should monitor the fetal heart tones and notify the physician, but only after stopping the oxytocin. The client should already be on her left side but the tonic contraction is more than likely due to the oxytocin.

CN: Physiological integrity; CNS: Reduction of risk potential; CL: Application

5. 3. A blood pressure of 146/90 mm Hg may indicate gestational hypertension. Over time, gestational hypertension reduces blood flow to the placenta and can cause intrauterine growth retardation and other problems that make the fetus less able to tolerate the stress of labor. A weight gain of 30 lb is within expected parameters for a healthy pregnancy. A woman at age 32 doesn't have a greater risk of complications if her general condition is healthy before pregnancy. Increased risk of complications begins around age 35. Syphilis that has been treated doesn't pose an additional risk.

CN: Physiological integrity; CNS: Reduction of risk potential; CL: Application

6. 1. The nurse should monitor fluid intake and output because prolonged oxytocin infusion may cause severe water intoxication, leading to seizure, coma, and death. Excessive thirst results from the work of labor and limited oral fluid intake, not oxytocin. Oxytocin has no nephrotoxic or diuretic effects; in fact, it produces an antidiuretic effect.

CN: Physiological integrity; CNS: Pharmacological therapies; CL: Knowledge

7. 2. Amniotomy increases the risk of umbilical cord prolapse, which would impair the fetal blood supply and tissue perfusion. Because the fetus's life depends on the oxygen carried by that blood, maintaining fetal tissue perfusion takes priority over goals related to increased knowledge, infection prevention, and pain relief.

CN: Safe, effective care environment; CNS: Safety and infection control; CL: Application

CN: Client needs category   CNS: Client needs subcategory   CL: Cognitive level

8. A client at 42-weeks' gestation is 3 cm dilated and 30% effaced with membranes intact and the fetus at +2 station. Fetal heart rate (FHR) is 140 to 150 beats/minute. After 2 hours, the nurse notes on the external fetal monitor that for the past 10 minutes the FHR ranged from 160 to 190 beats/minute. The client states that her baby has been extremely active. Uterine contractions are strong, occurring every 3 to 4 minutes and lasting 40 to 60 seconds. Which finding would indicate fetal hypoxia?

1. Abnormally long uterine contractions
2. Abnormally strong uterine intensity
3. Excessively frequent contractions, with rapid fetal movement
4. Excessive fetal activity and fetal tachycardia

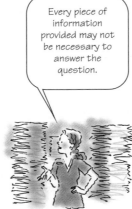

Every piece of information provided may not be necessary to answer the question.

8. 4. Fetal tachycardia and excessive fetal activity are the first signs of fetal hypoxia. The duration of uterine contractions is within normal limits. Uterine intensity can be mild to strong and still be within normal limits. The frequency of contractions is within the normal limits for the active phase of labor.

CN: Physiological integrity; CNS: Reduction of risk potential; CL: Analysis

9. A client at 33 weeks' gestation and leaking amniotic fluid is placed on an external fetal monitor. The monitor indicates uterine irritability, and contractions are occurring every 4 to 6 minutes. The physician orders terbutaline (Brethine) 0.25 mg to be given subcutaneously. Which teaching statement is appropriate for this client?

1. "This medicine will make you breathe better."
2. "You may feel a fluttering or tight sensation in your chest."
3. "This will dry your mouth and make you feel thirsty."
4. "You'll need to replace the potassium lost by this drug."

9. 2. A fluttering or tight sensation in the chest is a common adverse reaction to terbutaline. Although terbutaline relieves bronchospasm, this client is receiving it to reduce uterine motility. Dry mouth and thirst occur with the inhaled form of terbutaline but are unlikely with the subcutaneous form. Hypokalemia is a potential adverse reaction following large doses of terbutaline.

CN: Health promotion and maintenance; CNS: None; CL: Application

10. A 17-year-old primigravida with severe gestational hypertension has been receiving magnesium sulfate I.V. for 3 hours. The latest assessment reveals deep tendon reflexes (DTRs) of +1, blood pressure of 150/100 mm Hg, a pulse of 92 beats/minute, a respiratory rate of 10 breaths/minute, and urine output of 20 ml/hour. Which action would be <u>most appropriate</u>?

1. Continue monitoring per standards of care.
2. Stop the magnesium sulfate infusion.
3. Increase the infusion rate by 5 gtt/minute.
4. Decrease the infusion rate by 5 gtt/minute.

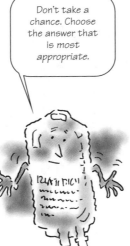

Don't take a chance. Choose the answer that is most appropriate.

10. 2. Magnesium sulfate should be withheld if the client's respiratory rate or urine output falls or if reflexes are diminished or absent, all of which are true for this client. The client also shows other signs of impending toxicity, such as flushing and feeling warm. Inaction won't resolve the client's suppressed DTRs and low respiratory rate and urine output. The client is already showing central nervous system depression because of excessive magnesium sulfate, so increasing the infusion rate is inappropriate. Impending toxicity indicates that the infusion should be stopped rather than just slowed down.

CN: Physiological integrity; CNS: Pharmacological therapies; CL: Application

CN: Client needs category   CNS: Client needs subcategory   CL: Cognitive level

11. During a vaginal examination of a client in labor, the nurse palpates the fetus's larger, diamond-shaped fontanel toward the anterior portion of the client's pelvis. Which statement best describes this situation?

1. The client can expect a brief and intense labor, with potential for lacerations.
2. The client is at risk for uterine rupture and needs constant monitoring.
3. The client may need interventions to ease her back labor and change the fetal position.
4. The client must be told that the fetus will be delivered using forceps or a vacuum extractor.

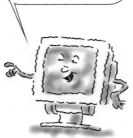

Be careful of the words will be in statement 4. They indicate an absolute, a rarity in health care.

11. 3. The fetal position is occiput posterior, a position that commonly produces intense back pain during labor. Most of the time, the fetus rotates during labor to occiput anterior position. Positioning the client on her side can facilitate this rotation. An occiput posterior position would most likely result in prolonged labor. Occiput posterior alone doesn't create a risk of uterine rupture. The fetus would be delivered with forceps or vacuum extractor only if it doesn't rotate spontaneously.

CN: Safe, effective care environment; CNS: Safety and infection control; CL: Analysis

12. The nurse-manager is meeting with the Director of Security and the staff to discuss ways to ensure client safety. Which instruction would be important to include in a plan for the maternity ward?

1. Keep the unit locked at all times.
2. Have spouses or significant others of the maternity clients wear identification bands.
3. Limit the number of visitors to two per client.
4. Limit visiting hours to 2 hours per day.

12. 2. Having the spouse or significant other of a maternity client wear an identification band is the most realistic and achievable instruction to include in the security plan for this client care area. Keeping the unit locked at all times isn't a viable suggestion for the security plan. Limiting the number of visitors to two per client may not be attainable. Limiting visiting hours to 2 hours per day is probably unrealistic.

CN: Safe, effective care environment; CNS: Safety and infection control; CL: Application

13. Which term would a nurse use to describe the thinning and shortening of the cervix that occurs just before and during labor?

1. Ballottement
2. Dilation
3. Effacement
4. Multiparous

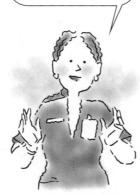

The long and short of it is—you probably know the answer to this question.

13. 3. Effacement is cervical shortening and thinning, while dilation is widening of the cervix; both facilitate opening the cervix in preparation for delivery. Ballottement is the ability of another individual to move the fetus by externally manipulating the maternal abdomen. A ballotable fetus hasn't yet engaged in the maternal pelvis. Multiparous refers to the number of live births a woman has had.

CN: Physiological integrity; CNS: Physiological adaptation; CL: Comprehension

14. Which fetal position is best for birth?
1. Vertex position
2. Transverse position
3. Frank breech position
4. Posterior position of the fetal head

14. 1. Vertex position (flexion of the fetal head) is the optimal position for passage through the birth canal. Transverse positioning generally results in poor labor contractions and an unacceptable fetal position for birth. Frank breech positioning, in which the buttocks present first, is a difficult delivery. Posterior positioning of the fetal head makes it difficult for the fetal head to pass under the maternal symphysis pubis bone.
CN: Physiological integrity; CNS: Reduction of risk potential; CL: Analysis

15. A nurse is preparing a client in the labor-and-delivery unit and is teaching her about the stages of labor. The client demonstrates understanding of these stages when stating that birth occurs during which stage?
1. First stage of labor
2. Second stage of labor
3. Third stage of labor
4. Fourth stage of labor

15. 2. The second stage of labor begins with complete dilation (10 cm) and ends with the expulsion of the fetus. The first stage of labor is the stage of dilation, which is divided into three distinct phases: latent, active, and transition. The third stage of labor begins immediately following the birth of the neonate and ends with the expulsion of the placenta. The fourth stage of labor is the first 1 to 4 hours after placental expulsion, in which the client's body begins the recovery process.
CN: Physiological integrity; CNS: Basic care and comfort; CL: Application

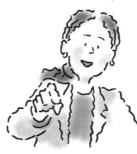

To answer question 16 correctly, it's critical that you understand you're being asked to consider only those laboratory values that are critical.

16. Which laboratory value would be <u>critical</u> for a client admitted to the labor-and-delivery unit?
1. Blood type
2. Calcium
3. Iron
4. Oxygen saturation

16. 1. Blood type would be a critical value to have because the risk of blood loss is always a potential complication during the labor-and-delivery process. Approximately 40% of a woman's cardiac output is delivered to the uterus; therefore, blood loss can occur quite rapidly in the event of uncontrolled bleeding. Calcium and iron aren't critical values and oxygen saturation isn't a laboratory value.
CN: Physiological integrity; CNS: Reduction of risk potential; CL: Analysis

17. A 34-year-old woman is in labor and the baby is full term. The nurse is checking the fetal heart rate. What range of fetal heart rates would reassure the nurse of appropriate fetal perfusion?
1. 80 to 100 beats/minute
2. 100 to 120 beats/minute
3. 110 to 160 beats/minute
4. 160 to 180 beats/minute

17. 3. A rate of 110 to 160 beats/minute in the fetal heart is appropriate for filling the heart with blood and pumping it out to the system. Faster or slower rates don't accomplish perfusion adequately.
CN: Health promotion and maintenance; CNS: None; CL: Analysis

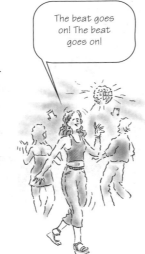

The beat goes on! The beat goes on!

CN: Client needs category   CNS: Client needs subcategory   CL: Cognitive level

18. A client in labor has external electronic fetal monitoring in place. Which data can be determined by examining the fetal heart rate strip produced by the external electronic fetal monitor?
1. Gender of the fetus
2. Fetal position
3. Labor progress
4. Oxygenation

18. 4. Oxygenation of the fetus may be indirectly determined through fetal monitoring by closely examining the fetal heart rate strip. Accelerations in the fetal heart rate indicate good oxygenation, whereas decelerations in the fetal heart rate sometimes indicate poor fetal oxygenation. The fetal heart rate strip can't determine the gender of the fetus or fetal position. Labor progress can be directly monitored only through cervical examination; although, commonly, the woman's body language can give some indication of the progression of labor.
CN: Physiological integrity; CNS: Reduction of risk potential; CL: Comprehension

19. Which nursing action is required before a client in labor receives an epidural?
1. Giving a fluid bolus of 500 ml
2. Checking for maternal pupil dilation
3. Testing maternal reflexes
4. Observing maternal gait

19. 1. One of the major adverse effects of epidural administration is hypotension. Therefore, a 500-ml fluid bolus is usually administered to help prevent hypotension in the client who wishes to receive an epidural for pain relief. Checking maternal reflexes, pupil response, and gait aren't necessary.
CN: Physiological integrity; CNS: Reduction of risk potential; CL: Analysis

20. Which complication is possible with an episiotomy?
1. Blood loss
2. Uterine disfigurement
3. Prolonged dyspareunia
4. Hormonal fluctuation postpartum

20. 3. Prolonged dyspareunia (painful intercourse) may result when complications such as infection interfere with wound healing. Minimal blood loss occurs when an episiotomy is performed. The uterus isn't affected by episiotomy; the perineum is cut to accommodate the fetus. Hormonal fluctuations that occur during the postpartum period aren't the result of an episiotomy.
CN: Physiological integrity; CNS: Basic care and comfort; CL: Analysis

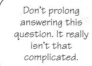

Don't prolong answering this question. It really isn't that complicated.

21. A client in labor notices a clear, milky discharge from both of her breasts. Which action by the nurse would be <u>most appropriate</u>?
1. Tell her that her milk is starting to come in because she's in labor.
2. Complete a thorough breast examination, and document the results in the chart.
3. Perform a culture on the discharge, and inform the client that she might have mastitis.
4. Inform the client that the discharge is colostrum, normally present after the 4th month of pregnancy.

21. 4. After the 4th month, colostrum may be noticed. The breasts normally produce colostrum for the first few days after delivery. Milk production begins 1 to 3 days postpartum. A clinical breast examination isn't usually indicated in the intrapartum setting. Although a culture may be indicated, it requires advanced assessment as well as a medical order.
CN: Health promotion and maintenance; CNS: None; CL: Application

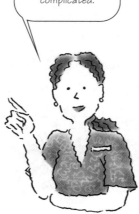

CN: Client needs category   CNS: Client needs subcategory   CL: Cognitive level

22. A nurse is participating in care planning for a client in labor. Which data may indicate a complication of labor?
   1. Urine output of 100 ml every 2 hours after epidural placement
   2. Increase in blood pressure to 154/96 mm Hg during contractions
   3. Decrease in respirations to 12 at the acme of contractions
   4. Increase in temperature from 98° F to 99.6° F (36.2° C to 37.6° C)

23. A client in early labor is concerned about the pinkish "stretch marks" on her abdomen. Which observation by the nurse shows an accurate understanding of the marks on the client's abdomen?
   1. Striae are common in pregnancy and will fade away completely after the uterus contracts to its prepregnant state.
   2. Striae are common in pregnancy, and will fade after delivery, but don't disappear.
   3. Striae are common in pregnancy and will fade away after application of an emollient cream.
   4. These marks are a sign of a separation of the rectus muscle and will require further assessment by the physician.

24. Which position increases cardiac output and stroke volume of a client in labor?
   1. Supine
   2. Sitting
   3. Side-lying
   4. Semi-Fowler's

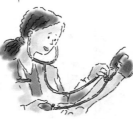

Monitoring blood pressure is an important component of intrapartum care.

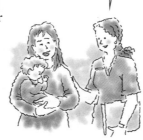

Stretch marks are yet another reminder of the joy of giving birth.

22. 2. During contractions, blood pressure increases and blood flow to the intervillous spaces changes, compromising the fetal blood supply. Therefore, the nurse should assess the client's blood pressure frequently to determine if it returns to precontraction level and allows adequate fetal blood flow again. A urine output of 100 ml every 2 hours, respirations of 12, and temperature changes are normal.

CN: Physiological integrity; CNS: Reduction of risk potential; CL: Analysis

23. 2. Striae are wavy, depressed streaks that may occur over the abdomen, breasts, or thighs as pregnancy progresses. They fade with time to a silvery color but won't disappear. Creams may soften the skin and reduce the appearance of striae, but won't remove the striae completely. Separation of the rectus muscle, diastasis, is a condition of pregnancy whereby the abdominal wall has difficulty stretching enough to accommodate the growing fetus, causing the muscle to separate.

CN: Health promotion and maintenance; CNS: None; CL: Knowledge

24. 3. In the side-lying position, cardiac output increases, stroke volume increases, and the pulse rate decreases. In the supine position, the blood pressure can drop severely, due to the pressure of the fetus on the vena cava, resulting in supine hypotensive syndrome or vena caval syndrome. Neither the sitting nor semi-Fowler's position increase cardiac output or stroke volume.

CN: Health promotion and maintenance; CNS: None; CL: Application

25. When caring for a client in the first stage of labor, the nurse documents cervical dilation of 9 cm and intense contractions that last 45 to 60 seconds and occur about every 2 minutes. Based on these findings, which action should the nurse perform next?
1. Notify the physician of the data collection results.
2. Begin the ordered oxytocin (Pitocin) to augment contractions.
3. Insert an intrauterine pressure catheter to accurately monitor contractions.
4. Continue to monitor the client and prepare equipment and supplies for delivery.

26. When assessing a client several minutes after vaginal delivery, the nurse notes blood gushing from the vagina, the umbilical cord lengthening, and a globe-shaped uterus. The nurse should monitor the client closely for which condition?
1. Uterine involution
2. Cervical laceration
3. Placental separation
4. Postpartum hemorrhage

27. A client in active labor believes in a holistic approach to health. Which strictly holistic approach is most realistic and might assist this client during the labor process?
1. A warm bath
2. A foot massage
3. Use of Reiki
4. Use of heated stones

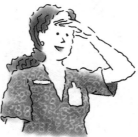

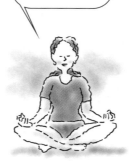

25. 4. The client is in the transition stage of labor. Labor is progressing normally; therefore, the nurse needs to set up for the delivery. The physician doesn't need to be notified until the client is fully dilated. Oxytocin isn't necessary because contractions are 2 minutes apart. There are no indications for an intrauterine contraction catheter. Placing the catheter isn't a nursing function.
CN: Physiological integrity; CNS: Physiological adaptation; CL: Application

26. 3. Placental separation causes a sudden gush or trickle of blood from the vagina, rise of the fundus in the abdomen, increased umbilical cord length at the introitus, and a globe-shaped uterus. Uterine involution causes a firmly contracted uterus, which can't occur until the placenta is delivered. Cervical lacerations produce a steady flow of bright red blood in a client with a firmly contracted uterus. Postpartum hemorrhage results in excessive vaginal bleeding and signs of shock, such as pallor and a rapid, thready pulse.
CN: Health promotion and maintenance; CNS: None; CL: Application

27. 3. The use of Reiki—a gentle technique focusing on the body's energy centers by loosening blocked energy, promoting total relaxation, and establishing spiritual equilibrium and mental well-being—is the most realistic holistic approach. A warm bath or foot massage might help any client, not just those who approach their health holistically. The use of heated stones might be difficult to obtain in a maternity unit.
CN: Physiological integrity; CNS: Basic care and comfort; CL: Analysis

CN: Client needs category   CNS: Client needs subcategory   CL: Cognitive level

28. Before discharging a client from the Antepartum Triage Unit, the nurse is reinforcing the teaching plan about the difference between Braxton Hicks contractions and true labor contractions. Which statement by the client indicates the teaching has been effective?
1. "Braxton Hicks contractions begin irregularly and become regular."
2. "Braxton Hicks contractions cause cervical dilation and effacement."
3. "Braxton Hicks contractions begin in the lower back and radiate to the abdomen."
4. "Braxton Hicks contractions begin in the abdomen and remain irregular."

29. Which description <u>best</u> fits the term effacement?
1. Enlargement of the cervical canal
2. Expulsion of the mucus plug
3. Shortening and thinning of the cervical canal
4. Downward movement of the fetal head

30. A client is in the first stage of labor and has progressed from 4 to 7 cm in cervical dilation. In which phase of the first stage does cervical dilation occur most rapidly?
1. Preparatory phase
2. Latent phase
3. Active phase
4. Transition phase

The question asks about rapid dilation.

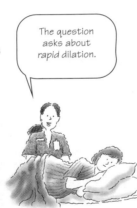

31. The nurse is teaching the stages of labor to a 26-year-old, pregnant client. The client would demonstrate appropriate comprehension when stating that crowning occurs during which stage of labor?
1. First
2. Second
3. Third
4. Fourth

28. 4. Braxton Hicks contractions begin and remain irregular. They're felt in the abdomen and remain confined to the abdomen and groin. They commonly disappear with ambulation and don't dilate the cervix. True contractions begin irregularly but become regular and predictable, causing cervical effacement and dilation. True contractions are felt initially in the lower back and radiate to the abdomen in a wavelike motion.
CN: Physiological integrity; CNS: Physiological adaptation; CL: Analysis

29. 3. With effacement, the cervical canal shortens and thins due to longitudinal traction from the contracting uterine fundus. Dilation is the enlargement of the cervical canal to approximately 10 cm. Show is the expulsion of the mucus plug, followed by a seepage of cervical capillary blood. Descent is a mechanism of labor whereby the biparietal diameter of the fetal head descends into the pelvic inlet.
CN: Health promotion and maintenance; CNS: None; CL: Knowledge

30. 3. Cervical dilation occurs more rapidly during the active phase than any of the previous phases. The active phase is characterized by cervical dilation that progresses from 4 to 7 cm. The preparatory, or latent, phase begins with the onset of regular uterine contractions and ends when rapid cervical dilation begins. Transition is defined as cervical dilation beginning at 8 cm and lasting until 10 cm or complete dilation.
CN: Health promotion and maintenance; CNS: None; CL: Comprehension

31. 2. The second stage of labor begins at full cervical dilation (10 cm) and ends when the infant is born. Crowning is present during this stage as the fetal head, pushed against the perineum, causes the vaginal introitus to open, allowing the fetal scalp to be visible. The first stage begins with true labor contractions and ends with complete cervical dilation. The third stage is from the time the infant is born until the delivery of the placenta. The fourth stage is the first 1 to 4 hours following delivery of the placenta.
CN: Health promotion and maintenance; CNS: None; CL: Application

CN: Client needs category   CNS: Client needs subcategory   CL: Cognitive level

32. A nurse suspects that a client in labor may have been physically abused by her male partner. Which intervention by the nurse would be most appropriate?
1. Confront the male partner.
2. Question the woman in front of her partner.
3. Contact hospital security.
4. Collaborate with the physician to make a referral to social services.

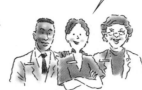

Consult other members of the medical team as needed.

32. 4. Collaborating with the physician to make a referral to social services will aid the client by creating a plan and providing support. Additionally, by law, the nurse or nursing supervisor must report the suspected abuse to the police and follow up with a written report. Although confrontation can be used therapeutically, this action will most likely provoke anger in the suspected abuser. Questioning the woman in front of her partner doesn't allow her the privacy required to address this issue and may place her in greater danger. If the woman isn't in imminent danger, there's no need to call hospital security.
CN: Physiological integrity; CNS: Reduction of risk potential; CL: Analysis

33. For a client in active labor, the physician plans to use an internal electronic fetal monitoring (EFM) device. What must occur before the internal EFM can be applied?
1. The membranes must rupture.
2. The fetus must be at 0 station.
3. The cervix must be dilated fully.
4. The client must receive anesthesia.

33. 1. Internal EFM can be applied only after the client's membranes have ruptured, when the fetus is at least at the −1 station, and when the cervix is dilated at least 2 cm. Although the client may receive anesthesia, it isn't required before application of an internal EFM device.
CN: Physiological integrity; CNS: Basic care and comfort; CL: Comprehension

34. The nurse has just admitted a client in the labor-and-delivery unit who has been diagnosed with diabetes mellitus. Which measure would be most appropriate for this situation?
1. Ask the client about her most recent blood glucose levels.
2. Prepare oral hypoglycemic medications for administration during labor.
3. Notify the neonatal intensive care unit that you'll be admitting a client with diabetes.
4. Prepare the client for cesarean delivery.

Stay on track by knowing the various fetal stations of labor. All aboard!

34. 1. As part of the history, asking about the client's most recent blood glucose levels will indicate how well her diabetes has been controlled. Oral hypoglycemic drugs are never used during pregnancy because they cross the placental barrier, stimulate fetal insulin production, and are potentially teratogenic. Plans to admit the neonate to the neonatal intensive care unit are premature. Cesarean delivery is no longer the preferred delivery for clients with diabetes. Vaginal birth is preferred and presents a lower risk to the mother and fetus.
CN: Physiological integrity; CNS: Reduction of risk potential; CL: Application

35. During a vaginal examination of a client in labor, the obstetrician determines that the biparietal diameter of the fetal head has reached the level of the ischial spines. How should the nurse document fetal station?
1. −1
2. 0
3. +1
4. +2

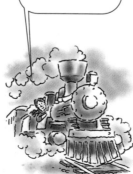

35. 2. When the largest diameter of the presenting part (typically the biparietal diameter of the fetal head) is level with the ischial spines, the fetus is at station 0. A station of −1 indicates that the fetal head is 1 cm above the ischial spines. At +1, it's 1 cm below the ischial spines. At +2, it's 2 cm below the ischial spines.
CN: Health promotion and maintenance; CNS: None; CL: Comprehension

CN: Client needs category   CNS: Client needs subcategory   CL: Cognitive level

36. A 30-year-old multiparous client admitted to the labor-and-delivery unit hasn't received prenatal care for this pregnancy. Which data is most relevant to the nursing assessment?
  1. Date of last menstrual period (LMP)
  2. Family history of sexually transmitted diseases (STDs)
  3. Name of insurance provider
  4. Number of siblings

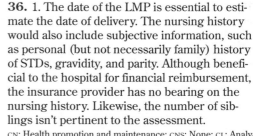

Careful. The question is looking for the most likely answer.

36. 1. The date of the LMP is essential to estimate the date of delivery. The nursing history would also include subjective information, such as personal (but not necessarily family) history of STDs, gravidity, and parity. Although beneficial to the hospital for financial reimbursement, the insurance provider has no bearing on the nursing history. Likewise, the number of siblings isn't pertinent to the assessment.
CN: Health promotion and maintenance; CNS: None; CL: Analysis

37. Which symptom, when observed in laboring clients with gestational hypertension, would most likely indicate a worsening condition?
  1. Decreasing blood pressure
  2. Increasing oliguria
  3. Decreasing edema
  4. Trace levels of protein in the urine

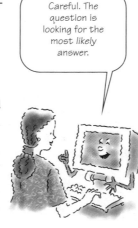

37. 2. Renal plasma flow and glomerular filtration are decreased in gestational hypertension, so increasing oliguria indicates a worsening condition. Blood pressure increases as a result of increased peripheral resistance. Increasing (not decreasing) edema would suggest a worsening condition. Trace levels to +1 proteinuria are acceptable; higher levels would indicate a worsening condition.
CN: Health promotion and maintenance; CNS: None; CL: Application

38. While in the first stage of labor, a client with active genital herpes is admitted to the labor-and-delivery area. Which type of birth should the nurse anticipate for this client?
  1. Mid-forceps
  2. Low forceps
  3. Induction
  4. Cesarean

38. 4. For a client with active genital herpes, cesarean delivery helps avoid infection transmission to the neonate, which could occur during a vaginal birth. Mid-forceps and low forceps are types of vaginal births that could transmit the herpes infection to the neonate. Induction is used only during vaginal birth; therefore, it's inappropriate for this client.
CN: Physiological integrity; CNS: Reduction of risk potential; CL: Application

39. A client is admitted to the labor-and-delivery unit in labor, with blood flowing down her legs. Which nursing intervention would be most appropriate?
  1. Placing an indwelling urinary catheter
  2. Monitoring fetal heart tones
  3. Performing a vaginal examination
  4. Preparing the client for cesarean delivery

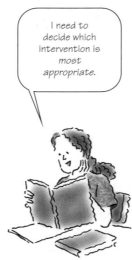

I need to decide which intervention is most appropriate.

39. 2. Monitoring fetal heart tones would be the first step because it's necessary to establish fetal well-being due to a possible placenta previa or abruptio placentae. Although an indwelling urinary catheter may be placed, it isn't an early intervention. Performing a vaginal examination would be contraindicated, as any agitation of the cervix with a previa can result in hemorrhage and death for the mother or fetus. Preparing the client for a cesarean delivery may not be indicated. An ultrasound should be performed to determine the cause of bleeding. If the diagnosis is a partial placenta previa, the client may still be able to deliver vaginally.
CN: Physiological integrity; CNS: Reduction of risk potential; CL: Application

40. A client in labor has been given an epidural anesthetic. Which nursing assessment finding is <u>most</u> important immediately following the administration of epidural anesthesia?
1. Maternal respirations decrease from 20 to 14 breaths/minute.
2. Maternal blood pressure decreases from 130/70 to 98/50 mm Hg.
3. Maternal pulse increases from 78 to 96 beats/minute.
4. Maternal temperature increases from 99° F (37.2° C) to 100° F (37.8° C).

41. Which drug would the nurse choose to use as an antagonist for magnesium sulfate?
1. Oxytocin (Pitocin)
2. Terbutaline (Brethine)
3. Calcium gluconate
4. Naloxone (Narcan)

I hope you know how many drops should drip.

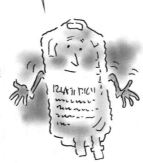

42. A physician has ordered an I.V. of 5% dextrose in lactated Ringer's solution at 125 ml/hour. The I.V. tubing delivers 10 drops per ml. How many drops per minute should fall into the drip chamber?
1. 10 to 11
2. 12 to 13
3. 20 to 21
4. 22 to 24

43. A nurse receives an order to start a rapid blood infusion for a client who's hemorrhaging from placenta previa. Which supplies will be needed?
1. Y tubing, normal saline solution, and a 20G catheter
2. Y tubing, normal saline solution, and an 18G catheter
3. Y tubing, lactated Ringer's solution, and an 18G catheter
4. Y tubing, lactated Ringer's solution, and a 16G catheter

40. 2. As the epidural anesthetic agent spreads through the spinal canal, it may produce hypotensive crisis, which is characterized by maternal hypotension, decreased beat-to-beat variability, and fetal bradycardia. The respiratory rate, pulse rate, and temperature are within normal limits for a laboring client.
CN: Physiological integrity; CNS: Physiological adaptation; CL: Analysis

41. 3. Calcium gluconate should be kept at the bedside while a client is receiving a magnesium infusion. If magnesium toxicity occurs, administer calcium gluconate as an antidote. Oxytocin is the synthetic form of the naturally occurring pituitary hormone used to initiate or augment uterine contractions. Terbutaline is a smooth muscle relaxant used to relax the uterus, especially for preterm labor and uterine hyperstimulation. Naloxone is an opiate antagonist administered to reverse the respiratory depression that sometimes follows doses of opiates.
CN: Physiological integrity; CNS: Pharmacological therapies; CL: Analysis

42. 3. Multiply the number of milliliters to be infused (125) by the drop factor (10); 125 × 10 = 1,250. Then divide the answer by the number of minutes to run the infusion (60). Use the following equation:
$$1,250 \div 60 = 20.83 \text{ (or 20 to 21 gtt/minute)}.$$
CN: Physiological integrity; CNS: Pharmacological therapies; CL: Knowledge

43. 2. Blood transfusions require Y tubing, normal saline solution to mix with the blood product, and an 18G catheter to avoid lysing (breaking) and to rapidly administer the red blood cells.
CN: Physiological integrity; CNS: Pharmacological therapies; CL: Comprehension

44. A laboring client in the latent stage of labor begins complaining of pain in the epigastric area, blurred vision, and a headache. The nurse knows that which medication should be prepared for administration?
1. Terbutaline (Brethine)
2. Oxytocin (Pitocin)
3. Magnesium sulfate
4. Calcium gluconate

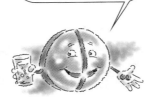

I'm the drug of choice to treat gestational hypertension. Do you know who I am?

44. 3. Magnesium sulfate is the drug of choice to treat gestational hypertension because it reduces edema by causing a shift from the extracellular spaces into the intestines. It also depresses the central nervous system, which decreases the incidence of seizures. Terbutaline is a smooth-muscle relaxant used to relax the uterus. Oxytocin is the synthetic form of the pituitary hormone used to stimulate uterine contractions. Calcium gluconate is the antagonist for magnesium toxicity.
CN: Physiological integrity; CNS: Pharmacological therapies; CL: Analysis

45. Which characteristic **best** describes variable decelerations?
1. Predictable response
2. Indicators of fetal well-being
3. Indicative of cord compression
4. Indicative of pressure on the fetal head

45. 3. Variable decelerations are commonly seen in labor when the membranes are ruptured, decreasing protection to the cord, especially as the fetus descends the birth canal. Variable decelerations are unpredictable. Atypical variable decelerations suggest fetal hypoxia. *Early* decelerations are related to pressure on the fetal head.
CN: Physiological integrity; CNS: Physiological adaptation; CL: Knowledge

46. A nurse is assisting in monitoring a client in labor. Which monitoring data are indicative of fetal well-being?
1. Fetal heart rate of 145 to 155 beats/minute with 15-second accelerations to 160
2. Fetal heart rate of 130 to 140 beats/minute with late decelerations to 110
3. Fetal heart rate of 110 to 120 beats/minute with variable decelerations to 90
4. Fetal heart rate of 165 to 175 beats/minute with late decelerations to 140

Only 4 more to go! It should be clear sailing from here.

46. 1. Accelerations of up to 15 beats/minute above baseline for a duration of 15 seconds are signs of fetal well-being. Decelerations initiated 30 to 40 seconds after the onset of the contraction are termed late decelerations and are due to uteroplacental insufficiency from decreased blood flow during uterine contractions. Variable decelerations are an indication of cord compression. Variable decelerations can occur with or without contractions.
CN: Physiological integrity; CNS: Physiological adaptation; CL: Analysis

47. A nurse is assisting in monitoring a client who's receiving oxytocin (Pitocin) to induce labor. The nurse should be alert to which maternal adverse reactions? Select all that apply:
1. Hypertension
2. Jaundice
3. Dehydration
4. Fluid overload
5. Uterine tetany
6. Bradycardia

47. 1, 4, 5. Adverse effects of oxytocin in the mother include hypertension, fluid overload, and uterine tetany. Oxytocin's antidiuretic effect increases renal reabsorption of water, leading to fluid overload, not dehydration. Jaundice and bradycardia are adverse effects that may occur in the neonate. Tachycardia, not bradycardia, is reported as a maternal adverse effect.
CN: Physiological integrity; CNS: Pharmacological therapies; CL: Application

CN: Client needs category   CNS: Client needs subcategory   CL: Cognitive level

48. A nurse is assigned to assist with the admission of a client in labor. Which actions are appropriate? Select all that apply:

1. Asking about the estimated date of delivery (EDD)
2. Estimating fetal size
3. Taking maternal and fetal vital signs
4. Asking about the woman's last menses
5. Administering an analgesic
6. Asking about the amount of time between contractions

49. Assessing a client progressing through labor reveals the findings below. Order them in the most likely sequence in which they would have occurred. Use all the options.

1. Uncontrollable urge to push
2. Cervical dilation of 7 cm
3. 100% cervical effacement
4. Strong Braxton Hicks contractions
5. Mild contractions lasting 20 to 40 seconds

48. 1, 3, 6. The nurse should ask about the EDD and then compare the response to the information in the prenatal record. If the fetus is preterm, special precautions and equipment are necessary. Maternal and fetal vital signs should be obtained to evaluate the well-being of the client and fetus. Determining how far apart the contractions are provides the health care team with valuable baseline information. The physician estimates the size of the fetus. It wouldn't be appropriate at this time for the nurse to ask about the client's last menses; this information would be collected at the first prenatal visit. It would be premature to administer an analgesic, which could slow or stop labor contractions.

CN: Health promotion and maintenance; CNS: None; CL: Application

49. Ordered response:

4. Strong Braxton Hicks contractions
5. Mild contractions lasting 20 to 40 seconds
2. Cervical dilation of 7 cm
3. 100% cervical effacement
1. Uncontrollable urge to push

Strong Braxton Hicks contractions typically occur before the onset of true labor and are considered a preliminary sign of labor. During the latent phase of the first stage of labor, contractions are mild, lasting about 20 to 40 seconds. As the client progresses through labor, contractions increase in intensity and duration, and cervical dilation occurs. Cervical dilation of 7 cm indicates that she has entered the active phase of the first stage of labor. Cervical effacement also occurs; effacement of 100% characterizes the transition phase of the first stage of labor. Progression into the second stage of labor is noted by the client's uncontrollable urge to push.

CN: Health promotion and maintenance; CNS: None: CL: Analysis

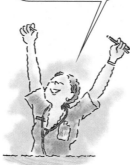

Congratulations! You finished! I knew you could do it.

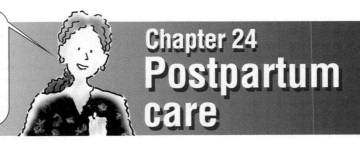

Before taking off through the chapter, why not spend a few minutes browsing the birthing stories at www.birthstories.com/? It will get you in just the right mood to tackle care of the postpartum client. Enjoy!

Chapter 24
Postpartum care

1. When completing the morning postpartum data collection, the nurse notices the client's perineal pad is completely saturated. Which action should be the nurse's <u>first</u> response?
1. Vigorously massage the fundus.
2. Immediately call the primary care provider.
3. Have the charge nurse review the assessment.
4. Ask the client when she last changed her perineal pad.

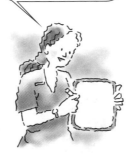

Be careful! The first question is asking for the nurse's first response.

1. 4. If the morning assessment is done relatively early, it's possible that the client hasn't yet been to the bathroom, in which case her perineal pad may have been in place all night. Secondly, her lochia may have pooled during the night, resulting in a heavy flow in the morning. Vigorous massage of the fundus, which is indicated for a boggy uterus, wouldn't be recommended as a *first* response until the client had gone to the bathroom, changed her perineal pad, and emptied her bladder. The nurse wouldn't want to call the primary care provider unnecessarily. If the nurse were uncertain, it would be appropriate to have another qualified individual check the client but only after a complete assessment of the client's status.
CN: Physiological integrity; CNS: Physiological adaptation; CL: Analysis

2. Which factor might result in a decreased supply of breast milk in a postpartum client?
1. Supplemental feedings with formula
2. Maternal diet high in vitamin C
3. An alcoholic drink
4. Frequent feedings

2. 1. Routine formula supplementation may interfere with establishing an adequate milk volume because decreased stimulation to the client's nipples affects hormonal levels and milk production. Vitamin C levels haven't been shown to influence milk volume. One drink containing alcohol generally tends to relax the client, facilitating letdown. Excessive consumption of alcohol may block letdown of milk to the infant, though supply isn't necessarily affected. Frequent feedings are likely to increase milk production.
CN: Physiological integrity; CNS: Physiological adaptation; CL: Application

3. Which intervention would be helpful to a bottle-feeding client who's experiencing hard or engorged breasts?
1. Applying ice
2. Restricting fluids
3. Applying warm compresses
4. Administering bromocriptine (Parlodel)

3. 1. Ice promotes comfort by decreasing blood flow (vasoconstriction), numbing the area, and discouraging further letdown of milk. Restricting fluids doesn't reduce engorgement and shouldn't be encouraged. Warm compresses will promote blood flow and hence, milk production, worsening the problem of engorgement. Bromocriptine has been removed from the market for lactation suppression.
CN: Physiological integrity; CNS: Basic care and comfort; CL: Application

CN: Client needs category   CNS: Client needs subcategory   CL: Cognitive level

4. A postpartum client who had a cesarean birth reports right calf pain to the nurse. The nurse observes that the client has nonpitting edema from her right knee to her foot. The nurse knows to prepare the client for which test <u>first</u>?
1. Venous duplex ultrasound of the right leg
2. Transthoracic echocardiogram
3. Venogram of the right leg
4. Noninvasive arterial studies of the right leg

4. 1. Right calf pain and nonpitting edema may indicate deep vein thrombosis (DVT). Postpartum clients and clients who have had abdominal surgery are at increased risk for DVT. Venous duplex ultrasound is a noninvasive test that visualizes the veins and assesses blood flow patterns. A venogram is an invasive test that utilizes dye and radiation to create images of the veins and wouldn't be the first choice. Transthoracic echocardiography looks at cardiac structures and isn't indicated at this time. Right calf pain and edema are symptoms of venous outflow obstruction, not arterial insufficiency.
CN: Physiological integrity; CNS: Reduction of risk potential; CL: Analysis

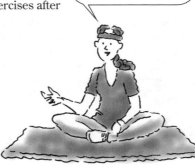

Performing Kegel exercises postpartum can aid in the healing process.

5. Which reason explains why women should be encouraged to perform Kegel exercises after delivery?
1. They assist with lochia removal.
2. They promote the return of normal bowel function.
3. They promote blood flow, enabling healing and muscle strengthening.
4. They assist the woman in burning calories for rapid postpartum weight loss.

5. 3. Exercising the pubococcygeal muscle increases blood flow to the area. The increased blood flow brings oxygen and other nutrients to the perineal area to aid in healing. Additionally, these exercises help strengthen the musculature, thereby decreasing the risk of future complications, such as incontinence and uterine prolapse. Performing Kegel exercises may assist with lochia removal, but that isn't their main purpose. Bowel function isn't influenced by Kegel exercises. Kegel exercises don't generate sufficient energy expenditure to burn many calories.
CN: Health promotion and maintenance; CNS: None; CL: Analysis

6. The nurse is monitoring a postpartum client who says she's concerned because she feels mildly depressed. The nurse recognizes that she's most likely experiencing "postpartum blues," and reassures the client that this symptom is experienced by approximately what percentage of women?
1. 25%
2. 50%
3. 75%
4. 100%

Be sure you know the clues to the postpartum blues!

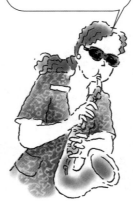

6. 3. Postpartum blues, or mild depression during the first 10 days after giving birth, affects 75% to 80% of women who give birth. More intense depression during this period is referred to as *postpartum depression,* which affects approximately 10% to 15% of postpartum clients. Postpartum depression can be severe with negative implications for maternal and neonatal well-being.
CN: Psychosocial integrity; CNS: None; CL: Application

7. Which practice would the nurse recommend to a client who has had a cesarean delivery?
1. Frequent douching after she's discharged
2. Coughing and deep-breathing exercises
3. Sit-ups for 2 weeks postoperatively
4. Side-rolling exercises

7. 2. As for any postoperative client, coughing and deep-breathing exercises should be taught to keep the alveoli open and prevent infection. Frequent douching isn't recommended and is contraindicated in clients who have just given birth. Sit-ups at 2 weeks postpartum could potentially damage the healing of the incision. Side-rolling exercises aren't an accepted medical practice.
CN: Physiological integrity; CNS: Reduction of risk potential; CL: Application

CN: Client needs category   CNS: Client needs subcategory   CL: Cognitive level

8. Which reason explains why a client might express disappointment after having a cesarean delivery instead of a vaginal delivery?
 1. Cesarean deliveries cost more.
 2. Depression is more common after a cesarean delivery.
 3. The client is usually more fatigued after cesarean delivery.
 4. The client may feel a loss for not having experienced a "normal" birth.

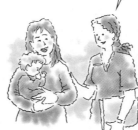

Remember to be sensitive to your postpartum client's needs.

9. The nurse is providing discharge instructions to a postpartum client after a vaginal birth. The nurse should inform the client that she may experience which <u>normal</u> finding?
 1. Redness or swelling in the calves
 2. A palpable uterine fundus beyond 6 weeks
 3. Vaginal dryness after the lochial flow has ended
 4. Dark red lochia for approximately 6 weeks after the birth

10. On completing fundal palpation, the nurse notes that the fundus is situated in the client's left abdomen. Which action is appropriate?
 1. Ask the client to empty her bladder.
 2. Straight-catheterize the client immediately.
 3. Call the client's primary health care provider for direction.
 4. Straight-catheterize the client for half of her urine volume.

11. The nurse is teaching a client with newly diagnosed mastitis about her condition. The nurse would inform the client that she <u>most likely</u> contracted the disorder from which organism?
 1. *Escherichia coli*
 2. Group beta-hemolytic streptococci (GBS)
 3. *Staphylococcus aureus*
 4. *Streptococcus pyogenes*

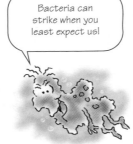

Bacteria can strike when you least expect us!

8. 4. Clients occasionally feel a loss after a cesarean delivery. They may feel they're inadequate because they couldn't deliver their infant vaginally. The cost of cesarean delivery doesn't generally apply because the client usually isn't directly responsible for payment. No conclusive studies support the theory that depression is more common after cesarean delivery than after vaginal delivery. Although clients are usually more fatigued after a cesarean delivery, fatigue hasn't been shown to cause feelings of disappointment over the method of delivery.
CN: Psychosocial integrity; CNS: None; CL: Analysis

9. 3. Vaginal dryness is a normal finding during the postpartum period due to hormonal changes. Redness or swelling in the calves may indicate thrombophlebitis. The fundus shouldn't be palpable beyond 6 weeks. Dark red lochia (indicating fresh bleeding) should only last 2 to 3 days postpartum.
CN: Physiological integrity; CNS: Physiological adaptation; CL: Application

10. 1. A full bladder may displace the uterine fundus to the left or right side of the abdomen. A straight catheterization is unnecessarily invasive if the client can urinate on her own. Nursing interventions should be completed before notifying the primary health care provider in a nonemergency situation.
CN: Physiological integrity; CNS: Physiological adaptation; CL: Application

11. 3. The most common cause of mastitis is *S. aureus*, transmitted from the neonate's mouth. Mastitis isn't harmful to the neonate. *E. coli*, GBS, and *S. pyogenes* aren't associated with mastitis. GBS infection *is* associated with neonatal sepsis and death.
CN: Health promotion and maintenance; CNS: None; CL: Analysis

CN: Client needs category   CNS: Client needs subcategory   CL: Cognitive level

12. The nurse is observing a client who gave birth yesterday. Where should the nurse expect to find the top of the client's fundus?
1. One fingerbreadth above the umbilicus
2. One fingerbreadth below the umbilicus
3. At the level of the umbilicus
4. Below the symphysis pubis

12. 2. After a client gives birth, the height of her fundus should decrease by about one fingerbreadth (about 1 cm) each day. So by the end of the first postpartum day, the fundus should be one fingerbreadth below the umbilicus. Immediately after birth, the fundus may be above the umbilicus; 6 to 12 hours after birth, it should be at the level of the umbilicus; 10 days after birth, it should be below the symphysis pubis.
CN: Physiological integrity; CNS: Physiological adaptation; CL: Application

13. The nurse receives a report on a client with type 1 diabetes mellitus whose delivery was complicated by polyhydramnios and macrosomia. The nurse is aware of these complications and knows to monitor the client closely for which of the following?
1. Postpartum mastitis
2. Increased insulin needs
3. Postpartum hemorrhage
4. Gestational hypertension

13. 3. The client is at risk for a postpartum hemorrhage from the overdistention of the uterus because of the extra amniotic fluid and the large neonate. The uterus may not be able to contract as well as it would normally. The diabetic client usually has decreased insulin needs for the first few days postpartum. Neither polyhydramnios nor macrosomia would increase the client's risk of gestational hypertension or mastitis.
CN: Physiological integrity; CNS: Reduction of risk potential; CL: Application

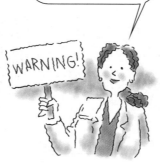

Beware of the special needs of a diabetic postpartum client.

WARNING!

14. The nurse is caring for a diabetic, postpartum client who has developed an infection. The nurse is aware that infections in diabetic clients tend to be more severe and can quickly lead to complications. Which complication should the nurse assess this client for?
1. Anemia
2. Ketoacidosis
3. Respiratory acidosis
4. Respiratory alkalosis

14. 2. Diabetic clients who become pregnant tend to become sicker and develop illnesses more quickly than pregnant clients without diabetes. Severe infections in diabetes can lead to diabetic ketoacidosis. Anemia, respiratory acidosis, and respiratory alkalosis aren't generally associated with infections in diabetic clients.
CN: Physiological integrity; CNS: Reduction of risk potential; CL: Analysis

15. The nurse is teaching a client about mastitis. Which statement should the nurse include in her teaching?
1. The most common pathogen is group A beta-hemolytic streptococci.
2. A breast abscess is a common complication of mastitis.
3. Mastitis usually develops in both breasts of a breast-feeding client.
4. Symptoms include fever, chills, malaise, and localized breast tenderness.

15. 4. Mastitis is an infection of the breast characterized by flulike symptoms, along with redness and tenderness in the breast. The most common causative agent is *Staphylococcus aureus*. Breast abscess is rarely a complication of mastitis if the client continues to empty the affected breast. Mastitis usually occurs in one breast, not bilaterally.
CN: Physiological integrity; CNS: Physiological adaptation; CL: Application

16. Which measurement best describes delayed postpartum hemorrhage?
   1. Blood loss in excess of 300 ml, occurring 24 hours to 6 weeks after delivery
   2. Blood loss in excess of 500 ml, occurring 24 hours to 6 weeks after delivery
   3. Blood loss in excess of 800 ml, occurring 24 hours to 6 weeks after delivery
   4. Blood loss in excess of 1,000 ml, occurring 24 hours to 6 weeks after delivery

17. The nurse receives a report on a client who delivered a healthy neonate 1 hour ago. What data should she monitor during the <u>immediate</u> postpartum period (first 2 hours) of this client?
   1. Blood glucose level
   2. Electrocardiogram (ECG)
   3. Height of fundus
   4. Stool test for occult blood

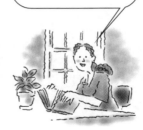

Remember: The question is asking for the most appropriate initial response.

18. When monitoring a postpartum client 2 hours after delivery, the nurse notices heavy bleeding with large clots. Which response is most appropriate <u>initially</u>?
   1. Massaging the fundus firmly
   2. Performing bimanual compressions
   3. Administering ergonovine (Ergotrate)
   4. Notifying the primary health care provider

Postpartum insulin requirements vary and are usually significantly different than prepregnancy requirements.

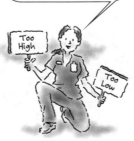

19. A nurse is about to give a client with type 2 diabetes insulin before breakfast on her first day postpartum. Which answer best describes insulin requirements immediately postpartum?
   1. Lower than during her pregnancy
   2. Higher than during her pregnancy
   3. Lower than before she became pregnant
   4. Higher than before she became pregnant

16. 2. Postpartum hemorrhage involves blood loss in excess of 500 ml. Most delayed postpartum hemorrhages occur between the fourth and ninth days postpartum. The most common causes of a delayed postpartum hemorrhage include retained placental fragments, intrauterine infection, and fibroids.
CN: Physiological integrity; CNS: Reduction of risk potential; CL: Knowledge

17. 3. A complete physical examination should be performed every 15 minutes for the first 1 to 2 hours postpartum, including determination of the fundus, lochia, perineum, blood pressure, pulse, and bladder function. A blood glucose level must be obtained only if the client has risk factors for an unstable blood glucose level or if she has symptoms of an altered blood glucose level. An ECG would be necessary only if the client is at risk for cardiac difficulty. A stool test for occult blood generally wouldn't be valid during the immediate postpartum period because it's difficult to sort out lochial bleeding from rectal bleeding.
CN: Health maintenance and promotion; CNS: None; CL: Analysis

18. 1. Initial management of excessive postpartum bleeding is firm massage of the fundus and administration of oxytocin (Pitocin). Bimanual compression is performed by a primary health care provider. Ergotrate should be used only if the bleeding doesn't respond to massage and oxytocin. The primary health care provider should be notified if the client doesn't respond to fundal massage, but other measures can be taken in the meantime.
CN: Physiological integrity; CNS: Physiological adaptation; CL: Analysis

19. 3. Postpartum insulin requirements are usually significantly lower than prepregnancy requirements. Occasionally, clients may require little to no insulin during the first 24 to 48 hours postpartum.
CN: Physiological integrity; CNS: Reduction of risk potential; CL: Knowledge

CN: Client needs category   CNS: Client needs subcategory   CL: Cognitive level

20. The nurse is caring for a 28-year-old client after the delivery of a healthy neonate. What would the nurse expect to find when assessing this client's fundus?
1. Fundus 1 cm above the umbilicus 1 hour postpartum
2. Fundus 1 cm above the umbilicus on postpartum day 3
3. Fundus palpable in the abdomen at 2 weeks postpartum
4. Fundus slightly to right; 2 cm above umbilicus on postpartum day 2

20. 1. Within the first 12 hours postpartum, the fundus is usually approximately 1 cm above the umbilicus. The fundus should be below the umbilicus by postpartum day 3. The fundus shouldn't be palpated in the abdomen after day 10. A uterus that isn't midline or is above the umbilicus on postpartum day 3 might be caused by a full, distended bladder or a uterine infection.
CN: Health promotion and maintenance; CNS: None; CL: Application

21. Which condition should the nurse look for in the client's history that may explain an increase in the severity of afterpains?
1. Bottle-feeding
2. Diabetes
3. Multiple gestation
4. Primiparity

21. 3. Multiple gestation, breast-feeding, multiparity, and conditions that cause overdistention of the uterus will increase the intensity of afterpains. Bottle-feeding and diabetes aren't directly associated with increasing severity of afterpains, unless the client has delivered a macrosomic neonate.
CN: Health promotion and maintenance; CNS: None; CL: Analysis

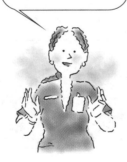

Question 22 is asking you to distinguish between heavy and excessive bleeding.

22. When giving a postpartum client self-care instructions, the nurse instructs her to report heavy or excessive bleeding. How should the nurse describe "heavy bleeding?"
1. Saturating 1 pad in 15 minutes
2. Saturating 1 pad in 1 hour
3. Saturating 1 pad in 4 to 6 hours
4. Saturating 1 pad in 8 hours

22. 2. Bleeding is considered heavy when a woman saturates 1 sanitary pad in 1 hour. Excessive bleeding occurs when a postpartum client saturates 1 pad in 15 minutes. Moderate bleeding occurs when the bleeding saturates less than 6″ (15 cm) of 1 pad in 1 hour.
CN: Health promotion and maintenance; CNS: None; CL: Application

23. The nurse is discharging a 34-year-old multiparous postpartum client 48 hours after a successful 16-hour vaginal delivery of an 8-lb, 14-oz (4,036-g) neonate. The nurse notes that the mother is rubella-immune with Rh-positive blood type. When formulating a discharge plan, the nurse should prioritize which objective first?
1. The client will receive Rh₀(D) immune globulin (RhoGAM) I.M. before discharge.
2. The client will understand the need for planned rest periods and identify a support system.
3. The client will understand and consent to a rubella vaccine before discharge.
4. The client will verbalize the importance of reporting any change in character of lochia.

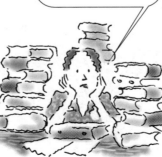

I can't remember why it's important for the client to report a change in lochia pattern.

23. 4. A multiparous client who has a history of prolonged labor and delivery of a large infant is at a higher risk for developing late postpartum hemorrhage. The nurse should ensure that the client understands the importance of reporting a change in lochia pattern, including increased amount, resumption of a brighter color, passage of clots, or foul odor. The client with Rh-positive blood doesn't require a RhoGAM injection. Postpartum hemorrhage instruction takes precedence over ensuring adequate rest. A client who is rubella-immune doesn't require immunization.
CN: Safe, effective care environment; CNS: Safety and infection control; CL: Analysis

CN: Client needs category   CNS: Client needs subcategory   CL: Cognitive level

24. A client and her neonate have a blood incompatibility, and the neonate has had a positive direct Coombs' test. Which nursing intervention is appropriate?
1. Because the client has been sensitized, give Rh_O(D) immune globulin (RhoGAM).
2. Because the client hasn't been sensitized, give RhoGAM.
3. Because the client has been sensitized, don't give RhoGAM.
4. Because the client hasn't been sensitized, don't give RhoGAM.

25. A client with a newly diagnosed puerperal infection asks the nurse to explain this condition. The nurse correctly defines the condition as which of the following?
1. An infection in the uterus of a postpartum client
2. An infection in the bladder of a postpartum client
3. An infection in the perineum of a postpartum client
4. An infection in the genital tract of a postpartum client

26. A nurse notes the progress note entry below and knows she must report the client's data because the client may be developing which condition?

Progress notes	
09/04/08 1030	Client is 5 hours post vaginal delivery with vacuum extraction. Fundus is firm; moderate lochia. VS: Temperature, 100.8° F (38.2° C) orally; heart rate, 10 beats/minute; respiratory rate, 22 breaths/minute; blood pressure, 110/78 mm Hg. _____ Barbara Smith L.V.N.

1. Urine retention
2. Pulmonary embolus
3. Shock from blood loss
4. Puerperal infection or endometritis

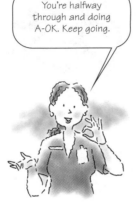

You're halfway through and doing A-OK. Keep going.

24. 3. A positive Coombs' test means that the Rh-negative client is now producing antibodies to the Rh-positive blood of the neonate. RhoGAM shouldn't be given to a sensitized client because it won't be able to prevent antibody formation.
CN: Physiological integrity; CNS: Reduction of risk potential; CL: Analysis

25. 4. A puerperal infection is an infection of the genital tract after delivery through the first 6 weeks postpartum. Endometritis is an infection of the mucous membrane or endometrium of the uterus. Cystitis is an infection of the bladder. Infection of the perineum or episiotomy site usually results in localized pain, low-grade fever, and redness and swelling at the wound edges.
CN: Physiological integrity; CNS: Reduction of risk potential; CL: Application

26. 4. The client's elevated temperature along with her prolonged labor and the instrumentalization associated with her delivery place her at risk for postpartum infection. Her temperature should be reported to the physician. At 5 hours postdelivery, the nurse wouldn't expect the client to have voided yet and wouldn't become concerned until after 8 hours had passed. Urine retention without infection wouldn't cause an elevation in temperature. The patient's respiratory rate is normal and there's no evidence to support pulmonary embolus. Shock from blood loss can be ruled out because the pulse rate is within normal limits and the firm fundus and moderate lochia are also normal.
CN: Psychosocial integrity; CNS: Reduction of risk potential; CL: Analysis

CN: Client needs category CNS: Client needs subcategory CL: Cognitive level

27. Which situation should concern the nurse treating a postpartum client within a few days of delivery?
1. The client is nervous about taking the baby home.
2. The client feels empty since she delivered the neonate.
3. The client would like to watch the nurse give the baby her first bath.
4. The client would like the nurse to take her baby to the nursery so she can sleep.

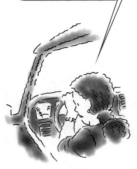

You need to be able to gauge the client's feelings of emptiness and respond appropriately. I should have done the same with my car.

28. A 30-year-old postpartum client has continuous seepage of blood from the vagina. Palpation of her uterus reveals a firm uterus, 1 cm below the umbilicus. A nurse who's aware of postpartum complications would monitor this client closely for which condition?
1. Retained placental fragments
2. Urinary tract infection
3. Cervical laceration
4. Uterine atony

29. A 29-year-old postpartum client is receiving anticoagulant therapy for deep venous thrombophlebitis. The nurse should include which instructions in her discharge teaching?
1. Avoid iron replacement therapy.
2. Avoid over-the-counter (OTC) salicylates.
3. Wear knee-high stockings when possible.
4. Shortness of breath is a common adverse effect of the medication.

30. TORCH is an acronym for maternal infections associated with congenital malformations and disorders. Which of the following disorders does the *H* represent?
1. Hemophilia
2. Hepatitis B virus
3. Herpes simplex virus
4. Human immunodeficiency virus

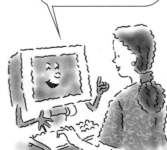

I hope you know what an acronym is. I don't, but I'm pretty sure it helps answer the question.

27. 2. A client experiencing postpartum blues may say she feels empty now that the infant is no longer in her uterus. She may also verbalize that she feels unprotected now. The other options are considered normal and wouldn't be cause for concern. Many first-time mothers are nervous about caring for their neonates by themselves after discharge. New mothers may want a demonstration before doing a task themselves. A client may want to get some uninterrupted sleep, so she may ask that the neonate be taken to the nursery.
CN: Psychosocial integrity; CNS: None; CL: Analysis

28. 3. Continuous seepage of blood may be due to cervical or vaginal lacerations if the uterus is firm and contracting. Retained placental fragments and uterine atony may cause subinvolution of the uterus, making it soft, boggy, and larger than expected. Urinary tract infection won't cause vaginal bleeding, although hematuria may be present.
CN: Physiological integrity; CNS: Reduction of risk potential; CL: Application

29. 2. Discharge teaching should include informing the client to avoid OTC salicylates, which may potentiate the effects of anticoagulant therapy. Iron won't affect anticoagulation therapy. Restrictive clothing should be avoided to prevent the recurrence of thrombophlebitis. Shortness of breath should be reported immediately because it may be a symptom of pulmonary embolism.
CN: Physiological integrity; CNS: Reduction of risk potential; CL: Application

30. 3. TORCH represents the following maternal infections: **t**oxoplasmosis; **o**thers, such as gonorrhea, syphilis, varicella, hepatitis, and human immunodeficiency virus; **r**ubella; **c**ytomegalovirus; and **h**erpes simplex virus. Hemophilia is a clotting disorder in which factors VII and X are deficient.
CN: Physiological integrity; CNS: Reduction of risk potential; CL: Knowledge

CN: Client needs category   CNS: Client needs subcategory   CL: Cognitive level

31. A 37-year-old client experienced a perinatal loss 3 days ago. The nurse, who's concerned about the possibility of <u>dysfunctional</u> grieving, should assess the client for which sign?
1. Lack of appetite
2. Denial of the death
3. Blaming herself
4. Frequent crying spells

32. Which condition in a postpartum client may cause fever not caused by infection?
1. Breast engorgement
2. Endometritis
3. Mastitis
4. Uterine involution

33. An Rh-positive client vaginally delivers a 6-lb, 10-oz neonate after 17 hours of labor. Which condition puts this client at risk for infection?
1. Length of labor
2. Maternal Rh status
3. Method of delivery
4. Size of the neonate

34. A client who gave birth by cesarean delivery 3 days ago is bottle-feeding her neonate. While collecting data the nurse notes that vital signs are stable, the fundus is four finger-breadths below the umbilicus, lochia are small and red, and the client complains of discomfort in her breasts, which are hard and warm to touch. The best nursing intervention based on this data would be:
1. encouraging the client to wear a supportive bra.
2. having the client stand facing in a warm shower.
3. informing the physician that the client is showing early signs of breast infection.
4. using a breast pump to facilitate removal of stagnant breast milk.

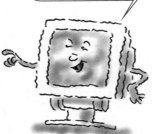

Don't deny that you know the answer to question 31.

31. 2. Denial of the perinatal loss is dysfunctional grieving in the client. Lack of appetite, blaming oneself, and frequent crying spells are part of a normal grieving process.
CN: Psychosocial integrity; CNS: None; CL: Analysis

32. 1. Breast engorgement and dehydration are noninfectious causes of postpartum fevers. Mastitis and endometritis are postpartum infections. Involution of the uterus won't cause temperature elevations.
CN: Health promotion and maintenance; CNS: None; CL: Knowledge

33. 1. A prolonged length of labor places the mother at increased risk for developing an infection. The average size of the neonate, vaginal delivery, and Rh status of the client don't place the mother at increased risk.
CN: Physiological integrity; CNS: Physiological adaptation; CL: Analysis

34. 1. These assessment findings are normal for the third postpartum day. Hard, warm breasts indicate engorgement, which occurs at about three days after birth. The client's vital signs are stable and don't indicate signs of infection. The client should be encouraged to wear a supportive bra which will help minimize engorgement and decrease nipple stimulation. Ice packs can reduce vasocongestion and relieve discomfort. Warm water and a breast pump will stimulate milk production.
CN: Physiological integrity; CNS: Basic care and comfort; CL: Application

CN: Client needs category   CNS: Client needs subcategory   CL: Cognitive level

35. What type of milk is present in the breasts 7 to 10 days postpartum?
1. Colostrum
2. Hind milk
3. Mature milk
4. Transitional milk

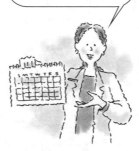

Timing is important in postpartum care.

35. 4. Transitional milk is present 7 to 10 days postpartum and lasts until 2 weeks postpartum. Colostrum is a thin, milky fluid released by the breasts before and up to a few days after parturition. Hind milk, which satisfies the neonate's hunger and promotes weight gain, arrives approximately 10 minutes after each feeding begins. Mature milk is white and thinner than transitional milk and arrives after 2 weeks postpartum.
CN: Health promotion and maintenance; CNS: None; CL: Knowledge

36. Which recommendation should be given to a client with mastitis who's concerned about breast-feeding her neonate?
1. She should stop breast-feeding until completing the antibiotic.
2. She should supplement feeding with formula until the infection resolves.
3. She shouldn't use analgesics because they aren't compatible with breast-feeding.
4. She should continue to breast-feed; mastitis won't infect the neonate.

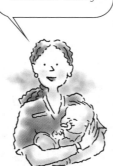

Mastitis shouldn't interfere with breast-feeding.

36. 4. The client with mastitis should be encouraged to continue breast-feeding while taking antibiotics for the infection. No supplemental feedings are necessary because breast-feeding doesn't need to be altered and actually encourages resolution of the infection. Analgesics are safe and should be administered as needed.
CN: Health promotion and maintenance; CNS: None; CL: Analysis

37. A client who had an emergency cesarean birth for fetal distress 3 days ago is preparing for discharge. When reviewing the home care instructions with the nurse, the client reveals she is saddened about her cesarean and feels let down that she wasn't able to have a vaginal delivery. When questioned further, the client states she feels "weepy about everything" and can't stop crying. What nursing action is indicated first?
1. Contact the physician to report the client's deteriorating mental status.
2. Discuss the client's potential depression with her family members.
3. Ask the client to elaborate on her feelings.
4. Document the conversation.

37. 3. The client's affect is consistent with postpartum blues, a transient source of sadness experienced during the first week after delivery. The nurse should offer support to the client and encourage her to discuss her concerns and feelings. The client's emotional state is normal and contacting the physician isn't indicated. Discussing the client's feelings with family members is a violation of confidentiality and isn't an appropriate action. Documenting the interaction is indicated but should take place after the encounter is completed.
CN: Psychosocial integrity; CNS: None; CL: Analysis

38. In which time period would the nurse most likely expect a client who has delivered twins to experience late postpartum hemorrhage?
1. 24 to 48 hours after delivery
2. 24 hours to 6 weeks after delivery
3. 6 weeks to 3 months after delivery
4. 6 weeks to 6 months after delivery

38. 2. Late or secondary postpartum hemorrhages occur more than 24 hours but less than 6 weeks postpartum. Early or primary postpartum hemorrhages occur within 24 hours of delivery.
CN: Physiological integrity; CNS: Reduction of risk potential; CL: Knowledge

CN: Client needs category   CNS: Client needs subcategory   CL: Cognitive level

39. Which complication is most likely responsible for a <u>late</u> postpartum hemorrhage?
  1. Cervical laceration
  2. Clotting deficiency
  3. Perineal laceration
  4. Uterine subinvolution

39. 4. Late postpartum bleeding is usually the result of subinvolution of the uterus. Retained products of conception or infection commonly cause subinvolution. Cervical or perineal lacerations can cause an immediate postpartum hemorrhage. A client with a clotting deficiency may have an immediate postpartum hemorrhage if the deficiency isn't corrected at the time of delivery.
CN: Physiological integrity; CNS: Physiological adaptation; CL: Knowledge

40. A client who gave birth vaginally 16 hours ago states she doesn't need to void at this time. The nurse reviews the documentation and finds that the client hasn't voided for 7 hours. Which response by the nurse is indicated?
  1. "If you don't attempt to void, I'll need to catheterize you."
  2. "It's not uncommon after delivery for you to have a full bladder even though you can't sense the fullness."
  3. "I'll contact your physician."
  4. "I'll check on you in a few hours."

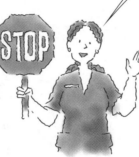

Make sure the client understands the necessary facts about the rubella vaccine.

40. 2. After a vaginal delivery, the client should be encouraged to void every 4 to 6 hours. As a result of anesthesia and trauma, the client may be unable to sense the filling bladder. It's premature to catheterize the client without allowing her to attempt to void first. There's no need to contact the physician at this time as the client is demonstrating common adaptations in the early postpartum period. Allowing the client's bladder to fill for another 2 to 3 hours might cause overdistention.
CN: Physiological integrity; CNS: Physiological adaptation; CL: Analysis

41. A nurse is reinforcing discharge teaching with a postpartum client who isn't immune to rubella. Which statement by the client indicates the need for further teaching?
  1. "I can continue to breast-feed my baby after taking the rubella vaccine."
  2. "There may be some soreness or tenderness at the injection site for a few days."
  3. "The immunization will be given at my 6-week postpartum examination."
  4. "Although I've had a tubal ligation, the rubella vaccine will still be needed."

41. 3. The rubella vaccine is administered at the time of discharge. It's safe for both bottle- and breast-feeding mothers. The medication is given as an intramuscular injection; there may be some localized tenderness, which will subside. To promote community health and wellness, the vaccine is administered to women who've had a tubal ligation.
CN: Health promotion and maintenance; CNS: None; CL: Analysis

42. A nurse has just received a client from the surgical suite following a cesarean birth. The report given reveals the client has received magnesium sulfate for management of gestational hypertension just before the emergency surgery. The nurse should monitor the client for adverse effects from the magnesium sulfate by checking which parameter?
  1. Consistency of the fundus
  2. Heart rate
  3. Homans' sign
  4. Gag reflex

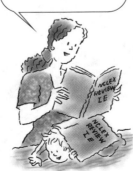

Magnesium sulfate. Magnesium sulfate. I know it's here somewhere.

42. 1. Magnesium sulfate has properties that act as a smooth-muscle relaxant; therefore, the uterus may fail to adequately contract after administration. Failure of the uterus to contract may result in excessive blood loss. The heart rate, Homans' sign, and gag reflex aren't affected by the administration of magnesium sulfate.
CN: Physiological integrity; CNS: Pharmacological therapies; CL: Application

CN: Client needs category   CNS: Client needs subcategory   CL: Cognitive level

43. A physician has prescribed magnesium sulfate for a client with premature labor. Data collection reveals the client's respiratory rate is 12 breaths/minute, and urine output is 30 ml/hour. The magnesium sulfate serum levels are 7 mg/dl. When questioned, the client reports feeling warm and flushed. Based upon the nurse's understanding of magnesium sulfate, what action is most appropriate?
1. The client is demonstrating early signs of toxicity and the dosage should be reduced.
2. The client is demonstrating an allergic reaction and the medication should be discontinued immediately.
3. The client's response is appropriate and within normal limits; therefore, no action is necessary.
4. The client is demonstrating potential complications and the physician should be notified.

44. Which change best describes the insulin needs of a client with type 1 diabetes mellitus who has just delivered an infant vaginally without complications?
1. Increased
2. Decreased
3. The same as before pregnancy
4. The same as during pregnancy

45. Which response is most appropriate for a client with diabetes who wants to breast-feed but is concerned about the effects of breast-feeding on her health?
1. Diabetic clients who breast-feed have a hard time controlling their insulin needs.
2. Diabetic clients shouldn't breast-feed because of potential complications.
3. Diabetic clients shouldn't breast-feed; insulin requirements are doubled.
4. Diabetic clients may breast-feed; insulin requirements may decrease from breast-feeding.

43. 3. Magnesium sulfate is associated with feelings of warmth and flushing; these symptoms do not indicate toxicity or allergic reaction. Respirations of 12 breaths/minute are considered normal. Urine output should be at least 30 ml/hour. Serum levels of magnesium sulfate should be between 4 and 8 mg/dl to promote a therapeutic response.
CN: Physiological integrity; CNS: Pharmacological therapies; CL: Analysis

44. 2. The placenta produces the hormone human placental lactogen, an insulin antagonist. After birth, the placenta, the major source of insulin resistance, is gone. Insulin needs decrease, and women with type 1 diabetes may need only one-half to two-thirds of the prenatal insulin dose during the first few postpartum days. Blood glucose levels should be monitored and insulin dosages adjusted as needed. The client should be encouraged to maintain appropriate dietary schedules, even if her infant is feeding on demand.
CN: Physiological integrity; CNS: Physiological adaptation; CL: Application

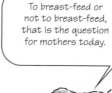

To breast-feed or not to breast-feed, that is the question for mothers today.

45. 4. Breast-feeding has an antidiabetic effect. Insulin needs are decreased because carbohydrates are used in milk production. Breast-feeding clients are at a higher risk for hypoglycemia in the first postpartum days after birth because glucose levels are lower. Diabetic clients should be encouraged to breast-feed.
CN: Physiological integrity; CNS: Pharmacological therapies; CL: Comprehension

CN: Client needs category   CNS: Client needs subcategory   CL: Cognitive level

46. A clinical pathway is being used to coordinate care for a postpartum client who had an uncomplicated vaginal delivery of an 8-lb, 2-oz (3,693-g) neonate over an intact perineum 24 hours ago. While planning care for this client, the registered nurse collaborates with the licensed practical nurse to achieve which priority outcome in the next 8 hours?
1. Encouraging high fiber foods to achieve a soft bowel movement
2. Encouraging the client to demonstrate an ability to breast-feed the neonate
3. Administering a rubella vaccination if the client isn't immune.
4. Completing an initial sitz bath

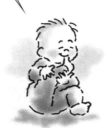

I sure hope you taught my mom what to do for me.

46. 2. With an uncomplicated vaginal birth, the average client will be hospitalized for 48 hours or less. By 24 hours postpartum, it's important for the client to start demonstrating the ability to care for her neonate. The first bowel movement occurs on average 2 to 3 days postpartum. The rubella vaccine is given, when indicated, on the day of discharge. This client delivered over an intact perineum, and although a sitz bath can provide comfort, it isn't a priority.
CN: Safe, effective care environment; CNS: Coordinated care; CL: Analysis

47. Which factor puts a multiparous client on her first postpartum day at risk for developing hemorrhage?
1. Hemoglobin level of 12 g/dl
2. Uterine atony
3. Thrombophlebitis
4. Moderate amount of lochia rubra

47. 2. Multiparous women typically experience a loss of uterine tone due to frequent distentions of the uterus from previous pregnancies. As a result, this client is also at higher risk for hemorrhage. Thrombophlebitis doesn't increase the risk of hemorrhage during the postpartum period. The hemoglobin level and lochia flow are within acceptable limits.
CN: Health promotion and maintenance; CNS: None; CL: Analysis

48. On the first postpartum night, a client requests that her neonate be sent back to the nursery so she can get some sleep. The client is most likely in which phase?
1. Depression phase
2. Letting-go phase
3. Taking-hold phase
4. Taking-in phase

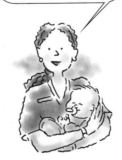

Always consider the needs of the client and the neonate when providing postpartum care.

48. 4. The taking-in phase occurs in the first 24 hours after birth. The client is concerned with her own needs and requires support from staff and relatives. The taking-hold phase occurs when the client is ready to take responsibility for her care as well as her neonate's care. The letting-go phase begins several weeks later, when the client incorporates the new infant into the family unit. The depression phase isn't an appropriate answer.
CN: Health promotion and maintenance; CNS: None; CL: Analysis

49. The nurse is performing a postpartum check on a 40-year-old client. Which nursing measure is appropriate?
1. Place the client in a supine position with her arms overhead for the examination of her breasts and fundus.
2. Instruct the client to empty her bladder before the examination.
3. Wear sterile gloves when assessing the pad and perineum.
4. Perform the examination as quickly as possible.

49. 2. An empty bladder facilitates the examination of the fundus. The client should be in a supine position with her arms at her sides and her knees bent. The arms-overhead position is unnecessary. Clean gloves should be used when assessing the perineum; sterile gloves aren't necessary. The postpartum examination shouldn't be done quickly. The nurse can take this time to teach the client about the changes in her body after delivery.
CN: Health promotion and maintenance; CNS: None; CL: Application

CN: Client needs category   CNS: Client needs subcategory   CL: Cognitive level

50. On examining a client who gave birth 3 hours ago, the nurse finds that the client has completely saturated a perineal pad within 15 minutes. Which actions should the nurse take? Select all that apply:

1. Begin an I.V. infusion of lactated Ringer's solution.
2. Assess the client's vital signs.
3. Palpate the client's fundus.
4. Place the client in high Fowler's position.
5. Administer a pain medication.

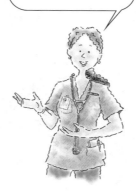

Think about what would make the client most comfortable.

50. 2, 3. Assessing vital signs provides information about the client's circulatory status and identifies significant changes to report to the physician. By palpating the client's fundus, the nurse also gains valuable assessment data. A boggy uterus may lead to excessive bleeding. Starting an I.V. infusion requires a physician's order. Placing the client in high Fowler's position may lower blood pressure and be harmful to the client. Administration of a pain medication doesn't address the current problem.
CN: Physiological integrity; CNS: Reduction of risk potential; CL: Application

51. The nurse observes several interactions between a mother and her new son. Which behaviors by the mother would the nurse identify as evidence of mother-infant attachment? Select all that apply:

1. Talks and coos to her son
2. Cuddles her son close to her
3. Doesn't make eye contact with her son
4. Requests the nurse to take the baby to the nursery for feedings
5. Encourages the father to hold the baby
6. Takes a nap when the baby is sleeping

51. 1, 2. Talking to, cooing to, and cuddling with her son are positive signs that the mother is adapting to her new role. Avoiding eye contact is a sign that the mother isn't bonding with her baby. Eye contact, touching, and speaking are important to establish attachment with an infant. Feeding a neonate is an important role of a new mother and facilitates attachment. Encouraging the dad to hold the baby facilitates attachment between the neonate and the father. Resting while the infant is sleeping conserves needed energy and allows the mother to be alert and awake when her infant is awake; however, it isn't evidence of bonding.
CN: Psychosocial integrity; CNS: None; CL: Analysis

52. The nurse is assisting in developing a care plan for a client who had an episiotomy. Which interventions would be included for the nursing diagnosis *Acute pain related to perineal sutures?* Select all that apply:

1. Apply an ice pack intermittently to the perineal area for 3 days.
2. Avoid the use of topical pain gels.
3. Administer sitz baths three to four times per day.
4. Encourage the client to do Kegel exercises.
5. Limit the number of times the perineal pad is changed.

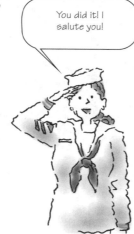

You did it! I salute you!

52. 3, 4. Sitz baths help decrease inflammation and tension in the perineal area. Kegel exercises improve circulation to the area and help reduce edema. Ice packs should be applied to the perineum for the first 24 hours only; after that time, heat should be used. Topical pain gels should be applied to the suture area to reduce discomfort, as ordered. The perineal pad should be changed frequently to prevent irritation caused by the discharge.
CN: Physiological integrity; CNS: Basic care and comfort; CL: Application

CN: Client needs category   CNS: Client needs subcategory   CL: Cognitive level

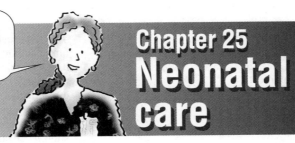

1. The use of breast milk for premature neonates helps prevent which condition?
1. Down syndrome
2. Hyaline membrane disease
3. Necrotizing enterocolitis
4. Turner's syndrome

2. A client asks the nurse what *surfactant* is. Which explanation would the nurse give as the <u>main role</u> of surfactant in the neonate?
1. Assists with ciliary body maturation in the upper airways
2. Helps maintain a rhythmic breathing pattern
3. Promotes clearing of mucus from the respiratory tract
4. Helps the lungs remain expanded after the initiation of breathing

3. The nurse observes that a 2-hour-old neonate has acrocyanosis. Which nursing action should be performed <u>immediately</u>?
1. Activate the code blue or emergency system.
2. Do nothing because acrocyanosis is normal in a neonate.
3. Immediately take the neonate's temperature according to facility policy.
4. Notify the physician of the need for genetic counseling.

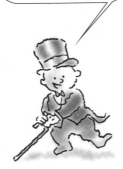

1. 3. Components specific to breast milk have been shown to lower the incidence of necrotizing enterocolitis in premature neonates. Hyaline membrane disease isn't directly influenced by breast milk or breast-feeding. Down syndrome and Turner's syndrome are genetic defects and aren't influenced by breast milk.
CN: Health promotion and maintenance; CNS: None; CL: Application

2. 4. Surfactant works by reducing surface tension in the lung, which allows the lung to remain slightly expanded, decreasing the amount of work required for inspiration. Surfactant hasn't been shown to influence ciliary body maturation, clearing of the respiratory tract, or regulation of the neonate's breathing pattern.
CN: Health promotion and maintenance; CNS: None; CL: Comprehension

3. 2. Acrocyanosis, or bluish discoloration of the hands and feet in the neonate (also called *peripheral cyanosis*), is a normal finding and shouldn't last more than 24 hours after birth. The other choices are inappropriate.
CN: Physiological integrity; CNS: Physiological adaptation; CL: Application

4. The nurse is caring for a neonate. Which is the <u>most</u> important step the nurse can take to prevent and control infection?
    1. Check frequently for signs of infection.
    2. Use sterile technique for all caregiving.
    3. Practice meticulous hand washing.
    4. Wear gloves at all times.

5. A woman with diabetes has just given birth. While caring for this neonate, the nurse is aware that he's <u>at risk</u> for which complication?
    1. Anemia
    2. Hypoglycemia
    3. Nitrogen loss
    4. Thrombosis

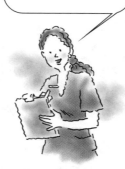

> Knowing your risk factors can help guide your data collection...

6. The nurse should be alert for which complication in neonates who receive prolonged mechanical ventilation following birth?
    1. Bronchopulmonary dysplasia
    2. Esophageal atresia
    3. Hydrocephalus
    4. Renal failure

7. Which finding indicates adequate hydration in a neonate?
    1. Soft, smooth skin
    2. A sunken fontanel
    3. Frequent spitting up
    4. No urine output in the first 24 hours of life

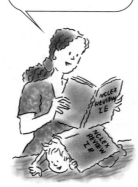

> ...knowing normal signs of development is also important.

4. 3. To prevent and control infection, the nurse should practice meticulous hand washing, scrubbing for 3 minutes before entering the nursery, washing frequently during caregiving activities, and scrubbing for 1 minute after providing care. Checking for signs of infection can detect, not *prevent,* infection. The nurse should use sterile technique for invasive procedures, not all caregiving. The nurse should wear gloves whenever contact with blood or body fluids is possible.
CN: Safe, effective care environment; CNS: Safety and infection control; CL: Comprehension

5. 2. Neonates of mothers with diabetes are at risk for hypoglycemia due to increased insulin levels. During gestation, an increased amount of glucose is transferred to the fetus through the placenta. The neonate's liver can't initially adjust to the changing glucose levels after birth. This inability may result in an overabundance of insulin in the neonate, causing hypoglycemia. Neonates of mothers with diabetes aren't at increased risk for anemia, nitrogen loss, or thrombosis.
CN: Physiological integrity; CNS: Reduction of risk potential; CL: Comprehension

6. 1. Bronchopulmonary dysplasia commonly results from the high pressures that must sometimes be used to maintain adequate oxygenation. Esophageal atresia, a structural defect in which the esophagus and trachea communicate with each other, doesn't relate to mechanical ventilation. Hydrocephalus and renal failure don't typically occur in these clients.
CN: Physiological integrity; CNS: Reduction of risk potential; CL: Analysis

7. 1. Soft, smooth skin is a sign of adequate hydration. A sunken fontanel and no urine output in the first 24 hours of life are signs of poor hydration. In the case of no urine output, kidney dysfunction would also be a concern. Frequent spitting up is normal in neonates. Excessive spitting up, however, may result in poor hydration.
CN: Physiological integrity; CNS: Physiological adaptation; CL: Analysis

CN: Client needs category   CNS: Client needs subcategory   CL: Cognitive level

8. Which sign is considered <u>normal</u> in a neonate?

　1. Doll eyes
　2. "Sunset" eyes
　3. Positive Babinski's sign
　4. Pupils that don't react to light

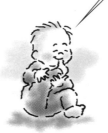

Question 8 asks what is considered normal in a neonate.

9. Which technique is <u>best</u> when bathing a 5-hour-old girl?

　1. Place her on a table covered with blankets, and give her a sponge bath.
　2. Bathe her in a tub of warm water.
　3. Keep her under a radiant warmer, and give her a sponge bath.
　4. Wash only her hands and head because her condition isn't stable enough for her to have a complete bath.

10. A mother asks the nurse why her neonate is getting an injection. The nurse answers that the neonate is receiving an injection of vitamin K. Which action of vitamin K explains why the drug is given to neonates?

　1. Assists with coagulation
　2. Assists the gut to mature
　3. Initiates the immunization process
　4. Protects the brain from excess fluid production

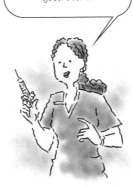

This can help the neonate get off to a good start.

8. 3. A positive Babinski's sign is present in infants until approximately age 1 and is normal in neonates, though abnormal in adults. Doll eyes is also a neurologic response but is noted in adults. The appearance of "sunset" eyes, in which the sclera is visible above the iris, results from cranial nerve palsies and may indicate increased intracranial pressure. A neonate's pupils normally react to light as an adult's would.

CN: Physiological integrity; CNS: Physiological adaptation; CL: Analysis

9. 3. During the first several hours after delivery, a neonate's thermal regulatory system is adapting to extrauterine life. When bathing a neonate under a radiant warmer, the external heat decreases the chances for cold stress by decreasing the number of internal mechanisms the neonate must use to stay warm. Bathing a neonate on a table, where she's exposed to air drafts and cooler air currents, can set her up for cold stress. Bathing the neonate in a tub and then removing her increases her heat loss and metabolism. Washing only the hands and head would chill the neonate and reduce thermoregulation because most heat is lost through the head.

CN: Physiological integrity; CNS: Physiological adaptation; CL: Application

10. 1. Vitamin K, deficient in the neonate, is needed to activate clotting factors II, VII, IX, and X. In the event of trauma, the neonate would be at risk for excessive bleeding. Vitamin K doesn't assist the gut to mature, but the gut produces vitamin K after maturity is achieved. Vitamin K doesn't influence fluid production in the brain or the immunization process.

CN: Physiological integrity; CNS: Reduction of risk potential; CL: Application

CN: Client needs category   CNS: Client needs subcategory   CL: Cognitive level

11. The nurse is caring for a neonate whose mother is infected with hepatitis B. The nurse should inform the mother that her son will receive which treatment?
1. Hepatitis B vaccine at birth and age 1 month
2. Hepatitis B immune globulin at birth; no hepatitis B vaccine
3. Hepatitis B immune globulin within 48 hours of birth and hepatitis B vaccine at age 1 month
4. Hepatitis B immune globulin within 12 hours of birth and hepatitis B vaccine at birth, age 1 month, and age 6 months

11. 4. Hepatitis B immune globulin should be given as soon as possible after birth but within 12 hours. Neonates should also receive hepatitis B vaccine at regularly scheduled intervals. This sequence of care has been determined as superior to the other options provided.
CN: Health promotion and maintenance; CNS: None; CL: Analysis

12. When a neonate is delivered with meconium staining in the amniotic fluid, which sequence of actions will <u>most</u> effectively decrease the risk of meconium aspiration?
1. Deliver the thorax; then suction the neonate's mouth.
2. Clamp the umbilical cord; then suction the mouth.
3. Deliver the head; then suction the mouth and then the nose.
4. Deliver the thorax; then suction the nose and then the mouth.

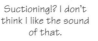

Suctioning!? I don't think I like the sound of that.

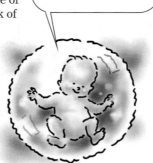

12. 3. To minimize the risk of meconium aspiration after delivery, the neonate's mouth, then nose, should be suctioned after delivery of the head. This suctioning shouldn't be delayed until after delivery of the thorax because the neonate will take its first breath with meconium in its mouth.
CN: Physiological integrity; CNS: Reduction of risk potential; CL: Analysis

13. Erythromycin ointment is administered to the neonate's eyes shortly after birth to prevent which disorder?
1. Cataracts
2. Diabetic retinopathy
3. Ophthalmia neonatorum
4. Strabismus

13. 3. Eye prophylaxis is administered to the neonate immediately or soon after birth to prevent ophthalmia neonatorum (conjunctivitis contracted during birth from passage through the birth canal). Cataracts are opacities of the lens of the eye in children with congenital rubella, galactosemia, or cortisone therapy. Diabetic retinopathy occurs in clients with diabetes when the retina bleeds into the vitreous humor causing scarring, after which neovascularization occurs. Strabismus is neuromuscular incoordination of the eye alignment.
CN: Health promotion and maintenance; CNS: None; CL: Comprehension

This question is looking for the major sign.

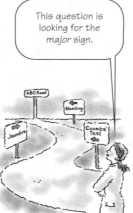

14. A client with group AB blood whose husband has group O blood has just given birth. Which complication or test result is a major sign of ABO blood incompatibility that the nurse should look for when assessing this neonate?
1. Negative Coombs' test
2. Bleeding from the nose or ear
3. Jaundice after the first 24 hours of life
4. Jaundice within the first 24 hours of life

14. 4. The neonate with an ABO blood incompatibility with its mother will have jaundice within the first 24 hours of life. The neonate would have a positive Coombs' test result. Jaundice after the first 24 hours of life is physiologic jaundice. Bleeding from the nose and ear should be investigated for possible causes but probably isn't related to ABO incompatibility.
CN: Health promotion and maintenance; CNS: None; CL: Analysis

CN: Client needs category   CNS: Client needs subcategory   CL: Cognitive level

15. Which condition of delivery would predispose a neonate to respiratory distress syndrome (RDS)?
1. Premature birth
2. Vaginal delivery
3. First born of twins
4. Postdate pregnancy

16. When caring for a male neonate on the day after he was circumcised, the nurse notices yellow-white exudate around the procedure site. What should the nurse do first?
1. Try to remove the exudate with a warm washcloth.
2. Take the neonate's temperature to check for infection.
3. Leave the area alone because it's part of the normal healing process.
4. Call the physician and notify him of the infection.

17. A client has just given birth at 42 weeks' gestation. What would the nurse expect to find during her assessment of the neonate?
1. A sleepy, lethargic neonate
2. Lanugo covering the neonate's body
3. Desquamation of the neonate's epidermis
4. Vernix caseosa covering the neonate's body

18. The small-for-gestation neonate is at increased risk for which complication during the transitional period?
1. Anemia probably due to chronic fetal hypoxia
2. Hyperthermia due to decreased glycogen stores
3. Hyperglycemia due to decreased glycogen stores
4. Polycythemia probably due to chronic fetal hypoxia

19. Which finding might be seen in a neonate suspected of having an infection?
1. Flushed cheeks
2. Increased temperature
3. Decreased temperature
4. Increased activity level

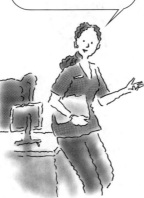

The color of an exudate helps determine its cause.

15. 1. Prematurity is the single most important risk factor for developing RDS. The second born of twins and neonates born by cesarean delivery are also at increased risk for RDS. Surfactant deficiency, which commonly results in RDS, isn't a problem for postdate neonates.
CN: Physiological integrity; CNS: Reduction of risk potential; CL: Analysis

16. 3. The yellow-white exudate is part of the granulating process. It isn't a sign of infection and shouldn't be removed. Explain to the parents that this exudate will disappear as the site heals.
CN: Health promotion and maintenance; CNS: None; CL: Application

17. 3. Postdate neonates lose the vernix caseosa, and the epidermis may become desquamated. A neonate at 42 weeks' gestation is usually very alert and missing lanugo.
CN: Health promotion and maintenance; CNS: None; CL: Analysis

18. 4. The small-for-gestation neonate is at risk for developing polycythemia during the transitional period in an attempt to decrease hypoxia. This neonate is also at increased risk for developing hypoglycemia and hypothermia due to decreased glycogen stores.
CN: Health promotion and maintenance; CNS: None; CL: Analysis

19. 3. A decreased temperature in the neonate may be a sign of infection. The neonate's color commonly changes with an infectious process but generally becomes ashen or mottled. The neonate with an infection will usually show a decrease in activity level or lethargy.
CN: Health promotion and maintenance; CNS: None; CL: Analysis

CN: Client needs category   CNS: Client needs subcategory   CL: Cognitive level

20. Which symptom would indicate the neonate was adapting <u>normally</u> to extrauterine life without difficulty?
1. Nasal flaring
2. Light, audible grunting
3. Respiratory rate of 40 to 60 breaths/minute
4. Respiratory rate of 60 to 80 breaths/minute

21. After reviewing the client's maternal history of receiving magnesium sulfate during labor, which condition should the nurse anticipate as a potential problem in the neonate?
1. Hypoglycemia
2. Twitching
3. Respiratory depression
4. Tachycardia

22. Which intervention is helpful for the neonate experiencing drug withdrawal?
1. Place the Isolette in a quiet area of the nursery.
2. Withhold all medication to help the liver metabolize drugs.
3. Dress the neonate in loose clothing so he won't feel restricted.
4. Place the Isolette near the nurses' station for frequent contact with health care workers.

23. While caring for a neonate of a diabetic mother, the nurse should monitor the neonate for which complication?
1. Atelectasis
2. Microcephaly
3. Pneumothorax
4. Macrosomia

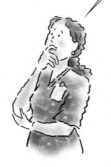

Which answer indicates a normal response?

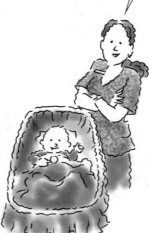

Some neonates need special interventions.

20. 3. A respiratory rate of 40 to 60 breaths/minute is normal for a neonate during the transitional period. Nasal flaring, respiratory rate of more than 60 breaths/minute, and audible grunting are signs of respiratory distress.
CN: Health promotion and maintenance; CNS: None; CL: Analysis

21. 3. Magnesium sulfate crosses the placenta, and adverse neonatal effects include respiratory depression, hypotonia, and bradycardia. The serum blood glucose level isn't affected by magnesium sulfate. The neonate would be floppy, not twitching.
CN: Physiological integrity; CNS: Pharmacological therapies; CL: Analysis

22. 1. Neonates experiencing drug withdrawal commonly have sleep disturbance. The neonate should be moved to a quiet area of the nursery to minimize environmental stimuli. Medications, such as phenobarbital and paregoric, should be given as needed. The neonate should be swaddled to prevent him from flailing and stimulating himself.
CN: Psychosocial integrity; CNS: None; CL: Analysis

23. 4. Neonates of diabetic mothers are at increased risk for macrosomia (excessive fetal growth) due to the increased supply of maternal glucose combined with an increase in fetal insulin. Along with macrosomia, neonates of diabetic mothers are at risk for respiratory distress syndrome, hypoglycemia, hypocalcemia, hyperbilirubinemia, and congenital anomalies. They aren't at greater risk for atelectasis or pneumothorax. Microcephaly is usually the result of cytomegalovirus or rubella virus infection.
CN: Health promotion and maintenance; CNS: None; CL: Application

24. A neonate is diagnosed with hemorrhagic disease. Which medication should have been administered as a preventative measure?
1. Vitamin K
2. Heparin
3. Iron
4. Warfarin

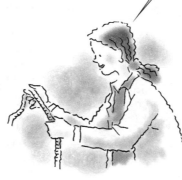

Which measure is preventive, rather than curative or restorative?

24. 1. Neonates have coagulation deficiencies because of a lack of vitamin K in the intestines, which helps the liver synthesize clotting factors II, VII, IX, and X. Heparin and warfarin are given as anticoagulant therapy, not to prevent hemorrhagic disease in the neonate. Iron is stored in the fetal liver; hemoglobin binds to iron and carries oxygen.
CN: Health promotion and maintenance; CNS: None; CL: Application

25. During the transition period, a neonate can lose heat in many different ways. A neonate who isn't completely dried immediately after birth or a bath loses heat through which method?
1. Conduction
2. Convection
3. Evaporation
4. Radiation

25. 3. Evaporation is the loss of heat that occurs when a liquid is converted to a vapor. In the neonate, heat loss by evaporation occurs as a result of vaporization of moisture from the skin. Convection is the flow of heat from the body surface to cooler air. Conduction is the loss of heat from the body surface to cooler surfaces in direct contact. Radiation is the loss of heat to a cooler surface that isn't in direct contact with the neonate.
CN: Health promotion and maintenance; CNS: None; CL: Knowledge

26. By keeping the nursery temperature warm and wrapping the neonate in blankets, the nurse is preventing which type of heat loss?
1. Conduction
2. Convection
3. Evaporation
4. Radiation

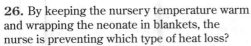

DO NOT DISTURB

26. 2. Convection heat loss is the flow of heat from the body surface to cooler air. Conduction is the loss of heat from the body surface to cooler surfaces in direct contact. Evaporation is the loss of heat that occurs when a liquid is converted to a vapor. Radiation is the loss of heat from the body surface to cooler solid surfaces not in direct contact but in relative proximity.
CN: Health promotion and maintenance; CNS: None; CL: Knowledge

27. A nurse is caring for a neonate and observes jaundice from physiologic hyperbilirubinemia. Which statement about this disorder is true?
1. The neonate usually also has a medical problem.
2. In full-term neonates, it usually appears after 24 hours.
3. It results in unusually elevated conjugated bilirubin levels.
4. It's usually progressive from the neonate's feet to his head.

27. 2. Physiologic hyperbilirubinemia, or jaundice, in full-term neonates first appears after 24 hours. Neonates with this condition are otherwise healthy and have no medical problems. Hyperbilirubinemia is caused almost exclusively by unconjugated bilirubin. Jaundice usually appears in a cephalocaudal progression from head to feet.
CN: Physiological integrity; CNS: Reduction of risk potential; CL: Application

28. A neonate has been diagnosed with caput succedaneum. What information should the nurse include while teaching the mother about caput succedaneum?
1. It usually resolves in 3 to 6 weeks.
2. It doesn't cross the cranial suture line.
3. It's a collection of blood between the skull and the periosteum.
4. It involves swelling of the tissue over the presenting part of the fetal scalp.

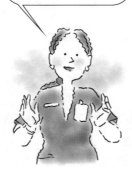

When you're teaching a new mom, it helps to know what to expect at each stage in a neonate's development!

29. The nurse teaches a postpartum client that her neonate's first stool will be meconium, which consists of intestinal secretions and cells. Which colors and consistencies should the nurse use to <u>best</u> describe the typical appearance of meconium?
1. Soft, pale yellow
2. Hard, pale brown
3. Sticky, greenish black
4. Loose, golden yellow

30. A 3-day-old neonate needs phototherapy for hyperbilirubinemia. Nursery care of a neonate receiving phototherapy includes which treatment?
1. Tube feedings
2. Mask over the mouth
3. Eye patches to prevent retinal damage
4. Temperature monitored every 6 hours during phototherapy

31. The nurse should carefully monitor which neonate for hyperbilirubinemia?
1. Black neonate
2. Neonate of an Rh-positive mother
3. Neonate with ABO incompatibility
4. Neonate with Apgar scores 9 and 10 at 1 and 5 minutes

28. 4. Caput succedaneum is the swelling of tissue over the presenting part of the fetal scalp due to sustained pressure. This boggy, edematous swelling is present at birth, crosses the suture line, and most commonly occurs in the occipital area. A cephalhematoma is a collection of blood between the skull and periosteum, doesn't cross cranial suture lines, and resolves in 3 to 6 weeks. Caput succedaneum resolves within 3 to 4 days.
CN: Physiological integrity; CNS: Reduction of risk potential; CL: Application

29. 3. Meconium collects in the GI tract during gestation and is initially sterile. Meconium is greenish black because of occult blood and is viscous. The stools of formula-fed babies are typically soft and pale yellow after feeding is well established. The stools of breast-fed neonates are loose and golden yellow after the transition to extrauterine life.
CN: Health promotion and maintenance; CNS: None; CL: Application

30. 3. The neonate's eyes must be covered with eye patches to prevent damage. The neonate can be removed from the lights and held for feeding. The mouth of the neonate doesn't need to be covered during phototherapy. The neonate's temperature should be monitored at least every 2 to 4 hours because of the risk of hyperthermia with phototherapy.
CN: Physiological integrity; CNS: Physiological adaptation; CL: Analysis

31. 3. The mother's blood type, which is different from the neonate's, has an impact on the neonate's bilirubin level due to the antigen-antibody reaction. Black neonates tend to have lower mean levels of bilirubin. Chinese, Japanese, Korean, and Greek neonates tend to have higher incidences of hyperbilirubinemia. Neonates of Rh-negative, not Rh-positive, mothers tend to have hyperbilirubinemia. Low Apgar scores may indicate a risk for hyperbilirubinemia.
CN: Physiological integrity; CNS: Physiological adaptation; CL: Analysis

32. A neonate has developed a major infection. Which gram-positive bacteria most likely contributed to this problem?
1. *Escherichia coli*
2. Group B streptococci
3. *Klebsiella* species
4. *Pseudomonas aeruginosa*

33. The <u>most common</u> neonatal sepsis and meningitis infections seen within 24 hours after birth are caused by which organism?
1. *Candida albicans*
2. *Chlamydia trachomatis*
3. *Escherichia coli*
4. Group B beta-hemolytic streptococci

34. The nurse observes a neonate delivered at 28 weeks' gestation. Which finding would the nurse expect to see?
1. The skin is pale, and no vessels show through it.
2. Creases appear on the interior two-thirds of the sole.
3. The pinna of the ear is soft and flat and stays folded.
4. The neonate has 7 to 10 mm of breast tissue.

35. When attempting to interact with a neonate experiencing drug withdrawal, which behavior would indicate that the neonate is willing to interact?
1. Gaze aversion
2. Hiccups
3. Quiet, alert state
4. Yawning

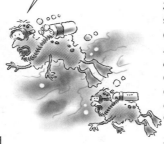

I'm positive we can be the cause of some neonatal infections. Let's find a good spot to colonize.

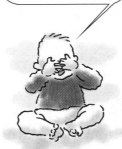

Go ahead and take a peek! You're halfway there and doing great!

32. 2. Group B streptococci are gram-positive cocci that the neonate is exposed to if these bacteria are colonized in the vaginal tract. *E. coli, Klebsiella* species, and *P. aeruginosa* are gram-negative rods that produce 78% to 85% of the bacterial infection in neonates.
CN: Physiological integrity; CNS: Physiological adaptation; CL: Application

33. 4. Transmission of group B beta-hemolytic streptococci to the fetus results in respiratory distress that can rapidly lead to septic shock. *E. coli* is the second most common cause. *Candida albicans* may be acquired from the birth canal. *C. trachomatis* infection causes neonatal conjunctivitis and pneumonia.
CN: Physiological integrity; CNS: Physiological adaptation; CL: Knowledge

34. 3. The ear has a soft pinna that's flat and stays folded. Pale skin with no vessels showing through and 7 to 10 mm of breast tissue are characteristic of a neonate at 40 weeks' gestation. Creases on the anterior two-thirds of the sole are characteristic of a neonate at 36 weeks' gestation.
CN: Health promotion and maintenance; CNS: None; CL: Analysis

35. 3. When caring for neonates experiencing drug withdrawal, the nurse must be alert for distress signals from the neonate. Stimuli should be introduced one at a time when the neonate is in a quiet, alert state. Gaze aversion, yawning, sneezing, hiccups, and body arching are distress signals that the neonate can't handle stimuli at that time.
CN: Psychosocial integrity; CNS: None; CL: Knowledge

CN: Client needs category   CNS: Client needs subcategory   CL: Cognitive level

36. The nurse is providing a mother with discharge instructions for her neonate's umbilical cord care. What information should she include in her instructions?

1. The stump should fall off 1 to 2 days after birth.
2. The stump should fall off 3 to 4 days after birth.
3. The stump should fall off 7 to 10 days after birth.
4. The stump should fall off 15 to 30 days after birth.

37. When caring for a neonate of a mother with diabetes, which physiologic finding is <u>most</u> indicative of a hypoglycemic episode?

1. Hyperalert state
2. Jitteriness
3. Excessive crying
4. Serum glucose level of 60 mg/dl

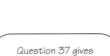

Question 37 gives me the jitters. By the way, that's a clue!

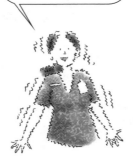

38. A neonate is born at 38 weeks' gestation. The mother asks what the thick, white, cheesy coating is on his skin. Which term is correct?

1. Lanugo
2. Milia
3. Nevus flammeus
4. Vernix

39. A nurse is giving care to a neonate. Which drug is <u>routinely</u> given to the neonate within 1 hour of birth?

1. Erythromycin ophthalmic ointment
2. Gentamycin
3. Nystatin
4. Vitamin A

I need my rest so I can mature.

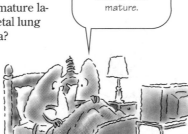

40. A nurse caring for a client in premature labor knows that the <u>best</u> indicator of fetal lung maturity is which of the following data?

1. Meconium in the amniotic fluid
2. Glucocorticoid treatment just before delivery
3. Lecithin to sphingomyelin ratio of more than 2:1
4. Absence of phosphatidylglycerol in amniotic fluid

36. 3. The umbilical stump deteriorates over the first 7 to 10 days postpartum due to dry gangrene and usually falls off by day 10. Wiping the base of the stump with alcohol helps dry the area, facilitating separation.
CN: Health promotion and maintenance; CNS: None; CL: Application

37. 2. Hypoglycemia in a neonate is expressed as jitteriness, lethargy, diaphoresis, and a serum glucose level below 40 mg/dl. A hyperalert state in a neonate is more suggestive of neuralgic irritability and has no correlation to blood glucose levels. Excessive crying isn't found in hypoglycemia. A serum glucose level of 60 mg/dl is a normal level.
CN: Physiological integrity; CNS: Physiological adaptation; CL: Analysis

38. 4. Vernix is a white, cheesy material present on the neonate's skin at birth. Lanugo is the fine body hair on a neonate at birth. Milia are small white papules on the skin. Nevus flammeus is a reddish discoloration of an area of skin.
CN: Health promotion and maintenance; CNS: None; CL: Knowledge

39. 1. Erythromycin ophthalmic ointment is given for prophylactic treatment of ophthalmia neonatorum. Gentamycin is an antibiotic used in the treatment of an infection in the neonate. Nystatin is used for treatment of thrush. Vitamin K, not vitamin A, is given.
CN: Physiological integrity; CNS: Pharmacological therapies; CL: Analysis

40. 3. Lecithin and sphingomyelin are phospholipids that help compose surfactant in the lungs; lecithin peaks at 36 weeks, and sphingomyelin concentrations remain stable. Meconium is released due to fetal stress before delivery, but it's chronic fetal stress that matures lungs. Glucocorticoids must be given at least 48 hours before delivery. The presence of phosphatidylglycerol indicates lung maturity.
CN: Physiological integrity; CNS: Physiological adaptation; CL: Application

CN: Client needs category   CNS: Client needs subcategory   CL: Cognitive level

41. Which condition would place a neonate at the least risk for developing respiratory distress syndrome (RDS)?
1. Second born of twins
2. Neonate born at 34 weeks
3. Neonate of a diabetic mother
4. Chronic maternal hypertension

41. 4. Chronic maternal hypertension is an unlikely factor because chronic fetal stress tends to increase lung maturity. Second twins may be prone to greater risk of asphyxia. Premature neonates younger than 35 weeks are associated with RDS. Even with a mature lecithin to sphingomyelin ratio, neonates of diabetic mothers may still develop respiratory distress.
CN: Physiological integrity; CNS: Physiological adaptation; CL: Analysis

42. Which finding is considered common in the healthy neonate?
1. Simian crease
2. Oral moniliasis
3. Cystic hygroma
4. Bulging fontanel

42. 2. Also known as *thrush,* oral moniliasis is a common finding in neonates, usually acquired from the mother during delivery. A Simian crease is present in 40% of neonates with trisomy 21. Cystic hygroma is a neck mass that can destruct the airway. Bulging fontanels are a sign of intracranial pressure.
CN: Health promotion and maintenance; CNS: None; CL: Analysis

43. When performing nursing care for a neonate after a birth, which intervention should be done immediately?
1. Obtain a Dextrostix.
2. Give the initial bath.
3. Give the vitamin K injection.
4. Cover the neonate's head with a cap.

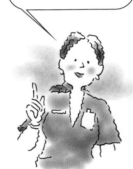

You should perform only one of these actions right away. Which one?

43. 4. Covering the neonate's head with a cap helps prevent cold stress due to excessive evaporative heat loss from a neonate's wet head. Initial baths aren't given until the neonate's temperature is stable. Dextrostix, appropriate for neonates with risk factors, are obtained at 30 minutes to 1 hour of age. Vitamin K can be given within 4 hours after birth.
CN: Health promotion and maintenance; CNS: None; CL: Analysis

44. The nurse observes small, white papules surrounded by erythematous dermatitis on a neonate's skin. This finding is characteristic of which condition?
1. Cutis marmorata
2. Epstein's pearls
3. Erythema toxicum
4. Mongolian spots

44. 3. Erythema toxicum has lesions that come and go on the face, trunk, and limbs. They're small, white or yellow papules or vesicles with erythematous dermatitis. Cutis marmorata is bluish mottling of the skin. Epstein's pearls, found in the mouth, are similar to facial milia. Mongolian spots are large macules or patches that are gray or blue green.
CN: Health promotion and maintenance; CNS: None; CL: Knowledge

45. Which nursing consideration is most important when giving a neonate his initial bath?
1. Giving a tub bath
2. Using water and mild soap
3. Giving the bath right after delivery
4. Using hexachlorophene soap

45. 2. Use only water and mild soap on a neonate to prevent drying out the skin. Tub baths are delayed until the umbilical cord falls off. The initial bath is given when the neonate's temperature is stable. Hexachlorophene soaps should be avoided; they're neurotoxic and may be absorbed through a neonate's skin.
CN: Health promotion and maintenance; CNS: None; CL: Analysis

CN: Client needs category   CNS: Client needs subcategory   CL: Cognitive level

46. The pediatric nurse is caring for neonates in a busy nursery. When weighing a neonate, which action should the nurse take?
 1. Leave the diaper on for comfort.
 2. Place a sterile scale paper on the scale for infection control.
 3. Keep a hand on the neonate's abdomen for safety.
 4. Weigh the neonate at the same time each day for accuracy.

47. A male neonate has just been circumcised. Which intervention is part of the initial care of a circumcised neonate?
 1. Apply alcohol to the site.
 2. Change the diaper as needed.
 3. Keep the neonate in the prone position.
 4. Apply petroleum gauze to the site for 24 hours.

48. The nurse is administering the initial bath to a neonate who's 4 hours old and weighs 7 lb, 2 oz. His vital signs before the bath were: pulse, 126 beats/minute, respiratory rate, 42 breaths/minute, and rectal temperature, 98.4° F (36.9° C). He has been crying lustily throughout the bath. As the nurse dries him, she notes that his color becomes slightly dusky. He cries weakly and he stops moving vigorously. What's the first action the nurse would take?
 1. Obtain a pulse oximetry reading and administer oxygen.
 2. Immediately place the neonate under the warmer.
 3. Use a bulb syringe to suction the neonate's nose and oropharynx.
 4. Cover the neonate's nose and mouth with the oxygen mask and deliver two rescue breaths.

49. Which intervention helps prevent evaporative heat loss in the neonate after birth?
 1. Administering warm oxygen
 2. Controlling the drafts in the room
 3. Immediately drying the neonate
 4. Placing the neonate on a warm, dry towel

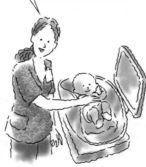

Consistency is the key to obtaining the accurate weight of a neonate.

46. 4. A neonate of any age should be weighed at the same time each day, using the same technique. A neonate should be weighed while undressed. Clean scale paper should be used when weighing the neonate. Sterile scale paper is unnecessary. The nurse should keep a hand above, not on, the abdomen when weighing the neonate.
CN: Health promotion and maintenance; CNS: None; CL: Application

47. 4. Petroleum gauze is applied to the site for the first 24 hours to prevent the skin edges from sticking to the diaper. Alcohol is contraindicated for circumcision care. Diapers are changed more frequently to inspect the site. Neonates are initially kept in the supine position.
CN: Health promotion and maintenance; CNS: None; CL: Application

48. 2. Because this neonate is receiving a bath, he's at risk for becoming cold and metabolizing brown fat. Immediately placing him under the warmer will help restore his body temperature and stop the acidosis that occurs with the metabolism of brown fat. After placing the neonate under the warmer, assessment will continue. If the neonate continues to deteriorate, the other actions may be necessary and should be performed under the warmer. There's no initial evidence that the neonate's respirations are compromised; he continues to cry, although weakly. His dusky color is not respiratory in origin but is due to metabolic acidosis. Based on the findings, there's no reason to suction him.
CN: Physiological integrity; CNS: Physiological adaptation; CL: Analysis

49. 3. Immediately drying the neonate decreases evaporative heat loss from his moist body from birth. Placing the neonate on a warm, dry towel decreases conductive losses. Controlling the drafts in the room and administering warmed oxygen help reduce convective loss.
CN: Health promotion and maintenance; CNS: None; CL: Analysis

CN: Client needs category   CNS: Client needs subcategory   CL: Cognitive level

50. A nurse is performing an assessment on a neonate. Which assessment finding would indicate a metabolic response to cold stress?
1. Arrhythmias
2. Hypoglycemia
3. Increase in liver function
4. Increase in blood pressure

51. Which goal should be placed <u>first</u> in regulating the temperature of a neonate?
1. Supply extra heat sources to the neonate.
2. Keep the ambient room temperature less than 100° F (37.8° C).
3. Minimize the energy needed for the neonate to produce heat.
4. Block radiant, convective, conductive, and evaporative losses.

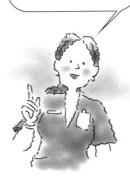

The word *first* is a clue to the answer!

52. A neonate undergoing phototherapy treatment must be monitored for which adverse effect?
1. Hyperglycemia
2. Increased insensible water loss
3. Severe decrease in platelet count
4. Increased GI transit time

53. A nurse is caring for a full-term neonate who's receiving phototherapy for hyperbilirubinemia. Which finding should the nurse report immediately?
1. Maculopapular rash
2. Absent Moro reflex
3. Greenish stool
4. Bronze-colored skin

54. Which clinical finding suggests physiologic hyperbilirubinemia?
1. Clinical jaundice before age 36 hours
2. Clinical jaundice lasting beyond 14 days
3. Bilirubin levels of 12 mg/dl by the third day of life
4. Serum bilirubin level increasing by more than 5 mg/dl/day

50. 2. Hypoglycemia occurs as the consumption of glucose increases with the increase in metabolic rate. Arrhythmias and increases in blood pressure occur due to cardiorespiratory manifestations. Liver function declines in cold stress.
CN: Health promotion and maintenance; CNS: None; CL: Analysis

51. 4. Prevention of heat loss is always the first goal in thermoregulation to avoid hypothermia. The second goal is to minimize the energy necessary for the neonate to produce heat. Adding extra heat sources is a means of correcting hypothermia. The ambient room temperature should be kept at approximately 100° F.
CN: Health promotion and maintenance; CNS: None; CL: Application

52. 2. Increased insensible water loss is due to absorbed photon energy from the lights. Hyperglycemia isn't a characteristic effect of phototherapy treatment. Phototherapy may cause a mild decrease in platelet count. GI transit time may decrease with use of phototherapy.
CN: Physiological integrity; CNS: Reduction of risk potential; CL: Analysis

53. 2. An absent Moro reflex, lethargy, and seizures are symptoms of bilirubin encephalopathy, which can be life-threatening. A maculopapular rash, greenish stools, and bronze-colored skin are minor adverse effects of phototherapy that should be monitored but don't require immediate intervention.
CN: Physiological integrity; CNS: Physiological adaptation; CL: Analysis

54. 3. Increased bilirubin levels in the liver usually cause bilirubin levels of 12 mg/dl by the third day of life. This rise results from the impaired conjugation and excretion of bilirubin and difficulty clearing bilirubin from plasma. The other answers suggest nonphysiologic jaundice.
CN: Health promotion and maintenance; CNS: None; CL: Analysis

55. When caring for a neonate receiving phototherapy, the nurse should remember to:
   1. decrease the amount of formula.
   2. dress the neonate warmly.
   3. massage the neonate's skin with lotion.
   4. reposition the neonate frequently.

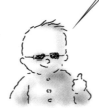

This isn't what I had in mind when I asked for bright lights.

55. 4. Phototherapy works by the chemical interaction between a light source and the bilirubin in the neonate's skin. Therefore, the larger the skin area exposed to light, the more effective the treatment. Changing the neonate's position frequently ensures maximum exposure. Because the neonate will lose water through the skin as a result of evaporation, the amount of formula or water may need to be increased. The neonate is typically undressed to ensure maximum skin exposure. The eyes are covered to protect them from light, and an abbreviated diaper is used to prevent soiling. The skin should be clean and patted dry. Use of lotions would interfere with phototherapy.

CN: Physiological integrity CNS: Physiological adaptation; CL: Application

56. A 2-day-old boy is scheduled for circumcision without anesthesia. Which measure should be included in the neonate's postcircumcision care plan?
   1. Chart the time of the neonate's voiding.
   2. Keep the neonate's penis exposed to air.
   3. Feed the neonate only clear fluids for the first 12 hours.
   4. Place a small ice cap on the neonate's penis.

56. 1. After a circumcision, urine retention may occur. Although the penis should be inspected for swelling and bleeding, further care is unnecessary. A petroleum dressing is commonly applied to the penis; then the neonate is diapered. Because no anesthetic was given, feeding restrictions are unnecessary.

CN: Safe, effective care environment; CNS: Safety and infection control; CL: Application

57. Which finding might be seen in a neonate suspected of having breast-milk jaundice?
   1. History of being a poor breast-feeder
   2. Decreased bilirubin level around day 3 of life
   3. Clinical jaundice evident after 96 hours
   4. Interruption of breast-feeding, resulting in increased bilirubin levels between 24 to 72 hours

57. 3. Breast-milk jaundice is an elevation of indirect bilirubin in a breast-fed neonate that develops following the first 4 to 7 days of life. History of being a poor breast-feeder and interruption of breast-feeding are indicative of breast-feeding jaundice, which occurs before the first 4 to 7 days of life and is caused by insufficient production or intake of breast milk. Jaundice is an elevation, not a decrease, in bilirubin.

CN: Health promotion and maintenance; CNS: None; CL: Analysis

58. A primiparous client who's ready for discharge after delivering 2 days ago is concerned because her neonate's birth weight has declined by 2 oz. She states that she'll continue to breast-feed, but will supplement after each breast-feeding with 4 oz of formula. What's the nurse's best response?
1. "That's a good idea. It's difficult to determine if the breast-fed baby is getting enough to eat."
2. "To determine if the baby is getting enough, you should weigh the baby before and after each feeding."
3. "It's normal for a neonate to lose 5% to 10% of its birth weight. While supplementing is acceptable, remember that a neonate's stomach can hold only about 3 oz."
4. "Supplementing is never recommended for breast-feeding infants."

59. Which sign appears <u>early</u> in a neonate with respiratory distress syndrome?
1. Bilateral crackles
2. Pale gray skin color
3. Tachypnea more than 60 breaths/minute
4. Poor capillary filling time (3 to 4 seconds)

60. Which respiratory disorder in a neonate is usually mild and runs a self-limited course?
1. Pneumonia
2. Meconium aspiration syndrome
3. Transient tachypnea
4. Persistent pulmonary hypertension

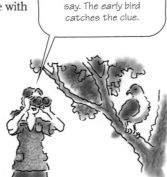

You know what they say. The early bird catches the clue.

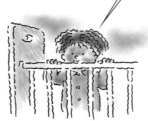

Only 10 more questions before your nap time.

58. 3. Normal neonatal weight loss can range from 5% to 10% of birth weight. The normal neonate's stomach holds about 3 oz (90 ml). A breast-fed neonate's continued weight gain is an indication of his getting enough to eat. While the premature or low-birth-weight neonate is weighed before and after eating in the clinical setting, this isn't an action that's ordinarily taken for the normal neonate in the home setting. Supplementing is an acceptable option for breast-feeding mothers; however, 4 oz would distend the neonate stomach and lead to regurgitation.
CN: Health promotion and maintenance; CNS: None; CL: Application

59. 3. Tachypnea and expiratory grunting occur early in respiratory distress syndrome to help improve oxygenation. Poor capillary filling time, a later manifestation, occurs if signs and symptoms aren't treated. Crackles occur as the respiratory distress progressively worsens. A pale gray skin color obscures earlier cyanosis as respiratory distress symptoms persist and worsen.
CN: Health promotion and maintenance; CNS: None; CL: Analysis

60. 3. Transient tachypnea has an invariably favorable outcome after several hours to several days. The outcome of pneumonia depends on the causative agent involved and may have complications. Meconium aspiration, depending on severity, may have long-term adverse effects. In persistent pulmonary hypertension, mortality is more than 50%.
CN: Physiological integrity; CNS: Physiological adaptation; CL: Analysis

CN: Client needs category   CNS: Client needs subcategory   CL: Cognitive level

61. A 10-hour-old neonate appears exceptionally irritable; he cries easily and startles when touched. The physician orders a drug screen test, which indicates that the neonate is positive for cocaine. Which nursing action would best help to soothe this neonate?
 1. Leaving the light beside the bassinet on at night
 2. Wrapping the neonate snugly in a blanket
 3. Providing multisensory stimulation while the neonate is awake
 4. Giving the neonate a warm bath

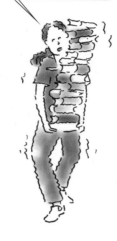

Avoid information overload. Pay attention to the most important facts to choose the correct answer.

61. 2. The practice of tightly wrapping, or swaddling, a cocaine-addicted neonate provides a safe, secure environment and maintains body warmth, which are soothing. A cocaine-addicted neonate typically experiences withdrawal 8 to 10 hours after birth; signs and symptoms include constant crying, jitteriness, poor feeding, emesis, respiratory distress, and seizures. To minimize or prevent these signs and symptoms, sensory stimulation is kept to a minimum and the neonate is typically kept in a quiet, dimly lit environment. A bath would necessitate the removal of clothing and exposure to changes in temperature, both of which are too stimulating.
CN: Physiological integrity; CNS: Basic care and comfort; CL: Application

62. Which immunoglobulin (Ig) provides immunity against bacterial and viral pathogens through passive immunity?
 1. IgA
 2. IgE
 3. IgG
 4. IgM

62. 3. IgG is a major Ig of serum and interstitial fluid that crosses the placenta. IgE has a major role in allergic reactions. IgM and IgA don't cross the placenta.
CN: Health promotion and maintenance; CNS: None; CL: Knowledge

63. Which facial change is characteristic in a neonate with fetal alcohol syndrome (FAS)?
 1. Macrocephaly
 2. Microcephaly
 3. Wide, palpebral fissures
 4. Well-developed philtrum

Maternal history may reveal important clues to the neonate's current condition.

63. 2. FAS infants are usually born with microcephaly. Their facial features include short, palpebral fissures and a thin upper lip.
CN: Physiological integrity; CNS: Physiological adaptation; CL: Knowledge

64. A 36-week neonate born weighing 1,800 g has microcephaly and microophthalmia. Based on these findings, which risk factor might be expected in the maternal history?
 1. Use of alcohol
 2. Use of marijuana
 3. Gestational diabetes
 4. Positive group B streptococci

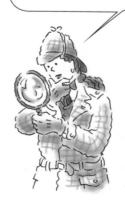

64. 1. The most common sign of the effects of alcohol on fetal development is retarded growth in weight, length, and head circumference. Intrauterine growth retardation isn't characteristic of marijuana use. Gestational diabetes usually produces large-for-gestational-age neonates. Positive group B streptococci isn't a relevant risk factor.
CN: Health promotion and maintenance; CNS: None; CL: Analysis

CN: Client needs category   CNS: Client needs subcategory   CL: Cognitive level

65. Which GI disorder is seen <u>exclusively</u> in neonates with cystic fibrosis?
1. Duodenal obstruction
2. Jejunal atresia
3. Malrotation
4. Meconium ileus

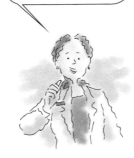

Pay close attention to the word exclusively.

66. A diabetic client delivers a full-term neonate who weights 10 lb, 1 oz (4.6 kg). While caring for this large-for-gestational age (LGA) neonate, the nurse palpates the clavicles for which reason?
1. Neonates of diabetic mothers have brittle bones.
2. Clavicles are commonly absent in neonates of diabetic mothers.
3. One of the neonate's clavicles may have been broken during delivery.
4. LGA neonates have glucose deposits on their clavicles.

67. A nurse is caring for a 4-hour-old male neonate. His heel stick hematocrit test result is 55%. Which statement is <u>true</u> concerning this finding?
1. It indicates serious anemia.
2. It's within normal limits.
3. It indicates the sample has been hemolyzed.
4. The test needs to be repeated using a venous blood sample.

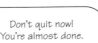

Don't quit now! You're almost done.

68. Which discharge instructions should the nurse provide to the parents of a neonate who has been circumcised? Select all that apply:
1. The infant must void before being discharged home.
2. Apply petroleum jelly to the glans of the penis with each diaper change.
3. Tub baths for the infant are acceptable while the circumcision heals.
4. Report blood on the front of the diaper.
5. The circumcision requires care for 2 to 4 days after discharge.

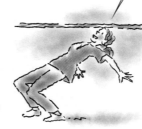

65. 4. Meconium ileus is a luminal obstruction of the distal small intestine by abnormal meconium seen in neonates with cystic fibrosis. Duodenal obstruction, jejunal atresia, and malrotation aren't characteristic findings in neonates with cystic fibrosis.
CN: Physiological integrity; CNS: Physiological adaptation; CL: Knowledge

66. 3. Because of the neonate's large size, clavicular fractures are common during delivery. The nurse should assess all LGA neonates for this occurrence. None of the other options are true.
CN: Physiological integrity; CNS: Physiological adaptation; CL: Application

67. 2. Hematocrit of 52% to 58% is normal in a neonate because of increased blood supply during intrauterine life. Hematocrit of 55% doesn't indicate serious anemia because the value is within the normal range for a neonate. If the heelstick blood test shows hematocrit greater than 58%, a venous blood sample is obtained for testing because hemolysis of the heelstick sample can show a false reading. Hematocrit greater than 58% requires treatment after the physician has been notified.
CN: Health promotion and maintenance; CNS: None; CL: Analysis

68. 1, 2, 5. It's necessary for a circumcised infant to void before discharge to ensure that the urethra isn't obstructed. Petroleum jelly should be applied to the glans with each diaper change. Typically, the penis heals within 2 to 4 days. Tub baths should be avoided until the circumcision heals to prevent infection. A small amount of blood is expected after circumcision; parents should report only large amounts to the physician.
CN: Safe, effective care environment; CNS: Coordinated care; CL: Application

CN: Client needs category   CNS: Client needs subcategory   CL: Cognitive level

69. The nurse is eliciting reflexes in a neonate during a physical examination. Identify the area the nurse would touch to elicit a plantar grasp reflex.

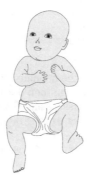

70. The nurse notes that, at 5 minutes after birth, a neonate is pink with acrocyanosis; his knees are flexed, his fists are clinched, he has a whimpering cry, and his heart rate is 128 beats/minute. He withdraws his foot to a slap on the sole. What 5-minute Apgar score should the nurse record for this neonate?

Sign	Apgar score		
	0	1	2
Heart rate	Absent	Less than 100 beats/minute (slow)	More than 100 beats/minute
Respiratory effort	Absent	Slow, irregular	Good crying
Muscle tone	Flaccid	Some flexion and resistance to extension of extremities	Active motion
Reflex irritability	No response	Grimace or weak cry	Vigorous cry
Color	Pallor, cyanosis	Pink body, blue extremities	Completely pink

69.

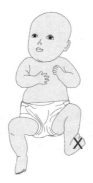

Touching the sole near the base of the digits elicits a plantar grasp reflex and causes flexion or grasping. This reflex disappears around age 9 months.

CN: Health promotion and maintenance; CNS: None; CL: Application

70. 8. The Apgar score quantifies neonatal heart rate, respiratory effort, muscle tone, reflexes, and color. Each category is assessed 1 minute after birth and again 5 minutes later. Scores in each category range from 0 to 2. This neonate has a heart rate above 100 beats/minute, which equals 2; is pink in color with acrocyanosis, which equals 1; is well-flexed, which equals 2; has a weak cry, which equals 1; and has a good response to slapping the soles, which equals 2. Therefore, the nurse should record a total Apgar score of 8.

CN: Physiological integrity; CNS: Physiological adaptation; CL: Analysis

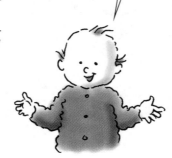

Success! You've proven you weren't born yesterday when it comes to neonatal care.

CN: Client needs category   CNS: Client needs subcategory   CL: Cognitive level

Part V Care of the child

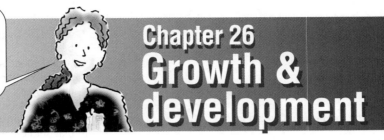

Here's a short but important chapter that covers the growth and development of children. Enjoy!

Chapter 26
Growth & development

1. A client tells the nurse that her 22-month-old child says "no" to everything. When scolded, the toddler becomes angry and starts crying loudly but then immediately wants to be held. What's the best interpretation of this behavior?
1. The toddler isn't coping effectively with stress.
2. The toddler's need for affection isn't being met.
3. It's normal behavior for a 2-year-old child.
4. It suggests the need for counseling.

2. The mother of a 12-month-old infant expresses concern about the effect of frequent thumb sucking on her child's teeth. After the nurse teaches her about this matter, which response by the mother indicates that the teaching has been effective?
1. "Thumb sucking should be discouraged at 12 months."
2. "I'll give the baby a pacifier instead."
3. "Sucking is important to the baby."
4. "I'll wrap the thumb in a bandage."

3. A 2-year-old child's mother is worried that her little girl may have attention deficit hyperactivity disorder because "she has so much energy, doesn't pay attention for long, and is always getting into things." Which response is best?
1. "Her behavior is normal. She's exploring and learning about the world around her."
2. "You should talk to your pediatrician. You have definite concerns."
3. "Keep her intake of sugar and treats to a minimum. This will help her settle down."
4. "I'd suggest taking her to a child psychologist. She probably needs evaluation."

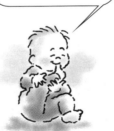

I have some important work to do.

1. 3. Toddlers are confronted with the conflict of achieving autonomy yet relinquishing the much-enjoyed dependence on—and affection of—others. As a result, their negativism is a necessary part of their growth and development. Nothing about this behavior indicates that the child is under stress, isn't receiving sufficient affection, or requires counseling.
CN: Health promotion and maintenance; CNS: None; CL: Comprehension

2. 3. Sucking is the infant's chief pleasure. However, thumb sucking can cause malocclusion if it persists after age 4. Many fetuses begin sucking their fingers in utero and, as infants, refuse a pacifier as a substitute. A young child is likely to chew on a bandage, which could lead to airway obstruction.
CN: Physiological integrity; CNS: Basic care and comfort; CL: Analysis

3. 1. It's normal for a 2-year-old child to eagerly explore her environment for new sensory experiences. Talking to the pediatrician is inappropriate because the nurse is assuming a corrective, parental role toward the mother without addressing her concerns. Restricting the child's intake of sugar and treats is incorrect because the nurse is making assumptions and recommendations that don't relate to the mother's concerns. Suggesting evaluation by a psychologist reinforces the mother's fear that something is wrong with her child.
CN: Safe, effective care environment; CNS: Safety and infection control; CL: Analysis

CN: Client needs category   CNS: Client needs subcategory   CL: Cognitive level

4. Which developmental milestones would the nurse expect a 10-month-old infant to display during a routine health maintenance visit? Select all that apply:
1. Holding his head erect
2. Self-feeding
3. Demonstrating good bowel and bladder control
4. Sitting on a firm surface without support
5. Bearing the majority of his weight on his legs
6. Walking alone

5. A 14-month-old is admitted to the pediatric floor with a diagnosis of croup. Which characteristics would the nurse expect the toddler to demonstrate if he's developing normally? Select all that apply:
1. Strong hand grasp
2. Tendency to hold one object while looking for another
3. Recognition of familiar voices (smiles in recognition)
4. Presence of Moro reflex
5. Weight that's triple his birth weight
6. Closed anterior fontanelle

6. When talking with 10- and 11-year-old children about death, the nurse should incorporate which guides? Select all that apply:
1. Logical explanations aren't appropriate.
2. The children will be curious about the physical aspects of death.
3. The children will know that death is inevitable and irreversible.
4. The children will be influenced by the attitudes of the adults in their lives.
5. Teaching about death and dying shouldn't start before age 11.
6. Telling children that death is the same as going to sleep as a way of relieving fear is appropriate.

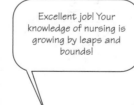

Excellent job! Your knowledge of nursing is growing by leaps and bounds!

4. 1, 4, 5. By age 10 months, an infant should be able to hold his head erect—a developmental milestone achieved by age 3 months. He should also be able to sit on a firm surface without support and bear the majority of his weight on his legs (for example, walking while holding on to furniture). Self-feeding and bowel and bladder control are developmental milestones of toddlers. By age 12 months, the infant should be able to stand alone and may take his first steps.
CN: Health promotion and maintenance; CNS: None; CL: Application

5. 1, 2, 3, 5. A strong hand grasp is demonstrated within the first month of life. Holding one object while looking for another is accomplished by the 20th week. Within the first year of life, the toddler masters smiling at familiar faces and voices, birth weight triples, and the Moro reflex disappears. The anterior fontanel closes at approximately age 18 months.
CN: Health promotion and maintenance; CNS: None; CL: Application

6. 2, 3, 4. School-age children are curious about the physical aspects of death and may wonder what happens to the body. By age 9 or 10, most children know that death is universal, inevitable, and irreversible. Their cognitive abilities are advanced and they respond well to logical explanations. They should be encouraged to ask questions. Because the adults in their environment influence their attitudes towards death, they should be encouraged to include children in the family rituals and be prepared to answer questions that may seem shocking. Teaching about death should begin early in childhood. Comparing death to sleep can be frightening for children and cause them to fear falling asleep.
CN: Psychosocial integrity; CNS: None; CL: Application

CN: Client needs category   CNS: Client needs subcategory   CL: Cognitive level

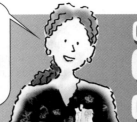

Chapter 27
Cardiovascular disorders

1. When auscultating heart sounds on a 2-year-old child, where would the nurse place the stethoscope to hear the first heart sound best?
 1. Third or fourth intercostal space
 2. The apex with the stethoscope bell
 3. Second intercostal space, midclavicular line
 4. Fifth intercostal space, left midclavicular line

2. The nurse auscultates the first heart sound, interpreting this sound as occurring:
 1. late in diastole.
 2. early in diastole.
 3. with closure of the mitral and tricuspid valves.
 4. with closure of the aortic and pulmonic valves.

3. Which characteristic best describes a grade 1 heart murmur?
 1. Equal to the heart sounds
 2. Softer than the heart sounds
 3. Can be heard with the naked ear
 4. Associated with a precordial thrill

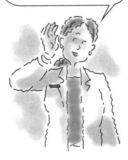

Listen carefully for the answer to question 3.

4. Which phrase best defines the term *stroke volume?*
 1. Volume of blood returning to the heart
 2. Ability of the cardiac muscle to act as an efficient pump
 3. Resistance against which the ventricles pump when ejecting blood
 4. Amount of blood ejected by the heart in any one contraction

1. 4. The first heart sound can best be heard at the fifth intercostal space, left midclavicular line. The second heart sound is heard at the second intercostal space. The third heart sound is heard with the stethoscope bell at the apex of the heart. The fourth heart sound can be heard at the third or fourth intercostal space.
CN: Health promotion and maintenance; CNS: None; CL: Application

2. 3. The first heart sound occurs during systole with closure of the mitral and tricuspid valves. The second heart sound occurs during diastole with closure of the aortic and pulmonic valves. The third heart sound is heard early in diastole. The fourth heart sound is heard late in diastole and may be a normal finding in children.
CN: Health promotion and maintenance; CNS: None; CL: Analysis

3. 2. A grade 1 heart murmur is usually difficult to hear and softer than the heart sounds. A grade 2 murmur is usually equal to the heart sounds. A grade 4 murmur can be associated with a precordial thrill. A thrill is a palpable manifestation associated with a loud murmur. A grade 6 murmur can be heard with the naked ear or with the stethoscope off the chest.
CN: Health promotion and maintenance; CNS: None; CL: Knowledge

4. 4. Stroke volume is the amount of blood ejected by the heart in any one contraction. It's influenced by preload, afterload, and contractility. Preload is the amount of blood returning to the heart. Contractility is the ability of the cardiac muscle to act as an efficient pump. Afterload is the resistance against which the ventricles pump when ejecting blood.
CN: Physiological integrity; CNS: Physiological adaptation; CL: Knowledge

CN: Client needs category   CNS: Client needs subcategory   CL: Cognitive level

5. A child is diagnosed with cardiogenic shock. The nurse understands this condition involves which of the following?
  1. Decreased cardiac output
  2. A reduction in circulating blood volume
  3. Overwhelming sepsis and circulating bacterial toxins
  4. Inflow or outflow obstruction of the main bloodstream

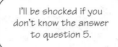

I'll be shocked if you don't know the answer to question 5.

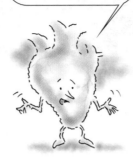

6. Which sign is considered a <u>late</u> sign of shock in children?
  1. Tachycardia
  2. Hypotension
  3. Delayed capillary refill
  4. Pale, cool, mottled skin

7. Which factor indicating a cardiac defect might be found when observing a 1-month-old infant?
  1. Weight gain
  2. Hyperactivity
  3. Poor nutritional intake
  4. Pink mucous membranes

8. A 2-year-old child is showing signs of shock. A 10-ml/kg bolus of normal saline solution is ordered. The child weighs 20 kg. How many milliliters should be administered?
  1. 20 ml
  2. 100 ml
  3. 200 ml
  4. 2,000 ml

Pick an arrhythmia, the *most common* arrhythmia.

9. In neonates and infants, the nurse would be alert for which arrhythmia as most common?
  1. Atrial fibrillation
  2. Bradyarrhythmia
  3. Premature atrial contractions
  4. Premature ventricular contractions

5. 1. Cardiogenic shock occurs when cardiac output is decreased and tissue oxygen needs aren't adequately met. Hypovolemic shock describes a reduction in circulating blood volume. Septic shock describes overwhelming sepsis and circulating bacterial toxins. Obstructive shock is seen with an inflow or outflow obstruction of the main bloodstream.
CN: Physiological integrity; CNS: Physiological adaptation; CL: Comprehension

6. 2. Hypotension is considered a late sign of shock in children. This represents a decompensated state and impending cardiopulmonary arrest. Tachycardia, delayed capillary refill, and pale, cool, mottled skin are earlier indicators of shock that may show compensation.
CN: Physiological integrity; CNS: Physiological adaptation; CL: Analysis

7. 3. Children with heart defects tend to have poor nutritional intake and weight loss, indicating poor cardiac output or hypoxemia. Hypoxemia causes lethargy and fatigue, not hyperactivity. Gray, pale, or mottled skin may indicate hypoxia or poor cardiac output. Pink, moist mucous membranes are normal.
CN: Health promotion and maintenance; CNS: None; CL: Analysis

8. 3. The child should receive 200 ml. Use the following equation:
$$10 \text{ ml/kg} \times 20 \text{ kg} = 200 \text{ ml.}$$
CN: Physiological integrity; CNS: Pharmacological therapies; CL: Analysis

9. 3. Premature atrial contractions are common in fetuses, neonates, and infants. They occur from increased automaticity of an atrial cell anywhere except the sinoatrial node. Atrial fibrillation is an uncommon arrhythmia in children occurring from a disorganized state of electrical activity in the atria. Bradyarrhythmias are usually congenital, surgically acquired, or caused by infection. Premature ventricular contractions are more common in adolescents.
CN: Physiological integrity; CNS: Physiological adaptation; CL: Comprehension

CN: Client needs category   CNS: Client needs subcategory   CL: Cognitive level

10. When reviewing a child's electrocardiogram, the nurse interprets which part as indicating ventricular depolarization and contraction?
1. P wave
2. PR interval
3. QRS complex
4. T wave

11. Which evaluation of cardiovascular status is <u>noninvasive</u>?
1. Echocardiogram
2. Cardiac enzyme levels
3. Cardiac catheterization
4. Transesophageal pacing

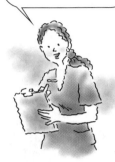

Noninvasive is a clue. So eliminate the invasive evaluations, and then choose the best answer.

12. A boy with a patent ductus arteriosus was delivered 6 hours earlier and is being held by his mother. As the nurse enters the room to assess the neonate's vital signs, the mother says, "The physician says that my baby has a heart murmur. Does that mean he has a bad heart?" Which response by the nurse would be most appropriate?
1. "He'll need more tests to determine his heart condition."
2. "He'll require oxygen therapy at home for awhile."
3. "He'll be fine. Don't worry about him."
4. "The murmur is caused by the natural opening, which can take a day or two to close. It's a normal part of your baby's transition."

13. Before a cardiac catheterization, which intervention is <u>most appropriate</u> for a child and his parents?
1. Supplying a map of the hospital
2. Limiting visitors to parents only
3. Offering a guided tour of the hospital and catheterization laboratory
4. Explaining that the child can't eat or drink for 1 to 2 days postoperatively

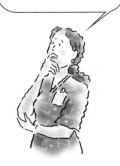

Which intervention is most appropriate at this time?

10. 3. The QRS complex reflects ventricular depolarization and contraction. The P wave represents atrial depolarization and contraction. The PR interval represents the time it takes an impulse to trace from the atrioventricular node to the bundle of His. The T wave represents repolarization of the ventricles.
CN: Physiological integrity; CNS: Physiological adaptation; CL: Analysis

11. 1. An echocardiogram is a noninvasive procedure to visualize the anatomy of the heart. Blood testing determines cardiac enzyme levels. Cardiac catheterization involves passing a catheter into the chambers of the heart for direct visualization of the heart and great vessels. Transesophageal pacing requires a probe to be placed in the esophagus for high-frequency ultrasound.
CN: Physiological integrity; CNS: Physiological adaptation; CL: Analysis

12. 4. Although the nurse may want to tell the client not to worry, the most appropriate response would be to explain the neonate's present condition, to relieve her, and to acknowledge an awareness of the condition. A neonate's vascular system changes with birth; certain factors help to reverse the flow of blood through the ductus and ultimately favor its closure. This closure typically begins within the first 24 hours after birth and ends within a few days after birth. The other responses don't adequately address the client's question.
CN: Health promotion and maintenance; CNS: None; CL: Analysis

13. 3. A guided tour will help minimize fears and allay anxieties for the child and his parents. It gives the opportunity for questions and teaching. A map of the hospital is helpful, but a tour provides the family with more information. The child will be able to start clear liquids and advance as tolerated after the procedure is completed and the child is fully awake. Visitors should include all significant others and siblings as part of the preoperative teaching.
CN: Physiological integrity; CNS: Physiological adaptation; CL: Analysis

CN: Client needs category   CNS: Client needs subcategory   CL: Cognitive level

14. Which statement about cardiac catheterization is correct?

1. It's a noninvasive procedure.
2. General anesthesia is required.
3. High-frequency sound waves produce an image of the heart in motion.
4. It provides visualization of the heart and great vessels with radiopaque dye.

14. 4. Cardiac catheterization provides visualization of the heart and great vessels. It's an invasive procedure in which a thin catheter is passed into the chambers of the heart through a peripheral vein or artery. Conscious sedation is usually given before cardiac catheterization. General anesthesia may be used for more complex catheterizations or procedures that place the child at greater risk. "High-frequency sound waves" describes ultrasound and echocardiography.
CN: Physiological integrity; CNS: Physiological adaptation; CL: Knowledge

15. Which nursing intervention is most appropriate when caring for a child in the immediate postcatherization phase?

1. Elevate the head of the bed 45 degrees.
2. Encourage the child to remain flat.
3. Assess vital signs every 2 to 4 hours.
4. Replace a bloody groin dressing with a new dressing.

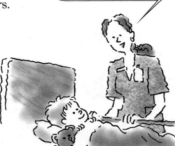

A child needs support and encouragement before and after any medical procedure.

15. 2. During recovery, the child should remain flat in bed, keeping the punctured leg straight for the prescribed time. The child should avoid raising the head, sitting, straining the abdomen, or coughing. Vital signs are taken every 15 minutes until the child is awake and stable, then every half hour, then hourly as ordered. If bleeding occurs at the insertion site, the nurse should reinforce the dressing and monitor for changes.
CN: Physiological integrity; CNS: Physiological adaptation; CL: Analysis

16. Which home care instruction is included for a child postcatheterization?

1. Encourage fluids and regular diet.
2. Encourage physical activities.
3. The child can routinely bathe after returning home.
4. The child may return to school the next day.

16. 1. A regular diet and increased fluids are encouraged postcatheterization. Increased fluids may flush the injected dyes out of the system. Normal activities may be resumed, but physical activities or sports should be avoided for about 3 days. Prolonged bathing can be resumed in about 2 days. A sponge bath is encouraged until then. The child may return to school in 2 to 3 days after discharge.
CN: Physiological integrity; CNS: Physiological adaptation; CL: Analysis

17. A 2-year-old child is being monitored after cardiac surgery. Which sign represents a decrease in cardiac output?

1. Hypertension
2. Increased urine output
3. Weak peripheral pulses
4. Capillary refill less than 2 seconds

17. 3. Signs of decreased cardiac output include weak peripheral pulses, low urine output, delayed capillary refill, hypotension, and cool extremities. Poor cardiac function leads to a decrease in cardiac output, so vasoactive and inotropic agents are needed to maintain adequate cardiac output.
CN: Physiological integrity; CNS: Physiological adaptation; CL: Analysis

18. A 3-year-old child is experiencing distress after having cardiac surgery. Which sign indicates cardiac tamponade?
1. Hypertension
2. Muffled heart sounds
3. Widened pulse pressures
4. Increased chest tube drainage

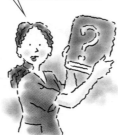

All of these signs may appear, but only one indicates cardiac tamponade. Which one?

19. A nurse is monitoring fluid and electrolyte balance in a child postoperatively. Which finding is expected?
1. Increased urine output
2. Increased sodium level
3. Decreased sodium level
4. Increased potassium level

20. A nurse is teaching wound care to parents after cardiac surgery. Which statement is <u>most</u> <u>appropriate</u>?
1. Lotions and powders are acceptable.
2. Your child can take a bath tomorrow.
3. Tingling, itching, and numbness are normal sensations at the wound site.
4. If the sterile adhesive strips over the incision fall off, call the physician.

21. Parents ask a nurse about a child's activity level after cardiac surgery. Which response would be best?
1. There are no exercise limitations.
2. The child may resume school in 3 days.
3. Encourage a balance of rest and exercise.
4. Climbing and contact sports are restricted for 1 week.

Teaching proper postoperative care is an important part of the nurse's responsibility.

22. Which home care instruction is <u>most</u> <u>appropriate</u> for a child after cardiac surgery?
1. Don't stop giving the child the prescribed drugs until the physician says so.
2. Maintain a sodium-restricted diet.
3. Routine dental care can be resumed.
4. Immunizations are delayed indefinitely.

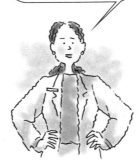

18. 2. Symptoms of cardiac tamponade include muffled heart sounds, hypotension, sudden cessation of chest tube drainage, and a narrowing pulse pressure. Cardiac tamponade occurs when a large volume of fluid interferes with ventricular filling and pumping and collects in the pericardial sac, decreasing cardiac output.
CN: Physiological integrity; CNS: Physiological adaptation; CL: Analysis

19. 2. In response to surgery and cardiopulmonary bypass, the body secretes aldosterone and antidiuretic hormone. This in turn increases water retention, increases sodium levels, and decreases potassium levels.
CN: Physiological integrity; CNS: Physiological adaptation; CL: Analysis

20. 3. As the area heals, tingling, itching, and numbness are normal sensations and will eventually go away. Lotions and powders should be avoided during the first 2 weeks after surgery. A complete bath should be delayed for the first week. Adhesive strips may loosen or fall off on their own. This is a common and normal occurrence.
CN: Physiological integrity; CNS: Physiological adaptation; CL: Analysis

21. 3. Activity should be increased gradually each day, allowing for a sensible balance of rest and exercise. School and large crowds should be avoided for at least 2 weeks to prevent exposure to people with active infections. Sports and contact activities should be restricted for about 6 weeks, giving the sternum enough time to heal.
CN: Physiological integrity; CNS: Physiological adaptation; CL: Analysis

22. 1. Drugs, such as digoxin (Lanoxin) and furosemide (Lasix), shouldn't be stopped abruptly. There are no diet restrictions, so the child may resume his regular diet. Routine dental care is usually delayed 4 to 5 months after surgery. Immunizations may be delayed 6 to 8 weeks after surgery.
CN: Physiological integrity; CNS: Physiological adaptation; CL: Analysis

CN: Client needs category   CNS: Client needs subcategory   CL: Cognitive level

23. A 4-year-old client with a chest tube is placed on water seal. Which statement is correct?
1. The water level rises with inhalation.
2. Bubbling is seen in the suction chamber.
3. Bubbling is seen in the water seal chamber.
4. Water seal is obtained by clamping the tube.

23. 1. The water seal chamber is functioning appropriately when the water level rises in the chamber with inhalation and falls with expiration. This shows that negative pressure required in the lung is being maintained. Bubbling in the suction chamber should only be seen when suction is being used. Bubbling in the water seal chamber generally indicates the presence of an air leak. The chest tube should never be clamped; a tension pneumothorax may occur. Water seal is activated when the suction is disconnected.
CN: Physiological integrity; CNS: Physiological adaptation; CL: Application

24. Which intervention is most appropriate when a chest tube falls out or becomes dislodged?
1. Place a dry gauze dressing over the insertion site.
2. Place a petroleum gauze dressing over the insertion site.
3. Wipe the tube with alcohol and reinsert it.
4. Call the physician immediately.

24. 2. Petroleum gauze should be placed over the insertion site immediately to prevent a pneumothorax. The physician should be notified after this step. A dry gauze dressing will allow air to escape, leading to a pneumothorax. The tube is only reinserted by a physician using a sterile thoracotomy tray.
CN: Physiological integrity; CNS: Physiological adaptation; CL: Application

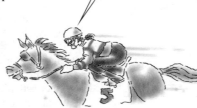

You're galloping right through these questions—good for you!

25. When observing a child with heart failure, which finding would the nurse expect?
1. Bradycardia
2. Weight gain
3. Gallop murmur
4. Strong, bounding pulses

25. 3. When the heart stretches beyond efficiency, an extra heart sound or S_3 gallop murmur may be audible. This is related to excessive preload and ventricular dilation. Tachycardia occurs as a compensatory mechanism to the decrease in cardiac output. It also attempts to increase the force and rate of myocardial contraction and increase oxygen consumption of the heart. Children with heart failure tend to have difficulty feeding and tire easily. They're commonly diagnosed as failure to thrive and are in the lower percentiles of their growth charts for weight. Pulses are usually weak and thready.
CN: Physiological integrity; CNS: Physiological adaptation; CL: Analysis

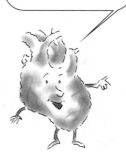

What happens when my left side isn't working properly?

26. A nurse is assessing a child with left-sided heart failure. Which symptom would be <u>most</u> indicative of this condition?
1. Weight gain
2. Peripheral edema
3. Neck vein distention
4. Tachypnea and dyspnea

26. 4. Respiratory symptoms, such as tachypnea and dyspnea, are seen due to pulmonary congestion. Weight gain, peripheral edema, and neck vein distention are seen with systemic venous congestion or right-sided failure. Fluid accumulates in the interstitial spaces due to blood pooling in the venous circulation.
CN: Physiological integrity; CNS: Physiological adaptation; CL: Application

CN: Client needs category   CNS: Client needs subcategory   CL: Cognitive level

27. Which intervention is <u>most appropriate</u> when caring for an infant with heart failure?
1. Limit fluid intake.
2. Avoid using infant seats.
3. Cluster nursing activities.
4. Place the infant in a prone or supine position.

28. Which diet plan is recommended for an infant with heart failure?
1. Restrict fluids.
2. Weigh once per week.
3. Use low-sodium formula.
4. Increase caloric content per ounce.

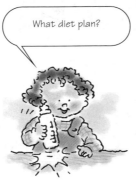

What diet plan?

29. Which statement is true about giving oxygen to a client with heart failure?
1. Oxygen is contraindicated in this situation.
2. Oxygen is given at high levels only.
3. Oxygen is a pulmonary bed constrictor.
4. Oxygen decreases the work of breathing.

30. A teenage client with heart failure is prescribed digoxin (Lanoxin) and asks the nurse, "What's the drug supposed to do?" The nurse responds to the teenager based on the understanding that this drug is classified as:
1. an angiotensin-converting enzyme (ACE) inhibitor.
2. a cardiac glycoside.
3. a diuretic.
4. a vasodilator.

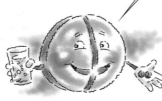

Knowing the classification of a drug can help you remember its actions.

27. 3. Energy expenditures need to be limited to reduce metabolic and oxygen needs. Nursing care should be clustered, followed by long periods of undisturbed rest. Fluid may be restricted in older children, but infants' nutritional requirements depend on fluid needs. Infants should be placed in the semi-Fowler or upright position. Infant seats help maintain an upright position. This facilitates lung expansion, provides less restrictive movement of the diaphragm, relieves pressure from abdominal organs, and decreases pulmonary congestion.
CN: Physiological integrity; CNS: Physiological adaptation; CL: Analysis

28. 4. Formulas with increased caloric content are given to meet the greater caloric requirements from the overworked heart and labored breathing. Fluid restriction and low-sodium formulas aren't recommended. An infant's nutritional needs depend on fluid. Daily weights at the same time of the day on the same scale before feedings are recommended to follow trends in nutritional stability and diuresis. Low-sodium formulas may cause hyponatremia.
CN: Physiological integrity; CNS: Physiological adaptation; CL: Application

29. 4. Oxygen decreases the work of breathing and increases arterial oxygen levels so it's indicated in this situation. Oxygen usually is administered at low levels with humidification. Oxygen is a pulmonary bed dilator, not constrictor, and can exacerbate the condition in which the lungs are overloaded.
CN: Physiological integrity; CNS: Physiological adaptation; CL: Analysis

30. 2. Digoxin is a cardiac glycoside. It decreases the workload of the heart and improves myocardial function. ACE inhibitors cause vasodilation and increase sodium excretion. Diuretics help remove excess fluid. Vasodilators enhance cardiac output by decreasing afterload.
CN: Physiological integrity; CNS: Pharmacological therapies; CL: Comprehension

31. Which toxic adverse reaction can be seen in a child taking digoxin (Lanoxin)?
1. Weight gain
2. Tachycardia
3. Nausea and vomiting
4. Purple tint around objects or halos

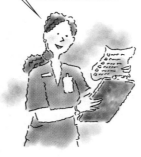

Pay attention to question 32. It's a math question but I know you can do it!

32. An 11-month-old infant with heart failure weighs 10 kg. Digoxin (Lanoxin) is prescribed as 0.01 mg/kg in divided doses every 12 hours. How much is given per dose?
1. 0.001 mg/dose
2. 0.05 mg/dose
3. 0.1 mg/dose
4. 0.5 mg/dose

33. A child with heart failure is given captopril (Capoten), an angiotensin-converting enzyme (ACE) inhibitor. Which action of captopril should the nurse teach the child's parents?
1. It increases vasoconstriction.
2. It increases sodium excretion.
3. It decreases sodium excretion.
4. It increases vascular resistance.

34. Which statement would the nurse need to keep in mind when assisting with the teaching plan for the parents of a child with patent ductus arteriosus?
1. Heart failure is uncommon.
2. The ductus normally closes completely by age 6 weeks.
3. An open ductus arteriosus causes decreased blood flow to the lungs.
4. It represents a cyanotic defect with decreased pulmonary blood flow.

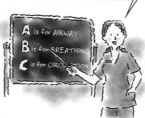

Teaching is an important part of the nurse's role.

A is for AIRWAY
B is for BREATHING
C is for CIRCULATION

35. During observation of a child who has undergone cardiac catheterization, the nurse notes significant bleeding from the percutaneous femoral catheterization site. Which action should be taken <u>first</u>?
1. Apply direct, continuous pressure.
2. Assess the pulse and blood pressure.
3. Seek the assistance of a registered nurse.
4. Check the pulses in the affected leg.

31. 3. Digoxin toxicity in infants and children may present with nausea, vomiting, anorexia, or a slow, irregular apical heart rate. Vision disturbances are described as a green or yellow tint to objects or green or yellow halos around objects or bright lights.
CN: Physiological integrity; CNS: Pharmacological therapies; CL: Analysis

32. 2. The child should receive 0.05 mg/dose. Use the following equations:
10 kg × 0.01 mg/kg = 0.1 mg;
24 hours/12 hours/dose = 2 doses;
0.1 mg/2 doses = 0.05 mg/dose.
CN: Physiological integrity; CNS: Pharmacological therapies; CL: Analysis

33. 2. ACE inhibitors block the conversion of angiotensin I to angiotensin II in the kidney. This causes decreased aldosterone, vasodilation, and increased sodium excretion. As a vasodilator, it also acts to reduce vascular resistance by the manipulation of afterload.
CN: Physiological integrity; CNS: Pharmacological therapies; CL: Application

34. 2. At birth, oxygenated blood normally causes the ductus to constrict, and the vessel closes completely by age 6 weeks. This defect is considered an acyanotic defect with increased pulmonary blood flow. Heart failure is common in premature infants with patent ductus arteriosus. The open ductus arteriosus can cause an excessive blood flow to the lungs because of the high pressure in the aorta.
CN: Physiological integrity; CNS: Physiological adaptation; CL: Comprehension

35. 1. Bleeding from a major vessel must be stopped immediately to prevent massive hemorrhage. Vital signs would be taken after bleeding control measures are instituted. Calling for help is important, but pressure on the site must be applied and maintained while help is found. Pulses would be checked after bleeding is controlled.
CN: Physiological integrity; CNS: Reduction of risk potential; CL: Application

CN: Client needs category   CNS: Client needs subcategory   CL: Cognitive level

36. Which intervention would be appropriate for an infant after cardiac catheterization?
1. Keep the leg on the operative site flexed to reduce bleeding.
2. Change the catheterization dressing immediately to reduce the risk of infection.
3. Apply pressure if oozing or bleeding is noted.
4. Keep the infant's temperature below normal to promote vasoconstriction and decrease bleeding.

36. 3. Applying pressure to the site is appropriate if bleeding is noted. The leg should be kept straight and immobile to prevent trauma and bleeding. The pressure dressing shouldn't be changed, but it may be reinforced if bleeding occurs. Hypothermia causes stress in infants and should be avoided.
CN: Physiological integrity; CNS: Reduction of risk potential; CL: Application

37. Which cardiovascular disorder is considered acyanotic?
1. Patent ductus arteriosus
2. Tetralogy of Fallot
3. Tricuspid atresia
4. Truncus arteriosus

37. 1. Patent ductus arteriosus represents an acyanotic heart defect with increased pulmonary blood flow. Tetralogy of Fallot and tricuspid atresia are cyanotic defects with decreased pulmonary blood flow. Truncus arteriosus is a cyanotic defect with increased pulmonary blood flow.
CN: Physiological integrity; CNS: Physiological adaptation; CL: Knowledge

38. Which finding is expected during an assessment of a child with an acyanotic heart defect?
1. Excess weight gain
2. Bradycardia
3. Hepatomegaly
4. Decreased respiratory rate

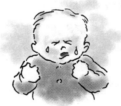

I'm telling you I'm not cyanotic!

38. 3. Hepatomegaly may result from blood backing up into the liver due to increased resistance in the right side of the heart. Poor growth and development, not excess weight gain, may be seen because of the increased energy required for breathing. The increase in blood flow to the lungs may cause tachycardia (not bradycardia) and increased respiratory rate to compensate.
CN: Physiological integrity; CNS: Physiological adaptation; CL: Application

39. A pediatric client is scheduled for echocardiography. The nurse is providing teaching to the client's mother. Which statement about echocardiography indicates the need for further teaching?
1. "I'm glad my child won't have an I.V. catheter inserted for this procedure."
2. "I'm glad my child won't need to have dye injected before the procedure."
3. "How am I ever going to explain to my son that he can't have anything to eat before the test?"
4. "I know my child may need to lie on his left side and breathe in and out slowly during the procedure."

39. 3. Echocardiography is a noninvasive procedure used to evaluate the size, shape, and motion of various cardiac structures. Therefore, it isn't necessary for the client to have an I.V. catheter, dye injected, or restrictions such as nothing by mouth, as would be the case with a cardiac catheterization. The child may need to lie on his left side and inhale and exhale slowly during the procedure.
CN: Physiological integrity; CNS: Reduction of risk potential; CL: Analysis

CN: Client needs category   CNS: Client needs subcategory   CL: Cognitive level

40. Which sign may be seen in a child with ventricular septal defect?
1. Clubbing of the fingers
2. Above average height on growth chart
3. Above average weight gain on growth chart
4. Pink nailbeds with capillary refill less than 2 seconds

41. When caring for a child diagnosed with a ventricular septal defect, which description would the nurse incorporate when talking with the parents about this condition?
1. Narrowing of the aortic arch
2. Failure of a septum to develop completely between the atria
3. Narrowing of the valves at the entrance of the pulmonary artery
4. Failure of a septum to develop completely between the ventricles

42. A 6-month-old infant with uncorrected tetralogy of Fallot suddenly becomes increasingly cyanotic and diaphoretic, with weak peripheral pulses and an increased respiratory rate. What should the nurse do <u>immediately</u>?
1. Administer oxygen.
2. Administer morphine sulfate.
3. Place the infant in a knee-chest position.
4. Place the infant in Fowler's position.

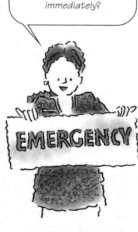

What should I do immediately?

43. A child with a ventricular septal repair is receiving dopamine (Intropin) postoperatively. The nurse should teach the child's parents that this medication is <u>most</u> likely to be given for which action?
1. To decrease the heart rate
2. To decrease urine output
3. To increase cardiac output
4. To decrease cardiac contractility

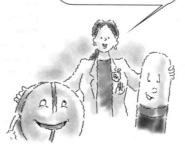

You know more about cardiac drugs than you realize!

40. 1. Clubbing and cyanotic nailbeds can be seen when shunting shifts right to left. These children usually show symptoms of poor growth and development, failure to thrive, and heart failure.
CN: Physiological integrity; CNS: Physiological adaptation; CL: Analysis

41. 4. Failure of a septum to develop between the ventricles results in a left-to-right shunt, which is noted as a ventricular septal defect. When the septum fails to develop between the atria, it's considered an atrial septal defect. The narrowing of the aortic arch describes coarctation of the aorta. Narrowing of the valves at the pulmonary artery describes pulmonary stenosis.
CN: Physiological integrity; CNS: Physiological adaptation; CL: Comprehension

42. 3. The knee-chest position reduces the workload of the heart by increasing the blood return to the heart and keeping the blood flow more centralized. Oxygen should be administered quickly but only after placing the infant in the knee-chest position. Morphine should be administered after positioning and oxygen administration are completed. Fowler's position wouldn't improve the situation.
CN: Physiological integrity; CNS: Physiological adaptation; CL: Application

43. 3. Dopamine stimulates $beta_1$ and $beta_2$ receptors. It's a selective cardiac stimulant that will increase cardiac output, heart rate, and cardiac contractility. Urine output increases in response to dilation of the blood vessels to the mesentery and kidneys.
CN: Physiological integrity; CNS: Pharmacological therapies; CL: Application

CN: Client needs category   CNS: Client needs subcategory   CL: Cognitive level

44. A child returns to his room after a cardiac catheterization. Which statement regarding mobility would be appropriate for the nurse to teach the child and parents?
1. The child may sit in a chair with the affected extremity immobilized.
2. The child will be maintained on bed rest with no further activity restrictions.
3. The child will be maintained on bed rest with the affected extremity immobilized.
4. The child may get out of bed to go to the bathroom, if necessary.

45. A nanny is taught to administer digoxin (Lanoxin) to a 6-month-old infant at home. Which statement by the nanny indicates the need for additional teaching?
1. "I'll count the baby's pulse before every dose."
2. "I'll make sure the pulse is regular before every dose."
3. "I'll measure the dose carefully."
4. "I'll withhold the medication if the pulse is below 60."

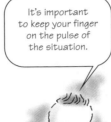

It's important to keep your finger on the pulse of the situation.

46. Which finding would concern the nurse who's caring for an infant after a right femoral cardiac catheterization?
1. Weak right dorsalis pedis pulse
2. Elevated temperature
3. Decreased urine output
4. Slight bloody drainage around catheterization site dressing

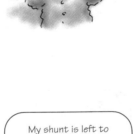

My shunt is left to right. How about yours?

47. Which cardiac anomaly produces a left-to-right shunt?
1. Atrial septal defect
2. Pulmonic stenosis
3. Tetralogy of Fallot
4. Total anomalous pulmonary venous return

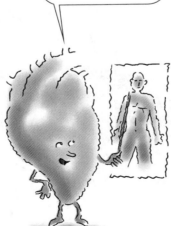

44. 3. The child should be maintained on bed rest with the affected extremity immobilized after cardiac catheterization to prevent hemorrhage. Allowing the child to sit in a chair with the affected extremity immobilized, to move the affected extremity while on bed rest, or to have bathroom privileges places him at risk for hemorrhage.
CN: Physiological integrity; CNS: Reduction of risk potential; CL: Application

45. 4. A pulse rate under 60 beats/minute is an indication for withholding digoxin from an adult. Withholding digoxin from an infant is appropriate if the infant's pulse is under 90 beats/minute. The pulse rate must be counted before each dose of digoxin is given to an infant. An irregular pulse may be a sign of digoxin toxicity; if this occurs, the physician should be consulted before the drug is given. The dose must be measured carefully to decrease the risk of toxicity.
CN: Physiological integrity; CNS: Pharmacological therapies; CL: Application

46. 1. The pulse below the catheterization site should be strong and equal to the unaffected extremity. A weakened pulse may indicate vessel obstruction or perfusion problems. Elevated temperature and decreased urine output are relatively normal findings after catheterization and may be the result of decreased oral fluids. A small amount of bloody drainage is normal; however, the site must be assessed frequently for increased bleeding.
CN: Physiological integrity; CNS: Reduction of risk potential; CL: Application

47. 1. Atrial septal defects shunt from left to right because pressures are greater on the left side of the heart. Pulmonary stenosis, tetralogy of Fallot, and total anomalous pulmonary venous return will show a right-to-left shunting of blood.
CN: Health promotion and maintenance; CNS: None; CL: Analysis

CN: Client needs category CNS: Client needs subcategory CL: Cognitive level

48. A child with an atrial septal repair is entering postoperative day 3. Which intervention would be <u>most appropriate</u>?
1. Give the child nothing by mouth.
2. Maintain strict bed rest.
3. Take vital signs every 8 hours.
4. Administer an analgesic as needed.

49. A 3-year-old child is on postoperative day 5 for an atrial septal repair. Which nursing diagnosis would be most appropriate?
1. *Activity intolerance*
2. *Chronic pain*
3. *Social isolation*
4. *Risk for imbalanced fluid volume*

50. Which condition best describes coarctation of the aorta?
1. Absent tricuspid valve
2. Narrowing in the area of the aortic valve
3. Localized constriction or narrowing of the aortic wall
4. Narrowing at some location along the right ventricular outflow tract

51. A client is diagnosed with coarctation of the aorta. Which finding would the nurse expect when observing this client?
1. Normal blood pressure
2. Increased blood pressure in the upper extremities
3. Decreased blood pressure in the upper extremities
4. Decreased or absent pulses in the upper extremities

48. 4. Pain management is always a priority and should be given on an as-needed basis. By day 3, the child should be advancing to a regular diet. Activity should be allowed as able in the step-down unit, with coughing and deep-breathing exercises. Vital signs should be performed routinely every 2 to 4 hours.
CN: Physiological integrity; CNS: Physiological adaptation; CL: Application

49. 4. Diuretics are still being used as needed at this point. By day 5, the child's activity level will be normal, and there will be little to no pain. The child isn't isolated from anyone and can usually attend the playroom on day 3 or 4.
CN: Physiological integrity; CNS: Physiological adaptation; CL: Analysis

50. 3. Coarctation of the aorta consists of a localized constriction or narrowing of the aortic wall. Tricuspid atresia is characterized by an absent tricuspid valve. Aortic stenosis is a narrowing in the area of the aortic valve. Pulmonary stenosis consists of a narrowing along the right ventricular outflow tract.
CN: Health promotion and maintenance; CNS: None; CL: Knowledge

51. 2. As blood is pumped from the left ventricle to the aorta, some blood flows to the head and upper extremities while the rest meets obstruction and jets through the constricted area. Pressures and pulses are greater in the upper extremities. Decreased or absent pulses are found in the lower extremities.
CN: Physiological integrity; CNS: Physiological adaptation; CL: Analysis

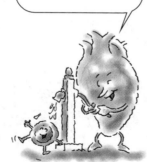

We're really pumped up about your progress on these practice questions.

52. A child with coarctation of the aorta experiences a postsurgical recoarctation. Which treatment should the nurse <u>expect</u> the physician to recommend?

1. Bypass graft repair
2. Patch aortoplasty
3. Balloon angioplasty
4. Left subclavian flap angioplasty

53. Which factor is an important part of observing a child with a possible cardiac anomaly?

1. Heart rate
2. Temperature
3. Blood pressure
4. Blood pressure in four extremities

54. Which intervention is recommended postoperatively for a client with repair of a coarctation of the aorta?

1. Give a vasoconstrictor.
2. Maintain hypothermia.
3. Maintain a low blood pressure.
4. Give a bolus of I.V. fluids.

55. Which observation is expected in a child with tetralogy of Fallot?

1. Machinelike murmur
2. Eisenmenger's complex
3. Increasing cyanosis with crying or activity
4. Higher pressure in the upper extremities than in the lower extremities

56. A child with tetralogy of Fallot has clubbing of the fingers and toes. The nurse understands that this finding is related to which condition?

1. Polycythemia
2. Chronic hypoxia
3. Pansystolic murmur
4. Abnormal growth and development

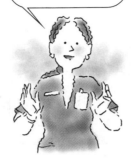

In question 52, pay attention to the word recoarctation.

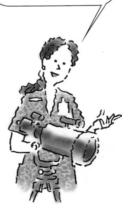

When it comes to observations, practice makes perfect!

52. 3. Balloon angioplasty is the treatment of choice for postsurgical recoarctation. Bypass graft repair, patch aortoplasty, and left subclavian flap angioplasty are surgical options to treat the original coarctation.
CN: Physiological integrity; CNS: Physiological adaptation; CL: Analysis

53. 4. Measuring blood pressure in all four extremities is necessary to document hypertension and the blood pressure gradient between the upper and lower extremities. Heart rate and temperature are also important observations.
CN: Physiological integrity; CNS: Physiological adaptation; CL: Application

54. 3. Blood pressure is tightly managed and kept low so there's no excessive pressure on the fresh suture lines. Normal body temperature is maintained, and diuretics may be given to decrease fluid volume.
CN: Physiological integrity; CNS: Physiological adaptation; CL: Analysis

55. 3. A child with tetralogy of Fallot will be mildly cyanotic at rest and have increasing cyanosis with crying, activity, or straining, as with a bowel movement. A machinelike murmur is a characteristic of patent ductus arteriosus. Eisenmenger's complex is a complication of ventricular resistance exceeding systemic pressure. Higher pressures in the upper extremities are characteristic of coarctation of the aorta.
CN: Physiological integrity; CNS: Physiological adaptation; CL: Application

56. 2. Chronic hypoxia causes clubbing of the fingers and toes when untreated. Hypoxia varies with the degree of pulmonary stenosis. Polycythemia is an increased number of red blood cells as a result of chronic hypoxemia. A pansystolic murmur is heard at the middle to lower left sternal border but has no impact on clubbing. Growth and development may appear normal.
CN: Physiological integrity; CNS: Physiological adaptation; CL: Comprehension

CN: Client needs category   CNS: Client needs subcategory   CL: Cognitive level

57. A child with tetralogy of Fallot may assume which position of comfort during exercise?
1. Prone
2. Semi-Fowler's
3. Side-lying
4. Squat

57. 4. A child may squat or assume a knee-chest position to reduce venous blood flow from the lower extremities and to increase systemic vascular resistance, which diverts more blood flow into the pulmonary artery. Prone, semi-Fowler's, and side-lying positions won't produce this effect.
CN: Physiological integrity; CNS: Physiological adaptation; CL: Analysis

58. A nurse is describing tetralogy of Fallot to a child's parents. Which statement by the parents demonstrates that the teaching has been effective?
1. "The condition is commonly referred to as 'blue tets.'"
2. "A child with this condition experiences hypercyanotic, or 'tet,' spells."
3. "A child with this condition experiences frequent respiratory infections."
4. "A child with this condition experiences decreased or absent pulses in the lower extremities."

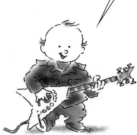

I don't think I have the blues today, but there's a spell that's over me...

58. 2. Hypercyanotic, or "tet" spells may occur due to increasing obstruction of right ventricular outflow, resulting in decreased pulmonary blood flow and increased right-to-left shunting. Infants with mild obstruction to blood flow have little or no right-to-left shunting and appear pink, or "pink tets." Frequent respiratory infections are seen in defects with increased pulmonary blood flow such as a patent ductus arteriosus. Decreased or absent pulses in the lower extremities are a sign of coarctation of the aorta.
CN: Physiological integrity; CNS: Physiological adaptation; CL: Analysis

59. Which test would show the direction and amount of shunting in a child with tetralogy of Fallot?
1. Chest radiography
2. Echocardiography
3. Electrocardiography
4. Cardiac catheterization

59. 4. Cardiac catheterization provides specific information about the direction and amount of shunting, coronary anatomy, and each portion of the heart defect. Chest radiographs will show right ventricular hypertrophy pushing the heart apex upward, resulting in a boot-shaped silhouette. Echocardiogram scans define such defects as large ventricular septal defects, pulmonary stenosis, and malposition of the aorta. Electrocardiograms show right ventricular hypertrophy with tall R waves.
CN: Physiological integrity; CNS: Physiological adaptation; CL: Knowledge

60. A nurse is teaching parents about tricuspid atresia. Which statement indicates the parents understand?
1. "There's a narrowing at the aortic outflow tract."
2. "The pulmonary veins don't return to the left atrium."
3. "There's a narrowing at the entrance of the pulmonary artery."
4. "There's no communication between the right atrium and the right ventricle."

60. 4. Tricuspid atresia is failure of the tricuspid valve to develop, leaving no communication between the right atrium and the right ventricle. Narrowing at the aortic outflow tract is aortic stenosis. Total anomalous pulmonary venous return is a defect in which the pulmonary veins don't return to the left atrium but abnormally return to the right side of the heart. Narrowing at the entrance of the pulmonary artery represents pulmonary stenosis.
CN: Physiological integrity; CNS: Physiological adaptation; CL: Analysis

CN: Client needs category   CNS: Client needs subcategory   CL: Cognitive level

61. Which characteristic can be noted when observing a child with tricuspid atresia?
1. Cyanosis
2. Machinelike murmur
3. Decreased respiratory rate
4. Capillary refill more than 2 seconds

61. 1. Cyanosis is the most consistent clinical sign of tricuspid atresia. A machinelike murmur is characteristic of a patent ductus arteriosus. Tricuspid atresia doesn't have a characteristic murmur. Tachypnea and dyspnea are typically present because of the pulmonary blood flow and right-to-left shunting. Decreased oxygenation would increase capillary refill time.
CN: Physiological integrity; CNS: Physiological adaptation; CL: Analysis

62. Which laboratory finding is expected in a child with tricuspid atresia?
1. Acidosis
2. Alkalosis
3. Normal red blood cell (RBC) count
4. Normal arterial oxygen saturation

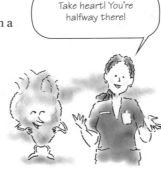

Take heart! You're halfway there!

62. 1. In tricuspid atresia, the tricuspid valve is completely closed so that no blood flows from the right atrium to the right ventricle. Therefore, no oxygenation of blood occurs. The child has chronic hypoxemia and acidosis, not alkalosis, due to decreased atrial oxygenation. This chronic hypoxemia leads to polycythemia, so a normal RBC wouldn't result. There's no normal arterial oxygenation as the blood bypasses the lungs and the step of oxygenation.
CN: Physiological integrity; CNS: Physiological adaptation; CL: Analysis

63. Which guideline should the nurse follow when administering digoxin (Lanoxin) to an infant?
1. Mix the digoxin with the infant's food.
2. Double the subsequent dose if a dose is missed.
3. Give the digoxin with antacids when possible.
4. Withhold the dose if the apical pulse rate is less than 90 beats/minute.

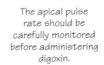

The apical pulse rate should be carefully monitored before administering digoxin.

63. 4. Digoxin is used to decrease heart rate; however, the apical pulse must be carefully monitored to detect a severe reduction. Administering digoxin to an infant with a heart rate of less than 90 beats/minute could further reduce the rate and compromise cardiac output. Mixing digoxin with other food may interfere with accurate dosing. Double-dosing should never be done. Antacids may decrease drug absorption.
CN: Physiological integrity; CNS: Pharmacological therapies; CL: Application

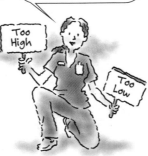

64. Which condition <u>best</u> describes total anomalous pulmonary venous return?
1. Pulmonary veins that don't return to the left atrium
2. A cyanotic defect with decreased pulmonary blood flow
3. An acyanotic defect with increased pulmonary blood flow
4. A single large vessel that arises from both ventricles astride a large ventricular septal defect

64. 1. Total anomalous pulmonary venous return is a condition in which the pulmonary veins don't return to the left atrium; instead, they abnormally return to the right side of the heart. This defect is classified as a cyanotic defect with increased pulmonary blood flow. A single large vessel arising from both ventricles astride a large ventricular septal defect describes truncus arteriosus.
CN: Health promotion and maintenance; CNS: None; CL: Knowledge

65. Of the four different ways the pulmonary veins may be abnormally routed with a total anomalous pulmonary venous return defect, which type would the nurse expect is most common?
1. Cardiac
2. Infracardiac
3. Supracardiac
4. Mixed combination of supracardiac, cardiac, and infracardiac

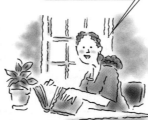

Question 65 asks about what occurs most commonly.

66. Which finding is common during an assessment of a child with a total anomalous pulmonary venous return defect?
1. Hypertension
2. Frequent respiratory infections
3. Normal growth and development
4. Above average weight gain on the growth chart

67. A child has undergone a repair of total anomalous pulmonary venous return. Which finding would the nurse be most likely to observe in a child with this condition?
1. Hypotension
2. Hypertension
3. Bradycardia
4. Tachypnea

68. Which statement about truncus arteriosus is correct?
1. It's classified as an acyanotic defect.
2. Systemic and pulmonary blood mix.
3. It can't be diagnosed until after birth.
4. There are two types of truncus arteriosus.

65. 3. Supracardiac, the most common type, is characterized by the pulmonary veins draining directly into the superior vena cava. With the cardiac type, the pulmonary veins drain into the coronary sinuses or directly flow into the right atrium. The infracardiac type shows the common pulmonary vein running below the diaphragm into the portal system. The fourth type is a mixed combination of less common types.
CN: Health promotion and maintenance; CNS: None; CL: Comprehension

66. 2. Children with total anomalous pulmonary venous return defects are prone to repeated respiratory infections due to increased pulmonary blood flow. Hypertension usually occurs with coarctation of the aorta, an acyanotic defect with obstructive flow. Poor feeding and failure to thrive are also signs. Infants look thin and malnourished.
CN: Physiological integrity; CNS: Physiological adaptation; CL: Application

67. 4. Pulmonary hypertension may result as a postoperative complication of this procedure and can cause hypoxia. Symptoms include tachypnea, cyanosis, chest retractions, and fatigue.
CN: Physiological integrity; CNS: Physiological adaptation; CL: Application

68. 2. Blood ejects from the left and right ventricles and enters a common trunk, mixing pulmonary and systemic blood. It's classified as a cyanotic defect with increased pulmonary blood flow. Diagnosis can be made in utero using echocardiography. Truncus arteriosus can be divided into four types or categories.
CN: Health promotion and maintenance; CNS: None; CL: Knowledge

69. Which finding would a nurse <u>expect</u> to observe in a child with truncus arteriosus?
1. Weak, thready pulses
2. Narrowed pulse pressure
3. Pink, moist mucous membranes
4. Harsh systolic ejection murmur

70. Treatment for truncus arteriosus includes digoxin (Lanoxin) and diuretics. Which technique would be <u>best</u> for giving these drugs to an infant?
1. Use a measuring spoon.
2. Use a graduated dropper.
3. Mix the drug with baby food.
4. Mix the drug in a bottle with juice or milk.

71. Which statement best describes transposition of the great arteries?
1. The body receives only saturated blood.
2. It's classified as an acyanotic defect with increased pulmonary blood flow.
3. The pulmonary artery leaves the left ventricle, and the aorta exits from the right ventricle.
4. The right atrium and the left atrium empty into one ventricular chamber.

72. Which statement about transposition of the great arteries is correct?
1. Electrocardiography will always show arrhythmias.
2. Diagnosis can be made in utero.
3. Chest X-ray can show an accurate view of the defect.
4. Heart failure isn't a related complication.

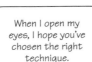

When I open my eyes, I hope you've chosen the right technique.

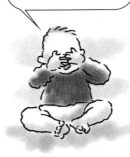

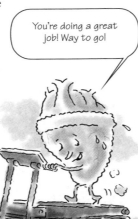

You're doing a great job! Way to go!

69. 4. As a result of the ventricular septal defect, a harsh systolic ejection murmur is heard along the left sternal border and is usually accompanied by a thrill. Increasing pulmonary blood flow causes bounding pulses and a widened pulse pressure. Pulmonary stenosis leads to mild or moderate cyanosis, so mucous membranes may appear dull or gray.
CN: Physiological integrity; CNS: Physiological adaptation; CL: Application

70. 2. Using a graduated dropper allows the exact dosage to be given. A teaspoon isn't as exact as a graduated dropper. Mixing drugs with juice, milk, or food may cause a problem because, if the child doesn't completely finish the meal, you can't determine the exact amount ingested. In addition, this may prevent the child from drinking or eating for fear of tasting the drug.
CN: Physiological integrity; CNS: Pharmacological therapies; CL: Application

71. 3. Transposition of the great arteries is a condition in which the pulmonary artery leaves the left ventricle and the aorta exits from the right ventricle. This type of circulation gives the body only desaturated blood. The mixing of blood characterizes this defect as a cyanotic defect with variable pulmonary blood flow or as a mixed defect. A single-ventricle defect is a condition in which the right and left atria empty into one ventricular chamber.
CN: Health promotion and maintenance; CNS: None; CL: Knowledge

72. 2. Echocardiography done by a fetal cardiologist can diagnose transposition of the great arteries in utero. The other defects associated with this condition include a patent foramen ovale and a ventricular septal defect that contribute to developing heart failure. Electrocardiography may or may not reveal arrhythmias. Chest X-ray can show cardiomegaly and pulmonary vascular markings only. Echocardiography or cardiac catheterization may be required preoperatively to show the coronary artery anatomy before surgical repair.
CN: Physiological integrity; CNS: Physiological adaptation; CL: Analysis

CN: Client needs category   CNS: Client needs subcategory   CL: Cognitive level

73. A nurse is caring for a child with transposition of the great arteries. Which associated defect should the nurse expect to see in this client?
1. Mitral atresia
2. Atrial septal defect
3. Patent foramen ovale
4. Hypoplasia of the left ventricle

73. 3. A patent foramen ovale, patent ductus arteriosus, and ventricular septal defect are associated defects related to transposition of the great arteries. An atrial septal defect is common in association with total anomalous pulmonary venous return. A patent foramen ovale is the most common and is necessary to provide adequate mixing of blood between the two circulations. Hypoplasia of the left ventricle and mitral atresia are two defects associated with hypoplastic left heart syndrome.
CN: Physiological integrity; CNS: Physiological adaptation; CL: Analysis

74. Which change would the nurse expect after administering oxygen to an infant with uncorrected tetralogy of Fallot?
1. Disappearance of the murmur
2. No evidence of cyanosis
3. Improvement of finger clubbing
4. Less agitation

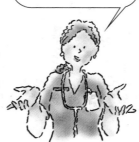

Don't get anxious about this question. Just take a deep breath and go for it!

74. 4. Supplemental oxygen will help the infant breathe more easily and feel less anxious or agitated. None of the other findings would occur as the result of supplemental oxygen administration.
CN: Physiological integrity; CNS: Basic care and comfort; CL: Application

75. Which surgical repair is recommended for a neonate whose aorta arises from the right ventricle and pulmonary artery arises from the left ventricle?
1. Jatene procedure
2. Fontan procedure
3. Balloon atrial septostomy
4. Blalock-Taussig operation

75. 1. Transposition of the great arteries occurs when the aorta arises from the right ventricle and the pulmonary artery arises from the left ventricle. The Jatene procedure involves transposing the great arteries and mobilizing and reimplanting the coronary arteries. The Fontan procedure is recommended for repair of tricuspid atresia. Balloon atrial septostomy is a palliative procedure used during cardiac catheterization for those children without a coexisting lesion. The Blalock-Taussig operation is used to palliate tricuspid atresia and pulmonic atresia.
CN: Physiological integrity; CNS: Physiological adaptation; CL: Application

76. Which statement best describes a characteristic of valvular pulmonic stenosis?
1. The valve is normal.
2. The right ventricle is hypoplastic.
3. Left ventricular hypertrophy develops.
4. Divisions between the cusps are fused.

76. 4. Blood flow through the pulmonic valve is restricted by fusion of the divisions between the cusps. The valve may be normal or malformed. Right ventricular hypertrophy, not hypoplasia, develops due to the increased resistance to blood flow. The left ventricle isn't affected.
CN: Physiological integrity; CNS: Physiological adaptation; CL: Analysis

77. The nurse is planning care for a 9-year-old male child with heart failure. Which nursing diagnosis should receive <u>priority</u>?
1. *Ineffective tissue perfusion (cardiopulmonary, renal) related to sympathetic response to heart failure*
2. *Imbalanced nutrition: Less than body requirements related to rapid tiring while feeding*
3. *Anxiety (parent) related to unknown nature of child's illness*
4. *Decreased cardiac output related to cardiac defect*

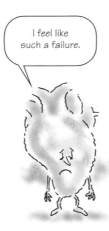

I feel like such a failure.

77. 4. The primary nursing diagnosis for a child with heart failure is *Decreased cardiac output related to cardiac defect.* The most common cause of heart failure in children is congenital heart defects. Some defects result from the blood being pumped from the left side of the heart to the right side of the heart. The heart can't manage the extra volume, resulting in the pulmonary system becoming overloaded. Ineffective tissue perfusion, imbalanced nutrition, and anxiety don't take priority over decreased cardiac output. The child's heart must produce cardiac output sufficient to meet the body's metabolic demands.
CN: Physiological integrity; CNS: Physiological adaptation; CL: Application

78. Which finding is seen during cardiac catheterization of a child with pulmonic stenosis?
1. Right-to-left shunting
2. Left-to-right shunting
3. Decreased pressure in the right side of the heart
4. Increased oxygenation in the left side of the heart

78. 1. Right-to-left shunting develops through a patent foramen ovale due to right ventricular failure and an increase in pressure in the right side of the heart. Decreased oxygenation in the left side of the heart is noted due to the right-to-left shunt.
CN: Physiological integrity; CNS: Physiological adaptation; CL: Analysis

79. Which finding is associated with aortic stenosis?
1. Hypotension
2. Right ventricular failure
3. Increased cardiac output
4. Loud systolic murmur with a thrill

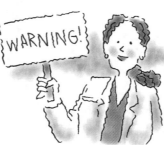

WARNING!

79. 1. Older children with aortic stenosis are at risk for hypotension, tachycardia, angina, syncope, left ventricular failure, dyspnea, fatigue, and palpitations. Poor left ventricular ejection leads to decreased cardiac output. Loud systolic murmurs are heard with ventricular septal defects.
CN: Physiological integrity; CNS: Physiological adaptation; CL: Knowledge

80. A nurse is teaching the parents of a child with congenital aortic stenosis. Which statement should the nurse include in her teaching about this disorder?
1. It can result from rheumatic fever (infection with group A streptococci).
2. It accounts for 25% of all congenital defects.
3. It causes an increase in cardiac output.
4. It's classified as an acyanotic defect with increased pulmonary blood flow.

80. 1. Aortic stenosis can result from rheumatic fever, which can damage the aortic valve in the first 8 weeks of pregnancy. It accounts for about 5% of all congenital heart defects. It causes a decrease in cardiac output. It's classified as an acyanotic defect with obstructed flow from the ventricles.
CN: Physiological integrity; CNS: Physiological adaptation; CL: Analysis

CN: Client needs category   CNS: Client needs subcategory   CL: Cognitive level

81. Which instruction would be <u>most appropriate</u> for a child with symptomatic aortic stenosis?
1. Restrict exercise.
2. Avoid prostaglandin E_1.
3. Avoid digoxin (Lanoxin) and diuretics.
4. Allow the child to exercise freely.

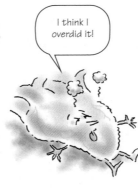

81. 1. Exercise should be restricted due to low cardiac output and left ventricular failure. Prostaglandin E_1 is recommended to maintain the patency of the ductus arteriosus in neonates. This allows for improved systemic blood flow. Digoxin and diuretics may be required for critically ill children experiencing heart failure as a result of severe aortic stenosis. Strenuous activity has been reported to result in sudden death from the development of myocardial ischemia.
CN: Physiological integrity; CNS: Physiological adaptation; CL: Application

82. Which statement is correct for hypoplastic left heart syndrome?
1. It can be diagnosed only at birth.
2. It includes a group of related anomalies.
3. It's classified as 25% of all congenital defects.
4. Surgical intervention is the only option for treatment.

82. 2. Hypoplastic left heart syndrome includes a group of related anomalies, such as hypoplasia of the left ventricle, mitral atresia, aortic atresia, and hypoplasia of the ascending aorta and aortic arch. It can be diagnosed prenatally with a level 2 ultrasound examination. It's classified as about 1% to 2% of all congenital defects. Treatment options include palliative surgery, cardiac transplantation, or no intervention, in which case death would occur.
CN: Health promotion and maintenance; CNS: None; CL: Knowledge

83. Which nursing diagnosis is the <u>most appropriate</u> when caring for an infant with hypoplastic left heart syndrome?
1. *Anticipatory grieving*
2. *Delayed growth and development*
3. *Deficient diversional activity*
4. *Risk for activity intolerance*

83. 1. Without intervention, death usually occurs within the first few days of life due to progressive hypoxia, acidosis, and shock as the ductus closes and systemic perfusion diminishes. If the parents choose cardiac transplantation, the child may die waiting for a donor heart. For those who choose surgery, the child may not survive the three stages of the surgery. The other three choices don't apply to this type of defect due to the low survival rates.
CN: Physiological integrity; CNS: Physiological adaptation; CL: Analysis

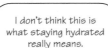

84. A 3-year-old client has a high red blood cell count and polycythemia. In planning care, the nurse would anticipate which goal to help prevent blood clot formation?
1. The child won't have signs of dehydration.
2. The child won't have signs of dyspnea.
3. The child will be pain-free.
4. The child will attain the 40th percentile of weight for his age.

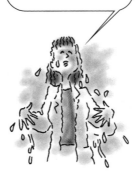

84. 1. When dehydration occurs, blood is thicker and more prone to clotting. Dyspnea would be a sign of hypoxia. Pain would be an indicator of nutritional status, not the risk of embolism. Weight gain wouldn't affect blood clot formation.
CN: Physiological integrity; CNS: Reduction of risk potential; CL: Application

85. A child receives prednisone after a heart transplant. Prednisone is in which drug classification?
1. Antibiotic
2. Cardiac glycoside
3. Corticosteroid
4. Diuretic

86. A child is given 0.5 mg/kg/day of prednisone divided into two doses. The child weighs 10 kg. How much is given in each dose?
1. 2.5 mg
2. 5 mg
3. 10 mg
4. 1.5 mg

87. Which adverse reaction of prednisone would a nurse expect to observe in a child who has received a heart transplant?
1. Weight loss
2. Hyperpyrexia
3. Anorexia
4. Poor wound healing

88. Which statement about bacterial/infective endocarditis is <u>most</u> accurate?
1. It's bacteria invading only tissues of the heart.
2. It's an infection of the valves and inner lining of the heart.
3. It's an inappropriate fusion of the endocardial cushions in fetal life.
4. It's caused by alterations in cardiac preload, afterload, contractility, or heart rate.

89. A child with suspected bacterial endocarditis arrives at the emergency department. Which finding is expected during data collection?
1. Weight gain
2. Bradycardia
3. Low-grade fever
4. Increased hemoglobin level

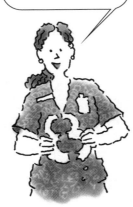

Math problems got you stumped? Just break each problem into manageable pieces, one by one.

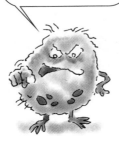

Hey, am I to blame for this or what?

85. 3. Prednisone is a corticosteroid used frequently during posttransplantation as part of antirejection therapy. The drug influences the immune system through its strong anti-inflammatory action and immunologic effect. The other three classes of drugs aren't indicated in this situation.
CN: Physiological integrity; CNS: Pharmacological therapies; CL: Knowledge

86. 1. The child should receive 2.5 mg/dose. Use the following equations:
0.5 mg/kg × 10 kg = 5 mg;
5 mg/2 doses = 2.5 mg/dose.
CN: Physiological integrity; CNS: Pharmacological therapies; CL: Analysis

87. 4. Common adverse reactions of prednisone include poor wound healing, weight gain, delayed temperature response, increased appetite, delayed sexual maturation, growth impairment, and a cushingoid appearance. The school-age child who has received prednisone is usually overweight and has a moon-shaped face.
CN: Physiological integrity; CNS: Physiological adaptation; CL: Application

88. 2. Bacterial/infective endocarditis is an infection of the valves and inner lining of the heart. It's usually caused by the bacteria *Streptococcus viridans* and frequently affects children with acquired or congenital anomalies of the heart or great vessels. Bacteria may grow into adjacent tissues and may break off and embolize elsewhere, such as the spleen, kidney, lung, skin, and central nervous system. Endocardial cushion defects represent inappropriate fusion of the endocardial cushions in fetal life. Alterations in preload, afterload, contractility, or heart rate refer to heart failure.
CN: Physiological integrity; CNS: Physiological adaptation; CL: Application

89. 3. Symptoms may include a low-grade intermittent fever, tachycardia, anorexia, weight loss, decreased activity level, and a decrease in hemoglobin level.
CN: Physiological integrity; CNS: Physiological adaptation; CL: Application

CN: Client needs category   CNS: Client needs subcategory   CL: Cognitive level

90. Which factor may lead to bacterial endocarditis in a child with underlying heart disease?

1. History of a cold for 3 days
2. Dental work pretreated with antibiotics
3. Peripheral I.V. catheter in place for 1 day
4. Indwelling urinary catheter for 2 days leading to a urinary tract infection

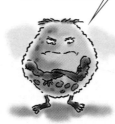

I'll find my way into the bloodstream one way or another.

90. 4. Bacterial organisms can enter the bloodstream from any site of infection such as a urinary tract infection. Gram-negative bacilli are common causative agents. A peripheral I.V. catheter is an entry site but only if signs and symptoms of infection are present. Colds are usually viral, not bacterial. Dental work is a common portal of entry if not pretreated with antibiotics. Long-term indwelling catheters pose a higher risk of infection. Heart surgery is also a common cause of endocarditis, especially if synthetic material is used.

CN: Physiological integrity; CNS: Physiological adaptation; CL: Analysis

91. Erythromycin (E-Mycin) is given to a 6-year-old child before dental work to prevent endocarditis. The child weighs 44 lb. The order is for 20 mg/kg by mouth 2 hours before the procedure. How many milligrams would that be?

1. 200 mg
2. 400 mg
3. 440 mg
4. 880 mg

91. 2. The child should receive 400 mg. Use the following equations:

$$44 \text{ lb}/2.2 \text{ kg} = 20 \text{ kg};$$
$$20 \text{ mg/kg} \times 20 \text{ kg} = 400 \text{ mg}.$$

CN: Physiological integrity; CNS: Pharmacological therapies; CL: Analysis

92. What would be the <u>most</u> common adverse reaction a nurse might <u>observe</u> after administering enteric-coated erythromycin (Ery-Tab)?

1. Weight gain
2. Constipation
3. Increased appetite
4. Nausea and vomiting

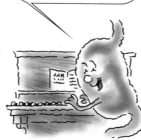

To avoid my playing off tune, be sure to take certain medications with a full glass of water.

92. 4. Erythromycin is an antibacterial antibiotic. Common adverse effects include nausea, vomiting, anorexia, diarrhea, and abdominal pain. It should be given with a full glass (8 ounces) of water and after meals or with food to lessen GI symptoms.

CN: Physiological integrity; CNS: Pharmacological therapies; CL: Application

93. A child is hospitalized with bacterial endocarditis. Which nursing diagnosis is <u>most appropriate</u>?

1. *Constipation*
2. *Excess fluid volume*
3. *Deficient diversional activity*
4. *Imbalanced nutrition: More than body requirements*

93. 3. Treatment for bacterial endocarditis requires long-term hospitalization or home care for I.V. antibiotics. Children may be bored and depressed, needing age-appropriate activities. *Diarrhea, Deficient fluid volume,* and *Imbalanced nutrition: Less than body requirements* may be possible nursing diagnoses related to such adverse reactions of antibiotics as GI upset.

CN: Physiological integrity; CNS: Physiological adaptation; CL: Analysis

CN: Client needs category   CNS: Client needs subcategory   CL: Cognitive level

94. When assessing a child with suspected Kawasaki disease, which symptom is common?
1. Low-grade fever
2. "Strawberry" tongue
3. Pink, moist mucous membranes
4. Abdominal pain

94. 2. Inflammation of the pharynx and oral mucosa develops, causing red, cracked lips and a "strawberry" tongue, in which the normal coating of the tongue sloughs off. A high fever of 5 or more days unresponsive to antibiotics and antipyretics is also part of the diagnostic criteria. Abdominal pain would suggest a possible GI problem.
CN: Physiological integrity; CNS: Physiological adaptation; CL: Knowledge

95. A nurse is teaching the parents of a child with Kawasaki disease. Which statement should the nurse include in her teaching about this disorder?
1. It mostly occurs in the summer and fall.
2. Diagnosis can be determined by laboratory testing.
3. It's an acute systemic vasculitis of unknown cause.
4. It manifests in two different stages: acute and subacute.

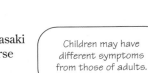

So much to know about one disease.

95. 3. Kawasaki disease can best be described as an acute systemic vasculitis of unknown cause. Most cases are geographic and seasonal, with most occurring in the late winter and early spring. Diagnosis is based on clinical findings of five of the six diagnostic criteria and associated laboratory results. There's no specific laboratory test for diagnosis. There are three stages: acute, subacute, and convalescent.
CN: Physiological integrity; CNS: Physiological adaptation; CL: Application

96. Which characteristic indicates a child with Kawasaki disease has entered the subacute phase?
1. Polymorphous rash
2. Normal blood values
3. Cervical lymphadenopathy
4. Desquamation of the hands and feet

96. 4. The subacute phase shows characteristic desquamation of the hands and feet. Blood values return to normal at the end of the convalescent phase. Polymorphous rash and cervical lymphadenopathy can be seen in the acute phase because of the onset of inflammation and fever.
CN: Physiological integrity; CNS: Physiological adaptation; CL: Analysis

97. A nurse is caring for a child with Kawasaki disease. Which symptom concerns the nurse the most?
1. Mild diarrhea
2. Pain in the joints
3. Abdominal pain with vomiting
4. Increased erythrocyte sedimentation rate

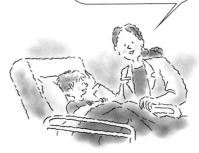

Children may have different symptoms from those of adults.

97. 3. The most serious complication of this disease is cardiac involvement. Abdominal pain, vomiting, and restlessness are the main symptoms of an acute myocardial infarction in children. Mild diarrhea can be treated with oral fluids. Pain in the joints is an expected sign of arthritis that usually occurs in the subacute phase. An increased erythrocyte sedimentation rate is a reflection of the inflammatory process and may be seen for 2 to 4 weeks after the onset of symptoms.
CN: Physiological integrity; CNS: Physiological adaptation; CL: Analysis

CN: Client needs category   CNS: Client needs subcategory   CL: Cognitive level

98. A nurse is caring for a 2-year-old toddler diagnosed with Kawasaki disease. The nurse must assess for which signs and symptoms in a child with Kawasaki disease?

1. Chest pain, dyspnea, fever, and headache
2. Fever, headache, and erythema marginatum
3. Bilateral conjunctivitis and strawberry tongue
4. Weight loss, abdominal pain, and cramping

99. Therapy for Kawasaki disease includes I.V. gamma globulin, prescribed at 400 mg/kg/day for 4 days. The child weighs 10 kg. What's the <u>daily</u> dose for this child?

1. 200 mg
2. 400 mg
3. 2,000 mg
4. 4,000 mg

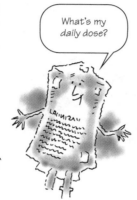

What's my daily dose?

100. A 2-month-old infant arrives in the emergency department with a heart rate of 180 beats/minute and a temperature of 103.1° F (39.5° C) rectally. Which intervention is <u>most</u> appropriate?

1. Give acetaminophen (Tylenol).
2. Encourage fluid intake.
3. Apply carotid massage.
4. Place the infant's hands in cold water.

101. A child is prescribed aspirin as part of the therapy for Kawasaki disease. The order is for 80 mg/kg/day orally in four divided doses until the child is afebrile. The child weighs 15 kg. How much is given in one dose?

1. 60 mg
2. 300 mg
3. 320 mg
4. 1,200 mg

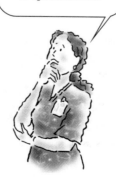

Let's see. Four daily doses. The child weighs 15 kg. I can do this.

98. 3. Bilateral conjunctivitis and redness of the oral mucosa (strawberry tongue) are typically observed early in the illness. Chest pain and dyspnea are sometimes observed in endocarditis. Erythema marginatum is a rash observed in rheumatic fever. Weight loss, abdominal pain, and cramping are characteristic of ulcerative colitis.

CN: Physiological integrity; CNS: Physiological adaptation; CL: Analysis

99. 4. The child should receive 4,000 mg. Use the following equation:

400 mg/kg × 10 kg = 4,000 mg (or 4 g).

CN: Physiological integrity; CNS: Pharmacological therapies; CL: Analysis

100. 1. Acetaminophen should be given first to decrease the temperature. A heart rate of 180 beats/minute is normal in an infant with a fever. Fluid intake is encouraged after the acetaminophen is given to help replace insensible fluid losses. Carotid massage is an attempt to decrease the heart rate as a vagal maneuver. This won't work in this infant because the source of the increased heart rate is fever. A tepid sponge bath may be given to help decrease the temperature and calm the infant.

CN: Physiological integrity; CNS: Physiological adaptation; CL: Application

101. 2. The child should receive 300 mg. Use the following equations:

80 mg/kg × 15 kg = 1,200 mg;
1,200 mg/4 doses = 300 mg/dose.

CN: Physiological integrity; CNS: Pharmacological therapies; CL: Analysis

CN: Client needs category   CNS: Client needs subcategory   CL: Cognitive level

102. A nurse is giving discharge instructions to the parents of a child with Kawasaki disease. Which statement shows an understanding of the treatment plan?
1. "A regular diet can be resumed at home."
2. "Black, tarry stools are considered normal."
3. "My child should use a soft-bristled toothbrush."
4. "My child can return to playing football next week."

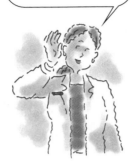

Listen for feedback to find out if your instructions were understood.

102. 3. Because of the anticoagulant effects of aspirin therapy, a soft-bristled toothbrush will prevent bleeding of the gums. A low-cholesterol diet should be followed until coronary artery involvement resolves, usually within 6 to 8 weeks. Black, tarry stools are abnormal and are signs of bleeding that should be reported to the physician immediately. Contact sports should be avoided because of the cardiac involvement and excessive bruising that may occur due to aspirin therapy.
CN: Physiological integrity; CNS: Physiological adaptation; CL: Analysis

103. A nurse is preparing the family of a client with Kawasaki disease for discharge. Which instruction is most appropriate?
1. Stop the aspirin when you return home.
2. Immunizations can be given in 2 weeks.
3. The child may return to school in 1 week.
4. Frequent echocardiography will be needed.

103. 4. Because of the risk of coronary artery involvement and possible aneurysm development, repeat echocardiography and electrocardiography will be required the first few weeks and at 6 months. Aspirin therapy may be continued for 2 weeks after the onset of symptoms. If signs of coronary artery involvement are present, aspirin therapy may be continued indefinitely. Live-virus vaccines should be avoided for at least 5 months after gamma globulin therapy because of an increased risk of a cross-sensitivity reaction to the antibodies found in the dose given. School should be avoided until cleared by the physician.
CN: Physiological integrity; CNS: Physiological adaptation; CL: Analysis

104. Which description of <u>acute</u> rheumatic fever is correct?
1. A progressive inflammation of the small vessels
2. A mucocutaneous lymph node syndrome
3. A serious infection of the endocardial surface of the heart
4. A sequela of group A beta-hemolytic streptococcal infections

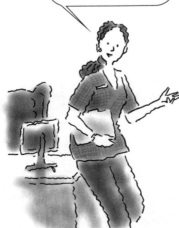

Question 104 asks about acute rheumatic fever, not chronic.

104. 4. Acute rheumatic fever is a multisystem disorder caused by group A beta-hemolytic streptococcal infections. It may involve the heart, joints, central nervous system, and skin. Kawasaki disease is a mucocutaneous lymph node syndrome characterized by a progressive inflammation of the small vessels. Endocarditis describes a serious infection of the endocardial surface of the heart.
CN: Health promotion and maintenance; CNS: None; CL: Knowledge

CN: Client needs category   CNS: Client needs subcategory   CL: Cognitive level

105. Which assessment finding is <u>expected</u> in a child with acute rheumatic fever?
1. Leukocyte count of 11,000/mm³
2. Normal electrocardiogram
3. High fever for 5 or more days
4. Normal erythrocyte sedimentation rate

106. Which criteria is required to establish a diagnosis of acute rheumatic fever?
1. Laboratory tests
2. Fever and four diagnostic criteria
3. Positive blood cultures for *Staphylococcus* organisms
4. Use of Jones criteria and presence of a streptococcal infection

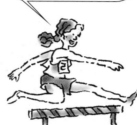

I'm just trying to keep up with the Joneses.

107. Which criteria would indicate the diagnosis of rheumatic fever?

Jones criteria for diagnosing rheumatic fever	
Major criteria	*Minor criteria*
• Carditis	• Fever
• Migratory polyarthritis	• Arthralgia
• Sydenham's chorea	• Elevated acute
• Subcutaneous nodules	phase reactants
• Erythema marginatum	• Prolonged PR
	interval

1. Carditis and fever
2. Carditis, fever, and arthralgia
3. Carditis and elevated acute phase reactants
4. Migratory polyarthritis and fever

Almost finished! Keep up the good work!

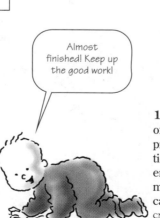

108. A nurse is caring for a child with acute rheumatic fever. Which symptom can be recognized as Sydenham's chorea, a major manifestation of acute rheumatic fever?
1. Cardiomegaly
2. Regurgitant murmur
3. Pericardial friction rubs
4. Involuntary muscle movements

105. 1. Leukocytosis can be seen as an immune response triggered by colonization of the pharynx with group A streptococci. The electrocardiogram will show a prolonged PR interval as a result of carditis. A low-grade fever is a minor manifestation. A high fever of 5 or more days may represent Kawasaki disease. The inflammatory response will cause an elevated erythrocyte sedimentation rate.
CN: Physiological integrity; CNS: Physiological adaptation; CL: Application

106. 4. Two major or one major and two minor manifestations from Jones criteria and the presence of a streptococcal infection justify the diagnosis of rheumatic fever. There's no single laboratory test for diagnosis. Fever and four diagnostic criteria are required to diagnose Kawasaki disease. Blood cultures would be positive for *Streptococcus*, not *Staphylococcus*, organisms.
CN: Physiological integrity; CNS: Physiological adaptation; CL: Analysis

107. 2. The Jones criteria are used to standardize the diagnosis of rheumatic fever. Diagnosis requires that either two major criteria, or one major criterion and two minor criteria be present, plus evidence of a previous group A hemolytic streptococcal infection.
CN: Physiological integrity; CNS: Physiological adaptation; CL: Analysis

108. 4. Sydenham's chorea is an involvement of the central nervous system by the rheumatic process. This is seen as muscular incoordination; purposeless, involuntary movements; and emotional lability. Cardiomegaly, a regurgitant murmur, and a pericardial friction rub are clinical signs of rheumatic carditis.
CN: Physiological integrity; CNS: Physiological adaptation; CL: Knowledge

CN: Client needs category   CNS: Client needs subcategory   CL: Cognitive level

109. Criteria for rheumatic fever are being discussed with parents. The nurse realizes that the parents understand chorea when they make which statement?
1. "My child may not be able to walk."
2. "Long movies may help for relaxation."
3. "My child might have difficulty in school."
4. "Many activities and visitors are recommended."

110. A 3-year-old child has a positive culture for *Streptococcus* organisms. Which intervention is <u>most appropriate</u>?
1. Give aspirin.
2. Give antibiotics.
3. Give corticosteroids.
4. Encourage fluid intake.

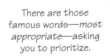

You better be sure you treat us right!

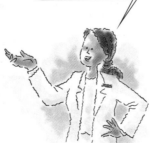

111. A nurse is preparing a child for discharge after being diagnosed with rheumatic fever without carditis. What instructions should the nurse give the parents?
1. Give aspirin for signs of chorea.
2. Give penicillin (Veetids) for 1 month total.
3. Only give penicillin for dental procedures.
4. It isn't necessary to give penicillin before dental procedures.

112. Which nursing diagnosis is <u>most appropriate</u> for a child with rheumatic fever?
1. *Imbalanced nutrition: More than body requirements*
2. *Risk for injury*
3. *Delayed growth and development*
4. *Impaired gas exchange*

There are those famous words—most appropriate—asking you to prioritize.

109. 3. Chorea may last 1 to 6 months. Central nervous system involvement contributes to a shortened attention span, so children might have difficulty learning in school. Muscle incoordination may cause the child to be more clumsy than usual when walking. A quiet environment is required for treatment.
CN: Physiological integrity; CNS: Physiological adaptation; CL: Analysis

110. 2. Infection caused by *Streptococcus* organisms is treated with antibiotics, mainly penicillin (Veetids). Antipyretics, such as acetaminophen (Tylenol), may be given for fever. Aspirin isn't recommended. Corticosteroids have no implication. Fluid intake is encouraged to prevent dehydration from decreased oral intake due to a sore throat or to replace fluids lost due to possible diarrhea from the antibiotics.
CN: Physiological integrity; CNS: Physiological adaptation; CL: Analysis

111. 4. Children who might benefit from prophylactic penicillin include those with unrepaired congenital heart defects, heart defects repaired with synthetic material, or prior infective endocarditis, and some children with heart transplants. Prophylactic antibiotic therapy isn't otherwise recommended.
CN: Physiological integrity; CNS: Pharmacological therapies; CL: Application

112. 2. Due to symptoms of chorea, safety measures should be taken to prevent falls or injury. There may be an imbalance in nutrition of less than body requirements because of a sore throat and dysphagia. Growth and development usually aren't delayed. Gas exchange usually isn't an issue unless the condition worsens with carditis and heart failure is present.
CN: Physiological integrity; CNS: Physiological adaptation; CL: Analysis

CN: Client needs category   CNS: Client needs subcategory   CL: Cognitive level

113. Sinus bradycardia can best be described as which condition?
1. Heart rate less than normal for age
2. Heart rate greater than normal for age
3. A variation of the normal cardiac rhythm
4. Increase in sinus node impulse formation

113. 1. Sinus bradycardia can best be described as a heart rate less than normal for age. Sinus tachycardia refers to a heart rate greater than normal for age or an increase in sinus node impulse formation. A sinus arrhythmia is a variation of the normal cardiac rhythm.
CN: Physiological integrity; CNS: Physiological adaptation; CL: Knowledge

114. In which condition or group is sinus bradycardia a <u>normal</u> finding?
1. Hypoxia
2. Hypothermia
3. Growth-delayed adolescent
4. Physically conditioned adolescent

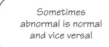

Sometimes abnormal is normal and vice versa!

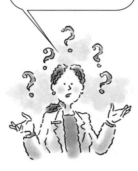

114. 4. A physically-conditioned adolescent might have a lower-than-normal heart rate, which is of no significance. Hypoxia and hypothermia are pathologic states in which a slow heart rate may produce a compromised hemodynamic state. Growth-delayed adolescents won't have bradycardia as a normal finding.
CN: Physiological integrity; CNS: Physiological adaptation; CL: Analysis

115. Treatment for a child with sinus bradycardia includes atropine 0.02 mg/kg. If the child weighs 20 kg, how much is given per dose?
1. 0.02 mg
2. 0.04 mg
3. 0.2 mg
4. 0.4 mg

115. 4. The child should receive 0.4 mg. Use the following equation:
$$0.02 \text{ mg/kg} \times 20 \text{ kg} = 0.4 \text{ mg}.$$
CN: Physiological integrity; CNS: Pharmacological therapies; CL: Analysis

116. Atropine, an anticholinergic agent, is being administered to a child with sinus bradycardia. Which statement is <u>most</u> accurate about the administration of this medication?
1. It increases heart rate.
2. It raises blood pressure.
3. It dilates bronchial tubes.
4. It decreases heart rate.

116. 1. Atropine blocks vagal impulses to the myocardium and stimulates the cardioinhibitory center in the medulla, thereby increasing hear rate and cardiac output. Atropine is not given to directly increase blood pressure or dilate the bronchial tubes.
CN: Physiological integrity; CNS: Pharmacological therapies; CL: Application

117. A nurse has given atropine to treat sinus bradycardia in an 11-month-old infant. Which <u>adverse reaction</u> is noted?
1. Lethargy
2. Diarrhea
3. No tears when crying
4. Increased urine output

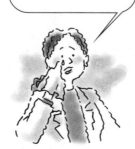

Don't have an adverse reaction to question 117.

117. 3. Atropine dries up secretions and also lessens the response of ciliary and iris sphincter muscles in the eye, causing mydriasis. It usually causes paradoxical excitement in children. Constipation and urinary retention can be seen because of a decrease in smooth-muscle contractions of the GI and genitourinary tracts.
CN: Physiological integrity; CNS: Pharmacological therapies; CL: Application

CN: Client needs category   CNS: Client needs subcategory   CL: Cognitive level

118. Which condition could cause sinus tachycardia?
1. Fever
2. Hypothermia
3. Hypothyroidism
4. Hypoxia

119. Which arrhythmia commonly seen in children involves heart rate changes related to respirations?
1. Sinus arrhythmia
2. Sinus block
3. Sinus bradycardia
4. Sinus tachycardia

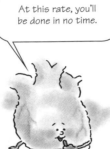

At this rate, you'll be done in no time.

120. Which condition <u>may</u> lead to sinus arrest or sinus pause in a child?
1. Hypokalemia
2. Hyperthermia
3. Valsalva's maneuver
4. Decreased intracranial pressure

I knew you could get the hang of math!

121. For temporary treatment of sinus arrest, isoproterenol (Isuprel) is given to increase the heart rate. The order is for 0.05 mcg/kg/minute. The child weighs 10 kg. How much should be given?
1. 0.05 mcg
2. 0.15 mcg
3. 0.25 mcg
4. 0.5 mcg

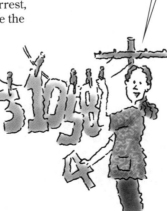

118. 1. Sinus tachycardia is commonly seen in children with a fever. It's usually a result of a noncardiac cause. Hypothermia, hypothyroidism, and hypoxia will result in sinus bradycardia.
CN: Physiological integrity; CNS: Physiological adaptation; CL: Analysis

119. 1. With respirations, intrathoracic pressures decrease on inhalation, which decreases vagal stimulation, and increase on expiration, which increases vagal stimulation. The result is the perfectly normal arrhythmia called *sinus arrhythmia,* a common occurrence in childhood and adolescence. Sinus block, sinus bradycardia, and sinus tachycardia are respiration-independent arrhythmias.
CN: Physiological integrity; CNS: Physiological adaptation; CL: Analysis

120. 3. Sinus arrest may occur in children when vagal tone is increased, such as during Valsalva's maneuver, vomiting, gagging, or straining during a bowel movement. This condition involves a failure of the sinoatrial node to generate an impulse. A straight line or pause occurs, indicating the absence of electrical activity. After the pause, another impulse will be generated and a cardiac complex will appear. Hyperkalemia, not hypokalemia; hypothermia, not hyperthermia; and increased rather than decreased intracranial pressure are pathologic conditions that may also produce sinus pause.
CN: Physiological integrity; CNS: Physiological adaptation; CL: Analysis

121. 4. The child should receive 0.5 mcg. Use the following equation:
0.05 mcg/kg × 10 kg = 0.5 mcg.
CN: Physiological integrity; CNS: Pharmacological therapies; CL: Analysis

CN: Client needs category   CNS: Client needs subcategory   CL: Cognitive level

122. The physician orders digoxin (Lanoxin) 0.1 mg orally every morning for a 6-month-old infant with heart failure. Digoxin is available in a 400 mcg/ml concentration. How many milliliters of digoxin should the nurse give? Record your answer using two decimal places.

_____ milliliters

123. The nurse is providing preoperative teaching to the parents of a 9-month-old infant who's having surgery to repair a ventricular septal defect. Identify the area of the heart where the defect is located.

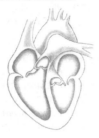

124. A 6-year-old boy arrives in the emergency department complaining of dizziness, and collapses before he can be taken into an examination room. Prioritize in ascending chronological order the steps to take during initial intervention. Use all the options.

1. Begin chest compressions.
2. Tilt the client's head back to open up the airway.
3. Look, listen, and feel for any signs of respiration.
4. Check the carotid pulse.
5. Give two rescue breaths.
6. Establish unresponsiveness and call for help.

You're finished! I knew you could do it—because you have heart!

122. 0.25. To convert mg to mcg:
1,000 mcg/1 mg = X mcg/0.1 mg;
X = 100 mcg.
To calculate drug dose:
Dose on hand/Quantity on hand = Dose desired/X.
400 mcg/ml = 100 mcg/X;
X = 0.25 ml.
CN: Physiological integrity; CNS: Pharmacological therapies; CL: Application

123.

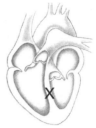

A ventricular septal defect is a hole in the septum between the ventricles. The defect can be anywhere along the septum but is most commonly located in the middle of the septum.
CN: Physiological integrity; CNS: Physiological adaptation; CL: Comprehension

124. Ordered response:

6. Establish unresponsiveness and call for help.
2. Tilt the client's head back to open up the airway.
3. Look, listen, and feel for any signs of respiration.
5. Give two rescue breaths.
4. Check the carotid pulse.
1. Begin chest compressions.

The first step is to establish unresponsiveness and call for help. Then position the head so that the airway is open, and then look, listen, and feel for respirations. If there are none, immediately give two breaths. If the breaths are administered without resistance in the airway, palpate the carotid artery to establish if there's a pulse. If there's no pulse, begin chest compressions.
CN: Safe, effective care environment; CNS: Coordinated care; CL: Application

CN: Client needs category   CNS: Client needs subcategory   CL: Cognitive level

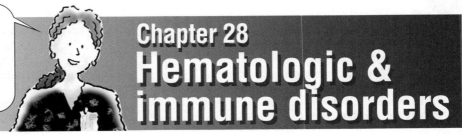

This chapter covers sickle cell disease, varicella, Rocky Mountain spotted fever, leukemia, and many other blood and immune system disorders in kids. It's a whopper of a chapter on a critical area. If you're ready, let's begin!

Chapter 28
Hematologic & immune disorders

1. A child is suspected of having Reye's syndrome. The nurse should monitor the child for which signs and symptoms?

1. Fever, profoundly impaired consciousness, and hepatomegaly
2. Fever, enlarged spleen, and hyperactive reflexes
3. Afebrile, intractable vomiting, and rhinorrhea
4. Malaise, cough, and sore throat

1. 1. Reye's syndrome is defined as toxic encephalopathy, characterized by fever, profoundly impaired consciousness, and disordered hepatic function. Reye's syndrome, commonly seen in children who have been given aspirin for flu symptoms, doesn't affect the spleen but causes fatty degeneration of the liver. Hyperactive reflexes occur with central nervous system involvement. Intractable vomiting may be noted. Malaise, cough, rhinorrhea, and sore throat are viral symptoms that commonly precede the illness.

CN: Physiological integrity; CNS: Physiological adaptation; CL: Application

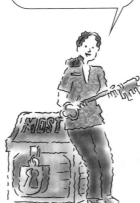

Early diagnosis is the key to treating Reye's syndrome.

2. Which medical intervention is <u>most important</u> for successful management of the child with Reye's syndrome?

1. Early diagnosis
2. Initiation of antibiotics
3. Isolation of the child
4. Staging of the illness

2. 1. Early diagnosis and therapy are essential because of the rapid clinical course of the disease and its high mortality. Reye's syndrome is associated with a viral illness, and antibiotic therapy isn't crucial to preventing the initial progression of the illness. Isolation isn't necessary because the disease isn't communicable. Staging, although important to therapy, occurs after a differential diagnosis is made.

CN: Physiological integrity; CNS: Reduction of risk potential; CL: Analysis

3. A child with Reye's syndrome is in stage I of the illness. Which measure will help prevent further progression of the illness?

1. Invasive monitoring
2. Endotracheal intubation
3. Hypertonic glucose solution
4. Pancuronium

3. 3. For children in stage I of Reye's syndrome, treatment is primarily supportive and directed toward restoring blood glucose levels and correcting acid-base imbalances. I.V. administration of dextrose solutions with added insulin helps to replace glycogen stores and may help prevent progression of the syndrome. Noninvasive monitoring is adequate to assess status at this stage. Endotracheal intubation may be necessary later. Pancuronium is used as an adjunct to endotracheal intubation and wouldn't be used in this stage of Reye's syndrome.

CN: Physiological integrity; CNS: Reduction of risk potential; CL: Application

CN: Client needs category   CNS: Client needs subcategory   CL: Cognitive level

4. Which laboratory results, along with the clinical manifestations, <u>establish</u> a diagnosis of Reye's syndrome?
1. Elevated liver enzyme levels
2. Increased serum glucose levels
3. Increased bilirubin levels
4. Increased alkaline phosphate levels

5. The nurse is caring for a 9-month-old boy with Reye's syndrome. It's most important that the nurse plans to:
1. check the skin for signs of breakdown every shift.
2. perform range-of-motion (ROM) exercises every 4 hours.
3. monitor the client's intake and output.
4. place the client in protective isolation.

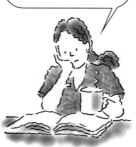

I hope the information that goes in my head comes back out as the correct answer.

6. Which change would indicate increased intracranial pressure (ICP) in a child acutely ill with Reye's syndrome?
1. Irritability and quick pupil response
2. Increased blood pressure and decreased heart rate
3. Decreased blood pressure and increased heart rate
4. Sluggish pupil response and decreased blood pressure

7. A child with Reye's syndrome is exhibiting signs of increased intracranial pressure (ICP). Which nursing intervention would be <u>most</u> appropriate for this child?
1. Position the child with the head elevated and the neck in a neutral position.
2. Maintain the child in the prone position.
3. Cluster together interventions that may be perceived as noxious.
4. Position the child in the supine position, with head turned to the side.

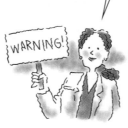

Warning: Note the word most.

4. 1. Reye's syndrome causes fatty degeneration of the liver, which results in elevated liver enzyme levels. Decreased serum glucose levels, with reduced insulin levels, occur secondary to dehydration caused by intractable vomiting. Serum bilirubin and alkaline phosphatase usually aren't affected.
CN: Physiological integrity; CNS: Physiological adaptation; CL: Analysis

5. 3. Monitoring intake and output alerts the nurse to the development of dehydration and cerebral edema, complications of Reye's syndrome. Although checking the skin for signs of breakdown is important because the child may not be as active as normal, it isn't as critical as monitoring the client's intake and output. Active ROM exercises may not be needed and aren't as important as monitoring the client's intake and output. Placing the client in protective isolation isn't necessary.
CN: Physiological integrity; CNS: Reduction of risk potential; CL: Application

6. 2. A marked increase in ICP will trigger the pressure response; increased ICP produces an elevation in blood pressure with a reflex slowing of the heart rate. Irritability is commonly an early sign, but pupillary response becomes more sluggish in response to increased ICP.
CN: Physiological integrity; CNS: Physiological adaptation; CL: Application

7. 1. Positioning the child with the head elevated and neck in the neutral position helps decrease ICP. The prone and supine positions cause increased ICP. Interventions that may be perceived as noxious should be spaced over time because if clustered together they may have a cumulative effect in increasing ICP. Turning the head to the side may impede venous return from the head and increase ICP.
CN: Physiological integrity; CNS: Physiological adaptation; CL: Application

CN: Client needs category   CNS: Client needs subcategory   CL: Cognitive level

8. A nurse is reinforcing the teaching plan with the father of a child who has asthma that's triggered by dust mite allergy. Which statement by the father indicates that teaching has been effective?
 1. "I'll wash all of the bedding in hot (130° F) water every week."
 2. "I'll use a humidifier in my child's room every night."
 3. "I'll replace my child's vinyl chair with an upholstered one."
 4. "I'll cover the hardwood bedroom floor with carpeting."

9. Which statement by the nurse most accurately explains the need for a child with pauciarticular juvenile rheumatoid arthritis (JRA) to have an annual eye exam?
 1. "Detached retinas are commonly associated with the disease."
 2. "Painless iritis (inflammation of the iris) is commonly seen with the disease."
 3. "Glaucoma is commonly seen with the disease."
 4. "Strabismus is commonly seen with the disease."

10. Which medication would the nurse include when discussing a connection to Reye's syndrome?
 1. Acetaminophen (Tylenol)
 2. Aspirin
 3. Ibuprofen (Motrin)
 4. Guaifenesin (Robitussin)

11. Which clinical manifestations should a nurse expect to see in a child in stage V of Reye's syndrome?
 1. Vomiting, lethargy, and drowsiness
 2. Seizures, flaccidity, and respiratory arrest
 3. Hyperventilation and coma
 4. Disorientation, aggressiveness, and combativeness

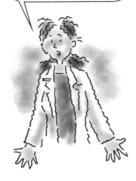

Stay calm when encountering NCLEX questions you're unsure about. That's what I do.

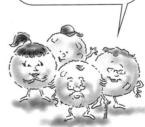

Rumor has it that one of us may be connected to Reye's syndrome.

8. 1. Washing all of the bedclothes (including the pillow) once a week in hot water will kill dust mites. Dust mites thrive in humid conditions, so using a dehumidifier in the child's room is recommended. Dust mites live on upholstery, fabric, and carpets, so these items should be replaced with nontextile surfaces when possible.
CN: Safe and effective care environment; CNS: Safety and infection control; CL: Analysis

9. 2. Painless iritis may be found in up to 75% of children with pauciarticular JRA. If it's not detected and is left untreated, permanent scarring in the anterior chamber of the eye may occur, with loss of vision. Children should have annual slit-lamp examinations by an ophthalmologist. Detached retinas, glaucoma, and strabismus aren't commonly associated with the disease.
CN: Health promotion and maintenance; CNS: None; CL: Application

10. 2. There's speculation regarding the relationship between aspirin administration and the development of Reye's syndrome; a child may receive salicylates for fever associated with prior viral infection, such as chickenpox or influenza. Acetaminophen, ibuprofen, and guaifenesin haven't been associated with the development of Reye's syndrome. In fact, there has been a decreased incidence of Reye's syndrome with the increased use of acetaminophen and ibuprofen for management of fevers in children.
CN: Physiological integrity; CNS: Pharmacological therapies; CL: Comprehension

11. 2. Staging criteria were developed to help evaluate the client's progress and to evaluate the efficacy of therapies. The clinical manifestations of stage V include seizures, loss of deep tendon reflexes, flaccidity, and respiratory arrest. Vomiting, lethargy, and drowsiness occur in stage I. Hyperventilation and coma occur in stage III. Disorientation and aggressive behavior occur in stage II.
CN: Physiological integrity; CNS: Physiological adaptation; CL: Analysis

CN: Client needs category   CNS: Client needs subcategory   CL: Cognitive level

12. An 8-year-old child is brought to the clinic with cold symptoms (watery eyes, clear nasal drainage) that have lasted more than 10 days, without fever. The nurse observes that the child has dark circles under his eyes and a crease above the tip of his nose. Which intervention should be the nurse's <u>priority</u>?
    1. Collect data about potential environmental allergy triggers.
    2. Prepare to administer amoxicillin (Amoxil) 25 mg/kg. P.O. every 12 hours.
    3. Prepare to administer trivalent inactivated influenza vaccine 0.5 ml P.O.
    4. Prepare the child for sinus X-rays.

13. A nurse is reinforcing the teaching plan with the mother of a 12-year-old child recently diagnosed with systemic juvenile rheumatoid arthritis (JRA). Which statement by the mother best indicates that teaching has been effective?
    1. "Maintaining an appropriate, regular exercise program is very important."
    2. "Systemic JRA typically appears at or before the age of 12."
    3. "High fevers that spike in the morning may be the first sign of the disease."
    4. "It's important to limit the amount of calcium in my child's diet."

14. A nurse is caring for a child with juvenile rheumatoid arthritis (JRA). The child has been ordered to begin oral prednisone (Orasone). The nurse knows that the drug will be given at the lowest possible dosage and for a short time in order to avoid which adverse effects?
    1. Growth retardation and increased risk of infection
    2. Deafness and severe weight loss
    3. Hypoglycemia and hypovolemia
    4. Fibrotic skin changes and increased muscle mass

15. Which immunizations should a healthy 4-month-old client receive?
    1. Measles and inactivated poliovirus vaccine (IPV)
    2. Measles, mumps, and rubella (MMR)
    3. Diphtheria, tetanus, and acellular pertussis (DTaP)
    4. DTaP and IPV

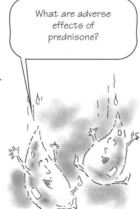

What are adverse effects of prednisone?

12. 1. Cold symptoms that last longer than 10 days without fever, circles under the eyes (from increased blood flow near the sinuses), and a crease near the tip of the nose (from upward nose wiping) are all signs and symptoms of perennial allergic rhinitis. The nurse's priority is to collect data about potential indoor and outdoor environmental triggers. Amoxicillin is used to treat bacterial infections, not allergies. Influenza vaccination is indicated annually. Sinus X-rays may be necessary to check for structural abnormalities, but they are not the priority at this time.
CN: Safe and effective care environment; CNS: Safety and infection control; CL: Analysis

13. 1. Maintaining a regular, appropriate exercise program is important to maintain muscle strength and joint flexibility. All types of JRA occur at or before the age of 16. High fevers that spike at night and then suddenly disappear typically may be the first sign of systemic JRA. It's important for a 12-year-old child to consume 1,300 mg of calcium daily to maintain bone health.
CN: Health promotion and maintenance; CNS: None; CL: Analysis

14. 1. Long-term prednisone use is associated with poor growth and immunosuppression; it may aggravate or mask serious infections. Prednisone is associated with weight gain and cataract formation, but not deafness. It may cause hyperglycemia, significant sodium and fluid retention, edema, and heart failure. Long-term use of prednisone may cause muscle wasting, weakness, and thin, fragile skin.
CN: Physiological integrity; CNS: Pharmacological therapies; CL: Analysis

15. 4. At age 4 months, DTaP and IPV are the recommended immunizations. DTaP is given again alone at age 6 months. MMR is given at age 12 months.
CN: Health promotion and maintenance; CNS: None; CL: Knowledge

16. Parents of a child with Reye's syndrome need a great deal of emotional support. Which nursing intervention would be helpful in reducing stress and alleviating fear?
1. Not accepting aggressive behavior from parents
2. Minimizing the expression of feelings and concerns
3. Letting parents interpret the child's behaviors and responses
4. Encouraging parents to talk about their feelings.

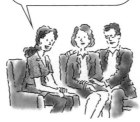

Encourage parents to talk about their feelings toward their child's illness.

16. 4. As the parents are encouraged to talk about their feelings, stress is reduced. Aggressive behavior shouldn't be tolerated, but recognized as a symptom of poor coping skills indicating their need for greater emotional support. It's critical to not minimize the feelings and concerns of the parents because this may increase their stress. It's important to explain the child's behavior to the parents so they don't misinterpret the meaning.
CN: Psychosocial integrity; CNS: None; CL: Application

17. Vaccinating a child against preventable diseases represents which type of immunity?
1. Acquired immunity
2. Active immunity
3. Natural immunity
4. Passive immunity

17. 2. Active immunity occurs when the individual forms immune bodies against certain diseases, either by having the disease or by the introduction of a vaccine into the individual. Acquired immunity results from exposure to the bacteria, virus, or toxins. Natural immunity is resistance to infection or toxicity. Passive immunity is a temporary immunity caused by transfusion of immune plasma proteins.
CN: Health promotion and maintenance; CNS: None; CL: Knowledge

18. Following the birth of a full-term, healthy newborn, the parents request information about when to begin immunizations. What information should the nurse reinforce when teaching the parents?
1. Immunizations will start before the child leaves the hospital.
2. Immunizations will begin when the child is 1 month old.
3. Immunizations will begin when the child is 6 months old.
4. Immunizations will begin when the child is weaned from breast-feeding.

18. 1. According to the American Academy of Pediatrics, birth is the recommended age for beginning primary immunizations, starting with hepatitis B vaccine. Breast-feeding has no impact on the recommended immunization schedule.
CN: Health promotion and maintenance; CNS: None; CL: Application

19. When teaching the parents of a newborn being discharged from the hospital, the nurse instructs them on administering acetaminophen to their child before immunizations at 2 months, 4 months, and 6 months of age. Which immunization would necessitate this action?
1. Diphtheria, tetanus, and acellular pertussis (DTaP)
2. *Haemophilus influenzae* type B (Hib)
3. Inactivated poliovirus vaccine (IPV)
4. Pneumococcal conjugate vaccine (PCV)

19. 1. Acetaminophen is recommended for prophylactic use at the time of DTaP immunization because of localized pain at the injection site. This isn't a standard recommendation for Hib, IPV, or PCV immunizations.
CN: Health promotion and maintenance; CNS: None; CL: Application

CN: Client needs category   CNS: Client needs subcategory   CL: Cognitive level

20. An infant with an immune deficiency should receive which type of polio vaccine?
1. Oral poliovirus vaccine
2. Inactivated poliovirus vaccine (IPV)
3. Either form
4. Neither form

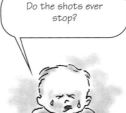

Do the shots ever stop?

20. 2. For all infants and children, an all-IPV schedule is recommended by the American Academy of Pediatrics for routine childhood polio vaccination in the United States. The four doses should be given at ages 2 months, 4 months, 6 to 18 months, and 4 to 6 years. The oral form is no longer given.
CN: Health promotion and maintenance; CNS: None; CL: Knowledge

21. A child is considered immunocompromised. What teaching should the nurse provide the parents concerning immunizations?
1. The immunization schedule should be followed as usual.
2. Immunizations should be delayed.
3. The child should be put on an accelerated immunization schedule.
4. The child should receive no further immunizations.

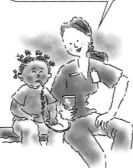

Avoid vaccinating a child who's already ill.

21. 2. Immunizations should be delayed until the physician has determined that the child is ready. The particular type and number of immunizations given at one time may vary for this child. The child may be put on a schedule to catch up eventually, but that would not be the first response. The child would not typically be excluded from having immunizations in the future.
CN: Health promotion and maintenance; CNS: None; CL: Application

22. Which schedule is recommended for immunization of normal infants and children in the first year of life?
1. Birth, 2 months, 4 months, 6 months, 12 months
2. 1 month, 3 months, 5 months, 9 months
3. 2 months, 6 months, 9 months, 12 months
4. 2 months, 4 months, 6 months, 12 to 15 months

22. 1. The nurse needs to be aware of the schedule for immunizations as well as the latest recommendations for their use. According to the American Academy of Pediatrics, the recommended age for beginning primary immunizations of normal infants is at birth.
CN: Health promotion and maintenance; CNS: None; CL: Application

23. Which direction is <u>most important</u> when administering immunizations?
1. Properly store the vaccine, and follow the recommended procedure for injection.
2. Monitor clients for approximately 1 hour after administration for adverse reactions.
3. Take the vaccine out of refrigeration 1 hour before administration.
4. Inject multiple vaccines at the same injection site.

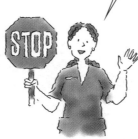

Stop and think: Immunizations commonly come as suspensions, don't they?

23. 1. Vaccines must be properly stored to ensure their potency. The nurse must be familiar with the manufacturer's directions for storage and reconstitution of the vaccine. Faulty refrigeration is a major cause of primary vaccine failure. It isn't necessary to monitor the clients, but the nurse should instruct parents to call the primary care provider and report any adverse effects. Taking the vaccine out of refrigeration too early can affect its potency. If more than one vaccine is to be administered, different injection sites should be used. The nurse should note which vaccine is given and at what site in case of a local reaction caused by the injection.
CN: Health promotion and maintenance; CNS: None; CL: Application

CN: Client needs category CNS: Client needs subcategory CL: Cognitive level

24. Which symptom would the nurse expect to find as most common in a child with severe combined immunodeficiency disease (SCID)?
    1. Increased bruising
    2. Failure to thrive
    3. Prolonged bleeding
    4. Susceptibility to infection

24. 4. SCID is characterized by absence of both humoral and cell-mediated immunity. The most common manifestation is susceptibility to infection early in life, most commonly by age 3 months. Increased bruising and prolonged bleeding aren't manifestations of SCID. Failure to thrive is a consequence of persistent illnesses.
CN: Physiological integrity; CNS: Physiological adaptation; CL: Comprehension

25. A child is admitted to the hospital for an asthma exacerbation. The nursing history reveals this client was exposed to chickenpox 1 week ago. When would this client require isolation if he were to remain hospitalized?
    1. Isolation isn't required.
    2. Immediate isolation is required.
    3. 10 days after exposure
    4. 12 days after exposure

25. 2. The incubation period for chickenpox is 2 to 3 weeks, commonly 13 to 17 days. A client is commonly isolated 1 week after exposure to avoid the risk of an earlier breakout. A person is infectious from 1 day before eruption of lesions until after the vesicles have formed crusts.
CN: Safe, effective care environment; CNS: Safety and infection control; CL: Application

26. While assessing a child's skin, the nurse notes a papular pruritic rash with some vesicles. The rash is profuse on the trunk and sparse on the distal limbs. The nurse interprets this as suggesting:
    1. measles.
    2. mumps.
    3. roseola.
    4. chickenpox.

26. 4. Chickenpox begins with a macule, rapidly progresses to a highly pruritic papule, then becomes a vesicle. All three stages are present in varying degrees at one time. Measles begin as an erythematous maculopapular eruption on the face and gradually spread downward. Mumps isn't associated with a skin rash. Roseola rash is nonpruritic and is described as discrete rose pink macules, appearing first on the trunk and then spreading to the neck, face, and extremities.
CN: Health promotion and maintenance; CNS: None; CL: Analysis

27. Which response would be appropriate to a parent inquiring, "When can my child with chickenpox return to school"?
    1. "When the child is afebrile"
    2. "When all vesicles have dried"
    3. "When vesicles begin to crust over"
    4. "When lesions and vesicles are gone"

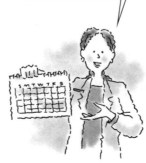

Chickenpox is highly contagious. Teach parents how to determine when it's safe to send their children back to school.

27. 2. Chickenpox is contagious. It's transmitted through direct contact, droplet spread, and contact with contaminated objects. Vesicles break open; therefore, the child is considered contagious until all vesicles have dried. A child may be fever-free but continue to have vesicles and remain contagious. Some vesicles may be crusted over, but new ones may have formed and the child remains contagious. It isn't necessary to wait until dried lesions have disappeared. Isolation is usually necessary only for about 1 week after the onset of the disease.
CN: Safe, effective care environment; CNS: Safety and infection control; CL: Application

28. A parent reports that his child has roseola. Which clinical manifestations would the nurse expect to find?
1. Apparent sickness, fever, and rash
2. Fever for 3 to 4 days, followed by rash
3. Rash, without history of fever or illness
4. Rash for 3 to 4 days, followed by high fevers

28. 2. Roseola is manifested by persistent high fever for 3 to 4 days followed by a rash. When the rash appears, a precipitous drop in fever occurs and the temperature returns to normal.
CN: Health promotion and maintenance; CNS: None; CL: Comprehension

29. Which finding is consistent with a roseola rash?
1. Maculopapular red spots on the torso
2. Pruritic papules and vesicles on the extremities
3. Rose pink macules that fade on pressure
4. Red maculopapular eruptions on the face

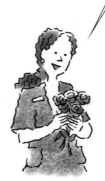

A rose-ola rash by any other name would still look the same.

29. 3. Roseola rashes are discrete, rose pink macules or maculopapules that fade on pressure and usually last 1 to 2 days. Chickenpox rash is macular, with papules and vesicles. Roseola isn't pruritic. Maculopapular red spots may be indicative of fifth disease. Measles begin as a maculopapular eruption on the face.
CN: Health promotion and maintenance; CNS: None; CL: Knowledge

30. The nurse would advise the child with chickenpox and his parents to avoid scratching and irritating open vesicles to prevent which condition?
1. Myocarditis
2. Neuritis
3. Obstructive laryngitis
4. Bacterial infection

30. 4. Bacterial infections can occur as a complication of chickenpox. Further irritation of skin lesions can lead to cellulitis or even an abscess. Myocarditis isn't considered a complication of chickenpox but has been noted as a complication of mumps. Neuritis has been associated with diphtheria. Obstructive laryngitis occurs as a complication of measles.
CN: Physiological integrity; CNS: Reduction of risk potential; CL: Application

31. Which characteristic <u>best</u> describes the cough of an infant admitted to the hospital with suspected pertussis?
1. Dry, hacking, more frequent on awakening
2. Loose and nonproductive
3. Occurring more frequently during the day
4. Harsh, associated with a high-pitched crowing sound

31. 4. The cough associated with pertussis is a harsh series of short, rapid coughs, followed by a sudden inspiration and a high-pitched crowing sound. Cheeks become flushed or cyanotic, eyes bulge, and the tongue protrudes. Paroxysm may continue until a thick mucus plug is dislodged. This cough occurs most commonly at night.
CN: Physiological integrity; CNS: Physiological adaptation; CL: Analysis

32. Which communicable disease requires isolating infected children from pregnant women?
1. Pertussis
2. Roseola
3. Rubella
4. Varicella

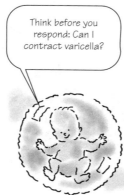

Think before you respond: Can I contract varicella?

32. 3. Rubella (German measles) has a teratogenic effect on the fetus. An infected child must be isolated from pregnant women. Pertussis, roseola, and varicella don't have any teratogenic effects on a fetus.
CN: Safe, effective care environment; CNS: Safety and infection control; CL: Application

CN: Client needs category   CNS: Client needs subcategory   CL: Cognitive level

33. The nurse would expect the physician to order which medication as the treatment of choice for scarlet fever?
1. Acyclovir (Zovirax)
2. Amphotericin B (Amphotec)
3. Ibuprofen (Motrin)
4. Penicillin (Veetids)

33. 4. The causative agent of scarlet fever is group A beta-hemolytic streptococci, which is susceptible to penicillin. Erythromycin (E-Mycin) is used for penicillin-sensitive children. Acyclovir is used in the treatment of herpes infections. Amphotericin B is used to treat fungal infections. Anti-inflammatory drugs, such as ibuprofen, aren't indicated for these clients.
CN: Physiological integrity; CNS: Pharmacological therapies; CL: Application

34. A 2-year-old hospitalized child is HIV positive with severe thrush. The child's anxious grandparents are at her bedside, continually calling the nurses with various concerns. The staff speaks disparagingly about them because they're tired of responding to the frequent call lights. What response to the staff would be appropriate in creating a more optimal care situation for the child?
1. "This situation will improve as you respond to the call light more promptly."
2. "This couple is demanding, but we need to handle things in a professional manner."
3. "It might be best to have the child transferred to a facility that's better staffed."
4. "If we stop by the room before the light goes on, they may be less anxious."

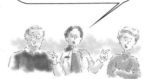

Be sensitive to the family's needs.

34. 4. Although the situation may improve with more prompt responses to the call light, stopping by the room before the light goes on addresses the needs of the family. This response encourages the staff to be proactive and compassionate, and provide prompt nursing intervention. Although the staff should handle the situation in a more professional manner, option 2 doesn't provide individualized care based on the needs of the family. Having the child transferred to a better-staffed facility is an inappropriate suggestion.
CN: Psychosocial integrity; CNS: None; CL: Analysis

35. Which instructions would the nurse include when teaching parents about caring for a child with chickenpox?
1. Administer antibiotics as ordered.
2. Administer antipruritics as ordered.
3. Provide peer interaction as a distraction.
4. Avoid varicella-zoster immunizations if the child has been taking aspirin.

35. 2. Chickenpox is highly pruritic. Preventing the child from scratching is necessary to prevent scarring and secondary infection caused by irritation of lesions. Antibiotics aren't usually used to treat chickenpox. Interaction with other children would be contraindicated due to the risk of disease transmission unless the other children have previously had chickenpox or have been immunized. Varicella-zoster immune globulin should be given to exposed children who are taking aspirin because of the possible risk of Reye's syndrome.
CN: Physiological integrity; CNS: Pharmacological therapies; CL: Application

36. Which period of isolation is indicated for a child with scarlet fever?
1. Until the associated diaper rash disappears
2. Until completion of antibiotic therapy
3. Until the child is fever-free for 24 hours
4. Until 24 hours after initiation of treatment

37. A client infected with human immunodeficiency virus (HIV) asks about breast-feeding her infant. Which response would be best?
1. "Don't breast-feed if you have HIV."
2. "Breast-feeding is safe if you have HIV."
3. "You can breast-feed your infant only if you are taking zidovudine (Retrovir)."
4. "It's best to supplement breast-feeding with formula to reduce exposure to HIV."

38. Which finding would the nurse expect to help diagnose human immunodeficiency virus (HIV) infection in children?
1. Excessive weight gain
2. Increased appetite
3. Intermittent diarrhea
4. Good tolerance of feedings

39. Which factor contributes to the difficulty in diagnosing human immunodeficiency virus infection during the first 15 months of life?
1. Presence of maternal antibody
2. Unavailability of proper testing
3. Onset of symptoms at age 2
4. Transmission occurring after birth

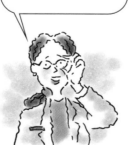

Antibody can see this is an important question. (Oops! I gave you a hint, didn't I?)

40. The nurse would suspect Kawasaki disease based on which finding?
1. Fever responsive to antipyretics
2. Vesicular rash on arms and legs
3. Edema and erythema of the hands and feet
4. Conjunctivitis with watery drainage

36. 4. A child requires respiratory isolation until 24 hours after initiation of treatment. Rash may persist for 3 weeks. It isn't necessary to wait until the end of treatment. The client usually becomes afebrile 24 hours after therapy has begun. It isn't necessary to maintain isolation for an additional 24 hours.
CN: Safe, effective environment; CNS: Safety and infection control; CL: Application

37. 1. Clients infected with HIV shouldn't breast-feed because the virus has been isolated in breast milk and can be transmitted to the infant. Taking zidovudine doesn't prevent transmission of the virus in breast milk, and supplementing breast-feeding with formula wouldn't reduce exposure of the infant to the HIV virus in breast milk.
CN: Health promotion and maintenance; CNS: None; CL: Application

38. 3. Findings that might help in the diagnosis of HIV infection in children include intermittent episodes of diarrhea, repeated respiratory infections, and the inability to tolerate feedings. Poor weight gain and failure to thrive are objective assessment findings that result from intolerance of feedings and frequent infections.
CN: Physiological integrity; CNS: Physiological adaptation; CL: Comprehension

39. 1. A confirmed diagnosis is difficult during the first 15 months because of the presence of maternal antibody. Onset of symptoms can occur before age 1, and the prognosis is poorer than if the onset of symptoms occurs between ages 2 and 3. Transmission of the virus occurs across the placenta in more than 50% of pregnancies in which the mother is infected.
CN: Health promotion and maintenance; CNS: None; CL: Application

40. 3. The clinical manifestations of Kawasaki disease include changes in the extremities, such as peripheral edema, peripheral erythema, and desquamation of the palms and the soles of the feet. Kawasaki disease is an acute febrile illness of unknown etiology that doesn't respond well to antipyretics. Rash associated with Kawasaki disease is usually located primarily on the trunk and is nonvesicular. Watery conjunctivitis is suggestive of viral conjunctivitis.
CN: Physiological integrity; CNS: Physiological adaptation; CL: Analysis

CN: Client needs category   CNS: Client needs subcategory   CL: Cognitive level

41. Sickle cell anemia occurs primarily in which ethnic group?
1. African-American
2. Asian
3. Caucasian
4. Hispanic

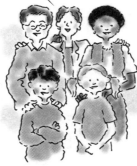

Ethnicity may increase the probability of certain diseases.

42. A child with sickle cell anemia comes to the emergency department suspected of being in vaso-occlusive crisis. Which assessment finding would indicate that the client is having a vaso-occlusive crisis?
1. Precipitous drop in blood volume
2. Decreased red blood cell (RBC) production
3. Anemia, jaundice, and reticulocytosis
4. Acute abdominal pain and hand-foot syndrome

43. A child tests positive for the sickle cell trait and his parents ask the nurse what this means. Which response by the nurse would be most appropriate?
1. Your child has sickle cell anemia.
2. Your child is a carrier but doesn't have the disease.
3. Your child is a carrier and will pass the disease to any offspring.
4. Your child doesn't have the disease now but may develop the disease as he gets older.

Know the difference between a positive test for a sickle cell trait and a positive test for sickle cell anemia.

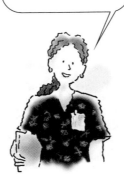

44. When caring for a child with sickle cell anemia in vaso-occlusive crisis, what's the priority?
1. Managing pain
2. Promoting activity
3. Promoting sickling
4. Preventing tissue oxygenation

41. 1. Sickle cell anemia is primarily found in African Americans. Uncommonly, it affects Whites, especially those of Mediterranean descent. It also affects Central Americans and people from Saudi Arabia and India, but in fewer numbers. Sickle cell anemia affects approximately 70,000 people in the United States. It's estimated that 1 in 12 African Americans carries the trait.

CN: Physiological integrity; CNS: Physiological adaptation; CL: Knowledge

42. 4. There are four types of episodic crises in sickle cell anemia: vaso-occlusive, splenic sequestration, aplastic, and hyperhemolytic. Vaso-occlusive crises are the most common and the only painful ones resulting from sickled cells obstructing the blood vessels. The major symptoms are fever, acute abdominal pain from visceral hypoxia, hand-foot syndrome, and arthralgia, without an exacerbation of anemia. A precipitous drop in blood volume is indicative of a splenic sequestration crisis. Aplastic crisis exhibits diminished RBC production. Hyperhemolytic crisis is characterized by anemia, jaundice, and reticulocytosis.

CN: Physiological integrity; CNS: Physiological adaptation; CL: Analysis

43. 2. A child with sickle cell trait is only a carrier and may never show any symptoms, except under special hypoxic conditions. A child with sickle cell trait doesn't have the disease and will never test positive for sickle cell anemia. Sickle cell anemia would be transmitted to offspring only as the result of a union between two individuals who are positive for the trait.

CN: Health promotion and maintenance; CNS: None; CL: Application

44. 1. Pain management is the priority in the care of a client with sickle cell anemia in vaso-occlusive crisis. The next priority is to prevent sickling. This can be accomplished by promoting tissue oxygenation, hydration, and rest, which minimize energy expenditure and oxygen utilization.

CN: Physiological integrity; CNS: Basic care and comfort; CL: Analysis

CN: Client needs category CNS: Client needs subcategory CL: Cognitive level

45. The nurse avoids palpating the abdomen of a child in vaso-occlusive crisis to prevent which complication?
1. Risk of splenic rupture
2. Risk of inducing vomiting
3. Increase of abdominal pain
4. Risk of blood cell destruction

45. 1. Palpating a child's abdomen in vaso-occlusive crisis should be avoided because sequestered red blood cells may precipitate splenic rupture. Abdominal pain alone wouldn't be a reason to avoid palpation. Vomiting or blood cell destruction wouldn't occur from palpation of the abdomen.
CN: Physiological integrity; CNS: Reduction of risk potential; CL: Application

46. Which intervention is most effective in maximizing tissue perfusion for a client in vaso-occlusive crisis?
1. Administering analgesics
2. Monitoring fluid restrictions
3. Encouraging activity as tolerated
4. Administering oxygen as prescribed

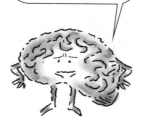

If I was *most* effective, I would know the answer.

46. 4. Administering oxygen is the most effective way to maximize tissue perfusion. Short-term oxygen therapy helps to prevent hypoxia, which leads to metabolic acidosis, causing sickling. Long-term oxygen therapy will depress erythropoiesis. Analgesics are used to control pain. Hydration is essential to promote hemodilution and maintain electrolyte balance. Bed rest should be promoted to reduce oxygen utilization.
CN: Physiological integrity; CNS: Reduction of risk potential; CL: Application

47. Which nursing measure is most important to decrease the risk of postoperative complications of a client with sickle cell anemia?
1. Increasing fluids
2. Preparing the child psychologically
3. Discouraging coughing
4. Limiting the use of analgesics

47. 1. The main surgical risk from anesthesia is hypoxia; however, emotional stress, demands of wound healing, and the potential for infection can each increase the sickling phenomenon. Increased fluids are encouraged because keeping the child well-hydrated is important for hemodilution to prevent sickling. Preparing the child psychologically to decrease fear will minimize undue emotional stress. Deep coughing is encouraged to promote pulmonary hygiene and prevent respiratory tract infection. Analgesics are used to control wound pain and to prevent abdominal splinting and decreased ventilation.
CN: Health promotion and maintenance; CNS: None; CL: Application

CN: Client needs category   CNS: Client needs subcategory   CL: Cognitive level

48. Which factor should be included as a <u>priority</u> in teaching parents about prevention of infection in children with sickle cell anemia?
1. Providing adequate nutrition and fluids
2. Avoiding emotional stress
3. Visiting the physician when sick
4. Avoiding strenuous physical exertion

49. In which ethnic group would the nurse most likely expect thalassemia to occur?
1. Blacks
2. Asians
3. Greeks
4. Hispanics

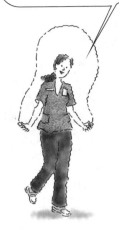

Don't let question 48 trip you up! It's asking you to prioritize.

50. When collecting data on a child with sickle cell anemia, which finding would indicate vaso-occlusive crisis?
1. Pain upon urination
2. Pain with ambulation
3. Throat pain
4. Fever with associated rash

51. The nurse is working overnight in the emergency department when a client is admitted in sickle cell crisis. Which intervention should the nurse expect to perform?
1. Giving blood transfusions
2. Giving antibiotics
3. Increasing fluid intake and giving analgesics
4. Preparing the client for a splenectomy

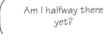

Am I halfway there yet?

52. What is the nurse's role with the parents of a client who has been diagnosed with sickle cell anemia?
1. Encouraging selective birth methods or abortion
2. Referring only sickle cell positive parents for counseling
3. Rendering support to parents of newly diagnosed clients
4. Telling the parents that the disease is unlikely in subsequent pregnancies

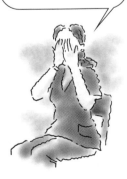

CN: Client needs category   CNS: Client needs subcategory   CL: Cognitive level

48. 1. The nurse must stress adequate nutrition and fluid intake. Frequent medical supervision can prevent infection, often a predisposing factor toward development of a crisis. Avoiding stress and strenuous physical exertion helps prevent sickling, but adequate nutrition remains a priority.
CN: Health promotion and maintenance; CNS: None;
CL: Application

49. 3. Thalassemia is highly prevalent in people living near the Mediterranean Sea (Greeks, Italians, and Syrians). Evidence suggests that the high prevalence among these groups is a result of selective damage of the trait as a result of malaria. Thalassemia isn't common among Blacks, Asians, and Hispanics.
CN: Health promotion and maintenance; CNS: None;
CL: Comprehension

50. 2. Bone pain is one of the major symptoms of vaso-occlusive crisis. Hand-foot syndrome, characterized by edematous painful extremities, is usually exhibited in the refusal of the child to bear weight and ambulate. Painful urination doesn't occur, but sickle cell anemia can cause kidney abnormalities. Throat pain isn't a symptom of vaso-occlusive crisis. Fever is one of the major symptoms of vaso-occlusive crisis but isn't associated with rash.
CN: Physiological integrity; CNS: Physiological adaptation;
CL: Analysis

51. 3. The primary therapy for sickle cell crisis is to increase fluid intake according to age and to give analgesics. Blood transfusions are only given conservatively to avoid iron overload. Antibiotics are given to clients with fever. Routine splenectomy isn't recommended. Splenectomy in clients with sickle cell anemia is controversial.
CN: Physiological integrity; CNS: Physiological adaptation;
CL: Application

52. 3. The nurse can be instrumental in providing support, encouragement, and correct information to the parents of newly diagnosed clients. Alternative birth methods are discussed, but parents make their own decisions. All heterozygous, or trait-positive, parents should be referred for genetic counseling. The risk of transmission in subsequent pregnancies remains the same.
CN: Health promotion and maintenance; CNS: None;
CL: Application

53. A 14-year-old girl is admitted for sickle cell crisis. Which nursing intervention would be the most important?

1. Gathering information about the child's ability to cope with this condition
2. Monitoring the child's temperature every 2 hours
3. Providing adequate oxygenation, hydration, and pain management
4. Making sure the family is involved in every step of the child's care

54. The nurse is administering a blood transfusion to a client with sickle cell anemia. Which assessment finding would indicate development of a transfusion reaction?

1. Diaphoresis and hot flashes
2. Urticaria, flushing, and wheezing
3. Fever, urticaria, and red, raised rash
4. Fever, disorientation, and abdominal pain

55. A mother asks the clinic nurse how often the influenza virus vaccine should be given to her child. Which response would be <u>most</u> accurate?

1. "The vaccine is usually given annually to children with certain risk factors."
2. "I wouldn't worry; your child doesn't need the vaccine."
3. "The vaccine is given monthly."
4. "The vaccine is given every 6 months."

56. A 3-year-old sister of a neonate is diagnosed with pertussis. The mother gives a history of having been immunized as a child. What should be included in teaching the mother about possible infection of her neonate?

1. The neonate will inevitably contract pertussis.
2. Immune globulin will protect the neonate.
3. The risk to the neonate is minimal.
4. Erythromycin will help prevent infection.

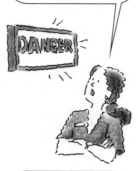

Know the critical needs of the client in sickle cell crisis.

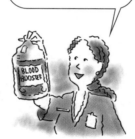

Be alert for allergic reactions to a blood transfusion.

53. 3. The most critical need of a client in sickle cell crisis is to provide adequate oxygenation, hydration, and pain management until the crisis passes. Obtaining a temperature every 2 hours would not be the priority intervention. While assessing the client's ability to cope and involving the family in the child's care are important, they aren't the priority interventions during a sickle cell crisis.
CN: Physiological integrity; CNS: Basic care and comfort; CL: Analysis

54. 2. Allergic reactions may occur when the recipient reacts to allergens in the donor's blood; this reaction causes urticaria, flushing, and wheezing. A febrile reaction can occur, causing fever and urticaria but it isn't accompanied by rash. Diaphoresis, hot flashes, disorientation, and abdominal pain aren't symptoms of a transfusion reaction.
CN: Physiological integrity; CNS: Reduction of risk potential; CL: Analysis

55. 1. The influenza virus vaccine is usually administered annually to children at risk, not at monthly or 6-month intervals. The vaccine isn't contraindicated in children but is targeted at clients with chronic cardiac, pulmonary, hematologic, and neurologic problems.
CN: Health promotion and maintenance; CNS: None; CL: Application

56. 4. In exposed, high-risk clients, such as neonates, erythromycin may be effective in preventing or lessening the severity of the disease if administered during the preparoxysmal stage. Immune globulin isn't indicated; it's used as an immunization against hepatitis A. Neonates exposed to pertussis are at considerable risk for infections, regardless of the mother's immune status; however, infection isn't inevitable.
CN: Health promotion and maintenance; CNS: None; CL: Application

CN: Client needs category CNS: Client needs subcategory CL: Cognitive level

57. A child has recently been admitted to the pediatric unit with laboratory values indicating an increase in hemoglobin A_2. Based on this finding, the nurse should expect to follow a care plan based on which condition?
1. Beta-thalassemia trait
2. Iron deficiency
3. Lead poisoning
4. Sickle cell anemia

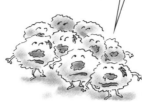

Somebody beta do something. It's getting awfully crowded in here.

57. 1. The concentration of hemoglobin A_2 is increased with beta-thalassemia trait. In severe iron deficiency, hemoglobin A_2 may be decreased. The hemoglobin A_2 level is normal in lead poisoning and sickle cell anemia.
CN: Physiological integrity; CNS: Reduction of risk potential; CL: Application

58. A 4-year-old client is asymptomatic but has a petechial rash. The platelet count is 20,000/µl and the hemoglobin level and white blood cell (WBC) count are normal. Which diagnosis would the nurse suspect as most likely?
1. Acute lymphoblastic leukemia (ALL)
2. Disseminated intravascular coagulation (DIC)
3. Idiopathic thrombocytopenic purpura (ITP)
4. Systemic lupus erythematosus (SLE)

58. 3. The onset of ITP typically occurs between ages 1 and 6. Clients are asymptomatic, except for petechial rash. ALL is associated with a low platelet count but an *abnormal* hemoglobin level and WBC count. DIC is secondary to a severe underlying disease. SLE is rare in a 4-year-old child.
CN: Physiological integrity; CNS: Physiological adaptation; CL: Analysis

59. Which of the following would the nurse incorporate in the discharge teaching for the parents of a neonate diagnosed with sickle cell anemia?
1. Stressing the importance of iron supplementation
2. Stressing the importance of monthly vitamin B_{12} injections
3. Demonstrating how to take an accurate temperature
4. Explaining that polyvalent pneumococcal vaccine is contraindicated

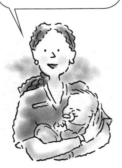

Make sure the parents of a neonate with sickle cell anemia are instructed in proper techniques.

59. 3. A temperature of 101.3° to 102.2° F (38.5° to 39° C) calls for emergency evaluation, even if the neonate appears well. Folic acid requirement is increased; therefore, supplementation is prudent. Vitamin B_{12} supplementation and iron supplementation aren't necessary. Pneumococcal vaccine is used because children with sickle cell anemia are prone to infection with *Streptococcus pneumoniae*.
CN: Health promotion and maintenance; CNS: None; CL: Application

60. Which finding yields a poor <u>prognosis</u> for a client with leukemia?
1. Presence of a mediastinal mass
2. Late central nervous system leukemia
3. Normal white blood cell (WBC) count at diagnosis
4. Disease presents between ages 2 and 10

60. 1. The presence of a mediastinal mass indicates a poor prognosis for clients with leukemia. Early central nervous system leukemia and a WBC count of 100,000/µl or higher indicate a poor prognosis for a client with leukemia. The prognosis is poorer if age at onset is less than 2 years or greater than 10 years.
CN: Physiological integrity; CNS: Physiological adaptation; CL: Analysis

CN: Client needs category   CNS: Client needs subcategory   CL: Cognitive level

61. A 1-year-old male infant is pale, but his physical examination is normal. Blood studies reveal his hematocrit is 24%. Which question would be most useful in helping to establish a diagnosis of anemia?
1. Is the infant on any medications?
2. What's the infant's usual daily diet?
3. Did the infant receive phototherapy for jaundice?
4. What's the pattern and appearance of bowel movements?

62. A nurse is teaching the parents of a child newly diagnosed with Hodgkin's disease. Which statement should the nurse include in her teaching?
1. "Staging laparotomy is mandatory for every client."
2. "Excessive weight gain can be a symptom."
3. "Hodgkin's disease is rare before age 5."
4. "The incidence of Hodgkin's disease peaks between ages 11 and 15."

63. A nurse counsels a client who has recently tested positive for human immunodeficiency virus (HIV). Which statement by the client indicates an understanding of the perinatal transmission of HIV?
1. "Drug therapy can reduce the incidence of perinatal infection."
2. "Since I have been recently diagnosed, the risk of infection is low."
3. "New drugs have eliminated the risk of perinatal infection."
4. "If you're really careful, there's no risk of infecting this child."

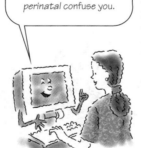

64. A 14-year-old female client is seen in the pediatrician's office with a history of mild sore throat, low-grade fever, and a diffuse maculopapular rash. She now complains of swelling of her wrists and redness in her eyes. The nurse interprets these findings as indications of which condition?
1. Rubella
2. Rubeola
3. Roseola
4. Varicella

61. 2. Iron deficiency anemia is the most common nutritional deficiency in infants between ages 9 months and 15 months. Anemia in a 1-year-old is mostly nutritional in origin, and its cause will be suggested by a detailed nutritional history. None of the other selections would be helpful in diagnosing anemia.
CN: Health promotion and maintenance; CNS: None; CL: Application

62. 3. Hodgkin's disease is rare before age 5. Staging laparotomy isn't recommended for clients who have obvious intra-abdominal disease easily diagnosed by noninvasive studies. Systemic symptoms of Hodgkin's disease include fever, night sweats, malaise, weight loss, and pruritus. The peak incidence of Hodgkin's disease occurs in late adolescence and young adulthood (ages 15 to 34).
CN: Physiological integrity; CNS: Physiological adaptation; CL: Analysis

63. 1. Transmission of HIV has decreased with the use of drugs given to the mother and the infant, but their use hasn't eliminated the transmission. There's no relationship between time of diagnosis and transmission.
CN: Health promotion and maintenance; CNS: None; CL: Analysis

64. 1. Rubella presents with a diffuse maculopapular rash, mild sore throat, low-grade fever and, occasionally, conjunctivitis, arthralgia, or arthritis. Rubeola is associated with high fever, which reaches its peak at the height of a generalized macular rash and typically lasts for 5 days. Roseola involves high fever and is abruptly followed by a rash. Varicella presents with fever, small erythematous macules on the trunk or scalp which progress to papules and clear vesicles on an erythematous base.
CN: Physiological integrity; CNS: Physiological adaptation; CL: Analysis

65. Which treatment would be the most appropriate for a child diagnosed with iron deficiency anemia?

1. Blood transfusion
2. Oral ferrous sulfate
3. An iron-fortified cereal
4. I.M. iron dextran

66. Which statement by a caregiver indicates that a 10-month-old client is at high risk for iron deficiency anemia?

1. "The baby is sleeping through the night without a bottle."
2. "The baby drinks about five 8-oz bottles of milk per day."
3. "The baby likes egg yolk in his cereal."
4. "The baby likes all vegetables except carrots."

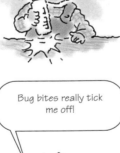

I'd like another bottle please.

67. A 6-year-old client has been diagnosed with Rocky Mountain spotted fever. In teaching the parents about the cause of the illness, the nurse would be correct in telling them that a bite by which animal or insect caused the illness?

1. Cat
2. Mosquito
3. Spider
4. Tick

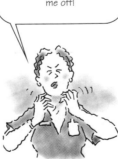

Bug bites really tick me off!

68. An iron dextran (DexFerrum) injection has been ordered for an 8-month-old client with iron deficiency anemia whose parents haven't been compliant with oral supplements. What's the correct method of injection for iron dextran?

1. Intradermally, using a small-gauge needle
2. Subcutaneously, using a small-gauge needle
3. I.M., at a 90-degree angle
4. I.M., using the Z-track method

65. 2. A prompt rise in hemoglobin level and hematocrit follows the administration of oral ferrous sulfate. Blood transfusion is rarely indicated unless a child becomes symptomatic or is further compromised by a superimposed infection. Dietary modifications are appropriate long-term measures, but they won't make enough iron available to replenish iron stores. I.M. iron dextran is reserved for use when compliance can't be achieved; it's expensive, painful, and no more effective than oral iron.
CN: Physiological integrity; CNS: Pharmacological therapies; CL: Application

66. 2. The recommended intake of milk, which doesn't contain iron, is 24 oz per day; 40 oz per day exceeds the recommended allotment and may reduce iron intake from solid food sources, risking iron deficiency anemia. Sleeping through the night without a bottle is an anticipated behavior at this age. Egg yolk is a good source of iron and would minimize any risk factor related to nutritional anemia. Because only dark green vegetables are good sources of iron, a dislike of carrots wouldn't be significant.
CN: Physiological integrity; CNS: Basic care and comfort; CL: Analysis

67. 4. Rocky Mountain spotted fever is caused by *Rickettsia rickettsii*, which is transmitted by the bite of a tick. Cat, mosquito, and spider bites haven't been known to transmit *R. rickettsii*.
CN: Safe, effective care environment; CNS: Safety and infection control; CL: Knowledge

68. 4. If iron dextran is ordered, it must be injected deeply into a large muscle mass, using the Z-track method to minimize skin staining and irritation. Neither a subcutaneous nor an intradermal injection would inject the dextran into the muscle. The Z-track method is preferred over a normal I.M. injection.
CN: Physiological integrity; CNS: Pharmacological therapies; CL: Application

69. When teaching parents about preventing nutritional iron deficiency, the nurse should emphasize which food as the most significant source of dietary iron?
1. Citrus fruits
2. Fish
3. Green vegetables
4. Milk products

70. Which instruction would the nurse incorporate into the teaching plan for parents about the proper administration of oral iron supplements?
1. Give the supplements with food.
2. Stop medication if vomiting occurs.
3. Decrease dose if constipation occurs.
4. Give the medicine via a dropper or through a straw.

71. While collecting client data, a nurse should recognize which symptom as the primary clinical manifestation of hemophilia?
1. Petechiae on the face
2. Prolonged bleeding time
3. Decreased clotting time
4. Decreased white blood cell (WBC) count

72. The nurse would be alert for signs and symptoms of internal bleeding <u>most commonly</u> at which site for a client with hemophilia?
1. Brain tissue
2. GI tract
3. Joint cavities
4. Spinal cord

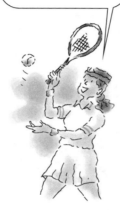

Be careful not to drop the ball on this question.

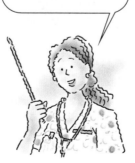

Careful! All of these answers may be accurate, but question 72 is asking for the most common site.

69. 3. Green vegetables are good sources of iron. Citrus foods aren't sources of iron but help with the absorption of iron. Fish isn't a good source of dietary iron. Milk is deficient in iron and should be limited in cases of nutritional anemia.
CN: Health promotion and maintenance; CNS: None; CL: Application

70. 4. Liquid iron preparations may temporarily stain the teeth; therefore, the drug should be given by dropper or through a straw. Supplements should be given between meals, when the presence of free hydrochloric acid is greatest. If vomiting occurs, supplementation shouldn't be stopped; instead, it should be administered with food. Constipation can be decreased by increasing intake of fruits and vegetables.
CN: Physiological integrity; CNS: Pharmacological therapies; CL: Application

71. 2. The effect of hemophilia is prolonged bleeding, anywhere from or within the body. With severe deficiencies, hemorrhage can occur as a result of minor trauma. Petechiae are uncommon in persons with hemophilia because repair of small hemorrhages depends on platelet function, not on blood clotting mechanisms. Clotting time is increased in a client with hemophilia. A decrease in WBCs is *not* indicative of hemophilia.
CN: Physiological integrity; CNS: Physiological adaptation; CL: Application

72. 3. The joint cavities, especially the knees, ankles, and elbows, are the most common site of internal bleeding. This bleeding typically results in bone changes and crippling, disabling deformities. Intracranial hemorrhage occurs less commonly than expected because the brain tissue has a high concentration of thromboplastin. Hemorrhage along the GI tract and spinal cord can occur but is less common.
CN: Physiological integrity; CNS: Physiological adaptation; CL: Application

CN: Client needs category   CNS: Client needs subcategory   CL: Cognitive level

73. Which measure should parents of a hemophilic client be taught to prepare them to initiate immediate treatment to prevent excessive blood loss?
 1. Applying heat to the area
 2. Not giving factor replacement
 3. Applying pressure for at least 5 minutes
 4. Immobilizing and elevating the affected area

74. A client with leukemia has an absolute granulocyte count of 400 µl. Which intervention would be the nurse's priority?
 1. Institute airborne precautions.
 2. Notify the physician immediately.
 3. Restrict anyone with active infections.
 4. Begin antibiotics per protocol.

75. Which measure is an important aid in prevention of the crippling effects of joint degeneration caused by hemophilia?
 1. Avoiding the use of analgesics
 2. Using aspirin for pain relief
 3. Administering replacement factor
 4. Using active range-of-motion (ROM) exercises

76. When comparing bleeding disorders, an increased tendency to bleed in which area differentiates von Willebrand's disease from hemophilia?
 1. Brain tissue
 2. GI tract
 3. Mucous membranes
 4. Spinal cord

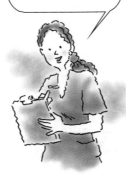

An ounce of prevention is worth a pound of cure.

73. 4. Elevating the area above the level of the heart will decrease blood flow. Cold, not heat, should be applied to promote vasoconstriction. Factor replacement should *not* be delayed. Pressure should be applied to the area for at least 10 to 15 minutes to allow clot formation.
CN: Physiological integrity; CNS: Physiological adaptation; CL: Application

74. 3. When the absolute granulocyte count is low, a client has difficulty fighting an infection. Anyone with active infections should be restricted to prevent the client from developing an infection. The client should be placed in a private room and fresh fruits, vegetables, and flowers should be restricted. Standard precautions are necessary and the client should wear a mask when out of the room, but airborne precautions aren't indicated because the client isn't infectious. The physician must be notified of the client's condition so that appropriate medical management is initiated. Antibiotics shouldn't be started without a septic workup first.
CN: Safe, effective care environment; CNS: Safety and infection control; CL: Application

75. 3. Prevention of bleeding is the ideal goal and is achieved by factor replacement therapy. Analgesics should be administered before physical therapy to control pain and provide the maximum benefit. Acetaminophen should be used for pain relief because aspirin has anticoagulant effects and has been linked to Reye's syndrome. Passive ROM exercises are usually instituted *after* the acute phase.
CN: Physiological integrity; CNS: Physiological adaptation; CL: Application

76. 3. The most characteristic clinical feature of von Willebrand's disease is an increased tendency to bleed from mucous membranes, which may be seen as frequent nosebleeds or menorrhagia. In hemophilia, the joint cavities are the most common site of internal bleeding. Bleeding into the GI tract, spinal cord, and brain tissue can occur, but these are *not* the most common sites for bleeding.
CN: Physiological integrity; CNS: Physiological adaptation; CL: Analysis

CN: Client needs category   CNS: Client needs subcategory   CL: Cognitive level

77. Which nursing measure is the priority for a client with von Willebrand's disease who's having <u>epistaxis</u>?
1. Lying the client in a supine position
2. Avoiding packing of nostrils
3. Avoiding pressure to the nose
4. Applying ice to the bridge of the nose

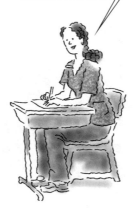

Epistaxis is a term from early in your schooling. Remember?

77. 4. Applying ice to the bridge of the nose is the priority because ice causes vasoconstriction and may stop bleeding. The client should be instructed to sit up and lean forward to avoid aspiration of blood. Pressure should then be maintained for at least 10 minutes to allow clotting to occur. Packing with tissue or cotton may be used to help stop bleeding, although care must be taken in removing packing to avoid dislodging the clot.
CN: Physiological integrity; CNS: Physiological adaptation; CL: Application

78. A nurse is teaching the parents of a child with acute lymphoblastic leukemia. The parents ask for information about what helps determine long-term survival. The nurse understands that the three most important prognostic factors are the:
1. histologic type of the disease, initial platelet count, and type of treatment.
2. type of treatment, stage at diagnosis, and age at diagnosis.
3. histologic type of the disease, initial white blood cell (WBC) count, and age at diagnosis.
4. progression of illness, initial WBC count, and age at diagnosis.

78. 3. The histologic type of the disease has the greatest prognostic value in determining long-term outcome. Clients with normal or low WBC counts at diagnosis tend to have much better prognoses than clients with high WBC counts. Clients diagnosed between the ages of 2 and 10 years consistently demonstrate better prognoses than clients who are younger than 2 years or older than 10 years when diagnosed.
CN: Physiological integrity; CNS: Physiological adaptation; CL: Analysis

79. Which complication would the nurse incorporate into a teaching plan about the three main consequences of leukemia?
1. Bone deformities, anemia, and infection
2. Anemia, infection, and bleeding tendencies
3. Pneumonia, thrombocytopenia, and alopecia
4. Polycythemia, decreased clotting time, and infection

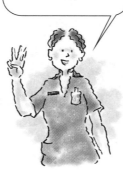

Do you know the three main consequences of leukemia?

79. 2. The three main consequences of leukemia are anemia, caused by decreased erythrocyte production, secondary to neutropenia; and infection and bleeding tendencies, from decreased platelet production. Bone deformities don't occur with leukemia. Pneumonia isn't a main consequence of leukemia. Alopecia occurs as an adverse effect of therapy. Anemia, not polycythemia, occurs. Clotting times would be prolonged.
CN: Physiological integrity; CNS: Physiological adaptation; CL: Application

80. A client is seen in the pediatrician's office for complaints of bone and joint pain. Which other signs and symptoms may suggest leukemia?
1. Abdominal pain
2. Increased activity level
3. Increased appetite
4. Petechiae

80. 4. The most common signs and symptoms of leukemia result from infiltration of the bone marrow. These include petechiae, fever, pallor, and joint pain with decreased activity level. Abdominal pain is caused by areas of inflammation from normal flora in the GI tract. Increased appetite can occur, but it usually isn't a presenting symptom.
CN: Physiological integrity; CNS: Physiological adaptation; CL: Application

81. Which findings in a client with leukemia would the nurse determine as indicating that the cancer has invaded the brain?
1. Headache and vomiting
2. Restlessness and tachycardia
3. Normal level of consciousness
4. Increased heart rate and decreased blood pressure

81. 1. The usual effect of leukemic infiltration of the brain is increased intracranial pressure. The proliferation of cells interferes with the flow of cerebrospinal fluid in the subarachnoid space and at the base of the brain. The increased fluid pressure causes dilation of the ventricles, which creates symptoms of severe headache, vomiting, irritability, lethargy, increased blood pressure, decreased heart rate and, eventually, coma.
CN: Physiological integrity; CNS: Physiological adaptation; CL: Analysis

82. Which type of leukemia carries the best prognosis?
1. Acute lymphoblastic leukemia
2. Acute myelogenous leukemia
3. Basophilic leukemia
4. Eosinophilic leukemia

82. 1. Acute lymphoblastic leukemia, which accounts for more than 80% of all childhood cases, carries the best prognosis. Acute myelogenous leukemia, with several subtypes, accounts for most of the other leukemias affecting children. Basophilic and eosinophilic leukemia are named for the specific cells involved. These are rarer and carry a poorer prognosis.
CN: Physiological integrity; CNS: Physiological adaptation; CL: Knowledge

83. The nurse prepares a client newly diagnosed with leukemia for a spinal tap based on the rationale that this procedure helps to:
1. rule out meningitis.
2. decrease intracranial pressure (ICP).
3. aid in classification of the leukemia.
4. assess for central nervous system infiltration.

83. 4. A spinal tap is performed to assess for central nervous system infiltration. A spinal tap can be done to rule out meningitis, but this isn't the indication for the test on a client with leukemia. It wouldn't be done to decrease ICP nor does it aid in the classification of the leukemia.
CN: Physiological integrity; CNS: Physiological adaptation; CL: Application

84. Which test would the nurse expect to be performed on a client with leukemia before initiation of therapy to evaluate his ability to metabolize chemotherapeutic agents?
1. Lumbar puncture
2. Liver function studies
3. Complete blood count (CBC)
4. Peripheral blood smear

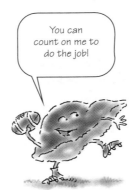

You can count on me to do the job!

84. 2. Liver and kidney function studies are done before initiation of chemotherapy to evaluate the child's ability to metabolize the chemotherapeutic agents. A lumbar puncture is performed to assess for central nervous system infiltration. A CBC is performed to assess for anemia. A peripheral blood smear is done to assess the level of immature white blood cells (blastocytes).
CN: Physiological integrity; CNS: Pharmacological therapies; CL: Application

85. Which type of leukemia accounts for most cases of childhood leukemia?
1. Acute lymphocytic leukemia (ALL)
2. Acute myelogenous leukemia (AML)
3. Chronic myelogenous leukemia (CML)
4. Chronic lymphocytic leukemia (CLL)

85. 1. The most common subtype, ALL, accounts for 75% to 80% of all childhood cases, with AML (myelocytic, myelogenous, or non-lymphoblastic) comprising approximately 20%, and CML approximately 2%. CLL occurs in older clients; 90% of cases are persons older than age 50.
CN: Physiological integrity; CNS: Physiological adaptation; CL: Knowledge

CN: Client needs category   CNS: Client needs subcategory   CL: Cognitive level

86. Which medication would the nurse expect the physician to order <u>most</u> commonly for a client with leukemia as prophylaxis against *Pneumocystis carinii* pneumonia?
1. Co-trimoxazole (Bactrim)
2. Oral nystatin suspension
3. Prednisone (Deltasone)
4. Vincristine (Oncovin)

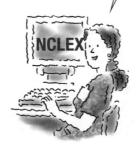

I'll have to choose one answer because they can't ALL be right!

86. 1. The most common cause of death from leukemia is overwhelming infection. *P. carinii* infection is lethal to a child with leukemia. As prophylaxis against *P. carinii* pneumonia, continuous low dosages of co-trimoxazole are usually prescribed. Oral nystatin suspension would be indicated for the treatment of thrush. Prednisone isn't an antibiotic and increases susceptibility to infection. Vincristine is an antineoplastic agent.
CN: Physiological integrity; CNS: Pharmacological therapies; CL: Application

87. A nurse is discussing the discharge plan for a child on methotrexate (Trexall) with his mother. The mother asks the nurse how the drug works. Which statement by the nurse is the <u>most</u> accurate?
1. "The drug interferes with the use of folic acid by cancer cells."
2. "The drug keeps the cancer cell wall from forming."
3. "The drug makes the cancer cells ineffective by massing them together."
4. "The drug interferes with mitochondrial activity."

87. 1. Methotrexate is an antimetabolite and antifolate. It prevents folic acid from being used to create nucleic acid. As a result, it interferes with mitosis, which prevents the cancer cells from multiplying. It doesn't interfere with the cell wall, cause massing of the cells, or interfere with mitochondrial activity.
CN: Physiological integrity; CNS: Pharmacological therapies; CL: Application

88. A 4-year-old child is diagnosed as having acute lymphocytic leukemia. His white blood cell (WBC) count, especially the neutrophil count, is low. Which intervention should the nurse teach the parents?
1. Protect the child from falls because of his increased risk of bleeding.
2. Protect the child from infections because his resistance to infection is decreased.
3. Provide rest periods because the oxygen-carrying capacity of the child's blood is diminished.
4. Treat constipation, which frequently accompanies a decrease in WBCs.

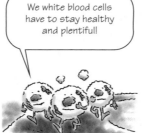

We white blood cells have to stay healthy and plentiful!

88. 2. One of the complications of both acute lymphocytic leukemia and its treatment is a decreased WBC count, specifically a decreased absolute neutrophil count. Because neutrophils are the body's first line of defense against infection, the child must be protected from infection. Bleeding is a risk factor if platelets or other coagulation factors are decreased. A decreased hemoglobin level, hematocrit, or both would reduce the oxygen-carrying capacity of the child's blood. Constipation isn't related to the WBC count.
CN: Safe, effective care environment; CNS: Safety and infection control; CL: Application

89. When teaching an adolescent with iron deficiency anemia about diet choices, which menu selection by the adolescent indicates that more instruction is necessary?
1. Caesar salad and pretzels
2. Cheeseburger and milkshake
3. Red beans and rice with sausage
4. Egg sandwich and snack peanuts

89. 1. Caesar salad and pretzels aren't foods high in iron and protein. Meats (especially organ meats), eggs, and nuts have high protein and iron.
CN: Health promotion and maintenance; CNS: None; CL: Analysis

CN: Client needs category   CNS: Client needs subcategory   CL: Cognitive level

90. Nausea and vomiting are common adverse effects of radiation and chemotherapy. When should a nurse administer antiemetics?
1. 30 minutes before initiation of therapy
2. With the administration of therapy
3. Immediately after nausea begins
4. When therapy is completed

91. A child is admitted to the pediatric unit with an unknown mass in her lower left abdomen. Which action should be the nurse's priority?
1. Obtain the history of the illness.
2. Place a "Do Not Palpate Abdomen" sign over the child's bed.
3. Obtain a complete set of vital signs.
4. Schedule a hemoglobin and hematocrit test for early morning.

> Question 91 describes a potentially dangerous situation, so prioritizing is important.

92. Which nursing measure is helpful when mouth ulcers develop as an adverse effect of chemotherapy?
1. Using lemon glycerin swabs
2. Administering milk of magnesia
3. Providing a bland, moist, soft diet
4. Frequently washing the mouth with alcohol-based mouthwash

> A nurse's keen observation is important.

93. Which condition assessed by the nurse would indicate an early warning sign of childhood cancer?
1. Difficulty in swallowing
2. Nagging cough or hoarseness
3. Slight change in bowel and bladder habits
4. Swellings, lumps, or masses anywhere on the body

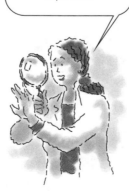

90. 1. Antiemetics are most beneficial if given before the onset of nausea and vomiting. To calculate the optimum time for administration, the first dose is given 30 minutes to 1 hour before nausea is expected, and then every 2, 4, or 6 hours for approximately 24 hours after chemotherapy. If the antiemetic were given with the medication or after the medication, it could lose its maximum effectiveness when needed.
CN: Physiological integrity; CNS: Pharmacological therapies; CL: Application

91. 2. The nurse must take measures to prevent palpation of the mass, if possible. If the mass is a malignant tumor, a do-not-palpate warning will help prevent trauma and rupture of the suspected tumor capsule. Rupture of the tumor capsule may cause seeding of cancer cells throughout the abdomen. Obtaining the history and vital signs and scheduling laboratory work are important but not the priority.
CN: Physiological integrity; CNS: Physiological adaptation; CL: Analysis

92. 3. Oral ulcers are red, eroded, and painful. Providing a bland, moist, soft diet will make chewing and swallowing less painful. The use of lemon glycerin swabs and milk of magnesia should be avoided. Glycerin, a trihydric alcohol, absorbs water and dries the membranes. Milk of magnesia also has a drying effect because unabsorbed magnesium salts exert an osmotic pressure on tissue fluids. Many children also find the taste unpleasant. Frequent mouthwashes consisting of ½ tsp of salt plus ½ tsp of baking soda dissolved in an 8-oz glass of water are recommended.
CN: Physiological integrity; CNS: Basic care and comfort; CL: Application

93. 4. By being aware of early signs of childhood cancer, nurses can refer children for further evaluation. Swellings, lumps, or masses anywhere on the body are early warning signals of childhood cancer. Difficulty swallowing, cough, and hoarseness are early signs of cancer in adults. Usually, there's also a marked change in bowel or bladder habits.
CN: Health promotion and maintenance; CNS: None; CL: Application

CN: Client needs category   CNS: Client needs subcategory   CL: Cognitive level

94. A mother of a child receiving the antineoplastic drug procarbazine (Mutalane) indicates that she understands her child's dietary requirements when she makes which statement?
  1. "I'll decrease his spicy food intake."
  2. "I'll decrease his fluid intake."
  3. "I'll include foods such as liver."
  4. "I'll keep him away from cheese and pepperoni pizza."

A careful diet is very important for a child receiving chemotherapy.

94. 4. Procarbazine has monoamine inhibitory activity. Foods high in tyramine, such as cheese and pepperoni, should be avoided. There's no chemotherapeutic or physiologic reason to restrict spicy foods. Increased fluid intake is essential to prevent calculi formation. Liver should be avoided because it contains tyramine, which can cause tremors, palpitations, and increased blood pressure.
CN: Physiological integrity; CNS: Pharmacological therapies; CL: Analysis

95. Which intervention can prevent hemorrhagic cystitis caused by bladder irritation from chemotherapeutic medications?
  1. Giving antacids
  2. Giving antibiotics
  3. Restricting fluid intake
  4. Increasing fluid intake

95. 4. Sterile hemorrhagic cystitis is an adverse effect of chemical irritation of the bladder from cyclophosphamide. It can be prevented by liberal fluid intake (at least 1½ times the recommended daily fluid requirement). Antacids wouldn't be indicated for treatment. Antibiotics don't aid in the prevention of sterile hemorrhagic cystitis. Restricting fluids would only increase the risk of developing cystitis.
CN: Physiological integrity; CNS: Reduction of risk potential; CL: Application

96. The parents of a child diagnosed with leukemia have stated that they'll give aspirin to their child for pain relief. Which statement by the nurse about aspirin would be <u>most</u> accurate?
  1. "It's contraindicated because it decreases platelet production."
  2. "It's contraindicated because it promotes bleeding tendencies."
  3. "It's not a strong enough analgesic."
  4. "It decreases the effects of methotrexate (Trexall)."

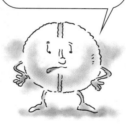

As much as I'd like to help, I'm not always the best choice.

96. 2. Aspirin would be contraindicated because it promotes bleeding. Aspirin use has also been associated with Reye's syndrome in children. For home use, acetaminophen (Tylenol) is recommended for mild to moderate pain. Aspirin enhances the effects of methotrexate and has no effect on platelet production. Nonopioid analgesia has been effective for mild to moderate pain in clients with leukemia.
CN: Physiological integrity; CNS: Pharmacological therapies; CL: Application

97. Which nursing measure helps prepare the parent and child for alopecia, a common adverse effect of several chemotherapeutic agents?
  1. Introducing the idea of a wig after hair loss occurs
  2. Explaining that hair begins to regrow in 6 to 9 months
  3. Stressing that hair loss during a second treatment with the same medication will be more severe
  4. Explaining that, as hair thins, keeping it clean, short, and fluffy may camouflage partial baldness

97. 4. The nurse must prepare parents and children for possible hair loss. Cutting the hair short lessens the impact of seeing large quantities of hair on bed linens and clothing. Sometimes, keeping the hair short and fuller can make a wig unnecessary. A child should be encouraged to pick out a wig similar to his own hair style and color before the hair falls out, to foster adjustment to hair loss. Hair regrows in 3 to 6 months. Hair loss during a second treatment with the same medication is usually less severe.
CN: Psychosocial integrity; CNS: None; CL: Application

CN: Client needs category   CNS: Client needs subcategory   CL: Cognitive level

98. A nurse is discussing childhood cancers with the parents of a child in an oncology unit. Which statement by the nurse would be <u>most</u> accurate?

1. "The most common site for children's cancer is the bone marrow."
2. "All childhood cancers have a high mortality rate."
3. "Children with leukemia have a higher survival rate if they're older than 17 when diagnosed."
4. "The prognosis for children with cancer isn't affected by treatment strategies."

99. Which nursing intervention helps to decrease the adverse effects of radiation therapy on the GI tract?

1. Avoiding the use of antispasmodics
2. Encouraging fluids and a soft diet
3. Giving antiemetics when nausea or vomiting occurs
4. Avoiding mouthwashes to prevent irritation of mouth ulcers

100. Short-term steroid therapy is used in clients with leukemia to promote which reaction?

1. Increased appetite
2. Altered body image
3. Increased platelet production
4. Decreased susceptibility to infection

101. The school nurse is conducting registration for a first grader. Which immunizations should the school nurse verify that the child has had before entering school? Select all that apply:

1. Hepatitis B series
2. Diphtheria-tetanus-pertussis series
3. Haemophilus influenzae type b series
4. Varicella zoster
5. Pneumonia vaccine
6. Inactivated polio vaccine

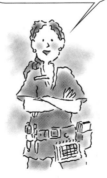

One hundred questions under your belt. Only a few more to go!

98. 1. Childhood cancers occur most commonly in tissue with rapid cell division such as bone marrow. Mortality depends on the time of diagnosis, the type of cancer, and the age at which the child was diagnosed. Children who are diagnosed between the ages of 2 and 9 consistently demonstrate a better prognosis. Treatment strategies are tailored to produce the most favorable prognosis.

CN: Physiological integrity; CNS: Physiological adaptation; CL: Application

99. 2. Radiation therapy can cause such adverse effects as nausea and vomiting, anorexia, mucosal ulceration, and diarrhea. Encouraging fluids and a soft diet will help with anorexia. Antispasmodics are used to help reduce diarrhea. Antiemetics should be given before the onset of nausea. Frequent mouthwashes are indicated to prevent mycosis.

CN: Physiological integrity; CNS: Pharmacological therapies; CL: Application

100. 1. Short-term steroid therapy produces no acute toxicities and results in two beneficial reactions: increased appetite and a sense of well-being. Physical changes, such as "moon-face," a result of steroid use, can cause alterations in body image and can be extremely distressing to children. Prednisone (steroid therapy) has no effect on platelet production but may increase susceptibility to infection.

CN: Physiological integrity; CNS: Pharmacological therapies; CL: Knowledge

101. 1, 2, 3, 6. Hepatitis B series, diphtheria-tetanus-pertussis series, *H. influenzae* type b series, and inactivated polio vaccine are immunizations that the child should receive before entering first grade. The varicella zoster vaccine is administered only if the child hasn't had chickenpox. Pneumonia vaccine isn't required or routinely given to children.

CN: Health promotion and maintenance; CNS: None; CL: Knowledge

CN: Client needs category   CNS: Client needs subcategory   CL: Cognitive level

102. The nurse is preparing a school-age child for a bone marrow biopsy to rule out leukemia. The nurse explains that the sample will be taken from the anterior iliac crest. Identify this area.

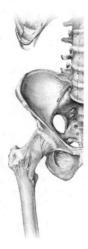

103. A child is admitted to the unit with a diagnosis of hemophilia. When assisting with the care plan, what facts about the disease should the nurse keep in mind? Select all that apply:
1. Hemophilia is a sex-linked genetic disorder.
2. Bleeding occurs most commonly in the joints.
3. The most common treatments include pressure and ice.
4. Hemophilia can be caused by a retrovirus.
5. Administration of whole blood is generally effective in stopping bleeding episodes.

102.

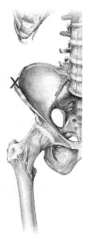

A bone marrow biopsy may be taken from the anterior or posterior iliac crests, sternum, vertebral spinous process, rib, or tibia.
CN: Physiological integrity; CNS: Physiological adaptation; CL: Comprehension

103. 1, 2. Hemophilia is a sex-linked genetic disorder and bleeding episodes most commonly occur in joints, such as the knee or elbow. Pressure and ice may be helpful, but these interventions don't have any effect on clotting factors in the blood, so bleeding may resume as soon as these interventions stop. Hemophilia isn't caused by a retrovirus and administration of clotting factors VIII and IX (not whole blood), is the treatment of choice.
CN: Safe, effective care environment; CNS: Coordinated care; CL: Analysis

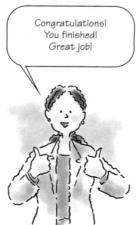

Congratulations! You finished! Great job!

CN: Client needs category   CNS: Client needs subcategory   CL: Cognitive level

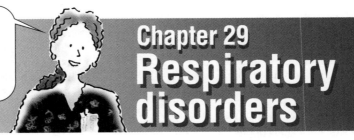

Chapter 29
Respiratory disorders

1. Which definition best describes the etiology of sudden infant death syndrome (SIDS)?
1. Cardiac arrhythmias
2. Apnea of prematurity
3. Unexplained death of an infant
4. Apparent life-threatening event

2. Which child has an increased risk of sudden infant death syndrome (SIDS)?
1. Premature infant with low birth weight
2. A healthy 2-year-old
3. Infant hospitalized for fever
4. Firstborn child

3. A 6-week-old infant who isn't breathing is brought to the emergency department; a preliminary finding of sudden infant death syndrome (SIDS) is made to the parents. Which intervention should the nurse take <u>initially</u>?
1. Call their spiritual advisor.
2. Explain the etiology of SIDS.
3. Allow them to see their infant.
4. Collect the infant's belongings and give them to the parents.

4. Which risk factor is related to sudden infant death syndrome (SIDS)?
1. Feeding habits
2. Gestational age of 42 weeks
3. Immunizations
4. Stomach sleeping

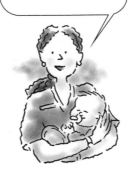

It's important to know the risk factors for SIDS.

1. 3. SIDS can best be defined as the sudden death of an infant younger than age 1 that remains unexplained after autopsy. Apnea of prematurity occurs in infants less than 32 weeks' gestation who have periodic breathing lapses for 20 seconds or more. Apparent life-threatening events usually have some combination of apnea, color change, marked change in muscle tone, choking, or gagging.
CN: Physiological integrity; CNS: Physiological adaptation; CL: Knowledge

2. 1. Premature infants, especially those with low birth weight, have an increased risk for SIDS. Infants with apnea, central nervous system disorders, or respiratory disorders also have a higher risk of SIDS. Peak age for SIDS is 2 to 4 months. Hospitalization for fever is insignificant. There's an increased risk of SIDS in subsequent siblings of two or more SIDS victims.
CN: Physiological integrity; CNS: Reduction of risk potential; CL: Knowledge

3. 3. The parents need time with their infant to assist with the grieving process. Calling their pastor and collecting the infant's belongings are also important steps in the care plan but aren't priorities. The parents will be too upset to understand an explanation of SIDS at this time.
CN: Physiological integrity; CNS: Physiological adaptation; CL: Application

4. 4. Studies have shown that stomach sleeping is the foremost risk factor for SIDS. Multiple births, prematurity, and low birth weight are also important risk factors. Feeding habits and a gestational age of 42 weeks aren't significant. Immunizations have been disproved to be associated with the disorder.
CN: Physiological integrity; CNS: Reduction of risk potential; CL: Knowledge

CN: Client needs category   CNS: Client needs subcategory   CL: Cognitive level

5. An infant is brought to the emergency department and pronounced dead with the preliminary finding of sudden infant death syndrome (SIDS). Which question to the parents is appropriate?

    1. Did you hear the infant cry out?
    2. Was the infant's head buried in a blanket?
    3. Were any of the siblings jealous of the new baby?
    4. How did the infant look when you found him?

5. 4. Only factual questions should be asked during the initial history in the emergency department. The other questions imply blame, guilt, or neglect.

CN: Physiological integrity; CNS: Physiological adaptation; CL: Application

6. Which diagnostic test should be included in the care plan for children with an increased risk of sudden infant death syndrome (SIDS)?

    1. Pulmonary function testing at regular intervals
    2. Home apnea monitoring
    3. Pulse oximetry while sleeping
    4. Chest X-ray at age 1 month

6. 2. A home apnea monitor is recommended for infants with an increased risk of SIDS. Diagnostic tests, such as pulmonary function tests, pulse oximetry, and chest X-rays, can't diagnose the risk of surviving or dying from SIDS.

CN: Physiological integrity; CNS: Reduction of risk potential; CL: Application

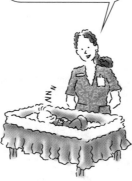

There's really only one way to monitor an infant for SIDS.

7. Which reaction is usually exhibited first by the family of an infant who has died from sudden infant death syndrome (SIDS)?

    1. Feelings of blame or guilt
    2. Acceptance of the diagnosis
    3. Requests for the infant's belongings
    4. Questions regarding the etiology of the diagnosis

7. 1. During the first few moments, the parents usually are in shock and have overwhelming feelings of blame or guilt. Acceptance of the diagnosis and questions regarding the etiology may not occur until the parents have had time to see the child. The infant's belongings are usually packaged for the family to take home but some parents may see this as a painful reminder.

CN: Psychosocial integrity; CNS: None; CL: Application

8. When talking with the parents of an infant who has died from sudden infant death syndrome (SIDS), which procedure would the nurse include as being used to confirm the diagnosis?

    1. Autopsy
    2. Chest X-ray
    3. Skeletal survey
    4. Laboratory analysis

8. 1. Autopsies reveal consistent pathologic findings, such as pulmonary edema and intrathoracic hemorrhages, that confirm the diagnosis of SIDS. Chest X-rays are used to diagnose respiratory complications. Skeletal surveys are used with cases of suspected child abuse. Laboratory analysis will show no characteristics to confirm the diagnosis of SIDS.

CN: Physiological integrity; CNS: Physiological adaptation; CL: Comprehension

9. Which plan is most appropriate for a discharge home visit to parents who lost an infant to sudden infant death syndrome (SIDS)?
1. One visit in 2 weeks
2. No visit is necessary
3. As soon after death as possible
4. One visit with parents only, no siblings

10. A few days after the death of an infant from sudden infant death syndrome (SIDS), which behavior would the nurse expect to observe in a parent?
1. Disorganized thinking
2. Feelings of guilt
3. Repressed thoughts
4. Structured thinking

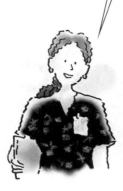

Make sure you understand the grieving process necessary for SIDS parents.

11. Which position is recommended for placing an infant to sleep?
1. Prone position
2. Supine position
3. Side-lying position
4. With head of bed elevated 30 degrees

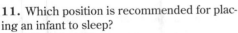

12. Which activity should be recommended for long-term support of parents who have lost an infant due to sudden infant death syndrome (SIDS)?
1. Attending support groups
2. Attending church regularly
3. Attending counseling sessions
4. Discussing feelings with family and friends

9. 3. When parents return home, a visit is necessary as soon after the death as possible. The nurse should assess what the parents have been told, what they think happened, and how they've explained this to the other siblings. Not all of these issues will be resolved in one visit. The number of visits and plan for intervention must be flexible. The needs of the siblings must always be considered.
CN: Psychosocial integrity; CNS: None; CL: Application

10. 1. Within a day or two of the infant's death, the parents enter the impact phase of crisis, which consists of disorganized thoughts in which they can't deal with the crisis in concrete terms. Almost immediately, at the time of death, parents may have repressed thoughts and feelings of guilt or blame. One week after the death, the parent of the infant would most likely be in the turmoil phase. In the turmoil phase, structured thinking is common.
CN: Psychosocial integrity; CNS: None; CL: Comprehension

11. 2. The American Academy of Pediatrics endorses placing infants only face-up in their cribs as a way to reduce the risk of sudden infant death syndrome (SIDS). Raising the head of the bed 30 degrees is recommended for infants with gastroesophageal reflux. The side-lying position promotes gastric emptying but the infant might roll to a prone position, predisposing him to SIDS. Placing infants on their stomachs is thought to make an attack of apnea harder to fight off but exactly how the sleeping position predisposes a child to SIDS is still unclear.
CN: Health promotion and maintenance; CNS: None; CL: Application

12. 1. The best support will come from parents who have had the same experience. Attending church and discussing feelings with family and friends can offer support, but they may not understand the experience. Counseling sessions are usually a short-term support.
CN: Psychosocial integrity; CNS: None; CL: Application

13. Which intervention is best to help a 2-year-old child adapt to a mist tent?
1. Tape the tent closed.
2. Place the child's favorite toys in the tent.
3. Allow the child to play with the tent first.
4. Ask one or both parents to stay with the child.

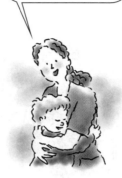

Encourage the parents of a hospitalized toddler to stay with the child as much as possible.

14. A 2-year-old child comes to the emergency department with inspiratory stridor and a barking cough. A preliminary diagnosis of croup has been made. Which action should be an initial intervention?
1. Administer I.V. antibiotics.
2. Provide oxygen by facemask.
3. Establish and maintain the airway.
4. Ask the mother to go to the waiting room.

15. Which is the best intervention for parents to take if their child is experiencing an episode of "midnight croup," or acute spasmodic laryngitis?
1. Give warm liquids.
2. Raise the heat on the thermostat.
3. Provide humidified air with cool mist.
4. Take the child into the bathroom with a warm, running shower.

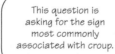

This question is asking for the sign most commonly associated with croup.

16. A child is admitted with a diagnosis of croup. Which sign, most characteristic of a child with croup, would the nurse expect?
1. "Barking" cough
2. High fever
3. Low heart rate
4. Severe respiratory distress

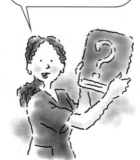

13. 4. The most important factor in helping a child cope with new and strange surroundings is to encourage feelings of security by having the parents present—the hallmark of family-centered care. Taping the tent closed is inappropriate. Placing the child's favorite toys in the tent provides distraction and allows the child to have something of his own with him but may *not* alleviate fears. Allowing the child to play with the tent may pose a safety hazard and isn't appropriate for a child in respiratory distress.
CN: Psychosocial integrity; CNS: None; CL: Application

14. 3. The initial priority is to establish and maintain the airway. Edema and accumulation of secretions may contribute to airway obstruction. Antibiotics aren't indicated for viral illnesses. Oxygen should be administered by tent as soon as possible to decrease the child's distress. Allowing the child to stay with the mother reduces anxiety and distress.
CN: Physiological integrity; CNS: Physiological adaptation; CL: Application

15. 3. High humidity with cool mist, such as from a cool mist humidifier, provides the most relief. Cool liquids would be best for the child. If unable to take liquid, the child needs emergency care. Raising the heat on the thermostat will result in dry, warm air, which may cause secretions to adhere to the airway wall. A warm, running shower provides a mist that may be helpful to moisten and decrease the viscosity of airway secretions and may also decrease laryngeal spasm.
CN: Physiological integrity; CNS: Physiological adaptation; CL: Application

16. 1. A resonant cough described as "barking" is the most characteristic sign of croup. Usually the heart rate is rapid. The child may present with a low-grade or high fever depending on whether the etiologic agent is viral or bacterial. The child may have varying degrees of respiratory distress related to swelling or obstruction.
CN: Physiological integrity; CNS: Physiological adaptation; CL: Comprehension

CN: Client needs category   CNS: Client needs subcategory   CL: Cognitive level

17. When describing croup to a child's parents, which characteristic would the nurse include?
1. Inflammation of the palatine tonsils
2. Acute, highly contagious respiratory infection
3. Infection of supraglottic area with involvement of the epiglottis
4. Clinical syndrome of laryngitis and laryngotracheobronchitis

18. Which intervention is the <u>most important</u> goal for a child with ineffective airway clearance?
1. Reducing the child's anxiety
2. Maintaining a patent airway
3. Providing adequate oral fluids
4. Administering medications as ordered

19. Which of the following would the nurse expect to find initially in a 2-year-old child with croup suffering respiratory distress?
1. Capillary refill time less than 3 seconds
2. Low temperature
3. Grunting or head bobbing
4. Respiratory rate of 28 breaths/minute

20. Which precaution is recommended when caring for children with respiratory infections such as croup?
1. Enforce hand washing.
2. Place the child in isolation.
3. Teach children to use tissues.
4. Keep siblings in the same room.

21. What's the best time to administer a nebulizer treatment to a hospitalized child with croup?
1. During naptime
2. During playtime
3. After the child eats
4. After the parents leave

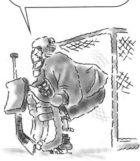

Question 18 is asking about the most important goal.

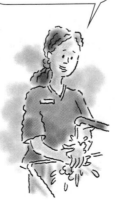

Hand washing helps prevent the spread of infection.

17. 4. Croup is a general term referring to acute infections affecting varying degrees of the larynx, trachea, and bronchi. Inflammation of the palatine tonsils is consistent with tonsillitis. Pertussis, or whooping cough, is an acute, highly contagious respiratory infection. Epiglottiditis is a form of croup affecting the supraglottic area.
CN: Physiological integrity; CNS: Physiological adaptation; CL: Comprehension

18. 2. The most important goal is to maintain a patent airway. Reducing anxiety and administering medications will follow after the airway is secure. The child shouldn't be allowed to eat or drink anything to avoid the risk of aspiration.
CN: Physiological integrity; CNS: Physiological adaptation; CL: Application

19. 3. Grunting or head bobbing is seen in a child in respiratory distress. Capillary refill time of less than 3 seconds and a respiratory rate of 28 breaths/minute are normal findings. The child's temperature may be elevated if infection is present.
CN: Physiological integrity; CNS: Physiological adaptation; CL: Comprehension

20. 1. Hand washing helps prevent the spread of infections. Ill children should be placed in separate bedrooms if possible but don't need to be isolated. Teaching children to use tissues properly is important, but the key is disposal and hand washing after use.
CN: Health promotion and maintenance; CNS: None; CL: Application

21. 1. The nurse should administer nebulizer treatments at prescribed intervals. During naptime allows for as little disruption as possible. Administering treatment during playtime will disrupt the child's daily pattern. A child should be given a treatment before eating so the airway will be open and the work of eating will be decreased. Parents are usually helpful when administering treatments. The child can sit on the parent's lap to help decrease anxiety or fear.
CN: Physiological integrity; CNS: Pharmacological therapies; CL: Application

CN: Client needs category   CNS: Client needs subcategory   CL: Cognitive level

22. During the recovery stages of croup, the nurse should explain which intervention to parents?

    1. Limiting oral fluid intake
    2. Recognizing signs of respiratory distress
    3. Providing three nutritious meals per day
    4. Allowing the child to go to the playground

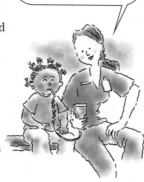

Adequate parent teaching is essential for managing a child with croup.

23. The nurse understands that which agent is related to acute epiglottiditis?

    1. Allergen
    2. Bacteria
    3. Virus
    4. Yeast

24. Which clinical observation would lead the nurse to suspect epiglottiditis?

    1. Decreased secretions
    2. Drooling
    3. Low-grade fever
    4. Spontaneous cough

25. Which strategy would be best to include in the care plan for a child with acute epiglottiditis?

    1. Encourage oral fluids for hydration.
    2. Maintain the client in semi-Fowler's position.
    3. Administer I.V. antibiotic therapy.
    4. Maintain respiratory isolation for 48 hours.

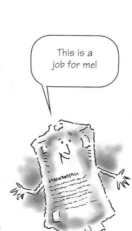

This is a job for me!

26. A 2-year-old child is found on the floor next to his toy chest. After first determining unresponsiveness and calling for help, which step should be taken <u>next</u>?

    1. Start mouth-to-mouth resuscitation.
    2. Begin chest compressions.
    3. Check for a pulse.
    4. Open the airway.

22. 2. Although most children recover without complications, the parents should be able to recognize signs and symptoms of respiratory distress and know how to access emergency services. Oral fluids should be encouraged because fluids help to thin secretions. Although nutrition is important, frequent small nutritious snacks are usually more appealing than an entire meal. Children should have optimal rest and engage in quiet play. A comfortable environment free of noxious stimuli lessens respiratory distress.

CN: Physiological integrity; CNS: Physiological adaptation; CL: Application

23. 2. *Haemophilus influenzae* type B is usually the bacterial agent responsible for acute epiglottiditis. Allergens and viral agents can be seen with acute laryngotracheobronchitis and acute spasmodic croup. Yeast infections in the oral cavity cause thrush.

CN: Physiological integrity; CNS: Physiological adaptation; CL: Comprehension

24. 2. Drooling is common due to the pain of swallowing, excessive secretions, and sore throat. The child usually has a high fever and the absence of a spontaneous cough. The classic picture is the child in a tripod position with mouth open and tongue protruding.

CN: Physiological integrity; CNS: Physiological adaptation; CL: Comprehension

25. 3. The etiologic agent for epiglottiditis is usually bacterial; therefore, the treatment consists of I.V. antibiotic therapy. The client shouldn't be allowed anything by mouth during the initial phases of the infection to prevent aspiration. The client should be placed in Fowler's position or any position that provides the most comfort and security. Respiratory isolation isn't required.

CN: Physiological integrity; CNS: Physiological adaptation; CL: Application

26. 4. The airway should be opened by using the head-tilt, chin-lift maneuver and breathlessness should be determined at the start of cardiopulmonary resuscitation. The sequence of airway, breathing, and circulation must be followed.

CN: Physiological integrity; CNS: Physiological adaptation; CL: Application

CN: Client needs category   CNS: Client needs subcategory   CL: Cognitive level

27. A 10-month-old infant is found in respiratory arrest and cardiopulmonary resuscitation is started. Which site is best to check for a pulse?
1. Brachial
2. Carotid
3. Femoral
4. Radial

27. 1. Palpation of the brachial artery is recommended. The short, chubby neck of infants makes rapid location of the carotid artery difficult. After age 1, the carotid or femoral would be used. The femoral pulse, commonly palpated in a hospital setting, may be difficult to assess because of the infant's position, fat folds, and clothing. The radial pulse isn't a good indicator of central artery perfusion.
CN: Physiological integrity; CNS: Physiological adaptation; CL: Application

28. A nurse is giving rescue breathing to an infant under age 1. What is the <u>ratio</u> of breaths per second?
1. One breath every 2 to 3 seconds
2. One breath every 3 to 5 seconds
3. One breath every 4 to 6 seconds
4. One breath every 5 to 7 seconds

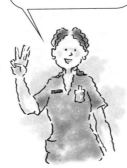

The next three questions ask you to think about procedures as they relate to infants or children, not adults.

28. 2. Rescue breathing should be performed once every 3 to 5 seconds until spontaneous breathing resumes. This provides approximately 12 to 20 breaths/minute. One breath every 2 to 3 seconds may cause gastric distention. One breath every 5 to 6 seconds is recommended for adults.
CN: Physiological integrity; CNS: Physiological adaptation; CL: Application

29. When performing chest compressions on a 2-year-old child, which depths is correct?
1. ½″ to 1″ (1 to 2.5 cm)
2. 1″ to 1½″ (2.5 to 4 cm)
3. 1½″ to 2″ (4 to 5 cm)
4. 2″ to 2½″ (5 to 6 cm)

29. 2. The chest compressions should equal approximately one-third to one-half the total depth of the chest. This corresponds to about 1″ to 1½″ in a child ages 1 to 8, ½″ to 1″ for an infant younger than age 1, and 1½″ to 2″ for an adult.
CN: Physiological integrity; CNS: Physiological adaptation; CL: Application

30. A nurse rescuer knows that chest compressions must be coordinated with ventilations. Which ratio should the nurse rescuer use for a 3-year-old child?
1. 15 compressions to 1 ventilation
2. 15 compressions to 2 ventilations
3. 30 compressions to 1 ventilation
4. 30 compressions to 2 ventilations

30. 4. A single health care provider rescuer should use a ratio of 30 chest compressions to 2 ventilations for children ages 1 year to the onset of adolescence. Ratios of 15:2 are indicated if there are two health care provider rescuers. Ratios of 15:1 and 30:1 won't provide optimal compression and ventilation.
CN: Physiological integrity; CNS: Physiological adaptation; CL: Application

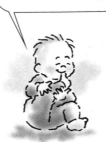

I put everything in my mouth. Do you want to take a peek?

31. A 10-month-old child is found choking and soon becomes unconscious. Which intervention should the nurse attempt <u>first</u> after opening the airway?
1. Look inside the infant's mouth for a foreign object.
2. Give five back blows and five chest thrusts.
3. Attempt a blind finger sweep.
4. Attempt rescue breathing.

31. 1. After the airway is open, the nurse should check for a foreign object and remove it with a finger sweep if it can be visualized. After this step, rescue breathing should be attempted. If ventilation is unsuccessful, the nurse should then give five back blows and five chest thrusts in an attempt to dislodge the object. Blind finger sweeps should never be performed because this may push the object further back into the airway.
CN: Physiological integrity; CNS: Physiological adaptation; CL: Application

CN: Client needs category   CNS: Client needs subcategory   CL: Cognitive level

32. Using which part of the hands is appropriate when performing chest compressions on a child between ages 1 and 8?
1. It depends on the size of the child and rescuer.
2. Heel of one hand
3. Index and middle fingers
4. Thumbs of both hands

32. 1. Children and rescuers vary widely in size. The rescuer should use one or two hands as needed to compress the chest one-half to one-third of its depth. Two hands are used for adult cardiopulmonary resuscitation. Chest thrusts administered with the middle and third fingers, and in some cases the thumbs of each hand, are used on infants younger than age 1.
CN: Physiological integrity; CNS: Physiological adaptation; CL: Application

33. A 3-year-old child who is unable to make a sound and is cyanotic and lethargic is brought to the emergency department. The mother states that she thinks he swallowed a penny. Which intervention should the nurse take <u>first</u>?
1. Give 100% oxygen.
2. Administer five back blows.
3. Attempt a blind finger sweep.
4. Administer abdominal thrusts.

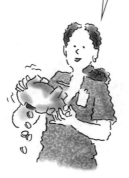

A penny for your thoughts...your first thought.

33. 4. A child between ages 1 and 8 should receive abdominal thrusts to help dislodge the object. Blind finger sweeps should never be performed because this could push the object further back into the airway. Administering 100% oxygen won't help if the airway is occluded. Infants younger than age 1 should receive back blows before chest thrusts.
CN: Physiological integrity; CNS: Physiological adaptation; CL: Application

34. A 1-year-old child is brought to the emergency department with a mild respiratory infection and a temperature of 101.3° F (38.5° C). Otitis media is diagnosed. Which sign would the nurse also expect to find?
1. Excessive drooling
2. Tugging on the ears
3. High-pitched, barking cough
4. Pearl-gray tympanic membrane

34. 2. Tugging on the ears is a common sign for a child with ear pain. Pearl-gray tympanic membranes are a normal finding. Excessive drooling, and a high-pitched, barking cough indicate croup. A child with otitis media usually exhibits a discolored membrane (bright red, yellow, or dull gray).
CN: Physiological integrity; CNS: Physiological adaptation; CL: Comprehension

35. A 7-month-old child is diagnosed with otitis media; the physician orders amoxicillin (Augmentin ES-600) 40 mg/kg/day to be administered three times per day. The child weighs 9 kg. How much amoxicillin should the child receive per dose?
1. 120 mg
2. 180 mg
3. 200 mg
4. 360 mg

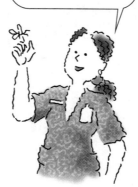

Make sure you remember this formula. You'll use it again later in this chapter.

35. 1. The child should receive 120 mg per dose. Use the following equations:
$$40 \text{ mg} \times 9 \text{ kg} = 360 \text{ mg/day};$$
$$360 \text{ mg/3 doses} = 120 \text{ mg/dose}.$$
CN: Physiological integrity; CNS: Pharmacological therapies; CL: Analysis

36. Children with chronic otitis media may require surgery for a myringotomy and ear tube placement. Which management strategy explains the purpose of the ear tubes?
1. To administer antibiotics
2. To flush the middle ear
3. To increase pressure
4. To drain fluid

36. 4. Ear tubes allow normal fluid to drain (not flush) from the middle ear. They also allow ventilation. The purpose isn't to administer medication. The tubes also allow pressure to equalize in the middle ear.
CN: Physiological integrity; CNS: Physiological adaptation; CL: Application

CN: Client needs category   CNS: Client needs subcategory   CL: Cognitive level

37. A nurse is teaching the parents of a 10-month-old infant the correct method for instilling eardrops prescribed for the infant when discharged. Which statement by the parents indicates understanding of the nurse's teaching?
1. "We should pull the earlobe upward."
2. "We should pull the earlobe up and back."
3. "We should pull the earlobe down and back."
4. "We should pull the earlobe down and forward."

38. A child is diagnosed as having right chronic otitis media. After the child returns from surgery for myringotomy and placement of ear tubes, which intervention is appropriate?
1. Apply gauze dressings.
2. Position the child on the left side.
3. Position the child on the right side.
4. Apply warm compresses to both ears.

39. A child is diagnosed with chronic otitis media. Which statement made by the mother indicates an understanding of this condition?
1. "I need to be sure the baby is dressed warmly."
2. "I must be sure he gets all of his DTaP vaccinations."
3. "I'll tell my relatives they can't smoke around the baby."
4. "I'll give him Tylenol once a day every week."

40. Which finding of otoscopy would the nurse identify as suggestive of acute otitis media?
1. Pearl-gray tympanic membrane
2. Red tympanic membrane
3. Dull gray membrane with fluid behind the eardrum
4. Bright red or yellow bulging or retracted tympanic membrane

37. 3. For infants, the parents should understand that they should gently pull the earlobe down and back to visualize the external auditory canal. For children older than age 3 and for adults, the earlobe is gently pulled slightly up and back.
CN: Physiological integrity; CNS: Pharmacological therapies; CL: Analysis

38. 3. The child should be positioned on the right side to facilitate drainage. The left side isn't an area of concern for drainage. Gauze dressings aren't necessary after surgery. Some physicians may prefer a loose cotton wick. Warm compresses may help to facilitate drainage only when used on the affected ear.
CN: Physiological integrity; CNS: Physiological adaptation; CL: Application

39. 3. Eliminating tobacco smoke and other allergens from the environment can help prevent otitis media. No extra clothing is needed. Diphtheria, tetanus, and pertussis aren't causes of otitis media. Tylenol should only be given when indicated for fever or pain.
CN: Health promotion and maintenance; CNS: None; CL: Analysis

40. 4. With acute otitis media, the tympanic membrane may present as bright red or yellow, bulging or retracted. A pearl-gray tympanic membrane is a normal finding. A red tympanic membrane isn't diagnostic for acute otitis media. Dull gray membrane with fluid is consistent with subacute or chronic otitis media.
CN: Physiological integrity; CNS: Physiological adaptation; CL: Comprehension

Acute, subacute, chronic. Do you know the difference?

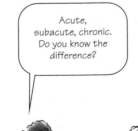

CN: Client needs category CNS: Client needs subcategory CL: Cognitive level

41. A nurse is teaching the parents of a 1-year-old infant with otitis media. Which statement regarding predisposing factors for otitis media would be <u>most</u> accurate for the nurse to make?
1. "The cartilage lining is overdeveloped."
2. "A sitting position contributes to the pooling of fluid."
3. "Humoral defense mechanisms decrease the risk of infection."
4. "Eustachian tubes are short, wide, and straight and lie in a horizontal plane."

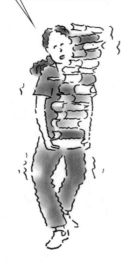

If you studied hard, you should be predisposed to doing well on these questions.

42. Which complication is most commonly related to acute otitis media?
1. Eardrum perforation
2. Hearing loss
3. Meningitis
4. Tympanosclerosis

43. Which statement by the parent of a child with otitis media indicates an understanding of the nurse's discharge instructions about the use of antibiotics?
1. "I'll give my child the full course of antibiotics."
2. "I'll stop the antibiotics when my child no longer has ear pain."
3. "I'll give the antibiotics when my child has ear pain."
4. "I'll put antibiotics in the affected ear."

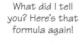

What did I tell you? Here's that formula again!

44. A 2-year-old child is diagnosed with epiglottiditis. Ampicillin is ordered 50 mg/kg/day in 6 divided doses. The client weighs 12 kg. How much ampicillin is given per dose?
1. 50 mg
2. 100 mg
3. 200 mg
4. 300 mg

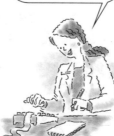

41. 4. In an infant or child, the eustachian tubes are short, wide, and straight and lie in a horizontal plane, allowing them to be more easily blocked by conditions such as large adenoids and infections. Until the eustachian tubes change in size and angle, children are more susceptible to otitis media. Cartilage lining is underdeveloped, making the tubes more distensible and more likely to open inappropriately. The usual lying-down position of infants contributes to the pooling of fluid such as formula in the pharyngeal cavity. Immature humoral defense mechanisms increase the risk of infection.
CN: Physiological integrity; CNS: Physiological adaptation; CL: Analysis

42. 1. Eardrum perforation is the most common complication of acute otitis media as the exudate accumulates and pressure increases. Hearing loss in most cases is conductive in nature and mild in severity but is less common than eardrum perforation. In addition, hearing tests aren't usually performed during episodes of otitis media. Meningitis and tympanosclerosis are possible but uncommon when adequate antibiotic therapy is implemented.
CN: Physiological integrity; CNS: Physiological adaptation; CL: Application

43. 1. Antibiotics should be given for the fully prescribed course of therapy, regardless of whether the child still has symptoms. Antibiotics are taken at prescribed intervals and not for episodes of ear pain. Oral antibiotics are used to treat otitis media.
CN: Physiological integrity; CNS: Pharmacological therapies; CL: Application

44. 2. The child should receive 100 mg per dose. Use the following equations:
50 mg × 12 kg = 600 mg/day;
600 mg/6 doses = 100 mg/dose.
CN: Physiological integrity; CNS: Pharmacological therapies; CL: Analysis

CN: Client needs category   CNS: Client needs subcategory   CL: Cognitive level

45. A 3-year-old child is receiving ampicillin for acute epiglottiditis. Which sign would lead the nurse to suspect that the child is experiencing a common adverse effect of this drug?
1. Constipation
2. Generalized rash
3. Increased appetite
4. Low-grade temperature

46. A 3-year-old child is given a preliminary diagnosis of acute epiglottiditis. Which nursing intervention is appropriate?
1. Obtain a throat culture immediately.
2. Place the child in a side-lying position.
3. Don't attempt to visualize the epiglottis.
4. Use a tongue depressor to look inside the throat.

47. Administration of which childhood vaccination assists in decreasing a child's incidence of developing of epiglottiditis?
1. Diphtheria vaccine
2. *Haemophilus influenzae* type B (Hib) vaccine
3. Measles vaccine
4. Inactivated polio vaccine (IPV)

48. In addition to an increasing respiratory rate, which sign in a 3-year-old child with acute epiglottiditis indicates that the client's respiratory distress is <u>increasing</u>?
1. Progressive, barking cough
2. Increasing irritability
3. Increasing heart rate
4. Productive cough

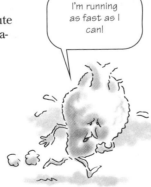

45. 2. Some clients may develop an erythematous or maculopapular rash after 3 to 14 days of therapy; however, this complication doesn't necessitate discontinuing the drug. Nausea, vomiting, epigastric pain, and diarrhea are adverse effects that may necessitate discontinuation of the drug.
CN: Physiological integrity; CNS: Pharmacological therapies; CL: Comprehension

46. 3. The nurse shouldn't attempt to visualize the epiglottis. The use of tongue blades or throat culture swabs may cause the epiglottis to spasm and totally occlude the airway. Throat inspection should be attempted only when immediate intubation or tracheostomy can be performed in the event of further or complete obstruction. The child should always remain in the position that provides the most comfort and security and ease of breathing.
CN: Physiological integrity; CNS: Physiological adaptation; CL: Application

47. 2. Epiglottiditis is caused by the bacterial agent *H. influenzae*. The American Academy of Pediatrics recommends that, beginning at age 2 months, children receive the Hib conjugate vaccine. A decline in the incidence of epiglottiditis has been seen as a result of this vaccination regimen. The diphtheria vaccine, measles vaccine, and IPV are preventive for those diseases, not epiglottiditis.
CN: Health promotion and maintenance; CNS: None; CL: Knowledge

48. 3. Increasing heart rate is an early sign of hypoxia. A progressive, barking cough is characteristic of spasmodic croup. A child in respiratory distress will be irritable and restless. As distress increases, the child will become lethargic related to the work of breathing and impending respiratory failure. A productive cough shows that secretions are moving and the child can effectively clear them.
CN: Physiological integrity; CNS: Physiological adaptation; CL: Application

CN: Client needs category   CNS: Client needs subcategory   CL: Cognitive level

49. While examining a child with acute epiglottiditis, the nurse should have which item available?

    1. Cool mist tent
    2. Intubation equipment
    3. Tongue depressors
    4. Viral culture medium

49. 2. Emergency intubation equipment should be at the bedside to secure the airway if examination precipitates further or complete obstruction. Tongue depressors are contraindicated and may cause the epiglottis to spasm. Cool mist tents and viral culture medium are recommended for the treatment and diagnosis of croup.

CN: Physiological integrity; CNS: Physiological adaptation; CL: Application

50. A 2-year-old child is brought to the emergency department in respiratory distress. The child is drooling, sitting upright, and leaning forward with the chin thrust out, mouth open, and tongue protruding. Which nursing action is most appropriate?

    1. Check the child's gag reflex with a tongue blade.
    2. Allow the child to cry to keep the lungs expanded.
    3. Check the airway for a foreign body obstruction.
    4. Support the child in an upright position on the parent's lap.

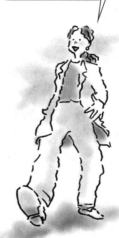

Congratulations! You've finished more than 50 questions! You're making great strides.

50. 4. The classic signs of epiglottiditis are drooling, sitting upright, and leaning forward with the chin thrust out, mouth open, and tongue protruding. The child should be kept in an upright position to ease the work of breathing, to avoid aspiration of secretions, and to help ease obstruction of the airway by the swollen epiglottis. Placing the child on the lap of a parent may help reduce the child's anxiety. The gag reflex of a child with epiglottiditis should never be checked unless emergency personnel and equipment are immediately available to perform a tracheotomy should the airway become obstructed by the swollen epiglottis. Crying and inspecting the airway for a foreign body may also cause complete airway obstruction.

CN: Physiological integrity; CNS: Reduction of risk potential; CL: Application

51. What's the best way for a nurse to position a 3-year-old child with right lower lobe pneumonia?

    1. Right side-lying
    2. Left side-lying
    3. Supine
    4. Prone

51. 2. The child with right lower lobe pneumonia should be placed on his left side. This places the unaffected left lung in a position that allows gravity to promote blood flow though the healthy lung tissue and improve gas exchange. Placing the child on his right side, back, or stomach doesn't promote circulation to the unaffected lung.

CN: Physiological integrity; CNS: Physiological adaptation; CL: Application

52. An 18-month-old boy is being evaluated at the clinic. In reviewing his chart, the nurse notices that he has missed many appointments and, consequently, his immunizations aren't up-to-date. While discussing communicable disease and the importance of immunizations with his mother, the nurse explains that the incidence of meningitis can be decreased with:
1. corticosteroid therapy.
2. tetanus toxoid vaccination.
3. tine testing.
4. *Haemophilus influenzae* vaccination.

I'm positive you'll do well on this question!

52. 4. *H. influenzae* vaccination is recommended for all children as a means of reducing the incidence of meningitis. Corticosteroids such as prednisone weaken the immune system and increase susceptibility to infectious disease. Tetanus toxoid vaccination provides immunity against tetanus or "lockjaw." A tine test is a screening measure for tuberculosis.
CN: Health promotion and maintenance; CNS: None; CL: Application

53. Which nursing action would relieve respiratory distress and dyspnea in a 2-year-old boy with laryngotracheobronchitis?
1. Stimulating the child to keep him awake
2. Providing an atmosphere of cool mist high humidity
3. Offering frequent oral feedings
4. Administering frequent sedatives

53. 2. Cool mist high humidity reduces mucosal edema and prevents drying of secretions, thus helping to maintain an open airway. Keeping the child calm, not stimulated, helps to reduce oxygen need. Oral feedings may need to be withheld in a child experiencing respiratory distress because eating may interfere with his ability to breathe. Sedation is generally contraindicated because it may cause respiratory depression and mask anxiety, a sign of respiratory distress.
CN: Physiological integrity; CNS: Physiological adaptation; CL: Application

54. When assessing a child for increased laryngotracheal edema and early signs of impending airway obstruction, the nurse should observe for which warning sign?
1. Decreased heart and respiratory rates and a high peak flow rate
2. Increased heart and respiratory rates, retractions, and restlessness
3. Decreased blood pressure
4. Increased temperature

Look for the classic warning signs.

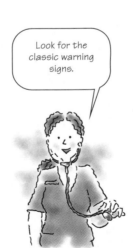

54. 2. Increased heart and respiratory rates, retractions, and restlessness are classic indicators of hypoxia. The heart and respiratory rates increase to enable increased oxygenation. Accessory breathing muscles are used, causing retractions in substernal, suprasternal, and intercostal areas. Reduced oxygen to the brain causes restlessness initially and altered level of consciousness later. A decrease in heart and respiratory rates would be a late ominous sign of decompensation. Peak flow rate is a test used in asthma. A decrease, not increase, in peak flow is diagnostic of disease. A drop in blood pressure would be a late sign of hypoxia. An increase in temperature is more indicative of infection or inflammation than respiratory distress.
CN: Physiological integrity; CNS: Physiological adaptation; CL: Application

55. Which strategy is recommended when caring for an infant with bronchopulmonary dysplasia?

1. Provide frequent playful stimuli.
2. Decrease oxygen during feedings.
3. Place the infant on a set schedule.
4. Place the infant in an open crib.

55. 3. Timing care activities with rest periods to avoid fatigue and to decrease respiratory effort is essential. Early stimulation activities are recommended but the infant will have limited tolerance for them because of the illness. Oxygen is usually increased during feedings to help decrease respiratory and energy requirements. Thermoregulation is important because both hypothermia and hyperthermia will increase oxygen consumption and may increase oxygen requirements. These infants are usually maintained on warmer beds or in Isolettes.

CN: Safe, effective care environment; CNS: Coordinated care; CL: Application

56. Which nursing diagnosis is the <u>priority</u> for an infant with bronchopulmonary dysplasia?

1. *Imbalanced nutrition: Less than body requirements*
2. *Ineffective infant feeding pattern*
3. *Impaired gas exchange*
4. *Risk for imbalanced fluid volume*

56. 3. The infant will have *Impaired gas exchange related to retention of carbon dioxide and borderline oxygenation secondary to fibrosis of the lungs.* Although the infant may require increased caloric intake and may have excess fluid volume, the other nursing diagnoses aren't the priority.

CN: Physiological integrity; CNS: Physiological adaptation; CL: Analysis

57. Which intervention is <u>most appropriate</u> for helping parents to cope with a child <u>newly diagnosed</u> with bronchopulmonary dysplasia?

1. Teach cardiopulmonary resuscitation.
2. Refer them to support groups.
3. Help parents identify necessary lifestyle changes.
4. Evaluate and assess parents' stress and anxiety levels.

57. 4. The emotional impact of bronchopulmonary dysplasia is clearly a crisis situation. The parents are experiencing grief and sorrow over the loss of a "healthy" child. The other strategies are more appropriate for long-term intervention.

CN: Psychosocial integrity; CNS: None; CL: Application

58. The care plan for an infant with bronchopulmonary dysplasia includes the nursing diagnosis of *Impaired gas exchange.* Which nursing action would be the <u>most</u> appropriate for the nurse to include?

1. Provide chest physiotherapy.
2. Provide enteral feedings.
3. Provide appropriate age-related activities.
4. Promote bonding between parents and child.

58. 1. All these activities are appropriate to include in the care of a child with bronchopulmonary dysplasia; however, providing chest physiotherapy is the nursing action that addresses the nursing diagnosis of *Impaired gas exchange.*

CN: Physiological integrity; CNS: Basic care and comfort; CL: Analysis

CN: Client needs category   CNS: Client needs subcategory   CL: Cognitive level

59. Theophylline (Elixophyllin) is ordered for a 1-year-old client with bronchopulmonary dysplasia. The recommended dosage is 24 mg/kg/day. The client weighs 10 kg. How much is given per dose when administered 4 times per day?
1. 60 mg/dose
2. 80 mg/dose
3. 120 mg/dose
4. 240 mg/dose

60. Infants with bronchopulmonary dysplasia require frequent, prolonged rest periods. Which sign indicates overstimulation?
1. Increased alertness
2. Good eye contact
3. Cyanosis
4. Lethargy

61. At discharge, which parental care outcome should be anticipated for a child with bronchopulmonary dysplasia?
1. Reports increased levels of stress
2. Only makes safe decisions with professional assistance
3. Participates in routine, but not complex, caretaking activities
4. Verbalizes the causes, risks, therapy options, and nursing care

62. Bronchopulmonary dysplasia can be classified into four categories. Which characteristic is noted during the early, or <u>first</u> stage of the disease?
1. Interstitial fibrosis
2. Signs of emphysema
3. Hyperexpansion on chest X-ray
4. Resemblance to respiratory distress syndrome

63. A child with bronchopulmonary dysplasia is receiving furosemide (Lasix). The nurse would <u>most</u> likely note which laboratory test result?
1. Serum potassium < 3.4 mEq/L
2. Serum calcium > 11 mg/dl
3. Serum sodium > 145 mEq/L
4. Serum potassium > 5 mEq/L

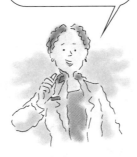

Pay close attention to the number of doses per day when calculating per dose amounts.

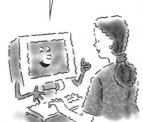

You're more than halfway finished. Now take a deep breath and keep going.

59. 1. The child should receive 60 mg/dose. Use the following equations:
$$24 \text{ mg/kg} \times 10 \text{ kg} = 240 \text{ mg/day};$$
$$240 \text{ mg/4 doses} = 60 \text{ mg/dose}.$$
CN: Physiological integrity; CNS: Pharmacological therapies; CL: Application

60. 3. Signs of overstimulation in an immature child include cyanosis, avoidance of eye contact, vomiting, diaphoresis, or falling asleep. The child may also become irritable and show signs of respiratory distress.
CN: Psychosocial integrity; CNS: None; CL: Application

61. 4. The parents should understand the causes, risks, therapy options, and care of their infant by the time of discharge. Having the parents verbalize this information is the only way to assess their understanding. The parents should report decreased levels of stress, be capable of making decisions independently, and participate in routine and complex care.
CN: Psychosocial integrity; CNS: None; CL: Application

62. 4. Stage I can be characterized by early interstitial changes and resembles respiratory distress syndrome. Stage III shows signs of the beginning of chronic disease with interstitial edema, signs of emphysema, and pulmonary hypertension. Stage IV shows interstitial fibrosis and hyperexpansion on chest X-ray.
CN: Physiological integrity; CNS: Physiological adaptation; CL: Analysis

63. 1. Furosemide can cause hypokalemia and hyponatremia from urinary diuresis. It may also cause hypocalcemia but not hypernatremia or hypercalcemia.
CN: Physiological integrity; CNS: Pharmacological therapies; CL: Application

64. A pediatric client is to receive furosemide (Lasix) 4 mg/kg/day in one daily dose. The client weighs 20 kg. How many milligrams should be administered in each dose?
1. 20 mg
2. 40 mg
3. 80 mg
4. 160 mg

65. A 2-year-old child with bronchopulmonary dysplasia is placed on furosemide (Lasix) once per day. The nurse is educating the parents on foods that are rich in potassium. Which food should the nurse recommend?
1. Apples
2. Oranges
3. Peaches
4. Raisins

66. Which scenario necessitates tracheostomy tube placement in long-term care of an infant with bronchopulmonary dysplasia?
1. Increased risk of tracheomalacia
2. Prolonged dependence on the ventilator
3. Need to allow for gastrostomy tube feedings
4. Increased signs of respiratory distress

67. A 1-year-old infant with bronchopulmonary dysplasia has just received a tracheostomy. Which intervention is <u>appropriate</u>?
1. Keep extra tracheostomy tubes at the bedside.
2. Secure ties at the back of the neck.
3. Change the tracheostomy tube 2 weeks after surgery.
4. Secure the tracheostomy ties tightly to prevent dislodgment of the tube.

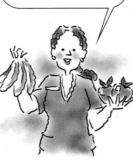

Might I recommend something from the fruit tray?

64. 3. The child should receive 80 mg per dose. Use the following equation:
$$4 \text{ mg/kg} \times 20 \text{ kg} = 80 \text{ mg}.$$
CN: Physiological integrity; CNS: Pharmacological therapies; CL: Application

65. 4. Raisins, dates, figs, and prunes are among the highest potassium-rich foods. They average 17 to 20 mEq of potassium. Apples, oranges, and peaches have very low amounts of potassium. They average 3 to 4 mEq.
CN: Physiological integrity; CNS: Pharmacological therapies; CL: Application

66. 2. Tracheostomy may be required after a child has been ventilator dependent and can't wean from the ventilator. Tracheomalacia can be a complication of prolonged tracheal intubation, not a condition that necessitates a tracheostomy. The need for gastrostomy feedings wouldn't necessitate putting in a tracheostomy tube. Increased signs of respiratory distress may indicate the need for endotracheal intubation and mechanical ventilation, not tracheostomy.
CN: Physiological integrity; CNS: Physiological adaptation; CL: Application

67. 1. Extra tracheostomy tubes should be kept at the bedside in case of an emergency, including one size smaller in case the appropriate size doesn't fit due to edema. The ties should be placed securely but allow the width of a little finger for room to prevent excessive pressure or skin breakdown. The first tracheostomy tube change is usually performed by the physician after 7 days. Ties are placed at the side of the neck to decrease the risk of skin breakdown.
CN: Physiological integrity; CNS: Physiological adaptation; CL: Application

CN: Client needs category   CNS: Client needs subcategory   CL: Cognitive level

68. An 11-month-old infant with bronchopulmonary dysplasia and a tracheostomy experiences a decline in oxygen saturation from 97% to 88%. He appears anxious and his heart rate is 180 beats/minute. Which intervention is most appropriate?

1. Change the tracheostomy tube.
2. Suction the tracheostomy tube.
3. Obtain an arterial blood gas (ABG) level.
4. Increase the oxygen flow rate.

69. Which intervention is most appropriate when suctioning a tracheostomy tube?

1. Hypoventilate the child before suctioning.
2. Repeat the suctioning process for two intervals.
3. Insert the catheter 1 to 2 cm below the tracheostomy tube.
4. Inject a small amount of normal saline solution into the tube before suctioning.

70. Which characteristic <u>distinguishes</u> allergies from colds?

1. Skin tests can diagnose a cold.
2. Allergies are accompanied by fever.
3. Colds cause itching of the eyes and nose.
4. Allergies trigger constant and consistent bouts of sneezing.

71. The parents of a child with asthma ask the nurse about the condition. Which description of asthma would be the <u>most</u> accurate?

1. Inflammation of the pulmonary parenchyma
2. Chronic lung disease caused by damaged alveoli
3. Infection of the lower airway, most commonly caused by a viral agent
4. Disease of the airways characterized by hyperactivity of the bronchi

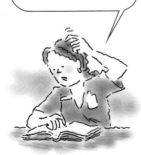

Asthma, asthma, oh here it is! So that's the correct definition.

68. 2. Tracheostomy tubes, particularly in small children, require frequent suctioning to remove mucus plugs and excessive secretions. The tracheostomy tube can be changed if suctioning is unsuccessful. Obtaining an ABG level may be beneficial if oxygen saturation remains low and the child appears to be in respiratory distress. Increasing the oxygen flow rate will only help if the airway is patent.
CN: Physiological integrity; CNS: Physiological adaptation; CL: Application

69. 4. Injecting a small amount of normal saline solution helps to loosen secretions for easier aspiration. Preservative-free normal saline solution should be used. The child should be hyperventilated before and after suctioning to prevent hypoxia. The suctioning process should be repeated until the trachea is clear. The catheter should be inserted 0.5 cm beyond the tracheostomy tube. If the catheter is inserted too far, it will irritate the carina and may cause blood-tinged secretions.
CN: Physiological integrity; CNS: Physiological adaptation; CL: Application

70. 4. Allergies elicit consistent bouts of sneezing, are seldom accompanied by fever, and tend to cause itching of the eyes and nose. Skin testing is performed to determine the client's sensitivity to specific allergens. Colds are accompanied by fever and are characterized by sporadic sneezing.
CN: Health promotion and maintenance; CNS: None; CL: Application

71. 4. Asthma is an obstructive disease that shows hyperactivity of the bronchi and edema of the mucous membranes. Pneumonia is characterized by an inflammation of the pulmonary parenchyma. Bronchopulmonary dysplasia is a chronic lung disease with damaged alveoli. Lower airway infection caused by a viral agent describes bronchitis.
CN: Health promotion and maintenance; CNS: None; CL: Application

CN: Client needs category CNS: Client needs subcategory CL: Cognitive level

72. A 2-year-old child has been diagnosed with asthma. Which allergen can be considered one of the <u>most common</u> asthma triggers?
1. Weather
2. Peanut butter
3. The cat next door
4. One parent with asthma

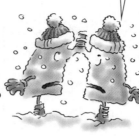

Some things trigger asthma in me more than others.

72. 1. Excessively cold air, wet or humid changes in weather and seasons, and air pollution are some of the most common asthma triggers. Food allergens are rarely responsible for airway reactions in children. Household pets are a trigger. Evidence suggests that asthma is partly hereditary in nature but heredity isn't an allergen.
CN: Physiological integrity; CNS: Physiological adaptation; CL: Knowledge

73. Which symptom would the nurse expect to find <u>most commonly</u> in a child with asthma?
1. Barking cough
2. Bradycardia
3. Dry, productive cough
4. Wheezing

There are various signs and symptoms of asthma. Do you know them?

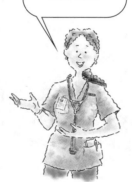

73. 4. Asthma commonly occurs with wheezing and coughing. Airway inflammation and edema increase mucus production. Other signs include dyspnea, tachycardia (not bradycardia), and tachypnea. A barking cough is associated with croup. A dry, nonproductive cough is an asthma variant commonly seen in older children and teenagers.
CN: Physiological integrity; CNS: Physiological adaptation; CL: Comprehension

74. Presence of which factor would place a child at increased risk for an asthma-related death?
1. Use of an inhaler at home
2. One admission for asthma last year
3. Prior admission to the general pediatric floor
4. Prior admission to an intensive care unit for asthma

74. 4. Asthma results in varying degrees of respiratory distress. A prior admission to an intensive care unit marks an increased severity and need of immediate therapy. Two or more hospitalizations for asthma, a recent hospitalization or emergency department visit in the past month, or three or more emergency department visits in the past year puts a child at high risk for asthma-related death. Although current use of systemic steroids would also be a risk factor, not all inhalers contain steroids.
CN: Physiological integrity; CNS: Reduction of risk potential; CL: Application

75. Which characteristic may be present in a client with status asthmaticus?
1. Several attacks per month
2. Less than 6 attacks per year
3. Increased response to bronchodilators
4. Constant attacks unrelieved by bronchodilators

75. 4. Status asthmaticus can best be described as constant attacks unrelieved by bronchodilators. Moderate asthma is characterized by several attacks per month. Mild asthma is less than 6 attacks per year. Little or no response to bronchodilators would describe severe asthma.
CN: Physiological integrity; CNS: Physiological adaptation; CL: Knowledge

76. A 2-year-old child with status asthmaticus is admitted to the pediatric unit and begins to receive continuous treatment with albuterol (Proventil), given by nebulizer. The nurse should observe for which adverse reaction?
1. Bradycardia
2. Lethargy
3. Tachycardia
4. Tachypnea

77. A 10-year-old child is admitted with asthma. The physician orders an aminophylline infusion. A loading dose of 6 mg/kg is ordered. The client weighs 30 kg. How much aminophylline is contained in the loading dose?
1. 60 mg
2. 90 mg
3. 120 mg
4. 180 mg

78. Which complication may be seen in a child receiving mechanical ventilation?
1. Pneumothorax
2. High cardiac output
3. Polycythemia
4. Hypovolemia

79. Which X-ray finding would you expect for a child with asthma?
1. Atelectasis
2. Hemothorax
3. Infiltrates
4. Pneumothoraces

80. Which intervention is <u>most</u> important for a client with atelectasis?
1. Perform chest physiotherapy.
2. Give increased I.V. fluids.
3. Administer oxygen.
4. Obtain arterial blood gas (ABG) levels.

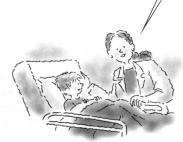

This question has really got me frazzled.

A child receiving mechanical ventilation should be closely monitored.

76. 3. Albuterol is a rapid-acting bronchodilator. Common adverse effects include tachycardia, nervousness, tremors, insomnia, irritability, and headache.
CN: Physiological integrity; CNS: Pharmacological therapies; CL: Application

77. 4. The child should receive 180 mg per dose. Use the following equation:
$$6 \text{ mg/kg} \times 30 \text{ kg} = 180 \text{ mg}.$$
CN: Physiological integrity; CNS: Pharmacological therapies; CL: Application

78. 1. Mechanical ventilation can cause barotrauma, as occurs with pneumothorax; a child receiving mechanical ventilation must be carefully monitored. Mechanical ventilation decreases, not increases, cardiac output. Polycythemia is the result of chronic hypoxia, not mechanical ventilation. Mechanical ventilation can cause fluid overload, not dehydration.
CN: Physiological integrity; CNS: Physiological adaptation; CL: Application

79. 1. Hyperexpansion, atelectasis, and a flattened diaphragm are typical X-ray findings for a child with asthma. Air becomes trapped behind the narrowed airways and the residual capacity rises, leading to hyperinflation. Hypoxemia results from areas of the lung not being well perfused. A hemothorax isn't a finding related to asthma. Infiltrates and pneumothoraces are uncommon.
CN: Physiological integrity; CNS: Physiological adaptation; CL: Application

80. 1. Chest physiotherapy and incentive spirometry help to enhance the clearance of mucus and open the alveoli. Although not the most important intervention, giving I.V. and oral fluids is recommended to help liquefy and thin secretions. Administration of oxygen won't provide enough pressure to open the alveoli. Obtaining ABG levels isn't necessary unless the client has signs of hypoxemia.
CN: Physiological integrity; CNS: Physiological adaptation; CL: Application

CN: Client needs category   CNS: Client needs subcategory   CL: Cognitive level

81. The parents of a 10-year-old child who was recently diagnosed with asthma ask if the child can continue to play sports. Which response is most appropriate?

1. Sports can cause asthma attacks.
2. You should limit activities to quiet play.
3. It's okay to play some sports but swimming isn't recommended.
4. Physical activity and sports are encouraged as long as the asthma is under control.

82. A client with thoracic water-seal drainage is on the elevator. The transport aide has placed the drainage system on the stretcher. What action should the nurse on the elevator take first?

1. Assist the aide in placing the drainage system lower than the client's chest.
2. Report the incident to the registered nurse when she returns to the unit.
3. Clamp the drainage tubing with a hemostat.
4. Immediately take the client's respiratory and pulse rates.

83. Which nursing intervention is appropriate to correct dehydration for a 2-year-old client with asthma?

1. Give warm liquids.
2. Give cold juice or ice pops.
3. Provide three meals and three snacks.
4. Provide small, frequent meals and snacks.

84. Which action by the parents decreases allergens in the home?

1. Covering floors with carpeting
2. Designating the basement as the play area
3. Dusting and cleaning the house thoroughly twice a month
4. Using foam rubber pillows and synthetic blankets

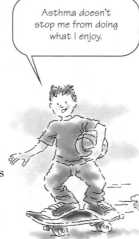

Asthma doesn't stop me from doing what I enjoy.

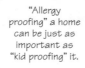

"Allergy proofing" a home can be just as important as "kid proofing" it.

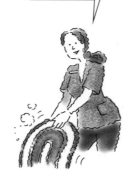

81. 4. Participation in sports is encouraged but should be evaluated on an individual basis as long as the asthma is under control. Exercise-induced asthma is an example of the airway hyperactivity common to asthmatics. Exclusion from sports or activities may hamper peer interaction. Swimming is well tolerated because of the type of breathing involved and the moisture in the air.

CN: Physiological integrity; CNS: Physiological adaptation; CL: Application

82. 1. The drainage device must be kept below the level of the chest to maintain straight gravity drainage. Placing it on the stretcher may cause a backflow of drainage into the thoracic cavity, which could collapse the partially expanded lung. Reporting the incident is indicated, but the immediate safety of the client takes priority. Clamping the tubing would place the client at risk for a tension pneumothorax. After the drainage system has been properly repositioned, the client's respiratory and pulse rates may be taken.

CN: Physiological integrity; CNS: Basic care and comfort; CL: Application

83. 1. Liquids are best tolerated if they're warm. Cold liquids may cause bronchospasm and should be avoided. Dehydration should be corrected slowly. Overhydration may increase interstitial pulmonary fluid and exacerbate small airway obstruction. Small, frequent meals should be provided to avoid abdominal distention that may interfere with diaphragm excursion, but these won't correct the dehydration.

CN: Physiological integrity; CNS: Physiological adaptation; CL: Application

84. 4. Bedding should be free from allergens and have nonallergenic covers. Unnecessary rugs should be removed, and floors should be bare and mopped a few times per week to reduce dust. Basements or cellars should be avoided to lessen the child's exposure to molds and mildew. Dusting and cleaning should occur daily or at least weekly.

CN: Physiological integrity; CNS: Physiological adaptation; CL: Application

CN: Client needs category   CNS: Client needs subcategory   CL: Cognitive level

85. Which nursing diagnosis is appropriate for a client with acute asthma?
1. *Imbalanced nutrition: More than body requirements*
2. *Excess fluid volume*
3. *Activity intolerance*
4. *Constipation*

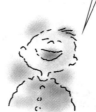

This is a cute question. Get it? A cute...just like me!

85. 3. Ineffective oxygen supply and demand may lead to activity intolerance. The nurse should promote rest and encourage developmentally appropriate activities. Nutrition may be decreased, not increased, due to respiratory distress and GI upset. Dehydration, not overhydration, is common due to diaphoresis, insensible water loss, and hyperventilation. Medications given to treat asthma may cause nausea, vomiting, and diarrhea, not constipation.
CN: Physiological integrity; CNS: Physiological adaptation; CL: Application

86. A nurse is explaining bronchiolitis to the parents of an infant admitted with the condition. Which explanation by the nurse would be the most accurate?
1. Acute inflammation and obstruction of the bronchioles
2. Airway obstruction from aspiration of a solid object
3. Inflammation of the pulmonary parenchyma
4. Acute highly contagious crouplike syndrome

86. 1. Bronchiolitis is an infection of the bronchioles, causing the mucosa to become edematous, inflamed, and full of mucus. Lower airway obstruction from a solid object is a form of foreign body aspiration. Pneumonia is characterized by inflammation of the pulmonary parenchyma. Croup syndromes are generally upper airway infections or obstructions.
CN: Physiological integrity; CNS: Physiological adaptation; CL: Application

87. A 2-month-old infant is given a preliminary diagnosis of bronchiolitis. Which symptom would the nurse expect to find?
1. Bradycardia
2. Increased appetite
3. Wheezing on auscultation
4. No signs of an upper respiratory infection

Consider the pathology of bronchiolitis when answering question 87.

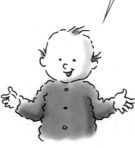

87. 3. In bronchiolitis, the bronchioles become narrowed and edematous, which can cause wheezing. These infants typically have a 2- to 3-day history of an upper respiratory infection and feeding difficulties with loss of appetite due to nasal congestion and increased work of breathing. This combination leads to respiratory distress with tachypnea and tachycardia.
CN: Physiological integrity; CNS: Physiological adaptation; CL: Application

88. In most cases, bronchiolitis is caused by a viral agent, most commonly respiratory syncytial virus (RSV). The nurse should keep in mind which statement regarding RSV infections?
1. It's more prevalent in the late summer and early fall months.
2. It's most likely to attack the respiratory tract mucosa.
3. It's more commonly seen in children older than age 5.
4. It's not particularly contagious.

88. 2. RSV attacks the respiratory tract mucosa. The virus is most prevalent in the winter and early spring months. Most children develop the infection between ages 2 and 6 months, and RSV generally occurs during the first 3 years of life. RSV is a highly contagious respiratory virus.
CN: Physiological integrity; CNS: Physiological adaptation; CL: Application

CN: Client needs category   CNS: Client needs subcategory   CL: Cognitive level

89. Which precaution should a nurse caring for a 2-month-old infant with respiratory syncytial virus (RSV) take to prevent the spread of infection?
1. Gloves only
2. Gown, gloves, and mask
3. No precautions are required; the virus isn't contagious
4. Proper hand washing between clients

90. Which test positively diagnoses respiratory syncytial virus (RSV)?
1. Blood test
2. Nasopharyngeal washings
3. Sputum culture
4. Throat culture

91. Which child would be at increased risk for a respiratory syncytial virus (RSV) infection?
1. 2-month-old child managed at home
2. 2-month-old child with broncho-pulmonary dysplasia
3. 3-month-old child requiring low-flow oxygen
4. 2-year-old child

92. Which nursing diagnosis would the nurse expect to find on the care plan of a 10-month-old infant to promote coping during hospitalization?
1. *Toileting self-care deficit related to the child's age*
2. *Powerlessness related to hospital environment*
3. *Deficient diversional activity related to hospital environment*
4. *Anxiety related to separation from parents*

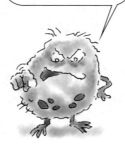

What precautions should you take when treating a highly contagious agent such as my none-too-lovable self?

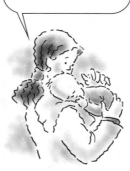

Can you identify the child at increased risk for RSV infection?

89. 2. RSV is highly contagious and is spread through direct contact with infectious secretions via hands, droplets, and fomites. Gown, gloves, and mask should be worn for client care to prevent the spread of infection.
CN: Safe, effective care environment; CNS: Safety and infection control; CL: Application

90. 2. RSV can only be diagnosed with direct aspiration of nasal secretions or nasopharyngeal washings. Positive identification is accomplished using the enzyme-linked immunosorbent assay. Blood, throat, and sputum cultures can't definitively diagnose RSV.
CN: Physiological integrity; CNS: Physiological adaptation; CL: Knowledge

91. 2. Infants with cardiac or pulmonary conditions are at highest risk for RSV. Because of their underlying conditions, they're more likely to require mechanical ventilation. Many infants can be managed at home; few require hospitalization. A 3-month-old on low-flow oxygen has some risks of progression but isn't at high risk. A 2-year-old child has built up the immune system and can tolerate the infection without major problems.
CN: Physiological integrity; CNS: Reduction of risk potential; CL: Application

92. 4. Attachment is critical in infancy, and prolonged separation has been well documented as a risk factor that compromises normal infant development. Toilet training wouldn't be an issue for a 10-month-old. Powerlessness is a concern after the toddler stage, when a child develops autonomy and independence. Diversion won't be an issue until the acute phase of the illness has passed. Providing diversion for infants is easily accomplished by the use of age-appropriate toys and play activities.
CN: Psychosocial integrity; CNS: None; CL: Application

CN: Client needs category CNS: Client needs subcategory CL: Cognitive level

93. Which medication is an antiviral agent used to treat bronchiolitis caused by respiratory syncytial virus (RSV)?
1. Albuterol (Proventil)
2. Aminophylline
3. Cromolyn sodium (Nasalcrom)
4. Ribavirin (Virazole)

93. 4. Ribavirin is an antiviral agent sometimes used to reduce the severity of bronchiolitis caused by RSV. Aminophylline and albuterol are bronchodilators and haven't been proven effective in treating viral bronchiolitis. Cromolyn sodium is an inhaled anti-inflammatory agent.
CN: Physiological integrity; CNS: Pharmacological therapies; CL: Application

94. Which intervention is <u>most important</u> when monitoring dehydration in an infant with bronchiolitis?
1. Measurement of intake and output
2. Blood levels every 4 hours
3. Urinalysis every 8 hours
4. Weighing each diaper

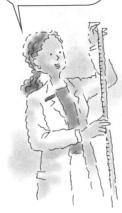

This one is tricky. Pay attention to the frequency of the measurements.

94. 1. Accurate measurement of intake and output is essential to assess for dehydration. Blood levels may be obtained daily or every other day. A urinalysis every 8 hours isn't necessary. Urine specific gravities are recommended but can be obtained with diaper changes. Weighing diapers is a way of measuring output only.
CN: Physiological integrity; CNS: Physiological adaptation; CL: Application

95. Which nursing diagnosis is appropriate for an infant with bronchiolitis?
1. *Imbalanced nutrition: More than body requirements*
2. *Deficient diversional activity*
3. *Impaired gas exchange*
4. *Social isolation*

95. 3. Infants with bronchiolitis will have impaired gas exchange related to bronchiolar obstruction, atelectasis, and hyperinflation. Nutrition may be seen as less than body requirements. If respiratory distress is present, these infants should have nothing by mouth and fluids given I.V. only. Deficient diversional activity and social isolation usually aren't priorities. These infants are too uncomfortable to respond to social stimuli and need quiet, soothing activities that minimize energy.
CN: Physiological integrity; CNS: Physiological adaptation; CL: Application

96. Which item is an essential skill for parents managing bronchiolitis at home?
1. Place the child in a prone position for comfort.
2. Use warm mist to replace insensible fluid loss.
3. Recognize signs of increasing respiratory distress.
4. Engage the child in many activities to prevent developmental delay.

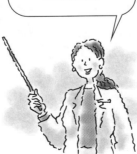

Parents must be taught to recognize the signs of respiratory distress in a child with bronchiolitis.

96. 3. It's essential for parents to be able to recognize signs of increasing respiratory distress and know how to count the respiratory rate. The child should be positioned with the head of the bed elevated for comfort and to facilitate removal of secretions. Use of cool mist may help to replace insensible fluid loss. Quiet play activities are required only as the child's energy level permits. These infants show clinical improvement in 3 to 4 days; therefore, developmental delay isn't an issue.
CN: Physiological integrity; CNS: Physiological adaptation; CL: Application

CN: Client needs category CNS: Client needs subcategory CL: Cognitive level

97. Which definition best describes pneumonia?
1. Inflammation of the large airways
2. Severe infection of the bronchioles
3. Inflammation of the pulmonary parenchyma
4. Acute viral infection with maximum effect at the bronchiolar level

98. Which organism is the <u>most common</u> causative agent for bacterial pneumonia?
1. *Mycoplasma*
2. Parainfluenza virus
3. Pneumococci
4. Respiratory syncytial virus (RSV)

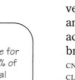

I'm responsible for about 90% of bacterial pneumonia.

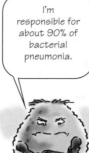

99. Which type of pneumonia is most common in children ages 5 to 12?
1. Enteric bacilli
2. *Mycoplasma* pneumonia
3. Staphylococcal pneumonia
4. Streptococcal pneumonia

100. A nurse knows to monitor a child with a diagnosis of pertussis for the development of which sign or symptom?
1. Barking cough
2. Whooping cough
3. Abrupt high fever
4. Inspiratory stridor

101. Which test is the <u>definitive</u> means of diagnosing tuberculosis (TB) in children?
1. Chest X-ray
2. Sputum specimen
3. Tuberculin test
4. Urine culture

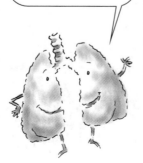

Psssst! Remember that definitive means best!

97. 3. Pneumonia is an inflammation of the pulmonary parenchyma. Bronchitis is inflammation of the large airways. Bronchiolitis is a severe infection of the bronchioles. Bronchiolitis and respiratory syncytial virus are types of acute viral infection with maximum effect at the bronchiolar level.
CN: Physiological integrity; CNS: Physiological adaptation; CL: Knowledge

98. 3. Pneumococcal pneumonia is the most common causative agent accounting for about 90% of bacterial pneumonia. *Mycoplasma* is a causative agent for primary atypical pneumonia. Parainfluenza virus and RSV account for viral pneumonia.
CN: Physiological integrity; CNS: Physiological adaptation; CL: Application

99. 2. *Mycoplasma* pneumonia is a primary atypical pneumonia seen in children between ages 5 and 12. Streptococcal pneumonia, enteric bacilli, and staphylococcal pneumonia are mostly seen in children in the 3-month to 5-year age-group.
CN: Physiological integrity; CNS: Physiological adaptation; CL: Knowledge

100. 2. Pertussis is characterized by consistent short, rapid coughs followed by a sudden inspiration with a high-pitched whooping sound. A barking cough and inspiratory stridor are noted with croup. Pertussis usually is accompanied by a low-grade fever.
CN: Physiological integrity; CNS: Physiological adaptation; CL: Application

101. 2. A sputum culture is the definitive test for TB in children. The tuberculin test is the most accurate but not necessarily the most reliable test for TB in children. X-rays usually appear normal in children with TB. Stool culture, not urine culture, and gastric washings will show positive results on acid-fast smears but aren't specific for *Mycobacterium tuberculosis*.
CN: Physiological integrity; CNS: Physiological adaptation; CL: Application

CN: Client needs category   CNS: Client needs subcategory   CL: Cognitive level

102. Which symptom is a characteristic sign of tuberculosis (TB) in children?
1. Chills
2. Hyperactivity
3. Lymphadenitis
4. Weight gain

103. Which adverse effect can be <u>expected</u> by the parents of a 2-year-old child who has been started on rifampin (Rifadin) after testing positive for tuberculosis?
1. Hyperactivity
2. Orange body secretions
3. Decreased bilirubin levels
4. Decreased levels of liver enzymes

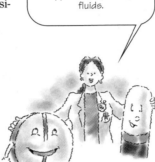

Certain medications can change the appearance of body fluids.

104. Children younger than age 3 are prone to aspirating foreign bodies. Which action is recommended to prevent aspiration?
1. Cut hot dogs in half.
2. Limit popcorn and peanuts.
3. Cut grapes into small pieces.
4. Limit hard candy to special occasions.

105. A child is admitted with a possible tracheal foreign body. Which findings would <u>most</u> likely indicate a foreign body in the trachea?
1. Cough, dyspnea, and drooling
2. Cough, stridor, and changes in phonation
3. Expiratory wheeze and inspiratory stridor
4. Cough, asymmetric breath sounds, and wheeze

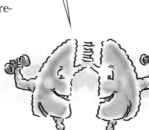

Keep pumping out those answers!

106. Which activity is recommended to prevent foreign body aspiration during meals?
1. Insist that children are seated.
2. Give children toys to play with.
3. Allow children to watch television.
4. Allow children to eat in a separate room.

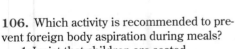

102. 3. Children with TB are usually asymptomatic and commonly don't manifest the usual pulmonary symptoms, but lymphadenitis is more likely in infants and children than in adults. Weight loss, anorexia, night sweats, fatigue, and malaise are general responses to the disease.
CN: Physiological integrity; CNS: Physiological adaptation; CL: Knowledge

103. 2. Rifampin and its metabolites will turn urine, feces, sputum, tears, and sweat an orange color. This isn't a serious adverse effect. Rifampin may also cause GI upset, headache, drowsiness, dizziness, vision disturbances, and fever. Liver enzyme and bilirubin levels increase because of hepatic metabolism of the drug. Parents should be taught the signs and symptoms of hepatitis and hyperbilirubinemia such as jaundice of the sclera or skin.
CN: Physiological integrity; CNS: Pharmacological therapies; CL: Application

104. 3. Grapes, hot dogs, and sausage should be cut into many small pieces. Hard candy, raisins, popcorn, and peanuts should be avoided for children age 4 and younger.
CN: Physiological integrity; CNS: Reduction of risk potential; CL: Application

105. 3. Expiratory and inspiratory noise indicates that the foreign body is in the trachea. Cough, dyspnea, drooling, and gagging indicate supraglottic obstruction. A cough with stridor and changes in phonation would occur if the foreign body were in the larynx. Asymmetric breath sounds indicate that the object may be located in the bronchi.
CN: Physiological integrity; CNS: Physiological adaptation; CL: Application

106. 1. Children should remain seated while eating. The risk of aspiration increases if children are running, jumping, or talking with food in their mouth. Toys and television are a dangerous distraction to toddlers and young children and should be avoided. Children need constant supervision and should be monitored while eating snacks and meals.
CN: Safe, effective care environment; CNS: Safety and infection control; CL: Application

CN: Client needs category CNS: Client needs subcategory CL: Cognitive level

107. Which diagnostic tool is <u>best</u> for general diagnosis of foreign body aspiration?
1. Bronchoscopy
2. Chest X-ray
3. Fluoroscopy
4. Lateral neck X-ray

108. A nurse is teaching the parents of a child newly diagnosed with cystic fibrosis. Which statement by the nurse concerning this condition is <u>most</u> accurate?
1. "It's an inflammation of the pulmonary parenchyma."
2. "It's a chromosomal abnormality inherited as an autosomal-dominant trait."
3. "It's a multisymptom disorder affecting the exocrine or mucus-producing glands."
4. "It's a chronic lung disease related to high concentrations of oxygen and ventilation."

109. Which clinical feature would be found in a child with cystic fibrosis?
1. Increase in pancreatic secretions of bicarbonate and chloride
2. Decrease in sodium and chloride in both saliva and sweat
3. Increased viscosity of mucous gland secretions
4. Decreased viscosity of mucous gland secretions

110. A nurse is performing an assessment on a newborn with a possible diagnosis of cystic fibrosis. Which of the following is an early sign of the disease?
1. Constipation
2. Decreased appetite
3. Hyperalbuminemia
4. Meconium ileus

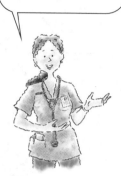

Question 107 has some good choices, but there's only one best answer.

107. 1. Bronchoscopy can give a definitive diagnosis of the presence of foreign bodies and is also the best choice for removal of the object with direct visualization. Chest X-ray and lateral neck X-ray may also be used but findings vary. Some films may appear normal or show changes such as inflammation related to the presence of the foreign body. Fluoroscopy is valuable in detecting and localizing foreign bodies in the bronchi.
CN: Physiological integrity; CNS: Physiological adaptation; CL: Knowledge

108. 3. Cystic fibrosis affects many organs as well as the exocrine or mucus-producing glands. In cystic fibrosis, an autosomal-recessive chromosomal abnormality, the child inherits defective genes from both parents. Inflammation of the pulmonary parenchyma describes pneumonia. Bronchopulmonary dysplasia is related to high concentrations of oxygen and ventilation.
CN: Physiological integrity; CNS: Physiological adaptation; CL: Application

109. 3. A primary feature of children with cystic fibrosis is the increased viscosity of mucous gland secretions. Instead of thin, free-flowing secretions, the mucous glands produce a thick mucoprotein that accumulates and dilates them. Pancreatic enzymes are decreased because mucus secretions block the pancreatic ducts. The electrolytes sodium and chloride are increased in sweat; this forms the basis of the diagnosis of the disorder.
CN: Physiological integrity; CNS: Physiological adaptation; CL: Knowledge

110. 4. Meconium ileus is a common early sign of cystic fibrosis. Thick, mucilaginous meconium blocks the lumen of the small intestine, causing intestinal obstruction, abdominal distention, and vomiting. Large-volume, loose, frequent, foul-smelling stool are common. The undigested food is excreted, increasing the bulk of feces. These infants may have an increased appetite related to poor absorption from the intestine. Hypoalbuminemia is a common result from the decreased absorption of protein.
CN: Physiological integrity; CNS: Physiological adaptation; CL: Application

CN: Client needs category   CNS: Client needs subcategory   CL: Cognitive level

111. Which tool is most commonly used to diagnose cystic fibrosis?
1. Chest X-ray
2. Pulmonary function test (PFT)
3. Stool culture
4. Sweat test

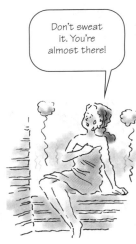

Don't sweat it. You're almost there!

112. Which is the best method to evaluate the success of the teaching plan for a 6-year-old child with cystic fibrosis who has been prescribed an aerosol inhaler?
1. Ask if the parents have any questions.
2. Ask the child to explain the procedure.
3. Ask the parents if they understand how to use the inhaler.
4. Ask the child to perform a return demonstration.

113. Which diet is recommended for a child with cystic fibrosis?
1. Fat-restricted diet
2. High-calorie diet
3. Low-protein diet
4. Sodium-restricted diet

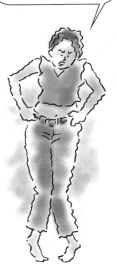

I apparently have been following the diet recommended in question 113.

114. Which statement concerning pancreatic enzymes for a cystic fibrosis client is correct?
1. Capsules may not be opened.
2. Microcapsules can be crushed.
3. Encourage eating throughout the day.
4. Administer enzymes at each meal and with snacks.

111. 4. A sweat test is the most reliable diagnostic procedure for cystic fibrosis. It involves stimulating the production of sweat, collecting the sweat, and measuring electrolytes in the sweat. Two separate samples are collected to assure reliability of the test. Chest X-rays can show characteristic atelectasis and obstructive emphysema. PFTs can show lung function and abnormal small airway function in cystic fibrosis. Stool analysis requires a 72-hour sample with an accurate food intake record.
CN: Physiological integrity; CNS: Physiological adaptation; CL: Knowledge

112. 4. A return demonstration is the best tool to evaluate the teaching. It will show if the child can demonstrate the steps taught and appropriately use the inhaler. The parents should understand how the inhaler should be used and ask questions, but the child must be able to correctly demonstrate usage first. A 6-year-old child may have difficulty verbalizing the procedure.
CN: Physiological integrity; CNS: Pharmacological therapies; CL: Application

113. 2. A well-balanced, high-calorie, high-protein diet is recommended for a child with cystic fibrosis due to impaired intestinal absorption. Fat restriction isn't required because digestion and absorption of fat in the intestine are impaired. The child usually increases enzyme intake when high-fat foods are eaten. Low-sodium foods can lead to hyponatremia; therefore, high-salt foods are recommended, especially during hot weather or when the child has a fever.
CN: Safe, effective care environment; CNS: Coordinated care; CL: Application

114. 4. Enzymes are administered with each feeding, meal, and snack to optimize absorption of the nutrients consumed. Microcapsules shouldn't be crushed due to the enteric coating. Regular capsules may be opened and the contents mixed with a small amount of applesauce or other nonalkaline food. Eating throughout the day should be discouraged. Three meals and two or three snacks per day are recommended.
CN: Physiological integrity; CNS: Physiological adaptation; CL: Application

115. Ranitidine (Zantac) is ordered for a 2-year-old child with cystic fibrosis. The nurse is aware that this medication falls within which drug class?
1. HMG-CoA inhibitor
2. Antacid
3. Anticholinergic
4. Histamine-receptor antagonist

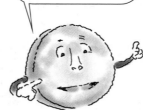

They say I'm an antagonist, but I'm actually a very pleasant guy.

115. 4. Ranitidine acts as a histamine-2 receptor antagonist. It helps to decrease duodenal acidity and enhance pancreatic enzyme activity. HMG-CoA inhibitors are antihyperlipidemics and help decrease serum cholesterol and low-density lipid levels. Antacids are used to neutralize gastric acid. Anticholinergics may be used to decrease gastric emptying and to decrease gastric acid secretions.
CN: Physiological integrity; CNS: Pharmacological therapies; CL: Application

116. The nurse is caring for a client with cystic fibrosis. Ranitidine (Zantac) 4 mg/kg/day every 12 hours is ordered. The child weighs 20 kg. How many milligrams are given per dose?
1. 16 mg
2. 20 mg
3. 40 mg
4. 80 mg

116. 3. The child should receive 40 mg per dose. Use the following equations:
20 kg × 4 mg/kg = 80 mg;
24 hours/12 hours = 2 doses;
80 mg/2 doses = 40 mg.
CN: Physiological integrity; CNS: Pharmacological therapies; CL: Application

117. Which intervention is appropriate for care of the child with cystic fibrosis?
1. Decrease exercise and limit physical activity.
2. Administer cough suppressants and antihistamines.
3. Administer chest physiotherapy two to four times per day.
4. Administer bronchodilator or nebulizer treatments after chest physiotherapy.

117. 3. Chest physiotherapy is recommended two to four times per day to help loosen and move secretions to facilitate expectoration. Exercise and physical activity are recommended to stimulate mucus secretion and to establish a good habitual breathing pattern. Cough suppressants and antihistamines are contraindicated. The goal is for the child to be able to cough and expectorate mucus secretions. Bronchodilator or nebulizer treatments are given before chest physiotherapy to help open the bronchi for easier expectoration.
CN: Safe, effective care environment; CNS: Coordinated care; CL: Application

118. Which statement is appropriate for the nurse to make to the parents of a child with cystic fibrosis who are planning to have a second child?
1. Genetic counseling is recommended.
2. There's a 50% chance that the child will be normal.
3. There's a 50% chance that the child will be affected.
4. There's a 25% chance that the child will only be a carrier.

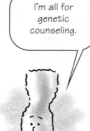

I'm all for genetic counseling.

118. 1. Genetic counseling should be recommended. Cystic fibrosis is an autosomal-recessive disease. Therefore, there's a 25% chance of the child having the disease, a 25% chance of the child being normal, and a 50% chance of the child being a carrier.
CN: Health promotion and maintenance; CNS: None; CL: Application

CN: Client needs category   CNS: Client needs subcategory   CL: Cognitive level

119. Which statement best describes an autosomal-recessive disorder such as cystic fibrosis?
  1. The genetic disorder is carried on the X chromosome.
  2. Both parents must pass the defective gene or set of genes.
  3. Only one defective gene or set of genes is passed by one parent.
  4. The child has an extra chromosome, resulting in an XXY karyotype.

120. Ceftazidime (Fortaz) has been ordered for a client with cystic fibrosis. The order states to give 40 mg/kg every 8 hours. The child is 2 years old and weighs 38½ lb. How many milligrams of the ceftazidime is given in one dose?
  1. 116 mg
  2. 233 mg
  3. 260 mg
  4. 466 mg

121. A nurse is teaching the parents of a 5-year-old male child admitted to the pediatric unit with cystic fibrosis. Which teaching statement concerning steatorrheaic stools is <u>most</u> accurate?
  1. They're black and tarry.
  2. They're frothy, foul-smelling, and fatty.
  3. They're clay-colored.
  4. They're orange or green.

122. A 3-year-old is admitted to the pediatric unit with pneumonia. He has a productive cough and appears to have difficulty breathing. The parents tell the nurse that the toddler hasn't been eating or drinking much and has been very inactive. Which interventions would be included in the care plan to improve airway clearance? Select all that apply:
  1. Restrict fluid intake.
  2. Perform chest physiotherapy as ordered.
  3. Encourage coughing and deep breathing.
  4. Keep the head of the bed flat.
  5. Perform postural drainage.
  6. Maintain humidification with a cool mist humidifier.

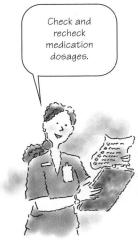

Check and recheck medication dosages.

119. 2. In recessive disorders such as cystic fibrosis, both parents must pass the defective gene or set of genes to the child. Dominant disorders are characterized by only one defective gene or set of genes passed by one parent. Sex-linked genetic disorders are carried on the X chromosome. A child with an XXY karyotype would have Klinefelter's syndrome.
CN: Health promotion and maintenance; CNS: None; CL: Knowledge

120. 2. The child should receive 233 mg per dose. Use the following equations:
  38.5 lb/2.2 kg = 17.5 kg (1 lb equals 2.2 kg);
  40 mg/kg × 17.5 kg = 700 mg;
  24 hours/8 hours = 3 doses;
  700 mg/3 doses = 233 mg.
CN: Physiological integrity; CNS: Pharmacological therapies; CL: Application

121. 2. Clients with cystic fibrosis have an abnormal electrolyte transport system in the cells that eventually blocks the pancreas, preventing the secretion of enzymes that digest certain foods such as protein and fats. This results in foul-smelling, fatty stool. Black, tarry stool is observed in clients who have upper GI bleeding, are on iron medications, or who consume diets high in red meat and dark-green vegetables. Clay-colored stool indicates possible bile obstruction. Orange or green stool may indicate intestinal infection.
CN: Physiological integrity; CNS: Physiological adaptation; CL: Application

122. 2, 3, 5, 6. Chest physiotherapy and postural drainage work together to break up congestion and then drain secretions. Coughing and deep breathing are also effective to remove congestion. A cool mist humidifier helps loosen thick mucus and relax airway passages. Fluids should be encouraged — not restricted. The child should be placed in semi-Fowler's or high Fowler's position to facilitate breathing and promote optimal lung expansion.
CN: Physiological integrity; CNS: Basic care and comfort; CL: Application

CN: Client needs category   CNS: Client needs subcategory   CL: Cognitive level

123. A nurse is caring for a 17-year-old female with cystic fibrosis who has been admitted to the hospital for treatment of a recurrent lung infection. The adolescent has many questions about her future and the consequences of her disease. Which statements about the course of cystic fibrosis are accurate? Select all that apply:
1. Breast development is frequently delayed.
2. The adolescent is at risk for developing diabetes.
3. Pregnancy and childbearing aren't affected.
4. Normal sexual relationships can be expected.
5. Only males carry the gene for the disease.
6. By age 20, the client should be able to decrease the frequency of respiratory treatment.

124. The nurse is to give ampicillin 125 mg I.M. every 6 hours to a 10-kg child with a respiratory tract infection. The label reads, "The recommended dose for a client weighing less than 40 kg is 25 mg to 50 mg/kg/day I.M. or I.V. in equally divided doses at 6- to 8-hour intervals." The drug concentration is 125 mg/5 ml. Which nursing intervention is appropriate? Select all that apply:
1. Draw up 10 ml of ampicillin to administer.
2. Administer the medication at 10:00 a.m., 2:00 p.m., 6:00 p.m., and 10:00 p.m.
3. Assess the client for allergies to penicillin.
4. Administer the medication; it's within dosing recommendations.
5. Question the physician about the order; it's more than the recommended dosage.
6. Obtain a sputum culture before administering the medication.

123. 1, 2, 4. Cystic fibrosis delays growth and the onset of puberty. Children with cystic fibrosis tend to be smaller-than-average size and develop secondary sexual characteristics later in life. In addition, clients with cystic fibrosis are at risk for developing diabetes mellitus because the pancreatic duct becomes obstructed as pancreatic tissue is damaged. Clients with cystic fibrosis can expect to have normal sexual relationships, but fertility may be affected because of changes in mucous membranes. Both males and females carry the gene for cystic fibrosis. Pulmonary disease commonly progresses as the client ages, requiring additional respiratory treatment, not less.

CN: Physiological integrity; CNS: Physiological adaptation; CL: Analysis

124. 3, 4, 6. Because ampicillin is a penicillin antibiotic, the client should be assessed for allergy to penicillin before the medication is administered. The dose of ampicillin is within the recommended range for a 10-kg client: 50 mg/kg × 10 kg = 500 mg. A dose of 500 mg divided by 4 (given every 6 hours) = 125 mg, which is within the recommended range. Cultures should be obtained before antibiotics are given. The nurse should draw up 5 ml to administer the correct dose, according to the concentration on the label. The dosing schedule of 4-hour intervals shouldn't be used because the recommended dosing is in 6- to 8-hour intervals.

CN: Physiological integrity; CNS: Pharmacological therapies; CL: Analysis

> You did it! Congratulations! Oh, you can breathe now. It's time to relax.

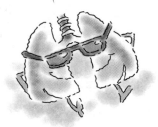

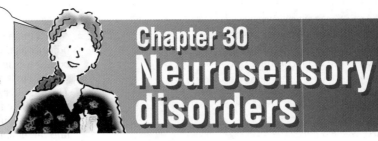

Chapter 30
Neurosensory disorders

Here are three Web sites for more information about neurosensory disorders in children: *www.chadd.org* (Children and Adults with Attention-Deficit Hyperactivity Disorder), *www.ndss.org* (National Down Syndrome Society), and *www.sbaa.org* (Spina Bifida Association of America).

1. The mother of a 3-year-old with a myelomeningocele is thinking about having another baby. The nurse should inform the woman that she should increase her intake of which acid?
   1. Folic acid to 0.4 mg/day
   2. Folic acid to 4 mg/day
   3. Ascorbic acid to 0.4 mg/day
   4. Ascorbic acid to 4 mg/day

2. Which nursing diagnosis is <u>most relevant</u> in the first 12 hours of life for a neonate born with a myelomeningocele?
   1. *Risk for infection*
   2. *Constipation*
   3. *Impaired physical mobility*
   4. *Delayed growth and development*

3. Which conditions would the nurse expect when assessing a neonate for hydrocephalus?
   1. Bulging fontanel, low-pitched cry
   2. Depressed fontanel, low-pitched cry
   3. Bulging fontanel, eyes rotated downward
   4. Depressed fontanel, eyes rotated downward

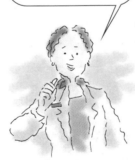

Most relevant — that's the key phrase for question 2.

1. 2. The American Academy of Pediatrics recommends that a woman who has had a child with a neural tube defect increase her intake of folic acid to 4 mg per day 1 month before becoming pregnant and continue this regimen through the first trimester. A woman who has no family history of neural tube defects should take 0.4 mg/day. All women of childbearing age should be encouraged to take a folic acid supplement because the majority of pregnancies in the United States are unplanned. Ascorbic acid hasn't been shown to have any effect on preventing neural tube defects.
CN: Health promotion and maintenance; CNS: None; CL: Application

2. 1. All of these diagnoses are important for a child with a myelomeningocele. However, during the first 12 hours of life, the most life-threatening event would be an infection. The other diagnoses will be addressed as the child develops.
CN: Physiological integrity; CNS: Reduction of risk potential; CL: Application

3. 3. Hydrocephalus is caused by an alteration in circulation of the cerebrospinal fluid (CSF). The amount of CSF increases, causing the fontanel to bulge. This also causes an increase in intracranial pressure. This increase in pressure causes the neonate's eyes to deviate downward (the "setting sun sign"), and the neonate's cry becomes high-pitched.
CN: Health promotion and maintenance; CNS: None; CL: Knowledge

CN: Client needs category   CNS: Client needs subcategory   CL: Cognitive level

4. A 2-year-old child is admitted to the hospital for revision of a ventriculoperitoneal shunt. Which complication is the <u>most common</u> reason for a revision?

1. Shunt infection
2. A broken shunt
3. Growth of the child
4. Heart failure

4. 3. This type of shunt has to be replaced periodically as the child grows and the tubing becomes too short. Shunt infection usually occurs within 2 to 3 months of insertion, not at 2 years. The shunts rarely break, unless there's head trauma. The fluid from a ventriculoperitoneal shunt goes into the peritoneal cavity and not into the heart; therefore, heart failure shouldn't occur.

CN: Health promotion and maintenance; CNS: None; CL: Knowledge

5. Which nursing action is <u>appropriate</u> to prevent injury when a child has a seizure?

1. Inserting a nasogastric tube to prevent emesis
2. Restraining the extremities with a pillow or blanket
3. Inserting a tongue blade to prevent injury to the tongue
4. Padding the side rails of the bed to protect the child from injury

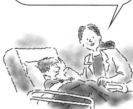

Remember, your first priority is to ensure the client's safety.

5. 4. A child having a seizure could fall out of bed or injure himself on anything, including the side rails of the bed. Attempts to insert anything into the child's mouth may injure the child. Attempting to restrain the child can't stop seizures. In fact, tactile stimulation may increase the seizure activity; therefore, it must be limited as much as possible.

CN: Safe, effective care environment; CNS: Safety and infection control; CL: Application

6. A mother brings her infant to the emergency department and says he had a seizure. While the nurse is obtaining a history, the mother says she was running out of formula so she stretched the formula by adding three times the normal amount of water. Electrolyte and blood glucose levels are drawn on the infant. The nurse would expect which laboratory value?

1. Blood glucose: 120 mg/dl
2. Chloride: 104 mmol/L
3. Potassium: 4 mmol/L
4. Sodium: 125 mmol/L

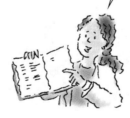

For the NCLEX, you need to be familiar with normal lab values.

6. 4. Diluting formula in a different manner from what's recommended alters the infant's electrolyte levels. Normal serum sodium for an infant is 135 to 145 mmol/L. When formula is diluted, the sodium in it is also diluted and will decrease the infant's sodium level. Hyponatremia is one of the causes of seizures in infants. The other values are all within normal limits.

CN: Physiological integrity; CNS: Physiological adaptation; CL: Application

7. For which signs and symptoms will the nurse monitor a neonate diagnosed with bacterial meningitis?

1. Hypothermia, irritability, and poor feeding
2. Positive Babinski's reflex, mottling, and pallor
3. Headache, nuchal rigidity, and developmental delays
4. Positive Moro embrace reflex, hyperthermia, and sunken fontanel

7. 1. The clinical appearance of a neonate with meningitis is different from that of a child or an adult. Neonates may be either hypothermic or hyperthermic. The irritation to the meninges causes the neonates to be irritable and to have a decreased appetite. They may be pale and mottled with a bulging, full fontanel. Normal neonates have positive Babinski's reflexes and Moros embrace. Older children and adults with meningitis have headaches, nuchal rigidity, and hyperthermia as clinical manifestations. Developmental delays, if present, would appear when the child was older.

CN: Physiological integrity; CNS: Physiological adaptation; CL: Comprehension

CN: Client needs category   CNS: Client needs subcategory   CL: Cognitive level

8. Which type of behavior demonstrated by a 6-year-old would help the nurse recognize a learning disability as opposed to attention deficit hyperactivity disorder (ADHD)?
1. The child reverses letters and words while reading.
2. The child is easily distracted and reacts impulsively.
3. The child is always getting into fights during recess.
4. The child has a difficult time reading a chapter book.

9. Which characteristic is true of cerebral palsy?
1. It's reversible.
2. It's progressive.
3. It results in mental retardation.
4. It appears at birth or during the first 2 years of life.

10. While assessing a full-term neonate, which symptom would cause the nurse to suspect a neurologic impairment?
1. A weak sucking reflex
2. A positive rooting reflex
3. A positive Babinski's reflex
4. Startle reflex in response to a loud noise

11. A mother reports that her school-age child has been reprimanded for daydreaming during class. This is a new behavior, and the child's grades are dropping. The nurse should suspect which problem?
1. The child may have a hearing problem and needs to have his ears checked.
2. The child may have a learning disability and needs referral to the special education department.
3. The child may have attention deficit hyperactivity disorder (ADHD) and needs medication.
4. The child may be having absence seizures and needs to see his primary health care provider for evaluation.

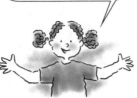

Welcome to the world of a school-age child! Guaranteed to keep you guessing and on your toes!

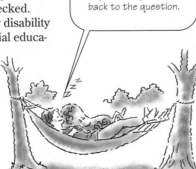

I better stop daydreaming and get back to the question.

8. 1. Children who reverse letters and words while reading have dyslexia. Two of the most common characteristics of children with ADHD include inattention and impulsiveness. Although aggressiveness may be common in children with ADHD, it isn't a characteristic that will aid in the diagnosis of this disorder. Six-year-old children aren't usually cognitively ready to read a chapter book.
CN: Health promotion and maintenance; CNS: None; CL: Application

9. 4. Cerebral palsy is an irreversible, nonprogressive disorder that results from damage to the developing brain during the prenatal, perinatal, or postnatal period. Although some children with cerebral palsy are mentally retarded, many have normal intelligence.
CN: Health promotion and maintenance; CNS: None; CL: Knowledge

10. 1. Normal neonates have a strong, vigorous sucking reflex. The rooting reflex is present at birth and disappears when the infant is between ages 3 and 4 months. A positive Babinski's reflex is present at birth and disappears by the time the infant is age 2. The startle reflex is present at birth and disappears when the infant is approximately age 4 months.
CN: Health promotion and maintenance; CNS: None; CL: Knowledge

11. 4. Absence seizures are commonly misinterpreted as daydreaming. The child loses awareness but no alteration in motor activity is exhibited. A mild hearing problem usually is exhibited as leaning forward, talking louder, listening to louder TV and music than usual, and a repetitive "what?" from the child. There isn't enough information to indicate a learning disability. ADHD is characterized by episodes of hyperactivity, not quietness.
CN: Physiological integrity; CNS: Physiological adaptation; CL: Application

CN: Client needs category CNS: Client needs subcategory CL: Cognitive level

12. A 2-month-old infant is brought to the well-baby clinic for a first checkup. On initial assessment, the nurse notes the infant's head circumference is at the 95th percentile. Which action would the nurse take <u>initially</u>?
   1. Assess vital signs.
   2. Measure the head again.
   3. Assess neurologic signs.
   4. Notify the primary health care provider.

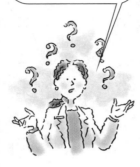

When in doubt, reassess data to make sure an error wasn't made.

12. 2. Whenever there's a question about vital signs or assessment data, the first logical step is to reassess to determine if an error has been made initially. Notifying the primary health care provider and assessing neurologic and vital signs are important and would follow the reassessment, if warranted.
CN: Health promotion and maintenance; CNS: None; CL: Comprehension

13. A nurse is teaching the parents of an 18-month-old infant diagnosed with bilateral otitis media about the prescribed medication amoxicillin and clavulanate potassium (Augmentin). Which statement by the parents indicates the teaching has been effective?
   1. "It can cause diarrhea."
   2. "It can cause headache."
   3. "It can cause petechiae."
   4. "It can cause a rash."

13. 1. Diarrhea is a common adverse effect of Augmentin suspension. Red rash and petechiae occur less commonly. Headache isn't a common adverse effect and would be difficult to determine in an 18-month-old infant.
CN: Physiological integrity; CNS: Pharmacological therapies; CL: Analysis

14. A 2-year-old child is admitted to the pediatric unit with the diagnosis of bacterial meningitis. Which <u>diagnostic</u> measure would be appropriate for the nurse to perform <u>first</u>?
   1. Obtain a urine specimen.
   2. Draw ordered laboratory tests.
   3. Place the toddler in respiratory isolation.
   4. Explain the treatment plan to the parents.

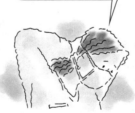

Be sure to protect yourself and others from infection.

14. 3. Nurses should take necessary precautions to protect themselves and others from possible infection from the bacterial organism causing meningitis. The affected child should immediately be placed in respiratory isolation; then the parents can be informed about the treatment plan. This should be done before laboratory tests are performed.
CN: Safe, effective care environment; CNS: Safety and infection control; CL: Application

15. A 10-month-old boy with bacterial meningitis was just started on antibiotic therapy. Which nursing action is <u>especially</u> important in this situation?
   1. Wearing a mask while providing care
   2. Flexing the child's neck every 4 hours to maintain range of motion
   3. Administering oral gentamicin (Garamycin)
   4. Encouraging the child to drink 3,000 ml of fluid per day

15. 1. With bacterial meningitis, respiratory isolation must be maintained for at least 24 hours after beginning antibiotic therapy. Wearing a mask is an important part of respiratory isolation. Moving the child's head would cause pain because his meninges are inflamed. Gentamicin is never administered orally. Encouraging 3,000 ml of fluid would cause overhydration in a 10-month-old infant and place him at risk for increased intracranial pressure.
CN: Safe, effective care environment; CNS: Safety and infection control; CL: Application

16. A preschool-age child has just been admitted to the pediatric unit with a diagnosis of bacterial meningitis. The nurse would include which recommendation in the nursing plan?
1. Take vital signs every 4 hours.
2. Monitor temperature every 4 hours.
3. Decrease environmental stimulation.
4. Encourage the parents to hold the child.

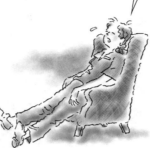

What I really need is some peace and quiet.

16. 3. A child with the diagnosis of meningitis is much more comfortable with decreased environmental stimuli. Noise and bright lights stimulate the child and can be irritating, causing the child to cry, in turn increasing intracranial pressure. Vital signs would be taken initially every hour and temperature monitored every 2 hours. Children with bacterial meningitis are usually much more comfortable if allowed to lie flat because this position doesn't cause increased meningeal irritation.
CN: Physiological integrity; CNS: Physiological adaptation; CL: Application

17. A child has just returned to the pediatric unit following ventriculoperitoneal shunt placement for hydrocephalus. Which intervention would the nurse perform <u>first</u>?
1. Monitor intake and output.
2. Place the child on the side opposite the shunt.
3. Offer fluids because the child has a dry mouth.
4. Administer pain medication by mouth as ordered.

17. 2. Following shunt placement surgery, the child should be placed on the side opposite the surgical site to prevent pressure on the shunt valve. Intake and output will be monitored, but that isn't the priority nursing intervention. Many children are nauseated after a general anesthetic, and ice chips or clear liquids would be introduced after the nurse had determined if the child was nauseated. Pain medication should initially be administered by an I.V. route postoperatively.
CN: Physiological integrity; CNS: Basic care and comfort; CL: Application

18. An otherwise healthy 18-month-old child with a history of febrile seizures is in the well-child clinic. Which statement by the father would indicate to the nurse that additional teaching should be done?
1. "I have ibuprofen available in case it's needed."
2. "My child will likely outgrow these seizures by age 5."
3. "I always keep phenobarbital with me in case of a fever."
4. "The most likely time for a seizure is when the fever is rising."

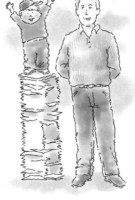

Sometimes, Father doesn't know what's best.

18. 3. Antiepileptics, such as phenobarbital (Luminal), are administered to children with prolonged seizures or neurologic abnormalities. Ibuprofen, not phenobarbital, is given for fever. Febrile seizures usually occur after age 6 months and are unusual after age 5. Treatment is to decrease the temperature because seizures occur as the temperature rises.
CN: Health promotion and maintenance; CNS: None; CL: Application

19. When checking a 5-month-old infant, which symptom would alert the nurse that the infant needs further follow-up?
1. Absent grasp reflex
2. Rolls from back to side
3. Balances head when sitting
4. Presence of Moro embrace reflex

19. 4. Moro embrace reflex should be absent at 4 months. Grasp reflex begins to fade at 2 months and should be absent at 3 months. A 4-month-old infant should be able to roll from back to side and balance his head when sitting.
CN: Health promotion and maintenance; CNS: None; CL: Application

CN: Client needs category CNS: Client needs subcategory CL: Cognitive level

20. An adolescent is started on valproic acid to treat seizures. Which statement should be included when educating the adolescent?
1. "This medication has no adverse effects."
2. "A common adverse effect is weight gain."
3. "Drowsiness and irritability commonly occur."
4. "Early morning dosing is recommended to decrease insomnia."

21. Which statement about cerebral palsy would be accurate?
1. "Cerebral palsy is a condition that runs in families."
2. "Cerebral palsy means there will be many disabilities."
3. "Cerebral palsy is a condition that doesn't get worse."
4. "Cerebral palsy occurs because of too much oxygen to the brain."

22. An older child has a craniotomy for removal of a brain tumor. Which statement would be appropriate for the nurse to say to the parents?
1. "Your child really had a close call."
2. "I'm sure your child will be back to normal soon."
3. "I'm so glad to hear your child doesn't have cancer."
4. "It may take some time for your child to return to normal."

23. A 6-month-old infant is admitted with a diagnosis of bacterial meningitis. The nurse would place the infant in which room?
1. A room with a 12-month-old infant with a urinary tract infection
2. A room with an 8-month-old infant with failure to thrive
3. A private room near the nurses' station
4. A two-bed room in the middle of the hall

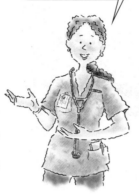

It's important to inform the client of possible adverse effects of a medication.

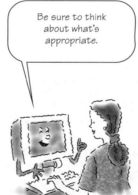

Be sure to think about what's appropriate.

20. 2. Weight gain is a common adverse effect of valproic acid. Drowsiness and irritability are adverse effects more commonly associated with phenobarbital. Felbamate (Felbatol) more commonly causes insomnia.
CN: Physiological integrity; CNS: Pharmacological therapies; CL: Application

21. 3. By definition, cerebral palsy is a nonprogressive neuromuscular disorder. It can be mild or quite severe and is believed to be the result of a hypoxic event during pregnancy or the birth process and doesn't run in families.
CN: Physiological integrity; CNS: Basic care and comfort; CL: Application

22. 4. After a craniotomy, it usually takes several weeks or longer before the child is back to normal. When comforting parents, it's best to first ascertain what the primary health care provider has told them about the tumor. Final pathology results won't be available for several days, so refrain from making premature statements about whether the tumor is malignant.
CN: Psychosocial integrity; CNS: None; CL: Application

23. 3. A child who has the diagnosis of bacterial meningitis will need to be placed in a private room until that child has received I.V. antibiotics for 24 hours because the child is considered contagious. Additionally, bacterial meningitis can be quite serious; therefore, the child should be placed near the nurses' station for close monitoring and easier access in case of a crisis.
CN: Safe, effective care environment; CNS: Coordinated care; CL: Application

CN: Client needs category CNS: Client needs subcategory CL: Cognitive level

24. In caring for a child immediately after a head injury, the nurse notes a blood pressure of 110/60, a heart rate of 78 beats/minute, dilated and nonreactive pupils, minimal response to pain, and slow response to name. Which symptom would cause the nurse the most concern?
  1. Vital signs
  2. Nonreactive pupils
  3. Slow response to name
  4. Minimal response to pain

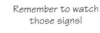
Remember to watch those signs!

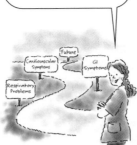

24. 2. Dilated and nonreactive pupils indicate that anoxia or ischemia of the brain has occurred. If the pupils are also fixed (don't move), then herniation of the brain through the tentorium has occurred. The vital signs are normal. Slow response to name can be normal after a head injury. Minimal response to pain is an indication of the child's level of consciousness.
CN: Physiological integrity; CNS: Basic care and comfort; CL: Application

25. Which nursing action should be included in the care plan to promote comfort in a 4-year-old child hospitalized with meningitis?
  1. Avoid making noise when in the child's room.
  2. Rock the child frequently.
  3. Have the child's 2-year-old brother stay in the room.
  4. Keep the lights on brightly so that he can see his mother.

25. 1. Meningeal irritation may cause seizures and heightens a child's sensitivity to all stimuli, including noise, lights, movement, and touch. Frequent rocking, presence of a younger sibling, and bright lights would increase stimulation.
CN: Physiological integrity; CNS: Basic care and comfort; CL: Application

26. Which developmental milestone would the nurse expect an 11-month-old infant to have achieved?
  1. Sitting independently
  2. Walking independently
  3. Building a tower of four cubes
  4. Turning a doorknob

26. 1. Infants typically sit independently, without support, by age 8 months. Walking independently may be accomplished as late as age 15 months and still be within the normal range. Few infants walk independently by age 11 months. Building a tower of three or four blocks is a milestone of an 18-month-old. Turning a doorknob is a milestone of a 24-month-old.
CN: Health promotion and maintenance; CNS: None; CL: Application

27. What's the nurse's priority when caring for a 10-month-old infant with meningitis?
  1. Maintaining an adequate airway
  2. Maintaining fluid and electrolyte balance
  3. Controlling seizures
  4. Controlling hyperthermia

If you're having trouble prioritizing, always go back to your basic ABCs.

27. 1. Maintaining an adequate airway is always a top priority. Maintaining fluid and electrolyte balance and controlling seizures and hyperthermia are all important but not as important as an adequate airway.
CN: Physiological integrity; CNS: Reduction of risk potential; CL: Application

28. Which intervention prevents a 17-month-old child with spastic cerebral palsy from going into a scissoring position?
  1. Keeping the child in leg braces 23 hours per day
  2. Letting the child lie down as much as possible
  3. Trying to keep the child as quiet as possible
  4. Placing the child on your hip

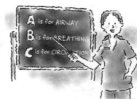
A is for AIRWAY
B is for BREATHING
C is for CIRCULATION

28. 4. To interrupt the scissoring position, flex the knees and hips. Placing the child on your hip is an easy way to stop this common spastic positioning. This child needs stimulation and movement to reach the goal of development to the fullest potential. Wearing leg braces 23 hours per day is inappropriate and doesn't allow the child to move freely. Trying to keep the child quiet and flat are inappropriate measures.
CN: Physiological integrity; CNS: Basic care and comfort; CL: Application

CN: Client needs category   CNS: Client needs subcategory   CL: Cognitive level

29. The mother of a child with a ventriculo-peritoneal shunt calls the nurse saying that her child has a temperature of 101.2° F (38.4° C), a blood pressure of 108/68 mm Hg, and a pulse of 100 beats/minute. The child is lethargic and vomited the night before. Other children in the family have had similar symptoms. Which nursing intervention is most appropriate?
1. Providing symptomatic treatment
2. Advising the mother that this is a viral infection
3. Consulting the primary health care provider
4. Having the mother bring the child to the primary health care provider's office

29. 4. One of the complications of a ventriculoperitoneal shunt is a shunt infection. Shunt infections can have similar symptoms as a viral infection so it's best to have the child examined. These symptoms may be due to the same viral infection that the siblings have, but it's better to rule out a shunt infection because infection can progress quickly to a very serious illness.
CN: Physiological integrity; CNS: Basic care and comfort; CL: Application

30. The mother of a 10-year-old child with attention deficit hyperactivity disorder says her husband won't allow their child to take more than 5 mg of methylphenidate (Ritalin) every morning. The child isn't doing better in school. Which recommendation would the nurse make to the mother?
1. Sneak the medication to the child anyway.
2. Put the child in charge of administering the medication.
3. Bring the child's father to the clinic to discuss the medication.
4. Have the school nurse give the child the rest of the medication.

30. 3. Bringing the father to the clinic for a teaching session about the medication should assist him in understanding why it's necessary for the child to receive the full dose. A nurse shouldn't advise dishonesty to a client or family. Putting a 10-year-old in charge of his medication is inappropriate. The father should be included in the treatment as much as possible. School nurses can only administer medications as per physician prescriptions.
CN: Physiological integrity; CNS: Pharmacological therapies; CL: Application

31. A hospitalized child is to receive 75 mg of acetaminophen (Tylenol) for fever control. How much will the nurse administer if the acetaminophen concentration is 40 mg per 0.4 ml?
1. 0.37 ml
2. 0.75 ml
3. 1.12 ml
4. 1.5 ml

31. 2. The nurse will administer 0.75 ml. Use the following equations:
$$40 \text{ mg}/0.4 \text{ ml} = 75 \text{ mg}/X \text{ ml};$$
$$40 \text{ mg} \times X \text{ ml} = 0.4 \text{ ml} \times 75 \text{ mg};$$
$$40X = 30;$$
$$X = 30/40; X = 0.75 \text{ ml}.$$
CN: Physiological integrity; CNS: Pharmacological therapies; CL: Application

You're looking for the correct findings in question 32.

32. The nurse is observing an infant who may have acute bacterial meningitis. Which finding might the nurse look for?
1. Flat fontanel
2. Irritability, fever, and vomiting
3. Jaundice, drowsiness, and refusal to eat
4. Negative Kernig's sign

32. 2. Findings associated with acute bacterial meningitis may include irritability, fever, and vomiting along with seizure activity. Fontanels would be bulging as intracranial pressure rises, and Kernig's sign would be present due to meningeal irritation. Jaundice, drowsiness, and refusal to eat indicate a GI disturbance rather than meningitis.
CN: Physiological integrity; CNS: Physiological adaptation; CL: Knowledge

CN: Client needs category   CNS: Client needs subcategory   CL: Cognitive level

33. A nurse notes the below chart entry concerning a school-age child who has had a brain tumor removed. Which nursing action should be performed <u>first</u>?

Progress Note	
10/14/08	Pupils equal and reactive to
1300	light; motor strength equal;
	aware of name, date, but
	not location. Complaining of
	headache.
	S. Jones, L.P.N

1. Provide medication for the headache.
2. Immediately notify the primary health care provider.
3. Check what the child's level of consciousness has been.
4. Call the child's parents to come and sit at the child's bedside.

34. The nurse is preparing a toddler for a lumbar puncture. For this procedure, the nurse should place the child in which position?
1. Lying prone, with the neck flexed
2. Sitting up, with the back straight
3. Lying on one side, with the back curved
4. Lying prone, with the feet higher than the head

35. Parents bring a toddler age 19 months to the clinic for a regular checkup. When palpating the toddler's fontanels, what should the nurse expect to find?
1. Closed anterior fontanel and open posterior fontanel
2. Open anterior fontanel and closed posterior fontanel
3. Closed anterior and posterior fontanels
4. Open anterior and posterior fontanels

36. A 10-year-old child with a concussion is admitted to the pediatric unit. The nurse would place this child in a room with which roommate?
1. A 6-year-old child with osteomyelitis
2. An 8-year-old child with gastroenteritis
3. A 10-year-old child with rheumatic fever
4. A 12-year-old child with a fractured femur

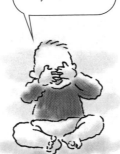

I can't wait to see if you know the correct answer to question 35.

33. 3. When there's an abnormality in current assessment data, it's vital to determine what the client's previous status was. Determine whether the status has changed or remained the same. Providing medication for the headache would be done after ascertaining the previous level of consciousness. Contacting the primary health care provider and the child's parents isn't necessary before a final assessment has been made.
CN: Physiological integrity; CNS: Physiological adaptation; CL: Application

34. 3. Lumbar puncture involves placing a needle between the lumbar vertebrae into the subarachnoid space. For this procedure, the nurse should position the client on one side with the back curved because curving the back maximizes the space between the lumbar vertebrae, facilitating needle insertion. Prone and seated positions don't achieve maximum separation of the vertebrae.
CN: Physiological integrity; CNS: Reduction of risk potential; CL: Application

35. 3. By age 18 months, the anterior and posterior fontanels should be closed. The diamond-shaped anterior fontanel normally closes between ages 9 and 18 months. The triangular posterior fontanel normally closes between ages 2 and 3 months.
CN: Health promotion and maintenance; CNS: None; CL: Application

36. 4. A child with a concussion should be placed with a roommate who's free from infection and close to the child's age. Osteomyelitis, gastroenteritis, and rheumatic fever involve infection.
CN: Safe, effective care environment; CNS: Coordinated care; CL: Application

CN: Client needs category CNS: Client needs subcategory CL: Cognitive level

37. A nurse is caring for a child with spina bifida. The child's mother asks the nurse what she did to cause the birth defect. Which statement would be the nurse's <u>best</u> response?
1. "Older age at conception is one of the major causes of the defect."
2. "It's a common complication of amniocentesis."
3. "It has been linked to maternal alcohol consumption during pregnancy."
4. "The cause is unknown and there are many environmental factors that may contribute to it."

38. An 11-year-old boy with a head injury has been in the hospital for 16 days. He's receiving physical, occupational, and speech therapies. He can swallow and has adequate oral intake; however, his speech is slow and he sometimes makes inappropriate statements. He's usually cooperative but occasionally has combative and violent outbursts. His parents are upset and want to know what's wrong with him. What's the best response by the nurse?
1. "He probably didn't receive enough discipline growing up and is throwing tantrums."
2. "He needs to be restrained during these episodes."
3. "This is a stage of healing for him."
4. "He'll need to be on life-long medication to control his temper."

39. Which mechanism causes the severe headache that accompanies an increase in intracranial pressure (ICP)?
1. Cervical hyperextension
2. Stretching of the meninges
3. Cerebral ischemia related to altered circulation
4. Reflex spasm of the neck extensors to splint the neck against cervical flexion

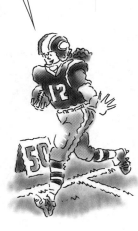

Congratulations. You're halfway there and headed in the right direction!

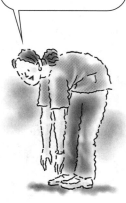

It's a stretch to come up with the correct answer for question 39.

37. 4. There is no one known cause of spina bifida, but scientists believe that it's linked to hereditary and environmental factors; neural tube defects, including spina bifida, have been strongly linked to low dietary intake of folic acid. Maternal age doesn't have an impact on spina bifida. An amniocentesis is performed to help diagnose spina bifida in utero but doesn't cause the disorder. Maternal alcohol intake during pregnancy has been linked to mental retardation, craniofacial defects, and cardiac abnormalities, but not spina bifida.
CN: Physiological integrity; CNS: Physiological adaptation; CL: Application

38. 3. Clients with head injuries may pass through eight stages during their recovery. Stage 1, marked by unresponsiveness, is the worst stage. Stage 8, characterized by purposeful, appropriate behavior, is the final stage of healing. This child is somewhere between stage 4 (confused, agitated behavior) and stage 6 (confused, appropriate behavior) because sometimes he can answer appropriately but at other times becomes confused and angry, resorting to violent behavior. Restraining the boy is inappropriate and can increase intracranial pressure. The other statements are inappropriate.
CN: Health promotion and maintenance; CNS: None; CL: Application

39. 2. The mechanism producing the headache that accompanies increased ICP may be the stretching of the meninges and pain fibers associated with blood vessels. Cerebral ischemia occurs because of vascular obstruction and decreased perfusion of the brain tissue. With nuchal rigidity, cervical flexion is painful due to the stretching of the inflamed meninges and the pain triggers a reflex spasm of the neck extensors to splint the area against further cervical flexion. It occurs in response to the pain; it doesn't cause it.
CN: Physiological integrity; CNS: Physiological adaptation; CL: Application

CN: Client needs category   CNS: Client needs subcategory   CL: Cognitive level

40. The nurse at a family health clinic is teaching a group of parents about normal infant development. What patterns of communication should the nurse tell parents to expect from an infant at age 1?
1. Squeals and makes pleasure sound
2. Understands "no" and other simple commands
3. Uses speechlike rhythm when talking with an adult
4. Uses multisyllabic babbling

41. A nurse is assessing a 3-year-old child with nuchal rigidity. Which sign would be documented on the chart to support this condition?
1. Positive Kernig's sign
2. Negative Brudzinski's sign
3. Positive Homans' sign
4. Negative Kernig's sign

42. The nurse is collecting data from a child who may have a seizure disorder. Which of the following is a description of an absence seizure?
1. Sudden, momentary loss of muscle tone, with a brief loss of consciousness
2. Muscle tone maintained and child frozen in position
3. Brief, sudden contracture of a muscle or muscle group
4. Minimal or no alteration in muscle tone, with a brief loss of consciousness

43. A child with a diagnosis of meningococcal meningitis develops sudden signs of sepsis and a purpuric rash over both lower extremities. The primary health care provider should be notified immediately because these signs could be indicative of which complication?
1. A severe allergic reaction to the antibiotic regimen with impending anaphylaxis
2. Onset of the syndrome of inappropriate antidiuretic hormone (SIADH)
3. Fulminant meningococcemia (Waterhouse-Friderichsen syndrome)
4. Adhesive arachnoiditis

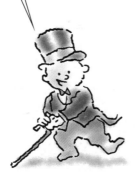

At 12 months old, I hope you're not expecting too much...I'm just beginning to get my act together.

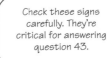

Check these signs carefully. They're critical for answering question 43.

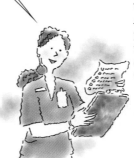

40. 2. At age 1, most babies understand the word "no" and other simple commands. Children at this age also learn one or two other words. Babies squeal, make pleasure sounds, and use multisyllabic babbling at age 3 to 6 months. Using speechlike rhythm when talking with an adult usually occurs between ages 6 to 9 months.
CN: Health promotion and maintenance; CNS: None; CL: Knowledge

41. 1. A positive Kernig's sign indicates nuchal rigidity, caused by an irritative lesion of the subarachnoid space. A positive Brudzinski's sign also is indicative of the condition. A positive Homans' sign may indicate venous inflammation of the lower leg.
CN: Physiological integrity; CNS: Physiological adaptation; CL: Application

42. 4. Absence seizures are characterized by a brief loss of responsiveness with minimal or no alteration in muscle tone. They may go unrecognized because the child's behavior changes very little. A sudden loss of muscle tone describes atonic seizures. A frozen position describes the appearance of someone having akinetic seizures. A brief, sudden contraction of muscles describes a myoclonic seizure.
CN: Physiological integrity; CNS: Physiological adaptation; CL: Knowledge

43. 3. Meningococcemia is a serious complication usually associated with meningococcal infection. When onset is severe, sudden, and rapid (fulminant), it's known as Waterhouse-Friderichsen syndrome. Anaphylactic shock would need to be differentiated from septic shock. SIADH can be an acute complication but wouldn't be accompanied by the purpuric rash. Adhesive arachnoiditis occurs in the chronic phase of the disease and leads to obstruction of the flow of cerebrospinal fluid.
CN: Physiological integrity; CNS: Reduction of risk potential; CL: Application

CN: Client needs category   CNS: Client needs subcategory   CL: Cognitive level

44. Which pathologic process is commonly associated with aseptic meningitis?
1. Ischemic infarction of cerebral tissue
2. Childhood virus, such as mumps
3. Brain abscess caused by various pyogenic organisms
4. Cerebral ventricular irritation from a traumatic brain injury

44. 2. Aseptic meningitis is caused principally by viruses and is commonly associated with other diseases, such as measles, mumps, herpes, and leukemia. Incidence of brain abscess is high in bacterial meningitis, and ischemic infarction of cerebral tissue can occur with tubercular meningitis. Traumatic brain injury could lead to bacterial (not viral) meningitis.
CN: Physiological integrity; CNS: Physiological adaptation; CL: Knowledge

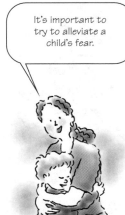

It's important to try to alleviate a child's fear.

45. To alleviate a child's pain and fear of lumbar puncture, which intervention should the nurse perform?
1. Sedate the child with an anxiolytic (midazolam).
2. Apply a topical anesthetic to the skin 5 to 10 minutes before the puncture.
3. Have a parent hold the child in her lap during the procedure.
4. Have the child inhale small amounts of nitrous oxide gas before the puncture.

45. 1. Sedation with an anxiolytic such as midazolam or other drugs can alleviate the pain and fear associated with a lumbar puncture. A topical anesthetic can be applied, but it should be done 30 minutes to 1 hour before the procedure to be fully effective. Having a parent hold a child in the lap increases the risk of neurologic injury due to the inability to assume and maintain the proper anatomic position required for a safe lumbar puncture. Use of nitrous oxide gas isn't recommended.
CN: Physiological integrity; CNS: Basic care and comfort; CL: Application

46. Antibiotic therapy to treat meningitis should be instituted <u>immediately after</u> which event?
1. Admission to the nursing unit
2. Initiation of I.V. therapy
3. Identification of the causative organism
4. Collection of cerebrospinal fluid (CSF) and blood for culture

46. 4. Antibiotic therapy should always begin immediately after the collection of CSF and blood cultures. After the specific organism is identified, bacteria-specific antibiotics can be administered if the initial choice of antibiotic therapy isn't appropriate. Admission and initiation of I.V. therapy aren't, by themselves, appropriate times to begin antibiotic therapy.
CN: Physiological integrity; CNS: Pharmacological therapies; CL: Application

47. Which description of the complications of bacterial meningitis is <u>most</u> accurate?
1. Complications occur most often when the disease is contracted during the first 2 months of life.
2. Complications occur most often in children with meningococcal meningitis.
3. Complications primarily involve the fourth ventricle of the brain.
4. Complications most commonly involve the facial nerve, leading to facial paralysis.

47. 1. Infants younger than age 2 months with bacterial meningitis commonly have such complications as hearing loss, impaired vision, seizures, and cardiac and renal abnormalities. Complications are seen less commonly among children diagnosed with meningococcal meningitis. Complications aren't isolated to the fourth ventricle of the brain. The facial nerve isn't commonly affected.
CN: Physiological integrity; CNS: Physiological adaptation; CL: Application

48. A 1-month-old infant is admitted to the pediatric unit and diagnosed with bacterial meningitis. Which assessment findings by the nurse support the diagnosis?
1. Hemorrhagic rash, first appearing as petechiae
2. Photophobia
3. Fever, change in feeding pattern, vomiting, or diarrhea
4. Fever, lethargy, and purpura or large necrotic patches

49. Which goal of nursing care is the most difficult to accomplish in caring for a child with meningitis?
1. Protecting self and others from possible infection
2. Avoiding actions that increase discomfort, such as lifting the head
3. Keeping environmental stimuli to a minimum, such as reduced light and noise
4. Maintaining I.V. infusion to administer adequate antimicrobial therapy

50. Which nursing assessment data should be given the highest priority for a child with clinical findings related to tubercular meningitis?
1. Onset and character of fever
2. Degree and extent of nuchal rigidity
3. Signs of increased intracranial pressure (ICP)
4. Occurrence of urine and fecal contamination

51. The clinical manifestations of acute bacterial meningitis are dependent on which factor?
1. Age of the child
2. Length of the prodromal period
3. Time span from bacterial invasion to onset of symptoms
4. Degree of elevation of cerebrospinal fluid (CSF) glucose compared to serum glucose level

48. 3. Fever, change in feeding patterns, vomiting, and diarrhea are commonly observed in children with bacterial meningitis. Hemorrhagic rashes, petechiae, photophobia, fever, lethargy, and purpura are common manifestations in older children with meningitis.
CN: Physiological integrity; CNS: Physiological adaptation; CL: Application

49. 4. One of the most difficult problems in the nursing care of children with meningitis is maintaining the I.V. infusion for the length of time needed to provide adequate therapy. All of the other options are important aspects in the provision of care for the child with meningitis, but they're secondary to antimicrobial therapy.
CN: Physiological integrity; CNS: Basic care and comfort; CL: Application

50. 3. Assessment of fever and evaluation of nuchal rigidity are important aspects of care, but assessment for signs of increasing ICP should be the highest priority due to the life-threatening implications. Urinary and fecal incontinence can occur in a child who's ill from nearly any cause but doesn't pose a great danger to life.
CN: Physiological integrity; CNS: Reduction of risk potential; CL: Application

51. 1. Clinical manifestations of acute bacterial meningitis depend largely on the age of the child. Clinical manifestations aren't dependent on the prodromal or initial period of the disease nor the time from invasion of the host to the onset of symptoms. The glucose level of the CSF is reduced, not elevated, in bacterial meningitis.
CN: Physiological integrity; CNS: Physiological adaptation; CL: Application

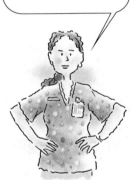

When you need to prioritize care based on assessment data, always treat the most life-threatening problems first.

52. The mother of a child with a history of closed head injury asks the nurse why her son would begin having seizures without warning. Which response by the nurse is the <u>most</u> accurate?

1. "Clonic seizure activity is usually interpreted as falling."
2. "It's not unusual to develop seizures after a head injury because of brain trauma."
3. "Focal discharge in the brain may lead to absence seizures that go unnoticed."
4. "The epileptogenic focus in the brain needs multiple stimuli before it will discharge to cause a seizure."

53. The nurse is assessing a 1-month-old male infant during a routine examination at a family health center. Which method does the nurse use to test for Babinski's sign?

1. Raise the child's leg with the knee flexed and then extend the child's leg at the knee to determine if resistance is noted.
2. With the knee flexed, dorsiflex the foot to determine if there's pain in the calf of the leg.
3. Flex the child's head while he's in a supine position to determine if the knees or hips flex involuntarily.
4. Stroke the bottom of the foot to determine if there's fanning and dorsiflexion of the big toe.

54. During the trial period to determine the efficacy of an anticonvulsant drug, which caution should be explained to the parents?

1. Plasma levels of the drug will be monitored on a daily basis.
2. Drug dosage will be adjusted depending on the frequency of seizure activity.
3. The drug must be discontinued immediately if even the slightest problem occurs.
4. The child shouldn't participate in activities that could be hazardous if a seizure occurs.

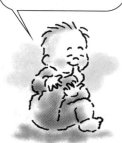

I don't know what this is a sign of, except that I'm awfully talented and cute!

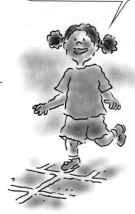

They say I need to take it easy for awhile because I started new medication. So, ya wanna play catch?

52. 2. Stimuli from an earlier injury may eventually elicit seizure activity, a process known as *kindling.* Atonic seizures, not clonic seizures, are commonly accompanied by falling. Focal seizures are partial seizures; absence seizures are generalized seizures. Focal seizures don't lead to absence seizures. The epileptogenic focus consists of a group of hyperexcitable neurons responsible for initiating synchronous, high-frequency discharges that lead to a seizure and don't need multiple stimuli.
CN: Physiological integrity; CNS: Physiological adaptation; CL: Application

53. 4. To test for Babinski's sign, stroke the bottom of the foot to determine if there's fanning and dorsiflexion of the big toe. Raising the child's leg with the knee flexed and then extending the leg at the knee to determine if resistance is noted tests for Kernig's sign. Dorsiflexion of the foot with the knee flexed to determine if there's pain in the calf of the leg tests for Homans' sign. Flexing the child's head while he's in a supine position to determine if the knees or hips flex involuntarily tests for Brudzinski's sign.
CN: Physiological integrity; CNS: Physiological adaptation; CL: Knowledge

54. 4. Until seizure control is certain, clients shouldn't participate in activities (such as riding a bicycle) that could be hazardous if a seizure were to occur. Plasma levels need to be monitored periodically over the course of drug therapy; daily monitoring isn't necessary. Dosage changes are usually based on plasma drug levels as well as seizure control. Anticonvulsant drugs should be withdrawn over a period of 6 weeks to several months, never immediately, as doing so could precipitate status epilepticus.
CN: Physiological integrity; CNS: Pharmacological therapies; CL: Application

55. What behavioral responses to pain would a nurse observe from an infant younger than age 1?

1. Localized withdrawal and resistance of the entire body
2. Passive resistance, clenching fists, and holding body rigid
3. Reflex withdrawal to stimulus and facial grimacing
4. Low frustration level and striking out physically

56. The parents of a child with a history of seizures who has been taking phenytoin (Dilantin) ask the nurse why it's difficult to maintain therapeutic plasma levels of this medication. Which statement by the nurse would be <u>most</u> accurate?

1. "A drop in the plasma drug level will lead to a toxic state."
2. "The capacity to metabolize the drug becomes overwhelmed over time."
3. "Small increments in dosage lead to sharp increases in plasma drug levels."
4. "Large increments in dosage lead to a more rapid stabilizing therapeutic effect."

57. Client teaching should stress which rule in relation to the differences in bioavailability of different forms of phenytoin (Dilantin)?

1. Use the cheapest formulation the pharmacy has on hand at the time of refill.
2. Shop around to get the least expensive formulation.
3. There's no difference between one formulation and another, regardless of price.
4. Avoid switching formulations without the primary health care provider's approval.

58. To detect complications as early as possible in a child with meningitis who's receiving I.V. fluids, monitoring for which condition should be the nurse's <u>priority</u>?

1. Cerebral edema
2. Renal failure
3. Left-sided heart failure
4. Cardiogenic shock

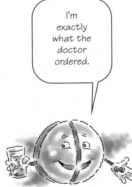

I'm exactly what the doctor ordered.

55. 3. Infants younger than age 1 become irritable and exhibit reflex withdrawal to the painful stimulus. Facial grimacing also occurs. Localized withdrawal is experienced by toddlers ages 1 to 3 in response to pain. The nurse would observe passive resistance in school-age children. Preschoolers show a low frustration level and strike out physically.
CN: Physiological integrity; CNS: Physiological adaptation; CL: Comprehension

56. 3. Within the therapeutic range for phenytoin, small increments in dosage produce sharp increases in plasma drug levels. The capacity of the liver to metabolize phenytoin is affected by slight changes in the dosage of the drug, not necessarily the length of time the client has been taking the drug. Large increments in dosage will greatly increase plasma levels, leading to drug toxicity.
CN: Physiological integrity; CNS: Pharmacological therapies; CL: Application

57. 4. Differences in bioavailability exist among different formulations (tablets and capsules) and among the same formulations produced by different manufacturers. Clients shouldn't switch from one formulation to another or from one brand to another without primary health care provider approval and supervision.
CN: Physiological integrity; CNS: Pharmacological therapies; CL: Application

58. 1. The child with meningitis is already at increased risk for cerebral edema and increased intracranial pressure due to inflammation of the meningeal membranes; therefore, the nurse should carefully monitor fluid intake and output to avoid fluid volume overload. Renal failure and cardiogenic shock aren't complications of I.V. therapy. The child with a healthy heart wouldn't be expected to develop left-sided heart failure.
CN: Physiological integrity; CNS: Pharmacological therapies; CL: Application

CN: Client needs category   CNS: Client needs subcategory   CL: Cognitive level

59. Which instruction should be included in client teaching specifically related to anticonvulsant drug efficacy?
   1. Wear a medical identification bracelet.
   2. Maintain a seizure frequency chart.
   3. Avoid potentially hazardous activities.
   4. Discontinue the drug immediately if adverse effects are suspected.

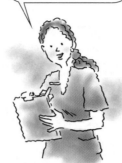

Keeping a frequency chart of all seizure activity can help evaluate drug efficacy.

59. 2. Ongoing evaluation of therapeutic effects can be accomplished by maintaining a frequency chart that indicates the date, time, and nature of all seizure activity. These data may be helpful in making dosage alterations and specific drug selection. Wearing a medical identification bracelet and avoiding hazardous activities are ways to minimize danger related to seizure activity, but these factors don't affect drug efficacy. Anticonvulsant drugs should never be discontinued abruptly due to the potential for development of status epilepticus.
CN: Physiological integrity; CNS: Pharmacological therapies; CL: Application

60. A 13-year-old with structural scoliosis has Harrington rods inserted. Which position would be best during the postoperative period?
   1. Supine in bed
   2. Side-lying
   3. Semi-Fowler's
   4. High Fowler's

60. 1. After placement of Harrington rods, the client must remain flat in bed. The gatch on a manual bed should be taped and electric beds should be unplugged to prevent the client from raising the head or foot of the bed. Other positions, such as the side-lying, semi-Fowler, and high Fowler positions, could prove damaging because the rods won't be able to maintain the spine in a straight position.
CN: Physiological integrity; CNS: Reduction of risk potential; CL: Application

61. At which time is seizure activity <u>most likely</u> to occur?
   1. During the rapid eye movement (REM) stage of sleep
   2. During long periods of excitement
   3. While falling asleep and on awakening
   4. While eating, particularly if the child is hurried

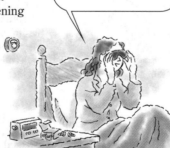

Seizure activity is most likely to occur during periods of functional instability of the brain.

61. 3. Falling asleep or awakening from sleep are periods of functional instability of the brain; seizure activity is more likely to occur during these times. Eating quickly, excitement without undo fatigue, and REM sleep haven't been identified as contributing factors.
CN: Physiological integrity; CNS: Physiological adaptation; CL: Knowledge

62. When educating the family of a child with seizures, it's appropriate to tell them to call emergency medical services in the event of a seizure if which complication occurs?
   1. Continuous vomiting for 30 minutes after the seizure
   2. Stereotypic or automatous body movements during onset
   3. Lack of expression, pallor, or flushing of the face during the seizure
   4. Unilateral or bilateral posturing of one or more extremities during onset

62. 1. Continuous vomiting after a seizure has ended can be a sign of an acute problem and indicates that the child requires an immediate medical evaluation. All of the other manifestations are normally present in various types of seizure activity and don't indicate a need for immediate medical evaluation.
CN: Physiological integrity; CNS: Reduction of risk potential; CL: Application

CN: Client needs category   CNS: Client needs subcategory   CL: Cognitive level

63. Identifying factors that trigger seizure activity could lead to which alteration in the child's environment or activities of daily living?
1. Avoiding striped wallpaper and ceiling fans
2. Having the child sleep alone to prevent sleep interruption
3. Including extended periods of intense physical activity daily
4. Allowing the child to drink soda only between noon and 5 p.m.

64. Which nursing intervention would be included to support the goal of avoiding injury, respiratory distress, or aspiration during a seizure?
1. Positioning the child with the head hyperextended
2. Placing a hand under the child's head for support
3. Using pillows to prop the child into the sitting position
4. Working a padded tongue blade or small plastic airway between the teeth

65. Which diagnostic measure is <u>most</u> accurate in detecting neural tube defects?
1. Flat plate of the lower abdomen after the 23rd week of gestation
2. Significant level of alpha-fetoprotein present in amniotic fluid
3. Amniocentesis for lecithin-sphingomyelin (L/S) ratio
4. Presence of high maternal levels of albumin after 12th week of gestation

66. A nurse is teaching the parents of a child who has been diagnosed with spina bifida. Which statement by the nurse would be the <u>most</u> accurate description of spina bifida?
1. "It has little influence on the intellectual and perceptual abilities of the child."
2. "It's a simple neurologic defect that's completely corrected surgically within 1 to 2 days after birth."
3. "Its presence indicates that many areas of the central nervous system (CNS) may not develop or function adequately."
4. "It's a complex neurologic disability that involves a collaborative health team effort for the entire first year of life."

CN: Client needs category   CNS: Client needs subcategory   CL: Cognitive level

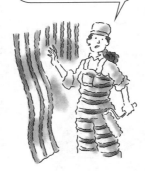

Yikes! All these stripes are starting to bother my eyes!

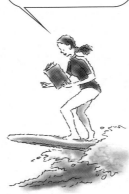

Hang on! You're almost finished!

63. 1. Striped wallpaper and ceiling fans can be triggers to seizure activity if the child is photosensitive. Sleep interruption hasn't been identified as a triggering factor. Avoidance of fatigue can reduce seizure activity; therefore, intense physical activity for extended periods of time should be avoided. Restricting caffeine intake by using caffeine-free soda is a dietary modification that may prevent seizures.
CN: Physiological integrity; CNS: Physiological adaptation; CL: Application

64. 2. Placing a hand or a small cushion or blanket under the child's head will help prevent injury. Position the child with the head in midline, not hyperextended, to promote a good airway and adequate ventilation. Don't attempt to prop the child up into a sitting position, but ease him to the floor to prevent falling and unnecessary injury. Don't put anything in the child's mouth because it could cause infection or obstruct the airway.
CN: Physiological integrity; CNS: Reduction of risk potential; CL: Application

65. 2. Screening for significant levels of alpha-fetoprotein is 90% effective in detecting neural tube defects. Prenatal screening includes a combination of maternal serum and amniotic fluid levels, amniocentesis, amniography, and ultrasonography and has been relatively successful in diagnosing the defect. Flat plate X-rays of the abdomen, L/S ratio, and maternal serum albumin levels aren't diagnostic for the defect.
CN: Health promotion and maintenance; CNS: None; CL: Application

66. 3. When a spinal cord lesion exists at birth, it commonly leads to altered development or function of other areas of the CNS. Spina bifida is a complex neurologic defect that heavily impacts the physical, cognitive, and psychosocial development of the child and involves collaborative, lifelong management due to the chronicity and multiplicity of the problems involved.
CN: Physiological integrity; CNS: Physiological adaptation; CL: Application

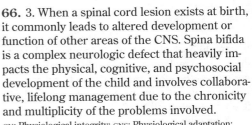

67. Common deformities occurring in the child with spina bifida are related to the muscles of the lower extremities that are active or inactive. These may include which complication?
1. Club feet
2. Hip extension
3. Ankylosis of the knee
4. Abduction and external rotation of the hip

68. A nurse notes that a 4-year-old child with cerebral palsy has a weight at the 30th percentile and a height at the 60th percentile. Which teaching information is appropriate for the child and parents?
1. The child should eat fewer calories.
2. The child's weight and height are within the normal range.
3. The child needs to increase his daily caloric intake.
4. The child is small for his age and will remain so through adolescence.

69. Infants with myelomeningocele must be closely observed for manifestations of Chiari II malformation, including which symptom?
1. Rapidly progressing scoliosis
2. Changes in urologic functioning
3. Back pain below the site of the sac closure
4. Respiratory stridor, apneic periods, and difficulty swallowing

70. A child with myelomeningocele and hydrocephalus may demonstrate problems related to damage of the white matter caused by ventricular enlargement. This damage may manifest itself in which condition?
1. Inability to speak
2. Early hand dominance
3. Impaired intellectual functions
4. Flaccid paralysis of the lower extremities

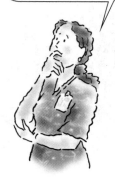

Question 67 is asking about spina bifida. What do you know about this congenital disorder?

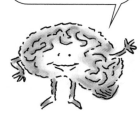

For question 70, it helps to know that my white matter is also known as the "association area."

67. 1. The type and extent of deformity in the lower extremities depends on the muscles that are active or inactive. Passive positioning in utero may result in deformities of the feet, such as equinovarus (club foot), knee flexion and extension contractures, and hip flexion with adduction and internal rotation leading to subluxation or dislocation of the hip.
CN: Physiological integrity; CNS: Physiological adaptation; CL: Application

68. 2. The weight and height are between the 25th and 75th percentiles, so the child is considered normal.
CN: Health promotion and maintenance; CNS: None; CL: Application

69. 4. Children with a myelomeningocele have a 90% chance of having a Chiari II malformation. This may lead to a possibility of respiratory function problems, such as respiratory stridor associated with paralysis of the vocal cords, apneic episodes of unknown cause, difficulty swallowing, and an abnormal gag reflex. Scoliosis and urologic function changes occur with myelomeningocele, but these complications aren't specifically related to Chiari II malformation. Lower back pain doesn't occur because the infant has a loss of sensory function below the level of the cord defect.
CN: Physiological integrity; CNS: Reduction of risk potential; CL: Knowledge

70. 3. Damage to the white matter (association area) caused by ventricular enlargement has been linked to impairment of intellectual and perceptual abilities commonly seen in children with spina bifida. It hasn't been related to hand dominance development, flaccid paralysis of the lower extremities, or the ability to speak, though it may affect the semantics of speech dependent upon the association areas.
CN: Physiological integrity; CNS: Physiological adaptation; CL: Application

CN: Client needs category   CNS: Client needs subcategory   CL: Cognitive level

71. One of the most important aspects of pre-operative care of an infant with myelomeningocele is the infant's positioning. Which position is the most appropriate for this infant?
1. Prone position with the head turned to the side for feeding
2. Side-lying position with the head elevated 30 degrees
3. Prone position with a nasogastric (NG) tube inserted for feeding
4. Supported by diaper rolls, both anterior and posterior, in the side-lying position

72. The nurse is preparing to administer antibiotic eardrops to a 2-year-old client with an infection of the external auditory canal. The order reads, "2 gtts right ear t.i.d." Which steps should the nurse take to administer this medication? Select all that apply:
1. Wash her hands and arrange supplies at the bedside.
2. Warm the medication to body temperature.
3. Lay the child on his right side with his left ear facing up.
4. Examine the client's ear canal for drainage.
5. Gently pull the pinna up and back and instill the drops into the external ear canal.

73. The nurse is caring for a 1-month-old infant who fell from the changing table during a diaper change. Which signs and symptoms of increased intracranial pressure (ICP) is the nurse likely to assess in this client? Select all that apply:
1. Bulging fontanels
2. Decreased blood pressure
3. Increased pulse
4. High-pitched cry
5. Headache
6. Irritability

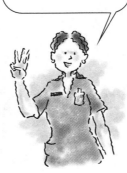

Oh, my. Only three questions left. One more turn of the page and you're home!

71. 1. The prone position is used preoperatively because it minimizes tension on the sac and the risk of trauma. The head is turned to one side for feeding. There's no advantage to elevating the head 30 degrees. Although feeding can be a problem in the prone position, it can be accomplished without an NG tube. Side-lying or partial side-lying positions are better used *after* the repair has been accomplished unless they permit undesirable hip flexion.
CN: Physiological integrity; CNS: Basic care and comfort; CL: Application

72. 1, 2, 4. The nurse should prepare to instill the eardrops by washing her hands, gathering the supplies, and arranging the supplies at the bedside. To avoid adverse effects resulting from eardrops that are too cold (such as vertigo, nausea, and pain), the medication should be warmed to body temperature in a bowl of warm water. The temperature of the drops should be tested by placing a drop on the wrist. Before instilling the drops, the ear canal should be examined for drainage that may reduce the medication's effectiveness. The child should be placed on his left side with his right ear facing up. For an infant or a child younger than age 3, gently pull the auricle down and back because the ear canal is straighter in children of this age-group.
CN: Physiological integrity; CNS: Pharmacological therapies; CL: Application

73. 1, 4, 6. Signs and symptoms of increased ICP in a 1-month-old infant include full, tense, bulging fontanels; a high-pitched cry; and irritability. With increased ICP, blood pressure rises while heart rate (pulse) falls. The infant may have a headache, but the nurse can't assess this finding in an infant.
CN: Physiological integrity; CNS: Physiological adaptation; CL: Analysis

CN: Client needs category CNS: Client needs subcategory CL: Cognitive level

74. An 11-month-old is diagnosed with an ear infection. Because it's his second ear infection, the mother asks why children experience more ear infections than adults. The nurse shows the mother a diagram of the ear and explains the differences in anatomy. Identify the portion of the infant's ear that allows fluid to stagnate and act as a medium for bacteria.

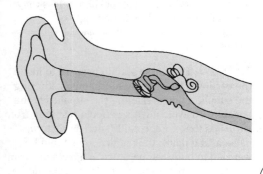

74.

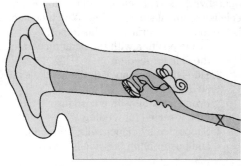

The eustachian tube in an infant is shorter and wider than in an adult or older child. It also slants horizontally. Because of these anatomical features, nasopharyngeal secretions can enter the middle ear more easily, stagnate, and tend to cause infections.

CN: Health promotion and maintenance; CNS: None; CL: Comprehension

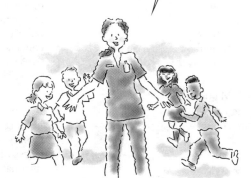

Congratulations! You finished! Now let's go out and play.

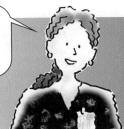

Chapter 31
Musculoskeletal disorders

1. Which definition best describes the form of clubfoot called *talipes varus*?
1. Inversion of the foot
2. Eversion of the foot
3. Plantar flexion
4. Dorsiflexion

2. Which type of clubfoot is most commonly treated by primary health care providers?
1. Talipes calcaneus
2. Talipes equinovarus
3. Talipes valgus
4. Talipes varus

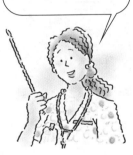

Knowing how to treat a disorder is only part of the NCLEX. Question 3 asks you for the *cause* of the disorder as well.

3. The mother of a neonate with clubfoot feels guilty because she believes she did something to cause the condition. The nurse should explain that the cause of clubfoot in neonates is due to which factor?
1. Unknown
2. Hereditary
3. Restricted movement in utero
4. Anomalous embryonic development

4. The nurse is preparing a teaching plan for the mother of a neonate with clubfoot. What information should the nurse include?
1. It's hereditary.
2. More girls than boys are affected.
3. More boys than girls are affected.
4. It occurs once in every 500 births.

5. The nurse would expect to find which muscle involvement in her client diagnosed with congenital torticollis?
1. Platysma
2. Lower trapezius
3. Middle trapezius
4. Sternocleidomastoid

1. 1. Talipes varus is an inversion of the foot. Talipes valgus is an eversion of the foot. Talipes equinus is plantar flexion of the foot and talipes calcaneus is dorsiflexion of the foot.
CN: Physiological integrity; CNS: Physiological adaptation; CL: Knowledge

2. 2. Ninety-five percent of treated clubfoot cases are for feet that point downward and inward (talipes equinovarus) in varying degrees. Talipes valgus, talipes calcaneus, and talipes varus aren't as common.
CN: Physiological integrity; CNS: Physiological adaptation; CL: Knowledge

3. 1. The definitive cause of clubfoot is unknown. In some families, there's an increased incidence. Some postulate that anomalous embryonic development or restricted fetal movement are the reasons. Currently, there's no way to predict the occurrence of clubfoot.
CN: Psychosocial integrity; CNS: None; CL: Comprehension

4. 3. Boys are affected twice as commonly as girls. It isn't known if the condition is hereditary. It occurs once in every 700 to 1,000 births.
CN: Physiological integrity; CNS: Physiological adaptation; CL: Application

5. 4. Congenital torticollis (wry neck) usually involves a shortening of the sternocleidomastoid muscle. Rotation is away from the side of shortening and side bending is toward the side of the contraction. The platysma muscle is involved in flexion and is shortened if the head is held in flexion, not contraction. The middle and lower trapezius aren't associated with torticollis.
CN: Physiological integrity; CNS: Physiological adaptation; CL: Comprehension

CN: Client needs category   CNS: Client needs subcategory   CL: Cognitive level

6. A nurse is teaching the parents of a 3-month-old infant who has severe torticollis, with the head rotated to the left and side bent to the right. Which statement by the parents indicates that the teaching has been effective?
1. "It involves shortening of the left upper trapezius."
2. "It involves shortening of the right middle trapezius."
3. "It involves shortening of the left sterno-cleidomastoid."
4. "It involves shortening of the right sterno-cleidomastoid."

7. A 9-month-old infant has torticollis with rotation of the head to the left and side bending to the right. Placing the infant in which position would be most effective for developing muscle lengthening?
1. Prone
2. Supine
3. Left side-lying
4. Right side-lying

8. The parents of a child with newly diagnosed scoliosis ask the nurse to describe this condition. Which response provides an accurate definition?
1. An increase in the lumbar lordosis
2. A decrease in the thoracic kyphosis
3. Lateral curves in the spinal column described as right or left concavities
4. Lateral curves in the spinal column described as right or left convexities

9. A child diagnosed with scoliosis is admitted for surgery. The nurse would expect to prepare the child for which intervention?
1. Segmental diskectomy
2. Austin Moore procedure
3. Segmented spine instrumentation
4. Thoracic and lumbar laminectomy

10. Upon physical examination, which condition would alert the nurse that her client may be developing scoliosis?
1. Scapula winging
2. Forward head posture
3. Raised right iliac crest
4. Forward flexion of the cervical spine

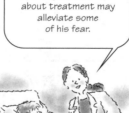

Talking with a child about treatment may alleviate some of his fear.

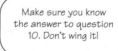

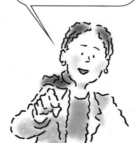

Make sure you know the answer to question 10. Don't wing it!

6. 4. The right sternocleidomastoid is shortened with the head in this position. The left upper trapezius isn't shortened. The middle trapezius isn't affected and the left sternocleidomastoid is lengthened.
CN: Physiological integrity; CNS: Physiological adaptation; CL: Application

7. 3. The left side-lying position will assist with lengthening of the muscles because this position will make it easier to stretch the sternocleidomastoid and upper trapezius. No other positions will assist in increasing muscle length.
CN: Physiological integrity; CNS: Reduction of risk potential; CL: Application

8. 4. Scoliosis is defined as "S" curves along the longitudinal axis of the body and curves are described according to the convexity, not the concavity. Lordosis and kyphosis describe the back in the frontal plane.
CN: Physiological integrity; CNS: Physiological adaptation; CL: Application

9. 3. In segmented spine instrumentation, flexible rods are placed on the transverse processes of the spine and wires are threaded through the laminae so the spinal column is stabilized. Austin Moore procedure is used in fractured hips. Thoracic and lumbar laminectomies are performed for herniated disks. Segmental diskectomy won't cure or help scoliosis.
CN: Physiological integrity; CNS: Basic care and comfort; CL: Application

10. 3. A raised iliac crest may be a warning sign of some curvature secondary to the attachment of the pelvis to the spine. Scapula winging could be caused by muscle paralysis. Forward head posture isn't a result of scoliosis. Forward flexion doesn't describe lateral curves in the spine.
CN: Physiological integrity; CNS: Physiological adaptation; CL: Analysis

CN: Client needs category   CNS: Client needs subcategory   CL: Cognitive level

11. Given her knowledge of corrective devices, the nurse would expect her client with scoliosis to be treated with which type of brace?
1. DonJoy braces
2. Long leg braces
3. Milwaukee brace
4. Knee-ankle-foot orthosis

11. 3. The Milwaukee brace is used to place lateral pressure on the back in hopes of halting or slowing the progression of the curves in the back. It isn't curative. DonJoy braces are used following knee reconstruction. Long leg braces are used for lower extremity weakness or partial paralysis. Knee-ankle-foot orthosis is used for lower extremity and foot weakness.
CN: Physiological integrity; CNS: Reduction of risk potential; CL: Application

12. The Milwaukee brace is commonly used in the treatment of scoliosis. Which position best describes the placement of the pressure rods?
1. Laterally on the convex portion of the curve
2. Laterally on the concave portion of the curve
3. Posteriorly on the convex portion of the curve
4. Posteriorly along the spinal column at the exact level of the curve

12. 1. Lateral pressure applied to the convex portion of the curve will help best in reducing the curvature. Pressure pads applied posteriorly will help maintain erect posture. Pressure applied to the concave portion of the curve will increase the lordosis.
CN: Physiological integrity; CNS: Reduction of risk potential; CL: Application

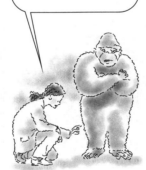

You've made tremendous progress with strengthening those evertor muscles...now, maybe, we can begin working on those six-pack abs.

13. Strengthening which muscle group is important in a client diagnosed with talipes equinovarus?
1. Evertors
2. Invertors
3. Plantar flexors
4. Plantar fascia musculature

13. 1. Because the foot is held in inversion, it's important to strengthen the evertors to counter the inversion present in the foot. Inversion is incorrect because the foot is already held in this position. Plantar musculature and plantar flexors aren't important because the foot is already in a plantar flexed position.
CN: Physiological integrity; CNS: Reduction of risk potential; CL: Analysis

14. Torticollis describes scoliosis in which area of the spine?
1. Cervical
2. Lumbar
3. Sacral
4. Thoracic

14. 1. Torticollis describes only the cervical spine. No other areas apply.
CN: Physiological integrity; CNS: Physiological adaptation; CL: Knowledge

15. A nurse receives a report on a client with structural scoliosis. What assessment finding should the nurse anticipate when examining the client?
1. Muscular dystrophy with muscle weakness
2. Cerebral palsy with muscle weakness
3. Leg length discrepancy
4. Spina bifida

15. 3. Leg length discrepancy is a structural deformity that can be associated with scoliosis. Cerebral palsy, muscular dystrophy, and spina bifida are disease processes that can cause scoliosis.
CN: Physiological integrity; CNS: Physiological adaptation; CL: Application

CN: Client needs category   CNS: Client needs subcategory   CL: Cognitive level

16. The parents of a child diagnosed with non-structural scoliosis ask the nurse how their child developed this condition. Which response by the nurse reflects the <u>most</u> likely cause of this condition?
1. Wedge vertebrae
2. Hemivertebrae
3. Poor posture
4. Tumor

17. Idiopathic scoliosis accounts for which percentage of cases of scoliosis?
1. 50% to 60%
2. 65% to 75%
3. 75% to 85%
4. 85% to 95%

18. Which technique may assist a 3-month-old client diagnosed with torticollis?
1. Lying supine
2. Gentle massage
3. Range-of-motion exercises
4. Lying on the side

19. A physical therapist has instructed the nursing staff in stretching exercises for an infant with torticollis. Which intervention should the nurse perform if she feels uncomfortable performing stretches that result in the infant's crying and grimacing?
1. Checking the primary health care provider's orders
2. Calling the primary health care provider
3. Calling the physical therapist
4. Discontinuing the exercises

20. A client has developed a right torticollis with side-bending to the right and rotation to the left. Which exercises may assist in reduction of the torticollis?
1. Rotation exercises to the right
2. Rotation exercises to the left
3. Cervical extension exercises
4. Cervical flexion exercises

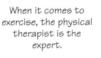

When it comes to exercise, the physical therapist is the expert.

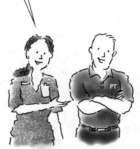

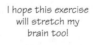

I hope this exercise will stretch my brain too!

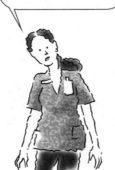

16. 3. Poor posture is a nonstructural problem that may be a cause of scoliosis. Wedge vertebrae, hemivertebrae, and tumor are all structural causes of scoliosis.
CN: Physiological integrity; CNS: Physiological adaptation; CL: Application

17. 3. Studies have shown that idiopathic scoliosis accounts for 75% to 85% of all cases.
CN: Physiological integrity; CNS: Physiological adaptation; CL: Knowledge

18. 4. Side-lying opposite the affected side may help elongate shortened muscles. Lying supine and gentle massage won't assist with elongation of muscles. Range-of-motion exercises won't assist with shortened muscles unless they're performed in specific patterns and with stretching.
CN: Health promotion and maintenance; CNS: None; CL: Application

19. 3. The only cure for the torticollis is exercise or surgery. The therapist is the expert in exercise and should be called for assistance in this situation. The primary health care provider would be called only if there was concern over the orders written or an abnormal development in the child.
CN: Physiological integrity; CNS: Physiological adaptation; CL: Application

20. 1. Performing rotation exercises to the right will help increase the length of the shortened right sternocleidomastoid. Rotation to the left will just add to the torticollis, as the head is already rotated in that direction. Cervical extension exercises won't lengthen tightened muscles. Cervical flexion will add to shortening of the muscles.
CN: Physiological integrity; CNS: Reduction of risk potential; CL: Application

21. A nurse who's aware of the most common complication of severe scoliosis would closely monitor for which complication?
1. Increased vital capacity
2. Increased oxygen uptake
3. Diminished vital capacity
4. Decreased residual volume

22. A 4-year-old child is diagnosed with thoracic scoliosis secondary to cerebral palsy. Which condition may be the cause of the scoliosis?
1. Hypotonia
2. Mental retardation
3. Increased thoracic kyphosis
4. Autonomic dysreflexia

23. Which disease process is <u>myopathic</u> in nature?
1. Cerebral palsy
2. Marfan syndrome
3. Muscular dystrophy
4. Spinal muscular atrophy

24. During a scoliosis screening, a school nurse examines a child and notes that she has a raised right iliac crest. The nurse should notify the child's parents and suggest further screening for which condition?
1. Forward head posture
2. Leg length discrepancy
3. Increased lumbar lordosis
4. Increased thoracic kyphosis

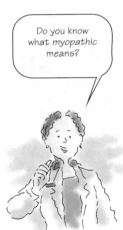

Do you know what *myopathic* means?

21. 3. Scoliosis of greater then 60 degrees can cause shifting of organs and decreased ability for the ribs to expand, thus decreasing vital capacity. An increase in vital capacity or oxygen uptake won't occur secondary to a decrease in chest expansion. Residual volume will increase secondary to decreased ability of the lungs to expel air.
CN: Physiological integrity; CNS: Physiological adaptation; CL: Application

22. 1. Cerebral palsy is usually associated with some degree of hypotonia or hypertonia. Poor muscle tone may result in scoliosis. Mental retardation isn't a cause of scoliosis. Increased thoracic kyphosis won't result in scoliosis. Autonomic dysreflexia occurs in spinal cord injury and involves abnormal muscle spasms secondary to abnormal inhibitory neurons present during stretch reflexes.
CN: Physiological integrity; CNS: Physiological adaptation; CL: Application

23. 3. Muscular dystrophy is myopathic (involves muscular tissue) in nature. Cerebral palsy occurs from prenatal, perinatal, or postnatal central nervous system damage. An upper motor neuron lesion may be the cause. Marfan syndrome is mesenchymal (involves connective tissue) in nature. Spinal muscular atrophy is related to lower motor neurons.
CN: Physiological integrity; CNS: Physiological adaptation; CL: Knowledge

24. 2. A raised iliac crest may be indicative of a leg length discrepancy or a curvature in the lumbar spine. It isn't indicative of forward head posture, lumbar lordosis, or thoracic kyphosis.
CN: Physiological integrity; CNS: Physiological adaptation; CL: Application

25. Given the predominence of scoliosis in certain age-groups, the school nurse should be sure to screen which group of students who most commonly develop the condition?
1. Preteenage girls
2. Preteenage boys
3. Adolescent girls
4. Adolescent boys

26. In caring for a child with a Harrington rod placement, which symptom would be of <u>greatest</u> concern two days postoperatively?
1. Fever of 99.5° F (37.5° C)
2. Pain along the incision
3. Decreased urine output
4. Hypoactive bowel sounds

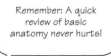
Remember: A quick review of basic anatomy never hurts!

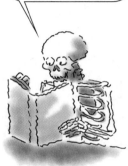

27. Observing which structure will serve the nurse best when screening a child for scoliosis?
1. Iliac crests
2. Spinous processes
3. Acromion processes
4. Posterior superior iliac spines

28. A nurse would expect her client with talipes equinovarus to be treated with which intervention?
1. Traction
2. Serial casting
3. Short leg braces
4. Inversion range-of-motion exercises

29. When performing stretches with a child who has scoliosis, which technique should be used?
1. Slow and sustained
2. Gradual, until a change in muscle length is seen
3. Quick movements to the end range of pain
4. Slow movements for brief, 3- to 4-second periods

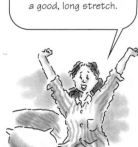
There's nothing like a good, long stretch.

25. 3. Scoliosis is eight times more prevalent in adolescent girls than boys.
CN: Physiological integrity; CNS: Physiological adaptation; CL: Analysis

26. 3. Due to extensive blood loss during surgery and possible renal hypoperfusion, decreased urine output could indicate decreased renal function. A fever of 99.5° F is of concern but may be due to decreased chest expansion secondary to anesthesia, surgery, and pain. A paralytic ileus is common after this surgery, and the client may have a nasogastric tube for the first 48 hours.
CN: Physiological integrity; CNS: Reduction of risk potential; CL: Application

27. 2. Spinous processes are the best bony landmark to identify when attempting to screen for scoliosis because this will show lateral deviation of the column. Abnormalities in the acromion process, iliac crests, and posterior superior iliac spines may not be indicative of scoliosis.
CN: Physiological integrity; CNS: Physiological adaptation; CL: Application

28. 2. Serial casting is a treatment choice in attempts to change the length of soft tissue. Traction isn't an option. Corrective shoes are used instead of short leg braces. Inversion exercises won't help; eversion exercises will.
CN: Physiological integrity; CNS: Reduction of risk potential; CL: Application

29. 1. Stretches should be slow and sustained. It's difficult to see changes in muscle length. Stretches shouldn't be performed with quick movements and should be performed for longer than a few seconds.
CN: Safe, effective care environment; CNS: Coordinated care; CL: Application

CN: Client needs category   CNS: Client needs subcategory   CL: Cognitive level

30. Developmental dysplasia of the hip (DDH) is most commonly found in which group?
1. Males
2. Females
3. First-born males
4. First-born females

31. The nurse would expect her client's suspected developmental dysplasia of the hip (DDH) to be confirmed by which diagnostic technique?
1. X-ray
2. Positive Ortolani's sign
3. Positive Trendelenburg gait
4. Audible clicking with adduction

32. Which hip position should be avoided in an 8-month-old infant who has been diagnosed with developmental dysplasia of the hip?
1. Extension
2. Abduction
3. Internal rotation
4. External rotation

33. Based on knowledge of the progression of muscular dystrophy, which activity would a nurse anticipate the client having difficulty with first?
1. Breathing
2. Sitting
3. Standing
4. Swallowing

34. Barlow's test is used to diagnose hip dysplasia in which age-group?
1. 0 to 3 months
2. 3 to 18 months
3. 18 to 36 months
4. 0 to 4 years

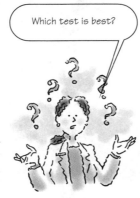

Which test is best?

30. 4. Studies have shown that first-born females are six times more likely to have DDH than males.
CN: Physiological integrity; CNS: Physiological adaptation; CL: Knowledge

31. 1. X-ray will confirm the diagnosis of DDH. All of the options are positive signs of DDH, but only the X-ray will confirm the diagnosis.
CN: Physiological integrity; CNS: Physiological adaptation; CL: Application

32. 3. Internal rotation of the hip is an unstable position and should be avoided in infants with hip instability. Hip extension is a relatively stable position. External rotation isn't necessarily an unstable position, as long as it isn't externally rotated too far. Typically, the child is placed in slight abduction while in a hip-spica cast.
CN: Physiological integrity; CNS: Reduction of risk potential; CL: Comprehension

33. 3. Muscular dystrophy usually affects postural muscles of the hip and shoulder first. Swallowing and breathing are usually affected last. Sitting may be affected, but a client would have difficulty standing before having difficulty sitting.
CN: Physiological integrity; CNS: Physiological adaptation; CL: Comprehension

34. 1. Barlow's test is most effective up to age 3 months. After 3 months, development of adduction contractures causes the hip "click" to disappear.
CN: Physiological integrity; CNS: Physiological adaptation; CL: Knowledge

35. The nurse is trying to weigh a 3-year-old child who's irritable and refuses to stand on the scale. What's the best way to obtain an accurate weight?
1. Ask the mother to approximate the weight.
2. Ask the mother to hold the child and record the combined weight.
3. Weigh the mother and child and subtract the mother's weight from the combined weight.
4. Obtain the admission weight and add 2 oz per day.

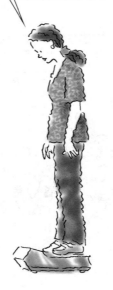

Can I subtract the 3-year-old's weight too?

35. 3. Subtracting the mother's weight from the combined weight will yield the child's weight. Weight is an important parameter used in calculating drug dosages based on kilograms per body weight. It also provides the most accurate information about a client's fluid balance. For these reasons, it should never be approximated. Combining the weights would be inaccurate.
CN: Health promotion and maintenance; CNS: None; CL: Application

36. A young child sustains a dislocated hip as well as a subcapital fracture. Which complication of greatest concern should the nurse assess for?
1. Avascular necrosis
2. Postsurgical infection
3. Hemorrhage during surgery
4. Poor postsurgical ambulation

36. 1. Avascular necrosis is common with fractures to the subcapital region secondary to possible compromise of blood supply to the femoral head. Postsurgical infection is always a concern but not a priority at first. Hemorrhage shouldn't occur. Poor postsurgical ambulation is of concern but not as much as the possibility of avascular necrosis.
CN: Physiological integrity; CNS: Reduction of risk potential; CL: Analysis

37. In a child with developmental dysplasia of the hip (DDH), how is the femur positioned in relation to the acetabulum?
1. Anterior
2. Inferior
3. Posterior
4. Superior

37. 1. The head of the femur is anterior to the acetabulum in DDH. All of the other positions are inaccurate.
CN: Physiological integrity; CNS: Physiological adaptation; CL: Comprehension

38. The nurse is planning to teach the parents of a child with newly diagnosed muscular dystrophy about the disease. Which definition should she use to best describe this condition?
1. A demyelinating disease
2. Lesions of the brain cortex
3. Upper motor neuron lesions
4. Degeneration of muscle fibers

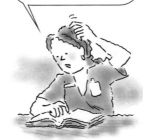

Muscular dystrophy affects the muscles. But which muscles does it affect first?

38. 4. Degeneration of muscle fibers with progressive weakness and wasting best describes muscular dystrophy. Demyelination of myelin sheaths is a description of multiple sclerosis. Lesions within the brain cortex and the upper motor neurons suggest a neurologic, not a muscular, disease.
CN: Physiological integrity; CNS: Physiological adaptation; CL: Application

39. When a child is suspected of having muscular dystrophy, a nurse should expect which muscles to be affected first?
1. Muscles of the hip
2. Muscles of the foot
3. Muscles of the hand
4. Muscles of respiration

39. 1. Positional muscles of the hip and shoulder are affected first. Progression later advances to muscles of the foot and hand. Involuntary muscles, such as the muscles of respiration, are affected last.
CN: Physiological integrity; CNS: Physiological adaptation; CL: Application

CN: Client needs category   CNS: Client needs subcategory   CL: Cognitive level

40. The nurse caring for a client with suspected muscular dystrophy would prepare her client for which diagnostic test?
1. X-ray
2. Muscle biopsy
3. EEG
4. Assessment of ambulation

41. The nurse caring for a client diagnosed with muscular dystrophy would expect which laboratory values to be most <u>abnormal</u>?
1. Bilirubin
2. Creatinine
3. Serum potassium
4. Sodium

42. Given her knowledge of muscular dystrophy, the nurse would expect to see which form of this condition <u>most commonly</u> in children?
1. Duchenne's
2. Becker's
3. Limb-girdle
4. Myotonic

43. Which condition would alert the nurse that a child may be suffering from muscular dystrophy?
1. Hypertonia of extremities
2. Increased lumbar lordosis
3. Upper extremity spasticity
4. Hyperactive lower extremity reflexes

44. Through which mechanism is Duchenne's muscular dystrophy acquired?
1. Virus
2. Heredity
3. Autoimmune factors
4. Environmental toxins

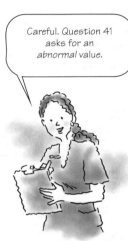

Careful. Question 41 asks for an abnormal value.

40. 2. A muscle biopsy shows the degeneration of muscle fibers and infiltration of fatty tissue. It's used for diagnostic confirmation of muscular dystrophy. X-ray is best for identifying an osseous deformity. Ambulation assessment alone wouldn't confirm diagnosis of this client's disorder. EEG wouldn't be appropriate in this case.
CN: Health promotion and maintenance; CNS: None; CL: Application

41. 2. Creatinine is a by-product of muscle metabolism as the muscle hypertrophies. Bilirubin is a by-product of liver function. Potassium and sodium levels can change due to various factors and aren't indicators of muscular dystrophy.
CN: Health promotion and maintenance; CNS: None; CL: Analysis

42. 1. Duchenne's accounts for 50% of all cases of muscular dystrophy.
CN: Physiological integrity; CNS: Physiological adaptation; CL: Analysis

43. 2. An increased lumbar lordosis would be seen in a child suffering from muscular dystrophy secondary to paralysis of lower lumbar postural muscles. Increased lower extremity support may also be seen. Hypertonia isn't seen in this disease. Upper extremity spasticity isn't seen because this disease isn't caused by upper motor neuron lesions. Hyperactive reflexes aren't indications of muscular dystrophy.
CN: Physiological integrity; CNS: Physiological adaptation; CL: Analysis

44. 2. Muscular dystrophy is hereditary and acquired through a recessive sex-linked trait. Therefore, it isn't caused by viral, autoimmune, or environmental factors.
CN: Physiological integrity; CNS: Physiological adaptation; CL: Knowledge

CN: Client needs category   CNS: Client needs subcategory   CL: Cognitive level

45. A client with muscular dystrophy has lost complete control of his lower extremities. He has some strength bilaterally in the upper extremities, but poor trunk control. Which mechanism would be the <u>most</u> important to have on the wheelchair?
1. Antitip device
2. Extended breaks
3. Headrest support
4. Wheelchair belt

46. When assessing a 2-year-old child with a history of muscular dystrophy, the nurse observes that the child's legs appear to be held together and the knees are touching. The nurse suspects contraction of which muscles?
1. Hip abductors
2. Hip adductors
3. Hip extensors
4. Hip flexors

47. A 12-year-old child diagnosed with muscular dystrophy is hospitalized secondary to a fall. Surgery is necessary as well as skeletal traction. Which complication would be of <u>greatest</u> concern to the nursing staff?
1. Skin integrity
2. Infection of pin sites
3. Respiratory infection
4. Nonunion healing of the fracture

48. Which problem is most commonly encountered by adolescent females with scoliosis?
1. Respiratory distress
2. Poor self-esteem
3. Poor appetite
4. Renal difficulty

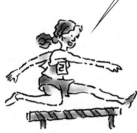

You're answering these questions by leaps and bounds. Good work!

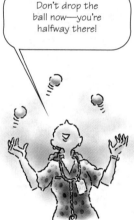

Don't drop the ball now—you're halfway there!

45. 4. This client has poor trunk control; a belt will prevent him from falling out of the wheelchair. Antitip devices, head rest supports, and extended breaks are all important options but aren't the most important options in this situation.
CN: Safe, effective care environment; CNS: Safety and infection control; CL: Application

46. 2. The hip adductors are in a shortened position. The abductors are in a lengthened position. This position isn't indicative of hip flexor or hip extensor shortening.
CN: Physiological integrity; CNS: Physiological adaptation; CL: Application

47. 3. Respiratory infection can be fatal for clients with muscular dystrophy due to poor chest expansion and decreased ability to mobilize secretions. Skin integrity, infection of pin sites, and nonunion healing are all causes for concern, but not as important as prevention of respiratory infection.
CN: Physiological integrity; CNS: Reduction of risk potential; CL: Application

48. 2. Poor self-esteem is a major issue with many adolescents. The use of orthopedic appliances such as those used to treat scoliosis make this issue much more significant for adolescents with scoliosis. Although respiratory distress and poor appetite may surface, they aren't as common as self-esteem problems. Renal problems aren't usually an issue in adolescents with scoliosis.
CN: Health promotion and maintenance; CNS: None; CL: Application

CN: Client needs category   CNS: Client needs subcategory   CL: Cognitive level

49. A nurse is examining the progress record of a 10-year-old girl with femur fractures who has had bilateral leg skeletal traction applied. The nurse teaches the child to perform Kegel exercises. What is the most important purpose of teaching these exercises?

Progress Notes	
09/22/08	Client ringing for nurse
1030	every 30 minutes for bed-
	pan. Voids 20 to 40 ml
	each time. Temperature,
	98° F; heart rate, 86 beats/
	minute; respiratory rate,
	16 breaths/minute; blood
	pressure, 102/60 mm Hg.
	_____ S. Jones, L.P.N.

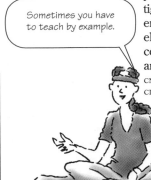

Sometimes you have to teach by example.

1. To strengthen the child's arms so that she can better use the trapeze to lift up for bedpan placement and removal
2. To strengthen the child's calf muscles so that she's less likely to get leg cramps
3. To distract the child
4. To maintain good perineal muscle tone by tightening the pubococcygeus muscle

49. 4. Because there's no evidence of a urinary tract infection, Kegel exercises are the appropriate intervention. Kegel exercises involve tightening the perineal muscles to help strengthen the pubococcygeus muscle and increase its elasticity. This helps to keep the child from becoming incontinent. None of the other options are related to Kegel exercises.
CN: Physiological integrity; CNS: Basic care and comfort; CL: Application

50. A child has developed difficulty ambulating and tends to walk on his toes. Which surgical technique may benefit the client?
1. Adductor release
2. Hamstring release
3. Plantar fascia release
4. Achilles tendon release

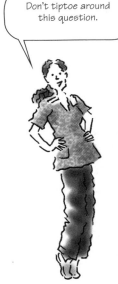

Don't tiptoe around this question.

50. 4. A shortened Achilles tendon may cause a child to walk on his toes. A release of the tendon may assist the child in walking. An adductor release is commonly performed if the legs are held together. A plantar fascia release won't help and a hamstring release is done only when there's a knee flexion contracture.
CN: Physiological integrity; CNS: Reduction of risk potential; CL: Application

51. Muscular dystrophy is a result of which cause?
1. Gene mutation
2. Chromosomal aberration
3. Unknown nongenetic origin
4. Genetic and environmental factors

51. 1. Muscular dystrophy is a result of a gene mutation. It isn't from a chromosome aberration or environmental factors. It's genetic and there's a known origin of the disease.
CN: Physiological integrity; CNS: Physiological adaptation; CL: Knowledge

CN: Client needs category   CNS: Client needs subcategory   CL: Cognitive level

52. A nurse is assessing the lower extremity strength of a child diagnosed with muscular dystrophy. Which muscle group would be the <u>most</u> important to assess when planning actions to maintain maximum lower extremity function?
1. Gastrocnemius
2. Gluteus maximus
3. Hamstrings
4. Quadriceps

53. Which of the following strategies would be the first choice in attempting to maximize function in a child with muscular dystrophy?
1. Long leg braces
2. Motorized wheelchair
3. Manual wheelchair
4. Walker

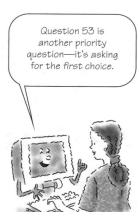

Question 53 is another priority question—it's asking for the first choice.

54. A child is having increased difficulty getting out of his chair at school. Which recommendation may the nurse make to assist the child?
1. A seat cushion
2. Long leg braces
3. Powered wheelchair
4. Removable arm rests on wheelchair

55. What finding would be expected while palpating the muscles of a child with muscular dystrophy?
1. Soft on palpation
2. Firm or woody on palpation
3. Extremely hard on palpation
4. No muscle consistency on palpation

56. Nurses should instruct wheelchair-bound clients with muscular dystrophy in which of the following exercises to best prevent skin breakdown?
1. Wheelchair push-ups
2. Leaning side-to-side
3. Leaning forward
4. Gluteal sets

52. 2. Gluteus maximus is the strongest muscle in the body and is important for standing as well as for transfers. All of the named muscles are important, but the maintenance of the gluteus maximus will enable maximum function.
CN: Health promotion and maintenance; CNS: None; CL: Application

53. 1. Long leg braces are functional assistive devices that provide increased independence and increased use of upper and lower body strength. Wheelchairs, both motorized and manual, provide less independence and less use of upper and lower body strength. Walkers are functional assistive devices that provide less independence than braces.
CN: Physiological integrity; CNS: Basic care and comfort; CL: Application

54. 1. A seat cushion will put the hip extensors at an advantage and make it somewhat easier to get up. Long leg braces wouldn't be the first choice. A powered wheelchair wouldn't be important in assisting with the transfer. Removable armrests have no bearing on assisting the client.
CN: Physiological integrity; CNS: Basic care and comfort; CL: Application

55. 2. Muscles will usually be firm on palpation secondary to the infiltration of fatty tissue and connective tissue into the muscle. The muscles won't be soft secondary to the infiltration and won't be hard upon palpation. There's some consistency to the muscle although, in advanced stages, atrophy is present.
CN: Physiological integrity; CNS: Physiological adaptation; CL: Analysis

56. 1. Wheelchair push-ups will alleviate the most pressure to the buttocks. Leaning side-to-side will help, but not as much as wheelchair push-ups. Gluteal sets won't help with pressure relief.
CN: Health promotion and maintenance; CNS: None; CL: Application

CN: Client needs category   CNS: Client needs subcategory   CL: Cognitive level

57. How would the nurse best describe Gowers' sign to the parents of a child with muscular dystrophy?
1. A transfer technique
2. A waddling-type gait
3. The pelvis position during gait
4. Muscle twitching present during a quick stretch

58. Which of the following most accurately describes pseudohypertrophy?
1. Increased muscle hypertrophy secondary to increased muscle mass
2. Increased muscle hypertrophy secondary to fat infiltration
3. Decreased muscle secondary to muscle degeneration
4. Decreased muscle mass secondary to disease

59. A 13-year-old boy admitted with a fractured femur had an open reduction and internal fixation 2 days ago and is currently in traction. He asks the nurse what would happen to him if a terrorist decided to bomb the hospital. What's the nurse's best response?
1. "I wouldn't worry about that. Spend your energy on getting well and going home."
2. "We have plans to call your parents and take care of you if there's a problem."
3. "What do you think might happen if terrorists attacked?"
4. "That's silly thinking. Why would anyone bomb a hospital?"

60. A client with bilateral fractured femurs is scheduled for a double–hip-spica cast. She says to the nurse, "Only 3 more months, and I can go home." Further investigation reveals that the client and her family believe she'll be hospitalized until the cast comes off. The nurse should explain to the client and her family that she:
1. may be hospitalized 2 to 4 months.
2. will go home 2 to 4 days after casting.
3. will go home 1 week after casting.
4. will go home as soon as she can move.

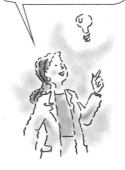

To remember Gower's sign, think going somewhere—that's a description of what the child is trying to do.

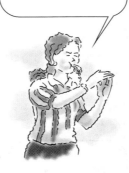

Time out! Think about the prefix pseudo to determine the correct definition.

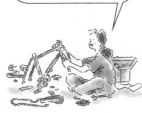

You'll be out of the hospital in less time than it takes me to reassemble my bike!

57. 1. Gowers' sign is a description of a transfer technique present during some phases of muscular dystrophy. The child turns on the side or abdomen, extends the knees, and pushes on the torso to an upright position by walking his hands up the legs. The child's gait is unrelated to the presence of Gowers' sign. Muscle twitching present after a quick stretch is described as clonus.
CN: Physiological integrity; CNS: Physiological adaptation; CL: Analysis

58. 2. Pseudohypertrophy is present secondary to fat infiltration. Increased muscle mass is called hypertrophy. Pseudohypertrophy isn't due to muscle degeneration or decreased muscle mass.
CN: Physiological integrity; CNS: Physiological adaptation; CL: Application

59. 3. Something prompted the child to ask such a question, and the nurse needs to take advantage of this opportunity to further explore his concerns and fears. Option 1 discounts the boy's feelings and may actually increase his anxiety. Although option 2 may be technically correct, it doesn't provide reassurance or help build a therapeutic relationship that can promote health and wellness. Option 4 is dismissive and chides the boy for asking the question.
CN: Psychosocial integrity; CNS: None CL: Analysis

60. 2. The cast will dry fairly rapidly with the use of fiberglass casting material. The time spent in the hospital after casting, typically 2 to 4 days, will be for teaching the client and her family how to care for her at home and for evaluating the client's skin integrity and neurovascular status before discharge. The time frames in the other options given are inaccurate for a double–hip-spica cast.
CN: Health promotion and maintenance; CNS: None; CL: Application

CN: Client needs category   CNS: Client needs subcategory   CL: Cognitive level

61. A toddler is hospitalized for treatment of multiple injuries. The parents state that the injuries occurred when their child fell down the stairs. However, inconsistencies between the history and physical findings suggest child abuse. What should the nurse do next?

1. Refer the parents to Parents Anonymous.
2. Prepare the child for foster care placement.
3. Prevent the parents from seeing their child.
4. Report the incident to proper authorities.

61. 4. The law requires the nurse to report all cases of suspected child abuse. Therefore, the nurse's first action should be to report this incident. After the authorities have been notified, steps can be taken toward protective custody, if appropriate, when the child is medically stable. Later, the nurse can refer the parents to Parents Anonymous, if needed. The nurse should give the parents opportunities to visit and help care for their child. During these visits, she can reinforce positive parenting behaviors.

CN: Safe, effective care environment; CNS: Coordinated care; CL: Application

62. The nurse receives a report on a child admitted with severe muscular dystrophy. The nurse suspects the child has been diagnosed with the most severe form of the disease, known as:

1. Duchenne's.
2. facioscapulohumeral.
3. limb-girdle.
4. myotonia.

62. 1. Studies have shown that Duchenne's is the most severe form of muscular dystrophy. Myotonia isn't a form of the disease; it's a symptom.

CN: Physiological integrity; CNS: Physiological adaptation; CL: Analysis

63. Which definition best describes acetabular dysplasia?

1. Partial dislocation of the head of the femur
2. Delay in acetabular development
3. Ligamentous laxity of the joint
4. Audible clicking of the femur

63. 2. Acetabular dysplasia is characterized by an underdevelopment of the acetabular ridge. Partial dislocation is described as a subluxation. Ligamentous laxity can be used to describe a ligament that's lacking stability but can also refer to a shoulder ligament, and therefore isn't specific to the acetabulum. Audible clicking is indicative of some degree of subluxation or dislocation.

CN: Physiological integrity; CNS: Physiological adaptation; CL: Knowledge

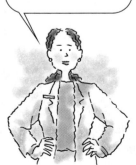

You'll get the greatest number of correct answers if you read each question carefully.

64. The parents of a child with newly diagnosed developmental dysplasia of the hip (DDH) ask the nurse how their child developed this condition. The nurse explains that the greatest number of cases are caused by which condition?

1. Dislocation
2. Subluxation
3. Acetabular dysplasia
4. Dislocation with fracture

64. 2. Studies show that subluxation accounts for the greatest number of cases of DDH.

CN: Physiological integrity; CNS: Physiological adaptation; CL: Application

CN: Client needs category   CNS: Client needs subcategory   CL: Cognitive level

65. Which finding would the nurse expect in a client with developmental dysplasia of the hip (DDH)?
1. Ligamentum teres is shortened.
2. Femoral head has lost contact with the acetabulum and is displaced inferiorly.
3. Femoral head has lost contact with the acetabulum and is displaced posteriorly.
4. Femoral head is in contact with acetabulum, but there's a noted capsular rupture.

66. The licensed practical nurse (LPN) is assigned to care for a 4-year-old client who had a Harrington rod inserted the day before. She notices the client is receiving antibiotics by a syringe pump. Although the nurse is I.V. certified, she's uncomfortable because she's unfamiliar with the equipment. What would be her best course of action?
1. Request another assignment.
2. Refuse the assignment for safety reasons.
3. Request in-service education for use of the syringe pump.
4. Read through the unit policy and procedure manual.

67. Which choice is best for handling a client's hip-spica cast that has been soiled?
1. Clean with damp cloth and dry cleanser.
2. Clean with soap and water.
3. Don't do anything.
4. Change the cast.

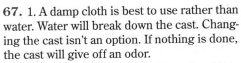

Sometimes all you need is a little soap and water.

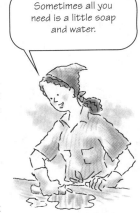

68. A child in a hip-spica cast who needs to be toileted should be assisted into what position?
1. Supine
2. Sitting in a toilet chair
3. Shoulder lower than buttocks
4. Buttocks lower than shoulder

69. Developmental dysplasia of the hip is most common among which ethnic group?
1. Blacks
2. Whites
3. Native Americans
4. Chinese

65. 3. In DDH, the femoral head loses contact with the acetabulum and is displaced posteriorly, not inferiorly, and the ligamentum teres is lengthened.
CN: Physiological integrity; CNS: Physiological adaptation; CL: Application

66. 3. Using this piece of equipment is within the LPN's scope of practice, so it's inappropriate to refuse the assignment. Reading the policy and procedure manual is a good first step, but not sufficient to insure that she'll be rendering safe care. Although she could request another assignment, option 3 is the best response because she's taking responsibility for what she doesn't know so that she can care for the child in a safe manner.
CN: Safe, effective care environment; CNS: Safety and infection control; CL: Analysis

67. 1. A damp cloth is best to use rather than water. Water will break down the cast. Changing the cast isn't an option. If nothing is done, the cast will give off an odor.
CN: Physiological integrity; CNS: Basic care and comfort; CL: Application

68. 4. The buttocks need to be lowered to toilet the child. This will keep the cast from being soiled. Supine positioning will cause soiling of the cast. The child can't use a toilet chair while in a hip-spica cast.
CN: Physiological integrity; CNS: Basic care and comfort; CL: Application

69. 3. Native Americans traditionally wrap their neonates in tight blankets that increase internal rotation in the hip. This condition isn't as common among other ethnic groups.
CN: Physiological integrity; CNS: Physiological adaptation; CL: Knowledge

CN: Client needs category   CNS: Client needs subcategory   CL: Cognitive level

70. A toddler is immobilized with traction to the legs. Which play activity would be appropriate for this child?
1. Pounding board
2. Tinker toys
3. Pull toy
4. Board games

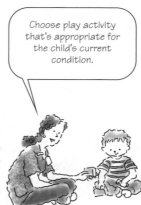

Choose play activity that's appropriate for the child's current condition.

70. 1. A pounding board is appropriate for an immobilized toddler because it promotes physical development and provides an acceptable energy outlet. Toys with small parts, such as tinker toys, aren't suitable because a toddler may swallow the parts. A pull toy is suitable for most toddlers, but not for one who's immobilized. Board games are usually too advanced for the developmental skills of a toddler.
CN: Health promotion and maintenance; CNS: None; CL: Application

71. Which complication involving leg length should a nurse anticipate in her client with developmental dysplasia of the hip?
1. Increased hip abduction
2. Increased leg length on the affected side
3. Decreased leg length on the affected side
4. No change in muscle length or leg length

71. 3. Internal rotation with subsequent dislocation will cause the affected leg to be shorter, not longer. Decreased, not increased, abduction as well as muscle and leg length changes commonly occur.
CN: Physiological integrity; CNS: Physiological adaptation; CL: Analysis

72. Which position should be <u>avoided</u> in a child suspected of developmental dysplasia of the hip?
1. Hip abduction
2. Knee extension
3. External rotation
4. Any position is fine, as long as he's wrapped tightly in blankets

72. 4. Tightly wrapped blankets force the hip into internal rotation. Abduction, external rotation, and knee extension won't increase the risk of dislocation.
CN: Health promotion and maintenance; CNS: None; CL: Application

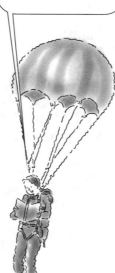

At the rate you're going, the sky's the limit!

73. The nurse would expect to see which activity level prescribed for a client immediately after a spinal fusion?
1. Supine bed rest
2. No weight bearing
3. No restriction
4. Limited weight bearing

73. 1. After a spinal fusion, the child is usually placed on bed rest and ordered to lie flat. In 2 to 4 days, the child is allowed to sit up in and get out of bed. Other activities are gradually reintroduced.
CN: Physiological integrity; CNS: Basic care and comfort; CL: Analysis

74. Which intervention would a nurse expect to use to prevent venous stasis after skeletal traction application?
1. Bed rest only
2. Convoluted foam mattress
3. Vigorous pulmonary care
4. Antiembolism stockings or an intermittent compression device

74. 4. To prevent venous stasis after skeletal traction application, antiembolism stockings or an intermittent compression device is used on the unaffected leg. Convoluted foam mattresses and pulmonary care don't prevent venous stasis. Bed rest can *cause* venous stasis.
CN: Health promotion and maintenance; CNS: None; CL: Application

CN: Client needs category   CNS: Client needs subcategory   CL: Cognitive level

75. A school nurse suspects that a 13-year-old girl has structural scoliosis. Asking the child to perform which maneuver would be the nurse's <u>priority</u> when assessing for this condition?
1. Bend over and touch her toes while the nurse observes from the back.
2. Stand sideways while the nurse observes her profile.
3. Assume a knee-chest position on the examination table.
4. Arch her back while the nurse observes her from the back.

76. At the scene of a trauma, which nursing intervention is appropriate for a child with a <u>suspected fracture</u>?
1. Don't move the child.
2. Sit the child up to facilitate breathing.
3. Move the child to a safe place immediately.
4. Immobilize the extremity and then move the child to a safe place.

77. Which statement should the nurse include in her teaching plan for a client about to undergo a fracture reduction?
1. "All fractures can be reduced."
2. "Fracture reduction restores alignment."
3. "Undisplaced fractures may be reduced."
4. "Fracture reduction is usually performed with minimal discomfort."

78. A child in skeletal traction for a fracture of the right femur reports new and constant left calf pain. Also, the nurse notes that the child's left calf is 1 inch larger than the right and that he has nonpitting edema below the left knee. The nurse knows these signs are <u>most</u> consistent with which condition?
1. A fat emboli
2. An infection
3. A pulmonary embolism
4. Deep vein thrombosis (DVT)

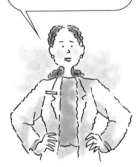

For questions involving a trauma scene, think safety first!

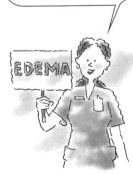

Know all the signs of DVT.

EDEMA

75. 1. As the child bends over, the curvature of the spine is more apparent. The scapula on one side becomes more prominent, and the opposite side hollows. Scoliosis can't be properly assessed from the side or the front. The knee-chest position is used for lumbar puncture, not assessment.
CN: Health promotion and maintenance; CNS: None; CL: Application

76. 4. At the scene of a trauma, the nurse should immobilize the extremity of a child with a suspected fracture and then move him to safety. If the child is already in a safe place, don't attempt to move him. Never try to sit the child up; this could make the fracture worse.
CN: Safe, effective care environment; CNS: Safety and infection control; CL: Application

77. 2. Fracture reduction restores alignment. Some fractures, such as undisplaced fractures, can't be reduced. Fracture reduction is usually painful.
CN: Physiological integrity; CNS: Reduction of risk potential; CL: Application

78. 4. Constant unilateral leg pain and significant edema should lead the nurse to suspect DVT. Symptoms of fat emboli include restlessness, tachypnea, and tachycardia and are more common in long-bone injuries. It's unlikely that an infection would occur on the opposite side of the fracture without cause. Tachycardia, chest pain, and shortness of breath may be symptoms of a pulmonary embolism.
CN: Physiological integrity; CNS: Reduction of risk potential; CL: Analysis

79. Nursing care for a child in traction may include which intervention?

1. Assessing pin sites every shift and as needed
2. Ensuring that the rope knots catch on the pulley
3. Adding and removing weights per the client's request
4. Placing all joints through range of motion every shift

80. After assisting the primary health care provider in applying a cast, the nurse should include which intervention in her immediate cast care?

1. Rest the cast on the bedside table.
2. Dispose of the plaster water in the sink.
3. Support the cast with the palms of her hand.
4. Wait until the cast dries before cleaning surrounding skin.

81. The parents of a child who just had a synthetic cast applied ask the nurse how long it takes for the cast to dry. Which response by the nurse is the <u>most</u> accurate?

1. Immediately
2. 20 minutes
3. 45 minutes
4. 2 hours

82. Which nursing intervention should be taken if, as a cast is drying, the child complains of heat from the cast?

1. Removing the cast immediately
2. Notifying the primary health care provider
3. Assessing the child for other signs of infection
4. Explaining to the child that this is a normal sensation

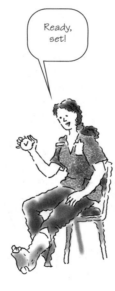

Ready, set!

79. 1. Nursing care for a child in traction may include assessing pin sites every shift and as needed and ensuring that the knots in the rope don't catch on the pulley. Weights should be added and removed per the primary health care provider's order, and all joints, except those immediately proximal and distal to the fracture, should be placed through range of motion every shift.
CN: Physiological integrity; CNS: Basic care and comfort; CL: Application

80. 3. After a cast has been applied, it should be immediately supported with the palms of the nurse's hands. Later, the nurse should dispose of the plaster water in a sink with a plaster trap or in a garbage bag, clean the surrounding skin before the cast dries, and make sure that the cast isn't resting on a hard or sharp surface.
CN: Safe, effective care environment; CNS: Coordinated care; CL: Application

81. 2. Synthetic casts take about 20 minutes to set.
CN: Safe, effective care environment; CNS: Coordinated care; CL: Application

82. 4. Normally, as the cast is drying, the child may complain of heat from the cast. The nurse should offer reassurance that this is a normal sensation. Notifying the primary health care provider or removing the cast is unneccesary. Heat from the cast isn't a sign of infection.
CN: Safe, effective care environment; CNS: Coordinated care; CL: Application

83. Which nursing intervention can best prevent foot drop in a casted leg?
1. Encourage bed rest.
2. Support the foot with 45 degrees of flexion.
3. Support the foot with 90 degrees of flexion.
4. Place a stocking on the foot to provide warmth.

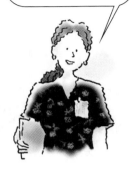

In question 83, you're trying to prevent a problem, not react to it.

83. 3. To prevent foot drop in a casted leg, the foot should be supported with 90 degrees of flexion. Bed rest can cause foot drop. Keeping the extremity warm won't prevent foot drop.
CN: Health promotion and maintenance; CNS: None; CL: Application

84. A nurse is instructing the family of a child who has recently had a hip-spica cast applied. As part of the teaching, the nurse states that the most important reason for the child to avoid eating gas-forming foods is:
1. to prevent flatus.
2. to prevent diarrhea.
3. to prevent constipation.
4. to prevent abdominal distention.

84. 4. A child with a hip-spica cast should avoid gas-forming foods to prevent abdominal distention. Gas-forming foods may cause flatus, but that isn't a reason to avoid them. Gas-forming foods don't generally cause diarrhea or constipation.
CN: Physiological integrity; CNS: Reduction of risk potential; CL: Application

85. A nurse determines that a child with a fractured left femur understands the instructions to perform only touch-down weight bearing when he makes which statement?
1. "I will place full weight on my left leg."
2. "I will place about 30% to 50% of my weight on my left leg."
3. "I will keep my left leg off the floor."
4. "I will allow my left leg to touch the floor without placing weight on it."

85. 4. Touch-down weight bearing allows the child to put no weight on the extremity, but the child may touch the floor with the affected extremity. Full weight bearing allows the child to bear all of his weight on the affected extremity. Partial weight bearing allows for only 30% to 50% weight bearing on the affected extremity. Non-weight bearing means bearing no weight on the extremity, and it must remain elevated.
CN: Safe, effective care environment; CNS: Coordinated care; CL: Application

86. Which strategy should a nurse teach an adolescent to help prevent sports-related injuries?
1. Warming up
2. Pacing activity
3. Building strength
4. Moderating intensity

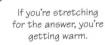

If you're stretching for the answer, you're getting warm.

86. 1. To prevent sports-related injuries, the nurse should teach the adolescent that the best prevention is warming up. Pacing activity, building strength, and using moderate intensity are other helpful preventive measures.
CN: Safe, effective care environment; CNS: Coordinated care; CL: Application

87. Which activity may be most therapeutic for a child who's allowed full activity after repair of a clubfoot?
1. Playing catch
2. Standing
3. Swimming
4. Walking

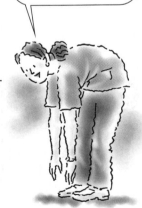

87. 4. Walking will stimulate all of the involved muscles and help with strengthening. All of the options are good exercises, but walking is the best choice.
CN: Physiological integrity; CNS: Physiological adaptation; CL: Application

CN: Client needs category   CNS: Client needs subcategory   CL: Cognitive level

88. Which history finding is <u>most significant</u> related to developmental dysplasia of the hip (DDH)?
1. Mother's activity during the third trimester
2. Breech presentation at birth
3. Infant's serum calcium level at birth
4. Apgar score of 4 at 1 minute and 6 at 5 minutes

89. Discharge planning for a child with Duchenne's muscular dystrophy should include teaching about which diet?
1. Low calorie, high protein, and high fiber
2. Low calorie, high protein, and low fiber
3. High calorie, high protein, and restricted fluids
4. High calorie, high protein, and high fiber

90. A nurse is teaching the parents of a child with structural scoliosis who has been fitted for a Milwaukee brace. The parents ask how many hours per day the child should wear the brace. Which teaching statement is <u>most</u> accurate?
1. 8 hours per day
2. 12 hours per day
3. 23 hours per day
4. 24 hours per day

91. A teenage boy suffers a broken leg as a result of a car accident and is taken to the emergency department. A plaster cast is applied. Before discharge, the nurse provides the client with instructions regarding cast care. Which instructions are most appropriate? Select all that apply:
1. Support the wet cast with pillows until it dries.
2. Use a hair dryer to speed the drying process.
3. Use the fingertips when moving the wet cast.
4. Apply powder to the inside of the cast after it dries.
5. Notify the physician if itching occurs under the cast.
6. Avoid putting straws or hangers inside the cast.

Remember to choose all of the correct responses with these questions...you can have more than one correct answer.

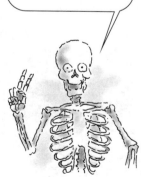

88. 2. Breech presentation is a factor commonly associated with DDH. The mother's activity during the third trimester, the infant's serum calcium level at birth, and Apgar scores have no bearing on DDH.
CN: Health promotion and maintenance; CNS: None; CL: Application

89. 1. A child with Duchenne's muscular dystrophy is prone to constipation and obesity, so dietary intake should include a diet low in calories, high in protein, and high in fiber. Adequate fluid intake should also be encouraged.
CN: Physiological integrity; CNS: Basic care and comfort; CL: Application

90. 3. The brace can be removed only 1 hour per day for bathing and hygiene; otherwise, it must remain in place. Wearing the brace for 8 or 12 hours per day isn't enough time to provide the necessary correction. Wearing the brace 24 hours per day doesn't allow for bathing or skin integrity checks.
CN: Physiological integrity; CNS: Reduction of risk potential; CL: Application

91. 1, 6. Supporting the wet cast with pillows prevents the cast from changing shape and interfering with the alignment of the fractured bone. The nurse should instruct the client not to place sharp objects, such as straws or hangers, down the inside of the cast to avoid the risk of impairing the skin and causing infection. Using a hair dryer isn't advised because it dries the cast unevenly, can cause burns to the tissue, and can crack the cast, causing poor alignment to the injured bone. The palms, not the fingertips, should be used when handling the wet cast because fingertips can dent the cast, thus causing pressure points that can affect the skin's integrity. Powder shouldn't be used because it can cake under the cast. Itching is a common occurrence with casts because the skin cells can't slough as they normally would and the dry skin causes itching. The physician isn't usually called for this problem.
CN: Physiological integrity; CNS: Basic care and comfort; CL: Application

Chapter 32
Gastrointestinal disorders

1. A nurse is caring for a 17-year-old girl who's receiving parenteral nutrition in 25% dextrose solution. How should this solution be administered?
1. Directly into a superficial vein
2. Directly into the superior vena cava
3. Through a gastrostomy tube
4. Orally as part of the prescribed diet

2. What goal should the nurse make her <u>highest</u> priority when teaching the parents of a child diagnosed with celiac disease?
1. Promote a normal life for the child.
2. Stress the importance of good health in preventing infection.
3. Introduce the parents and child to a peer with celiac disease.
4. Help the parents and child follow the prescribed dietary restrictions.

3. A nurse reviewing the chart of a child diagnosed with celiac disease would expect to find which characteristic or condition noted in her medical records?
1. Constipation
2. Pleasant disposition
3. Proper weight gain
4. Diarrhea

It's important to discuss dietary restrictions with a client with celiac disease.

4. A client with celiac disease is being discharged from the hospital. Which food item would be included in his diet?
1. Cereal
2. Luncheon meat
3. Pizza
4. Rice

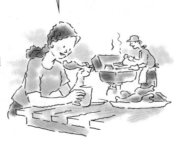

1. 2. Solutions that contain more than 12.5% dextrose are administered through a central venous access device directly into the superior vena cava by way of the jugular or subclavian vein. Special tubing is used that contains an in-line filter to remove bacteria and particulate material. A superficial vein, gastrostomy tube, and the oral route are never used for this type of solution.
CN: Physiological integrity; CNS: Pharmacological therapies; CL: Application

2. 4. It takes a long time to describe the disease process, the specific role of gluten, and the foods that must be restricted. Gluten is added to many foods but is obscurely listed on labels. To avoid hidden sources of gluten, parents need to read labels carefully. Promoting a normal life for the child, stressing good health in preventing infection, and meeting a peer with celiac disease are also important nursing considerations but would come after education about the dietary means of dealing with this chronic disease.
CN: Psychosocial integrity; CNS: None; CL: Application

3. 4. Diarrhea is common due to the child's inability to absorb the protein gluten. Profuse watery diarrhea, not constipation, is usually a sign of celiac crisis. Behavior changes, such as irritability, uncooperativeness, and apathy, are common and they usually aren't pleasant. Poor weight gain would be a symptom of celiac disease because impaired absorption leads to malnutrition.
CN: Physiological integrity; CNS: Physiological adaptation; CL: Analysis

4. 4. Sources of gluten found in wheat, rye, barley, and oats should be avoided. Rice and corn are suitable substitutes because they don't contain gluten. Pizza, luncheon meat, and cereal contain gluten and, when broken down, can't be digested by people with celiac disease.
CN: Physiological integrity; CNS: Reduction of risk potential; CL: Application

CN: Client needs category   CNS: Client needs subcategory   CL: Cognitive level

5. To help promote a normal life for children with celiac disease, which intervention should the parents use?
1. Treating the child differently from other siblings
2. Focusing on restrictions that make him feel different
3. Introducing the child to another peer with celiac disease
4. Not allowing the child to express doubt in keeping with dietary restrictions

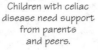

Children with celiac disease need support from parents and peers.

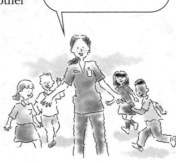

6. Which condition would be considered a malabsorption disease of the GI system?
1. Addison's disease
2. Celiac disease
3. Crohn's disease
4. Hirschsprung's disease

7. Within a day or two after starting their prescribed diet, most children with celiac disease show which characteristic?
1. Diarrhea
2. Foul-smelling stools
3. Improved appetite
4. Weight loss

8. In caring for a neonate with cleft lip and palate, which issue is <u>first</u> encountered by the nurse?
1. Feeding difficulties
2. Operative care
3. Pain management
4. Parental reaction

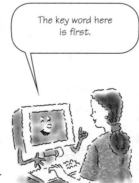

The key word here is first.

9. To prevent trauma to the suture line of an infant who underwent cleft lip repair, the nurse would perform which intervention?
1. Placing mittens on the infant's hands
2. Maintaining arm restraints
3. Not allowing the parents to touch the infant
4. Removing the lip device from the infant after surgery

5. 3. Introducing the child to another child with celiac disease will let him know he isn't alone. It will show him how other people live a normal life with similar restrictions. Instead of focusing on restrictions that make him feel different, the parents should focus on ways he can be normal. They should treat the child no differently from other siblings but stress appropriate limit setting. Allow the child with celiac disease to express his feelings about dietary restrictions.
CN: Psychosocial integrity; CNS: None; CL: Application

6. 2. In celiac disease, the absorptive surface of the small intestine is impaired. Addison's disease involves dysfunction of the adrenal cortex. Crohn's disease is an inflammatory disease of the bowel. Hirschsprung's disease is an obstructive defect in part of the intestine.
CN: Physiological integrity; CNS: Physiological adaptation; CL: Knowledge

7. 3. Within a day or two of starting their diet, most children show improved appetite, weight gain, and disappearance of diarrhea. Steatorrhea (fatty, oily, foul-smelling stool) disappearance is a good indicator that the child's ability to absorb nutrients is improving.
CN: Physiological integrity; CNS: Physiological adaptation; CL: Application

8. 4. Parents usually show strong negative responses to this deformity. They may mourn the loss of the perfect child. Helping the parents cope with their child's condition is the first step. Feeding issues are important, but parents must first cope with the reality of their neonate's condition. Surgical repair of the lip is performed between birth and age 3 months. This deformity isn't painful.
CN: Psychosocial integrity; CNS: None; CL: Application

9. 2. Arm restraints are used to prevent the infant from rubbing the sutures. Placing mittens alone won't prevent the infant from rubbing the suture line. Parental contact will increase the infant's comfort. The lip device shouldn't be removed.
CN: Physiological integrity; CNS: Reduction of risk potential; CL: Analysis

CN: Client needs category   CNS: Client needs subcategory   CL: Cognitive level

10. To prevent tissue infection and breakdown after cleft palate or lip repair, the nurse would use which intervention?
1. Keeping the suture line moist at all times
2. Allowing the infant to suck on his pacifier
3. Rinsing the infant's mouth with water after each feeding
4. Following orders from the physician to not feed the infant by mouth

11. The nurse would expect use of the Logan bow in a postoperative client after which structural defect repair?
1. Cleft lip or palate
2. Esophageal atresia
3. Hiatal hernia
4. Tracheoesophageal fistula

12. When bottle-feeding an infant with a cleft palate or lip, gentle steady pressure should be applied to the base of the bottle for which reason?
1. To reduce the risk of choking or coughing
2. To prevent further damage to the affected area
3. To decrease the amount of formula lost while eating
4. To decrease the amount of noise the infant makes when eating

13. Which nursing intervention should be used when feeding an infant with cleft lip and palate?
1. Burping the infant often
2. Limiting the amount the infant eats
3. Feeding the infant at scheduled times
4. Removing the nipple if the infant is making loud noises

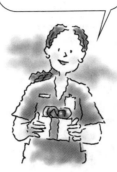

I can make a bow— but I don't think it's a Logan bow.

10. 3. To prevent formula buildup around the suture line, the mouth is usually rinsed. The sutures should be kept dry at all times. Objects placed in the mouth are generally avoided after surgery. Infants are fed by mouth using a catheter-tipped plunger–type syringe.
CN: Physiological integrity; CNS: Physiological adaptation; CL: Application

11. 1. Immediately after surgery for cleft lip or palate, the Logan bow, a thin arched metal device, is used to protect the suture line from tension. Esophageal atresia, hiatal hernia, or tracheoesophageal fistula repairs don't need a device to protect sutures after surgery.
CN: Physiological integrity; CNS: Reduction of risk potential; CL: Comprehension

12. 1. Children with cleft palate or lip have a greater risk of choking while eating, so all measures are used to reduce this risk. Steady pressure creates a seal when the nipple is against the cleft palate or lip, reducing the risk of aspiration. The nurse can't cause more damage to an infant's cleft lip or palate unless proper precautions aren't followed postoperatively. If the nipple is cut correctly and proper procedures are followed, the infant won't lose a lot of formula during a feeding. Infants with cleft palate or lip usually make more noise while eating.
CN: Physiological integrity; CNS: Reduction of risk potential; CL: Comprehension

13. 1. Infants with cleft lip and palate have a tendency to swallow an excessive amount of air. The amount of formula they eat at each feeding is the same as an infant without cleft lip or palate, and scheduled feedings aren't necessary. Loud noises are common when these infants eat.

CN: Physiological integrity; CNS: Physiological adaptation;
CL: Application

14. Which intervention is essential in the nursing care of an infant with cleft lip or palate?
1. Discouraging breast-feeding
2. Holding the infant flat while feeding
3. Involving the parents as soon as possible
4. Using a normal nursery nipple for feedings

15. The parents of an infant born with cleft lip and palate are seeing the infant for the first time. The nurse caring for the infant should focus on which area?
1. The infant's positive features
2. Irritation with how the infant eats
3. Ambivalence in caring for an infant with this defect
4. Dissatisfaction with the infant's physical appearance

16. The parents of a child who has had cleft palate surgery should be educated about which potential long-term physical problem?
1. Deviated septum
2. Recurring tonsillitis
3. Tooth decay
4. Varying degrees of hearing loss

17. The mother of a neonate born with a cleft lip and palate is preparing to feed him for the first time. Which intervention should the nurse teach the mother <u>first</u>?
1. Burping the neonate
2. Cleaning the mouth
3. Holding the neonate in an upright position
4. Preparing the bottle using a normal nursery nipple

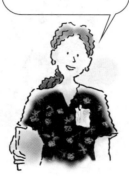

The parents of an infant born with cleft lip and palate need support and encouragement.

14. 3. The sooner the parents become involved, the quicker they can determine the method of feeding best suited for them and the infant. Breast-feeding, like bottle-feeding, may be difficult but can be facilitated if the mother intends to breast-feed. Sometimes, especially if the cleft isn't severe, breast-feeding may be easier because the human nipple conforms to the shape of the infant's mouth. Feedings are usually given in the upright position to prevent formula from coming through the nose. Various special nipples have been devised for infants with cleft lip or palate; a normal nursery nipple isn't effective.
CN: Physiological integrity; CNS: Physiological adaptation;
CL: Application

15. 1. To relieve the parents' anxiety, positive aspects of the infant's physical appearance need to be emphasized. Showing optimism toward surgical correction and showing a photograph of possible cosmetic improvements may be helpful. The other responses are inappropriate.
CN: Psychosocial integrity; CNS: None; CL: Application

16. 4. Improper draining of the middle ear causes recurrent otitis media and scarring of the tympanic membrane, which lead to varying degrees of hearing loss. The septum remains intact with cleft palate repair. Cleft palate doesn't cause problems with the tonsils. Improper tooth alignment, not tooth decay, is common.
CN: Physiological adaptation; CNS: Reduction of risk potential;
CL: Analysis

17. 3. When neonates are held in the upright position, the formula is less likely to leak out the nose or mouth. Neonates need to be burped frequently but not before a feeding. There's no need to clean the mouth before eating. After surgical repair, the mouth is cleaned at the suture site to prevent infection. The bottle should be prepared using a special nipple or feeding device.
CN: Physiological integrity; CNS: Physiological adaptation;
CL: Application

18. An infant returns from surgery after repair of a cleft palate. Which nursing intervention should be done first?
 1. Offering a pacifier for comfort
 2. Positioning the infant on his side
 3. Suctioning all secretions from the mouth and nose
 4. Removing the arm restraints placed on the infant after surgery

18. 2. The infant should be positioned on his side to allow oral secretions to drain from the mouth so suctioning is avoided. Pacifiers shouldn't be used because they can damage the suture line. Arm restraints should be kept on to protect the suture line. The restraints should be removed periodically to allow for full range of motion during this time. Only one restraint should be removed at a time, and the infant should be closely supervised.
CN: Physiological integrity; CNS: Reduction of risk potential; CL: Application

19. A small child has just had surgical repair of a cleft palate. Which instruction should be included in the discharge teaching to the parents?
 1. Continue a normal diet.
 2. Continue using arm restraints at home.
 3. Don't allow the child to drink from a cup.
 4. Establish good mouth care and proper brushing.

> Client teaching includes the family.

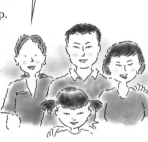

19. 2. Arm restraints are also used at home to keep the child's hands away from the mouth until the palate is healed. A soft diet is recommended. No food harder than mashed potatoes can be eaten. Fluids are best taken from a cup. Proper mouth care is encouraged after the palate is healed.
CN: Physiological integrity; CNS: Physiological adaptation; CL: Application

20. Most cleft palates are repaired at what age?
 1. Immediately after birth
 2. 1 to 2 months
 3. 3 to 4 months
 4. 12 to 15 months

20. 4. Most surgeons will correct the cleft at age 12 to 15 months, before faulty speech patterns develop. To take advantage of palatal changes, surgical repair is usually postponed until this time.
CN: Physiological integrity; CNS: Physiological adaptation; CL: Knowledge

21. After an infant with a cleft lip has surgical repair and heals, the parents can expect to see which result?
 1. A large scar
 2. An abnormally large upper lip
 3. Distorted jaw
 4. Some scarring

21. 4. If there's no trauma or infection to the site, healing occurs with little scar formation. There may be some inflammation right after surgery, but after healing, the lip is a normal size. No jaw malformation occurs with cleft lip repair.
CN: Physiological integrity; CNS: Physiological adaptation; CL: Comprehension

22. The nurse would expect which specialist to be involved in the management of a neonate born with cleft lip or palate?
 1. Cardiologist
 2. Neurologist
 3. Nutritionist
 4. Otolaryngologist

> Ear infections and hearing loss are common in infants with cleft lip or palate.

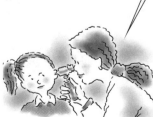

22. 4. An otolaryngologist is used because ear infections are common, along with hearing loss. Brain and cardiac function are usually normal. A nutritionist isn't needed unless the neonate becomes malnourished.
CN: Safe, effective care environment; CNS: Coordinated care; CL: Comprehension

CN: Client needs category   CNS: Client needs subcategory   CL: Cognitive level

23. Esophageal atresia and tracheoesophageal fistula can be attributed to which condition or factor?

1. Genetics
2. Prematurity
3. Poor nutrition during pregnancy
4. Unknown causes

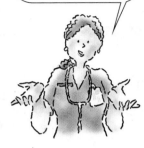

It's OK to say "I don't know." Maybe no one else does either.

24. Which type of tracheoesophageal fistula and esophageal atresia is <u>most commonly</u> encountered?

1. A cleft from the trachea to the upper esophagus
2. A normal trachea and esophagus connected by a common fistula
3. A blind pouch at each end, widely separated, with no involvement of the trachea
4. Proximal esophageal segment terminated in a blind pouch, distal segment connected to the trachea

25. A nurse examining a neonate born with esophageal atresia should be alert to which <u>common</u> finding?

1. Cyanosis
2. Decreased production of saliva
3. Inability to cough
4. Inadequate swallow

26. A definitive diagnostic evaluation that includes radiographic examination of a neonate suspected of having esophageal atresia would also include which finding?

1. Decreased breath sounds
2. Absent bowel sounds
3. Inability to tolerate feeding
4. Inability to aspirate gastric contents

23. 4. The cause of these malformations is unknown. Genetics isn't an issue with these structural defects. A premature neonate isn't necessarily born with either malformation. These defects occur much earlier in the process of development than viability (23 to 24 weeks' gestation). Poor nutrition could contribute to other factors in a neonate such as iron deficiency anemia.
CN: Physiological integrity; CNS: Physiological adaptation; CL: Application

24. 4. In 80% to 90% of all cases, these malformations have the proximal esophageal segment terminated in a blind pouch and the distal segment connected to the trachea. A cleft doesn't occur in the trachea. A normal trachea and esophagus connected by a common fistula represents the rarest form. A blind pouch at each end, widely separated, with no involvement of the trachea is the second most common type of tracheoesophageal fistula, making up 5% to 8% of all cases.
CN: Physiological integrity; CNS: Physiological adaptation; CL: Knowledge

25. 1. Cyanosis occurs when fluid from the blind pouch is aspirated into the trachea. Increased drooling is common, along with choking, coughing, and sneezing. The ability to swallow isn't affected by this disorder.
CN: Physiological integrity; CNS: Physiological adaptation; CL: Application

26. 4. A catheter will meet resistance and not reach the stomach if the esophagus is blocked. If the esophagus is patent, the catheter will pass unobstructed to the stomach. Breath sounds and bowel sounds aren't affected in esophageal atresia. The neonate who doesn't tolerate feedings might have any number of other conditions.
CN: Physiological integrity; CNS: Physiological adaptation; CL: Application

27. For a neonate diagnosed with a tracheo-esophageal fistula, which intervention would be needed?
1. Initiating antibiotic therapy
2. Keeping the neonate lying flat
3. Continuing feedings
4. Removing the diagnostic catheter from the esophagus

28. When tracheoesophageal fistula or esophageal atresia is suspected, which nursing intervention would be done <u>first</u>?
1. Giving oxygen
2. Telling the parents
3. Putting the neonate in an Isolette or on a radiant warmer
4. Reporting the suspicion to the physician

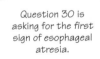

Remember the nurse is part of the team and responsible for notifying the physician as needed.

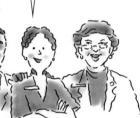

29. Which complication may follow the surgical repair of a tracheoesophageal fistula?
1. Atelectasis
2. Choking during feeding attempts
3. Damaged vocal cords
4. Infection

30. A nurse caring for a neonate should suspect esophageal atresia with distal tracheoesophageal fistula if the neonate develops which sign <u>first</u>?
1. Abdominal distention
2. Decreased oral secretions
3. Normal respiratory effort
4. Scaphoid abdomen

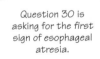

Question 30 is asking for the first sign of esophageal atresia.

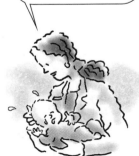

27. 1. Antibiotic therapy is started because aspiration pneumonia is inevitable and appears early. The neonate's head is usually kept in an upright position to prevent aspiration. I.V. fluids are started, and the neonate isn't allowed oral intake. The catheter is left in the upper esophageal pouch to easily remove fluid that collects there.
CN: Physiological integrity; CNS: Pharmacological therapies; CL: Application

28. 4. The physician needs to be told so immediate diagnostic tests can be done for a definitive diagnosis and surgical correction. Oxygen should be given only after notifying the physician, except in the case of an emergency. It isn't the nurse's responsibility to inform the parents of the suspected finding. By the time tracheoesophageal fistula or esophageal atresia is suspected, the neonate would have already been placed in an Isolette or a radiant warmer.
CN: Physiological integrity; CNS: Physiological adaptation; CL: Application

29. 1. Respiratory complications (atelectasis) are a threat to the neonate's life preoperatively and postoperatively due to the continual risk of aspiration. Choking is more likely to occur preoperatively, although careful attention is paid postoperatively when neonates begin to eat to make sure they can swallow without choking. Vocal cord damage isn't common after this repair. The neonate is generally given antibiotics preoperatively to prevent infection.
CN: Physiological integrity; CNS: Physiological adaptation; CL: Application

30. 1. Crying may force air into the stomach, causing distention. Secretions in a client with this condition may be more visible, though normal in quantity, due to the client's inability to swallow effectively. Respiratory effort is usually more difficult. When no distal fistula is present, the abdomen will appear scaphoid.
CN: Physiological integrity; CNS: Physiological adaptation; CL: Application

CN: Client needs category CNS: Client needs subcategory CL: Cognitive level

31. Dietary management in a child diagnosed with ulcerative colitis would include which diet?
1. High-calorie
2. High-residue
3. Low-protein
4. Low-sodium

32. A neonate returns from the operating room after surgical repair of a tracheoesophageal fistula and esophageal atresia. Which intervention is done <u>immediately</u>?
1. Maintaining a patent airway
2. Starting feedings right away
3. Letting the parents hold the neonate right away
4. Suctioning the trachea and stopping when resistance is met

33. Before discharging a neonate with a repaired tracheoesophageal fistula and esophageal atresia, the nurse would give the parents or caregivers instructions in which area?
1. Giving antibiotics
2. Preventing infection
3. Positioning techniques
4. Giving solid food as soon as possible

34. Which nursing intervention would be done postoperatively for a neonate after repair of tracheoesophageal fistula and esophageal atresia?
1. Withholding mouth care
2. Offering a pacifier frequently
3. Decreasing tactile stimulation
4. Using restraints to prevent injury to the repair

35. A client is admitted with a history of tracheoesophageal fistula and esophageal atresia repair. The nurse should evaluate this client for which potential <u>long-term</u> postoperative complication?
1. Oral aversion
2. Gastroesophageal reflux
3. Inability to tolerate feedings
4. Strictures

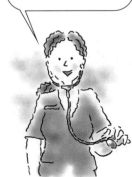

Pay close attention to the clues: history of and long-term.

31. 1. A high-calorie diet is given to combat weight loss and restore nitrogen balance. A low-residue or residue-free diet is encouraged to decrease bowel irritation. A high-protein diet is encouraged. Sodium intake isn't a factor in this disease.
CN: Physiological integrity; CNS: Physiological adaptation; CL: Analysis

32. 1. Maintaining a patent airway is essential until sedation from surgery wears off. Feedings usually aren't started for at least 48 hours after surgery. Parents are encouraged to participate in the neonate's care, but not immediately after surgery. Tracheal suctioning should be done only with a premeasured catheter to avoid injury to the surgical site.
CN: Physiological integrity; CNS: Physiological adaptation; CL: Application

33. 3. Positioning instructions should be given during hospitalization and before the neonate returns home. Antibiotics are usually discontinued before discharge. Preventing infection, especially at the operative sites, is a responsibility of the nurse postoperatively. For optimum effective respiration and because gastroesophageal reflux is a common complication, solid food usually isn't started until liquid feedings are tolerated and isn't given during the neonatal period.
CN: Psychosocial integrity; CNS: None; CL: Comprehension

34. 2. Meeting the neonate's oral needs is important because he can't drink from a bottle. The nurse should give mouth care to these neonates and provide tactile stimulation. Restraints should be avoided if possible.
CN: Physiological integrity; CNS: Physiological adaptation; CL: Application

35. 4. Strictures of the anastomosis occur in 40% to 50% of cases. Oral aversion can be a problem, but it occurs quickly after surgery. Reflux is a common complication but appears when feedings are started. If the neonate is having problems tolerating feedings, it's quickly noted.
CN: Physiological integrity; CNS: Physiological adaptation; CL: Application

CN: Client needs category   CNS: Client needs subcategory   CL: Cognitive level

36. A nurse is reviewing the following progress note entry in a neonate's chart and suspects the neonate has which structural defect?

Progress Notes	
09/29/08 1300	4-day-old neonate male ad- mitted with coughing, choking, and sneezing fol- lowing feedings. Neonate's mother states, "He seems to have a lot of saliva in his mouth and drools quite a bit." —S. Jones, L.P.N.

1. Cleft lip
2. Cleft palate
3. Gastroschisis
4. Tracheoesophageal fistula and esophageal atresia

37. Which nursing diagnosis takes the <u>highest</u> priority during the first 24 hours following surgical repair of esophageal atresia and tracheoesophageal fistula?
    1. *Ineffective airway clearance*
    2. *Imbalanced nutrition: Less than body requirements*
    3. *Risk for impaired parenting*
    4. *Ineffective infant feeding pattern*

38. Which structural defect involves a portion of an organ protruding through an abnormal opening?
    1. Cleft lip
    2. Cleft palate
    3. Gastroschisis
    4. Tracheoesophageal fistula

39. When an infant is diagnosed with a diaphragmatic hernia on the <u>left side</u>, which abdominal organ may be found in the thorax?
    1. Appendix
    2. Descending colon
    3. Right kidney
    4. Spleen

Hmmm. Now where did that organ go?

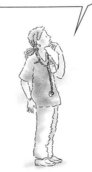

36. 4. Because of an ineffective swallow, saliva and secretions appear in the mouth and around the lips. Coughing, choking, and sneezing occur for the same reason and usually after an attempt at eating. Cleft lip and palate don't produce excessive salivation. None of these symptoms occur with gastroschisis.
CN: Physiological integrity; CNS: Physiological adaptation; CL: Analysis

37. 1. The nursing diagnosis that takes the highest priority for the first postoperative day is *Ineffective airway clearance*. The nurse must assess the infant's airway for the buildup of mucus and other secretions. The nurse must also carefully monitor the infant's respiratory status and keep suction equipment and a laryngoscope immediately available. Although the other nursing diagnoses are all important in the immediate postoperative period, they don't take the highest priority.
CN: Physiological integrity; CNS: Reduction of risk potential; CL: Analysis

38. 3. Gastroschisis is a herniation of the bowel through an abnormal opening in the abdominal wall. Tracheoesophageal fistula is a malformation of the trachea and esophagus. Cleft lip and palate are facial malformations, not herniations.
CN: Physiological integrity; CNS: Physiological adaptation; CL: Knowledge

39. 4. The spleen has commonly been seen in the thorax of infants with this defect. The appendix and descending colon usually don't protrude into the thorax due to limited space from the other organs present. The right kidney wouldn't be seen with a left-sided defect.
CN: Physiological integrity; CNS: Physiological adaptation; CL: Application

CN: Client needs category   CNS: Client needs subcategory   CL: Cognitive level

40. In which direction does the mediastinum shift in an infant diagnosed with a diaphragmatic hernia?
   1. No shifting occurs
   2. Shifts to the affected side
   3. Shifts to the unaffected side
   4. Partially shifts to the affected or unaffected sides

41. Which action confirms that a nasogastric (NG) tube is properly positioned in a client's stomach?
   1. Inverting the tube into a glass of water and observing for bubbling
   2. Examining the aspirate with a pH test strip
   3. Clamping the tube for 10 minutes and listening with a stethoscope for increased peristalsis
   4. Instilling 30 ml of normal saline solution and observing the client's response

42. A nurse is preparing a preoperative care plan for a neonate scheduled for diaphragmatic hernia repair. Which nursing action would help decrease gastric and bowel distention?
   1. Feeding the infant
   2. Providing tactile stimulation
   3. Preventing the infant from crying
   4. Placing the infant on the unaffected side

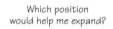

Which position would help me expand?

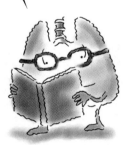

43. Which action by the nurse is <u>essential</u> when caring for a neonate with an omphalocele?
   1. Keeping the malformation dry
   2. Not letting the parents see the malformation
   3. Carefully positioning and handling the neonate
   4. Touching the malformation often to assess changes

40. 3. The increased volume in the chest cavity from the abdominal organs causes the mediastinum to shift to the unaffected side, which causes a partial collapse of that lung. Due to the increased volume on the affected side, the mediastinum can't shift that way.
CN: Physiological integrity; CNS: Physiological adaptation; CL: Application

41. 2. To verify positioning, the gastric aspirate should be tested with a pH test strip. Probability of gastric placement is increased if the aspirate has a typical gastric fluid appearance (grassy-green, clear and colorless with mucus shreads, or brown) and the pH is ≤ 5.0. Inverting the tube into a glass of water and observing for bubbling would be done to verify that an NG tube is in the respiratory tract. Clamping the tube and listening for increased peristalsis provides no information on the location of the tube. If the tube is in the respiratory tract, instilling normal saline will cause respiratory distress.
CN: Physiological integrity; CNS: Reduction of risk potential; CL: Comprehension

42. 3. The stomach and intestine in the chest cavity become distended with swallowed air from crying. Negative pressure from crying pulls the intestines into the chest cavity, increasing the amount of distention. The infant usually isn't fed until after surgery. Tactile stimulation is limited because it may disturb the infant's fragile condition. The infant is always placed on the affected side.
CN: Physiological integrity; CNS: Physiological adaptation; CL: Application

43. 3. Careful positioning and handling of the neonate prevents infection and rupture of the sac. The omphalocele is kept moist until the neonate is taken to the operating room. The parents should be allowed to see the defect if they choose. Touching the malformation often increases the risk of infection.
CN: Physiological integrity; CNS: Physiological adaptation; CL: Application

CN: Client needs category   CNS: Client needs subcategory   CL: Cognitive level

44. Which treatment option would the nurse anticipate for an infant with a diagnosed omphalocele?
　1. Immediate surgical repair
　2. Surgical repair after the sac ruptures
　3. Sterile technique and manual manipulation
　4. No treatment (it goes away by itself)

44. 1. Surgical repair is done immediately to prevent infection and possible tissue damage. The omphalocele is covered and kept moist until the infant goes to the operating room. Careful positioning and handling techniques are used to prevent rupture of the sac and damage to the abdominal contents. The disorder doesn't disappear by itself.
CN: Physiological integrity; CNS: Physiological adaptation; CL: Application

45. Which abdominal defect <u>isn't</u> covered by a protective sac and <u>doesn't</u> cause damage to the umbilical cord?
　1. Diaphragmatic hernia
　2. Gastroschisis
　3. Omphalocele
　4. Umbilical hernia

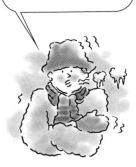

Oh! I thought I was searching for an *abominable* defect. No wonder I was having such a tough time!

45. 2. Gastroschisis is always located to the right of an intact umbilical cord and isn't enclosed in a protective sac. Diaphragmatic hernia is a protrusion of abdominal organs into the thoracic cavity. The omphalocele is covered by only a translucent sac of amnion. Umbilical hernia is a protrusion of the intestine into the umbilicus, which is covered by skin.
CN: Physiological integrity; CNS: Physiological adaptation; CL: Knowledge

46. Which statement should the nurse include when teaching the family of an infant diagnosed with pyloric stenosis about this condition?
　1. "It's more common in girls."
　2. "It's diagnosed by severe diarrhea."
　3. "It's more common in Blacks and Asians."
　4. "It's more common in full-term neonates."

46. 4. Pyloric stenosis is more likely to affect a full-term neonate than a preterm one. It's more common in boys and is usually diagnosed by vomiting. It occurs more commonly in White neonates.
CN: Physiological integrity; CNS: Physiological adaptation; CL: Application

47. The mother of an infant with pyloric stenosis expresses feelings of guilt and fear that she may have caused her child's condition. Which would be an accurate response by the nurse?
　1. "The cause of pyloric stenosis is unknown."
　2. "The cause of pyloric stenosis is believed to be hereditary."
　3. "Pyloric stenosis is typically caused by poor nutrition in pregnancy."
　4. "Pyloric stenosis is directly related to poor muscle development in the stomach."

47. 1. The cause of the narrowing of the pyloric musculature is unknown. A hereditary factor hasn't been established. Poor nutrition in pregnancy and poor muscle development in the stomach may relate to this defect, but haven't been established as a definitive cause.
CN: Physiological integrity; CNS: Physiological adaptation; CL: Analysis

My pyloric canal is really putting the squeeze on me.

48. In which area does the pyloric canal narrow in clients with pyloric stenosis?
　1. Stomach and esophagus
　2. Stomach and duodenum
　3. Both the stomach and esophagus and the stomach and duodenum
　4. Neither the stomach and esophagus nor the stomach and duodenum

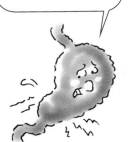

48. 2. The narrowing of the pyloric canal occurs between the stomach and duodenum, where the pyloric sphincter is located. Hyperplasia and hypertrophy cause narrowing and possibly obstruction of the circular muscle of the pylorus.
CN: Physiological integrity; CNS: Physiological adaptation; CL: Knowledge

CN: Client needs category　CNS: Client needs subcategory　CL: Cognitive level

49. The nurse caring for an infant with pyloric stenosis should be alert for which classic sign or symptom?
1. Loss of appetite
2. Chronic diarrhea
3. Projectile vomiting
4. Occasional nonprojectile vomiting

49. 3. The obstruction doesn't allow food to pass through to the duodenum. When the stomach becomes full, the infant vomits for relief. Occasional nonprojectile vomiting may occur initially if the obstruction is only partial. Chronic hunger is commonly seen. There's no diarrhea because food doesn't pass the stomach.
CN: Physiological integrity; CNS: Physiological adaptation; CL: Analysis

50. When assessing a neonate, the nurse notes visible <u>peristaltic waves</u> across the epigastrium. This characteristic is indicative of which disorder?
1. Hypertrophic pyloric stenosis
2. Imperforate anus
3. Intussusception
4. Short-gut syndrome

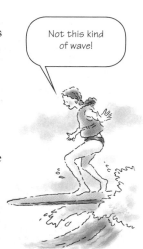

Not this kind of wave!

50. 1. The diagnosis of pyloric stenosis can be established from a finding of hypertrophic pyloric stenosis. Imperforate anus, intussusception, and short-gut syndrome are diagnosed by other characteristics.
CN: Physiological integrity; CNS: Physiological adaptation; CL: Analysis

51. After surgical repair of pyloric stenosis, the nurse should expect an infant's <u>normal</u> feeding regimen to resume after what timeframe?
1. 4 to 6 hours
2. 24 hours
3. 48 hours
4. 1 week

51. 3. Small, frequent feedings of clear fluids are usually started 4 to 6 hours after surgery. If clear fluids are tolerated, formula feedings are started 24 hours after surgery, in gradually increasing amounts. It usually takes 48 hours to reach a normal full feeding regimen in this manner. The infant usually goes home on the fourth postoperative day.
CN: Physiological integrity; CNS: Physiological adaptation; CL: Application

52. A nurse admits an infant diagnosed with pyloric stenosis. Which nursing intervention would most likely be done <u>first</u>?
1. Weighing the infant
2. Checking urine specific gravity
3. Placing an I.V. catheter
4. Changing the infant and weighing the diaper

52. 1. Weighing the infant would be done first so a baseline weight can be established and weight changes can be assessed. After a baseline weight is obtained, an I.V. catheter can be placed because oral feedings generally aren't given. These infants are usually dehydrated, so while checking the diaper and specific gravity are important tools to help assess their status, they aren't the first priority.
CN: Physiological integrity; CNS: Physiological adaptation; CL: Application

53. A nurse is caring for an infant with pyloric stenosis. After feeding the infant, he should be placed in which position?
1. Prone in Fowler's position
2. On his back without elevation
3. On his left side in Fowler's position
4. Slightly on his right side in high Fowler's position

53. 4. Positioning the infant slightly on his right side in high Fowler's position will help facilitate gastric emptying. The other positions won't facilitate gastric emptying and may cause the infant to vomit.
CN: Physiological integrity; CNS: Physiological adaptation; CL: Application

54. When preparing to feed an infant with pyloric stenosis, which intervention is important?
1. Giving feedings quickly
2. Burping the infant frequently
3. Discouraging parental participation
4. Not giving more feedings if the infant vomits

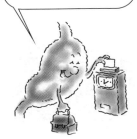

I must be the luckiest guy in the world...I actually get paid to stretch out my feeding times. Time to go to work!

54. 2. These infants usually swallow a lot of air from sucking on their hands and fingers because of their intensive hunger (feedings aren't easily tolerated). Burping often will lessen gastric distention and increase the likelihood the infant will retain the feeding. Feedings are given slowly with the infant lying in a semiupright position. Parental participation should be encouraged and allowed to the extent possible. Record the type, amount, and character of the vomit as well as it's relation to the feeding. The amount of feeding volume lost is usually refed.
CN: Physiological integrity; CNS: Physiological adaptation; CL: Application

55. Which <u>common</u> symptom would the nurse expect in an infant up to 48 hours after surgical repair of pyloric stenosis?
1. Dysuria
2. Oral aversion
3. Scaphoid abdomen
4. Vomiting

55. 4. Even with successful surgery, most infants have some vomiting during the first 24 to 48 hours after surgery. Dysuria isn't a complication with this surgical procedure. Oral aversion doesn't occur because these infants may be fed until surgery. Scaphoid abdomen isn't characteristic of this condition. The abdomen may appear distended, not scaphoid.
CN: Physiological integrity; CNS: Physiological adaptation; CL: Analysis

56. Which intervention should the nurse perform to help prevent vomiting in an infant diagnosed with pyloric stenosis?
1. Holding the infant for 1 hour after feeding
2. Handling the infant minimally after feedings
3. Spacing out feedings and giving large amounts
4. Laying the infant prone with the head of the bed elevated

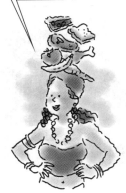

So many of my clients require small, frequent feedings...I thought I'd give this a try.

56. 2. Minimal handling, especially after a feeding, will help prevent vomiting. Holding the infant would provide too much stimulation, which might increase the risk of vomiting. Feedings are given frequently and slowly in small amounts. An infant should be positioned in semi-Fowler's position and slightly on the right side after a feeding.
CN: Physiological integrity; CNS: Physiological adaptation; CL: Application

57. It's an important nursing function to give support to the parents of an infant diagnosed with pyloric stenosis. Which nursing intervention best serves that purpose?
1. Keeping the parents informed of the infant's progress
2. Providing all care for the infant, even when the parents visit
3. Telling the parents to minimize handling of the infant at all times
4. Telling the physician to keep the parents informed of the infant's progress

57. 1. Keeping the parents informed will decrease their anxiety. The nurse should encourage the parents to be involved with the infant's care. Telling the parents to minimize handling of the infant isn't appropriate because parent-child contact is important. The physician is responsible for updating the parents on the infant's medical condition, and the nurse is responsible for updating the parents on the day-to-day activities of the infant and his improvement with the day's activities.
CN: Psychosocial integrity; CNS: None; CL: Analysis

CN: Client needs category   CNS: Client needs subcategory   CL: Cognitive level

58. Which symptom would be likely in an infant diagnosed with pyloric stenosis?
1. Apathy
2. Arrhythmia
3. Dry lips and skin
4. Hypothermia

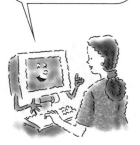

Question 59 is asking what's normally found with a disease, not what's normal in a healthy infant?

58. 3. Dry lips and skin are signs of dehydration, which is common in infants with pyloric stenosis. These infants are constantly hungry due to their inability to retain feedings. Apathy, arrhythmias, and hypothermia aren't clinical findings with pyloric stenosis.
CN: Physiological integrity; CNS: Physiological adaptation; CL: Application

59. When assessing an infant diagnosed with pyloric stenosis, which finding would the nurse consider <u>normal</u>?
1. Decreased or diminished bowel sounds
2. Heart murmur
3. Normal respiratory effort
4. Increased bowel sounds

59. 1. Bowel sounds decrease because food can't pass into the intestines. Normal respiratory effort is affected due to the abdominal distention that pushes the diaphragm up into the pleural cavity. Heart murmurs may be present but aren't directly associated with pyloric stenosis.
CN: Physiological integrity; CNS: Physiological adaptation; CL: Analysis

60. Which abdominal organs are directly affected when pyloric stenosis is diagnosed?
1. Colon and rectum
2. Stomach and duodenum
3. Stomach and esophagus
4. Liver and bile ducts

60. 2. This defect occurs at the pyloric sphincter, which is located between the stomach and duodenum. The stomach and esophagus, liver and bile ducts, and colon and rectum aren't affected by this obstructive disorder.
CN: Physiological integrity; CNS: Physiological adaptation; CL: Knowledge

61. Which nursing intervention is the <u>most important</u> in dealing with a child who has been poisoned?
1. Stabilizing the child
2. Notifying the parents
3. Identifying the poison
4. Determining when the poisoning took place

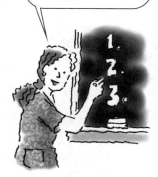

Practice setting priorities because it's part of nursing practice.

61. 1. Stabilization and the initial emergency treatment of the child (such as respiratory assistance, circulatory support, or control of seizures) will prevent further damage to the body from the poison. If the parents didn't bring the child in, they can be notified as soon as the child is stabilized or treated. Although identification of the poison is crucial and should begin at the same time as the stabilization of the child, the initial assessment of airway, breathing, and circulation should occur first. Determining when the poisoning took place is an important consideration, but emergency stabilization and treatment are priorities.
CN: Physiological integrity; CNS: Physiological adaptation; CL: Application

62. For a child who has ingested a poisonous substance, the initial step in emergency treatment is to stop the exposure to the substance. Which method would best achieve this?
1. Inducing vomiting
2. Calling 911 as soon as possible
3. Giving large amounts of water to flush the system
4. Emptying the mouth of pills, plant parts, or other material

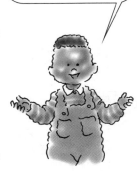

I'm not going to look so happy after reading the next few questions!

63. The Poison Control Center reports that the poison a child has ingested can be removed by inducing vomiting. Which method for inducing vomiting is best?
1. Giving syrup of ipecac
2. Having the child smell something offensive to cause vomiting
3. Putting a finger down the throat of the child who ingested the poison
4. Doing nothing because ingesting the poison may cause vomiting in some children

64. Emetic agents are indicated for the treatment of poisoning under which circumstance?
1. When the poison is a salicylate (aspirin)
2. When the child is in severe shock
3. When the child is experiencing seizures
4. When the poison is a low-viscosity hydrocarbon

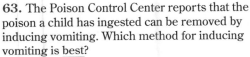

I think it should be smooth sailing from here!

65. Which inflammatory disease most commonly affects the terminal ileum?
1. Acute appendicitis
2. Crohn's disease
3. Meckel's diverticulum
4. Ulcerative colitis

62. 4. Emptying the mouth of pills, plant parts, or other material will stop exposure to the poison. Inducing vomiting is important, but won't remove exposure to the substance; it's also contraindicated with some poisons. Calling 911 is important, but removing any further sources of the poison would come first. Only small amounts of water are recommended so the poison is confined to the smallest volume. Large amounts of water will let the poison pass the pylorus. The small intestines absorb fluid rapidly, increasing the risk of toxicity.
CN: Physiological integrity; CNS: Physiological adaptation; CL: Application

63. 1. If vomiting is indicated, syrup of ipecac should be given instead of waiting for the child to vomit by himself. This syrup causes stimulation of the vomiting center and an irritant effect on gastric mucosa. Vomiting should occur within 20 minutes. Smelling something offensive may not work because it's difficult to get the child to comply. Putting a finger down his throat could cause damage to the oropharynx. Waiting for the child to vomit may allow the poison to enter the systemic circulation.
CN: Physiological integrity; CNS: Pharmacological therapies; CL: Application

64. 1. If the child has ingested a salicylate (aspirin), inducing vomiting with an emetic is indicated. Severe shock increases the risk of aspiration, so emetic treatment is contraindicated when a child is in severe shock. An emetic shouldn't be administered to a child experiencing seizures because the child could aspirate the poison if he vomits while having a seizure. If the poison is a low-viscosity hydrocarbon, it can cause severe chemical pneumonitis if aspirated; therefore, inducing vomiting is contraindicated.
CN: Physiological integrity; CNS: Physiological adaptation; CL: Application

65. 2. Crohn's disease affects the terminal ileum. Acute appendicitis affects the blind sac at the end of the cecum. Ulcerative colitis affects the entire large bowel. Meckel's diverticulum is a sac that becomes inflamed.
CN: Physiological integrity; CNS: Physiological adaptation; CL: Knowledge

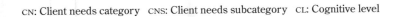

CN: Client needs category   CNS: Client needs subcategory   CL: Cognitive level

66. If a child ingests poisonous hydrocarbons, what would be an important nursing intervention?
1. Inducing vomiting
2. Keeping the child calm and relaxed
3. Scolding the child for the wrongdoing
4. Keeping the parents away from the child

66. 2. Keeping the child calm and relaxed will help prevent vomiting. If vomiting occurs, there's a great chance the esophagus will be damaged from regurgitation of the gastric poison. Additionally, the risk of chemical pneumonitis exists if vomiting occurs. Scolding the child may upset him. The parents should remain with the child to help keep him calm.
CN: Physiological integrity; CNS: Physiological adaptation; CL: Application

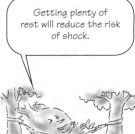

Getting plenty of rest will reduce the risk of shock.

67. Shock is a complication of several types of poisoning. Which measure should the nurse implement to help reduce the risk of shock?
1. Keeping the child on his right side
2. Letting the child maintain normal activity as possible
3. Elevating the head and legs to the level of the heart
4. Keeping the head flat and raising the legs to the level of the heart

67. 3. Elevating the head and legs to the level of the heart will promote venous drainage and decrease the chance of the child going into shock. The child may safely lie on the side he prefers. The child should be encouraged to get plenty of rest.
CN: Physiological integrity; CNS: Physiological adaptation; CL: Application

68. A 7-year-old child ingested several leaves of a poinsettia plant. After arrival in the emergency department, which intervention would be the <u>main</u> nursing function for this client?
1. Beginning teaching accident prevention
2. Providing emotional support to the child
3. Preparing for immediate intervention
4. Providing emotional support to the parents

68. 3. Time and speed are critical factors in recovery from poisonings. The remaining three answers are important nursing functions but don't require the immediate attention that first stabilizing the child does.
CN: Physiological integrity; CNS: Reduction of risk potential; CL: Application

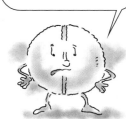

Why do you think my bottle reads "Keep out of the reach of children"?

69. A child is being admitted through the emergency department with a diagnosis of suspected accidental poisoning by medication. The nurse is aware that which class of medication is the <u>most</u> likely cause of accidental poisoning in children?
1. Pain medications
2. Vitamins
3. Laxatives
4. Antibiotics

69. 1. According to the Centers for Disease Control and Prevention, the most common accidentally ingested class of drugs is pain medications, followed by cardiovascular drugs. The most common pain medications ingested are acetaminophen (Tylenol)-containing drugs, nonsteroidal anti-inflammatory drugs, and opioids. The other classes of drugs are less commonly ingested.
CN: Physiological integrity; CNS: Physiological adaptation; CL: Analysis

70. A client is undergoing testing for a diagnosis of ulcerative colitis. Which symptom would the nurse most likely idenfity during this <u>initial</u> diagnosis?
1. Constipation
2. Diarrhea
3. Vomiting
4. Weight loss

70. 2. Recurrent or persistent diarrhea is a common feature of ulcerative colitis. Constipation doesn't occur because the bowel becomes smooth and inflexible. Vomiting isn't common in this disease. Weight loss will occur after or during the episode but not initially.
CN: Physiological integrity; CNS: Physiological adaptation; CL: Analysis

CN: Client needs category   CNS: Client needs subcategory   CL: Cognitive level

71. A child arrives in the emergency department after ingesting poisonous amounts of salicylates. How soon after ingestion should the nurse look for <u>obvious</u> signs of toxicity?
1. Immediately
2. 2 to 4 hours after ingestion
3. 6 hours after ingestion
4. 18 hours after ingestion

72. The nurse caring for a client with an extreme case of salicylate poisoning should anticipate, or prepare the client for, which treatment?
1. Gastric lavage
2. Hypothermia blankets
3. Peritoneal dialysis
4. Vitamin K injection

73. When a child has been poisoned, identifying the ingested poison is an important treatment goal. Which action would help determine which poison was ingested?
1. Call the local poison control center.
2. Ask the child.
3. Ask the parents.
4. Save all evidence of poison.

74. A nurse is educating parents about salicylate poisoning. What teaching information is the <u>most</u> important?
1. Identifying the salicylate overdose level
2. Teaching children the hazards of ingesting nonfood items
3. Decreasing curiosity; teaching parents to keep aspirin and drugs in clear view
4. Teaching parents to keep large amounts of drugs on hand but out of reach of children

The adage, "Timing is everything," holds true in nursing practice, too.

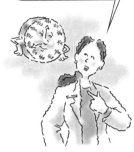

It's the nurse's responsibility to teach children the hazards of ingesting poisonous substances.

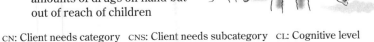

71. 3. There's usually a delay of 6 hours before evidence of toxicity is noted. Toxic evidence is rarely immediate. Aspirin will exert its peak effect in 2 to 4 hours. The effect of aspirin may last as long as 18 hours.
CN: Health promotion and maintenance; CNS: None; CL: Application

72. 3. Peritoneal dialysis is usually reserved for cases of life-threatening salicylism. Gastric lavage is the immediate treatment for salicylate poisoning because the stomach contents and salicylates will move from the stomach to the remainder of the GI tract, where vomiting will no longer result in the removal of the poison. Hypothermia blankets may be used to reduce the possibility of seizures. Vitamin K may be used to decrease bleeding tendencies, but if evidence of this exists.
CN: Physiological integrity; CNS: Physiological adaptation; CL: Analysis

73. 4. Saving all evidence of poison (container, vomitus, urine) will help determine which drug was ingested and how much. Calling the local poison control center may help get information on specific poisons or if a certain household placed a call, although rarely can they help determine which poison has been ingested. Asking the child may help, but the child may fear punishment and may not be honest about the incident. The parent may be helpful in some instances, although the parent may not have been home or with the child when the ingestion occurred.
CN: Physiological integrity; CNS: Reduction of risk potential; CL: Application

74. 2. Teaching children the hazards of ingesting nonfood items will help prevent ingestion of poisonous substances. Identifying the overdose level won't prevent it from occurring. Aspirin and drugs should be kept out of the sight and reach of children. Parents should be warned about keeping large amounts of drugs on hand.
CN: Health promotion and maintenance; CNS: None; CL: Analysis

CN: Client needs category   CNS: Client needs subcategory   CL: Cognitive level

75. A nurse is aware that which condition is the <u>most</u> likely to develop as a result of an acute overdose of acetaminophen?
1. Brain damage
2. Heart failure
3. Hepatic damage
4. Kidney damage

76. A client is diagnosed with acetaminophen poisoning. Which sign would the nurse expect when assessing the client 12 to 24 hours after ingestion?
1. Hyperthermia
2. Increased urine output
3. Profuse sweating
4. Rapid pulse

77. A nurse is evaluating the effectiveness of therapy with acetylcysteine (Mucomyst) in a child with acetaminophen poisoning. Which laboratory values would be <u>most</u> important for the nurse to monitor?
1. Serum alanine aminotransferase (ALT) and aspartate aminotransferase (AST) levels
2. Serum calcium levels
3. Serum methemoglobin (MetHb) levels
4. Serum platelet count

78. Which ethnic group has the highest prevalence of lead poisoning in children?
1. Black
2. Hispanic
3. Asian
4. White

79. The ingestion of lead-containing substances is <u>mostly</u> influenced by which risk factor?
1. Child's age
2. Child's gender
3. Child's nationality
4. A parent with the same habit

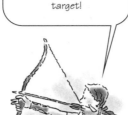

You're right on target!

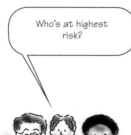

Who's at highest risk?

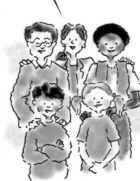

75. 3. The damage to the hepatic system isn't from the drug but from one of its metabolites. This metabolite binds to liver cells in large quantities. Brain damage, heart failure, and kidney damage may develop but not initially.
CN: Physiological integrity; CNS: Physiological adaptation; CL: Application

76. 3. During the first 12 to 24 hours, profuse sweating is a significant sign of acetaminophen poisoning. Weak pulse, hypothermia, and decreased urine output are also common findings.
CN: Physiological integrity; CNS: Physiological adaptation; CL: Analysis

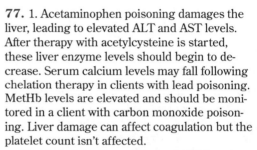

77. 1. Acetaminophen poisoning damages the liver, leading to elevated ALT and AST levels. After therapy with acetylcysteine is started, these liver enzyme levels should begin to decrease. Serum calcium levels may fall following chelation therapy in clients with lead poisoning. MetHb levels are elevated and should be monitored in a client with carbon monoxide poisoning. Liver damage can affect coagulation but the platelet count isn't affected.
CN: Physiological integrity; CNS: Pharmacological therapies; CL: Analysis

78. 1. Black children have a six times greater risk of lead poisoning than White children. Lead poisoning isn't as common among Asian or Hispanic populations.
CN: Health promotion and maintenance; CNS: None; CL: Knowledge

79. 1. The highest risk of lead poisoning occurs in young children who tend to put things in their mouths. In older homes that contain lead-based paint, paint chips may be eaten directly by the child or they may cling to toys or hands that are then put into the child's mouth. Poisoning isn't gender-related. Blacks have a higher incidence of lead poisoning, but it can happen in any race. Children of low socioeconomic status are more likely to eat lead-based paint chips. Most parents don't eat lead-based paint on purpose.
CN: Health promotion and maintenance; CNS: None; CL: Application

CN: Client needs category   CNS: Client needs subcategory   CL: Cognitive level

80. Lead retained in the body is largely stored in which organ?
1. Bone
2. Brain
3. Kidney
4. Liver

81. When monitoring a child with lead poisoning, the nurse should be alert for which condition that commonly appears <u>first</u>?
1. Anemia
2. Diarrhea
3. Overeating
4. Paralysis

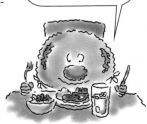

Excuse me...I think someone forgot my heme!

82. The most serious and irreversible adverse effects of lead poisoning affect which body system?
1. Central nervous system (CNS)
2. Hematologic system
3. Renal system
4. Respiratory system

83. Black lines along the gums indicate which type of poisoning?
1. Acetaminophen
2. Lead
3. Plants
4. Salicylates

84. Which procedure is the main treatment for lead poisoning?
1. Blood transfusion
2. Bone marrow transplant
3. Chelation therapy
4. Dialysis

Think about what would be most important to prepare a child for chelation therapy.

85. Which nursing objective would be the <u>most important</u> for a child with lead poisoning who must undergo chelation therapy?
1. Preparing the child for complete bed rest
2. Preparing the child for I.V. fluid therapy
3. Preparing the child for an extended hospital stay
4. Preparing the child for a large number of injections

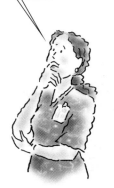

80. 1. Ingested lead is initially absorbed by bone. If chronic ingestion occurs, then the hematologic, renal, and central nervous systems are affected.
CN: Physiological integrity; CNS: Physiological adaptation; CL: Knowledge

81. 1. Lead is dangerously toxic to the biosynthesis of heme. The reduced heme molecule in red blood cells causes anemia. Constipation, not diarrhea, and a poor appetite and vomiting, not overeating, are signs of lead poisoning. Paralysis may occur as toxic damage to the brain progresses, but it isn't an initial sign.
CN: Physiological integrity; CNS: Physiological adaptation; CL: Analysis

82. 1. Damage that occurs to the CNS is difficult to repair. Damage to the renal and hematologic systems can be reversed if treated early. The respiratory system isn't affected until coma and death occur.
CN: Physiological integrity; CNS: Physiological adaptation; CL: Application

83. 2. One diagnostic characteristic of lead poisoning is black lines along the gums. Black lines don't occur along the gums with acetaminophen, plant, or salicylate poisoning.
CN: Physiological integrity; CNS: Physiological adaptation; CL: Knowledge

84. 3. Chelation therapy involves the removal of metal by combining it with another substance. Sometimes exchange transfusions are used to rid the blood of lead quickly. Bone marrow transplants usually aren't needed. Dialysis usually isn't part of treatment.
CN: Physiological integrity; CNS: Physiological adaptation; CL: Knowledge

85. 4. Chelation therapy involves receiving a large number of injections in a relatively short period. It's traumatic to most children, and they need some preparation for the treatment. The other components of the treatment plan are important but not as likely to cause the same anxiety as multiple injections. Receiving I.V. fluid isn't as traumatizing as multiple injections. Physical activity is usually limited. Allowing adequate rest to not aggravate the painful injection sites is important.
CN: Physiological integrity; CNS: Physiological adaptation; CL: Application

CN: Client needs category   CNS: Client needs subcategory   CL: Cognitive level

86. A nurse is caring for a 5-year-old child who exhibits signs of lead poisoning. The nurse should assess the child for which of the following signs?
   1. Nausea, vomiting, seizures, and coma
   2. Jaundice, confusion, and coagulation abnormalities
   3. Insomnia, weight loss, diarrhea, and gingivitis
   4. General fatigue, difficulty concentrating, tremors, and headache

87. Which intervention is the best way to prevent lead poisoning in children?
   1. Educating the child
   2. Educating the public
   3. Identifying high-risk groups
   4. Providing home chelation kits

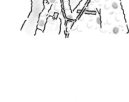

You know the routine; keep on teachin'.

88. Which term describes a purposeful ingestion of a nonfood substance?
   1. PDA
   2. RDSI
   3. Pica
   4. Plumbism

89. Certain forms of pica are caused by a nutrient deficiency. Which nutrient is most commonly deficient?
   1. Minerals
   2. Vitamin B complex
   3. Vitamin C
   4. Vitamin D

90. Which helminthic infection caused by nematodes is the most common?
   1. Flukes
   2. Hookworms
   3. Roundworms
   4. Tapeworms

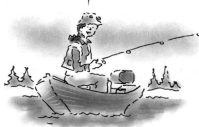

I didn't realize nursing would require knowledge of worms.

86. 4. Signs and symptoms of lead poisoning depend on the degree of toxicity. General fatigue, difficulty concentrating, tremors, and headache indicate moderate toxicity. Nausea, vomiting, seizures, and coma are observed in salicylate and iron poisoning. Jaundice, confusion, and coagulation abnormalities are observed in acetaminophen poisoning. Insomnia, weight loss, diarrhea, and gingivitis are observed in mercury poisoning.
CN: Physiological integrity; CNS: Physiological adaptation; CL: Analysis

87. 2. By educating others about lead poisoning, including danger signs, symptoms, and treatment, identification can be determined quickly. Young children may not understand the dangers of lead poisoning. Identifying high-risk groups will help but won't prevent the poisoning. Home chelation kits currently aren't available.
CN: Health promotion and maintenance; CNS: None; CL: Application

88. 3. *Pica* is a Latin word for magpie, a bird with a voracious appetite. Today, pica refers to the purposeful ingestion of a nonfood substance. PDA stands for patent ductus arteriosus, a term for a heart murmur. RDSI stands for revised developmental screening inventory, a developmental screening test. Plumbism is another term for lead poisoning.
CN: Health promotion and maintenance; CNS: None; CL: Knowledge

89. 1. Eating clay is related to zinc deficiency, and eating chalk to calcium deficiency. Vitamin deficiencies aren't related to pica.
CN: Health promotion and maintenance; CNS: None; CL: Analysis

90. 3. Roundworms are caused by nematodes. Hookworm is caused by *Necator americanus*. Tapeworms are caused by cestodes, and flukes by trematodes; both live throughout North America.
CN: Health promotion and maintenance; CNS: None; CL: Knowledge

CN: Client needs category CNS: Client needs subcategory CL: Cognitive level

91. Which advice should a nurse give over the phone to the mother of a 7-year-old child with right lower abdominal pain, fever, and vomiting?
1. "Give prune juice to relieve constipation."
2. "Test for rebound tenderness in the left lower abdominal quadrant."
3. "Encourage fluids to prevent dehydration."
4. "Seek immediate emergency medical care."

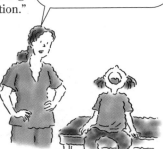

Abdominal pain is just one of the symptoms of appendicitis.

91. 4. The mother of a child with abdominal pain, fever, and vomiting (the cardinal signs of appendicitis) should be urged to seek immediate emergency care to reduce the risk of complications from potential appendix rupture. Prune juice has laxative effects and shouldn't be given because laxatives increase the risk of rupture of the appendix. Testing for rebound tenderness may elicit McBurney's sign in the right lower quadrant (an indication of appendicitis); however, the nurse shouldn't rely on the mother's findings. The child should be given nothing by mouth in case surgery is needed.
CN: Physiological integrity; CNS: Reduction of risk potential; CL: Application

92. Which symptom is the most common for acute appendicitis?
1. Bradycardia
2. Fever
3. Pain descending to the lower left quadrant
4. Pain radiating down the legs

92. 2. Fever, abdominal pain, and tenderness are the first symptoms of appendicitis. Tachycardia, not bradycardia, is seen. Pain can be generalized or periumbilical. It usually descends to the lower right quadrant, not to the left and not to the legs.
CN: Physiological integrity; CNS: Physiological adaptation; CL: Application

93. Which nursing intervention would be important to do preoperatively in a child with appendicitis?
1. Giving clear fluids
2. Applying heat to the abdomen
3. Maintaining complete bed rest
4. Administering an enema, if ordered

93. 3. Bed rest will prevent aggravating the condition. Clients with appendicitis aren't allowed anything by mouth. Cold applications are placed on the abdomen as heat would increase blood flow to the area and possibly spread infectious disease. Enemas may aggravate the condition.
CN: Physiological integrity; CNS: Physiological adaptation; CL: Application

94. Postoperative care of a child with peritonitis from a ruptured appendix would include which intervention?
1. Giving a liquids-only diet
2. Giving oral antibiotics for 7 to 10 days
3. Positioning the child on his left side
4. Giving parenteral antibiotics for 7 to 10 days

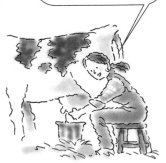

Believe me, position counts.

94. 4. Parenteral antibiotics are used for 7 to 10 days postoperatively to help prevent the spread of infection. The child is kept on I.V. fluids and isn't allowed anything by mouth. Oral antibiotics may continue after the parenteral antibiotics are discontinued. The child is positioned on his right side after surgery.
CN: Physiological integrity; CNS: Physiological adaptation; CL: Application

95. After surgical repair of a ruptured appendix, which position would be the <u>most</u> appropriate?
1. High Fowler's position
2. Left side-lying
3. Semi-Fowler's position
4. Supine

95. 3. Using the semi-Fowler or right side-lying position will facilitate drainage from the peritoneal cavity and prevent the formation of a subdiaphragmatic abscess. High Fowler's, left side-lying, and supine positions won't facilitate drainage from the peritoneal cavity.
CN: Physiological integrity; CNS: Physiological adaptation; CL: Application

CN: Client needs category   CNS: Client needs subcategory   CL: Cognitive level

96. In which inflammatory disease do most children show signs of painless bright or dark red rectal bleeding?
1. Crohn's disease
2. Meckel's diverticulum
3. Ruptured appendix
4. Ulcerative colitis

97. The nurse is assessing the laboratory results for a 9-year-old child hospitalized with severe vomiting and diarrhea. What's the <u>normal</u> serum potassium range in a child?
1. 4.5 to 7.2 mmol/L
2. 3.7 to 5.2 mmol/L
3. 3.5 to 5.8 mmol/L
4. 3.5 to 5.5 mmol/L

98. A 5-year-old child is admitted with diarrhea and vomiting for the last 2 days. Her vital signs are: temperature, 98.8° F (37.1° C); pulse, 132 beats/minute; respirations, 28 breaths/minute; and blood pressure, 88/56 mm Hg. The nurse notes poor skin turgor, dry mucous membranes, and tearless crying. What should be the next step in this child's care?
1. Obtain a stool specimen, along with hemocrit (HCT), complete blood count (CBC), and chemistries.
2. Implement nothing-by-mouth (NPO) status and begin an I.V. stat.
3. Begin offering an oral electrolyte solution.
4. Obtain a culture and sensitivity test before starting I.V. antibiotics.

99. A neonate is suspected of having a tracheoesophageal fistula (type III/C). Which sign would be seen on the <u>initial</u> assessment?
1. Excessive drooling
2. Excessive vomiting
3. Mottling
4. Polyhydramnios

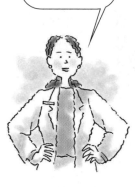

It's normal to have to give question 97 some serious thought.

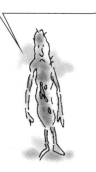

Thank you, thank you, thank you, for knowing the signs of severe dehydration.

96. 2. Acute and sometimes massive hemorrhage may occur in Meckel's diverticulum. There's no rectal bleeding with a ruptured appendix or Crohn's disease. Children with ulcerative colitis present with recurring diarrhea.
CN: Physiological integrity; CNS: Physiological adaptation; CL: Knowledge

97. 3. The normal potassium level in children ranges from 3.5 to 5.8 mmol/L. Levels of 4.5 to 7.2 mmol/L are observed in premature infants. Potassium levels of 3.7 to 5.2 mmol/L are observed in full-term infants. Potassium levels of 3.5 to 5.5 mmol/L are usually seen in adults.
CN: Physiological integrity; CNS: Reduction of risk potential; CL: Knowledge

98. 2. This child is showing signs of severe dehydration. The child should be put on NPO status in order to rest the bowel, and an I.V. should be started immediately to begin the rehydration process. A stool specimen, HCT, CBC, and chemistries, and I.V. antibiotics may be ordered, but these aren't the priority intervention. There's no reason to suspect that the child will need a blood culture at this time because her temperature isn't elevated.
CN: Physiological integrity; CNS: Basic care and comfort; CL: Analysis

99. 1. In type III/C tracheoesophageal fistula, the proximal end of the esophagus ends in a blind pouch and a fistula connects the distal end of the esophagus to the trachea. Saliva will pool in this pouch and cause the child to drool. Because the distal end of the esophagus is connected to the trachea, the neonate can't vomit, but he can aspirate, and stomach acid may go into the lungs through this fistula, causing pneumonitis. Mottling is a netlike reddish blue discoloration of the skin usually due to vascular contraction in response to hypothermia. The mother of a neonate with tracheoesophageal fistula may have had polyhydramnios.
CN: Physiological integrity; CNS: Physiological adaptation; CL: Application

CN: Client needs category   CNS: Client needs subcategory   CL: Cognitive level

100. When assessing a client suspected of having pyloric stenosis, which finding should the nurse expect?

1. An "olive" mass in the right upper quadrant
2. An "olive" mass in the left upper quadrant
3. A "sausage" mass in the right upper quadrant
4. A "sausage" mass in the left upper quadrant

101. The nurse caring for an infant with pyloric stenosis would expect which laboratory values?

1. pH, 7.30; chloride, 120 mEq/L
2. pH, 7.38; chloride, 110 mEq/L
3. pH, 7.43; chloride, 100 mEq/L
4. pH, 7.49; chloride, 90 mEq/L

102. Which nursing diagnosis has the <u>highest</u> priority in a 1-month-old infant admitted with projectile vomiting after feeding?

1. *Risk for deficient fluid volume*
2. *Risk for impaired parenting*
3. *Interrupted breast-feeding*
4. *Risk for infection*

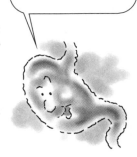

All this talk about "olives" and "sausages" is suddenly making me very hungry!

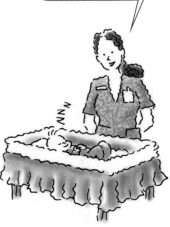

Question 102 is looking for the highest priority.

100. 1. Pyloric stenosis involves hypertrophy of the circular muscle fibers of the pylorus. This hypertrophy is palpable in the right upper quadrant of the abdomen. A "sausage" mass is palpable in the right upper quadrant in children with intussusception. A "sausage" mass in the left upper quadrant wouldn't indicate pyloric stenosis.

CN: Physiological integrity; CNS: Physiological adaptation; CL: Analysis

101. 4. Infants with pyloric stenosis vomit hydrochloric acid. This causes them to become alkalotic and hypochloremic. Normal serum pH is 7.35 to 7.45; levels above 7.45 represent alkalosis. The normal serum chloride level is 99 to 111 mEq/L; levels below 99 mEq/L represent hypochloremia.

CN: Physiological integrity; CNS: Physiological adaptation; CL: Application

102. 1. Projectile vomiting in an infant is a sign of pyloric stenosis, a condition that requires surgical intervention to correct. Because the infant has been vomiting, he is at risk for deficient fluid volume and fluid and electrolyte imbalances that must be corrected before surgery. Whenever an infant is hospitalized, the nursing diagnoses of *Risk for impaired parenting* and *Interrupted breast-feeding* may apply; however, they don't take priority over the diagnosis of *Risk for deficient fluid volume*. Following surgery, the infant is at risk for infection because the incision is near the diaper area.

CN: Physiological integrity; CNS: Reduction of risk potential; CL: Analysis

103. The nurse is teaching the parents of an infant undergoing repair for a cleft lip. Which instructions should the nurse give? Select all that apply:
1. Offer a pacifier as needed.
2. Lay the infant on his back or side to sleep.
3. Sit the infant up for each feeding.
4. Loosen the arm restraints every 4 hours.
5. Clean the suture line after each feeding by dabbing it with saline solution.
6. Give the infant extra care and support.

103. 2, 3, 5, 6. An infant with a repaired cleft lip should be put to sleep on his back or side to prevent trauma to the surgery site. He should be fed in the upright position with a syringe and attached tubing to prevent stress to the suture line from sucking. To prevent crusts and scarring, the suture line should be cleaned after each feeding by dabbing it with half-strength hydrogen peroxide or saline solution. The infant should receive extra care and support because he can't meet emotional needs by sucking. Extra care and support may also prevent crying, which stresses the suture line. Pacifiers shouldn't be used during the healing process because they stress the suture line. Arm restraints are used to keep the infant's hands away from the mouth and should be loosened every 2 hours.
CN: Physiological integrity; CNS: Reduction of risk potential; CL: Application

104. A 13-month-old is admitted to the pediatric unit with a diagnosis of gastroenteritis. The toddler has experienced vomiting and diarrhea for the past 3 days, and laboratory tests reveal that he's dehydrated. Which nursing interventions are correct to prevent further dehydration? Select all that apply:
1. Encouraging the child to eat a balanced diet
2. Giving clear liquids in small amounts
3. Giving milk in small amounts
4. Encouraging the child to eat nonsalty soups and broths
5. Monitoring the I.V. solution per the physician's order
6. Withholding all solid food and liquids until the symptoms pass

104. 2, 4, 5. A child experiencing nausea and vomiting wouldn't be able to tolerate a regular diet. He should be given sips of clear liquids, and the diet should be advanced as tolerated. Unsalted soups and broths are appropriate clear liquids. I.V. fluids should be monitored to maintain the fluid status and help to rehydrate the child. Milk shouldn't be given because it can worsen the child's diarrhea. Solid foods may be withheld throughout the acute phase; however, clear fluids should be encouraged in small amounts (3 to 4 tablespoons every half hour).
CN: Physiological integrity; CNS: Basic care and comfort; CL: Application

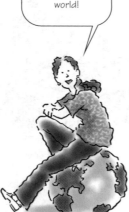

You're finished! You should feel on top of the world!

105. A 5-year-old is admitted to the hospital for a tonsillectomy. After the surgery, the physician orders a clear liquid diet. The nurse is correct in giving the child which items? Select all that apply:
1. Cream of chicken soup
2. Orange juice
3. Ice cream
4. Apple juice
5. Lime gelatin
6. Chicken broth

105. 4, 5, 6. Clear liquids include clear broth, gelatin, clear juices, water, and ice chips. Cream of chicken soup, orange juice, and ice cream are included in a full liquid diet.
CN: Physiological integrity; CNS: Basic care and comfort; CL: Application

CN: Client needs category   CNS: Client needs subcategory   CL: Cognitive level

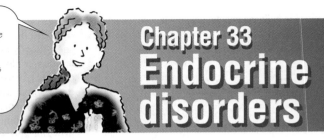

Caring for a child with an endocrine system disorder can be overwhelming. To get started on the right track, check out the Web site of the Juvenile Diabetes Research Foundation at *www.jdrf.org/*. Go for it!

Chapter 33
Endocrine disorders

1. After explaining the causes of hypothyroidism to the parents of a newly diagnosed infant, the nurse should recognize that further education is needed when the parents ask which question?
1. "So, hypothyroidism can be only temporary, right?"
2. "Are you saying that hypothyroidism is caused by a problem in the way the thyroid gland develops?"
3. "Do you mean that hypothyroidism may be caused by a problem in the way the body makes thyroxine?"
4. "So, hypothyroidism can be treated by exposing our baby to a special light, right?"

2. The nurse understands that transient hypothyroidism can result from which factor?
1. Intrauterine transfer of insulin
2. Placental transfer of antibodies
3. Placental transfer of teratogens
4. Intrauterine transfer of expectorants

3. When a nurse is teaching parents of a neonate newly diagnosed with hypothyroidism, which statement should be included?
1. A large goiter in a neonate doesn't present a problem.
2. Preterm neonates usually aren't affected by hypothyroidism.
3. Usually, the neonate exhibits obvious signs of hypothyroidism.
4. The severity of the disorder depends on the amount of thyroid tissue present.

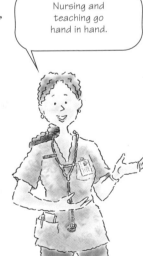

Nursing and teaching go hand in hand.

1. 4. Congenital hypothyroidism can be permanent or transient and may result from a defective thyroid gland or an enzymatic defect in thyroxine synthesis. Only the last question, which refers to phototherapy for physiologic jaundice, indicates that the parents need more information.
CN: Psychosocial integrity; CNS: None; CL: Analysis

2. 4. Intrauterine transfer of antithyroid drugs and expectorants given for asthma are factors associated with transient hypothyroidism. The other choices don't affect hypothyroidism.
CN: Health promotion and maintenance; CNS: None; CL: Knowledge

3. 4. The severity of the disorder depends on the amount of thyroid tissue present. The more thyroid tissue present, the less severe the disorder. Usually, the neonate doesn't exhibit obvious signs of the disorder because of maternal circulation. A large goiter in a neonate could possibly occlude the airway and lead to obstruction. Preterm neonates are usually affected by hypothyroidism as a result of hypothalamic and pituitary immaturity.
CN: Physiological integrity; CNS: Physiological adaptation; CL: Application

CN: Client needs category   CNS: Client needs subcategory   CL: Cognitive level

4. When collecting data on an infant, which condition would alert the nurse as a subtle sign of hypothyroidism?
1. Diarrhea
2. Lethargy
3. Severe jaundice
4. Tachycardia

5. When observing a neonate with congenital hypothyroidism, the nurse would be alert for which complication as the <u>most serious</u> consequence of this condition?
1. Anemia
2. Cyanosis
3. Retarded bone age
4. Delayed central nervous system (CNS) development

6. When counseling parents of a neonate with congenital hypothyroidism, the nurse understands that the severity of the intellectual deficit is related to which parameter?
1. Duration of the condition before treatment
2. Degree of hypothermia
3. Cranial malformations
4. Thyroxine (T$_4$) level at diagnosis

7. Which statement should be included in an explanation of the diagnostic evaluation of neonates for congenital hypothyroidism?
1. Tests are mandatory in all states.
2. An arterial blood test is preferred.
3. Tests shouldn't be performed until after discharge.
4. Blood tests should be done after the first month of life.

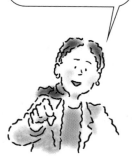

In question 5, the phrase *most serious* means you must prioritize.

4. 2. Subtle signs of this disorder that may be seen shortly after birth include lethargy, poor feeding, prolonged jaundice, respiratory difficulty, cyanosis, constipation, and bradycardia. Diarrhea in the neonate isn't normal and isn't associated with this disorder. Severe jaundice needs immediate attention by the primary health care provider and isn't a subtle sign. Tachycardia typically occurs in hyperthyroidism, not hypothyroidism.
CN: Physiological integrity; CNS: Physiological adaptation; CL: Comprehension

5. 4. The most serious consequence of congenital hypothyroidism is delayed development of the CNS, which leads to severe mental retardation. The other choices occur but aren't the most serious consequences.
CN: Safe, effective care environment; CNS: Coordinated care; CL: Comprehension

6. 1. The severity of the intellectual deficit is related to the degree of hypothyroidism and the duration of the condition before treatment. Cranial malformations don't affect the severity of the intellectual deficit, nor does the degree of hypothermia as it relates to hypothyroidism. It isn't the specific T$_4$ level at diagnosis that affects the intellect but how long the client has been hospitalized.
CN: Health promotion and maintenance; CNS: None; CL: Application

7. 1. Heelstick blood tests are mandatory in all states and are usually done on neonates between ages 2 and 6 days. Typically, specimens are taken before the neonate is discharged from the hospital; the test is included with other tests that screen the neonate for errors of metabolism.
CN: Health promotion and maintenance; CNS: None; CL: Application

CN: Client needs category   CNS: Client needs subcategory   CL: Cognitive level

8. Which results would indicate to the nurse the possibility that a neonate has congenital hypothyroidism?
1. High thyroxine (T_4) level and low thyroid-stimulating hormone (TSH) level
2. Low T_4 level and high TSH level
3. Normal TSH level and high T_4 level
4. Normal T_4 level and low TSH level

9. The nurse is teaching parents about therapeutic management of their neonate diagnosed with congenital hypothyroidism. Which response by a parent would indicate the need for further teaching?
1. "My baby will need regular measurements of his thyroxine levels."
2. "Treatment involves lifelong thyroid hormone replacement therapy."
3. "Treatment should begin as soon as possible after diagnosis is made."
4. "As my baby grows, his thyroid gland will mature and he won't need medications."

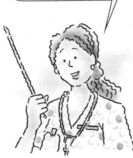

In question 9, the phrase *further teaching* indicates that you're looking for an incorrect statement.

10. Which comment made by the mother of a neonate at her 2-week office visit should alert the nurse to suspect congenital hypothyroidism?
1. "My baby is unusually quiet and good."
2. "My baby seems to study my face during feeding time."
3. "After feedings, my baby pulls her legs up and cries."
4. "My baby seems to be a yellowish color."

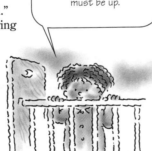

If I'm too quiet and too good, something must be up.

11. Which statement should be included when educating a mother about giving levothyroxine (Synthroid) to her neonate after a diagnosis of hypothyroidism is made?
1. The drug has a bitter taste.
2. The pill shouldn't be crushed.
3. Never put the medication in formula or juice.
4. If a dose is missed, double the dose the next day.

8. 2. Screening results that show a low T_4 level and a high TSH level indicate congenital hypothyroidism and the need for further tests to determine the cause of the disease.
CN: Physiological integrity; CNS: Reduction of risk potential; CL: Application

9. 4. Treatment involves lifelong thyroid hormone replacement therapy that begins as soon as possible after diagnosis to abolish all signs of hypothyroidism and to reestablish normal physical and mental development. The drug of choice is synthetic levothyroxine (Synthroid or Levothroid). Regular measurements of thyroxine levels are important in ensuring optimum treatment.
CN: Physiological integrity; CNS: Physiological adaptation; CL: Application

10. 1. Parental remarks about an unusually "quiet and good" neonate together with any of the early physical manifestations should lead to a suspicion of hypothyroidism, which requires a referral for specific tests. The neonate likes looking at the human face and should show this interest at age 2 weeks. If the neonate is pulling her legs up and crying after feedings, she might be showing signs of colic. If a neonate begins to look yellow in color, hyperbilirubinemia may be the cause.
CN: Health promotion and maintenance; CNS: None; CL: Application

11. 4. If a dose is missed, twice the dose should be given the next day. The importance of compliance with the drug regimen must be emphasized in order for the neonate to achieve normal growth and development. Because the drug is flavorless, it can be crushed and added to formula, water, or food.
CN: Physiological integrity; CNS: Pharmacological therapies; CL: Application

CN: Client needs category   CNS: Client needs subcategory   CL: Cognitive level

12. When teaching the parents about signs that indicate levothyroxine (Synthroid) overdose, which comment by a parent indicates the need for <u>further teaching</u>?
1. "Irritability is a sign of overdose."
2. "If my baby's heartbeat is fast, I should count it."
3. "If my baby loses weight, I should be concerned."
4. "I shouldn't worry if my baby doesn't sleep very much."

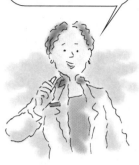

Watch out! Question 12 is another further teaching question.

12. 4. Parents need to be aware of signs indicating overdose, such as rapid pulse, dyspnea, irritability, insomnia, fever, sweating, and weight loss. The parents would be given acceptable parameters for the heart rate and weight loss or gain. If the baby is experiencing a heart rate or weight loss outside of the acceptable parameters, the primary health care provider should be called.
CN: Physiological integrity; CNS: Pharmacological therapies; CL: Analysis

13. A nurse should recognize that exophthalmos (protruding eyeballs) may occur in children with which condition?
1. Hypothyroidism
2. Hyperthyroidism
3. Hypoparathyroidism
4. Hyperparathyroidism

13. 2. Exophthalmos occurs when there's an overproduction of thyroid hormone. This sign should alert the primary health care provider to follow up with further testing.
CN: Health promotion and maintenance; CNS: None; CL: Application

14. A nurse would be alert for which symptom as a common clinical manifestation of juvenile hypothyroidism?
1. Accelerated growth
2. Diarrhea
3. Dry skin
4. Insomnia

14. 3. Children with hypothyroidism have dry skin. The other choices aren't evident in children with juvenile hypothyroidism.
CN: Health promotion and maintenance; CNS: None; CL: Comprehension

15. A nurse is observing an infant with thyroid hormone deficiency. Which signs would the nurse <u>commonly</u> observe?
1. Tachycardia, profuse perspiration, and diarrhea
2. Lethargy, feeding difficulties, and constipation
3. Hypertonia, small fontanels, and moist skin
4. Dermatitis, dry skin, and round face

Question 16 is asking for the *most appropriate* behavior that should be encouraged. In other words, *prioritize!*

15. 2. Hypothyroidism results from inadequate thyroid production to meet an infant's needs. Clinical signs include feeding difficulties, prolonged physiologic jaundice, lethargy, and constipation.
CN: Physiological integrity; CNS: Physiological adaptation; CL: Analysis

16. When counseling parents of a neonate with congenital hypothyroidism, the nurse should encourage which behavior as the <u>most appropriate</u>?
1. Seeking professional genetic counseling
2. Retracing the family tree for others born with this condition
3. Talking to relatives who have gone through a similar experience
4. Waiting until the neonate is age 1 year before obtaining counseling

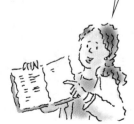

16. 1. Seeking professional genetic counseling is the best option for parents who have a neonate with a genetic disorder. Retracing the family tree and talking to relatives won't help the parents to become better educated about the disorder. Education about the disorder should occur as soon as the parents are ready so they'll understand the genetic implications for future children.
CN: Safe, effective care environment; CNS: Coordinated care; CL: Application

CN: Client needs category CNS: Client needs subcategory CL: Cognitive level

17. A nurse is teaching an adolescent with type 1 diabetes about the disease. Which instruction by the nurse about how to prevent hypoglycemia would be most appropriate for the adolescent?
　　1. "Limit participation in planned exercise activities that involve competition."
　　2. "Carry crackers or fruit to eat before or during periods of increased activity."
　　3. "Increase the insulin dosage before planned or unplanned strenuous exercise."
　　4. "Check your blood glucose level before exercising, and eat a protein snack if the level is elevated."

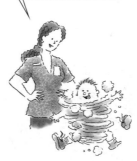

Caring for children with diabetes can be a real challenge.

18. When caring for a child with diabetes, the nurse would be alert for which change when the child is more physically active?
　　1. Increased food intake
　　2. Decreased food intake
　　3. Decreased risk of insulin shock
　　4. Increased risk of hyperglycemia

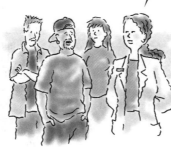

Always consider the age of your client and how diabetes may affect his lifestyle.

19. When helping the adolescent deal with diabetes, the nurse understands which characteristic about this age-group?
　　1. Want to be an individual
　　2. Need to be like their peers
　　3. Are preoccupied with future plans
　　4. Able to teach peers about the seriousness of the disease

20. An adolescent with diabetes tells the community nurse that he has recently started drinking alcohol on the weekends. Which action would be most appropriate for the nurse to take?
　　1. Recommend referral to counseling.
　　2. Make the adolescent promise to stop drinking.
　　3. Discuss with the adolescent why he has started drinking.
　　4. Teach the adolescent about the effects of alcohol on diabetes.

17. 2. Hypoglycemia can usually be prevented if an adolescent with diabetes eats more food before or during exercise. Because exercise with adolescents isn't commonly planned, carrying additional carbohydrate foods is a good preventive measure.
CN: Health promotion and maintenance; CNS: None; CL: Application

18. 1. If a child is more active at one time of the day than another, food or insulin should be altered to meet the child's activity pattern. Food intake should be increased when a child with diabetes is more physically active. Exercise lowers blood sugar by increasing carbohydrate metabolism as well as sensitivity to insulin. There would be an increased risk of insulin shock if the child didn't take in more food, and the child would become hypoglycemic, not hyperglycemic.
CN: Physiological integrity; CNS: Reduction of risk potential; CL: Comprehension

19. 2. Adolescents appear to have the most difficulty adjusting to diabetes. Adolescence is a time when being "perfect" and being like one's peers are emphasized and, to adolescents, having diabetes means they're different.
CN: Health promotion and maintenance; CNS: None; CL: Comprehension

20. 4. Ingestion of alcohol inhibits the release of glycogen from the liver, resulting in hypoglycemia. Teens who drink alcohol may become hypoglycemic. Manifesting behaviors that are similar to intoxication include shakiness, combativeness, slurred speech, and loss of consciousness. Recommending that he see a counselor is a good option but you should first teach about the effects of his alcohol consumption. You can't stop an adolescent from doing something if he doesn't understand why it's wrong. Discussing the reason for the adolescent's drinking should be left up to the counselor.
CN: Health promotion and maintenance; CNS: None; CL: Application

CN: Client needs category　CNS: Client needs subcategory　CL: Cognitive level

21. A child has experienced symptoms of hypoglycemia and has eaten sugar cubes. The nurse expects to follow this rapid-releasing sugar with which food?
1. Fruit juices
2. Six glasses of water
3. Foods that are high in protein
4. Complex carbohydrates and protein

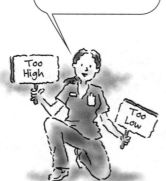

If you know the definitions of hypo and hyper, it can help you with a bunch of questions.

22. Which symptom would lead the nurse to suspect possible hypoglycemia?
1. Irritability
2. Drowsiness
3. Abdominal pain
4. Nausea and vomiting

23. Which observation about diabetic ketoacidosis is most accurate?
1. It's a normal outcome of diabetes.
2. It's a life-threatening situation.
3. It's a situation that can easily be treated at home.
4. It's a situation that's best treated in the pediatrician's office.

24. Which guideline is appropriate when teaching an 11-year-old child recently diagnosed with diabetes about insulin injections?
1. The parents don't need to be involved in learning this procedure.
2. Self-injection techniques aren't usually taught until the child reaches age 16.
3. At age 11, the child should be old enough to give most of his own injections.
4. Self-injection techniques should be taught only when the child can reach all injection sites.

21. 4. When a child exhibits signs of hypoglycemia, most cases can be treated with a simple concentrated sugar, such as honey or sugar cubes, that can be held in the mouth for a short time. This will elevate the blood glucose level and alleviate the symptoms. The simpler the carbohydrate, the more rapidly it will be absorbed. A complex carbohydrate and protein, such as a slice of bread or a cracker spread with peanut butter, should follow the rapid-releasing sugar or the client may become hypoglycemic again.
CN: Health promotion and maintenance; CNS: None; CL: Application

22. 1. Signs of hypoglycemia include irritability, shaky feeling, hunger, headache, and dizziness. Drowsiness, abdominal pain, nausea, and vomiting are signs of *hyper*glycemia.
CN: Physiological integrity; CNS: Physiological adaptation; CL: Comprehension

23. 2. Diabetic ketoacidosis, the most complete state of insulin deficiency, is a life-threatening situation. The child should be admitted to an intensive care facility for management, which consists of rapid assessment, adequate insulin to reduce the elevated blood glucose level, fluids to overcome dehydration, and electrolyte replacement (especially potassium).
CN: Physiological integrity; CNS: Reduction of risk potential; CL: Comprehension

24. 3. The parents must supervise and manage the child's therapeutic program, but the child should assume responsibility for self-management as soon as he can. Children can learn to collect their own blood for glucose testing at a relatively young age (4 to 5 years), and most can check their blood glucose level and administer insulin at about age 9. Some children can do it earlier.
CN: Health promotion and maintenance; CNS: None; CL: Application

25. Which blood glucose value would alert the nurse to the possibility of diabetic ketoacidosis?
1. 150 mg/dl
2. 300 mg/dl
3. 450 mg/dl
4. 600 mg/dl

26. A nurse should recognize which symptom as a cardinal sign of diabetes mellitus?
1. Nausea
2. Seizure
3. Hyperactivity
4. Frequent urination

27. The parent of a child with diabetes asks a nurse why blood glucose monitoring is needed. The nurse should base her reply on which premise?
1. This is an easier method of testing.
2. This is a less expensive method of testing.
3. This allows children the ability to better manage their diabetes.
4. This gives children a greater sense of control over their diabetes.

28. To increase the adolescent's compliance with treatment for diabetes mellitus, the nurse should attempt which strategy?
1. Provide for a special diet in the high school cafeteria.
2. Clarify the adolescent's values to promote involvement in care.
3. Identify energy requirements for participation in sports activities.
4. Educate the adolescent about long-term consequences of poor metabolic control.

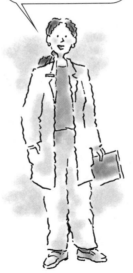

Teaching clients how to help manage their own conditions is a common subject on the NCLEX.

25. 2. Diabetic ketoacidosis is determined by the presence of hyperglycemia (blood glucose measurement of 300 mg/dl or higher), accompanied by acetone breath, dehydration, weak and rapid pulse, and decreased level of consciousness.
CN: Physiological integrity; CNS: Physiological adaptation; CL: Comprehension

26. 4. Polyphagia, polyuria, polydipsia, and weight loss are cardinal signs of diabetes mellitus. Other signs include irritability, shortened attention span, lowered frustration tolerance, fatigue, dry skin, blurred vision, sores that are slow to heal, and flushed skin.
CN: Health promotion and maintenance; CNS: None; CL: Knowledge

27. 3. Blood glucose monitoring improves diabetes management and is used successfully by children from the onset of their diabetes. By testing their own blood, children can change their insulin regimen to maintain their glucose level in the normoglycemic range of 80 to 120 mg/dl. This allows them to better manage their diabetes.
CN: Health promotion and maintenance; CNS: None; CL: Application

28. 2. Adolescent compliance with diabetes management may be hampered by dependence versus independence conflicts and ego development. Attempts to have the adolescent clarify personal values fosters compliance. Providing for a special meal in the school cafeteria isn't feasible and doesn't guarantee that the adolescent would eat it. The question doesn't provide sufficient information about the adolescent's sports activity. An adolescent is usually concerned only with the present, not the future.
CN: Health promotion and maintenance; CNS: None; CL: Application

CN: Client needs category   CNS: Client needs subcategory   CL: Cognitive level

29. A child with type 1 diabetes tells the nurse she feels shaky. The nurse assesses the child's skin to be pale and sweaty. Which action should the nurse initiate <u>immediately</u>?
   1. Give supplemental insulin.
   2. Have the child eat a glucose tablet.
   3. Administer glucagon subcutaneously.
   4. Offer the child a complex carbohydrate snack.

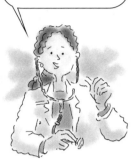

The word *immediately* signals a need for you to prioritize.

30. The parents of a child diagnosed with diabetes ask the nurse about maintaining metabolic control during a minor illness with loss of appetite. Which nursing response is appropriate?
   1. "Decrease the child's insulin by one-half of the usual dose during the course of the illness."
   2. "Call your primary health care provider to arrange hospitalization."
   3. "Give increased amounts of clear liquids to prevent dehydration."
   4. "Substitute calorie-containing liquids for uneaten solid food."

31. Which criteria would the nurse use to measure good metabolic control in a child with diabetes mellitus?
   1. Five to eight episodes of severe hyperglycemia in a month
   2. Infrequent occurrences of mild hypoglycemia reactions
   3. Hemoglobin A values less than 12%
   4. Growth below the 15th percentile

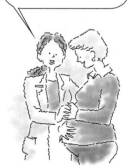

Poorly controlled maternal diabetes can result in congenital anomalies.

32. Which congenital anomaly is most commonly associated with poorly controlled maternal diabetes?
   1. Cataracts
   2. Low-set ears
   3. Cardiac malformations
   4. Cleft lip and palate deformities

29. 2. These are symptoms of hypoglycemia. Rapid treatment involves giving the alert child a glucose tablet (4 mg dextrose) or, if unavailable, a glass of glucose-containing liquid. Either would be followed by a complex carbohydrate snack and protein. Giving supplemental insulin would be contraindicated because that would lower the blood glucose even more. Glucagon would be given only if there were a risk of aspiration with oral glucose, such as if the child were semiconscious.
CN: Safe, effective care environment; CNS: Coordinated care; CL: Application

30. 4. Calorie-containing liquids can help to maintain more normal blood glucose levels as well as decrease the danger of dehydration. The child with diabetes should always take *at least* the usual dose of insulin during an illness based on more frequent blood glucose checks. During an illness that involves vomiting or loss of appetite, NPH insulin is cut in half or stopped altogether and regular insulin is given according to home glucose monitoring results. Minor illnesses usually don't require hospitalization. Giving increased amounts of clear liquids may prevent dehydration but he should try to maintain his caloric intake during illness.
CN: Safe, effective care environment; CNS: Coordinated care; CL: Application

31. 2. Criteria for good metabolic control generally includes few episodes of hypoglycemia or hyperglycemia, hemoglobin A values less than 8%, and normal growth and development.
CN: Health promotion and maintenance; CNS: None; CL: Application

32. 3. Cardiac and central nervous system anomalies, along with neural tube defects, skeletal abnormalities, and GI anomalies, are most likely to occur in uncontrolled maternal diabetes.
CN: Health promotion and maintenance; CNS: None; CL: Knowledge

CN: Client needs category   CNS: Client needs subcategory   CL: Cognitive level

33. Which condition could possibly cause <u>hypoglycemia</u>?
1. Too little insulin
2. Mild illness with fever
3. Excessive exercise without a carbohydrate snack
4. Eating ice cream and cake to celebrate a birthday

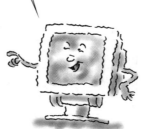

Comparing signs of hypoglycemia and hyperglycemia is a common NCLEX subject.

33. 3. Excessive exercise without a carbohydrate snack could cause hypoglycemia. The other options describe situations that cause *hyper*glycemia.

CN: Health promotion and maintenance; CNS: None; CL: Application

34. Which assessment factor is the <u>best</u> indicator of a client's diabetic control during the preceding 2 to 3 months?
1. Fasting glucose level
2. Oral glucose tolerance test
3. Glycosylated hemoglobin level
4. The client's record of glucose monitoring

34. 3. A glycosylated hemoglobin level provides an overview of a person's blood glucose level over the previous 2 to 3 months. Glycosylated hemoglobin values are reported as a percentage of the total hemoglobin within an erythrocyte. The time frame is based on the fact that the usual life span of an erythrocyte is 2 to 3 months; a random blood sample, therefore, will theoretically give samples of erythrocytes for this same period. The other options won't indicate a true picture of the person's blood glucose level over the previous 2 to 3 months.

CN: Health promotion and maintenance; CNS: None; CL: Application

35. A client has received diet instruction as part of his treatment plan for type 1 diabetes. Which statement by the client indicates to the nurse that he needs <u>additional instructions</u>?
1. "I will need a bedtime snack because I take an evening dose of NPH insulin."
2. "I can eat whatever I want as long as I cover the calories with sufficient insulin."
3. "I can have an occasional low-calorie drink as long as I include it in my meal plan."
4. "I should eat meals as scheduled, even if I'm not hungry, to prevent hypoglycemia."

Additional instructions is another way of saying further teaching. Both types of questions ask you to find an incorrect statement.

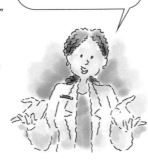

35. 2. The goal of diet therapy in diabetes mellitus is to attain and maintain ideal body weight. Each client will be prescribed a specific caloric intake and insulin regimen to help accomplish this goal.

CN: Physiological integrity; CNS: Basic care and comfort; CL: Analysis

36. Which symptom is a sign of <u>hyperglycemia</u>?
1. Rapid heart rate
2. Headache
3. Hunger
4. Thirst

36. 4. Thirst (polydipsia) is one of the symptoms of hyperglycemia. Rapid heart rate, headache, and hunger are signs and symptoms of *hypo*glycemia.

CN: Physiological integrity; CNS: Physiological adaptation; CL: Knowledge

37. A client is learning to mix regular insulin and NPH insulin in the same syringe. Which action, if performed by the client, would indicate the need for <u>further teaching</u>?
1. Withdraws the NPH insulin first
2. Injects air into the NPH insulin bottle first
3. After drawing up the first insulin, removes air bubbles from the syringe
4. Injects an amount of air equal to the desired dose of insulin

38. A client is diagnosed with type 1 diabetes. The primary health care provider prescribes an insulin regimen of regular insulin and NPH insulin administered subcutaneously each morning. How soon after administration will the onset of regular insulin begin?
1. Within 5 minutes
2. 30 minutes to 1 hour
3. 1 to 1½ hours
4. 4 to 8 hours

39. When collecting data on a neonate for signs of diabetes insipidus, a nurse should recognize which symptom as a sign of this disorder?
1. Hyponatremia
2. Jaundice
3. Polyuria and polydipsia
4. Hypochloremia

40. Which sign or symptom would a nurse commonly observe <u>first</u> in an infant with diabetes insipidus?
1. Dehydration
2. Inability to be aroused
3. Extreme hunger relieved by frequent feedings of milk
4. Irritability relieved with feedings of water but not milk

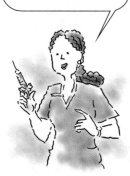

It's important to know how and when different types of insulin react.

37. 1. Regular insulin is *always* withdrawn first so it won't become contaminated with NPH insulin. The client is instructed to inject air into the NPH insulin bottle equal to the amount of insulin to be withdrawn because there will be regular insulin in the syringe and he won't be able to inject air when he needs to withdraw the NPH. It's necessary to remove the air bubbles from the syringe to ensure a correct dosage before drawing up the second insulin.
CN: Physiological integrity; CNS: Pharmacological therapies; CL: Application

38. 2. Regular insulin's onset is 30 minutes to 1 hour, peak is 2 to 4 hours, and duration is 8 to 12 hours. Lispro insulin has an onset within 5 minutes. NPH insulin has an onset within 1 to 1½ hours, and extended insulin zinc suspension (Ultralente) is the longest acting, with an onset of 4 to 8 hours.
CN: Physiological integrity; CNS: Pharmacological therapies; CL: Application

39. 3. The cardinal signs of diabetes insipidus are polyuria and polydipsia. Hypernatremia, not hyponatremia, occurs with diabetes insipidus. Jaundice occurs because of abnormal bilirubin metabolism, not diabetes insipidus. Hyperchloremia, not hypochloremia, occurs with diabetes insipidus.
CN: Physiological integrity; CNS: Physiological adaptation; CL: Application

40. 4. An initial symptom of diabetes insipidus in an infant is irritability relieved with feedings of water but not milk. Dehydration and the inability to be aroused are late signs.
CN: Health promotion and maintenance; CNS: None; CL: Application

41. A nurse is helping parents understand when treatments of growth hormone replacement will end. Which statement should be included?

1. The dosage of growth hormone will decrease as the child's age increases.
2. The dosage of growth hormone will increase as the time of epiphyseal closure nears.
3. After giving growth hormone replacement for 1 year, the dose will be tapered.
4. Growth hormone replacement can't be abruptly stopped. Decreasing growth hormone replacement must be spread out over several months.

42. The nurse is explaining diabetes insipidus to an infant's parents. When explaining the diagnostic test that's used, which comment by the parents would indicate an <u>understanding</u> of the diagnostic test?

1. "Fluids will be offered every 2 hours."
2. "My infant's fluid intake will be restricted."
3. "I won't change anything about my infant's intake."
4. "Formula will be restricted, but glucose water is OK."

43. A nurse should anticipate which physiologic response in an infant being tested for diabetes insipidus?

1. Increase in urine output
2. Decrease in urine output
3. No effect on urine output
4. Increase in urine specific gravity

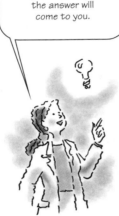

Think about question 42 and the answer will come to you.

41. 2. Dosage of growth hormone is increased as the time of epiphyseal closure nears to gain the best advantage of the growth hormone. The medication is then stopped. There's no tapering of the dose.
CN: Physiological integrity; CNS: Pharmacological therapies; CL: Application

42. 2. The simplest test used to diagnose diabetes insipidus is restriction of oral fluids and observation of consequent changes in urine volume and concentration. A weight loss of 3% to 5% indicates severe dehydration, and the test should be terminated at this point. This is done in the hospital, and the infant is watched closely.
CN: Health promotion and maintenance; CNS: None; CL: Application

43. 3. In diabetes insipidus, fluid restriction for diagnostic testing has little or no effect on urine formation but causes weight loss from dehydration.
CN: Physiological integrity; CNS: Physiological adaptation; CL: Application

44. If an infant has a positive test result for diabetes insipidus, the nurse should expect the primary health care provider to order a test dose of which medication?

1. Human placental lactogen (HPL)
2. Glucose loading test
3. Corticotropin
4. Aqueous vasopressin (Pitressin)

45. In teaching the parents of an infant diagnosed with diabetes insipidus, the nurse should include which treatment?

1. The need for blood products
2. Antihypertensive medications
3. Hormone replacement
4. Fluid restrictions

46. When providing information about treatment of diabetes insipidus to parents, a nurse explains the use of nasal spray and injections. Which indication might <u>deter</u> a parent from choosing nasal spray treatment?

1. Applications must be repeated every 8 to 12 hours.
2. Applications must be repeated every 2 to 4 hours.
3. Nasal sprays can't be used in infants.
4. Measurements are too difficult.

We're nearing the halfway point. Keep moving toward the goal.

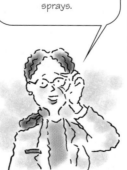

Look closely. Although the word *deter* sounds like a negative, question 46 actually asks you to identify a true characteristic of nasal sprays.

44. 4. If the fluid restriction test is positive, the child should be given a test dose of injected aqueous vasopressin, which should alleviate the polyuria and polydipsia. Unresponsiveness to exogenous vasopressin usually indicates nephrogenic diabetes insipidus. The other choices are used to determine other types of endocrine disorders. HPL is a hormone secreted by the placenta, and its level in the blood assesses placental function. Glucose loading test or growth hormone suppression test evaluates baseline levels of growth hormone. Administration of corticotropin measures pituitary gland function.
CN: Physiological integrity; CNS: Pharmacological therapies; CL: Knowledge

45. 3. The usual treatment for diabetes insipidus is hormone replacement with vasopressin or desmopressin acetate (DDAVP). Blood products shouldn't be needed. No problem with hypertension is associated with this condition, and fluids shouldn't be restricted.
CN: Physiological integrity; CNS: Pharmacological therapies; CL: Knowledge

46. 1. Applications of nasal spray used to treat diabetes insipidus must be repeated every 8 to 12 hours; injections, although quite painful, last for 48 to 72 hours. The nasal spray must be timed for adequate night sleep. Nasal sprays have been used in infants with diabetes insipidus and are dispensed in premeasured intranasal inhalers, eliminating the need for measuring doses.
CN: Physiological integrity; CNS: Pharmacological therapies; CL: Analysis

47. A nurse is teaching the parents of an infant with diabetes insipidus about an injectable drug used to treat the disorder. Which statement made by a parent would indicate the need for further teaching?
1. "I must hold the medication under warm running water for 10 to 15 minutes before administering it."
2. "The medication must be shaken vigorously before being drawn up into the syringe."
3. "Small brown particles must be seen in the suspension."
4. "I will store this medication in the refrigerator."

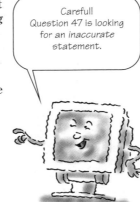

Careful!
Question 47 is looking for an inaccurate statement.

47. 4. The medication should be stored at room temperature. When giving injectable vasopressin, it must be thoroughly resuspended in the oil by being held under warm running water for 10 to 15 minutes and shaken vigorously before being drawn into the syringe. If this isn't done, the oil may be injected minus the drug. Small brown particles, which indicate drug dispersion, must be seen in the suspension.
CN: Physiological integrity; CNS: Pharmacological therapies; CL: Application

48. When teaching parents of an infant newly diagnosed with diabetes insipidus, which statement by a parent indicates a good understanding of this condition?
1. " When my infant stabilizes, I won't have to worry about giving hormone medication."
2. " I don't have to measure the amount of fluid intake that I give my infant."
3. " I realize that treatment for diabetes insipidus is lifelong."
4. "My infant will outgrow this condition."

48. 3. Diabetes insipidus requires lifelong treatment. The amount of fluid intake is important and must be measured with the infant's output to monitor the medication regimen. The infant won't outgrow this condition.
CN: Safe, effective care environment; CNS: Coordinated care; CL: Application

49. The nurse understands that diabetes insipidus involves which glandular dysfunction?
1. Thyroid hyperfunction
2. Pituitary hypofunction
3. Pituitary hyperfunction
4. Parathyroid hypofunction

49. 2. Diabetes insipidus is the principal disorder caused by posterior pituitary hypofunction, not hyperfunction. The disorder results from hyposecretion of antidiuretic hormone, producing a state of uncontrolled diuresis. Diabetes insipidus doesn't involve the thyroid or parathyroid glands.
CN: Health promotion and maintenance; CNS: None; CL: Knowledge

50. After the nurse has explained the causes of diabetes insipidus to the parents, which statement made by a parent indicates the need for further teaching?

1. "This condition could be familial or congenital."
2. "Drinking alcohol during my pregnancy caused this condition."
3. "My child might have a tumor that's causing these symptoms."
4. "An infection such as meningitis may be the reason my child has diabetes insipidus."

50. 2. Drinking alcohol during pregnancy can lead to a neonate born with fetal alcohol syndrome but has no known effect on diabetes insipidus. The other options are possible causes of diabetes insipidus.

CN: Physiological integrity; CNS: Physiological adaptation; CL: Application

51. Which assessment finding would alert the nurse to <u>change</u> the intranasal route for vasopressin administration?

1. Mucous membrane irritation
2. Severe coughing
3. Nosebleeds
4. Pneumonia

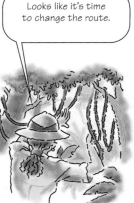

Looks like it's time to change the route.

51. 1. Mucous membrane irritation caused by a cold or allergy renders the intranasal route unreliable. Severe coughing, pneumonia, or nosebleeds shouldn't interfere with the intranasal route.

CN: Physiological integrity; CNS: Pharmacological therapies; CL: Application

52. The nurse should include which in-home management instruction for a child who's receiving desmopressin acetate (DDAVP) for symptomatic control of diabetes insipidus?

1. Give DDAVP only when urine output begins to decrease.
2. Clean skin with alcohol before applying the DDAVP dermal patch.
3. Increase the DDAVP dose if polyuria occurs just before the next scheduled dose.
4. Call the primary health care provider for an alternate route of DDAVP when the child has an upper respiratory infection (URI) or allergic rhinitis.

52. 4. Excessive nasal mucus associated with URI or allergic rhinitis may interfere with DDAVP absorption because it's given intranasally. Parents should be instructed to contact the primary health care provider for advice in altering the hormone dose during times when nasal mucus may be increased. To avoid over-medicating the child, the DDAVP dose should remain unchanged, even if there's polyuria just before the next dose.

CN: Safe, effective care environment; CNS: Coordinated care; CL: Application

53. A nurse is caring for a client with suspected hypopituitarism. Which sign or symptom of this condition would the nurse <u>most</u> commonly observe?

1. Sleep disturbance
2. Polyuria
3. Polydipsia
4. Short stature

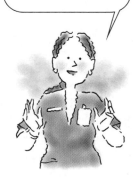

The long and short of it is... you're doing great.

53. 4. The most common sign in most instances of hypopituitarism is short stature. Sleep disturbance may indicate thyrotoxicosis. Polydipsia and polyuria may be indications of diabetes mellitus or diabetes insipidus.

CN: Physiological integrity; CNS: Physiological adaptation; CL: Application

CN: Client needs category   CNS: Client needs subcategory   CL: Cognitive level

54. Which statement made to the nurse by the parents of a child with hypopituitarism would indicate the need for <u>further teaching</u>?
1. "This disorder may be familial."
2. "There's no genetic basis for this disorder."
3. "This disorder may be secondary to hypothalamic deficiency."
4. "There may be other disorders related to pituitary hormone deficiencies."

55. A nurse is teaching health to a class of fifth graders. Which statement related to growth should be included?
1. "There's nothing that you can do to influence your growth."
2. "Intensive physical activity that begins before puberty might stunt growth."
3. "Children who are short in stature also have parents who are short in stature."
4. "Because this is a time of tremendous growth, being concerned about calorie intake isn't important."

56. While teaching the parents of a child with short stature, the nurse discusses familial short stature. Which statement by the nurse about this condition is <u>most</u> correct?
1. "It occurs in children who are members of a very large family with limited resources."
2. "It occurs in children who have no siblings who moved a great deal during their early childhood."
3. "It occurs in children with delayed linear growth and skeletal and sexual maturation that's behind that of age-mates."
4. "It occurs in children who have ancestors with adult height in the lower percentiles and whose height during childhood is appropriate."

54. 2. The cause of idiopathic growth hormone deficiency is unknown. The condition is typically associated with other pituitary hormone deficiencies, such as deficiencies of thyroid stimulating hormone and corticotropin, and so may be secondary to hypothalamic deficiency. There's also a higher-than-average occurrence of the disorder in some families, which indicates a possible genetic cause.
CN: Psychosocial integrity; CNS: None; CL: Application

55. 2. Intensive physical activity (greater than 18 hours per week) that begins before puberty may stunt growth so that the child doesn't reach full adult height. During the school-age years, growth slows and doesn't accelerate again until adolescence. Children who are short in stature don't necessarily have parents who are short in stature. Nutrition and environment influence a child's growth.
CN: Health promotion and maintenance; CNS: None; CL: Application

56. 4. Familial short stature refers to otherwise healthy children who have ancestors with adult height in the lower percentiles and whose height during childhood is appropriate for genetic background. Children with delayed linear growth and skeletal and sexual maturation behind that of age-mates are said to have constitutional growth delay. Children who are members of very large families with limited resources or who are only children don't fit the description of familial short stature.
CN: Physiological integrity; CNS: Physiological adaptation; CL: Application

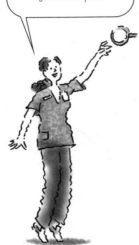

I know practicing for the NCLEX will make me feel good in the long run. I just have to keep my eyes on the prize!

57. When evaluating a 2-year-old child, which finding would indicate to the nurse the possibility of growth hormone deficiency?
1. The child had normal growth during the first year of life but showed a slowed growth curve below the 3rd percentile for the 2nd year of life.
2. The child fell below the 5th percentile for growth during the first year of life but, at this checkup, only falls below the 50th percentile.
3. There has been a steady decline in growth over the 2 years of this infant's life that has accelerated during the past 6 months.
4. There was delayed growth below the 5th percentile for the first and second years of life.

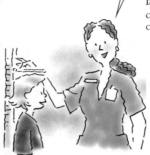

A child's growth pattern can tell you a lot about his overall health.

58. When collecting data on a child with growth hormone deficiency, the nurse would expect to observe which characteristic?
1. Decreased weight with no change in height
2. Decreased weight with increased height
3. Increased weight with decreased height
4. Increased weight with increased height

59. The nurse should find which characteristic in her observations of a child with growth hormone deficiency?
1. Normal skeletal proportions
2. Abnormal skeletal proportions
3. Child appearing older than his age
4. Longer than normal upper extremities

Children with growth hormone deficiency should be directed to size-appropriate sports.

60. When counseling the parents of a child with growth hormone deficiency, the nurse should encourage which sport?
1. Basketball
2. Field hockey
3. Football
4. Gymnastics

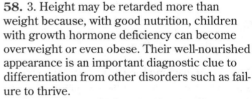

57. 1. Children with growth hormone deficiency generally grow normally during the first year and then follow a slowed growth curve that's below the 3rd percentile. Growth consistently below the 5th percentile may be an indication of failure to thrive.
CN: Health promotion and maintenance; CNS: None; CL: Application

58. 3. Height may be retarded more than weight because, with good nutrition, children with growth hormone deficiency can become overweight or even obese. Their well-nourished appearance is an important diagnostic clue to differentiation from other disorders such as failure to thrive.
CN: Physiological integrity; CNS: Physiological adaptation; CL: Knowledge

59. 1. Skeletal proportions are normal for the age, but these children appear younger than their chronological age. However, later in life, premature aging is evident.
CN: Physiological integrity; CNS: Physiological adaptation; CL: Application

60. 4. Children with growth hormone deficiency can be no less active than other children if directed to size-appropriate sports, such as gymnastics, swimming, wrestling, or soccer.
CN: Psychosocial integrity; CNS: None; CL: Application

CN: Client needs category   CNS: Client needs subcategory   CL: Cognitive level

61. In explaining to parents the social behavior of children with hypopituitarism, a nurse should recognize which statement as a need for further teaching?
1. "I realize that my child might have school anxiety and low self-esteem."
2. "Because my child is short in stature, people expect less of him than of his peers."
3. "Because of my child's short stature, he may not be pushed to perform at his chronological age by others."
4. "My child's vocabulary is very well developed, so even though he's short in stature, no one will treat him differently."

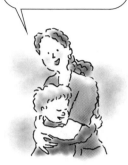

It's important that parents have realistic expectations about their child's disorder.

61. 4. Height discrepancy has been significantly correlated with emotional adjustment problems and may be a valuable predictor of the extent to which growth hormone–delayed children will have trouble with anxiety, social skills, and positive self-esteem. Also, academic problems aren't uncommon. These children aren't usually pushed to perform at their chronological age but are typically subjected to juvenilization (related to an infantile or childish manner).
CN: Psychosocial integrity; CNS: None; CL: Application

62. The mother of a child diagnosed with hypopituitarism states to the nurse that she feels guilty because she feels that she should have recognized this disorder. Which statement by the nurse about children with hypopituitarism would be the most helpful?"
1. "They're usually large for gestational age at birth."
2. "They're usually small for gestational age at birth."
3. "They usually exhibit signs of this disorder soon after birth."
4. "They're usually of normal size for gestational age at birth."

62. 4. Children with hypopituitarism are usually of normal size for gestational age at birth. Clinical features develop slowly and vary with the severity of the disorder and the number of deficient hormones.
CN: Physiological integrity; CNS: Physiological adaptation; CL: Application

63. When plotting height and weight on a growth chart, which observation would indicate that a child who's 4 years old has a growth hormone deficiency?
1. Upward shift of 1 percentile or more
2. Upward shift of 5 percentiles or more
3. Downward shift of 2 percentiles or more
4. Downward shift of 5 percentiles or more

63. 3. When the primary health care provider evaluates the results of plotting height and weight, upward or downward shifts of 2 percentiles or more in children older than age 3 may indicate a growth abnormality.
CN: Health promotion and maintenance; CNS: None; CL: Analysis

64. When reviewing the results of radiographic examinations of a child with hypopituitarism, which characteristic should the nurse expect to observe?
1. Bone age near normal
2. Epiphyseal maturation normal
3. Epiphyseal maturation retarded
4. Bone maturation greatly retarded

64. 3. Epiphyseal maturation is retarded in hypopituitarism consistent with retardation in height. This is in contrast to hypothyroidism, in which bone maturation is greatly retarded, or Turner's syndrome, in which bone age is near normal.
CN: Physiological integrity; CNS: Physiological adaptation; CL: Knowledge

CN: Client needs category   CNS: Client needs subcategory   CL: Cognitive level

65. A nurse should understand that which test is used for a definitive diagnosis of hypopituitarism?

1. Hypersecretion of thyroid hormone
2. Increased reserves of growth hormone
3. Hyposecretion of antidiuretic hormone
4. Decreased reserves of growth hormone

66. The parents of a child who's going through testing for hypopituitarism ask the nurse what test results they should expect. The nurse's response should be based on which factor?

1. Measurement of growth hormone will occur only one time.
2. Growth hormone levels are decreased after strenuous exercise.
3. There will be increased overnight urine growth hormone concentration.
4. Growth hormone levels are elevated 45 to 90 minutes following the onset of sleep.

67. Which method is considered the definitive treatment for hypopituitarism due to growth hormone deficiency?

1. Treatment with desmopressin acetate (DDAVP)
2. Replacement of antidiuretic hormone
3. Treatment with testosterone or estrogen
4. Replacement with biosynthetic growth hormone

68. When obtaining information about a child, which comment made by a parent to the nurse would indicate the possibility of hypopituitarism in a child?

1. "I can pass down my child's clothes to his younger brother."
2. "Usually my child wears out his clothes before his size changes."
3. "I have to buy bigger-sized clothes for my child about every 2 months."
4. "I have to buy larger shirts more frequently than larger pants for my child."

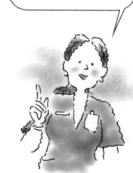

You definitely know the answer to question 67.

65. 4. Definitive diagnosis is based on absent or subnormal levels of pituitary growth hormone. Antidiuretic hormone and thyroid hormone levels aren't affected.
CN: Physiological integrity; CNS: Reduction of risk potential; CL: Knowledge

66. 4. Growth hormone levels are elevated 45 to 90 minutes following the onset of sleep. Low growth hormone levels following the onset of sleep would indicate the need for further evaluation. Exercise is a natural and benign stimulus for growth hormone release, and elevated levels can be detected after 20 minutes of strenuous exercise in normal children. Also, growth hormone levels will need to be checked frequently related to the type of therapy instituted.
CN: Physiological integrity; CNS: Physiological adaptation; CL: Application

67. 4. The definitive treatment of growth hormone deficiency is replacement of growth hormone and is successful in 80% of affected children. DDAVP is used to treat diabetes insipidus. Antidiuretic hormone deficiency causes diabetes insipidus and isn't related to hypopituitarism. Testosterone or estrogen may be given during adolescence for normal sexual maturation but neither is the definitive treatment for hypopituitarism.
CN: Physiological integrity; CNS: Pharmacological therapies; CL: Application

68. 2. Parents of children with hypopituitarism usually comment that the child wears out clothes before growing out of them or that, if the clothing fits the body, it's typically too long in the sleeves or legs.
CN: Physiological integrity; CNS: Physiological adaptation; CL: Application

69. A nurse is teaching parents who are planning to give growth hormone at home to their child. The nurse should teach the parents that the best time to administer growth hormone to achieve optimal dosing is:
1. at bedtime.
2. after dinner.
3. in the middle of the day.
4. first thing in the morning.

70. In educating parents of a child with hypopituitarism about realistic expectations of height for their child who's successfully responding to growth hormone replacement, a nurse should include which statement?
1. "Your child will never reach a normal adult height."
2. "Your child will attain his eventual adult height at a faster rate."
3. "Your child will attain his eventual adult height at a slower rate."
4. "The rate of your child's growth will be the same as children without this disorder."

71. Which statement made by a parent of a child with short stature would indicate to the nurse the need for further teaching?
1. "Obtaining blood studies won't aid in proper diagnosis."
2. "A history of my child's growth patterns should be discussed."
3. "X-rays should be included in my child's diagnostic procedures."
4. "A family history is important information for me to share with my primary health care provider."

72. If hypersecretion of growth hormone occurs after epiphyseal closure, which condition might be observed by the nurse?
1. Acromegaly
2. Cretinism
3. Dwarfism
4. Gigantism

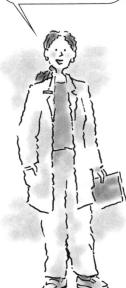

Careful—here's another further teaching question.

69. 1. Optimal dosing is usually achieved when growth hormone is administered at bedtime. Pituitary release of growth hormone occurs during the first 45 to 90 minutes after the onset of sleep, so normal physiological release is mimicked with bedtime dosing.
CN: Physiological integrity; CNS: Pharmacological therapies; CL: Application

70. 3. Even when hormone replacement is successful, these children attain their eventual adult height at a slower rate than their peers do; therefore, they need assistance in setting realistic expectations regarding improvement.
CN: Health promotion and maintenance; CNS: None; CL: Application

71. 1. A complete diagnostic evaluation should include a family history, a history of the child's growth patterns and previous health status, physical examination, physical evaluation, radiographic survey, and endocrine studies that may involve blood samples.
CN: Physiological integrity; CNS: Reduction of risk potential; CL: Application

72. 1. If excessive growth hormone is evident after epiphyseal closure, growth is in the transverse direction, producing a condition known as *acromegaly.* The other options aren't seen as a result of excess growth hormone after epiphyseal closure.
CN: Physiological integrity; CNS: Physiological adaptation; CL: Knowledge

CN: Client needs category   CNS: Client needs subcategory   CL: Cognitive level

73. Which metabolic alteration characteristic might be associated with growth hormone deficiency?
1. Galactosemia
2. Homocystinuria
3. Hyperglycemia
4. Hypoglycemia

73. 4. The development of hypoglycemia is a characteristic finding related to growth hormone deficiency. Galactosemia is a rare autosomal recessive disorder with an inborn error of carbohydrate metabolism. Homocystinuria is an indication of amino acid transport or metabolism problems. Hyperglycemia isn't a problem in hypopituitarism.
CN: Physiological integrity; CNS: Physiological adaptation; CL: Application

74. A child is admitted to the medical-surgical unit with complaints of weight loss and lack of energy. The child's ears and cheeks are flushed, and the nurse observes an acetone odor to the client's breath. The blood glucose level is 325 mg/dl. The blood pressure is 104/60 mm Hg, pulse is 88 beats/minute, and respirations are 16 breaths/minute. Which does the nurse expect the physician to order first?
1. Subcutaneous (subQ) administration of glucagon
2. Administration of regular insulin by continuous infusion pump
3. Administration of regular insulin subQ every 4 hours as needed by sliding scale insulin
4. Administration of I.V. fluids in boluses of 20 ml/kg

74. 2. Weight loss, lack of energy, acetone odor to the breath, and a blood glucose level of 325 mg/dl indicate diabetic ketoacidosis. Insulin is given by continuous infusion pump at a rate not to exceed 100 mg/dl/hour. Faster reduction of hypoglycemia could be related to the development of cerebral edema. Glucagon is administered for mild hypoglycemia. Sliding scale insulin isn't as effective as the administration of insulin by continuous infusion pump in the treatment of diabetic ketoacidosis. Administration of I.V. fluids in boluses of 20 mg/kg is recommended for the treatment of shock.
CN: Physiological integrity; CNS: Physiological adaptation; CL: Application

75. When assessing a neonate diagnosed with diabetes insipidus, which finding would indicate the need for intervention?
1. Edema
2. Increased head circumference
3. Weight gain
4. Weight loss

A normal neonate should gain weight as he grows.

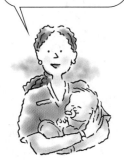

75. 4. Diabetes insipidus usually appears gradually. Weight loss from a large loss of fluid occurs. A normal neonate should gain weight as he grows. There should be an increase in his head circumference with treatment. Edema isn't evident in the neonate with diabetes insipidus.
CN: Physiological integrity; CNS: Reduction of risk potential; CL: Application

76. In a client with diabetes insipidus, a nurse could expect which characteristics of the urine?
1. Pale; specific gravity less than 1.006
2. Concentrated; specific gravity less than 1.006
3. Concentrated; specific gravity less than 1.030
4. Pale; specific gravity more than 1.030

76. 1. With diabetes insipidus, the client has difficulty with excessive urine output; therefore, the urine will be pale and the specific gravity will fall below the low normal of 1.010.
CN: Physiological integrity; CNS: Physiological adaptation; CL: Analysis

77. In a child with diabetes insipidus, which characteristic would most likely be present in the child's health history?

1. Delayed closure of the fontanels, coarse hair, and hypoglycemia in the morning
2. Gradual onset of personality changes, lethargy, and blurred vision
3. Vomiting early in the morning, headache, and decreased thirst
4. Abrupt onset of polyuria, nocturia, and polydipsia

78. A client is on fluid restriction before diagnostic testing for diabetes insipidus. Which condition would indicate to the nurse the need to discontinue fluid restriction?

1. Weight gain of 3% to 5%
2. Weight loss of 3% to 5%
3. Increase in urine output
4. Generalized edema

79. When a child with diabetes insipidus has a viral illness that includes congestion, nausea, and vomiting, the nurse should instruct the parents to take which action?

1. Make no changes in the medication regimen.
2. Give medications only once per day.
3. Obtain an alternate route for desmopressin acetate (DDAVP) administration.
4. Give medication 1 hour after vomiting has occurred.

80. A nurse is preparing to discharge a child with diabetes insipidus who'll be taking injectable vasopressin. Which teaching strategy is best for the nurse regarding injection techniques?

1. Teach injection techniques to the primary caregiver.
2. Teach injection techniques to anyone who'll provide care for the child.
3. Teach injection techniques to anyone who'll provide care for the child as well as to the child if he's old enough to understand.
4. Provide information about the nearest home health agency so the parents can arrange for the home health nurse to come and give the injection.

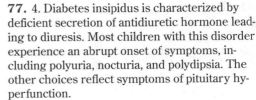

Question 78 is asking for an adverse reaction.

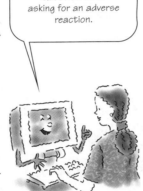

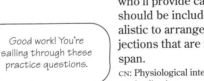

Good work! You're sailing through these practice questions.

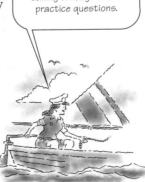

77. 4. Diabetes insipidus is characterized by deficient secretion of antidiuretic hormone leading to diuresis. Most children with this disorder experience an abrupt onset of symptoms, including polyuria, nocturia, and polydipsia. The other choices reflect symptoms of pituitary hyperfunction.

CN: Physiological integrity; CNS: Physiological adaptation; CL: Application

78. 2. A weight loss of 3% to 5% indicates significant dehydration and requires termination of fluid restriction. Weight gain would be a good sign. Generalized edema wouldn't occur with fluid restriction, nor would increased urine output.

CN: Physiological integrity; CNS: Physiological adaptation; CL: Analysis

79. 3. An alternate route for administration of DDAVP would be needed for absorption due to nasal congestion. The other options reflect actions that need to be covered by a medical order.

CN: Physiological integrity; CNS: Pharmacological therapies; CL: Application

80. 3. The best strategy is to teach all those who'll provide care for the child. The child should be included if age-appropriate. It's unrealistic to arrange home health nurses to give injections that are required throughout the life span.

CN: Physiological integrity; CNS: Pharmacological therapies; CL: Application

CN: Client needs category   CNS: Client needs subcategory   CL: Cognitive level

81. When providing care for a school-age client with diabetes insipidus, the nurse understands that which behavior might be difficult related to this child's growth and development?
1. Taking his medication at school
2. Taking his medication before bedtime
3. Letting his mother administer his medication
4. Giving himself a vasopressin injection before school starts

82. Which monitoring method would be <u>best</u> for a child newly diagnosed with diabetes insipidus?
1. Measuring abdominal girth every day
2. Measuring intake, output, and urine specific gravity
3. Checking daily weight and measuring intake
4. Checking for pitting edema in the lower extremities

83. A nurse is caring for a neonate with congenital hypothyroidism. Which assessment finding should the nurse anticipate observing in the neonate?
1. Hyperreflexia
2. Long forehead
3. Puffy eyelids
4. Small tongue

84. Which factor is most significant in <u>adversely</u> affecting eventual intelligence of a neonate with hypothyroidism?
1. Overtreatment
2. Inadequate treatment
3. Educational level of the parents
4. Socioeconomic level of the family

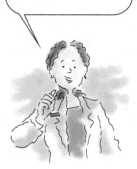

I know you'll try your best on these last few questions.

81. 1. Anything that singles out a child and makes him feel different from his peers will result in possible noncompliance with the medical regimen. It's important for the nurse to help the client schedule the need for medications around the times he'll be in school.
CN: Health promotion and maintenance; CNS: None; CL: Application

82. 2. Measuring intake and output with related specific gravity results will enable the nurse to closely monitor the child's condition along with daily weight. All other options aren't as accurate for a child with diabetes insipidus.
CN: Physiological integrity; CNS: Reduction of risk potential; CL: Application

83. 3. Assessment findings would include depressed nasal bridge, short forehead, puffy eyelids, and large tongue; thick, dry, mottled skin that feels cold to the touch; coarse, dry, lusterless hair; abdominal distention; umbilical hernia; hyporeflexia; bradycardia; hypothermia; hypotension; anemia; and wide cranial sutures.
CN: Physiological integrity; CNS: Physiological adaptation; CL: Application

84. 2. The most significant factor adversely affecting eventual intelligence is inadequate treatment, which may be related to noncompliance. Although overtreatment could cause physical problems and, possibly, death, these adverse reactions would occur before the intellect was affected. Parental factors, such as educational and socioeconomic level, affect only the environmental stimulation, not the child's basic intellect.
CN: Physiological integrity; CNS: Physiological adapation; CL: Application

85. Which nursing objective is <u>most important</u> when working with neonates who are suspected of having congenital hypothyroidism?
1. Early identification
2. Promoting bonding
3. Allowing rooming in
4. Encouraging fluid intake

86. When the parents of an infant diagnosed with hypothyroidism have been taught to count the pulse, which intervention should the nurse teach them in case they obtain a high pulse rate?
1. Allow the infant to take a nap and then give the medication.
2. Withhold the medication and give a double dose the next day.
3. Withhold the medication and call the primary health care provider.
4. Give the medication and then consult the primary health care provider.

87. In an infant receiving inadequate treatment for congenital hypothyroidism, the nurse would expect to observe which symptom?
1. Irritability and jitteriness
2. Fatigue and sleepiness
3. Increased appetite
4. Diarrhea

88. Which characteristic best describes congenital hypothyroidism?
1. It's sex-linked.
2. It has no genetic basis.
3. It's an autosomal dominant gene.
4. It's caused by an inborn error of metabolism.

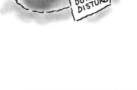

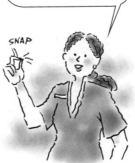

It should be a snap now. Just a few more questions to go!

85. 1. The most important nursing objective is early identification of the disorder. Nurses caring for neonates must be certain that screening is performed, especially in neonates who are preterm, discharged early, or born at home. Promoting bonding, allowing rooming in, and encouraging fluid intake are all important but are less important than early identification.
CN: Physiological integrity; CNS: Basic care and comfort; CL: Application

86. 3. If parents have been taught to count the infant's pulse, they should be instructed to withhold the dose and consult their primary health care provider if the pulse rate is above a certain value.
CN: Physiological integrity; CNS: Reduction of risk potential; CL: Application

87. 2. Signs of inadequate treatment are fatigue, sleepiness, decreased appetite, and constipation.
CN: Physiological integrity; CNS: Reduction of risk potential; CL: Application

88. 4. The disorder is caused by an inborn error of thyroid hormone synthesis, which is autosomal recessive. Therefore, genetic counseling is important. There's no evidence that this disorder is sex-linked.
CN: Physiological integrity; CNS: Physiological adaptation; CL: Knowledge

CN: Client needs category   CNS: Client needs subcategory   CL: Cognitive level

89. When collecting data from a child with Cushing's syndrome, which would the nurse be <u>most</u> likely to find? Select all that apply:
   1. Obesity
   2. Moon-shaped face
   3. Hypotension
   4. Emotional instability
   5. Quickened healing
   6. Loss of hair

90. Which signs and symptoms would the health care team most commonly use as a basis for determining appropriate priorities and interventions for a child with type 1 diabetes mellitus? Select all that apply:
   1. Polyuria
   2. Weakness
   3. Abdominal pain
   4. Weight loss
   5. Postprandial nausea
   6. Orthostatic hypertension

89. 1, 2, 4. Cushing's syndrome occurs as a result of excessive cortisol exposure (through corticosteroid medications) or production by the adrenal glands. Common findings include obesity, moon-shaped face, and emotional instability. Hypertension, excessive hair growth, and slower healing are additional findings, making the other options incorrect.
CN: Physiological integrity; CNS: Physiological adaptation; CL: Analysis

90. 1, 2, 4, 5. Polyuria, weakness, weight loss, and postprandial nausea are commonly seen in diabetes mellitus. The health care team would plan care to manage these signs and symptoms. Abdominal pain isn't a symptom in this disease, and orthostatic hypotension rather than orthostatic hypertension would be a significant finding.
CN: Safe, effective care environment; CNS: Coordinated care; CL: Analysis

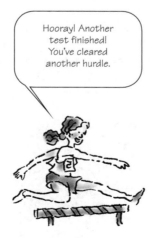

Hooray! Another test finished! You've cleared another hurdle.

CN: Client needs category   CNS: Client needs subcategory   CL: Cognitive level

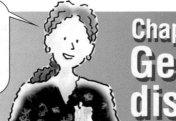

This chapter covers altered patterns of urinary elimination in children and includes glomerulonephritis, hypospadias, and—oh, a whole lot of other conditions. Ready? Let's go!

Chapter 34
Genitourinary disorders

1. A child with acute glomerulonephritis has a nursing diagnosis of *Impaired urinary elimination related to fluid retention and impaired glomerular filtration.* The child should have which expected outcome?

 1. Exhibits no evidence of infection
 2. Engages in activities appropriate to capabilities
 3. Demonstrates no periorbital, facial, or body edema
 4. Maintains a fluid intake of more than 2,000 ml in 24 hours

2. An important nursing intervention to support the therapeutic management of the child with acute glomerulonephritis would include which measure?

 1. Measuring daily weight
 2. Increasing oral fluid intake
 3. Providing sodium supplements
 4. Monitoring the client for signs of hypokalemia

3. A child has been diagnosed with acute glomerulonephritis. Based on the results of the routine urinalysis below, which component is <u>most</u> consistent with this diagnosis?

Laboratory results	
Urinalysis	
Color:	Straw
Appearance:	Clear
Specific gravity:	1.032
pH:	5.5
Protein:	Negative
Blood:	Negative
RBC casts:	Present
Crystals:	Negative

 1. Specific gravity
 2. Protein
 3. Blood
 4. Red blood cell (RBC) casts

CN: Client needs category   CNS: Client needs subcategory   CL: Cognitive level

1. 3. The goal of this diagnosis involves interventions, such as decreased fluid and salt intake, designed to minimize or prevent fluid retention and edema. These interventions may be evaluated through observations for edema. The other options are appropriate outcomes for other nursing diagnoses, not the diagnosis in question.
CN: Health promotion and maintenance; CNS: None; CL: Analysis

2. 1. The child with acute glomerulonephritis should be monitored for fluid imbalance, which is done through daily weights. Increasing oral intake, providing sodium supplements, and monitoring for hypokalemia aren't part of the therapeutic management of acute glomerulonephritis.
CN: Physiological integrity; CNS: Basic care and comfort; CL: Application

If you're having trouble deciding on an answer, begin by eliminating the ones you know are incorrect.

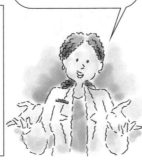

3. 4. Urinalysis findings consistent with acute glomerulonephritis would include a specific gravity less than 1.030, proteinuria, hematuria, and the presence of RBC casts. The presence of crystals in the urine typically indicates a congenital metabolic problem.
CN: Physiological integrity; CNS: Physiological adaptation; CL: Application

4. A nurse is taking frequent blood pressure readings on a child diagnosed with acute glomerulonephritis. The parents ask the nurse why this is necessary. When implementing nursing care, which teaching statement by the nurse is <u>most</u> accurate?

1. Blood pressure fluctuations are a sign that the condition has become chronic.
2. Blood pressure fluctuations are a common adverse effect of antibiotic therapy.
3. Hypotension leading to sudden shock can develop at any time.
4. Acute hypertension must be anticipated and identified.

5. When evaluating the urinalysis report of a child with <u>acute</u> glomerulonephritis, the nurse would expect which result?

1. Proteinuria and decreased specific gravity
2. Bacteriuria and increased specific gravity
3. Hematuria and proteinuria
4. Bacteriuria and hematuria

6. Which statement by the nurse would be the <u>best</u> response to a mother who wants to know the first indication that acute glomerulonephritis is improving?

1. Urine output will increase.
2. Urine will be protein-free.
3. Blood pressure will stabilize.
4. The child will have more energy.

7. Which statement regarding acute glomerulonephritis indicates that the parents of a child with this diagnosis understand the teaching provided by the nurse?

1. "This disease occurs after a urinary tract infection."
2. "This disease is associated with renal vascular disorders."
3. "This disease occurs after a streptococcal infection."
4. "This disease is associated with structural anomalies of the genitourinary tract."

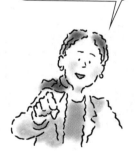

More than one answer may seem correct. It's your job to choose the best answer.

4. 4. Regular measurement of vital signs, body weight, and intake and output is essential to monitor the progress of the disease and to detect complications that may appear at any time during the course of the disease. Blood pressure fluctuations don't indicate that the condition has become chronic and aren't common adverse reactions to antibiotic therapy. Hypertension is more likely to occur with glomerulonephritis than hypotension.

CN: Safe, effective care environment; CNS: Coordinated care; CL: Application

5. 3. Urinalysis during the acute phase of this disease characteristically shows hematuria, proteinuria, and increased specific gravity.

CN: Physiological integrity; CNS: Physiological adaptation; CL: Analysis

6. 1. One of the first signs of improvement during the acute phase of glomerulonephritis is an increase in urine output. It will take time for the urine to be protein-free. Antihypertensive drugs may be needed to stabilize blood pressure. Children generally don't have much energy during the acute phase of this disease.

CN: Physiological integrity; CNS: Reduction of risk potential; CL: Analysis

7. 3. Acute glomerulonephritis is an immune-complex disease that occurs as a by-product of an antecedent streptococcal infection. Certain strains of the infection are usually beta-hemolytic streptococci.

CN: Physiological integrity; CNS: Physiological adaptation; CL: Analysis

8. When obtaining a client's daily weight, the nurse notes that the child has lost 6 lb (2.7 kg) after 3 days of hospitalization for acute glomerulonephritis. This is most likely the result of which factor?
1. Poor appetite
2. Reduction of edema
3. Decreased salt intake
4. Restriction to bed rest

9. A nurse should make which dietary recommendation to a client who has been newly diagnosed with acute glomerulonephritis?
1. Reduce calories.
2. Increase potassium.
3. Severely restrict sodium.
4. Moderately restrict sodium.

10. The nurse is evaluating a group of children for acute glomerulonephritis. Which client would be most likely to develop the disease?
1. A client who had pneumonia a month ago
2. A client who was bitten by a brown spider
3. A client who shows no signs of periorbital edema
4. A client who had a streptococcal infection 2 weeks ago

11. At which age would the nurse observe a higher incidence of acute glomerulonephritis?
1. 1 to 2 years
2. 6 to 7 years
3. 12 to 13 years
4. 18 to 20 years

12. In understanding the recurrence of glomerulonephritis, the nurse should understand which characteristic?
1. Second attacks are quite common.
2. A recessive gene transfers this disease.
3. Multiple cases tend to occur in families.
4. Overcrowding in the schoolroom leads to higher incidence.

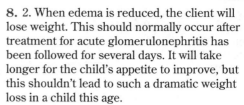

10 questions down! That's a good start!

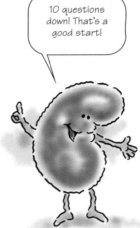

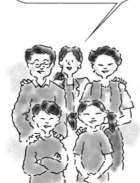

Sometimes it's a family affair.

8. 2. When edema is reduced, the client will lose weight. This should normally occur after treatment for acute glomerulonephritis has been followed for several days. It will take longer for the child's appetite to improve, but this shouldn't lead to such a dramatic weight loss in a child this age.
CN: Physiological integrity; CNS: Basic care and comfort; CL: Application

9. 4. Moderate sodium restriction with a diet that has no added salt after cooking is usually effective. Reduced calorie consumption and increased potassium consumption aren't necessary because of the decrease in urine output. Severe sodium restriction isn't needed and will make it more difficult to ensure adequate nutrition.
CN: Physiological integrity; CNS: Basic care and comfort; CL: Application

10. 4. A latent period of 10 to 14 days occurs between the streptococcal infection of the throat or skin and the onset of clinical manifestations. The peak incidence of disease corresponds to the incidence of streptococcal infections. Pneumonia isn't a precursor to glomerulonephritis, nor is a bite from a brown spider. A sign of periorbital edema would lead the nurse to investigate the possibility of glomerulonephritis, especially if reported to be worse in the morning.
CN: Safe, effective care environment; CNS: Coordinated care; CL: Analysis

11. 2. Acute glomerulonephritis can occur at any age, but it primarily affects early-school-age children with a peak age of onset of 6 to 7 years. It's uncommon in children younger than 2 years old.
CN: Health promotion and maintenance; CNS: None; CL: Knowledge

12. 3. Multiple cases of glomerulonephritis tend to occur in families. Second attacks are rare. Acute glomerulonephritis isn't transmitted through a recessive gene, and overcrowding in the schoolroom should have no influence on this disease.
CN: Health promotion and maintenance; CNS: None; CL: Application

CN: Client needs category   CNS: Client needs subcategory   CL: Cognitive level

13. When teaching families of children with acute glomerulonephritis about complications, which comment made by a parent would indicate to the nurse the need for <u>further education</u>?

1. "Dizziness is expected and I should have my child lie down."
2. "I should let the nurse know every time my child urinates."
3. "I need to ask my child if he has a headache."
4. "I shouldn't force my child to eat."

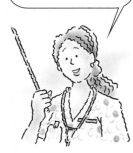

The phrase further education indicates that question 13 is looking for an inaccurate statement.

13. 1. Dizziness is a sign of encephalopathy and must be reported to the nurse. Hypertensive encephalopathy, acute cardiac decompensation, and acute renal failure are the major complications that tend to develop during the acute phase of glomerulonephritis. Reporting each urination, assessing headache, and avoiding forced food intake are measures that should be performed.

CN: Physiological integrity; CNS: Reduction of risk potential; CL: Application

14. Which test is the most familiar and most readily available test for streptococcal antibodies?

1. Antistreptolysin-O titer (ASOT)
2. Blood culture
3. Blood urea nitrogen (BUN)
4. Mono spot

14. 1. ASOT is the most familiar and most readily available test for streptococcal antibodies. ASO appears in the serum approximately 10 days after the initial infection; however, there's no correlation between the degree of elevation and the severity or prognosis of the glomerulonephritis. Blood cultures are drawn to determine sepsis, and a BUN will indicate renal function. The mono spot test is done to detect mononucleosis.

CN: Physiological integrity; CNS: Physiological adaptation; CL: Comprehension

15. When teaching an 8-year-old child to obtain a clean-catch urine specimen, which technique should be included by the nurse?

1. Collect the specimen right after a nap.
2. Discard the first voided specimen of the day.
3. Collect the specimen at the beginning of urination.
4. You don't need to wash your perineal area before collecting the specimen.

Don't a-void this question. You're doing great!

15. 2. When collecting a clean-catch urine specimen, the first voided specimen of the day should never be used because of urinary stasis; this also applies after a nap. The specimen should be collected midstream, not at the beginning of urination. Washing the perineal area before collecting a specimen is important to make sure there are no contaminants from the skin in the specimen.

CN: Physiological integrity; CNS: Reduction of risk potential; CL: Application

16. In explaining treatment for glomerulo-nephritis, the nurse should include which statement?
 1. All children who have signs of glomerulonephritis are hospitalized for approximately 1 week.
 2. Parents should expect children to have a normal energy level during the acute phase.
 3. Children who have normal blood pressure and a satisfactory urine output can generally be treated at home.
 4. Children with gross hematuria and significant oliguria should be brought to the primary health care provider's office about every 2 days for monitoring.

17. Which reason accounts for why bed rest is not typically prescribed during the acute phase of glomerulonephritis?
 1. It's too difficult to keep a child on bed rest.
 2. Children on bed rest lose too much muscle tone because of lack of movement.
 3. Parents find enforcing bed rest causes them to feel guilty about the disease.
 4. Ambulation doesn't seem to have an adverse effect on the course of the disease.

18. Which food should the nurse eliminate from the diet of a child who's diagnosed with acute glomerulonephritis?
 1. Turkey sandwich with mayonnaise
 2. Hot dog with ketchup and mustard
 3. Chocolate cake with white icing
 4. Apple with peanut butter

19. Which therapy should the nurse expect to incorporate into the care of the child with acute glomerulonephritis?
 1. Antibiotic therapy
 2. Dialysis therapy
 3. Diuretic therapy
 4. Play therapy

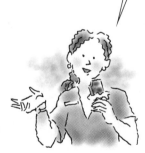

Question 18 asks what foods the client with acute glomerulonephritis should avoid.

16. 3. Children who have normal blood pressure and a satisfactory urine output can generally be treated at home. Those with gross hematuria and significant oliguria will probably be hospitalized for monitoring. Parents should expect children to have a decrease in energy levels during the acute phase of the disease.
CN: Physiological integrity; CNS: Reduction of risk potential; CL: Comprehension

17. 4. Ambulation doesn't seem to have an adverse effect on the course of the disease after the gross hematuria, edema, hypertension, and azotemia have abated. Because they're generally listless and experience fatigue and malaise, most children voluntarily restrict their activities during the most active phase of the disease. Children on short-term bed rest don't lose muscle tone because they usually move around in the bed. Parents don't feel guilty enforcing bed rest, but they may find it challenging.
CN: Physiological integrity; CNS: Reduction of risk potential; CL: Application

18. 2. Foods that are high in sodium should be eliminated from the child's diet. Such snacks as pretzels and potato chips should be discouraged. Any other foods that the child likes should be encouraged. Because hot dogs contain a great deal of sodium, they should be eliminated from the child's diet.
CN: Physiological integrity; CNS: Basic care and comfort; CL: Application

19. 4. Play therapy is a very important aspect of care to help the child understand what's happening to him. Unless the child can express concerns and fears, he may have night terrors and regress in his stage of growth and development. Antibiotic and diuretic therapy aren't routine treatments for acute glomerulonephritis. Dialysis may be indicated with chronic glomerulonephritis.
CN: Health promotion and maintenance; CNS: None; CL: Application

CN: Client needs category   CNS: Client needs subcategory   CL: Cognitive level

20. After the acute phase of glomerulonephritis is over, which discharge instructions should the nurse include?

1. Every 6 months, a cystogram will be needed for evaluation of progress.
2. Weekly visits to the primary health care provider may be needed for evaluation.
3. It will be acceptable to keep the regular yearly checkup appointment for the next evaluation.
4. There's no need to worry about further evaluations by the primary health care provider related to this disease.

21. The nurse understands that the term *hypospadias* refers to which condition?

1. Absence of a urethral opening
2. Penis shorter than usual for age
3. Urethral opening along the dorsal surface of the penis
4. Urethral opening along the ventral surface of the penis

22. The nurse understands that the term *chordee* refers to which condition?

1. Ventral curvature of the penis
2. Dorsal curvature of the penis
3. No curvature of the penis
4. Misshapen penis

23. Which anomaly commonly accompanies hypospadias?

1. Undescended testes
2. Ambiguous genitalia
3. Umbilical hernias
4. Inguinal hernias

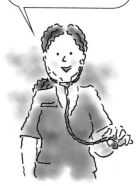

Part of the nurse's role is to make sure the client understands discharge instructions.

20. 2. Weekly or monthly visits to the primary health care provider will be needed for evaluation of improvement and will usually involve the collection of a urine specimen for urinalysis. A cystogram isn't helpful in determining the progression of this disease; it's used to review the anatomic structures of the urinary tract.

CN: Physiological integrity; CNS: Reduction of risk potential; CL: Application

21. 4. Hypospadias refers to a condition in which the urethral opening is located below the glans penis or anywhere along the ventral surface of the penile shaft. Hypospadias refers to a malposition of the opening, not absence of the opening, and has nothing to do with the size of the penis.

CN: Physiological integrity; CNS: Physiological adaptation; CL: Knowledge

22. 1. Chordee, or ventral curvature of the penis, results from the replacement of normal skin with a fibrous band of tissue and usually accompanies more severe forms of hypospadias.

CN: Physiological integrity; CNS: Physiological adaptation; CL: Knowledge

23. 1. Because undescended testes may also be present, the small penis may appear to be an enlarged clitoris. This shouldn't be mistaken for ambiguous genitalia. If there's any doubt, more tests should be performed. Hernias don't generally accompany hypospadias.

CN: Physiological integrity; CNS: Reduction of risk potential; CL: Knowledge

CN: Client needs category   CNS: Client needs subcategory   CL: Cognitive level

24. Which reason explains why surgical repair of hypospadias is done as early as possible?
1. To prevent separation anxiety
2. To prevent urinary complications
3. To promote acceptance of hospitalization
4. To promote development of normal body image

24. 4. Whenever there are defects of the genitourinary tract, surgery should be performed early to promote development of a normal body image, not acceptance of hospitalization. A child with normal emotional development shows separation anxiety at 7 to 9 months. Within a few months, he understands the mother's permanence, and anxiety diminishes. Hypospadias doesn't put the child at a greater risk for urinary complications.
CN: Physiological integrity; CNS: Reduction of risk potential; CL: Application

25. A child is undergoing hypospadias repair. Which statement made by the child's parents about the principal objective of surgical correction implies a need for <u>further teaching</u>?
1. "The purpose is to improve the physical appearance of the genitalia for psychological reasons."
2. "The purpose is to enhance the child's ability to void in the standing position."
3. "The purpose is to decrease the chances of urinary tract infections."
4. "The purpose is to preserve a sexually adequate organ."

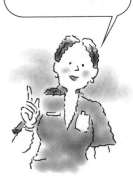

Question 25 is looking for the one inaccurate statement.

25. 3. A child with hypospadias isn't at greater risk for urinary tract infections. The principal objectives of surgical corrections are to enhance the child's ability to void in the standing position with a straight stream, to improve the physical appearance of the genitalia for psychological reasons, and to preserve a sexually adequate organ.
CN: Physiological integrity; CNS: Reduction of risk potential; CL: Application

26. The nurse should counsel parents to postpone which action until after their son's hypospadias has been repaired?
1. Circumcision
2. Infant baptism
3. Getting hepatitis B vaccine
4. Checking blood for inborn errors of metabolism

26. 1. Circumcision shouldn't be performed until after the hypospadias has been repaired. The foreskin might be needed to help in the repair of hypospadias. None of the other choices has any bearing on the repair of hypospadias.
CN: Physiological integrity; CNS: Reduction of risk potential; CL: Application

27. Which nursing intervention should be included in the care plan for a male infant following surgical repair of hypospadias?
1. Sterile dressing changes every 4 hours
2. Frequent inspection of the tip of the penis
3. Removal of the suprapubic catheter on the 2nd postoperative day
4. Urethral catheterization if voiding doesn't occur over an 8-hour period

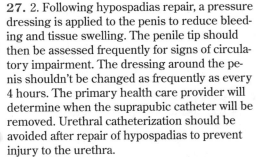

Looks like you're doing fine so far.

27. 2. Following hypospadias repair, a pressure dressing is applied to the penis to reduce bleeding and tissue swelling. The penile tip should then be assessed frequently for signs of circulatory impairment. The dressing around the penis shouldn't be changed as frequently as every 4 hours. The primary health care provider will determine when the suprapubic catheter will be removed. Urethral catheterization should be avoided after repair of hypospadias to prevent injury to the urethra.
CN: Physiological integrity; CNS: Basic care and comfort; CL: Application

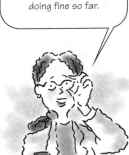

CN: Client needs category   CNS: Client needs subcategory   CL: Cognitive level

28. When explaining to the parents the optimal time for repair of hypospadias, the nurse should indicate which as the age of choice?
1. 1 week
2. 6 to 18 months
3. 2 years
4. 4 years

29. After a nurse has provided discharge teaching to the parents of a child with hypospadias, which statement by the mother indicates that additional teaching is needed?
1. "I'll need to learn irrigation techniques."
2. "I should bathe my child in the tub daily."
3. "Proper catheter care helps prevent infection."
4. "It's important to keep the catheter free of kinks and blockages."

30. When providing discharge instructions to parents of an older child who has had hypospadias repair, which activity should be avoided?
1. Finger painting
2. Playing in sandboxes
3. Increased fluid intake
4. Playing with the family pet

31. The mother of a neonate born with hypospadias is sharing her feelings of guilt about this anomaly with a nurse. The nurse should explain which fact about the defect?
1. It occurs around the third month of fetal development.
2. It occurs around the sixth month of fetal development.
3. It's carried by an autosomal recessive gene.
4. It's hereditary.

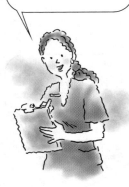

Be careful! Question 29 is looking for an incorrect statement.

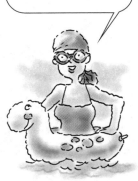

After hypospadias repair, certain activities should be avoided.

28. 2. The preferred time for surgical repair is ages 6 to 18 months, before the child has developed body image and castration anxiety. Surgical repair of hypospadias as early as age 3 months has been successful but with a high incidence of complications.
CN: Physiological integrity; CNS: Reduction of risk potential; CL: Comprehension

29. 2. A tub bath should be avoided to prevent infection until the stent has been removed. Parents are taught to care for the indwelling catheter or stent and irrigation techniques if indicated. They need to know how to empty the urine bag and how to avoid kinking, twisting, or blockage of the catheter or stent.
CN: Safe, effective care environment; CNS: Coordinated care; CL: Analysis

30. 2. Sandboxes, straddle toys, swimming, and rough activities are avoided until allowed by the surgeon. The family is advised to encourage the child to increase fluid intake. Quiet, nonstrenuous activities are encouraged.
CN: Physiological integrity; CNS: Physiological adaptation; CL: Application

31. 1. The defect of hypospadias occurs around the end of the third month of fetal development. This defect isn't hereditary, nor is it carried by an autosomal recessive gene.
CN: Physiological integrity; CNS: Physiological adaptation; CL: Application

32. The discovery of hypospadias is <u>usually</u> made by which individual?

1. By the primary health care provider when doing a neonatal assessment
2. By the primary health care provider just before circumcision
3. By the mother when she sees her neonate for the first time
4. By the nurse doing the neonatal assessment

33. A 1-year-old underwent hypospadias repair yesterday; he has a suprapubic catheter in place and an I.V. Which rationale is appropriate for administering propantheline (Pro-Banthine) on an as-needed basis?

1. To decrease the chance of infection at the suture line
2. To decrease the number of organisms in the urine
3. To prevent bladder spasms while the catheter is present
4. To increase urine flow from the kidney to the ureters

34. Which intervention by the nurse would be <u>most helpful</u> when discussing hypospadias with the parents of an infant with this defect?

1. Refer the parents to a counselor.
2. Be there to listen to the parents' concerns.
3. Notify the primary health care provider, and have him talk to the parents.
4. Suggest a support group of other parents who have gone through this experience.

35. The nurse should understand that hypospadias defects take the greatest emotional toll on which person?

1. The father
2. The mother
3. The grandfather
4. The grandmother

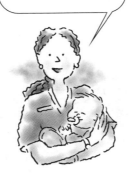

Question 32 asks you to think about the typical sequence of events for a neonate.

32. 4. After delivery, neonates bond with their mothers for a period of time and then are taken to the neonate nursery. The nurse who admits the neonate does a thorough assessment and should recognize hypospadias and alert the primary health care provider. The pediatrician who examines the neonate may not come to the nursery for hours after the delivery.

CN: Physiological adaptation; CNS: Reduction of risk potential; CL: Knowledge

33. 3. Propantheline is an antispasmodic that works effectively on children. It isn't an antibiotic and therefore won't decrease the chance of infection or the number of organisms in the urine. The drug has no diuretic effect and won't increase urine flow.

CN: Physiological integrity; CNS: Pharmacological therapies; CL: Application

34. 2. The nurse must recognize that parents are going to grieve the loss of the normal child when they have a neonate born with a birth defect. Initially, the parents need to have a nurse who will listen to their concerns for their neonate's health. Suggesting a support group or referring the parents to a counselor might be good actions, but not initially. The primary health care provider will need to spend time with the parents but, again, the nurse is in the best position to allow the parents to vent their grief and anger.

CN: Psychosocial integrity; CNS: None; CL: Application

35. 1. Because the penis is involved, studies have shown that fathers have a great deal of difficulty dealing with a birth defect like hypospadias.

CN: Psychosocial integrity; CNS: None; CL: Knowledge

36. The difference between hypospadias and epispadias is defined by which characteristic?
1. Epispadias defects can only occur in males.
2. The difference between the defects is the length of the urethra.
3. Hypospadias is an abnormal opening on the ventral side of the penis; epispadias is an abnormal opening on the dorsal side.
4. Hypospadias is an abnormal opening on the dorsal side of the penis; epispadias is an abnormal opening on the ventral side.

37. Which nursing diagnosis would be most appropriate for a client with hypospadias?
1. *Deficient fluid volume*
2. *Impaired urinary elimination*
3. *Delayed growth and development*
4. *Risk for infection*

38. When a nurse is teaching a parent how to care for her son's penis after hypospadias repair with a skin graft, which statement made by the parent would indicate the need for <u>further teaching</u>?
1. "My infant will be able to take baths after the repair has healed."
2. "I'll change the dressing around his penis daily."
3. "I'll make sure I change my infant's diaper often."
4. "If there's a color change in his penis, I'll notify my primary care provider."

39. The nurse is preparing the parents of an infant with hypospadias for surgery. Which statement made by the parents would indicate the need for <u>further teaching</u>?
1. "Skin grafting might be involved in my infant's repair."
2. "After surgery, my infant's penis will look perfectly normal."
3. "Surgical repair may need to be performed in several stages."
4. "My infant will probably be in some pain after the surgery and might need to take some medication for relief."

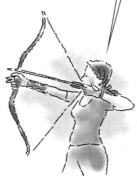

Don't alter your course. You're right on target!

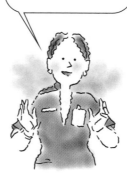

Remember to look for the incorrect statement.

36. 3. Hypospadias results from the incomplete closure of the urethral folds along the ventral surface of the developing penis. Epispadias results when the urinary meatus is on the dorsal surface of the penis. Epispadias defects can occur in males and females. The difference is where the opening of the urinary meatus is located, not the urethra's length.
CN: Physiological integrity; CNS: Physiological adaptation; CL: Comprehension

37. 2. The most appropriate diagnosis for a client with hypospadias is *Impaired urinary elimination*. A client with hypospadias should have no problems with the ingestion of fluids. The child's growth and development isn't affected with this defect, and he shouldn't have any problem with infection until possibly after hypospadias repair is performed.
CN: Physiological integrity; CNS: Physiological adaptation; CL: Analysis

38. 2. Dressing changes after a hypospadias repair with a skin graft are generally performed by the primary health care provider and aren't performed every day because the skin graft needs time to heal and adhere to the penis. Changing the infant's diapers usually helps keep the penis dry. Baths aren't given until postoperative healing has taken place. If the penis color changes, it might be evidence of circulation problems and should be reported.
CN: Psychosocial integrity; CNS: None; CL: Analysis

39. 2. It's important to stress to the parents that, even after a repair of hypospadias, the outcome isn't a completely "normal-looking" penis. The goals of surgery are to allow the child to void from the tip of his penis, void with a straight stream, and stand up while voiding.
CN: Psychosocial integrity; CNS: None; CL: Application

CN: Client needs category CNS: Client needs subcategory CL: Cognitive level

40. Which data collected by the nurse would indicate to the primary care provider the need for a staged repair of a hypospadias rather than a single repair?

1. Chordee is present with the hypospadias.
2. The urinary meatus opens close to the scrotum.
3. The urinary meatus is just below the tip of the penis.
4. The infant had been circumcised before the defect was discovered.

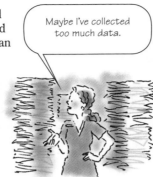

Maybe I've collected too much data.

40. 2. Increased surgical experience and improvements in technique have reduced the number of staged procedures applied to hypospadias defects; however, a staged procedure is indicated in particularly severe defects with marked deficits of available skin for mobilization of flaps. If an infant has a relatively minor hypospadias or has been circumcised, the repair can still occur in one stage. Having chordee present doesn't require a staged hypospadias repair.

CN: Physiological integrity; CNS: Physiological adaptation; CL: Analysis

41. A nurse is planning to teach a female adolescent about pelvic inflammatory disease (PID). Which teaching statement best reflects the focus of preventative teaching needs for this age-group?

1. Poor hygiene practices increase the risk of PID.
2. The use of hormonal contraceptives decreases the risk of PID.
3. There are long-term complications related to reproductive tract infections.
4. There are risks of defects in future infants born to adolescents with PID.

41. 3. Long-term complications of PID include abscess formation in the fallopian tubes and adhesion formation leading to an increased risk of ectopic pregnancy or infertility. PID isn't prevented by proper personal hygiene or by any form of contraception, even though some forms of contraception, such as the male or female condom, do help to decrease the incidence. PID does not increase the risk of birth defects in infants born to adolescents with PID.

CN: Health promotion and maintenance; CNS: None CL: Application

42. After the nurse has completed discharge teaching, which statement made by the client treated for a sexually transmitted disease would indicate that discharge instructions were understood?

1. "I don't need those condoms because I'm not allergic to penicillin and I'll come for a shot at the first sign of infection."
2. "I will notify my sex partners and not have unprotected sex from now on."
3. "I will be careful not to have intercourse with someone who isn't clean."
4. "I don't think it will happen to me again."

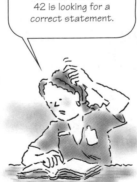

Hmmm. Question 42 is looking for a correct statement.

42. 2. Goal achievement is indicated by the client's ability to describe preventive behaviors and health practices. The other options indicate that the client doesn't understand the need to take preventive measures.

CN: Health promotion and maintenance; CNS: None; CL: Analysis

43. Besides the fact that it's highly infectious, the nurse should teach a client with gonorrhea about which characteristic?

1. It occurs rarely.
2. It can produce sterility.
3. It's always easily cured.
4. It's limited to the external genitalia.

43. 2. Gonorrhea may destroy the epididymis in a male or the tubal mucosa in a female, which can cause sterility. Gonorrhea, a common sexually transmitted disease, occasionally affects the rectum, pharynx, and eyes. Treatment is effective when the client complies.

CN: Physiological integrity; CNS: Physiological adaptation; CL: Knowledge

CN: Client needs category   CNS: Client needs subcategory   CL: Cognitive level

44. Before a client with syphilis can be treated, the nurse must determine which factor?
  1. Portal of entry
  2. Size of the chancre
  3. Names of sexual contacts
  4. Existence of medication allergies

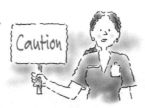

44. 4. The treatment of choice for syphilis is penicillin; clients allergic to penicillin must be given another antibiotic. The other choices aren't necessary before treatment can begin.
CN: Physiological integrity; CNS: Pharmacological therapies; CL: Comprehension

45. Which statement regarding chlamydial infections is correct?
  1. The treatment of choice is oral penicillin.
  2. The treatment of choice is nystatin (Nilstat) or miconazole (Monistat).
  3. Clinical manifestations include dysuria and urethral itching in males.
  4. Clinical manifestations include small, painful vesicles on genital areas.

45. 3. Clinical manifestations of chlamydia include meatal erythema, tenderness, itching, dysuria, and urethral discharge in the male and mucopurulent cervical exudate with erythema, edema, and congestion in the female. The treatment of choice is doxycycline (Vibramycin) or azithromycin (Zithromax). Small, painful vesicles in the genital area refer to herpes.
CN: Physiological integrity; CNS: Physiological adaptation; CL: Application

46. Which technique should the nurse consider when she's discussing sex and sexual activities with adolescents?
  1. Break down all the information into scientific terminology.
  2. Refer adolescents to their parents for sexual information.
  3. Only answer questions that are asked; don't present any other content.
  4. Present sexual information using the proper terminology and in a straightforward manner.

The NCLEX tests your ability to teach clients at different life stages.

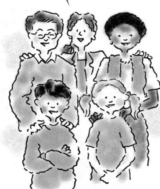

46. 4. Although many adolescents have received sex education from parents and school throughout childhood, they aren't always adequately prepared for the impact of puberty. A large portion of their knowledge is acquired from peers, television, movies, and magazines. Consequently, much of the sex information they have is incomplete, inaccurate, riddled with cultural and moral values, and not very helpful. The public perceives nurses as having authoritative information and being willing to take time with adolescents and their parents. To be effective teachers, nurses need to be honest and open with sexual information.
CN: Health promotion and maintenance; CNS: None; CL: Application

47. Without proper treatment, anogenital warts caused by the human papillomavirus (HPV) increase the risk of which illness in adolescent females?
  1. Gonorrhea
  2. Cervical cancer
  3. Chlamydial infections
  4. Urinary tract infections

47. 2. All external lesions are treated because of concern regarding the relationship of HPV to cancer. HPV doesn't increase the risk of gonorrhea, chlamydia, or urinary tract infections.
CN: Physiological integrity; CNS: Reduction of risk potential; CL: Application

48. Which statement should the nurse include when teaching an adolescent about gonorrhea?
1. It's caused by *Treponema pallidum.*
2. Treatment of sexual partners is an essential part of treatment.
3. It's usually treated by multidose administration of penicillin.
4. It may be contracted through contact with a contaminated toilet seat.

49. When planning sex education and contraceptive teaching for adolescents, which factor should the nurse consider?
1. Neither sexual activity nor contraception requires planning.
2. Most teenagers today are knowledgeable about reproduction.
3. Most teenagers use pregnancy as a way to rebel against their parents.
4. Most teenagers are open about contraception but inconsistently use birth control.

50. A sexually active teenager seeks counseling from the school nurse about prevention of sexually transmitted diseases (STDs). Which contraceptive measure should the nurse recommend?
1. Rhythm method
2. Withdrawal method
3. Prophylactic antibiotic use
4. Condom and spermicide use

51. The nurse understands that which developmental rationale explains risk-taking behavior in adolescents?
1. Adolescents are concrete thinkers and concentrate only on what's happening at the time.
2. Belief in their own invulnerability persuades adolescents that they can take risks safely.
3. Risk of parents' anger and disappointment usually deters adolescents from risky behavior.
4. Peer pressure usually doesn't play an important part in an adolescent's decision to become sexually active.

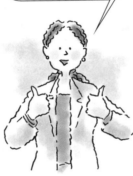

Nice work! You've finished nearly 50 questions already!

48. 2. Adolescents should be taught that treatment is needed for all sexual partners. *Treponema pallidum* is the causative organism of syphillis, not gonorrhea. The medication of choice is a single dose of I.M. ceftriaxone (Rocephin) in males and a single oral dose of cefixime (Suprax) in females. Gonorrhea can't be contracted from a contaminated toilet seat.
CN: Health promotion and maintenance; CNS: None; CL: Application

49. 4. Most teenagers today are very open about discussing contraception and sexuality, but they may get caught up in the moment of sexuality and forget about birth control measures. Adolescents receive most of their information on reproduction and sexuality from their peers, who generally don't have correct information. Teenagers generally become pregnant because they fail to use birth control for other reasons than rebelling against their parents. Contraception should always be part of sex education and requires planning.
CN: Physiological integrity; CNS: Reduction of risk potential; CL: Analysis

50. 4. Prevention of STDs is the primary concern of health care professionals. Barrier contraceptive methods, such as condoms with the addition of spermicide, seem to offer the best protection for preventing STDs and their serious complications. The other contraceptive choices don't prevent the transmission of an STD. Antibiotics can't be taken throughout the life span.
CN: Health promotion and maintenance; CNS: None; CL: Application

51. 2. Understanding the growth and development of adolescents helps the nurse see that they feel they're invulnerable. Peer pressure plays an important role in risk-taking behaviors, more so than fear of parents' anger or disappointment. Adolescents can and do think about the future but are willing to take risks that more mature adults might not take.
CN: Health promotion and maintenance; CNS: None; CL: Analysis

CN: Client needs category   CNS: Client needs subcategory   CL: Cognitive level

52. Statistics about sexually transmitted diseases (STDs) may not be reliable for which reason?
1. Most adolescents seek out treatment for their STD.
2. Adolescents are usually honest with their parents about their sexual behavior.
3. All STDs must be reported to the Centers for Disease Control and Prevention (CDC).
4. Human papillomavirus (HPV) infections aren't required to be reported to the CDC.

52. 4. HPV infections aren't required to be reported to the CDC. Most teenagers are afraid to seek out health care for sexual diseases or are unaware of the signs and symptoms of STDs. Teenagers find this a very difficult topic to discuss with their parents and will usually seek out a peer or another adult to obtain information.
CN: Safe, effective care environment; CNS: Safety and infection control; CL: Application

53. Which statement by an adolescent would alert the nurse that <u>more education</u> about sexually transmitted diseases (STDs) <u>is needed</u>?
1. "You always know when you've got gonorrhea."
2. "The most common STD in kids my age is chlamydia infection."
3. "Most of the girls who have chlamydia don't even know it."
4. "If you have symptoms of gonorrhea, they can show up a day or a couple of weeks after you got the infection to begin with."

53. 1. Gonorrhea can occur with or without symptoms. There are four main forms of the disease: asymptomatic, uncomplicated symptomatic, complicated symptomatic, and disseminated disease. All of the other statements are accurate.
CN: Health promotion and maintenance; CNS: None; CL: Application

54. Which approach describes primary prevention of sexually transmitted diseases (STDs) by avoiding exposure?
1. The least accepted and most difficult approach
2. The least expensive and most effective approach
3. The most expensive and least effective approach
4. The most difficult and most time-consuming approach

54. 2. Primary prevention of STDs by avoiding exposure is the least expensive and most effective approach. The nurse can play a role in offering this education to young people before they initiate sexual intercourse.
CN: Safe, effective care environment; CNS: Safety and infection control; CL: Application

Keep at it! You're more than halfway finished!

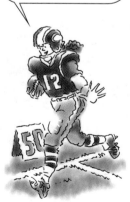

55. It's very important for the nurse to include which statement in discharge education for the client who's taking metronidazole (Flagyl) to treat trichomoniasis?
1. Sexual intercourse should stop.
2. Alcohol shouldn't be consumed.
3. Milk products should be avoided.
4. Exposure to sunlight should be limited.

55. 2. While taking metronidazole to treat trichomoniasis, clients shouldn't consume alcohol for at least 48 hours following the last dose. The other choices have no effect on the client while taking this medication.
CN: Physiological integrity; CNS: Pharmacological therapies; CL: Application

CN: Client needs category   CNS: Client needs subcategory   CL: Cognitive level

56. The nurse should include which fact when teaching an adolescent group about the human immunodeficiency virus (HIV)?

1. The incidence of HIV in the adolescent population has declined since 1995.
2. The virus can be spread through many routes, including sexual contact.
3. Knowledge about HIV spread and transmission has led to a decrease in the spread of the virus among adolescents.
4. About 50% of all new HIV infections in the United States occurs in people younger than age 22.

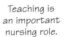

Teaching is an important nursing role.

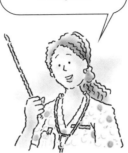

56. 2. HIV can be spread through many routes, including sexual contact and contact with infected blood or other body fluids. The incidence of HIV in the adolescent population has *increased* since 1995, even though more information about the virus is targeted to reach the adolescent population. Only about 25% of all new HIV infections in the United States occurs in people younger than age 22.

CN: Health promotion and maintenance; CNS: None; CL: Application

57. When planning a program to teach adolescents about acquired immunodeficiency syndrome (AIDS), which action might lead to better success of the program?

1. Surveying the community to evaluate the level of education
2. Obtaining peer educators to provide information about AIDS
3. Setting up clinics in community centers and having condoms readily available
4. Having primary health care providers host workshops in community centers

57. 2. Peer education programs have noted that teens are more likely to ask questions of peer educators than of adults and that peer education can change personal attitudes and the perception of the risk of HIV infection. The other approaches would be helpful but wouldn't necessarily make the outreach program more successful.

CN: Safe, effective care environment; CNS: Coordinated care; CL: Analysis

58. Which client would the nurse consider at greater risk for developing acquired immunodeficiency syndrome (AIDS)?

1. A client who lives in crowded housing with poor ventilation
2. A young sexually active client with multiple partners
3. A homeless adolescent who lives in a shelter
4. A young sexually active client with one partner

58. 2. The younger the client when sexual activity begins, the higher the incidence of human immunodeficiency virus and AIDS. Also, the more sexual partners, the higher the incidence. Neither crowded living environments nor homeless environments by themselves lead to an increase in the incidence of AIDS.

CN: Health promotion and maintenance; CNS: None; CL: Knowledge

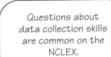

Questions about data collection skills are common on the NCLEX.

59. When collecting data from an adolescent with pelvic inflammatory disease (PID), which signs and symptoms should the nurse expect to see?

1. A hard, painless, red defined lesion
2. Small vesicles on the genital area with itching
3. Cervical discharge with redness and edema
4. Lower abdominal pain

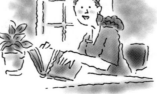

59. 4. PID is an infection of the upper female genital tract most commonly caused by sexually transmitted diseases. Initial symptoms in the adolescent may be generalized, with fever and abdominal pain. Small vesicles on the genital area with itching indicate herpes genitalis. Cervical discharge with redness and edema indicates chlamydia. A hard, painless, red defined lesion indicates syphilis.

CN: Physiological integrity; CNS: Physiological adaptation; CL: Application

CN: Client needs category   CNS: Client needs subcategory   CL: Cognitive level

60. After a nurse completes teaching an adolescent about syphilis, which statement by the adolescent indicates the need for further teaching?
1. "The disease is divided into four stages: primary, secondary, latent, and tertiary."
2. "Affected persons are most infectious during the first year."
3. "Syphilis is easily treated with penicillin or doxycycline."
4. "Syphilis is rarely transmitted sexually."

60. 4. About 95% of the cases of syphilis are transmitted sexually. There are four stages to syphilis, although some people may only experience the first three stages. Affected persons are most contagious in the first year of the disease. The drug of choice for treating syphilis is penicillin or doxycycline.
CN: Health promotion and maintenance; CNS: none; CL: Analysis

61. In teaching a group of parents about monitoring for urinary tract infection (UTI) in preschoolers, which symptom would indicate that a child should be evaluated?
1. Voids only twice in any 6-hour period
2. Exhibits incontinence after being toilet trained
3. Has difficulty sitting still for more than a 30-minute period of time
4. Urine smells strongly of ammonia after standing for more than 2 hours

61. 2. A child who exhibits incontinence after being toilet trained should be evaluated for UTI. Most urine smells strongly of ammonia after standing for more than 2 hours, so this doesn't necessarily indicate UTI. The other options aren't reasons for parents to suspect problems with their child's urinary system.
CN: Safe, effective care environment; CNS: Coordinated care; CL: Application

62. Which instructions should a nurse include in the teaching plan for the parents of a child receiving co-trimoxazole (Septra) for a repeated urinary tract infection with *Escherichia coli*?
1. "For the drug to be effective, keep your child's urine acidic by having him drink at least a quart of cranberry juice per day."
2. "Make sure your child takes the medication for 10 days even if his symptoms improve in a few days."
3. "Wake your child during the night to void to prevent urinary stasis."
4. "Give your child two pills each day, but keep the rest of the pills to give if the symptoms reappear within 2 weeks."

Teaching about medications—that's another common NCLEX subject.

62. 2. Discharge instructions for parents of children receiving an anti-infective medication should include taking all of the prescribed medication for the prescribed time. It isn't necessary to wake the child during the night to void. Drinking highly acidic juices, such as cranberry juice, may help maintain urinary health, but won't get rid of an infection already present.
CN: Physiological integrity; CNS: Pharmacological therapies; CL: Application

63. The nurse should include which fact when teaching parents about handling a child with recurrent urinary tract infection (UTI)?
1. Antibiotics should be discontinued 48 hours after symptoms subside.
2. Recurrent symptoms should be treated by renewing the antibiotic prescription.
3. Complicated UTIs are related to poor perineal hygiene practice.
4. Follow-up urine cultures are necessary to detect recurrent infections and antibiotic effectiveness.

63. 4. A routine follow-up urine specimen is usually obtained 2 or 3 days after the completion of the antibiotic treatment. All of the antibiotic should be taken as ordered and not stopped when symptoms disappear. If recurrent symptoms appear, a urine culture should be obtained to see whether the infection is resistant to antibiotics. Simple, not complicated, UTIs are generally caused by poor perineal hygiene.
CN: Health promotion and maintenance; CNS: None; CL: Application

CN: Client needs category   CNS: Client needs subcategory   CL: Cognitive level

64. When monitoring a child with vesicoureteral reflux, the nurse should understand that this client is at risk for developing which complication?
1. Glomerulonephritis
2. Hemolytic uremia syndrome
3. Nephrotic syndrome
4. Renal damage

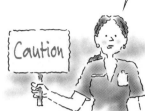

Be aware of possible complications.

64. 4. Reflux of urine into the ureters and then back into the bladder after voiding sets up the client for a urinary tract infection, which can lead to renal damage due to scarring of the parenchyma. Glomerulonephritis is an autoimmune reaction to a beta-hemolytic streptoccocal infection. Eighty percent of nephrotic syndrome cases are idiopathic. Hemolytic uremia syndrome may be the result of genetic factors.
CN: Physiological integrity; CNS: Reduction of risk potential; CL: Knowledge

65. A nurse is reviewing a child's clean-voided urine specimen results. The nurse understands that which result indicates a urinary tract infection?
1. A specific gravity of 1.020
2. Cloudy color without odor
3. A large amount of casts present
4. 100,000 bacterial colonies per milliliter

65. 4. The diagnosis of UTI is determined by the detection of bacteria in the urine. Infected urine usually contains more than 100,000 colonies/ml, usually of a single organism. The urine is usually cloudy, hazy, and may have strands of mucus. It also has a foul, fishy odor even when fresh. Casts and increased specific gravity aren't specific to UTI.
CN: Physiological integrity; CNS: Physiological adaptation; CL: Application

66. Nurses should understand which factor as contributing to the increased incidence of urinary tract infections (UTI) in girls?
1. Vaginal secretions are too acidic.
2. Girls can't be protected by circumcision like boys can.
3. The urethra is in close proximity to the anus.
4. Girls touch their genitalia more often than boys do.

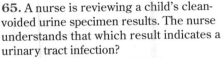

Boys and girls have basic anatomical differences.

66. 3. Girls are especially at risk for bacterial invasion of the urinary tract because of basic anatomical differences; the urethra is shorter and closer to the anus. Vaginal secretions are normally acidic, which decreases the risk of infection; circumcision doesn't protect boys from UTI; and there's no documented research that supports that girls touch their genitalia more often than boys do.
CN: Health promotion and maintenance; CNS: None; CL: Knowledge

67. A nurse is teaching the parents of a child with a urinary tract infection. Which factor should the nurse indicate contributes to urinary tract infection?
1. Increased fluid intake
2. Short urethra
3. Ingestion of highly acidic juices
4. Frequent emptying of the bladder

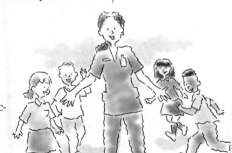

67. 2. A short urethra contributes to infection because bacteria have to travel a shorter distance to the urinary tract. The risk of infection is higher in women because women have shorter urethras than men (¾″ [1.9 cm] in young women, 1½″ [3.8 cm] in mature women, 7¾″ [19.7 cm] in adult men). Increased fluid intake would help flush the urinary tract system and frequent emptying of the bladder would decrease the risk of urinary tract infection. Drinking highly acidic juices, such as cranberry juice, may help maintain urinary health.
CN: Health promotion and maintenance; CNS: None; CL: Application

CN: Client needs category   CNS: Client needs subcategory   CL: Cognitive level

68. A child has been sent to the school nurse for wetting her pants three times in the past 2 days. The nurse should recommend that this child be evaluated for which complication?
1. School phobia
2. Emotional trauma
3. Urinary tract infection
4. Structural defect of the urinary tract

69. Which intervention should a nurse recommend to parents of young girls to help prevent urinary tract infections (UTIs)?
1. Limit bathing as much as possible.
2. Increase fluids and decrease salt intake.
3. Have the child wear cotton underpants.
4. Have the child clean her perineum from back to front.

70. The nurse understands that which characteristic is the single most important factor influencing the occurrence of urinary tract infections (UTI)?
1. Urinary stasis
2. Frequency of baths
3. Type of clothing worn
4. Amount of fluid intake

71. When the nurse is teaching parents of children about recurrent urinary tract infections, which goal should be included as the most important?
1. Detection
2. Education
3. Prevention
4. Treatment

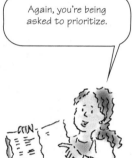

Again, you're being asked to prioritize.

Question 71 should be a slam dunk!

68. 3. Frequent urinary incontinence should be evaluated by the primary health care provider, with the first action being checking the urine for infection. Children exhibit signs of school phobia by complaining of an ailment before school starts and getting better after they're allowed to miss school. After infection, structural defect, and diabetes mellitus have been ruled out, emotional trauma should be investigated.
CN: Health promotion and maintenance; CNS: None; CL: Application

69. 3. Cotton is a more breathable fabric and allows for dampness to be absorbed from the perineum. Increasing fluids would be helpful, but decreasing salt isn't necessary. Bathing shouldn't be limited; however, the use of bubble bath or whirlpool baths should. However, if the child has frequent UTIs, taking a bath should be discouraged and taking a shower encouraged. The perineum should always be cleaned from front to back.
CN: Health promotion and maintenance; CNS: None; CL: Knowledge

70. 1. Ordinarily, urine is sterile. However, at 98.6° F (37° C), it provides an excellent culture medium. Under normal conditions, the act of completely and repeatedly emptying the bladder flushes away organisms before they have an opportunity to multiply and invade surrounding tissue. Tight jeans and pants may contribute to UTI, but aren't the most important factor. Baths and fluid intake are factors in the development of UTI but aren't the most important ones.
CN: Physiological integrity; CNS: Reduction of risk potential; CL: Application

71. 3. Prevention is the most important goal in primary and recurrent infection; most preventive measures are simple, ordinary hygienic habits that should be a routine part of daily care. Treatment, detection, and education are all important goals but not the most important ones.
CN: Physiological integrity; CNS: Reduction of risk potential; CL: Analysis

CN: Client needs category   CNS: Client needs subcategory   CL: Cognitive level

72. When evaluating infants and young toddlers for signs of urinary tract infections (UTIs), a nurse should know that which symptom would be most common?
1. Abdominal pain
2. Feeding problems
3. Frequency
4. Urgency

73. When obtaining a urine specimen for culture and sensitivity, the nurse should understand that which method of collection is best?
1. Bagged urine specimen
2. Clean-catch urine specimen
3. First-voided urine specimen
4. Catheterized urine specimen

74. After collecting a urine specimen, which action by the nurse is the <u>most appropriate</u>?
1. Take the specimen to the laboratory immediately.
2. Send the specimen to the laboratory on the scheduled run.
3. Take the specimen to the laboratory on the nurse's next break.
4. Keep the specimen in the refrigerator until it can be taken to the laboratory.

75. When teaching the parents of a child with a urinary tract infection (UTI) about fluid intake, which statement by a parent would indicate the need for further teaching?
1. "I should encourage my child to drink about 50 ml per pound of body weight daily."
2. "Clear liquids should be the primary liquids that my child drinks."
3. "I should offer my child carbonated beverages about every 2 hours."
4. "My child should avoid drinking caffeinated beverages."

72. 2. In infants and children younger than age 2, the signs are characteristically nonspecific, and feeding problems are usually the first indication. Symptoms more nearly resemble GI tract disorders. Abdominal pain, urgency, and frequency are signs that would be observed in the older child with a UTI.
CN: Physiological integrity; CNS: Physiological adaptation; CL: Application

73. 4. The most accurate tests of bacterial content are suprapubic aspiration (for children younger than age 2) and properly performed bladder catheterization. The other methods of obtaining a specimen have a high incidence of contamination not related to infection.
CN: Physiological integrity; CNS: Basic care and comfort; CL: Application

74. 1. Care of urine specimens obtained for culture is an important nursing aspect related to diagnosis. Specimens should be taken to the laboratory for culture immediately. If the culture is delayed, the specimen can be placed in the refrigerator, but storage can result in a loss of formed elements, such as blood cells and casts.
CN: Physiological integrity; CNS: Basic care and comfort; CL: Application

75. 3. Carbonated or caffeinated beverages are avoided because of their potentially irritating effect on the bladder mucosa. Adequate fluid intake is always indicated during an acute UTI. It's recommended that a person drink approximately 50 ml/lb of body weight daily. The client should primarily drink clear liquids.
CN: Physiological integrity; CNS: Basic care and comfort; CL: Analysis

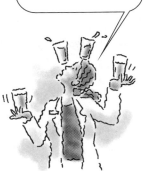

When it comes to fluid intake, it's a real balancing act!

CN: Client needs category   CNS: Client needs subcategory   CL: Cognitive level

76. Which treatment should the nurse anticipate in a child who has a history of recurrent urinary tract infections (UTIs)?
1. Frequent catheterizations
2. Prophylactic antibiotics
3. Limited activities
4. Surgical intervention

76. 2. Children who experience recurrent UTI may require antibiotic therapy for months or years. Recurrent UTI would be investigated for anatomic abnormalities and surgical intervention may be indicated, but the client would also be placed on antibiotics before the tests. The child's activities aren't limited, and frequent catheterization predisposes a child to infection.
CN: Physiological integrity; CNS: Basic care and comfort; CL: Application

77. When teaching parents about giving medications to children for recurrent urinary tract infections, which instructions should be included?
1. The medication should be given first thing in the morning.
2. The medication should be given right before bedtime.
3. The medication is generally given four times per day.
4. It doesn't matter when the medication is given.

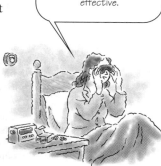

Teach clients to take medication when it will be most effective.

77. 2. Medication is commonly administered once per day, and the client and parents are advised to give the antibiotic before sleep because this represents the longest period without voiding.
CN: Physiological integrity; CNS: Pharmacological therapies; CL: Application

78. A nurse is providing education to a group of parents about urinary tract infections (UTIs). The nurse knows teaching has been effective when the parents state that which situation has the greatest impact on the potential for progressive renal injury after UTIs?
1. A school-age child who must get permission to go to the bathroom
2. An adolescent female who has started menstruation
3. Children who participate in competitive sports
4. Infections occurring in young infants and toddlers

78. 4. The hazard of progressive renal injury is greatest when infection occurs in young children, especially those under age 2. The first two options might lead to a simple UTI that would need to be treated. Competitive sports have no bearing on a UTI.
CN: Safe, effective care environment; CNS: Safety and infection control; CL: Application

79. Which statement should the nurse make to help parents understand the recovery period after a child has had surgery to remove a Wilms' tumor?
1. "Children will easily lie in bed and restrict their activities."
2. "Recovery is usually fast in spite of the abdominal incision."
3. "Recovery usually takes a great deal of time because of the large incision."
4. "Parents need to perform activities of daily living for about 2 weeks after surgery."

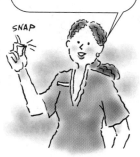

The answer to question 79 should be a snap!

SNAP

79. 2. Children generally recover very quickly from surgery to remove a Wilms' tumor, even though they may have a large abdominal incision. Children like to get back into the normalcy of being a child, which is through play. Parents need to encourage their children to do as much for themselves as possible, although some regression is expected.
CN: Psychosocial integrity; CNS: None; CL: Analysis

CN: Client needs category   CNS: Client needs subcategory   CL: Cognitive level

80. When teaching parents about administering co-trimoxazole (Septra) to a child for treatment of a urinary tract infection, the nurse should include which instructions?
1. Give the medication with food.
2. Give the medication with water.
3. Give the medication with a cola beverage.
4. Give the medication 1 hour after a meal.

81. The nurse understands that which characteristic is <u>true</u> of the incidence of Wilms' tumor?
1. Peak incidence occurs at age 10.
2. It's the least common type of renal cancer.
3. It's the most common type of renal cancer.
4. It has a decreased incidence among siblings.

82. Which initial sign is most common with Wilms' tumor?
1. Pain in the abdomen
2. Fever greater than 104° F (40° C)
3. Decreased blood pressure
4. Swelling within the abdomen

83. When the nurse is explaining the diagnosis of Wilms' tumor to parents, which statement by a parent would indicate the need for further teaching?
1. "Wilms' tumor usually involves both kidneys."
2. "Wilms' tumor is slightly more common in the left kidney."
3. "Wilms' tumor is staged during surgery for treatment planning."
4. "Wilms' tumor stays encapsulated for an extended time."

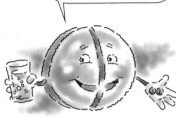

It's important to tell your client how and when to take me.

80. 2. When giving Septra, the medication should be administered with a full glass of water on an empty stomach. If nausea and vomiting occur, giving the drug with food may decrease gastric distress. Carbonated beverages should be avoided because they irritate the bladder.
CN: Physiological integrity; CNS: Pharmacological therapies; CL: Application

81. 3. Wilms' tumor is the most common intra-abdominal tumor of childhood and the most common type of renal cancer. The peak incidence is age 3, and there's an increased incidence among siblings and identical twins.
CN: Physiological integrity; CNS: Physiological adaptation; CL: Knowledge

82. 4. The most common initial sign is a swelling or mass within the abdomen. The mass is characteristically firm, nontender, confined to one side, and deep within the flank. A high fever isn't an initial sign of Wilms' tumor. Blood pressure is characteristically increased, not decreased.
CN: Physiological integrity; CNS: Physiological adaptation; CL: Application

83. 1. Wilms' tumor usually involves only one kidney and is usually staged during surgery so that an effective course of treatment can be established. Wilms' tumor has a slightly higher occurrence in the left kidney, and it stays encapsulated for an extended time.
CN: Physiological integrity; CNS: Physiological adaptation; CL: Knowledge

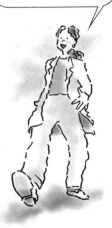

Keep it up! You're making great strides.

84. A parent asks the nurse about the prognosis of her child diagnosed with Wilms' tumor. The nurse should base her response on which factor?
1. Usually children with Wilms' tumor needs only surgical intervention.
2. Survival rates for Wilms' tumor are the lowest among childhood cancers.
3. Survival rates for Wilms' tumor are the highest among childhood cancers.
4. Children with localized tumor have only a 30% chance of cure with multimodal therapy.

85. If <u>both kidneys</u> are involved with Wilms' tumor, the nurse should understand that treatment before surgery might include which method?
1. Peritoneal dialysis
2. Abdominal gavage
3. Radiation and chemotherapy
4. Antibiotics and I.V. fluid therapy

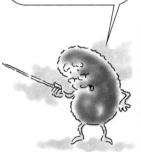

Hmmm, might the treatment for both kidneys differ from that for one?

86. When caring for the child with Wilms' tumor <u>preoperatively</u>, which nursing intervention would be most important?
1. Avoiding abdominal palpation
2. Closely monitoring arterial blood gas (ABG) values
3. Preparing the child and family for long-term dialysis
4. Preparing the child and family for renal transplantation

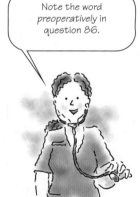

Note the word preoperatively in question 86.

87. A child is scheduled for surgery to remove a Wilms' tumor from one kidney. The parents ask the nurse what treatment, if any, they should expect after their child recovers from surgery. Which response would be most accurate?
1. "Chemotherapy may be necessary."
2. "Kidney transplant is indicated eventually."
3. "No additional treatments are usually necessary."
4. "Chemotherapy with or without radiation therapy is indicated."

84. 3. Survival rates for Wilms' tumor are the highest among childhood cancers. Usually, children with Wilms' tumor who have stage I or II localized tumor have a 90% chance of cure with multimodal therapy.
CN: Physiological integrity; CNS: Physiological adaptation; CL: Application

85. 3. If both kidneys are involved, the child may be treated with radiation therapy or chemotherapy preoperatively to shrink the tumor, allowing more conservative therapy. Peritoneal dialysis would be needed only if the kidneys weren't functioning. Abdominal gavage wouldn't be indicated. Antibiotics aren't needed because Wilms' tumor isn't an infection.
CN: Safe, effective care environment; CNS: Coordinated care; CL: Application

86. 1. After the diagnosis of Wilms' tumor is made, the abdomen shouldn't be palpated. Palpation of the tumor might lead to rupture, which would cause the cancerous cells to spread throughout the abdomen. ABG values shouldn't be affected. If surgery is successful, there won't be a need for long-term dialysis or renal transplantation.
CN: Physiological integrity; CNS: Reduction of risk potential; CL: Application

87. 4. Because radiation therapy and chemotherapy are usually begun immediately after surgery, parents need an explanation of what to expect, such as major benefits and adverse effects. Kidney transplant isn't usually necessary.
CN: Safe, effective care environment; CNS: Coordinated care; CL: Application

88. A toddler is admitted to the hospital with nephrotic syndrome. The nurse carefully monitors the toddler's fluid intake and output and checks urine specimens regularly with a reagent strip (Labstix). Which finding is the nurse most likely to report?

1. Proteinuria
2. Glucosuria
3. Ketonuria
4. Polyuria

89. The parent of a child with Wilms' tumor asks the nurse about surgery. Which statement best explains the need for surgery for Wilms' tumor?

1. Surgery isn't indicated in children with Wilms' tumor.
2. Surgery is usually performed within 24 to 48 hours of admission.
3. Surgery is the least favorable therapy for the treatment of Wilms' tumor.
4. Surgery will be delayed until the client's overall health status improves.

90. A 3-year-old client has had surgery to remove a Wilms' tumor. Which action should the nurse take first when the mother asks for pain medication for the child?

1. Get the pain medication ready for administration.
2. Assess the client's pain using a pain scale of 1 to 10.
3. Assess the client's pain using a smiley face pain scale.
4. Check for the last time pain medication was administered.

91. A child has been diagnosed with Wilms' tumor. Because of the parents' religious beliefs, they choose not to treat the child. Which statement by the nurse indicates the need for further discussion?

1. "I know this is a lot of information in a short period of time."
2. "I don't think parents have the legal right to make these kinds of decisions."
3. "These parents just don't understand how easily treated a Wilms' tumor is."
4. "I think the parents are in shock."

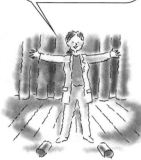

Your performance so far has been outstanding!

88. 1. In nephrotic syndrome, the glomerular membrane of the kidneys becomes permeable to proteins. This results in massive proteinuria, which the nurse can detect with a reagent strip. Nephrotic syndrome typically doesn't cause glucosuria or ketonuria. Because the syndrome causes fluids to shift from plasma to interstitial spaces, it's more likely to decrease urine output than to cause polyuria (excessive urine output).
CNS: Physiological integrity; CN: Reduction of risk potential; CL: Application

89. 2. Surgery is the preferred treatment and is scheduled as soon as possible after confirmation of a renal mass, usually within 24 to 48 hours of admission, to make sure the encapsulated tumor remains intact.
CN: Safe, effective care environment; CNS: Coordinated care; CL: Comprehension

90. 3. The first action of the nurse should be to assess the client for pain. A 3-year-old child is too young to use a pain scale from 1 to 10 but can easily use the smiley face pain scale. After assessing the pain, the nurse should then investigate the time the pain medication was last given and administer the medication accordingly.
CN: Physiological integrity; CNS: Pharmacological therapies; CL: Application

91. 2. Parents *do* have the legal right to make decisions regarding the health issues for their child. Religion plays an important role in many people's lives, and decisions about surgery and treatment for cancer are sometimes made that scientifically don't make sense to the health care provider. The parents are probably in a state of shock because a lot of information has been given, and this is a cancer that requires decisions to be made quickly, especially surgical intervention.
CN: Psychosocial integrity; CNS: None; CL: Analysis

CN: Client needs category   CNS: Client needs subcategory   CL: Cognitive level

92. A child with a Wilms' tumor has had surgery to remove a kidney and has received chemotherapy. The nurse should include which instructions at discharge?
1. Avoid contact sports.
2. Decrease fluid intake.
3. Decrease sodium intake.
4. Avoid contact with other children.

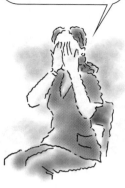

I think you're almost done, but I just can't look!

93. A 3-year-old child has nephrotic syndrome. As the amount of protein loss in the urine decreases, what response would the nurse expect?
1. Weight gain
2. Increased hyperlipidemia
3. Decreased edema
4. Decreased appetite

94. When caring for a child after removal of a Wilms' tumor, which finding would indicate the need to notify the primary care provider?
1. Fever of 100° F (37.8° C)
2. Absence of bowel sounds
3. Slight congestion in the lungs
4. Complaints of pain when moving

95. A child with nephrotic syndrome develops generalized edema as a result of his nephrosis. Which goal would be included in the care plan to prevent complications of edema?
1. Continually support the scrotum.
2. Change the child's position every 2 hours.
3. The child's skin will remain intact during hospitalization.
4. Maintain continuous bed rest.

92. 1. Because the child is left with only one kidney, certain precautions, such as avoiding contact sports, are recommended to prevent injury to the remaining kidney. Decreasing fluid intake wouldn't be indicated; fluid intake is essential for renal function. The child's sodium intake shouldn't be reduced. Avoiding other children is unnecessary and will make the child feel self-conscious and may lead to regressive behavior.
CN: Physiological integrity; CNS: Reduction of risk potential; CL: Application

93. 3. The loss of protein in the urine results in decreased osmotic pressure in the vascular system, causing a fluid shift to the extravascular compartments and producing edema. As the proteinuria decreases, the edema decreases. Weight gain is consistent with proteinuria and a fluid shift from the vascular to the interstitial spaces. Hyperlipidemia and anorexia are associated with nephrotic syndrome but decrease as the disease resolves.
CN: Physiological integrity; CNS: Reduction of risk potential; CL: Comprehension

94. 2. After tumor removal, the child is at risk for intestinal obstruction. GI abnormalities require notification of the primary health care provider. A slight fever following surgery isn't uncommon, nor are slight congestion in the lungs and complaints of pain.
CN: Physiological integrity; CNS: Reduction of risk potential; CL: Application

95. 3. This is the only option written as a goal. The other options are interventions recommended to maintain skin integrity, not goals.
CN: Physiological integrity; CNS: Basic care and comfort; CL: Application

96. In providing psychosocial care to a 6-year-old client who has had abdominal surgery for Wilms' tumor, which activity initiated by the nurse would be the <u>most appropriate</u>?

1. Allowing the child to watch a 2-hour movie without interruptions
2. Giving the child a puzzle with five pieces to encourage him to move while in bed
3. Telling the child that you can give him enough medication so that he feels no pain
4. Providing the child with supplies and asking him to draw how he feels

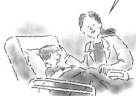

This item is looking for the *most appropriate* answer. In other words, prioritize.

96. 4. A movie is a good diversion, but giving supplies and encouraging the child to draw his feelings is a better outlet. Many procedures have been performed on this client since admission. You probably can't give enough pain medication so that a person who has had surgery will feel no pain. A puzzle with only five pieces is too basic for a 6-year-old child and wouldn't hold his interest.
CN: Psychosocial integrity; CNS: None; CL: Application

97. A nurse should understand that staging of a Wilms' tumor helps to determine which parameter?

1. Size of tumor
2. Level of treatment
3. Length of incision
4. Amount of anesthesia

97. 2. Staging the tumor helps to determine the level of treatment because it provides information about the level of involvement. The other choices aren't influenced by staging the tumor.
CN: Physiological integrity; CNS: Physiological adaptation; CL: Knowledge

98. The nurse is educating parents about Wilms' tumor. Which statement made by a parent would indicate the need for <u>further teaching</u>?

1. "My child could have inherited this disease."
2. "Wilms' tumor can be associated with other congenital anomalies."
3. "This disease could have been a result of trauma to the baby in utero."
4. "There's no method to identify gene carriers of Wilms' tumor."

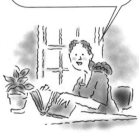

You didn't think you'd finish these practice questions without another further teaching question, did you?

98. 3. Wilms' tumor isn't a result of trauma to the fetus in utero. Wilms' tumor can be genetically inherited and is associated with other congenital anomalies. There is, however, no method to identify gene carriers of Wilms' tumor at this time.
CN: Psychosocial integrity; CNS: None; CL: Application

99. A 6-year-old boy's indwelling urinary catheter was removed at 6 a.m. At noon, the child still hasn't voided. He appears uncomfortable, and the nurse palpates slight bladder distention. Which action should the nurse take first?

1. Insert a straight catheter, as ordered, for urine retention.
2. Consult the physician about replacing the indwelling urinary catheter.
3. Wait awhile longer to see whether the client can void on his own.
4. Turn on the water faucet and provide privacy.

99. 4. Urine retention can result from many factors, including stress and use of opiates. Initially, the nurse should use independent nursing actions, such as providing the client with privacy, placing him in a sitting or standing position to enlist the aid of gravity and increase intra-abdominal pressure, and turning on the water faucet. If these measures are unsuccessful and the physician has left standing orders for straight catheterization, the nurse can proceed with the catheterization. Consulting the physician would involve the use of a dependent nursing action; independent actions should be attempted first. Waiting longer will only increase the child's distention and pain.
CN: Physiological integrity; CNS: Basic care and comfort; CL: Application

CN: Client needs category   CNS: Client needs subcategory   CL: Cognitive level

100. A nurse has orders to notify the physician if a 44-lb preschooler's urine output drops below 3 ml/kg/hr. The urine output for the previous hour was 30 ml. Which nursing intervention would be the <u>priority</u>?

1. Continue to monitor the child's urine output.
2. Encourage the child to drink more fluids.
3. Wait another 30 minutes and then notify the physician.
4. Notify the physician of the child's urine output.

100. 4. First, convert the child's weight to kg. There are 2.2 kg in 1 lb; thus, 44 divided by 2.2 = 20 kg. 3 ml × 20 kg = 60 ml/hr. This is the minimum urine output for a child of 20 kg. Since the child had only a 30-ml urine output in the previous hour, it's crucial for the nurse to notify the physician. The nurse should continue to monitor the urine output after notifying the physician. Fluid should be encouraged as long as the child isn't on fluid restrictions. The nurse should not wait another 30 minutes before notifying the physician because the lack of urine output could indicate a complication.
CN: Physiological integrity; CNS: Reduction of risk potential; CL: Analysis

101. A mother reports that her 6-year-old girl recently started wetting the bed and running a low-grade fever. A urinalysis is positive for bacteria and protein. A diagnosis of a urinary tract infection (UTI) is made, and the child is prescribed antibiotics. Which interventions are appropriate? Select all that apply:

1. Limit fluids for the next few days to decrease the frequency of urination.
2. Assess the mother's understanding of UTI and its causes.
3. Instruct the mother to administer the antibiotic as prescribed—even if the symptoms diminish.
4. Provide instructions solely to the mother, not the child.
5. Discourage taking bubble baths.
6. Advise wiping from the back to the front after voiding and defecation.

101. 2, 3, 5. Assessing the mother's understanding of UTI and its causes provides the nurse with a baseline for teaching. The full course of antibiotics must be given to eradicate the organism and prevent recurrence, even if the child's signs and symptoms decrease. Bubble baths can irritate the vulva and urethra and contribute to the development of a UTI. Fluids should be encouraged, not limited, in order to prevent urinary stasis and help flush the organism out of the urinary tract. Instructions should be given to the child at her level of understanding to help her better understand the treatment and promote compliance. The child should wipe from the front to the back, not back to front, to minimize the risk of contamination after elimination.
CN: Health promotion and maintenance; CNS: None; CL: Application

102. When describing enuresis to a child's parents, which statements would the nurse include in the description? Select all that apply:

1. The child may experience involuntary urination after age 5.
2. Episodes primarily occur when the child is awake and playing.
3. The child may suffer deep feelings of shame and may withdraw from peers because of ridicule.
4. The condition may respond to tricyclic antidepressants and antidiuretics.
5. The condition may become permanent without appropriate intervention.

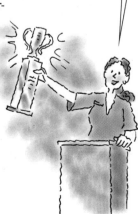

Congratulations! You finished all 102 questions! Fantastic!

102. 1, 3, 4. Enuresis is a condition in which there's involuntary urination after age 5. It generally occurs while the child is sleeping. There can be long-lasting emotional trauma resulting from peer ridicule and feelings of shame and embarrassment. The condition may be treated with the use of tricyclic antidepressants and antidiuretics. With support and understanding, the condition generally resolves in time.
CN: Physiological integrity; CNS: Physiological adaptation; CL: Analysis

CN: Client needs category   CNS: Client needs subcategory   CL: Cognitive level

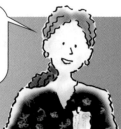

Skin diseases in children and teens are common and varied. This chapter covers common and uncommon skin disorders among these populations.

1. A 3-year-old child gets a burn at the angle of the mouth from chewing on an electrical cord. Which finding should the nurse expect to inspect <u>10 days</u> after the injury?
1. Normal granular tissue
2. Contracture of the injury site
3. Ulceration with serous drainage
4. Profuse bleeding from the injury site

2. Providing adequate nutrition is essential for a burn client. Which statement <u>best</u> describes the nutritional needs of a child who has burns?
1. A child needs 100 cal/kg during hospitalization.
2. The hypermetabolic state after a burn injury leads to poor healing.
3. Caloric needs can be lowered by controlling environmental temperature.
4. Maintaining a hypermetabolic rate will lower the child's risk of infection.

Limit your answer to the correct time span.

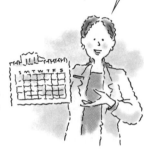

3. A 7-year-old child is brought to the emergency department with burns to the back of the head and the back of the right thigh. According to the Lund-Browder classifications, what percentage of body surface area is affected and should be recorded?
1. 9½%
2. 9¾%
3. 8½%
4. 9%

Measuring burns in children is different from measuring them in adults.

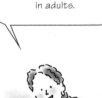

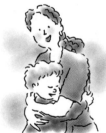

1. 4. Ten days after oral burns from electrical cords, the eschar falls off, exposing arteries and veins. Burns to the oral cavity heal rapidly, but with contractures and scarring. Although contractures are likely, they aren't seen 10 days postinjury.

CN: Physiological integrity; CNS: Physiological adaptation; CL: Application

2. 2. A burn injury causes a hypermetabolic state leading to protein and lipid catabolism, which affects wound healing. Caloric intake should be 1½ to 2 times the basal metabolic rate, with a minimum of 1.5 to 2 g/kg of body weight of protein daily. High metabolic rates increase the risk of infection. Keeping the temperature within a normal range lets the body function efficiently and use calories for healing and normal physiological processes. If the temperature is too warm or too cold, energy must be used for warming or cooling, taking energy away from tissue repair.

CN: Physiological integrity; CNS: Basic care and comfort; CL: Analysis

3. 2. The back of the head in a 7-year-old is 5½%. The back of the right thigh is 4¼%. Therefore, the total is 9¾%.

CN: Physiological integrity; CNS: Physiological adaptation; CL: Application

CN: Client needs category   CNS: Client needs subcategory   CL: Cognitive level

4. An 18-month-old child is admitted to the hospital for full-thickness burns to the anterior chest. The mother asks how the burn will heal. Which statement would the nurse incorporate in the response?

1. Surgical closure and grafting are usually needed.
2. Healing takes 10 to 12 days, with little or no scarring.
3. Pigment in a black client will return to the injured area.
4. Healing can take up to 6 weeks, with a high incidence of scarring.

5. Which finding would the nurse associate with a deep partial-thickness burn in a 9-year-old child?

1. Erythema and pain
2. Minimal damage to the epidermis
3. Necrosis through all layers of skin
4. Tissue necrosis through most of the dermis

6. A 4-year-old child is admitted to the burn unit with a <u>circumferential</u> burn to the left forearm. Which <u>finding</u> would alert the nurse to a potential complication that should be reported to the physician?

1. Numbness of fingers
2. +3 radial and ulnar pulses
3. Full range of motion and no pain
4. Bilateral capillary refill less than 2 seconds

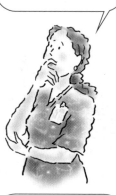

What do I know about the healing time of full-thickness burns?

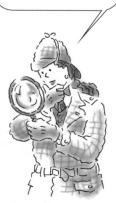

The word *circumferential* is the clue to question 6.

4. 1. Full-thickness burns usually need surgical closure and grafting for complete healing. Deep partial-thickness burns heal in 6 weeks, with scarring. Healing in 10 to 12 weeks with little or no scarring is associated with superficial partial-thickness burns. With superficial partial-thickness burns, pigment is expected to return to the injured area after healing.
CN: Physiological integrity; CNS: Physiological adaptation; CL: Application

5. 4. A client with a deep partial-thickness burn will have tissue necrosis to the epidermis and dermis layers. Necrosis through all skin layers is seen with full-thickness injuries. Erythema and pain are characteristic of superficial injury. With deep burns, the nerve fibers are destroyed and the client won't feel pain in the affected area. Superficial burns are characteristic of slight epidermal damage.
CN: Physiological integrity; CNS: Physiological adaptation; CL: Application

6. 1. Circumferential burns can compromise blood flow to an extremity, causing numbness. Capillary refill less than 2 seconds indicates a normal vascular blood flow. Absence of pain and full range of motion imply good tissue oxygenation from intact circulation. +3 pulses indicate normal circulation.
CN: Physiological integrity; CNS: Physiological adaptation; CL: Analysis

7. When talking with the parents of a child with erythema infectiosum (fifth disease), the nurse should include which statement?
1. There's a possible reappearance of the rash for up to 1 week.
2. Isolation of high-risk contacts should be avoided for 4 to 10 days.
3. Pregnant clients are at risk for fetal death if infected with fifth disease.
4. Children with fifth disease are contagious only while the rash is present.

8. A mother is concerned that her 3-year-old daughter has been exposed to erythema infectiosum (fifth disease). Which characteristic finding would the nurse incorporate in the response to the mother?
1. A fine, erythematous rash with a texture-like sandpaper
2. Intense redness of both cheeks that may spread to the extremities
3. Low-grade fever, followed by vesicular lesions of the trunk, face, and scalp
4. Three- to five-day history of sustained fever, followed by a diffuse erythematous maculopapular rash

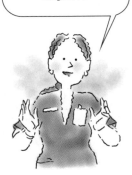

Different symptoms indicate different diagnoses.

9. A family that recently went camping brings their child to the clinic with a complaint of a rash after a tick bite. Lyme disease is suspected. Which assessment finding should the nurse expect to see in a child with Lyme disease?
1. Erythematous rash surrounding a necrotic lesion
2. Bright rash with red outer border circling the bite site
3. Onset of a diffuse rash over the entire body 2 months after exposure
4. A linear rash of papules and vesicles that occur 1 to 3 days after exposure

7. 3. There's a 3% to 5% risk of fetal death from hydrops fetalis if a pregnant client is exposed during the first trimester. The cutaneous eruption of fifth disease can reappear for up to 4 months. A child with fifth disease is contagious during the first stage, when symptoms of headache, body aches, fever, and chills are present, not after the rash. The child should be isolated from pregnant women, immunocompromised clients, and clients with chronic anemia for up to 2 weeks.
CN: Safe, effective care environment; CNS: Safety and infection control; CL: Application

8. 2. The classic symptoms of erythema infectiosum begin with intense redness of both cheeks. An erythematous rash after a fever is characteristic of roseola. Children with varicella typically have vesicular lesions of the trunk, face, and scalp after a low-grade fever. An erythematous rash with a sandpaper-like texture is associated with scarlet fever, which is a bacterial infection.
CN: Physiological integrity; CNS: Physiological adaptation; CL: Application

9. 2. A bull's eye rash is a classic symptom of Lyme disease. Necrotic, painful rashes are associated with the bite of a brown recluse spider. In Lyme disease, the rash is located primarily at the site of the bite. A linear, papular, vesicular rash indicates exposure to the leaves of poison ivy.
CN: Physiological integrity; CNS: Physiological adaptation; CL: Application

10. When administering a Mantoux test for a 6-year-old child, which procedure would the nurse expect to follow?
1. Read results within 24 hours.
2. Read results 48 to 72 hours later.
3. Use the large muscle of the upper leg.
4. Massage the site to increase absorption.

11. When teaching the parents of a child with Kawasaki disease, which information would the nurse keep in mind?
1. It's highly contagious.
2. It's an afebrile condition with cardiac involvement.
3. It usually occurs in children older than 5 years.
4. Prolonged fever, with peeling of the fingers and toes, are the initial symptoms.

12. A 22-lb child is diagnosed with Kawasaki disease and started on gamma globulin therapy. The physician orders an I.V. infusion of gamma globulin, 2 g/kg, to run over 12 hours. Which dose is correct?
1. 11 g
2. 20 g
3. 22 g
4. 44 g

13. A mother is concerned because her child was exposed to varicella in day care. Which statement by the nurse would be <u>most</u> accurate?
1. "The rash is nonvesicular."
2. "The treatment of choice is aspirin."
3. "Varicella has an incubation period of 5 to 10 days."
4. "A child is no longer contagious once the rash has crusted over."

10. 2. The test should be read 48 to 72 hours after placement by measuring the diameter of the induration that develops at the site. The purified protein derivative is injected intradermally on the volar surface of the forearm. Massaging the site could cause leakage from the injection site.
CN: Physiological integrity; CNS: Reduction of risk potential; CL: Application

11. 4. To be diagnosed with Kawasaki disease, the child must have a fever for 5 days or more, plus four of the following five symptoms: bilateral conjunctivitis, changes in the oral mucosa, changes in the peripheral extremities, rash, and lymphadenopathy. Kawasaki disease is more likely to occur in children younger than age 5. It isn't contagious.
CN: Physiological integrity; CNS: Physiological adaptation; CL: Comprehension

12. 2. One kilogram equals 2.2 lb, so a 22-lb child weighs 10 kg. Use the following equations to convert the weight to kilograms and calculate the dose:
22 (lb) ÷ 2.2 = 10 (kg);
2 g × 10 = 20 g.
CN: Physiological integrity; CNS: Pharmacological therapies; CL: Application

13. 4. When every varicella lesion is crusted over, the child is no longer considered contagious. The incubation period is 10 to 20 days. Use of aspirin has been associated with Reye's syndrome and is contraindicated in varicella. The rash is typically a maculopapular vesicular rash.
CN: Physiological integrity; CNS: Physiological adaptation; CL: Application

---

CN: Client needs category   CNS: Client needs subcategory   CL: Cognitive level

14. Which statement is correct about the rash associated with varicella?
1. It's diagnostic in the presence of Koplik's spots in the oral mucosa.
2. It's a maculopapular rash starting on the scalp and hairline and spreading downward.
3. It's a vesicular maculopapular rash that appears abruptly on the trunk, face, and scalp.
4. It appears as yellow ulcers surrounded by red halos on the surface of the hands and feet.

15. Which statement would the nurse keep in mind when describing frostbite to the parents of a child brought to the emergency department after an extended period of sledding?
1. The skin is white.
2. The skin looks deeply flushed and red.
3. Frostbite is helped by rubbing to increase circulation.
4. Slow gradual rewarming of the extremities with hot water is needed.

16. A mother brings her child to the physician's office because the child complains of pain, redness, and tenderness of the left index finger. The child is diagnosed with paronychia. Which organism is the most likely cause of this superficial abscess of the cuticle?
1. *Borrelia burgdorferi*
2. *Escherichia coli*
3. *Pseudomonas* species
4. *Staphylococcus* species

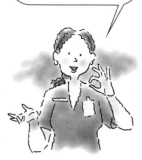

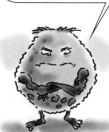

14. 3. In varicella, teardrop vesicles on an erythematous base generally begin on the trunk, face, and scalp, with minimal involvement of the extremities. A descending maculopapular rash is characteristic of rubeola, and Koplik's spots are diagnostic of the disease. Yellow ulcers of the hands and feet are associated with Coxsackie virus or hand-foot-and-mouth disease.
CN: Physiological integrity; CNS: Physiological adaptation; CL: Knowledge

15. 1. Signs and symptoms of frostbite include tingling, numbness, burning sensation, and white skin. Treatment includes very gentle handling of the affected area. Rubbing is contraindicated as it can damage fragile tissue. Gradual rewarming by exposure to hot water can lead to more tissue damage.
CN: Physiological integrity; CNS: Physiological adaptation; CL: Comprehension

16. 4. Paronychia is a localized infection of the nail bed caused by either staphylococci or streptococci. *B. burgdorferi* is responsible for Lyme disease. *E. coli* is associated with urinary tract infections. *Pseudomonas* species are associated with ecthyma.
CN: Physiological integrity; CNS: Physiological adaptation; CL: Knowledge

CN: Client needs category   CNS: Client needs subcategory   CL: Cognitive level

17. Which treatment for paronychia would be the most appropriate?
1. Drain the abscess and give warm soaks.
2. Splint and put ice on the affected finger.
3. Allow the infection to resolve without treatment.
4. Admit the child to the hospital for I.V. antibiotic therapy.

18. Which finding would alert the nurse to suspect a scabies infestation?
1. Diffuse pruritic wheals
2. Oval white dots stuck to the hair shafts
3. Pain, erythema, and edema with an embedded stinger
4. Pruritic papules, pustules, and linear burrows of the finger and toe webs

19. A child has severe cellulitis of the lower leg with a great deal of purulent drainage. The physician performed an incision and debridement and inserted a drain. The nurse is performing a dressing change when there's an overhead page announcing the hospital code for a security situation. What would be the most appropriate course of action?
1. Close the door to the room and stay with the client.
2. Immediately report to the site of the security alert to demonstrate a show of force.
3. Reassure the client as the dressing is completed; then report to the charge nurse.
4. Reassure the client and report to the charge nurse.

20. The mother of a 5-month-old infant is planning a trip to the beach and asks for advice about sunscreen. Which instruction would the nurse incorporate into the teaching plan?
1. The sun protection factor (SPF) of the sunscreen should be at least 10.
2. Sunscreen is applied to the exposed areas of the skin.
3. Sunscreen shouldn't be applied to infants younger than age 6 months.
4. Sunscreen needs to be applied heavily only once, 30 minutes before going out in the sun.

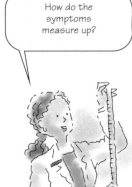

How do the symptoms measure up?

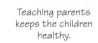

Teaching parents keeps the children healthy.

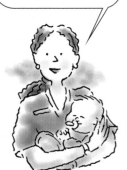

17. 1. Draining the abscess and giving warm soaks is the treatment of choice for paronychia. Splinting and icing aren't indicated. Untreated, the local abscess can spread beneath the nail bed, called secondary lymphangitis. I.V. antibiotic therapy isn't needed if the abscess is kept from spreading.
CN: Physiological integrity; CNS: Physiological adaptation; CL: Knowledge

18. 4. Pruritic papules, vesicles, and linear burrows are diagnostic for scabies. Urticaria is associated with an allergic reaction. Nits, seen as white oval dots, are characteristic of head lice. Bites from honeybees are associated with a stinger, pain, and erythema.
CN: Physiological integrity; CNS: Physiological adaptation; CL: Analysis

19. 3. A security alert notifies everyone in the hospital that there may be a dangerous situation occurring that indicates a trained show of force. The nurse should complete the dressing change, reassure the client, and then report to the charge nurse for further instructions. Simply closing the door and remaining with the client would not appropriately address the security situation and could potentially place the nurse and client in danger. The nurse shouldn't leave the room with the wound uncovered, nor would it be appropriate to leave the room without first reassuring the client.
CN: Safe, effective care environment; CNS: Safety and infection control; CL: Analysis

20. 3. Sunscreen isn't recommended for use in infants younger than age 6 months. These children should be dressed in cool light clothes and kept in the shade. On children older than age 6 months, sunscreen should be applied evenly throughout the day and each time the child is in the water. The SPF for children should be 15 or greater. Sunscreen should be applied to all areas of the skin.
CN: Health promotion and maintenance; CNS: None; CL: Application

CN: Client needs category   CNS: Client needs subcategory   CL: Cognitive level

21. An infant is being treated with antibiotic therapy for otitis media and develops an erythematous, fine, raised rash in the groin and suprapubic area. Which explanation would the nurse suspect?

1. The infant most likely has candidiasis.
2. The brand of diapers should be changed.
3. An over-the-counter diaper remedy is best to use.
4. The antibiotic therapy must be stopped immediately.

22. The skin in the diaper area of a 6-month-old infant is excoriated and red. Which instructions would the nurse give to the mother?

1. Change the diaper more often.
2. Apply talcum powder with diaper changes.
3. Wash the area vigorously with each diaper change.
4. Decrease the infant's fluid intake to decrease saturating diapers.

23. A 9-year-old child is being discharged from the hospital after severe urticaria caused by an allergy to nuts. Which instructions would be included in discharge teaching for the child's parents?

1. Use emollient lotions and baths.
2. Apply topical steroids to the lesions as needed.
3. Apply over-the-counter products such as diphenhydramine (Benadryl).
4. Follow up with an allergist and instruct the client on how to use an epinephrine administration kit.

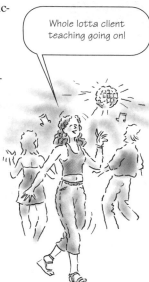

Whole lotta client teaching going on!

21. 1. Candidiasis, caused by yeastlike fungi, can occur with the use of antibiotics. Changing the brand of diapers or suggesting that the parent use an over-the-counter remedy would be appropriate for treating diaper rash, not candidiasis. The treatment for candidiasis is topical nystatin ointment. Antibiotic therapy shouldn't be stopped.

CN: Physiological integrity; CNS: Physiological adaptation; CL: Analysis

22. 1. Simply decreasing the amount of time the skin comes in contact with wet, soiled diapers will help heal the irritation. Talc is contraindicated in children because of the risks associated with inhalation of the fine powder. Gentle cleaning of the irritated skin should be encouraged. Infants shouldn't have fluid intake restrictions.

CN: Safe, effective care environment; CNS: Safety and infection control; CL: Application

23. 4. Children who have urticaria in response to nuts, seafood, or bee stings should be warned about the possibility of anaphylactic reactions to future exposure. The use of epinephrine pens should be taught to the parents and to older children. Other treatment choices, such as emollients, topical steroids, and Benadryl, are for the treatment of mild urticaria.

CN: Physiological integrity; CNS: Reduction of risk potential; CL: Application

24. When examining a nursery school–age child, the nurse finds multiple contusions over the body. Child abuse is suspected. Which statement indicates the findings that should be documented?

1. Contusions confined to one body area are typically suspicious.
2. All lesions, including location, shape, and color, should be documented.
3. Natural injuries usually have straight linear lines, while injuries from abuse have multiple curved lines.
4. The depth, location, and amount of bleeding that initially occurs is constant, but the sequence of color change is variable.

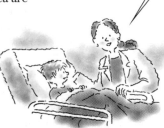

Be aware of the signs of child abuse. It's the nurse's responsibility to report it.

24. 2. An accurate precise examination must be properly documented as a legal document. Contusions that result from falls are typically confined to a single body area and are considered a reasonable finding of a child still learning to walk. Injuries from normal falls are usually not linear in nature. Bleeding can cause variations, but color change is consistent.

CN: Psychosocial integrity; CNS: None; CL: Application

25. A 5-year-old girl is admitted to the emergency department with a broken clavicle. Her mother indicates she fell down the stairs while playing. The nurse notices bruises in various stages of healing on the girl's torso and extremities. The mother and child stiffen as the child's father enters the room. He angrily demands to take the child home. Which action is most appropriate?

1. Tell the man that his little girl has a broken bone and can't leave.
2. Ask the father whether he knows how the child received the bruises.
3. Step out of the room, notify the charge nurse, and then call security.
4. Take the child out of the room and call security.

25. 3. In order to ensure the nurse's safety as well as the safety of the child and her mother, the best course of action would be to leave the room and immediately notify the charge nurse, and then call security. The nurse wouldn't want to further anger the father and create the potential for violence by taking the child out of the room. Asking for personal information and telling the father he can't take his child are also neither wise nor appropriate actions.

CN: Physiological integrity; CNS: Physiological adaptation; CL: Knowledge

26. For which reason is lindane (Kwell) shampoo used only as a second-line treatment for lice?

1. Lindane causes alopecia.
2. Lindane causes hypertension.
3. Lindane is associated with seizures.
4. Lindane increases liver function test (LFT) results.

What do you need to know about lice treatment?

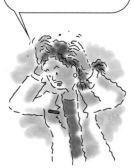

26. 3. Lindane is associated with seizures after absorption with topical use. Alopecia, hypertension, and increased LFT results aren't associated with the use of lindane.

CN: Physiological integrity; CNS: Pharmacological therapies; CL: Knowledge

CN: Client needs category CNS: Client needs subcategory CL: Cognitive level

27. Which instructions would the nurse include for the parents about the <u>treatment</u> of hair lice?
1. The treatment should be repeated in 7 to 12 days.
2. Treatment should be repeated every day for 1 week.
3. If treated with a shampoo, combing to remove eggs isn't necessary.
4. All contacts with the infested child should be treated even without evidence of infestation.

28. A mother reports that her 4-year-old child has been scratching at his rectum recently. Which infestation or condition would the nurse suspect as most likely?
1. Anal fissure
2. Lice
3. Pinworms
4. Scabies

29. Diagnosing pinworms by the clear cellophane tape test is preferred. How many tests are necessary to detect infestations at virtually 100% accuracy?
1. One
2. Three
3. Five
4. Ten

30. Each member of the family of a child diagnosed with pinworms is prescribed a single dose of pyrantel (Antiminth). Which statement would the nurse incorporate into the teaching plan?
1. The drug may stain the feces red.
2. The dose may be repeated in 2 weeks.
3. Fever and rash are common adverse effects.
4. The medicine will kill the eggs in about 48 hours.

31. A large dog bit the hand of a child. The nurse would expect to find which type of injury?
1. Abrasion
2. Crush injury
3. Fracture
4. Puncture wound

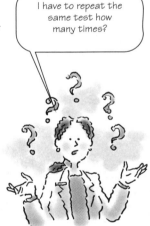

I have to repeat the same test how many times?

27. 1. Treatment should be repeated in 7 to 12 days to ensure that all eggs are killed. Combing the hair thoroughly is necessary to remove the lice eggs. People exposed to head lice should be examined to assess the presence of infestation before treatment.
CN: Physiological integrity; CNS: Physiological adaptation; CL: Application

28. 3. The clinical sign of pinworms is perianal itching that increases at night. Anal fissures are associated with rectal bleeding and pain with bowel movements. Lice are infestations of the hair. Scabies are associated with a pruritic rash characterized as linear burrows of the webs of the fingers and toes.
CN: Physiological integrity; CNS: Physiological adaptation; CL: Analysis

29. 3. Detection is virtually 100% accurate with five tests. Three tests should detect infestations at about 90% accuracy. One test is only 50% accurate.
CN: Physiological intergrity; CNS: Reduction of risk potential; CL: Application

30. 2. Pyrantel is effective against the adult worms only, so treatment can be repeated to eradicate any emerging parasites in 2 weeks. Staining the feces isn't associated with pyrantel. Common adverse effects are headaches and abdominal complaints.
CN: Physiological integrity; CNS: Pharmacological therapies; CL: Application

31. 2. Although the bite of a large dog can exert pressure of 150 to 400 lb per square inch, the bite causes crush injuries, not fractures. Abrasions are associated with friction injuries. Puncture wounds are associated with smaller animals such as cats.
CN: Physiological integrity; CNS: Physiological adaptation; CL: Application

CN: Client needs category   CNS: Client needs subcategory   CL: Cognitive level

32. The nurse understands that bites from dogs heighten the risk of infection. Which intervention should be done to help prevent infection?

1. Give the rabies vaccine.
2. Give antibiotics immediately.
3. Clean and irrigate the wounds.
4. Nothing; bites from dogs have a low incidence of infection.

33. When collecting data from a 6-year-old burn client who has a 20% deep partial-thickness (second-degree) burn of the arms and trunk, the nurse understands that the client has damage to what layers of skin?

1. Epidermis
2. Epidermis and part of the dermis
3. Epidermis and all of the dermis
4. Dermis and subcutaneous tissue

34. A child is brought to the office for multiple scratches and bites from a kitten and is being evaluated for cat-scratch disease. While collecting data, which symptom would the nurse expect to find?

1. Abdominal pain
2. Adenitis
3. Fever
4. Pruritus

35. In which child population would the nurse be alert for giardiasis, the most common parasitic intestinal infection in the United States?

1. Children riding a school bus
2. Children playing on a playground
3. Children attending a sporting event
4. Children attending group day care or nursery school

36. Which finding should the nurse expect to observe if a child has papules?

1. Palpable elevated masses
2. Loss of the epidermal layer
3. Fluid-filled elevations of the skin
4. Nonpalpable flat changes in skin color

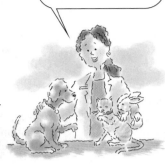

All injuries involving a break in the skin require cleaning the wound.

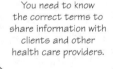

You need to know the correct terms to share information with clients and other health care providers.

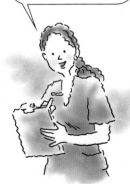

32. 3. Not every dog bite requires antibiotic therapy, but cleaning the wound is necessary for all injuries involving a break in the skin. Rabies vaccine is used if the dog is suspected of having rabies. The infection rate for dog bites has been reported to be as high as 50%.
CN: Physiological integrity; CNS: Reduction of risk potential; CL: Application

33. 2. A deep partial-thickness burn affects the epidermis and part of the dermis. A superficial partial-thickness (first-degree) burn affects the epidermis and all the dermis; it may also affect the subcutaneous tissue.
CN: Physiological integrity; CNS: Physiological adaptation; CL: Application

34. 2. Adenitis (inflammation of a gland or lymph node) is the primary feature of cat-scratch disease. Although low-grade fever has been associated with cat-scratch disease, it's present only 25% of the time. Pruritus and abdominal pain aren't symptoms of cat-scratch disease.
CN: Physiological integrity; CNS: Physiological adaptation; CL: Comprehension

35. 4. The most common intestinal parasitic infection in the United States is giardiasis, prevalent among children attending group day care or nursery school. Playgrounds, sporting events, and school buses don't present unusual risk of giardiasis.
CN: Safe, effective care environment; CNS: Safety and infection control; CL: Comprehension

36. 1. Papules are elevated up to 0.5 cm. Nodules and tumors are elevated more than 0.5 cm. Erosions are characterized as loss of the epidermal layer. Fluid-filled lesions are vesicles and pustules. Macules and patches are described as nonpalpable flat changes in skin color.
CN: Health promotion and maintenance; CNS: None; CL: Application

CN: Client needs category CNS: Client needs subcategory CL: Cognitive level

37. When collecting data on a child diagnosed with impetigo, which symptom would the nurse identify as the primary manifestation?
1. Lesion filled with pus
2. Superficial area of localized edema
3. Serous-filled lesion less than 0.5 cm
4. Serous-filled lesion greater than 0.5 cm

38. A 5-year-old male sustained third-degree burns to the right upper extremity after tipping over a frying pan. Which skin structures would the nurse include when explaining a third-degree burn to the child's mother?
1. Epidermis only
2. Epidermis and dermis
3. All skin layers and nerve endings
4. Skin layers, nerve endings, muscles, tendons, and bone

39. A child is brought to the physician's office for treatment of a rash. Many petechiae are seen over his entire body. The nurse would suspect which condition?
1. Bleeding disorder
2. Scabies
3. Varicella
4. Vomiting

40. A child fell at camp and sustained a bruise to his thigh. Which description would accurately describe the bruise after 1 week?
1. Resolved
2. Reddish blue
3. Greenish yellow
4. Dark blue to bluish brown

41. Which factor would lead the nurse to suspect child abuse?
1. Multiple contusions of the shins
2. Contusions of the back and buttocks
3. Contusions at the same stages of healing
4. Large contusion and hematoma of the forehead

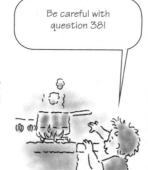

Be careful with question 38!

37. 1. Pustules, the primary lesions with impetigo, are pus-filled lesions, such as acne and impetigo. Bullae are serous-filled lesions greater than 0.5 cm in diameter. A wheal is a superficial area of localized edema. Vesicles are serous-filled lesions up to 0.5 cm in diameter.
CN: Physiological integrity; CNS: Physiological adaptation; CL: Application

38. 3. A third-degree burn involves all of the skin layers and the nerve endings. First-degree burns involve only the epidermis. Second-degree burns affect the epidermis and dermis. Fourth-degree burns involve all skin layers, nerve endings, muscles, tendons, and bone.
CN: Physiological integrity; CNS: Physiological adaptation; CL: Application

39. 1. Petechiae are caused by blood outside a vessel, associated with low platelet counts and bleeding disorders. Petechiae aren't found with varicella disease or scabies. Petechiae can be associated with vomiting, but they would be present on the face, not the entire body.
CN: Physiological integrity; CNS: Physiological adaptation; CL: Analysis

40. 3. After 7 to 10 days, the bruise becomes greenish yellow. Resolution can take up to 2 weeks. Initially after the fall, there's a reddish blue discoloration, followed by dark blue to bluish brown at days 1 to 3.
CN: Physiological integrity; CNS: Physiological adaptation; CL: Application

41. 2. Contusions of the back and buttocks are highly suggestive of abuse related to punishment. Contusions at various stages of healing are red flags to potential abuse. Contusions of the shins and forehead are usually related to an active toddler falling and bumping into objects.
CN: Psychosocial integrity; CNS: None; CL: Analysis

CN: Client needs category   CNS: Client needs subcategory   CL: Cognitive level

42. Which statement would the nurse include when teaching a new mother about salmon patches (stork bites)?
   1. They're benign and usually fade in adult life.
   2. They're usually associated with syndromes of the neonate.
   3. They can cause mild hypertrophy of the muscle associated with the lesion.
   4. They're treatable with laser pulse surgery in late adolescence and adulthood.

43. When inspecting a neonate, the nurse notes a blue-black macular lesion over the lower lumbar sacral region. The nurse interprets this as:
   1. café-au-lait spots.
   2. Mongolian spots.
   3. nevus of Ota.
   4. stork bites.

44. Which finding would alert the nurse to severe dehydration in a child?
   1. Gray skin and decreased tears
   2. Capillary refill less than 2 seconds
   3. Mottling and tenting of the skin
   4. Pale skin with dry mucous membranes

45. Isotretinoin (Accutane) is associated with which adverse effect?
   1. Diarrhea
   2. Gram-negative folliculitis
   3. Teratogenesis
   4. Vaginal candidiasis

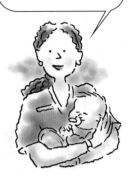

Know what to tell a family when a neonate is born with salmon patches.

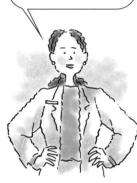

Read question 43 carefully and you'll spot the correct answer.

42. 1. Salmon patches occur over the back of the neck in 40% of neonates and are harmless, needing no intervention. Port-wine stains are associated with syndromes of neonates, such as Sturge-Weber syndrome. Port-wine stains found on the face or extremities may be associated with soft tissue and bone hypertrophy. Laser pulse surgery isn't recommended for salmon patches because they typically fade on their own in adulthood.

CN: Health promotion and maintenance; CNS: None; CL: Application

43. 2. Mongolian spots are large blue-black macular lesions generally located over the lumbosacral areas, buttocks, and limbs. Café-au-lait spots occur between ages 2 and 16, not in infancy. Nevus of Ota is found surrounding the eyes. Stork bites, or salmon patches, occur at the neck and hairline area.

CN: Health promotion and maintenance; CNS: None; CL: Analysis

44. 3. Severe dehydration is associated with mottling and tenting of the skin. Malnutrition is characterized by gray skin. Capillary refill less than 2 seconds is normal. Pale skin with dry mucous membranes is a sign of mild dehydration.

CN: Physiological integrity; CNS: Physiological adaptation; CL: Analysis

45. 3. The use of even small amounts of isotretinoin has been associated with severe birth defects. Most female clients are prescribed oral contraceptives. Clindamycin (Cleocin T), another medicine used in the treatment of acne, is associated with both diarrhea and gram-negative folliculitis. Tetracycline (Sumycin) is associated with yeast infections.

CN: Physiological integrity; CNS: Pharmacological therapies; CL: Knowledge

46. The nurse is developing a teaching plan for adolescents about acne. The nurse incorporates which of the following as commonly responsible for the failure of treatment of acne in teenagers?

1. Topical treatment
2. Systemic treatment
3. A dominant parent who wants treatment and a passive teenager who doesn't
4. A dominant teenager who wants treatment and a passive, uninterested parent

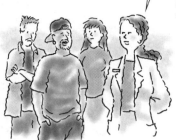

Encourage teens to participate actively in treatment.

46. 3. The active participation of a teenager is needed for the successful treatment of acne. Systemic and topical therapy are needed in most acne treatment.

CN: Health promotion and maintenance; CNS: None; CL: Application

47. Which cause would the nurse include when describing the cause of acne to a group of adolescents?

1. Diet
2. Gender
3. Poor hygiene
4. Hormonal changes

47. 4. Acne is caused by hormonal changes in sebaceous gland anatomy and the biochemistry of the glands. These changes lead to a blockage in the follicular canal and cause an inflammatory response. Diet, hygiene, and the client's gender don't cause acne.

CN: Health promotion and maintenance; CNS: None; CL: Application

48. When teaching a client about tetracycline (Achromycin) for severe inflammatory acne, which instructions must be given?

1. Take the drug with or without meals.
2. Take the drug with milk and milk products.
3. Take the drug on an empty stomach with small amounts of water.
4. Take the drug 1 hour before or 2 hours after meals with large amounts of water.

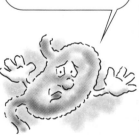

I'm really running on empty!

48. 4. Tetracycline must be taken on an empty stomach to increase absorption and with ample water to avoid esophageal irritation. Milk products impede absorption.

CN: Physiological integrity; CNS: Pharmacological therapies; CL: Application

49. When advising parents about the prevention of burns from tap water, which instructions would the nurse include in the teaching plan?

1. Set the water-heater temperature at 130° F (54.4° C) or less.
2. Run the hot water first; then adjust the temperature with cold water.
3. Before you put your infant in the tub, first test the water with your hand.
4. Supervise an infant in the bathroom, only leaving him for a few seconds if needed.

49. 3. The cold water should be run first and then adjusted with hot water. Instruct the parents to fill the tub with water first and then test all of the water in the tub with their hand for hot spots. Water heaters should be set at 120° F (48.9° C). Never leave a infant alone in the bathroom, even for a second.

CN: Physiological integrity; CNS: Reduction of risk potential; CL: Application

50. A 14-year-old male client is brought to the hospital with smoke inhalation because of a house fire. The nurse's major intervention for this client is to:
1. check the oral mucous membranes.
2. check for any burned areas.
3. obtain a medical history.
4. ensure a patent airway.

51. A 15-month-old child is diagnosed with pediculosis of the eyebrows. Which intervention would the nurse expect to be included in the treatment?
1. Using lindane
2. Using petroleum jelly
3. Shaving the eyebrows
4. Doing nothing; no treatment is needed

52. A 13-year-old client has received third-degree burns over 20% of his body. When observing this client 72 hours after the burn, which finding should the nurse expect?
1. Increased urine output
2. Severe peripheral edema
3. Respiratory distress
4. Absent bowel sounds

53. Which change in the mouth is consistent with Kawasaki disease?
1. Koplik's spots
2. Tonsillar exudate
3. Vesicular lesions
4. Dry, cracked lips; strawberry tongue

54. The nurse is assessing a 3-month-old male infant of Mediterranean descent during a routine examination in a family health center. The nurse notes the presence of bluish discolorations of the skin and interprets these as:
1. milia.
2. Mongolian spots.
3. lanugo.
4. vernix caseosa.

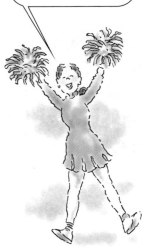

Hip! Hip! Hurray for you! You're about halfway there.

50. 4. The nurse's top priority is to make sure the airway is open and the client is breathing. Checking the mucous membranes and burned areas is important but not as vital as maintaining a patent airway. Obtaining a medical history can be pursued after ensuring a patent airway.
CN: Physiological integrity; CNS: Physiological adaptation; CL: Application

51. 2. Petroleum jelly should be applied twice daily for 8 days, followed by manual removal of nits. Lindane is contraindicated because of the risk of seizures. The eyebrow should never be shaved because of the uncertainty of hair return.
CN: Physiological integrity; CNS: Physiological adaptation; CL: Application

52. 1. During the resuscitative-emergent phase of a burn, fluids shift back into the interstitial space, resulting in the onset of diuresis. Edema resolves during the emergent phase, when fluid shifts back to the intravascular space. Respiratory rate increases during the first few hours as a result of edema. When edema resolves, respirations return to normal. Absent bowel sounds occur in the initial stage.
CN: Physiological integrity; CNS: Physiological adaptation; CL: Application

53. 4. Oral changes associated with Kawasaki disease include an injected pharynx, injected lips, dry fissured lips, and strawberry tongue. Koplik's spots are consistent with measles. Tonsillar exudate is consistent with pharyngitis caused by group A beta-hemolytic streptococci. Vesicular lesions are associated with Coxsackie virus.
CN: Physiological integrity; CNS: Physiological adaptation; CL: Knowledge

54. 2. Bluish discolorations of the skin, which are common in babies of Black, Native American, and Mediterranean races, are called *Mongolian spots*. Pinpoint pimples caused by obstruction of sebaceous glands are called *milia*. The fine hair covering the body of a neonate is called *lanugo*. Vernix caseosa is a cheeselike substance that covers the skin of a neonate.
CN: Health promotion and maintenance; CNS: None; CL: Analysis

CN: Client needs category   CNS: Client needs subcategory   CL: Cognitive level

55. Topical treatment with 2.5% hydrocortisone is prescribed for a 6-month-old infant with eczema. The nurse advises the mother to use the cream for no more than 1 week based on which rationale?
1. The drug loses its efficacy after prolonged use.
2. Excessive use can have adverse effects, such as skin atrophy and fragility.
3. If no improvement is seen, a stronger concentration will be prescribed.
4. If no improvement is seen after 1 week, an antibiotic will be prescribed.

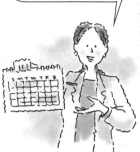

Teach the parents why the time limit is important.

55. 2. Hydrocortisone cream should be used for brief periods to decrease adverse effects such as atrophy of the skin. The drug doesn't lose efficacy after prolonged use, a stronger concentration may not be prescribed if no improvement is seen, and an antibiotic would be inappropriate in this instance.
CN: Physiological integrity; CNS: Pharmacological therapies; CL: Application

56. A 1-year-old infant is hospitalized with a diagnosis of eczema. Which signs and symptoms does the nurse expect to observe?
1. Exudative, crusty, papulovesicular, erythematous lesions on the cheeks, scalp, forehead, and arms
2. Erythematous, dry, scaly, papular, thickened, well-circumscribed, and lichenified pruritic lesions on the wrists, hands, and neck
3. Large, thickened, lichenified plaques on the face, neck, and back
4. Erythematous papules with oozing, crusting, and edema

56. 1. Exudative, crusty, papulovesicular, erythematous lesions on the cheeks, scalp, forehead, and arms are observed in children ages 2 months to 2 years with a diagnosis of eczema. Erythematous, dry, scaly, well-circumscribed, papular, thickened, lichenified, pruritic lesions on the wrists, hands, and neck are observed in children ages 2 years to puberty. In adolescents, lesions on the face, neck, and back consist of large plaques that are thickened and lichenified. Erythematous papules with oozing, crusting, and edema are characteristic of contact dermatitis.
CN: Physiological integrity; CNS: Physiological adaptation; CL: Comprehension

57. A 4-year-old child had a subungual hemorrhage of the toe after a jar fell on his foot. Electrocautery is performed. Which teaching statement regarding the rationale for using electrocautery to treat the injury is <u>most</u> accurate?
1. It's used to prevent loss of nail growth.
2. It's used to prevent loss of the nail.
3. It's used to relieve pain and reduce the risk of infection.
4. It's used to prevent permanent discoloration of the nail bed.

57. 3. The hematoma is treated with electrocautery to relieve pain and reduce the risk of infection. Electrocautery doesn't prevent the loss of the nail. The discoloration seen with subungual hemorrhage is from the collection of blood under the nail bed. It isn't permanent and doesn't affect nail growth.
CN: Physiological integrity; CNS: Physiological adaptation; CL: Application

58. The nurse is caring for a 12-year-old child with a diagnosis of eczema. Which nursing interventions are appropriate for a child with eczema?
1. Administering antibiotics as prescribed
2. Administering antifungals as ordered
3. Administering tepid baths and patting dry or air-drying the affected areas
4. Administering hot baths and using moisturizers immediately after the bath

58. 3. Tepid baths and moisturizers are indicated to keep the infected areas clean and minimize itching. Antibiotics are given only when superimposed infection is present. Antifungals aren't usually administered in the treatment of eczema. Hot baths can exacerbate the condition and increase itching.
CN: Physiological integrity; CNS: Physiological adaptation; CL: Application

CN: Client needs category   CNS: Client needs subcategory   CL: Cognitive level

59. A 9-year-old child is brought to the emergency department with extensive burns received in a restaurant fire. What's the <u>most important</u> aspect of caring for the burned child?
1. Administering antibiotics to prevent superimposed infections
2. Conducting wound management
3. Administering liquids orally to replace fluid
4. Administering frequent small meals to support nutritional requirements

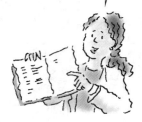

Number 59 is asking you to prioritize!

59. 2. The most important aspect of caring for a burned child is wound management. The goals of wound care are to speed debridement, protect granulation tissue and new grafts, and conserve body heat and fluids. Antibiotics aren't always administered prophylactically. Fluids are administered I.V. according to the child's body weight to replace volume. Enteral feedings, rather than meals, are initiated within the first 24 hours after the burn to support the child's increased nutritional requirements.
CN: Physiological integrity; CNS: Physiological adaptation; CL: Application

60. The mother of a 4-month-old infant asks about the strawberry hemangioma on his cheek. Which statement would the nurse include when responding to the mother?
1. The lesion will continue to grow for 3 years, then need surgical removal.
2. If the lesion continues to enlarge, referral to a pediatric oncologist is warranted.
3. Surgery is indicated before age 12 months if the diameter of the lesion is greater than 3 cm.
4. The lesion will continue to grow until age 12 months, then begin to resolve by age 2 to 3 years.

60. 4. These rapidly growing vascular lesions reach maximum growth by age 1 year. The growth period is then followed by an involution period of 6 to 12 months. Lesions show complete involution by age 2 or 3 years. These benign lesions don't need surgical or oncologic referrals.
CN: Health promotion and maintenance; CNS: None; CL: Application

61. A 3-year-old child is being discharged from the emergency department after receiving three sutures for a scalp laceration. The nurse should tell the family to return for suture removal in how many days?
1. 1 to 3 days
2. 5 to 7 days
3. 8 to 10 days
4. 10 to 14 days

61. 2. The recommended healing time for this type of laceration is 5 to 7 days. Sutures need longer than 1 to 3 days to form an effective bond. Sutures of the fingertips and feet need 8 to 10 days, and 10 to 14 days is the recommended time for extensor surfaces of the knees and elbows.
CN: Physiological integrity; CNS: Physiological adaptation; CL: Application

CN: Client needs category   CNS: Client needs subcategory   CL: Cognitive level

62. The nurse is caring for a 16-year-old female admitted for poor insulin regulation. When the nurse walks into her room and sees her eating a hamburger and fries brought in by a friend, the client looks at the nurse with an expression of guilt. Which response by the nurse would be most appropriate?

1. Firmly tell the client that she's never allowed to eat this kind of food.
2. Have a frank talk about eating food that isn't on her diet.
3. Politely suggest removing the food; then ask how she feels the disease is changing her life.
4. Have all visitors come to the nurse's station before visiting the client to search them for food.

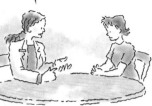

Open communication is key to a good nurse-client relationship.

62. 3. Politely suggesting removal of the food and then asking how the client feels about the disease and her life would be the best approach. The nurse is taking the appropriate action from a dietary and health perspective, but she's also fostering a relationship and encouraging open communication with the client. The first two options are inappropriate because of their scolding tone, which may create more resistance than dietary compliance. Having visitors check into the nurses' station isn't an appropriate use of the nurses' time, nor does it encourage the client to take responsibility for her disease.

CN: Physiological integrity; CNS: Reduction of risk potential; CL: Analysis

63. The nurse is teaching a 17-year-old client who'll be discharged soon how to change a sterile dressing on the right leg. During the teaching session, the nurse notices redness, swelling, and induration at the wound site, interpreting these as suggesting:

1. infection.
2. dehiscence.
3. hemorrhage.
4. evisceration.

63. 1. Infection produces such signs as redness, swelling, induration, warmth and, possibly, drainage. Dehiscence may cause unexplained fever and tachycardia, unusual wound pain, prolonged paralytic ileus, and separation of the surgical incision. Hemorrhage can result in increased pulse and respiratory rate, decreased blood pressure, restlessness, thirst, and cold, clammy skin. Evisceration produces visible protrusion of organs, usually through an incision.

CN: Physiological integrity; CNS: Physiological adaptation; CL: Analysis

64. When being examined, a 6-year-old child is noted to have a papulovesicular eruption on the left anterior lateral chest, with complaints of pain and tenderness of the lesion. The nurse interprets this finding as suggestive of:

1. contusion.
2. herpes zoster.
3. scabies.
4. varicella.

64. 2. Herpes zoster is caused by the varicella zoster virus. It has papulovesicular lesions that erupt along a dermatome, usually with hyperesthesia, pain, and tenderness. Contusions aren't found with papulovesicular lesions. Scabies appear as linear burrows of the fingers and toes caused by a mite. The papulovesicular lesions of varicella are distributed over the entire trunk, face, and scalp and don't follow a dermatome.

CN: Physiological integrity; CNS: Physiological adaptation; CL: Analysis

65. During an examination of a 5-month-old infant, a flat, dull pink, macular lesion is noted on the infant's forehead. The nurse suspects which condition?
1. Cavernous hemangioma
2. Nevus flammeus
3. Salmon patch
4. Strawberry hemangioma

65. 3. Salmon patches are common vascular lesions in infants. They appear as flat, dull pink, macular lesions in various regions of the face and head. When they appear on the nape of the neck, they're commonly called *stork bites*. These lesions fade by the first year of life. Nevus flammeus, or port-wine stains, are reddish purple lesions that don't fade. Strawberry and cavernous hemangiomas are raised lesions.
CN: Physiological integrity; CNS: Physiological adaptation; CL: Analysis

66. A child's parents ask for advice on the use of an insect repellent that contains DEET. Which statement would the nurse incorporate in the response?
1. Spray the child's clothing instead of the skin.
2. The repellent works better as the temperature increases.
3. The repellent isn't effective against the ticks responsible for Lyme disease.
4. Apply insect repellent as you would sunscreen, with frequent applications during the day.

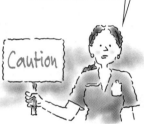

DEET-containing products should be used sparingly on children.

Caution

66. 1. DEET spray has been approved for use on children. It should be used sparingly on all skin surfaces. By concentrating the spray on clothing and camping equipment, the adverse effects and potential toxic buildup is significantly reduced. Repellent is lost to evaporation, wind, heat, and perspiration. With each 10° F increase in temperature, it leads to as much as a 50% reduction in protection time. DEET is very effective as a tick repellent.
CN: Physiological integrity; CNS: Reduction of risk potential; CL: Application

67. A nurse is teaching a parent about which DEET-containing insect repellant to use on his child. Which concentration should she instruct him to use on the child's skin for optimal results?
1. 10%
2. 15%
3. 20%
4. 30%

67. 1. The highest concentration approved by the Food and Drug Administration for children is 10%. Because of thinner skin and a greater surface-area-to-mass ratio in children, parents should use DEET products sparingly.
CN: Physiological integrity; CNS: Reduction of risk potential; CL: Application

68. Which statement about warts would the nurse incorporate when assisting with a community health teaching program on common skin problems?
1. Cutting the wart is the preferred treatment for children.
2. No treatment exists that specifically kills the wart virus.
3. Warts are caused by a virus affecting the inner layer of skin.
4. Warts are harmless and usually last 2 to 4 years if untreated.

68. 2. The goal of treatment is to kill the skin that contains the wart virus. Cutting the wart is likely to spread the virus. The virus that causes warts affects the outer layer of the skin. Warts are harmless and last 1 to 2 years if untreated.
CN: Physiological integrity; CNS: Physiological adaptation; CL: Application

69. The nurse is assisting with a teaching program for new parents that focuses on oral hygiene promotion. Which factor would the nurse include as causing tooth decay and gum disease when allowed to remain on the teeth for prolonged periods?

1. Breast milk
2. Pacifiers
3. Thumb or other fingers
4. Formula

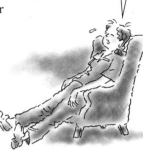

What I need is a prolonged period of rest.

70. When collecting data on a child with cellulitis, which symptoms would the nurse expect to find?

1. Pale, irritated, and cold to touch
2. Vesicular blisters at the site of the injury
3. Fever, edema, tenderness, and warmth at the site
4. Swelling and redness with well-defined borders

71. A 2-year-old child has cellulitis of the finger. Which organism or condition is the most likely cause of the infection?

1. Parainfluenza virus
2. Respiratory syncytial virus
3. *Escherichia coli*
4. *Streptococcus*

72. A child has a desquamative rash of the hands and feet. Which additional finding should the nurse expect to observe with this rash?

1. Peeling skin
2. Thin, reddened layers of epidermis
3. Thick skin with deep, visible burrows
4. Thinning skin that may appear translucent

73. Which instructions would the nurse include for the parents of a child who is to receive nystatin oral solution?

1. Give the solution immediately after feedings.
2. Give the solution immediately before feedings.
3. Mix the solution with small amounts of the feeding.
4. Give half the solution before and half the solution after the feeding.

69. 4. Tooth decay and gum disease result when the carbohydrates in commercial formula, cow's milk, and fruit juices are allowed to remain on the teeth for a prolonged period. Studies have shown that breast milk only contributes to dental caries when sugar is already present on the teeth. Breast milk alone actually promotes enamel growth. Pacifiers and fingers don't cause tooth decay and gum disease, although they may contribute to malocclusion.
CN: Health promotion and maintenance; CNS: None;
CL: Application

70. 3. Cellulitis is a deep, locally diffuse infection of the skin. It's associated with redness, fever, edema, tenderness, and warmth at the site of the injury. Vesicular blisters suggest impetigo. Cellulitis has no well-defined borders.
CN: Physiological integrity; CNS: Physiological adaptation;
CL: Analysis

71. 4. *Streptococcus* causes most cases of cellulitis. Parainfluenza and respiratory syncytial virus cause infections of the respiratory tract. *E. coli* is a cause of bladder infections.
CN: Physiological integrity; CNS: Physiological adaptation;
CL: Knowledge

72. 1. Desquamation is characteristic in diseases such as Stevens-Johnson syndrome. Scaling is thin, reddened layers of epidermis. Thickening of the skin with burrows is defined as lichenification. Thinning skin is best described as atrophy of the skin.
CN: Physiological integrity; CNS: Physiological adaptation;
CL: Application

73. 1. Nystatin oral solution should be swabbed onto the mouth after feedings to allow for optimal contact with mucous membranes. Before meals and with meals don't give the best contact with the mucous membranes.
CN: Physiological integrity; CNS: Pharmacological therapies;
CL: Application

CN: Client needs category   CNS: Client needs subcategory   CL: Cognitive level

74. An infant is examined and found to have a petechial rash. The nurse documents a description of this rash as:
1. purple macular lesions larger than 1 cm in diameter.
2. purple to brown bruises, macular or papular, of various sizes.
3. a collection of blood from ruptured blood vessels and larger than 1 cm in diameter.
4. pinpoint, pink to purple, nonblanching, macular lesions that are 1 to 3 mm in diameter.

75. A child has a red rash in a circular shape on his legs. The lesions aren't connected. Which classification is the most appropriate for this rash?
1. A linear rash
2. A diffuse rash
3. An annular rash
4. A confluent rash

76. A mother reports that her teenager is losing hair in small round areas on the scalp. The nurse interprets this as suggesting which condition?
1. Alopecia
2. Amblyopia
3. Exotropia
4. Seborrhea dermatitis

77. When inspecting the <u>palms</u> of a child, with which rash would the nurse expect to find no changes?
1. Coxsackie virus
2. Measles
3. Rocky Mountain spotted fever
4. Syphilis

78. A mother of a toddler diagnosed with atopic dermatitis is concerned about how her child acquired the disease. The nurse should explain that the cause of atopic dermatitis is a:
1. fungal infection.
2. hereditary disorder.
3. sex-linked disorder.
4. viral infection.

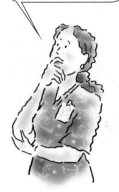

Petechiae. Even the word sounds small, doesn't it?

74. 4. Petechiae are small 1- to 3-mm macular lesions. Purple macular lesions greater than 1 cm are defined as purpura. A bruise is defined as ecchymosis. A hematoma is a collection of blood.
CN: Physiological integrity; CNS: Physiological adaptation; CL: Application

75. 3. An annular rash is ring-shaped. Linear rashes are lesions arranged in a line. A diffuse rash usually has scattered, widely distributed lesions. Confluent rash has lesions that are touching or adjacent to each other.
CN: Physiological integrity; CNS: Physiological adaptation; CL: Knowledge

76. 1. Alopecia is the correct term for thinning hair loss. Amblyopia and exotropia are eye disorders. Seborrhea dermatitis is cradle cap and occurs in infants.
CN: Physiological integrity; CNS: Physiological adaptation; CL: Application

77. 2. The rash in measles occurs on the face, trunk, and extremities. Rocky Mountain spotted fever, syphilis, and Coxsackie virus show changes on the palms and soles.
CN: Physiological integrity; CNS: Physiological adaptation; CL: Analysis

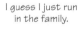

I guess I just run in the family.

78. 2. Atopic dermatitis is a hereditary disorder associated with a family history of asthma, allergic rhinitis, or atopic dermatitis. Fungal and viral infections don't cause atopic dermatitis.
CN: Physiological integrity; CNS: Physiological adaptation; CL: Application

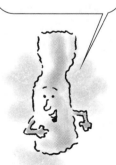

79. The mother of a 6-month-old infant with atopic dermatitis asks for advice on bathing the child. Which instructions or information should be given to her?
1. Bathe the infant twice daily.
2. Bathe the infant every other day.
3. Use bubble baths to decrease itching.
4. The frequency of the infant's baths isn't important in atopic dermatitis.

80. Discharge instructions for a child with atopic dermatitis include keeping the fingernails cut short. Which statement would explain the reason for this intervention?
1. To prevent infection of the nail bed
2. To prevent the spread of the disorder
3. To prevent the child from causing a corneal abrasion
4. To reduce breaks in skin from scratching that may lead to secondary bacterial infections

81. A 10-year-old child being treated for common warts asks about the cause. The nurse would incorporate which virus as the cause?
1. Coxsackie virus
2. Human herpesvirus (HHV)
3. Human immunodeficiency virus (HIV)
4. Human papillomavirus (HPV)

82. The nurse is caring for an 11-year-old client with cerebral palsy with a pressure ulcer on the sacrum. When teaching the mother about dietary intake, which foods should the nurse plan to emphasize?
1. Legumes and cheese
2. Whole grain products
3. Fruits and vegetables
4. Lean meats and low-fat milk

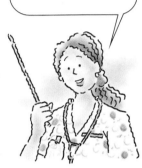

Here's another question pointing out the importance of client teaching.

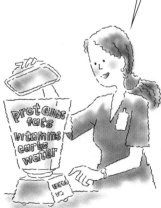

Protein helps build and repair body tissue, which promotes healing.

79. 2. Bathing removes lipoprotein complexes that hold water in the stratum corneum and increase water loss. Decreasing bathing to every other day can help prevent the removal of lipoprotein complexes. Soap and bubble bath should be used sparingly while bathing the child.
CN: Physiological integrity; CNS: Basic care and comfort; CL: Application

80. 4. Keeping fingernails cut short will prevent breaks in the skin when a child scratches. Cutting fingernails too short or cutting the skin around the nail can increase the risk of infection. Atopic dermatitis can be found in various areas of the skin but isn't spread from one area to another. Keeping fingernails short is a good way to reduce corneal abrasions but doesn't apply to atopic dermatitis
CN: Physiological integrity; CNS: Physiological adaptation; CL: Knowledge

81. 4. HPV is responsible for various forms of warts. Coxsackie virus is associated with hand-foot-and-mouth disease. HHV is associated with varicella and herpes zoster. HIV infections aren't associated with epithelial tumors known as warts.
CN: Physiological integrity; CNS: Physiological adaptation; CL: Application

82. 4. Although the client should eat a balanced diet with foods from all food groups, the diet should emphasize foods that supply complete protein, such as lean meats and low-fat milk. Protein helps build and repair body tissue, which promotes healing. Legumes provide incomplete protein. Cheese contains complete protein but also fat, which should be limited to 30% or less of caloric intake. Whole grain products supply incomplete proteins and carbohydrates. Fruits and vegetables provide mainly carbohydrates.
CN: Physiological integrity; CNS: Basic care and comfort; CL: Application

CN: Client needs category   CNS: Client needs subcategory   CL: Cognitive level

83. An adolescent says his feet itch, sweat a lot, and have a foul odor. The nurse suspects which condition?
1. Candidiasis
2. Tinea corporis
3. Tinea pedis
4. Molluscum contagiosum

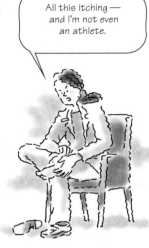

All this itching — and I'm not even an athlete.

83. 3. Tinea pedis is a superficial fungal infection on the feet, commonly called *athlete's foot.* Candidiasis is a fungal infection of the skin or mucous membranes commonly found in the oral, vaginal, and intestinal mucosal tissue. Tinea corporis, or ringworm, is a flat, scaling, papular lesion with raised borders. Molluscum contagiosum is a viral skin infection with lesions that are small, red papules.
CN: Physiological integrity; CNS: Physiological adaptation; CL: Analysis

84. A nurse is explaining treatment to the parents of a child with hypertrophic scarring. Which method would be the best for controlling this condition?
1. Compression garments
2. Moisturizing creams
3. Physiotherapy
4. Splints

84. 1. Compression garments are worn for up to 1 year to control hypertrophic scarring. Moisturizing creams help decrease hyperpigmentation. Physiotherapy and splints help keep joints and limbs supple.
CN: Physiological integrity; CNS: Physiological adaptation; CL: Application

85. During a physical examination, a child is noted to have nails with "ice-pick" pits and ridges. The nails are thick and discolored and have splintered hemorrhages easily separated from the nail bed. Which condition would cause this to occur?
1. Paronychia
2. Psoriasis
3. Scabies
4. Seborrhea

85. 2. Psoriasis is a chronic skin disorder with an unknown cause that shows these characteristic skin changes. A paronychia is a bacterial infection of the nail bed. Scabies are mites that burrow under the skin, usually between the webbing of the fingers and toes. Seborrhea is a chronic inflammatory dermatitis or cradle cap.
CN: Physiological integrity; CNS: Physiological adaptation; CL: Knowledge

86. A neonate is examined and noted to have bruising on the scalp, along with diffuse swelling of the soft tissue that crosses over the suture line. The nurse interprets this finding as:
1. caput succedaneum.
2. cephalohematoma.
3. craniotabes.
4. hydrocephalus.

86. 1. Caput succedaneum originates from trauma to the neonate while descending through the birth canal. It's usually a benign injury that spontaneously resolves over time. Cephalohematoma is a collection of blood in the periosteum of the scalp that doesn't cross over the suture line. Craniotabes is the thinning of the bone of the scalp. Hydrocephalus is an increased volume of cerebrospinal fluid (CSF) or the obstruction of the flow of the CSF and isn't related to soft-tissue swelling.
CN: Physiological integrity; CNS: Physiological adaptation; CL: Analysis

CN: Client needs category   CNS: Client needs subcategory   CL: Cognitive level

87. A child has a healed wound from a traumatic injury. A lesion formed over the wound is pink, thickened, smooth, and rubbery in nature. Which condition best describes this wound?
1. Erosion
2. Fissure
3. Keloids
4. Striae

88. An infant's mother gives a history of poor feeding for a few days. A complete physical examination shows white plaques in the infant's mouth with an erythematous base. The plaques stick to the mucous membranes tightly and bleed when scraped. Which condition best describes the plaques?
1. Chickenpox
2. Herpes lesions
3. Measles
4. Oral candidiasis

89. A child was found unconscious at home and brought to the emergency department by the fire and rescue unit. While collecting data, the nurse notes cherry-red mucous membranes, nail beds, and skin. Which cause is the most likely explanation for the child's condition?
1. Aspirin ingestion
2. Carbon monoxide poisoning
3. Hydrocarbon ingestion
4. Spider bite

90. A teenager asks advice about getting a tattoo. Which statement about tattoos is a common <u>misperception</u>?
1. Human immunodeficiency virus (HIV) is a possible risk factor.
2. Hepatitis B is a possible risk factor.
3. Tattoos are easily removed with laser surgery.
4. Allergic response to pigments is a possible risk factor.

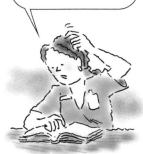

Hmmm, white plaques with an erythematous base. What could that mean?

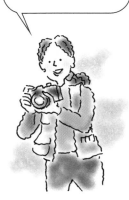

Be sure to clearly focus on question 90. It asks for what isn't correct.

87. 3. Keloids are an exaggerated connective tissue response to skin injury. Striae are linear depressions of the skin. An erosion is a depressed vesicular lesion. A fissure is a cleavage in the surface of skin.
CN: Physiological integrity; CNS: Physiological adaptation; CL: Knowledge

88. 4. Oral candidiasis, or *thrush,* is a painful inflammation that can affect the tongue, soft and hard palates, and buccal mucosa. Chickenpox, or *varicella,* causes open ulcerations of the mucous membranes. Herpes lesions are usually vesicular ulcerations of the oral mucosa around the lips. Measles that form Koplik's spots can be identified as pinpoint, white, elevated lesions.
CN: Physiological integrity; CNS: Physiological adaptation; CL: Knowledge

89. 2. Cherry-red skin changes are seen when a child has been exposed to high levels of carbon monoxide. Nausea and vomiting and pale skin are symptoms of aspirin ingestion. A hydrocarbon or petroleum ingestion usually results in respiratory symptoms and tachycardia. Spider-bite reactions are usually localized to the area of the bite.
CN: Physiological integrity; CNS: Physiological adaptation; CL: Knowledge

90. 3. The removal of tattoos isn't easily done, and most people are left with a significant scar. The cost is expensive and not covered by insurance. Because of the moderate amount of bleeding with a tattoo, both hepatitis B and HIV are potential risks if proper techniques aren't followed. Allergic reactions have been seen when establishments don't use Food and Drug Administration–approved pigments for tattoo coloring.
CN: Health promotion and maintenance; CNS: None; CL: Knowledge

CN: Client needs category   CNS: Client needs subcategory   CL: Cognitive level

91. Which term describes a fungal infection found on the upper arm?
1. Tinea capitis
2. Tinea corporis
3. Tinea cruris
4. Tinea pedis

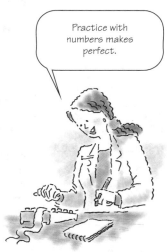

Practice with numbers makes perfect.

91. 2. Tinea corporis describes fungal infections of the body. Tinea capitis describes fungal infections of the scalp. Tinea cruris is used to describe fungal infections of the inner thigh and inguinal creases. Tinea pedis is the term for fungal infections of the foot.
CN: Physiological integrity; CNS: Physiological adaptation; CL: Application

92. A 15-kg toddler is started on amoxicillin and clavulanate (Augmentin) therapy, 200 mg/5 ml, for cellulitis. The dose is 40 mg/kg over 24 hours given three times daily. How many milliliters would be given for each dose?
1. 2.5 ml
2. 5 ml
3. 15 ml
4. 20 ml

92. 2. 5 ml should be given. The dose is first calculated by multiplying the weight and the milligrams and then dividing into three even doses. The milligrams are then used to determine the milliliters based on the concentration of the medicine. Use the following equation:
$$40 \text{ mg} \times 15 \text{ kg} = 600/3 \text{ doses} = 200 \text{ mg/dose};$$
The concentration is 200 mg in every 5 ml.
CN: Physiological integrity; CNS: Pharmacological therapies; CL: Application

93. At what stage of acquired syphilis are chancres found?
1. Tertiary syphilis
2. Primary acquired syphilis
3. Secondary acquired syphilis
4. Not found in syphilis

93. 2. A chancre is a painless, shallow ulcer that develops in primary syphilis and appears 3 weeks after exposure. In secondary syphilis, nodular, pustular, and annular lesions are seen. Tertiary stages are rare in children.
CN: Physiological integrity; CNS: Physiological adaptation; CL: Knowledge

94. A 4-year-old child has a tick embedded in the scalp. Which method is the preferred way of removing the tick?
1. Burning the tick at the skin surface
2. Surgically removing the tick
3. Grasping the tick with tweezers and applying slow, outward pressure
4. Grasping the tick with tweezers and quickly pulling the tick out

94. 3. Applying gentle outward pressure prevents injuring the skin and leaving parts of the tick in the skin. Surgical removal is indicated if portions of the tick remain in the skin. Burning the tick and quickly pulling the tick out may injure the skin and should be avoided.
CN: Physiological integrity; CNS: Physiological adaptation; CL: Knowledge

95. An infant with hives is prescribed diphenhydramine (Benadryl) 5 mg/kg over 24 hours in divided doses every 6 hours. The child weighs 8 kg. How many milligrams should be given with each dose?
1. 4.5 mg
2. 10 mg
3. 22 mg
4. 40 mg

95. 2. 10 mg should be given. Multiplying 5 mg by the weight (8 kg) gives the amount of milligrams for 24 hours (40 mg). Divide this by the number of doses per day (4), giving 10 mg/dose. Use the following equation:
$$5 \text{ mg} \times 8 \text{ kg} = 40 \text{ mg}/4 \text{ doses} = 10 \text{ mg/dose}.$$
CN: Physiological integrity; CNS: Pharmacological therapies; CL: Application

CN: Client needs category   CNS: Client needs subcategory   CL: Cognitive level

96. An 8-year-old child arrives at the emergency department with chemical burns to both legs. Which nursing action should the nurse perform first?
1. Dilute the burns.
2. Apply sterile dressings.
3. Apply topical antibiotics.
4. Debride and graft the burns.

97. A 7-year-old client is admitted to the hospital for treatment of facial cellulitis. He's admitted for observation and for administration of a 10-day course of I.V. antibiotics. Which interventions would help this client cope with the insertion of a peripheral I.V. line? Select all that apply:
1. Explain the procedure to the child immediately before the procedure.
2. Apply a topical anesthetic to the I.V. site before the procedure.
3. Ask the child which hand he uses for drawing.
4. Explain the procedure to the child using abstract terms.
5. Don't let the child see the equipment to be used in the procedure.
6. Tell the child that the procedure won't hurt.

98. A 14-year-old diagnosed with acne vulgaris asks what causes it. Which factors should the nurse identify for this client? Select all that apply:
1. Chocolates and sweets
2. Increased hormone levels
3. Growth of anaerobic bacteria
4. Caffeine
5. Heredity
6. Fatty foods

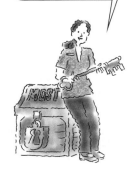

The key to question 96 is the word first.

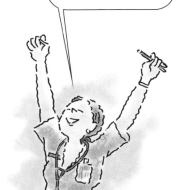

Success! And you thought you couldn't do it. Super job!

96. 1. Diluting the chemical is the first treatment. It will help remove the chemical and stop the burning process. The remaining treatments are initiated after dilution.
CN: Physiological integrity; CNS: Physiological adaptation; CL: Analysis

97. 2, 3. Topical anesthetics reduce the pain of a venipuncture. The cream should be applied about 1 hour before the procedure and requires a physician's order. Asking which hand the child draws with helps to identify the dominant hand. The I.V. should be inserted into the opposite extremity so that the child can continue to play and to do homework with a minimum amount of disruption. Younger school-age children don't have the capability for abstract thinking. The procedure should be explained using simple words. Definitions of unfamiliar terms should be provided. The child should have the procedure explained to him well before it takes place so that he has time to ask questions. Although the topical anesthetic will relieve some pain, there's usually some pain or discomfort involved in venipuncture, so the child shouldn't be told otherwise.
CN: Psychosocial integrity; CNS: None; CL: Application

98. 2, 3, 5. Acne vulgaris is characterized by the appearance of comedones (blackheads and whiteheads). Comedones develop for various reasons, including increased hormone levels, heredity, irritation or application of irritating substances (such as cosmetics), and growth of anaerobic bacteria. A direct relationship between acne vulgaris and consumption of chocolates, caffeine, or fatty foods hasn't been established.
CN: Physiological integrity; CNS: Physiological adaptation; CL: Application

CN: Client needs category   CNS: Client needs subcategory   CL: Cognitive level

Part VI Coordinated care

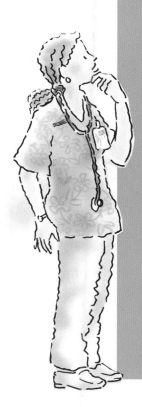

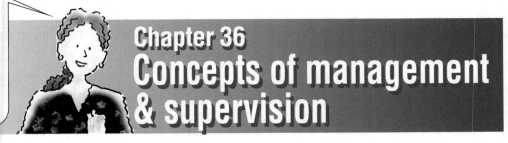

> Knowing key concepts of management and supervision is just as important as your clinical knowledge for a successful nursing career. Test your knowledge of these concepts with the following questions.

Chapter 36
Concepts of management & supervision

1. The nurse and a new licensed practical nurse she's supervising are reviewing proper procedures for administering medications. The new nurse is correct in stating which procedure as the 5 "rights" of medication administration?
1. Right client, right medication, right dose, right time, and right route
2. Right client, right medication, right dose, right time, and right reason
3. Right client, right medication, right dose, right time, and right physician
4. Right client, right medication, right dose, right time, and right quantity

2. The nurse is caring for a 52-year-old female client diagnosed with right-sided stroke who has expressive aphasia and left-sided weakness. When planning care for this client, which intervention should the nurse delegate to a nursing assistant?
1. Accompany the client to speech therapy.
2. Perform active range-of-motion (ROM) exercises for the client's upper extremities.
3. Turn and position the client every 2 hours.
4. Begin teaching the client simple sign language phrases.

3. The nurse finds a suicidal client trying to hang himself in his room. In order to preserve self-esteem and safety, the nurse should:
1. place the client in seclusion with checks every 15 minutes.
2. assign a nursing staff member to remain with the client at all times.
3. make the client stay with the group at all times.
4. refuse to let the client in his room.

> It's important to know the limits of a nursing assistant's skills and responsibilities.

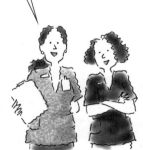

1. 1. Before administering medication, the nurse should make sure she has the right client by checking the identification band, check the physician's order for dosage and frequency, check that the medication is ordered for the right route, and make sure she administers the medication at the right time. The right reason, right physician, and right quantity aren't part of this process.
CN: Physiological integrity; CNS: Pharmacological therapies; CL: Knowledge

2. 3. Nursing assistants are taught proper positioning skills, although this activity should still be supervised. It isn't necessary to accompany the client to speech therapy and would take the assistant off the unit, reducing available help. Not all nursing assistants are taught to perform active ROM exercises. It wouldn't be necessary to teach the client sign language.
CN: Safe, effective care environment; CNS: Coordinated care; CL: Analysis

3. 2. Implementing a one-on-one staff-to-client ratio is the nurse's highest priority. This allows the client to maintain his self-esteem and keeps him safe. Seclusion would damage the client's self-esteem. Forcing the client to stay with the group and refusing to let him in his room don't guarantee his safety.
CN: Safe, effective care environment; CNS: Coordinated care; CL: Application

CN: Client needs category   CNS: Client needs subcategory   CL: Cognitive level

4. The staff of an outpatient clinic has formed a task force to develop new procedures for swift, safe evacuation of the unit. These new procedures haven't yet been reviewed, approved, or shared with all personnel. The nurse-manager has been informed of a bomb threat, and her task force members are pushing her to evacuate the unit using the new procedures. The nurse-manager should:

1. determine that the procedures currently in place must be followed and direct staff to follow them without question.
2. tell staff members to use whatever procedures they feel are best.
3. ask staff members to quickly meet among themselves and decide what procedures to follow.
4. tell staff members to assemble in the staff lounge to quickly offer their opinions about evacuation procedures before deciding what to do.

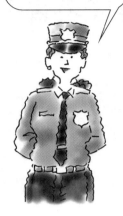

Just like when there's a fire, in an emergency situation, the nurse-manager must act quickly and decisively.

4. 1. In an emergency situation, the nurse-manager must determine the best course of action for the safety and welfare of clients and staff. In this particular situation, there's no time for hesitation. Allowing staff members to do whatever they think best will cause confusion and inefficient client evacuation because following different procedures won't allow them to function effectively as a team during this crisis. Taking the time to have staff meet with one another and the nurse-manager is wasting valuable time during a life-or-death crisis.
CN: Safe, effective care environment; CNS: Coordinated care; CL: Analysis

5. The nursing assistant reports to the nurse that a client became short of breath while being bathed but is breathing better now. Which approach should the nurse take initially?

1. Instruct the nursing assistant to observe the client for any further shortness of breath.
2. Check the client and gather subjective and objective data related to shortness of breath.
3. Tell the physician about the client's episode of shortness of breath.
4. Instruct the nursing assistant to complete the bath after allowing the client to rest.

5. 2. The nurse must assess the client herself to determine what might have precipitated the episode and obtain a pulse oximetry reading if indicated. Instructing the nursing assistant to observe the client for further shortness of breath would be appropriate after the nurse has checked the client. It wouldn't be necessary to call the physician about the client's episode of shortness of breath, but he should be informed and this should be documented. After checking the client, the nurse may ask the nursing assistant to complete the bath after allowing the client to rest.
CN: Safe, effective care environment; CNS: Coordinated care; CL: Application

6. While discussing a client's care with a nursing assistant, the nurse detects an odor of alcohol on the assistant's breath. The nurse should plan to:

1. report her observations to the charge nurse.
2. monitor the assistant closely to determine whether performance is impaired.
3. tell the assistant she'll have to leave the unit immediately.
4. warn the assistant that she could lose her certification.

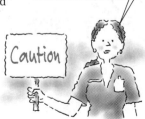

Don't gamble with client safety when you suspect your coworker of substance abuse.

Caution

6. 1. The nurse is obligated to report suspected substance abuse. Allowing the assistant to continue to work could jeopardize client care. It isn't the practical nurse's role to decide that the assistant must leave the unit immediately. Warning the assistant that she could lose her certification doesn't address the issue sufficiently.
CN: Safe, effective care environment; CNS: Coordinated care; CL: Comprehension

CN: Client needs category   CNS: Client needs subcategory   CL: Cognitive level

7. The nurse notices that a 33-year-old male client with borderline personality disorder is very manipulative and plays one staff member against another. The best way to deal with this behavior is to:
1. consistently enforce limits when the client attempts to manipulate.
2. seek the client's approval for any change in routine on the unit.
3. allow the client to bend the unit rules rather than entering into power struggles.
4. assign the client to the same staff member to maintain consistency.

8. The nurse is concerned about another nurse's relationship with the members of a family and their ill preschooler. Which behavior would be most worrisome and should be brought to the attention of the nurse-manager?
1. The nurse keeps communication channels open among herself, the family, physicians, and other health care providers.
2. The nurse attempts to influence the family's decisions by presenting her own thoughts and opinions.
3. The nurse works with the family members to find ways to decrease their dependence on health care providers.
4. The nurse has developed teaching skills to instruct the family members so they can accomplish tasks independently.

9. The manager of an outpatient clinic is explaining the various health care delivery systems to a client. The client is interested in joining a system that has a reasonable fixed capitation rate. The manager realizes that the client is primarily interested in joining:
1. a preferred provider organization (PPO).
2. a managed care organization.
3. a health maintenance organization (HMO).
4. a privately funded insurance company.

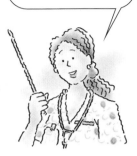

Eliminating the wrong answers can be as important as selecting the right one.

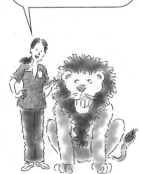

Fixed capitation sounds scarier than it is, although the teeth are pretty sharp!

7. 1. The staff must be consistent in setting limits on negative behaviors. Situations can escalate to crisis level when limit setting is inconsistent. The nurse should inform the client about changes in unit routines but shouldn't seek his approval. Allowing the client to bend the unit rules is a form of manipulation and shouldn't be allowed. Staff members should be rotated so that the client can learn to relate to more than one person.
CN: Safe, effective care environment; CNS: Coordinated care; CL: Application

8. 2. When a nurse attempts to influence a family's decision with her own opinions and values, the situation becomes one of overinvolvement on the nurse's part and a nontherapeutic relationship. When a nurse keeps communication channels open, works with family members to decrease their dependence on health care providers, and instructs family members so they can accomplish tasks independently, she has developed an appropriate therapeutic relationship.
CN: Safe, effective care environment; CNS: Coordinated care; CL: Analysis

9. 3. An HMO provides comprehensive health services for a fixed rate of payment or capitation. A PPO pays healthcare expenses for members if they use a provider who's under contract to that PPO. Managed care provides beneficiaries with various services for an established, agreed-upon payment. A privately funded insurance company won't offer services for a fixed rate.
CN: Safe, effective care environment; CNS: Coordinated care; CL: Application

CN: Client needs category   CNS: Client needs subcategory   CL: Cognitive level

10. A 2-year-old female is admitted for pneumonia secondary to a positive human immunodeficiency virus (HIV) status. Her condition is stable, and the nurse asks the nursing assistant to give the child a bed bath. The nursing assistant is reluctant to bathe the child for fear that she'll contract the virus. Which statements would be most appropriate for the nurse to include in the response? Select all that apply:

1. "As a nursing assistant, you should already know that there's little chance you will acquire HIV from bathing anyone."
2. "I know you're frightened, but by taking proper precautions there's little to no risk of acquiring HIV."
3. "I'm in charge, and you need to follow through on this assignment."
4. "The purpose of using standard precautions is to prevent the inadvertent transmission of HIV and other diseases in situations where you may come in contact with blood, body fluids or secretions."
5. "If you don't bathe the child as I requested, I'll have to write up an incident report."

10. 2, 4. Recognizing that the nursing assistant is frightened and then clarifying information about the use of standard precautions provides her with guidance and education to allay her fears. Option 1 is demeaning and doesn't encourage the nursing assistant to take appropriate precautions. Options 3 and 5 are threatening and don't address the nursing assistant's fears.
CN: Safe, effective care environment; CNS: Coordinated care; CL: Analysis

11. A nursing assistant frequently disappears from the floor without telling anyone. When she returns, her clothing smells strongly of smoke. This behavior is creating a problem with the staff and some clients on the unit and must be addressed. What steps should be taken? Place the following steps in ascending chronological order. Use all the options.

| 1. Report the nursing assistant to the charge nurse if the behavior remains unchanged. |
| 2. Approach the nursing assistant privately to discuss the issue. |
| 3. Keep notes with dates and times this behavior is observed. |
| 4. Try to work with the nursing assistant to schedule daily breaks. |
| 5. Observe the nursing assistant's behavior for signs of improvement. |

11. Ordered response:

| 3. Keep notes with dates and times this behavior is observed. |
| 2. Approach the nursing assistant privately to discuss the issue. |
| 4. Try to work with the nursing assistant to schedule daily breaks. |
| 5. Observe the nursing assistant's behavior for signs of improvement. |
| 1. Report the nursing assistant to the charge nurse if the behavior remains unchanged. |

Keeping notes listing dates and times the inappropriate behavior is observed will be helpful to verify facts. Then approach the nursing assistant privately and confidentially to discuss the issue. Work to schedule defined break times, and request that she contact you before leaving the unit. Observe the nursing assistant's behavior for signs of improvement, and bring the issue to the attention of the charge nurse for further action if it continues unimproved.
CN: Safe, effective care environment; CNS: Coordinated care; CL: Analysis

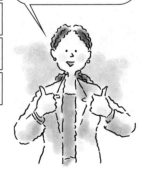

Congratulations! You're done with the chapter and you managed to ace it!

CN: Client needs category   CNS: Client needs subcategory   CL: Cognitive level

Ethical and legal issues are a daily challenge in nursing practice. Ace them on the NCLEX, and you'll be able to face each challenge with confidence! Let's go!

1. An elderly client has been admitted to the medical-surgical unit from the postanesthesia care unit. While the nurse is off the floor, the client falls out of bed, resulting in a fracture of his right leg and right wrist. The nurse finding him states that the "side rails were left down and the bed was in the high position." Legal charges are filed against the nurse and the hospital. What's the most likely charge for her actions?
   1. Collective liability
   2. Comparative negligence
   3. Battery
   4. Negligence

2. The time frame in which a client's attorney has to file a lawsuit is known as:
   1. discovery rule.
   2. statute of limitation.
   3. grace period.
   4. alternative dispute resolution.

Here's a hint: Only three of these four choices refer to "time frames." Even eliminating one option makes choosing the correct answer easier.

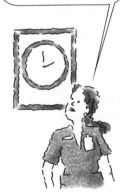

3. What elements must be proven by a client's attorney in the case of a professional negligence action?
   1. Duty, breach of duty, damages, and causation
   2. Duty, damages, and causation
   3. Duty, breach of duty, and damages
   4. Breach of duty, damages, and causation

1. 4. *Negligence* is a general term that denotes conduct lacking in due care and is commonly interpreted as a deviation from the standard of care that a reasonable person would use in a particular set of circumstances. Collective liability stems from cooperation by several manufacturers in a wrongful activity that by its nature requires group participation. Comparative negligence is a defense that holds injured parties accountable for their fault in the injury. Battery involves a harmful or unwarranted contact with the client.
CN: Safe, effective care environment; CNS: Safety and infection control; CL: Analysis

2. 2. Statute of limitation is the time interval during which a case must be filed or the injured party is barred from bringing the lawsuit. The statute of limitations typically gives clients 2 years from the time of discovery to file a lawsuit; however, this may vary from state to state. Statutes of limitations are set by state legislatures. *Discovery rule* is the term for when the client has discovered the injury. A grace period refers to any period specified in a contract during which payment is permitted without penalty, beyond the due date of the debt. Alternative dispute resolution refers to any means of settling disputes outside the courtroom setting.
CN: Safe, effective care environment; CNS: Safety and infection control; CL: Knowledge

3. 1. Any professional negligence action must meet these demands in order to be considered negligence and result in legal action. They're commonly known as the four D's: duty of the health care professional to provide care to the person making the claim, a dereliction (breach) of that duty, damages resulting from that breach of duty, and evidence that damages were directly due to negligence (causation).
CN: Safe, effective care environment; CNS: Coordinated care; CL: Application

CN: Client needs category   CNS: Client needs subcategory   CL: Cognitive level

4. The scope of nursing professional practice defines what a nurse can and can't do. What defines and regulates the scope of nursing professional practice?
1. Nursing process
2. Facilities' policies and procedures
3. Standards of care
4. Nurse Practice Act

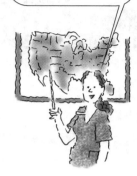

The Nurse Practice Act is specific to each state.

4. 4. The Nurse Practice Act is a series of statutes enacted by each state to outline the legal scope of nursing practice within that state. State boards of nursing oversee this statutory law. Nurse practice acts set educational requirements for the nurse, distinguish between nursing practice and medical practice, and define the scope of nursing practice. Nursing process is an organizational framework for nursing practice, encompassing all major steps a nurse takes when caring for a patient. Facility policies govern the practice in that particular facility. Standards of care are criteria that serve as a basis for comparison when evaluating the quality of nursing practice. Standards of care are established by federal, state, professional, and accreditation organizations.
CN: Safe, effective care environment; CNS: Coordinated care; CL: Application

5. A Jehovah's Witness client refuses a blood transfusion based on his religious beliefs and practices. His decision must be followed based on what ethical principle?
1. The right to die
2. Advance directive
3. The right to refuse treatment
4. Substituted judgment

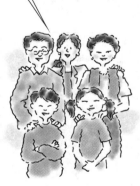

It's important to respect the religious beliefs and cultural practices of all clients.

5. 3. The right to refuse treatment is grounded in the ethical principle of respect for autonomy of the individual. The client has the right to refuse treatment as long as he's competent and is made aware of the risks and complications associated with refusal of treatment. Substituted judgment is an ethical principle used when the decision is made for an incapacitated client based on what's best for the client. An advance directive is a document used as a guideline for life-sustaining medical care of a client with a terminal disease or disability who can no longer indicate his own wishes.
CN: Safe, effective care environment; CNS: Coordinated care; CL: Application

6. A nurse gives a client the wrong medication. After assessment of the client, the nurse completes an incident report. Which scenario describes what should occur next?
1. The incident would be reported to the state board of nursing for disciplinary action.
2. The incident would be documented in the nurse's personnel file.
3. The medication error would result in the nurse being suspended and possibly terminated from employment at the facility.
4. The incident report would be used to promote quality care and risk management.

6. 4. Unusual occurrences and deviations from care are documented on incident reports. Incident reports are internal to the facility and are used to evaluate the care, determine potential risks, and identify possible system problems that could have attributed to the error. This type of error wouldn't result in suspension of the nurse or reporting to the state board of nursing. Some facilities do trend and track the number of errors that take place on particular units or by individual nurses for educational purposes and as a way to improve the process.
CN: Safe, effective care environment; CNS: Coordinated care; CL: Analysis

CN: Client needs category   CNS: Client needs subcategory   CL: Cognitive level

7. A client has suffered an extensive brain injury and can't make his own treatment choices. Which document would be least likely to provide directions concerning the provision of care in this situation?
1. Advance directive
2. Living will
3. Durable power of attorney
4. Occurrence policy

7. 4. An occurrence policy is a professional liability policy that protects against an error of omission that occurs during a policy period, which doesn't involve provision of care. A living will is a document prepared by a competent adult that provides direction regarding medical care in the event the person can't make his own decisions. A durable power of attorney is an authorization that enables any competent individual to name someone to exercise decision-making authority on the individual's behalf under specific circumstances. A living will and a durable power of attorney are examples of advance directives.
CN: Safe, effective care environment; CNS: Coordinated care; CL: Comprehension

8. In what way do nurses play a key role in error prevention?
1. Identifying incorrect dosages or potential interactions of prescribed medications
2. Never questioning the order of a physician because he's ultimately responsible for the client outcome
3. Notifying the Occupational Safety and Health Association (OSHA) of violations in the workplace
4. Informing the client of his rights as a client

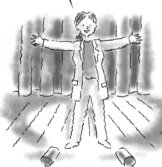

Nurses have lots of roles and responsibilities, but question 8 is asking specifically about error prevention. Which answer fits best?

8. 1. Nurses must be knowledgeable about drug dosages and possible interactions when administering medications and be able to follow the appropriate policy to correct the situation. The nurse is responsible for questioning an unclear or ambiguous order from the physician and should never carry out an order she's uncomfortable with. Notifying OSHA doesn't solve medication errors. OSHA establishes comprehensive safety and health standards, inspects workplaces, and orders employers to eliminate safety hazards. The client should be aware of his rights as a client, but that doesn't play a key role in error prevention.
CN: Safe, effective care environment; CNS: Safety and infection control; CL: Application

9. Which statement is true concerning informed consent?
1. Minors are permitted to give informed consent.
2. The professional nurse and physician may both obtain informed consent.
3. The client must be fully informed regarding treatment, tests, surgery, risks, and benefits before obtaining informed consent.
4. Mentally competent and incompetent clients can legally give informed consent.

9. 3. When the professional nurse is involved in the informed consent process, the nurse is only witnessing the consent process and doesn't actually obtain the consent. Only a minor who's married or emancipated can give informed consent. Obtaining the consent is the physician's responsibility. Legally, the client must be mentally competent to give consent for procedures.
CN: Safe, effective care environment; CNS: Coordinated care; CL: Comprehension

CN: Client needs category CNS: Client needs subcategory CL: Cognitive level

10. The Omnibus Reconciliation Act of 1986 states that:

1. all families of clients who are nearing death, or have died, must be approached with the option of organ and tissue donation.
2. the medical examiner should be notified of all potential organ donors.
3. a request must be made to the family regarding release or remains of donors.
4. hospitals aren't responsible for establishing designated requesters for donation.

10. 1. The federal Omnibus Reconciliation Act of 1986 mandates that hospitals establish written protocols for the identification of potential organ and tissue donors. This law was enacted to attempt to correct the disparity between the organs that could be transplanted and the number of people waiting for them. The medical examiner should be notified if the client is a potential organ or tissue donor only in the event that the medical examiner is involved in the case. Requesters for donation are health care professionals who have received special training on how to properly approach family members regarding organ or tissue donation.
CN: Safe, effective care environment; CNS: Coordinated care; CL: Comprehension

11. When approaching a family for organ or tissue donation, it's important that:

1. it's done with a physician's approval and written order.
2. the requester doesn't have to believe in the benefits of organ donation or support the process with a positive attitude.
3. the requester is knowledgeable about the basics of organ and tissue donation and can educate the family members about brain death early in the organ donation process.
4. the family is offered an opportunity to speak with an organ procurement coordinator.

11. 4. The family should be offered an opportunity to speak with an organ procurement coordinator. An organ procurement coordinator is very knowledgeable about the organ donation process and dealing with grieving family members. Physician support in the process is desirable, but consent or written orders aren't necessary for a referral to the organ procurement organization. The requester has to believe in the benefits of organ donation and support the process. Approaching the family should only occur when the family members are made aware of the client's condition and prognosis. Approaching a family member when he believes that there's still hope for recovery will only result in a negative outcome.
CN: Safe, effective care environment; CNS: Coordinated care; CL: Analysis

> Question 12 asks about stages—in other words, a progression. Only one of these answer choices offers a logical progression. Can you figure it out?

12. A nurse is discussing the stages of grief with family members. Which statement is the most accurate regarding the stages of grief?

1. The stages of grief include acceptance, depression, anger, bargaining, and denial.
2. The stages of grief include denial, anger, decreased interaction, depression, and mourning.
3. The stages of grief include acceptance, anger, denial, and bargaining.
4. The stages of grief include denial, anger, bargaining, depression, and acceptance.

12. 4. Denial is the avoidance of death's inevitability and is the first step of the grieving process. Anger, the most intense grief reaction, arises when people realize that death and loss will actually occur or has occurred for a family member. Bargaining happens when family members attempt to stall or to manipulate the outcome or death. Depression is a response to loss that's expressed as profound sadness or deep suffering. Acceptance, the final stage, is the ability to overcome the grief and accept what has happened.
CN: Psychosocial integrity; CNS: None; CL: Application

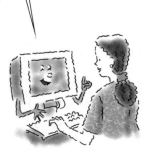

CN: Client needs category   CNS: Client needs subcategory   CL: Cognitive level

13. There are reports that morphine has been missing from the medication cart several times during the last 3 months. As the nurse walks into the medication room, she witnesses another nurse quickly slipping something into her pocket from the controlled substance drawer. Place the following steps in ascending chronological sequence. Use all the options.

1. If directed, fill out a confidential incident report describing what was seen.
2. Approach the charge nurse privately and discuss the matter.
3. Do not share any observations with others on the unit.
4. Continue to observe this nurse in question for signs of unusual behavior.
5. Carefully review and document what was observed.

13. Ordered response:

5. Carefully review and document what was observed.
2. Approach the charge nurse privately and discuss the matter.
1. If directed, fill out a confidential incident report describing what was seen.
3. Do not share any observations with others on the unit.
4. Continue to observe this nurse in question for signs of unusual behavior.

A premature conclusion shouldn't be drawn based on one suspicious incident. It's best to first review and carefully document in detail what was seen. Then speak with the charge nurse privately, and if directed, fill out a confidential incident report describing what was observed. At this point, the charge nurse will follow through and investigate the situation further. It's important to not speak to others on the unit to maintain professionalism and to avoid spreading potentially unfounded rumors. The reporting nurse should remain alert for repeated suspicious behavior.

CN: Safe, effective care environment; CNS: Coordinated care; CL: Analysis

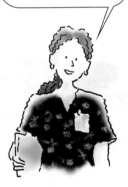

Know what to do if you see something suspicious.

14. A nurse observes her coworker administering a medication several hours after it's scheduled. When confronted, the coworker simply makes a dismissive joke and then charts the medication as given at the scheduled time even though it was late. Place the following steps in ascending chronological sequence. Use all the options.

1. Request a private meeting to discuss the incident.
2. Encourage her to take responsibility for her actions.
3. Express concern and clearly inform her that her behavior is unethical.
4. Report the incident to the charge nurse if resistance is noted.
5. Approach the coworker in a calm and professional manner.

14. Ordered response:

5. Approach the coworker in a calm and professional manner.
1. Request a private meeting to discuss the incident.
3. Express concern and clearly inform her that her behavior is unethical.
2. Encourage her to take responsibility for her actions.
4. Report the incident to the charge nurse if resistance is noted.

The nurse must maintain a calm and professional demeanor and talk with her coworker privately. It's important to discuss ethical concerns and encourage the coworker to take responsibility for her actions. The charge nurse should be informed of the incident if resistance is noted.

CN: Safe, effective care environment; CNS: Coordinated care; CL: Analysis

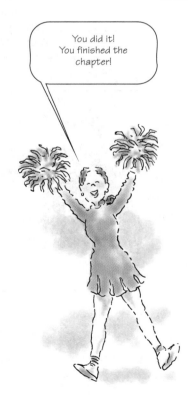

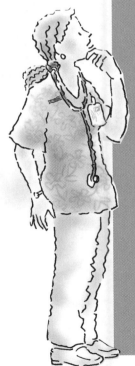

Appendices and index

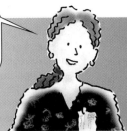

This comprehensive test, the first of four, is just like a real NCLEX exam. It's a great way to practice!

COMPREHENSIVE
Test 1

1. A 43-year-old client with blunt chest trauma from a motor vehicle accident has sinus tachycardia, is hypotensive, and has developed muffled heart sounds. There are no obvious signs of bleeding. Which condition is suspected?
1. Heart failure
2. Pneumothorax
3. Cardiac tamponade
4. Myocardial infarction (MI)

1. 3. Cardiac tamponade results in signs of obvious shock and muffled heart sounds. Heart failure would result in inspiratory crackles, pulmonary edema, and jugular vein distention. Pneumothorax would result in diminished breath sounds in the affected lung, respiratory distress, and tracheal displacement. In an MI, the client may complain of chest pain. An electrocardiogram could confirm changes consistent with an MI.
CN: Physiological integrity; CNS: Physiological adaptation; CL: Analysis

2. Which type of shock would the nurse be alert for in a client with tamponade?
1. Anaphylactic
2. Cardiogenic
3. Hypovolemic
4. Septic

2. 2. Fluid accumulates in the pericardial sac, hindering motion of the heart muscle and causing it to pump inefficiently, resulting in signs of cardiogenic shock. Anaphylactic and septic shock are types of distributive shock in which fluid is displaced from the capillaries and leaks into surrounding tissues. Hypovolemic shock involves the actual loss of fluid.
CN: Physiological integrity; CNS: Physiological adaptation; CL: Application

3. Which diagnostic test is best at detecting cardiac tamponade?
1. Chest X-ray
2. Echocardiography
3. Electrocardiogram (ECG)
4. Pulmonary artery pressure monitoring

Which test best helps diagnose cardiac tamponade?

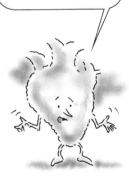

3. 2. Echocardiography measures pericardial effusion and can detect signs of right ventricular and atrial compression. Chest X-rays show a slightly widened mediastinum and enlarged cardiac silhouette. An ECG can rule out other cardiac disorders. Pulmonary artery pressure monitoring shows increased right atrial or central venous pressure and right ventricular diastolic pressure.
CN: Physiological integrity; CNS: Reduction of risk potential; CL: Application

CN: Client needs category   CNS: Client needs subcategory   CL: Cognitive level

4. The nurse is caring for a client with cardiac tamponade. Which of the following treatments would the nurse anticipate for this client?
1. Surgery
2. Dopamine (Intropin)
3. Blood transfusion
4. Pericardiocentesis

4. 4. Pericardiocentesis, or needle aspiration of the pericardial cavity, is done to relieve tamponade. An opening is created surgically if the client continues to have recurrent episodes of tamponade. Dopamine is used to restore blood pressure in normovolemic individuals. Blood transfusions may be given if the client is hypovolemic from blood loss.
CN: Physiological integrity; CNS: Physiological adaptation; CL: Application

5. A nurse is teaching a 50-year-old client how to decrease risk factors for coronary artery disease. He's an executive who smokes, has a type A personality, and is hypertensive. Which risk factor can't be changed?
1. Age
2. Hypertension
3. Personality
4. Smoking

5. 1. Age is a risk factor that can't be changed. Hypertension, type A personality, and smoking factors can be controlled.
CN: Health promotion and maintenance; CNS: None; CL: Comprehension

6. A client says he's stressed by his job but enjoys the challenge. Which suggestion is best to help the client?
1. Switch job positions.
2. Take stress management classes.
3. Spend more time with his family.
4. Don't take his work home with him.

6. 2. Stress management classes will teach the client how to better manage the stress in his life, after identifying the factors that contribute to it. Alternatives may be found to leaving his job, which he enjoys. Not spending enough time with his family and not taking his job home with him haven't yet been identified as contributing factors.
CN: Physiological integrity; CNS: Reduction of risk potential; CL: Application

7. Which nursing diagnosis is correctly worded?
1. *Anger related to terminal illness*
2. *Pain related to alteration in comfort*
3. *Red sacrum related to improper positioning*
4. *Social isolation related to laryngectomy evidenced by inability to speak*

7. 4. The fourth option is a correctly worded nursing diagnosis. The first option identifies anger as an unhealthy response when it may be an appropriate and socially acceptable response. The second option is incorrect because both parts of this diagnosis relate to pain and say the same thing. The third option is improperly written; it's a legally inadvisable statement. Also, the first three diagnoses are not part of the North American Nursing Diagnosis Association (NANDA) Taxonomy II Codes.
CN: Safe, effective care environment; CNS: Coordinated care; CL: Application

CN: Client needs category   CNS: Client needs subcategory   CL: Cognitive level

8. A 28-year-old client with human immunodeficiency virus is admitted to the hospital with flu-like symptoms. He has dyspnea and a cough. He's placed on a 100% nonrebreather mask and arterial blood gases are drawn. Which results indicate the client needs intubation?
  1. Pao_2, 90 mm Hg; $Paco_2$, 40 mm Hg
  2. Pao_2, 85 mm Hg; $Paco_2$, 45 mm Hg
  3. Pao_2, 80 mm Hg; $Paco_2$, 45 mm Hg
  4. Pao_2, 70 mm Hg; $Paco_2$, 55 mm Hg

9. Which substance most commonly transmits the human immunodeficiency virus (HIV)?
  1. Blood
  2. Feces
  3. Saliva
  4. Urine

10. Which opportunistic disease is caused by protozoa in clients with acquired immunodeficiency syndrome?
  1. Tuberculosis (TB)
  2. Histoplasmosis
  3. Kaposi's sarcoma
  4. *Pneumocystis carinii* infection

11. A client with acquired immunodeficiency syndrome is intubated, leaving him prone to skin breakdown from the endotracheal (ET) tube. Which intervention is best to prevent this?
  1. Using lubricant on the lips
  2. Providing oral care every 2 hours
  3. Suctioning the oral cavity every 2 hours
  4. Repositioning the ET tube every 24 hours

12. A client requiring the highest possible concentration of oxygen will need which delivery system?
  1. Face tent
  2. Venturi mask
  3. Nasal cannula
  4. Mask with reservoir bag

8. 4. A decreasing partial pressure of arterial oxygen (Pao_2) and an increasing partial pressure of arterial carbon dioxide ($Paco_2$) indicate poor oxygen perfusion. Normal Pao_2 levels are 80 to 100 mm Hg and normal $Paco_2$ levels are 35 to 45 mm Hg.
CN: Physiological integrity; CNS: Physiological adaptation; CL: Analysis

9. 1. HIV is most commonly transmitted by contact with infected blood. It exists in all body fluids but transmission through feces, saliva, and urine is much less likely to occur.
CN: Safe, effective care environment; CNS: Safety and infection control; CL: Knowledge

10. 4. *P. carinii* infection is caused by protozoa. TB is caused by bacteria. Histoplasmosis is a fungal infection. Kaposi's sarcoma is a neoplasm.
CN: Physiological integrity; CNS: Physiological adaptation; CL: Knowledge

11. 4. Pressure causes skin breakdown. However, repositioning the ET tube from one side of the mouth to the other or to the center of the mouth can relieve pressure in one area for a time. Extreme care must be taken to move the tube only laterally; it must not be pushed in or pulled out. The tape securing the tube must be changed daily. Two nurses should perform this procedure. Lubricant, oral care, and suctioning help keep skin clean and intact and reduce the risk of further infection.
CN: Physiological integrity; CNS: Basic care and comfort; CL: Application

12. 4. A mask with a reservoir bag administers 70% to 100% oxygen at flow rates of 8 to 10 L/minute. The nasal cannula maximum rate is 44% at 6 L/minute, the Venturi mask maximum rate is 24% to 55%, and a face tent maximum delivery is 22% to 34%.
CN: Physiological integrity; CNS: Pharmacological therapies; CL: Comprehension

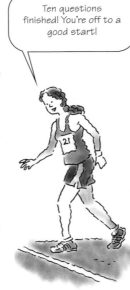

Ten questions finished! You're off to a good start!

13. A client with difficulty breathing has a respiratory rate of 34 breaths/minute and seems anxious. She's refusing all her medications, claiming they're making her worse. Which nursing action is best?
  1. Notify the physician of the status of this client.
  2. Hold the medication until the next scheduled dose.
  3. Encourage the client to take some of her medications.
  4. Put the medicine in applesauce to give it without the client's knowledge.

14. A nurse caring for a client with acquired immunodeficiency syndrome is working with a nursing student. She notes the student doesn't attempt to suction or assist with care of the client. Which action is appropriate?
  1. Talk to the student.
  2. Talk to the charge nurse.
  3. Address a coworker with the concerns.
  4. Seek advice from the student's instructor.

15. A client's significant other is tearful over the client's condition and lack of improvement. He says he feels very powerless and unable to help his friend. Which response by the nurse is the best?
  1. Agree with the client.
  2. Tell the client there's nothing he can do.
  3. State she understands how he must feel.
  4. Ask if the client would like to help with some comfort measures.

16. A 31-year-old client is admitted to the hospital with respiratory failure. He's intubated in the emergency department, placed on 100% F_{IO_2}, and is coughing up copious secretions. Which intervention has priority?
  1. Getting an X-ray
  2. Suctioning the client
  3. Restraining the client
  4. Obtaining an arterial blood gas (ABG) analysis

13. 1. Notifying the physician of the client's condition and her refusal to take her medications allows the physician to decide what alternatives should be instituted. Holding a medication requires the physician to be notified. Even if the client takes some of the medications, the physician will still need to be notified. Giving medications in applesauce destroys trust between the nurse and client. It needs to be explored why the client believes the medications are making her worse.
CN: Physiological integrity; CNS: Pharmacological therapies; CL: Application

14. 1. The nurse should approach the student to determine her feelings and experience in caring for this client. The charge nurse and coworkers aren't familiar with the student's abilities, but the instructor may be approached if the nurse can't communicate with the student.
CN: Safe, effective care environment; CNS: Coordinated care; CL: Analysis

15. 4. The significant other expresses a need to help and the nurse can encourage him to do whatever he feels comfortable with, such as putting lubricant on lips, moist cloth on forehead, or lotion on skin. The nurse may not understand his situation, and agreeing with a person doesn't diminish powerlessness. There are many ways the significant other can assist.
CN: Psychosocial integrity; CNS: None; CL: Analysis

16. 2. Secretions can cut off the oxygen supply to the client and result in hypoxia. X-rays are a priority to check placement of the endotracheal tube. Restraints are warranted only if the client is a threat to his safety. After the client has acclimated to his ventilator settings, ABG levels can be drawn.
CN: Physiological integrity; CNS: Reduction of risk potential; CL: Analysis

CN: Client needs category   CNS: Client needs subcategory   CL: Cognitive level

17. A client with an endotracheal tube has copious, brown-tinged secretions. Which intervention is a priority?
1. Using a trap to obtain a specimen
2. Instilling saline to break up secretions
3. Culturing the specimen with a culturette swab
4. Obtaining an order for a liquefying agent for the sputum

17. 1. Suspicious secretions should be sent for culture and sensitivity testing using a sterile technique such as a trap. Saline would dilute the specimen. Swab culturettes are useful for wound cultures—not endotracheal cultures. Various agents are available to help break up secretions, and respiratory therapists can usually help recommend the right agent, but this isn't a priority.
CN: Safe, effective care environment; CNS: Safety and infection control; CL: Analysis

18. An X-ray shows that an endotracheal (ET) tube is ¾″ (2 cm) above the carina, and there are nodular lesions and patchy infiltrates in the upper lobe. Based on this report, the nurse can expect which conclusion?
1. The X-ray is inconclusive.
2. The client has a disease process going on.
3. The ET tube needs to be advanced.
4. The ET tube needs to be pulled back.

18. 2. The X-ray is conclusive and suggests tuberculosis. At ¾″, the ET tube is at an adequate level in the trachea and doesn't have to be advanced or pulled back.
CN: Health promotion and maintenance; CNS: None; CL: Analysis

19. The X-ray results of a client who has copious secretions indicate tuberculosis. Which of the following procedures is most conclusive in diagnosing tuberculosis?
1. Repeat X-ray
2. Tracheostomy
3. Bronchoscopy
4. Arterial blood gas (ABG) analysis

19. 3. Bronchoscopy can help diagnose TB and obtain specimens while clearing the bronchial tree of secretions. X-rays may be repeated periodically to determine lung and endotracheal tube status. Tracheostomy may be done if the client remains on the ventilator for a prolonged period. A change in condition or treatment may require an ABG analysis.
CN: Physiological integrity; CNS: Reduction of risk potential; CL: Application

20. A nurse is aware that staff and family members of a client diagnosed with tuberculosis may have been exposed to the disease. A tuberculin skin test may show which condition?
1. Active disease
2. Recent infection
3. Extent of the infection
4. Infection at some point

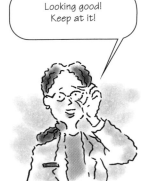

Looking good! Keep at it!

20. 4. A tuberculin skin test shows the presence of infection at some point; however, a positive skin test doesn't guarantee that an infection is *currently* present. Some people have false-positive results. Active disease may be viewed on a chest X-ray. Computed tomography scan or magnetic resonance imaging can evaluate the extent of lung damage.
CN: Safe, effective care environment; CNS: Safety and infection control; CL: Knowledge

CN: Client needs category   CNS: Client needs subcategory   CL: Cognitive level

21. A client is diagnosed with tuberculosis (TB). In addition to recommending skin testing of the family members, TB must be reported to which individual or agency?
1. Centers for Disease Control and Prevention (CDC)
2. Local health department
3. Infection-control nurse
4. Client's physician

21. 2. The local health department must be informed of an outbreak of TB because it's a reportable disease. They, in turn, inform the CDC. The infection-control nurse or local health department may request that staff be tested if exposed. Generally, the client's family can inform his physician.

CN: Safe, effective care environment; CNS: Safety and infection control; CL: Application

22. The usual treatment for tuberculosis (TB) includes the use of isoniazid (INH) and which therapy?
1. Theophylline (Slo-Phyllin)
2. I.M. penicillin
3. Three other antibacterial agents
4. Aerosol treatments with pentamidine (NembuPent)

22. 3. Because TB has become resistant to many antibacterial agents, the initial treatment includes the use of multiple antitubercular or antibacterial drugs. These may include rifampin (Rifadin), ethambutol (Myambutol), pyrazinamide, cycloserine (Seromycin), and streptomycin. Theophylline is a bronchodilator used to treat asthma and chronic obstructive pulmonary disease. Penicillins are used to treat *Staphylococcus aureus* infection—not TB. Pentamidine is used in the treatment of *Pneumocystis carinii* pneumonia.

CN: Physiological integrity; CNS: Pharmacological therapies; CL: Knowledge

23. How long do most clients receive treatment for tuberculosis (TB)?
1. 2 to 4 months
2. 9 to 12 months
3. 18 to 24 months
4. More than 2 years

23. 2. Treatment for TB is usually continued for 9 to 12 months. Option 1 isn't adequate time for treatment to be successful. Options 3 and 4 are treatment times that are beyond therapeutic value.

CN: Physiological integrity; CNS: Pharmacological therapies; CL: Knowledge

24. A nurse teaches a client with tuberculosis that he is still considered infectious up to what time period after treatment is started?
1. 72 hours
2. 1 week
3. 2 weeks
4. 4 weeks

24. 4. After 4 weeks, the disease is no longer infectious but the client must continue to take the medication.

CN: Safe, effective care environment; CNS: Safety and infection control; CL: Application

CN: Client needs category   CNS: Client needs subcategory   CL: Cognitive level

25. A client tells his nurse that his tuberculosis medications are so expensive that he can't afford them. Which intervention by the nurse is best?
1. Referring the client to social services
2. Telling the client to apply for Medicaid
3. Referring the client to the local or county health department
4. Telling the client to follow his insurance rules and regulations

25. 3. The local and county health departments provide treatment and follow-up free of charge for all residents to ensure proper care. Social services can help seek alternative methods of payment and reimbursement but would probably first refer the client to the local and county health departments. Insurance can be an alternative source to help pay for treatment, but the client may not be insured or the policy may not cover prescriptions. Medicaid or medical assistance is another avenue for the client, if he qualifies.
CN: Safe, effective care environment; CNS: Coordinated care; CL: Analysis

26. A 62-year-old client is admitted to the hospital with pneumonia. He has a history of Parkinson's disease, which his family says is progressively worsening. Which assessment is expected?
1. Impaired speech
2. Muscle flaccidity
3. Pleasant and smiling demeanor
4. Tremors in the fingers that increase with purposeful movement

26. 1. In Parkinson's disease, dysarthria (impaired speech) is due to a disturbance in muscle control. Muscle rigidity results in resistance to passive muscle stretching. The client may have a masklike appearance. Tremors should decrease with purposeful movement and sleep.
CN: Physiological integrity; CNS: Physiological adaptation; CL: Application

27. Which term describes a clinical judgment that an individual, family, or community is more vulnerable to develop a certain problem than others in the same or similar situation?
1. Risk nursing diagnosis
2. Actual nursing diagnosis
3. Possible nursing diagnosis
4. Wellness nursing diagnosis

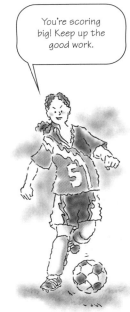

You're scoring big! Keep up the good work.

27. 1. Risk nursing diagnosis refers to the vulnerability of a client, family, or community to health problems. An actual nursing diagnosis describes a human response to a health problem being manifested. Possible nursing diagnoses are made when there isn't enough evidence to support the presence of the problem, but the nurse believes the problem is highly probable and wants to collect more data. A wellness nursing diagnosis is a diagnostic statement describing the human response to levels of wellness in an individual, family, or community that have a potential for enhancement to a higher state.
CN: Safe, effective care environment; CNS: Coordinated care; CL: Knowledge

28. Which intervention is best to decrease a client's risk of skin breakdown?
1. Using a specialty mattress
2. Positioning the client in alignment
3. Repositioning the client every 4 hours
4. Massaging bony prominences every shift

28. 1. Specialty beds, such as fluid, air, and convoluted foam mattresses, can protect pressure areas on the client. Pressure areas on the client should be padded to prevent skin breakdown. Positioning the client in alignment is important, but pressure areas still need to be protected. The client should be turned every 2 hours. Massaging bony prominences causes friction and may irritate tissues.
CN: Physiological integrity; CNS: Reduction of risk potential; CL: Application

CN: Client needs category   CNS: Client needs subcategory   CL: Cognitive level

29. A male client with Parkinson's disease is frequently incontinent of urine. Which intervention is appropriate?
    1. Diapering the client
    2. Applying a condom catheter
    3. Inserting an indwelling urinary catheter
    4. Providing skin care every 4 hours

29. 2. A condom catheter uses a condom-type device to drain urine away from the client. Diapering the client may keep urine away from the body but may also be demeaning if the client is alert or the family objects. Because the client with Parkinson's disease is prone to urinary tract infections, an indwelling urinary catheter should be avoided because it may promote this. Skin care must be provided as soon as the client is incontinent to prevent skin maceration and breakdown.
CN: Physiological integrity; CNS: Basic care and comfort; CL: Analysis

30. Family members report exhaustion and difficulty taking care of a dependent family member. Which approach is in the client's best interest?
    1. Ask the client what he wishes.
    2. Have the family members discuss it among themselves.
    3. Tell the family the client should go to a nursing care facility.
    4. Call a family conference and ask social services for assistance.

30. 4. A family conference with social services can enlighten the family to all prospects of care available to them. The client should supply input if he can but this may not help solve the problems of exhaustion and care difficulties. The family may not be aware of alternative care measures for the client so a discussion among themselves may not be helpful. The client may not qualify for a nursing care facility because of stringent criteria.
CN: Safe, effective care environment; CNS: Coordinated care; CL: Analysis

31. A 30-year-old primagravida in her second trimester tells a nurse her fingers feel tight and sometimes she feels as though her heart skips a beat. She has a history of rheumatic fever. Which symptom indicates the client may be experiencing cardiovascular disease?
    1. Clear breath sounds
    2. Sinus tachycardia
    3. Increasing dyspnea on exertion
    4. Runs of paroxysmal atrial tachycardia

31. 3. Increasing dyspnea on exertion should alert the nurse to cardiovascular compromise. Cardiac arrhythmias (other than sinus tachycardia or paroxysmal atrial tachycardia) and persistent crackles at the bases are also symptoms of cardiovascular disease, not clear breath sounds.
CN: Health promotion and maintenance; CNS: None; CL: Analysis

32. Which diagnostic test determines the extent of cardiovascular disease during pregnancy?
    1. Stress test
    2. Chest X-ray
    3. Echocardiography
    4. Cardiac catheterization

32. 3. Echocardiography is less invasive than X-rays and other methods and provides the information needed to determine cardiovascular disease, especially valvular disorders. Cardiac catheterization and stress tests may be postponed until after delivery.
CN: Physiological integrity; CNS: Physiological adaptation; CL: Knowledge

CN: Client needs category   CNS: Client needs subcategory   CL: Cognitive level

33. A nurse who is caring for a client in labor with a history of rheumatic heart disease should perform which of the following assessments in order to determine fetal well-being?
1. Urinalysis
2. Fetal heart tones
3. Laboratory test results of the mother
4. Other signs and symptoms of the client

34. Which factor is an example of subjective data in a nursing assessment?
1. Laboratory study results
2. Physical assessment data
3. Report of a diagnostic procedure
4. Client's feelings and statements about health problems

35. Which classification of medication may be used safely for a pregnant client with cardiovascular disease?
1. Antibiotics
2. Warfarin (Coumadin)
3. Cardiac glycosides
4. Diuretics

36. While the nurse is assisting a 350-lb client with diabetes with her personal hygiene measures, the client states, "I've heard the charge nurse and others joking about me. I know you're from a registry, but you've helped me so much. Could you be my nurse tomorrow?" Which response by the nurse would be most appropriate?
1. "I can't promise that, but I'll make sure those nurses know how you feel."
2. "I'll check with the charge nurse."
3. "I'll make sure the other nurses don't talk about you anymore."
4. "I'm going to report your concerns to my supervisor, and if I return I'll come see how you are"

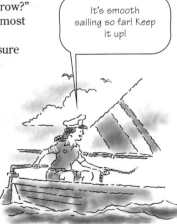

It's smooth sailing so far! Keep it up!

33. 2. Fetal heart tones show how the fetus is responding to the environment. Assessing other signs and symptoms of the mother, including laboratory test results and urinalysis, can only determine the effect on the mother, not the fetus.
CN: Health promotion and maintenance; CNS: None; CL: Application

34. 4. Subjective data, also known as *symptoms* or *covert cues,* include the client's own verbatim statements about health problems. Laboratory study results, physical assessment data, and diagnostic procedure reports are observable, perceptible, and measurable and can be verified and validated by others.
CN: Safe, effective care environment; CNS: Coordinated care; CL: Comprehension

35. 3. Cardiac glycosides and common antiarrhythmics such as procainamide hydrochloride (Procanbid) and quinidine may be used. Prophylactic antibiotics are reserved for clients susceptible to endocarditis. If anticoagulants are needed, heparin is the drug of choice—not warfarin. Diuretics should be used with extreme caution, if at all, because of the potential for causing uterine contractions.
CN: Physiological integrity; CNS: Pharmacological therapies; CL: Comprehension

36. 4. Option 4 acknowledges the client's feelings and indicates care and concern. It's best to go through the proper chain of command and inform the nursing supervisor of this situation. Telling the client that she'll make sure the others know how the client feels only increases the client's embarrassment. Checking with the charge nurse is incorrect because there's no assurance that, as a registry nurse, the nurse will return to this agency. The nurse can't guarantee the other nurses won't talk about the client.
CN: Safe, effective care environment; CNS: Coordinated care; CL: Analysis

CN: Client needs category CNS: Client needs subcategory CL: Cognitive level

37. After assessing vital signs and applying an external monitor, which intervention is a priority for a client with suspected placenta previa?
   1. Inserting an indwelling urinary catheter
   2. Planning for an immediate cesarean delivery
   3. Placing the client in Trendelenburg's position
   4. Starting I.V. catheters and obtaining blood work

38. A pregnant client with vaginal bleeding asks a nurse how the fetus is doing. Which response is best?
   1. "I don't know for sure."
   2. "I can't answer that question."
   3. "It's too early to tell anything."
   4. "I'll tell you what the monitors show."

39. A client with placenta previa is hospitalized, and a cesarean delivery is planned. In addition to the routine neonatal assessment, the neonate should be assessed for which condition?
   1. Prematurity
   2. Congenital anomalies
   3. Respiratory distress
   4. Aspiration pneumonia

40. The nursing staff is developing a care plan for a client who's receiving palliative care for end-stage leukemia. The client is experiencing breakthrough pain, which she rates as a 5 on a pain scale of 1 to 10. Which action by the nurse should be included in the client's care plan?
   1. Meeting with the pain management team to devise a better pain control plan
   2. Explaining that pain relief may not be possible because she's receiving maximum doses of pain medications
   3. Assessing whether the client is abusing the pain medications
   4. Providing nonpharmacologic pain measures only, because maximum doses of pain medications are ineffective

37. 4. Blood for hemoglobin analysis, hematocrit, type, and crossmatch should be collected and I.V. catheters inserted. Depending on the degree of bleeding and fetal maturity, a cesarean delivery may be required. The nurse shouldn't attempt Trendelenburg's positioning or urinary catheterization. The client may be placed on her left side.
CN: Physiological integrity; CNS: Reduction of risk potential; CL: Application

38. 4. The client deserves a truthful answer and the nurse should be objective without giving opinions. Vague answers may be misleading and aren't therapeutic.
CN: Psychosocial integrity; CNS: None; CL: Analysis

39. 3. Hypoxia, resulting in respiratory distress, is a potential risk due to decreased blood volume and prematurity. The age of maturity can be determined through established maternal dates. Congenital anomalies aren't necessarily associated with placenta previa. Aspiration pneumonia isn't considered a threat unless the amniotic fluid is meconium-stained.
CN: Physiological integrity; CNS: Reduction of risk potential; CL: Application

40. 1. Patient comfort is top priority in palliative care. The nurse should meet with the pain management team to devise a plan to control the client's pain. Typically, doses are increased above the normal maximum doses to meet the client's needs. Clients who require opioids long term develop drug tolerance so it's necessary to increase dosages. There's no need to assess the client for drug abuse. The nursing staff should also incorporate nonpharmacologic measures to relieve pain into the client's care plan; but they shouldn't be the only measures used to control pain.
CN: Physiological integrity; CNS: Basic care and comfort; CL: Application

CN: Client needs category   CNS: Client needs subcategory   CL: Cognitive level

41. A nurse working in the triage area of an emergency department sees that several pediatric clients arrive simultaneously. Which client is treated first?

1. A crying 4-year-old child with a laceration on his scalp
2. A 3-year-old child with a barking cough and flushed appearance
3. A 3-year-old child with Down syndrome who's pale and asleep in his mother's arms
4. A 2-month-old infant with stridorous breath sounds, sitting up in his mother's arms and drooling

41. 4. The 2-month-old infant with the airway emergency should be treated first because of the risk of epiglottiditis. The 3-year-old with the barking cough and fever should be suspected of having croup and should be seen promptly, as should the child with the laceration. The nurse would need to gather information about the child with Down syndrome to determine the priority of care.

CN: Safe, effective care environment; CNS: Coordinated care; CL: Analysis

42. A 2-year-old child is being examined in the emergency department for epiglottiditis. Which assessment finding supports this diagnosis?

1. Mild fever
2. Clear speech
3. Tripod position
4. Gradual onset of symptoms

42. 3. The tripod position (sitting up and leaning forward) facilitates breathing. Epiglottiditis presents with a sudden onset of symptoms, high fever, and muffled speech. Additional symptoms are inspiratory stridor and drooling.

CN: Physiological integrity; CNS: Physiological adaptation; CL: Application

43. Which method is best when approaching a 2-year-old child to listen to breath sounds?

1. Tell the child it's time to listen to his lungs now.
2. Tell the child to lie down while the nurse listens to his lungs.
3. Ask the caregiver to wait outside while the nurse listens to his lungs.
4. Ask the child if he would like the nurse to listen to the front or the back of his chest first.

43. 4. The 2-year-old child needs to feel in control, and this approach best supports the child's independence. Giving the child no choice may make him uncooperative. The child should be allowed to remain in the tripod position to facilitate breathing. The caregiver should be allowed to remain with the child because fear of separation is common in 2-year-olds.

CN: Health promotion and maintenance; CNS: None; CL: Application

44. A mother says a 2-year-old child is up to date with his vaccines. Which immunization should be included?

1. Diphtheria-tetanus-pertussis (DTaP), inactivated poliovirus (IPV), measles-mumps-rubella (MMR), and pneumococcal vaccine (PCV)
2. DTaP, IPV, MMR, hepatitis B, *Haemophilus influenzae* type b (Hib), varicella, PCV, rotavirus (Rota), and influenza
3. DTaP, hepatitis B, and IPV
4. MMR, IPV, hepatitis B, and varicella

Way to go! You're more than halfway finished!

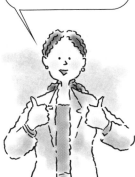

44. 2. By the age of 2, the DTaP, IPV, MMR, hepatitis B, Hib, varicella, PCV, Rota, and influenza vaccines should have been received. The nurse should clarify this with the mother or caregiver.

CN: Safe, effective care environment; CNS: Safety and infection control; CL: Application

CN: Client needs category   CNS: Client needs subcategory   CL: Cognitive level

45. A child with epiglottiditis is at risk for which condition?
1. Airway obstruction
2. Dehydration
3. Malnutrition
4. Seizures

45. 1. The biggest threat to the child is airway obstruction because of the inflammation and swelling of the epiglottis and surrounding tissue. Dehydration can be prevented with I.V. therapy and seizures averted by decreasing the fever. Malnutrition is least likely to occur because epiglottiditis is a short-lived situation.
CN: Physiological integrity; CNS: Reduction of risk potential; CL: Comprehension

46. A pregnant client being seen in the clinic is complaining of increasing leg cramps. Which response by the nurse is most appropriate?
1. "Have you asked the doctor to prescribe a muscle relaxant for the cramps?"
2. "Sometimes gently stretching the legs helps relieve leg cramps."
3. "Relax! Everyone who's pregnant has leg cramps."
4. "Don't worry about them. They go away after you deliver."

46. 2. Leg cramps are a common discomfort of pregnancy. Gentle stretching may be effective in relieving the cramps. Typically, muscle relaxants aren't used for leg cramps associated with pregnancy. Telling the client to relax or not to worry, or that everyone has them or that they go away after delivery ignores the client's concern and minimizes the client's feelings.
CN: Physiological integrity; CNS: Basic care and comfort; CL: Analysis

47. A nurse is assessing a child with epiglottiditis. Which action by the nurse is appropriate?
1. Obtaining a flashlight and tongue blade
2. Obtaining a sterile tongue blade and culturette swab
3. Asking the registered nurse to visualize the child's throat
4. Waiting for visualization to be done by the anesthesiologist

47. 4. Direct visualization of the epiglottis can trigger a complete airway obstruction and should only be done in a controlled environment by an anesthesiologist or a physician skilled in pediatric intubation.
CN: Physiological integrity; CNS: Basic care and comfort; CL: Analysis

48. The mother of a 2-year-old child with epiglottiditis says she needs to pick up her older child from school. The 2-year-old child begins to cry and appears more stridorous. Which intervention by the nurse is best?
1. Asking the mother how long she may be gone
2. Telling the 2-year-old everything will be all right
3. Telling the 2-year-old the nurse will stay with him
4. Asking the mother if someone else can meet the older child

48. 4. Increased anxiety and agitation should be avoided in the child to prevent airway obstruction. A 2-year-old child fears separation from parents, so the mother should be encouraged to stay. Other means of picking up the older child need to be found. The mother is the primary caregiver and important to the child for emotional and security reasons. Asking the mother how long she'll be gone doesn't emphasize that she shouldn't leave. A 2-year-old can't understand that all will be okay. Telling the 2-year-old that the nurse will stay with him won't comfort the child as much as the mother being there.
CN: Health promotion and maintenance; CNS: None; CL: Analysis

CN: Client needs category   CNS: Client needs subcategory   CL: Cognitive level

49. A father arrives in a busy emergency department and is upset with his wife for bringing their 2-year-old child with epiglottiditis in for treatment. Which intervention by the nurse is best?
1. Leaving the room
2. Calling for security
3. Recognizing the father's behavior as his attempt to cope with the situation
4. Telling both parents to leave because they're upsetting the child

50. A 40-year-old client is being treated for GI bleeding. On his fifth day of hospitalization, he begins to have tremors, is agitated, and is experiencing hallucinations. These signs suggest which condition?
1. Alcohol withdrawal
2. Allergic response
3. Alzheimer's disease
4. Hypoxia

51. If a nurse suspects a client is experiencing alcohol withdrawal syndrome, which action is appropriate?
1. Verify it with family.
2. Inform social services.
3. Ask the client about his drinking.
4. Tell the client everything will be all right.

52. A client experiencing alcohol withdrawal syndrome says he sees cockroaches on the ceiling. Which response is appropriate?
1. Ask the client where he sees them.
2. Ask the client if the cockroaches are still there.
3. Tell the client there are no cockroaches on the ceiling.
4. Tell the client it's dim in the room and turn on the overhead lights.

49. 3. Lack of control over his child's situation results in irrational behavior. The nurse should try to calm both parents and let them know they did the right thing due to the seriousness of their child's situation. Leaving the room, calling for security, or sending the parents out won't help the child, nor will it reduce frustration or inappropriate behavior.
CN: Psychosocial integrity; CNS: None; CL: Analysis

50. 1. These are signs of alcohol withdrawal syndrome, which can occur 5 to 10 hours after the last drink or even 7 to 10 days later. An allergic reaction would cause difficulty breathing, skin rash, or edema as primary symptoms. Alzheimer's disease occurs in older individuals and has other psychosocial signs, such as a masklike face and altered mentation. Hypoxia would cause symptoms of respiratory distress.
CN: Psychosocial integrity; CNS: None; CL: Analysis

51. 3. Confirming suspicions with the client is the most beneficial way to help in diagnosis and treatment. If the client isn't cooperative, verification can be sought with the family. Social services aren't required at this time but may be helpful in discharge planning. Giving false reassurance isn't therapeutic for the client.
CN: Psychosocial integrity; CNS: None; CL: Application

52. 4. Try to reorient the client to reality and minimize distortions. Don't support the client's hallucinations or place the client on the defensive. Try to present reality gently without agitating the client.
CN: Psychosocial integrity; CNS: None; CL: Application

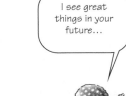

I see great things in your future...

CN: Client needs category   CNS: Client needs subcategory   CL: Cognitive level

53. A client experiencing alcohol withdrawal syndrome says he's itching everywhere from the bugs on his bed. Which response is appropriate?
  1. Examine the client's skin.
  2. Ask what kind of bugs he thinks they are.
  3. Tell the client there are no bugs on his bed.
  4. Tell the client he's having tactile hallucinations.

53. 1. Make sure the client doesn't have a rash, skin allergy, or something on his skin (such as food crumbs) causing his discomfort. Reality should then be presented to the client gently without being derogatory. The nurse shouldn't support the client's hallucinations.
CN: Psychosocial integrity; CNS: None; CL: Application

54. A client with alcohol withdrawal syndrome is pulling at his central venous catheter saying he's swatting the spiders crawling over him. Which intervention is appropriate?
  1. Encouraging the client to rest
  2. Protecting the client from harm
  3. Telling the client there are no spiders
  4. Telling the client he's pulling the I.V. tubing

54. 2. During periods of alcohol withdrawal, the nurse must take necessary measures to protect the client from harming himself, including preventing the dislodgment of his central venous catheter, which can cause a life-threatening embolus. Although encouraging the client to rest and presenting reality are important, the client may not heed the nurse's attempts to calm and reassure him in this situation.
CN: Psychosocial integrity; CNS: None; CL: Analysis

55. A client who experienced alcohol withdrawal syndrome is no longer having hallucinations or tremors and says he would like to enter a rehabilitation facility to stop drinking. Which intervention is appropriate?
  1. Asking about his insurance
  2. Telling him he should talk with his family
  3. Referring him to Alcoholics Anonymous (AA)
  4. Promoting participation in a treatment program

55. 4. The client should be encouraged to enter a facility if that's in his best interest. Arrangements can be made and discussed with the social service coordinator and his physician as well as having social services discuss insurance concerns. The client can inform his family, and support should be encouraged. Referral to AA should be considered after rehabilitation takes place.
CN: Psychosocial integrity; CNS: None; CL: Application

56. A 72-year-old male client with cirrhosis is admitted to the hospital in a hepatic coma. Which assessment would be the nurse's priority?
  1. Performing a neurologic check
  2. Completing the client admission
  3. Orienting the client to his environment
  4. Checking airway, breathing, and circulation

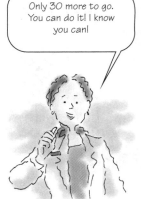

Only 30 more to go. You can do it! I know you can!

56. 4. Priorities include checking the client's airway, breathing, and circulation. After these are ensured, a neurologic check is needed to determine status. General orientation and completing the admission may require the help and affirmation of family members. The ability of the nurse to orient the client depends on his level of consciousness..
CN: Physiological integrity; CNS: Reduction of risk potential; CL: Application

CN: Client needs category   CNS: Client needs subcategory   CL: Cognitive level

57. A client with cirrhosis is restless and at times tries to climb out of bed. Which intervention is best to promote safety?
1. Leather restraints
2. Soft wrist restraints
3. Vest restraint device
4. Sheet tied across the client's chest

57. 3. The client may require gentle reminders not to get out of bed to prevent a fall. The vest restraint would help in this endeavor. Leather restraints are only warranted for extremely combative and unsafe clients. Soft wrist restraints may not stop the client from sitting up or trying to swing his legs over the bed rails. A sheet tied across the client's chest can hamper breathing or may asphyxiate the client if he slides down in the bed.
CN: Safe, effective care environment; CNS: Coordinated care; CL: Analysis

58. The nurse knows that which of the following condition is consistent with a late stage of cirrhosis?
1. Constipation
2. Diarrhea
3. Hypoxia
4. Vomiting

58. 3. In the later stage of cirrhosis, fluid in the lungs and weak chest expansion can lead to hypoxia. Constipation, diarrhea, and vomiting are early signs and symptoms of cirrhosis.
CN: Physiological integrity; CNS: Physiological adaptation; CL: Analysis

59. A client with cirrhosis is jaundiced and edematous. He's experiencing severe itching and dryness. Which intervention is best to help the client?
1. Putting mitts on his hands
2. Using alcohol-free body lotion
3. Lubricating the skin with baby oil
4. Washing the skin with soap and water

59. 2. Alcohol-free body lotion applied to the skin can help relieve dryness and is absorbed without oiliness. Mitts may help keep the client from scratching his skin open. Baby oil doesn't allow excretions through the skin and may block pores. Soap dries out the skin.
CN: Physiological integrity; CNS: Basic care and comfort; CL: Application

60. A 20-year-old client with a spinal cord injury sustained in a previous motorcycle accident is hospitalized for renal calculi. To reduce the client's risk for developing recurrent renal calculi, which instruction is correct?
1. Eat yogurt daily.
2. Drink cranberry juice.
3. Eat more fresh fruits and vegetables.
4. Increase the intake of dairy products.

60. 2. Acid urine decreases the potential for renal calculi. Most renal calculi form in alkaline urine. Cranberries, prunes, and plums promote acidic urine. Yogurt helps restore pH balance to secretions in yeast infections. Fruits and vegetables increase fiber in the diet and promote alkaline urine. Dairy products may contribute to the formation of renal calculi.
CN: Physiological integrity; CNS: Reduction of risk potential; CL: Application

61. A client with a spinal cord injury says he has difficulty recognizing the symptoms of urinary tract infection (UTI) before it's too late. Which symptom is an early sign of UTI?
1. Lower back pain
2. Burning on urination
3. Frequency of urination
4. Fever and change in the clarity of urine

61. 4. The client with a spinal cord injury should recognize fever and change in the clarity of urine as early signs of UTI. Lower back pain is a late sign. The client with a spinal cord injury may not have burning or frequency of urination.
CN: Physiological integrity; CNS: Reduction of risk potential; CL: Application

CN: Client needs category   CNS: Client needs subcategory   CL: Cognitive level

62. A client tells a nurse he boils his urinary catheters to keep them sterile. Which question should the nurse ask?
1. "What technique do you use for sterilization?"
2. "What temperature are the catheters boiled at?"
3. "Why aren't prepackaged sterile catheters used?"
4. "Are the catheters dried and stored in a clean, dry place?"

63. A 60-year-old client had a colostomy 4 days ago due to rectal cancer and is having trouble adjusting to it. Which condition is most common?
1. Anxiety
2. Low self-esteem
3. Alteration in comfort
4. Alteration in body image

64. A nurse approaches a client who recently had a colostomy and finds him crying. Which action is appropriate?
1. Stating she'll come back another time
2. Asking the client if he's having pain or discomfort
3. Telling the client she needs to take his vital signs
4. Sitting down with the client and asking if he'd like to talk about anything

65. After a review of colostomy care, a client says she doesn't know if she can care for herself at home without help. Which nursing intervention is most appropriate?
1. Reviewing care with the client again
2. Providing written instructions for the client
3. Asking the client if there's anyone who can help
4. Arranging for home health care to visit the client

66. A client is experiencing mild diarrhea through his colostomy. Which instruction is correct?
1. Eat prunes.
2. Drink apple juice.
3. Increase lettuce intake.
4. Increase intake of bananas.

62. 1. The client should describe his procedure to make sure sterile technique is used. Water boils at 212° F (100° C), but the nurse should make sure the client is boiling the catheters for an appropriate amount of time. Catheters should be boiled just before use and allowed to cool before using. Prepackaged sterile catheters aren't necessary if the proper sterilization techniques are used.
CN: Physiological integrity; CNS: Reduction of risk potential; CL: Analysis

63. 4. Alteration in body image is most common with a new colostomy and dealing with its care. The client shouldn't have signs of anxiety, but he may not be comfortable caring for the colostomy. Low self-esteem may also be a concern for the client. The client should be having less discomfort postoperatively.
CN: Psychosocial integrity; CNS: None; CL: Comprehension

64. 4. Asking open-ended questions and appearing interested in what the client has to say will encourage verbalization of feelings. Leaving the client may make him feel unaccepted. Asking closed-ended questions won't encourage verbalization of feelings. Ignoring the client's present state isn't therapeutic for the client.
CN: Psychosocial integrity; CNS: None; CL: Application

65. 4. Home health care should be contacted to ensure continuity of appropriate care. Follow a detailed teaching plan to educate the client before discharge. Because of the complexity of care, family members can help if possible and should be present for teaching.
CN: Safe, effective care environment; CNS: Coordinated care; CL: Application

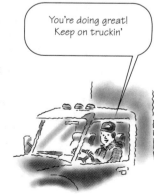

You're doing great! Keep on truckin'

66. 4. Bananas help make formed stool and aren't irritating to the bowel. Apple juice and prunes can increase the frequency of diarrhea. Lettuce acts as a fiber and can increase the looseness of stool.
CN: Physiological integrity; CNS: Basic care and comfort; CL: Application

CN: Client needs category CNS: Client needs subcategory CL: Cognitive level

67. A client reports a lot of gas in her colostomy bag. Which instruction is best?
1. Burp the bag.
2. Eat fewer beans.
3. Replace the bag.
4. Put a tiny hole in the top of the bag.

67. 1. Letting air out of the bag by opening it and burping it is the best solution. The client can be encouraged to note which foods are causing gas and to eat fewer gas-forming foods. Replacing the bag is costly. Putting a hole in the bag will cause fluids to leak out.
CN: Physiological integrity; CNS: Basic care and comfort; CL: Knowledge

68. A postpartum client recovering from spinal anesthesia with morphine complains that her nose itches. The nurse would suspect which of the following?
1. The client may be having a reaction to a material she encountered in the delivery room.
2. Postpartum itching is common after delivery because of hormonal changes.
3. The client may be still be partially sedated and imagining this feeling.
4. The client is experiencing a common effect due to a morphine-based anesthetic.

68. 4. Morphine has a relatively high incidence of itching when used in spinal anesthesia. The itching usually begins at the tip of the nose, possibly becoming more generalized. Antipruritics, such as diphenhydramine (Benadryl) or hydroxyzine (Atarax), may be prescribed after the use of morphine. Itching on the tip of the nose isn't typical of an allergic reaction nor is it caused by postpartum hormonal changes. The client is awake and speaking appropriately, so it's incorrect to assume that she isn't alert.
CN: Physiological integrity; CNS: Pharmacological therapies; CL: Analysis

69. A client recently diagnosed with pre-diabetes asks the nurse about the risk factors for developing diabetes mellitus. The nurse identifies which of the following factors as the client's greatest risk for developing diabetes mellitus?
1. Obesity
2. Japanese descent
3. A great-grandparent with diabetes mellitus
4. Delivery of a neonate weighing more than 10 lb

69. 1. Obesity is the risk factor that puts the client at greatest risk for developing diabetes mellitus. Other leading risk factors include delivery of a neonate weighing more than 9 lb, a family history of diabetes mellitus (specifically a mother, father, or sibling), and Native American, Black, Asian, or Hispanic descent.
CN: Health promotion and maintenance; CNS: None; CL: Analysis

70. A 52-year-old client had gastric bypass surgery, is on nothing-by-mouth (NPO) status, and is in pain. The nurse gives meperidine (Demerol) 75 mg I.M. as ordered. In 20 minutes, he's feeling nauseous. What would the nurse suspect as the most likely cause?
1. The surgery is causing his nausea.
2. Because he's NPO, the increase in gastric secretions is precipitating this symptom.
3. Meperidine, which was given for his pain, has a tendency to cause nausea.
4. He may be reacting to blood still remaining in his mouth after extubation.

70. 3. Although gastric bypass surgery may precipitate some feelings of nausea, the timing of this symptom after the administration of meperidine is suspicious. Most likely, this client is experiencing a very common adverse effect of the analgesic meperidine. The status of being NPO wouldn't cause an increase in gastric secretions. It's possible that there may be some blood in his mouth after extubation, but the chances of this happening are minimal and less likely to be the cause of the client's complaint.
CN: Physiological integrity; CNS: Pharmacological therapies; CL: Analysis

71. A physician's order reads: Amoxicillin (Amoxil) 500 mg capsules x 2 P.O. now, followed by 500 mg P.O. every 6 hours. How many grams of amoxicillin would the nurse administer as the initial dose?
1. 0.5
2. 1
3. 1.5
4. 2

71. 2. The order states you are giving two 500 mg capsules now. This would give you a total of 1000 mg or 1 gram followed by 500 mg or 0.5 grams every 6 hours. Therefore the correct answer is 2.
CN: Physiological integrity; CNS: Pharmacological therapies; CL: Analysis

72. A client with a family history of diabetes asks the nurse what measures he can practice to decrease his chances of developing the disease. Which of the following would be the nurse's best response?
1. "Eat only poultry and fish."
2. "Omit carbohydrates from your diet."
3. "Start a moderate exercise program."
4. "Check blood glucose levels every month."

72. 3. Exercise and weight control are the goals in preventing and treating diabetes mellitus. Red meat can be eaten but should be limited because it contributes to cardiovascular disease. Complex carbohydrates, especially whole grains, are necessary for a healthy diet. Fiber intake of 14 g/1,000 kcal is recommended. Checking blood glucose levels will help monitor the development of diabetes mellitus but won't prevent or decrease the chance of it occurring.
CN: Physiological integrity; CNS: Reduction of risk potential; CL: Application

73. An 83-year-old client fractured a hip after a fall in her home. Because of her extensive cardiac history and chronic obstructive pulmonary disease, surgery isn't an option. The client tells a nurse she doesn't know how she's going to get better. Which response is best?
1. "You're doing fine."
2. "What's your biggest concern right now?"
3. "Just give it some time and you'll be okay."
4. "You don't believe you're doing well?"

73. 2. Open-ended questions allow the client to have control over what she wants to discuss and help the nurse determine care needs. Telling the client she's doing fine or that she just needs more time doesn't encourage her to verbalize concerns. A reiteration of the client's concerns may not be helpful in encouraging the client to verbalize feelings.
CN: Health promotion and maintenance; CNS: None; CL: Comprehension

74. A client says she slipped on a throw rug while going to the bathroom at night. Which factor needs assessment?
1. If the home is safe
2. If the client is confused
3. If the client hit her head
4. If the client has a urinary tract infection (UTI)

74. 1. A safety assessment of the home can determine if changes need to be made to ensure the client doesn't fall again. The nurse may determine if the client has experienced a head injury or confusion by asking how the accident occurred. Going to the bathroom at night isn't necessarily a sign of a UTI.
CN: Safe, effective care environment; CNS: Safety and infection control; CL: Application

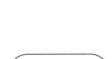

You're entering the home stretch!

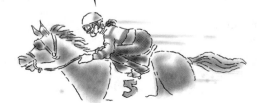

CN: Client needs category   CNS: Client needs subcategory   CL: Cognitive level

75. A client in her third trimester of pregnancy is having contractions 5 minutes apart that began suddenly. The nurse identifies that it's the client's seventh month. She's admitted directly to the obstetric department. Which intervention has priority?
1. Calling the obstetrician
2. Timing the contractions
3. Checking fetal heart tones
4. Calling the client's husband

76. The nurse is monitoring the following clients' vitals signs. Which client's vital signs would be the priority to report to the physician?
1. A healthy male client who is undergoing elective surgery with a blood pressure of 120/72 mm Hg
2. A postoperative client with a pulse of 110 beats/minute on awakening in the morning
3. A healthy female client undergoing elective surgery with a blood pressure of 110/68 mm Hg
4. A client with a pulse of 120 beats/minute after 30 minutes of aerobic exercise in physical therapy

77. A nurse is collecting data on a 40-year-old client undergoing elective facial surgery and notes that he has a pulse rate of 130 beats/minute with a regular rhythm. Which of the following factors would be the most likely explanation for the tachycardia?
1. Age
2. Anxiety
3. Exercise
4. Pain

78. A client on a psychiatric unit asks a nurse about the medications another client takes. Which response is best?
1. "How close are the two of you?"
2. "I can't give you that information, I must protect her privacy."
3. "Let me ask her if it's OK for me to tell you about her condition and medications."
4. "The client is taking insulin for her diabetes and digoxin for her heart condition."

75. 3. The nurse should check fetal heart tones and assess the client's vital signs. The client should be placed on a monitor to check contractions and for continuous fetal monitoring. The obstetrician and husband should be notified as soon as possible.
CN: Health promotion and maintenance; CNS: None; CL: Application

76. 2. The normal range for a pulse is 60 to 100 beats/minute and, in the morning, the rate is at its lowest. Blood pressures of 120/72 mm Hg for a healthy man and 110/68 mm Hg for a healthy woman are normal. Aerobic exercise increases the heart rate over the normal range of 60 to 100 beats/minute.
CN: Physiological integrity; CNS: Physiological adaptation; CL: Analysis

77. 2. Anxiety tends to increase heart rate, temperature, and respirations. The normal heart rate for a client this age is 60 to 100 beats/minute. Exercise will increase the heart rate but most likely won't occur preoperatively. The client shouldn't be in any pain preoperatively.
CN: Physiological integrity; CNS: Physiological adaptation; CL: Application

78. 2. Revealing one client's medication to another client is violating procedures of client confidentiality and directly violates the Health Insurance Portability and Accountability Act. Seeking the client's permission to release confidential information is an inappropriate action. Asking the client the nature of his relationship to the other client won't help the client understand the purpose of protecting confidentiality. Assuring the client that the facility has an obligation to protect not only his confidentiality but that of others will provide the client with a sense of comfort.
CN: Psychosocial integrity; CNS: None; CL: Application

CN: Client needs category   CNS: Client needs subcategory   CL: Cognitive level

79. The vital signs of a 56-year-old client are: temperature, 98.6° F (37° C) orally; pulse, 80 beats/minute; and respirations, 30 breaths/minute. Which interpretation of these values is correct?
1. Pulse is above normal range.
2. Temperature is above normal range.
3. Respirations are above normal range.
4. Respirations and pulse are above normal range.

80. The nurse is monitoring a client's pulse notes that it's easily palpable at 84 beats/minute and regular. Which term would the nurse use in charting the pulse assessment?
1. Arrhythmia
2. Bradycardia
3. Regular
4. Tachycardia

81. Which action is correct for performing tracheal suctioning?
1. Apply suction during insertion of the catheter.
2. Limit suctioning to 10 to 15 seconds' duration.
3. Resterilize the suction catheter in alcohol after use.
4. Repeat suctioning intervals every 15 minutes until clear.

82. Which position is optimal for a client having a nasogastric tube inserted?
1. Fowler's
2. Prone
3. Side-lying
4. Supine

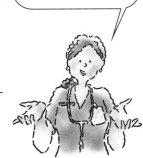

Five more to go! Now it wasn't that bad, was it?

79. 3. Normal vital signs for an adult client are: temperature, 96.6° to 99° F (35.9° to 37.2° C); pulse, 60 to 100 beats/minute; respirations, 16 to 20 breaths/minute.
CN: Health promotion and maintenance; CNS: None; CL: Application

80. 3. The pulse is regular when it's rhythmic, easily palpable, and between the rate of 60 and 100 beats/minute. Tachycardia is a heart rate faster than 100 beats/minute. Arrhythmia is a heart rate with either irregular rate or rhythm. Bradycardia is a heart rate slower than 60 beats/minute.
CN: Health promotion and maintenance; CNS: None; CL: Application

81. 2. The length of time a client should be able to tolerate the suction procedure is 10 to 15 seconds. Any longer may cause hypoxia. Suctioning during insertion can cause trauma to the mucosa and removes oxygen from the respiratory tract. Suction catheters are disposed of after each use and are cleaned in normal saline solution after each pass. Suctioning intervals with supplemental oxygen between suctions is performed after at least 1-minute intervals to allow the client to rest.
CN: Physiological integrity; CNS: Physiological adaptation; CL: Application

82. 1. The upright position is more natural for swallowing and protects against aspiration. Positioning on the client's back, stomach, or side places the client at risk for aspiration if he should gag. It's also difficult to swallow in these positions.
CN: Physiological integrity; CNS: Basic care and comfort; CL: Comprehension

CN: Client needs category   CNS: Client needs subcategory   CL: Cognitive level

83. The nurse is completing the intake and output record for a client who was restarted on his regular diet after being on nothing-by-mouth status for laboratory studies. It reads: Intake: 4 oz of cranberry juice, ½ cup of oatmeal, 2 slices of toast, 8 oz of black decaffeinated coffee, tuna fish sandwich, ½ cup of fruit-flavored gelatin, 1 cup of cream of mushroom soup, 6 oz. of 1% milk, 16 oz of water.
Output: 1,300 ml of urine
How many milliliters should the nurse document as the client's intake? Record the answer using a whole number.

_____ ml.

84. The nurse is collecting data on a newly admitted client. When filling out the family assessment, who would the nurse consider to be a part of the client's family? Select all that apply:
1. People related by blood or marriage
2. All the people whom the client views as family
3. People who live in the same house
4. People who the nurse thinks are important to the client
5. People who live in the same house with the same racial background as the client
6. People who provide for the physical and emotional needs of the client

85. When caring for a client who sustained a chemical burn in his right eye, the nurse is preparing to irrigate the eye with sterile normal saline solution. Which steps are appropriate when performing the procedure? Select all that apply:
1. Tilt the client's head toward his left eye.
2. Place absorbent pads in the area of the client's shoulder.
3. Wash hands and put on gloves.
4. Place the irrigation syringe directly on the cornea.
5. Direct the solution onto the exposed conjunctival sac from the inner to outer canthus.
6. Irrigate the eye for 1 minute.

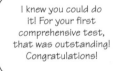

I knew you could do it! For your first comprehensive test, that was outstanding! Congratulations!

83. 1,380. There are 30 ml in each ounce and 240 ml in each cup. The fluid intake for this client includes 4 oz (120 ml) of cranberry juice, 8 oz (240 ml) of coffee, ½ cup (120 ml) of fruit-flavored gelatin, 1 cup (240 ml) of cream of mushroom soup, 6 oz (180 ml) of milk, and 16 oz (480 ml) of water, for a total of 1,380.
CN: Physiological integrity; CNS: Basic care and comfort; CL: Application

84. 2, 6. When providing care to a client, the nurse should consider family members to be all the people whom the client views as family. Family members may also include those people who provide for the physical and emotional needs of the client. The traditional definition of a family has changed and may include people not related by blood or marriage, those of a different racial background, and those who may not live in the same house as the client. Family members are defined by the client, not by the nurse.
CN: Health promotion and maintenance; CNS: None; CL: Analysis

85. 2, 3, 5. The nurse should place absorbent pads on the client's shoulder area to prevent saturating the client's clothing and bed linens. She should also wash her hands and put on gloves to reduce the transmission of microorganisms. The solution should be directed from the inner to outer canthus of the eye to prevent contamination of the unaffected eye. The head should be tilted toward the affected (right) eye to facilitate drainage and to prevent irrigating solution from entering the left eye. The irrigation syringe should be held about 1 inch (2.5 cm) above the eye to prevent injury to the cornea. In a chemical exposure, the eye should be irrigated for at least 10 minutes.
CN: Physiological integrity; CNS: Reduction of risk potential; CL: Application

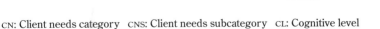

CN: Client needs category   CNS: Client needs subcategory   CL: Cognitive level

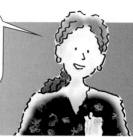

Here's another comprehensive test to help you get ready to take the NCLEX exam. Good luck!

COMPREHENSIVE
Test 2

1. A newly hired LPN is helping the charge nurse admit a client. The charge nurse asks the LPN if she understands the facility's rules of ethical conduct. Which statement by the LPN indicates the need for further teaching?
   1. "I make sure that I do everything in my client's best interest."
   2. "I maintain client confidentiality always."
   3. "I'll support the Client's Bill of Rights."
   4. "I don't discuss advance directives unless the client initiates the conversation."

2. Which diagnostic test is performed first to detect transposition of the great vessels (TGV)?
   1. Blood cultures
   2. Cardiac catheterization
   3. Chest X-ray
   4. Echocardiogram

3. Four 6-month-old children arrive at the clinic for diphtheria-pertussis-tetanus (DPT) immunization. Which child can safely receive the immunization at this time?
   1. The child with a temperature of 103° F (39.4° C)
   2. The child with a runny nose and cough
   3. The child taking prednisone for the treatment of leukemia
   4. The child with difficulty breathing after the last immunization

4. A nurse is giving discharge instructions to the parents of a child who had a tonsillectomy. Which instruction is the most important?
   1. The child should drink extra milk.
   2. The child shouldn't drink from straws.
   3. Orange juice should be given to provide pain control.
   4. Rinse the mouth with salt water to provide pain relief.

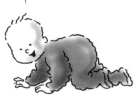

You're going to do great on this test.

1. 4. The law mandates that health care agencies ask all clients if they have an advance directive. Therefore, the nurse must address this question regardless of whether the client initiates a conversation about it. Nurses need to always act in the best interest of their clients, maintain confidentiality, and support the Client's Bill of Rights.
CN: Safe, effective care environment; CNS: Coordinated care; CL: Analysis

2. 3. Chest X-ray would be done first to visualize congenital heart diseases such as TGV. Blood cultures won't diagnose TGV. Cardiac catheterization and an echocardiogram would be done after TGV is seen on the chest X-ray.
CN: Health promotion and maintenance; CNS: None; CL: Application

3. 2. Children with cold symptoms can safely receive DPT immunization. Children with a temperature more than 102° F (38.9° C), serious reactions to previous immunizations, or those receiving immunosuppressive therapy shouldn't receive DPT immunization.
CN: Health promotion and maintenance; CNS: None; CL: Analysis

4. 2. Straws and other sharp objects inserted into the mouth could disrupt the clot at the operative site. Extra milk wouldn't promote healing and may encourage mucus production. Although drinking orange juice and rinsing with salt water will irritate the tissue at the operative site, irritation doesn't pose the same level of danger as clot disruption.
CN: Physiological adaptation; CNS: Basic care and comfort; CL: Application

CN: Client needs category   CNS: Client needs subcategory   CL: Cognitive level

5. A 2-year-old child is diagnosed with bronchiolitis caused by respiratory syncytial virus (RSV). The client has an 8-year-old sibling. Which statement is correct?
1. RSV isn't highly communicable in infants.
2. RSV isn't communicable to older children and adults.
3. The 2-year-old client must be admitted to the hospital for isolation.
4. The children should be separated to prevent the spread of the infection.

6. A child with asthma uses a peak expiratory flowmeter in school. The results indicate his peak flow is in the yellow zone. Which intervention by the school nurse is appropriate?
1. Following the child's routine asthma treatment plan
2. Monitoring for signs and symptoms of an acute attack and reviewing the child's treatment plan
3. Calling 911 and preparing for transport to the nearest emergency department
4. Calling the child's mother to take the child to the family physician immediately

7. Parents of a child with asthma are trying to identify possible allergens in their household. Which inhaled allergen is the most common?
1. Perfume
2. Dust mites
3. Passive smoke
4. Dog or cat dander

8. A nurse is verifying orders from a physician. Which diet is correct for a child newly diagnosed with celiac disease?
1. Low-fat diet
2. No-gluten diet
3. High-protein diet
4. No-phenylalanine diet

5. 4. RSV is communicable among children and adults, so the children should be separated to prevent the spread of the infection. Older children and adults may have mild symptoms of the disorder. Hospitalization is indicated only for children who need oxygen and I.V. therapy.
CN: Safe, effective care environment; CNS: Safety and infection control; CL: Analysis

6. 2. The routine treatment plan may be insufficient when the peak flow is in the yellow zone (50% to 80% of personal best). The child should be monitored to determine if an asthma attack is imminent and his treatment plan should be reviewed to see if revisions are needed. There's no immediate need to see the physician if the child is asymptomatic. This isn't an emergency situation.
CN: Safe, effective care environment; CNS: Coordinated care; CL: Application

7. 2. The household dust mite is the most commonly inhaled allergen that can cause an asthma attack. Perfume, passive smoke, and animal dander are allergens that can cause asthma attacks but aren't as common as dust mites.
CN: Physiological integrity; CNS: Reduction of risk potential; CL: Application

8. 2. The intestinal cells of individuals with celiac disease become inflamed when the child eats products containing gluten, such as wheat, rye, barley, or oats. The child with celiac disease needs normal amounts of fat and protein in the diet for growth and development. Omitting phenylalanine products would be appropriate for the client with phenylketonuria.
CN: Physiological integrity; CNS: Reduction of risk potential; CL: Application

CN: Client needs category   CNS: Client needs subcategory   CL: Cognitive level

9. A client is undergoing a bedside thoracentesis. The nurse assists the client to an upright position with a table and pillow in front of him supporting his arms. Which of the following is the correct rationale for using this position?
1. Fluid will accumulate at the base of the lung.
2. There's less chance to injure lung tissue.
3. It allows for better expansion of the lung.
4. It's less painful for the client in this position.

10. Which leisure activity would the nurse include in the care plan for a school-age child with hemophilia?
1. Baseball
2. Cross-country running
3. Football
4. Swimming

11. Which finding is important for an infant in sickle cell crisis?
1. The infant has no bruises.
2. The infant has normal skin turgor.
3. The infant participates in exercise.
4. The infant maintains bladder control.

12. A nurse is caring for a dyspneic client who has a resting respiratory rate of 44 breaths/minute and dusky nail beds. Arterial blood gases are obtained and the results are as follows: pH, 7.52; PaO_2, 50 mm Hg; $PaCO_2$, 28 mm Hg; HCO_3^-, 24 mEq/L. The nurse knows these results are consistent with which condition?
1. Metabolic acidosis
2. Metabolic alkalosis
3. Respiratory acidosis
4. Respiratory alkalosis

13. A client with chronic alcohol abuse is admitted to the hospital for detoxification. Later that day, his blood pressure increases and he's given lorazepam (Ativan) to prevent which complication?
1. Stroke
2. Seizure
3. Fainting
4. Anxiety reaction

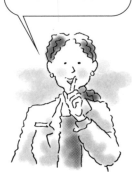

Don't tell anybody, but you're doing great!

9. 1. Fluids will drain and collect in the dependent positions. There's a risk of pneumothorax regardless of the client's position. The position doesn't allow for better expansion of the lung because the fluid in the pleural space is preventing this. This procedure is done using local anesthesia, so it isn't painful.
CN: Physiological integrity; CNS: Physiological adaptation; CL: Analysis

10. 4. Swimming is a noncontact sport with low risk of traumatic injury. Baseball, cross-country running, and football all involve a risk of trauma from falling, sliding, or contact.
CN: Physiological integrity; CNS: Physiological adaptation; CL: Application

11. 2. Normal skin turgor indicates the infant isn't severely dehydrated. Dehydration may cause sickle cell crisis or worsen a crisis. Bruising isn't associated with sickle cell crisis. Bed rest is preferable during a sickle cell crisis. Bladder control may be lost when oral or I.V. fluid intake is increased during a sickle cell crisis.
CN: Physiological integrity; CNS: Physiological adaptation; CL: Analysis

12. 4. A pH greater than 7.45 and a partial pressure of arterial carbon dioxide ($PaCO_2$) less than 35 mm Hg indicate respiratory alkalosis. A pH less than 7.35 and a bicarbonate (HCO_3^-) less than 22 mEq/L indicate metabolic acidosis. A pH greater than 7.45 and an HCO_3^- greater than 24 mEq/L indicate metabolic alkalosis. A pH less than 7.35 and a $PaCO_2$ greater than 45 mm Hg indicate respiratory acidosis.
CN: Physiological integrity; CNS: Physiological adaptation; CL: Application

13. 2. During detoxification from alcohol, changes in the client's physiologic status, especially an increase in blood pressure, may indicate an increased risk for seizure. Clients are treated with benzodiazepines to prevent this occurrence. Stroke, fainting, and anxiety aren't the primary concerns when withdrawing from alcohol.
CN: Physiological integrity; CNS: Pharmacological therapies; CL: Application

CN: Client needs category   CNS: Client needs subcategory   CL: Cognitive level

14. An adolescent client ingests a large number of acetaminophen tablets in an attempt to commit suicide. Which of the following laboratory results are most consistent with an acetaminophen overdose?
1. Metabolic acidosis
2. Elevated liver enzyme levels
3. Increased serum creatinine level
4. Increased white blood cell (WBC) count

15. A nurse is caring for a client recently diagnosed with acute pancreatitis. Which statement indicates that a short-term goal of nursing care has been met?
1. The client denies abdominal pain.
2. The client doesn't complain of thirst.
3. The client denies pain at McBurney's point.
4. The client swallows liquids without coughing.

16. A physician prescribes acetaminophen gr X (10 grains) as necessary every 4 hours for pain for a client in a long-term care facility. How many milligrams of acetaminophen should the nurse give?
1. 10 mg
2. 325 mg
3. 650 mg
4. 1,000 mg

17. A man stepped on a piece of sharp glass while walking barefoot. He comes to the emergency department with a deep laceration on the bottom of his foot. Which question is the most important for the nurse to ask?
1. "Was the glass dirty?"
2. "Are you immune to tetanus?"
3. "When did you have your last tetanus shot?"
4. "How many diphtheria-pertussis-tetanus (DPT) shots did you receive as a child?"

14. 2. Elevated liver enzyme levels, which could indicate liver damage, are associated with acetaminophen overdose. Metabolic acidosis isn't associated with acetaminophen overdose. An increased serum creatinine level may indicate renal damage. An increased WBC count indicates infection.
CN: Physiological integrity; CNS: Pharmacological therapies; CL: Application

15. 1. Pancreatitis is accompanied by acute pain from autodigestion by pancreatic enzymes. When the client denies abdominal pain, the short-term goal of pain control is met. Clients with acute pancreatitis receive I.V. fluids and may not have a sensation of thirst. Pain at McBurney's point accompanies appendicitis. Clients with acute pancreatitis receive nothing by mouth during initial therapy.
CN: Physiological integrity; CNS: Physiological adaptation; CL: Application

16. 3. The nurse should give 650 mg. Use the following equation:
One grain = 65 mg;
$10 \times 65 = 650$ mg.
CN: Physiological integrity; CNS: Pharmacological therapies; CL: Application

17. 3. Questioning the client about the date of his last tetanus immunization is important because the booster immunization should be received every 10 years in adulthood or at the time of the injury if the last booster immunization was given more than 5 years before the injury. Whether the client noticed dirt on the glass is immaterial because all deep lacerations require a tetanus immunization or booster. A client wouldn't know his tetanus immune status. DPT immunizations in childhood don't give lifelong immunization to tetanus.
CN: Safe, effective care environment; CNS: Safety and infection control; CL: Application

CN: Client needs category   CNS: Client needs subcategory   CL: Cognitive level

18. A postmenopausal client asks a nurse how to prevent osteoporosis. Which response is best?
1. "Take a multivitamin daily."
2. "After menopause, there's no way to prevent osteoporosis."
3. "Drink two glasses of milk each day and swim three times per week."
4. "Do weight-bearing exercises regularly."

18. 4. Weight-bearing exercises are recommended for the prevention of osteoporosis. Telling the patient that there's no way to prevent osteoporosis would be an incorrect statement. A multivitamin doesn't provide adequate calcium for a postmenopausal woman, and calcium alone won't prevent osteoporosis. Two glasses of milk per day don't provide the daily requirements for adult women, and swimming isn't a weight-bearing exercise.
CN: Health promotion and maintenance; CNS: None; CL: Application

19. A client diagnosed with cardiomyopathy saw a posting on the Internet describing research about a new herbal treatment for the disorder. When the client asks about this research, which response is most appropriate?
1. "Herbs are commonly used to treat cardiomyopathy."
2. "Cardiomyopathy can be treated only by heart surgery."
3. "The Internet is a reliable source of research, so try this treatment."
4. "Research found on the Internet should be verified with a physician."

19. 4. Although the Internet contains some valid medical research, there's no control over the validity of information posted. The research should be discussed with a physician, who can verify the accuracy of the information. Herbs aren't standard treatment for cardiomyopathy. Cardiomyopathy is treatable with drugs or surgery.
CN: Safe, effective care environment; CNS: Coordinated care; CL: Application

20. A young adult client received her first chemotherapy treatment for breast cancer. Which statement by the client requires further exploration by the nurse?
1. "I'm thinking about joining a dance club."
2. "I don't think I'm going to work tomorrow."
3. "I don't care about the adverse effects of the drugs."
4. "I want to return to school for a college degree."

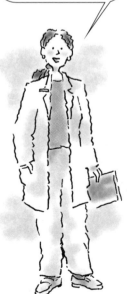

You've finished 20 questions already? Super!

20. 3. Adverse effects of chemotherapy may occur after treatment and should be discussed with the client because some can be treated, controlled, or prevented. The nurse needs to explore what the client means by this statement. The client may feel poorly after chemotherapy and may want to take time off from work until feeling better. Joining social clubs and returning to school is typical behavior for a young adult.
CN: Health promotion and maintenance; CNS: None; CL: Analysis

21. A client with long-standing rheumatoid arthritis has frequent complaints of joint pain. The nurse's care plan is based on the understanding that chronic pain is most effectively relieved when analgesics are administered in which way?
1. Conservatively
2. I.M.
3. On an as-needed basis
4. At regularly scheduled intervals

21. 4. To control chronic pain and prevent cycled pain, regularly scheduled intervals are most effective. As-needed and conservative methods aren't effective means to manage chronic pain because the pain isn't relieved regularly. I.M. administration isn't practical on a long-term basis.
CN: Physiological integrity; CNS: Pharmacological therapies; CL: Application

CN: Client needs category   CNS: Client needs subcategory   CL: Cognitive level

22. Which nursing intervention is appropriate for an adult client with chronic renal failure?

1. Weighing the client daily before breakfast
2. Offering foods high in calcium and phosphorus
3. Serving the client large meals and a bedtime snack
4. Encouraging the client to drink large amounts of fluids

23. A client with a recent history of a stroke has been discharged from the rehabilitation facility with a walker. On a return visit to the physician's office, the nurse assesses his gait. Which observation indicates the need for further client teaching about walker use?

1. The client moves his weak leg forward with the walker.
2. The client moves his hands to the chair armrests before lowering himself into the chair.
3. The client's arms are fully extended when using the walker.
4. The client backs up to the chair until his legs touch the chair, then sits down.

24. Which finding indicates an increased risk of skin cancer?

1. A deep sunburn
2. A dark mole on the client's back
3. An irregular scar on the client's abdomen
4. White irregular patches on the client's arm

25. Which behavior is consistent with the diagnosis of conduct disorder in a child?

1. Enuresis
2. Suicidal ideation
3. Cruelty to animals
4. Fear of going to school

22. 1. Daily weights are obtained to monitor fluid retention. Calcium intake is encouraged, but clients with chronic renal failure have difficulty excreting phosphorus. Therefore, phosphorus must be restricted. To improve food intake, meals and snacks should be given in small portions. Fluids should be restricted for the client with chronic renal failure.

CN: Physiological integrity; CNS: Physiological adaptation; CL: Application

23. 3. When using a walker, the client's arms should be slightly bent at the elbow, allowing maximum support from the arms while ambulating. The weak leg is always moved forward first with the walker to provide the maximum support. The client should use the armrests of the chair for support, because the armrests are more stable than the walker. When sitting, the client should always back up to the chair and feel the chair with his legs before sitting.

CN: Physiological integrity; CNS: Basic care and comfort; CL: Analysis

24. 1. A deep sunburn is a risk factor for skin cancer. A dark mole or an irregular scar are benign findings. White irregular patches are abnormal but aren't a risk factor for skin cancer.

CN: Health promotion and maintenance; CNS: None; CL: Application

25. 3. Cruelty to animals is a symptom of conduct disorder. Enuresis and suicidal ideation aren't usually associated with conduct disorder. Fear of going to school is school phobia.

CN: Psychosocial integrity; CNS: None; CL: Application

CN: Client needs category   CNS: Client needs subcategory   CL: Cognitive level

26. A client has been admitted to the hospital with signs of dehydration. Which intervention would be most effective in increasing the client's oral fluid intake?
  1. Explaining the need for increased fluid intake
  2. Placing his choice of beverages at the bedside
  3. Serving small amounts of fluids at frequent intervals
  4. Serving fluids in large amounts at mealtimes

27. Which outcome is appropriate for a client with a diagnosis of depression and attempted suicide?
  1. The client will never feel suicidal again.
  2. The client will find a group home to live in.
  3. The client will remain hospitalized for at least 6 months.
  4. The client will verbalize an absence of suicidal ideation, plan, and intent.

28. The nurse is reviewing the proper technique in obtaining a urine specimen from an indwelling urinary catheter. When collecting the urine, which would be the most appropriate technique to use?
  1. Collect urine from the drainage collection bag.
  2. Disconnect the catheter from the drainage tubing to collect urine.
  3. Remove the indwelling catheter and insert a sterile straight catheter to collect urine.
  4. Insert a sterile needle with syringe through a tubing drainage port cleaned with alcohol to collect the specimen.

26. 3. Fluids should be served in small amounts spread out at frequent intervals. Teaching the client about the need for fluid increase and including the client in the selection of beverages will aid in compliance. It's overwhelming for the client to have large amounts of fluids to drink.
CN: Physiological integrity; CNS: Basic care and comfort; CL: Application

27. 4. An appropriate outcome is that the client will verbalize that he no longer feels suicidal. It's unrealistic to ask that he'll never feel suicidal. There's no reason for a group home or 6 months of hospitalization.
CN: Psychosocial integrity; CNS: None; CL: Application

28. 4. Wearing clean gloves, cleaning the port with alcohol, and then obtaining the specimen with a sterile needle ensures the specimen and the closed urinary drainage system won't be contaminated. A urine specimen must be new urine, and the urine in the bag could be several hours old and growing bacteria. The urinary drainage system must be kept closed to prevent microorganisms from entering. A straight catheter is used to relieve urine retention, obtain sterile urine specimens, measure the amount of postvoid residual urine, and empty the bladder for certain procedures. It isn't necessary to remove an indwelling catheter to obtain a sterile urine specimen unless the physician requests that the whole system be changed.
CN: Safe, effective care environment; CNS: Safety and infection control; CL: Application

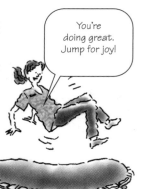

You're doing great. Jump for joy!

CN: Client needs category   CNS: Client needs subcategory   CL: Cognitive level

29. A registered nurse (RN) is supervising a licensed practical nurse (LPN). The LPN is caring for a client diagnosed with a terminal illness. Which statement by the LPN should be corrected by the RN?

1. "Some clients write a living will indicating their end-of-life preferences."
2. "The law says you have to write a new living will each time you go to the hospital."
3. "You could designate another person to make end-of-life decisions when you can't make them yourself."
4. "Some people choose to tell their physician they don't want to have cardiopulmonary resuscitation."

30. An elderly client's husband tells the nurse he's concerned because his wife insists on talking about events that happened to her years ago. The nurse finds the client alert, oriented, and answering questions appropriately. Which statement made to the husband is correct?

1. "Your wife is reviewing her life."
2. "A spiritual advisor should be notified."
3. "Your wife should be discouraged from talking about the past."
4. "Your wife is regressing to a more comfortable time in the past."

31. A client with a new colostomy asks the nurse how to avoid leakage from the ostomy bag. Which instruction is correct?

1. Limit fluid intake.
2. Eat more fruits and vegetables.
3. Empty the bag when it's about half full.
4. Tape the end of the bag to the surrounding skin.

32. A nurse must obtain the blood pressure of a client on airborne precautions. Which method is best to prevent transmission of infection to other clients by the equipment?

1. Dispose of the equipment after each use.
2. Wear gloves while handling the equipment.
3. Use the equipment only with other clients in airborne isolation.
4. Leave the equipment in the room for use only with that client.

29. 2. One living will is sufficient for all hospitalizations unless the client wishes to make changes. The "No Code" or "Do Not Resuscitate" status is discussed with the physician, who then enters this in the client's chart. A living will explains a person's end-of-life preferences. A durable power of attorney for health care can be written to designate who will make health care decisions for the client in the event the client can't make decisions for himself.
CN: Safe, effective care environment; CNS: Coordinated care; CL: Analysis

30. 1. Life review or reminiscing is characteristic of elderly people and the dying. A spiritual advisor might comfort the client but isn't necessary for a life review. Discouraging the client from talking would block communication. Regression occurs when a client returns to behaviors typical of another developmental stage.
CN: Health promotion and maintenance; CNS: None; CL: Application

31. 3. Emptying the bag when partially full will prevent the bag from becoming heavy and detaching from the skin or skin barrier. Limiting fluids may cause constipation but won't prevent leakage. Increasing fruits and vegetables in the diet will help prevent constipation, not leakage. Taping the bag to the skin will secure the bag to the skin but won't prevent detachment.
CN: Physiological integrity; CNS: Basic care and comfort; CL: Application

32. 4. Leaving equipment in the room is appropriate to avoid organism transmission by inanimate objects. Disposing of equipment after each use prevents the transmission of organisms but isn't cost-effective. Wearing gloves protects the nurse, not other clients. Using equipment for other clients spreads infectious organisms among clients.
CN: Safe, effective care environment; CNS: Safety and infection control; CL: Application

CN: Client needs category　CNS: Client needs subcategory　CL: Cognitive level

33. To prevent circulatory impairment in an arm when applying an elastic bandage, which method is best?
1. Wrap the bandage around the arm loosely.
2. Stretch the bandage slightly while wrapping toward the heart.
3. Apply heavy pressure with each turn of the bandage.
4. Start applying the bandage at the upper arm and work toward the lower arm.

34. A client needs to use an incentive spirometer after abdominal surgery. Which statement about incentive spirometry is correct?
1. It's a substitute for early postoperative ambulation.
2. It's better than deep breathing to prevent atelectasis.
3. It causes less discomfort for the client than deep breathing.
4. It helps the client visualize deep breathing to prevent atelectasis.

35. A client complains of an inability to sleep while on the medical unit. Which intervention to promote sleep has priority?
1. Offering a sedative routinely at bedtime
2. Giving the client a backrub before bedtime
3. Questioning the client about his sleeping habits
4. Moving the client to a bed farthest from the nurses' station

36. To test the function of the optic nerve, which tool is used?
1. Finger, to test the cardinal fields
2. Flashlight, to test corneal reflexes
3. Snellen chart, to test visual acuity
4. Piece of cotton, to test corneal reflexes

37. A client is to be placed in the prone position. The nurse would place the client:
1. sitting upright.
2. lying on the side.
3. lying on the back.
4. lying on the abdomen.

33. 2. Stretching the bandage slightly maintains uniform tension on the bandage. Wrapping toward the heart promotes venous return to the heart. Wrapping the bandage loosely wouldn't secure the bandage on the arm. Using heavy pressure would cause circulatory impairment. Beginning the wrapping at the upper arm would cause uneven application of the bandage. For example, elastic stockings are applied distal to proximal to promote venous return.
CN: Physiological integrity; CNS: Reduction of risk potential; CL: Application

34. 4. Incentive spirometry helps the client see inspiratory effort using floating balls, lights, or bellows. Early ambulation is still indicated for this postoperative client. Incentive spirometry is no more effective than deep breathing without equipment. Deep breathing and incentive spirometry cause equal discomfort during inspiration.
CN: Physiological integrity; CNS: Reduction of risk potential; CL: Comprehension

35. 3. Interviewing the client about sleeping habits may give more information about the causes of the inability to sleep. Sedatives should be given as a last option. A backrub may promote sleep but may not address this client's problem. Moving the client may not address the client's specific problem.
CN: Physiological integrity; CNS: Basic care and comfort; CL: Application

36. 3. The Snellen chart is used to test the function of the optic nerve. Testing the cardinal fields assesses the oculomotor, trochlear, and abducens nerves. Corneal light reflex indicates the function of the oculomotor nerve. Corneal sensitivity is controlled by the trigeminal and facial nerves.
CN: Physiological integrity; CNS: Basic care and comfort; CL: Comprehension

37. 4. Prone position is lying on the abdomen. Sitting upright is known as *Fowler's* or *high-Fowler's* position. Side lying is also known as the *lateral position.* Lying on the back is the supine position.
CN: Safe, effective care environment; CNS: Coordinated care; CL: Comprehension

CN: Client needs category   CNS: Client needs subcategory   CL: Cognitive level

38. Which intervention is best to prevent bladder infections for a client with an indwelling urinary catheter?
1. Limiting fluid intake
2. Encouraging showers rather than tub baths
3. Opening the drainage system to obtain a urine specimen
4. Irrigating the catheter twice daily with sterile saline solution

38. 2. A shower would prevent bacteria in the bath water from sustaining contact with the urinary meatus and the catheter, whereas a tub bath may allow easier transit of bacteria into the urinary tract. Increased—not limited—fluid intake is recommended for a client with an indwelling urinary catheter. Opening the drainage system would provide a pathway for the entry of bacteria. Catheter irrigation is performed only with an order from the physician to keep the catheter patent.
CN: Physiological integrity; CNS: Reduction of risk potential; CL: Comprehension

39. A nurse wants to use a waist restraint for a client who wanders at night. Which factor or intervention should be considered before applying the restraint?
1. The nurse's convenience
2. The client's reason for getting out of bed
3. A sleeping medication ordered as needed at bedtime
4. The lack of nursing assistants on the night shift

39. 2. The nurse should question the client's reason for getting out of bed because the client may be looking for a bathroom. Lack of adequate staffing and convenience aren't reasons for applying restraints. Sleeping medications are chemical restraints that should be used only if the client can't go to sleep and stay asleep.
CN: Safe, effective care environment; CNS: Safety and infection control; CL: Application

Give yourself a pat on the back. You're doing great!

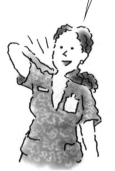

40. Six months after the death of her infant son, a client is diagnosed with dysfunctional grieving. Which behavior would the nurse expect to find?
1. She goes to the infant's grave weekly.
2. She cries when talking about the loss.
3. She's overactive without a sense of loss.
4. She states the infant will always be part of the family.

40. 3. One of the signs of dysfunctional grieving is overactivity without a sense of loss. Going to the grave, tears, and including the infant as a part of the family are all normal responses.
CN: Psychosocial integrity; CNS: None; CL: Comprehension

41. A nurse notices a client has been crying. Which response is the most therapeutic?
1. None; this is a private matter.
2. "You seem sad. Would you like to talk?"
3. "Why are you crying and upsetting yourself?"
4. "It's hard being in the hospital, but you must keep your chin up."

41. 2. Therapeutic communication is a primary tool of nursing. The nurse must recognize the client's nonverbal behaviors indicate a need to talk. Asking "why" might be interpreted as an accusation. Ignoring the client's nonverbal cues or giving opinions and advice are barriers to communication.
CN: Psychosocial integrity; CNS: None; CL: Application

CN: Client needs category   CNS: Client needs subcategory   CL: Cognitive level

42. A nurse gives the wrong medication to a client. Another nurse employed by the hospital as a risk manager will expect to receive which communication?

1. Incident report
2. Oral report from the nurse
3. Copy of the medication Kardex
4. Order change signed by the physician

42. 1. Incident reports are tools used by risk managers when a client might be harmed. They're used to determine how future problems can be avoided. An oral report won't serve as legal documentation. A copy of the medication Kardex wouldn't be sent with the incident report to the risk manager. A physician won't change an order to cover the nurse's mistake.

CN: Safe, effective care environment; CNS: Coordinated care; CL: Application

43. Performing a procedure on a client in the absence of informed consent can lead to which charge?

1. Fraud
2. Harassment
3. Assault and battery
4. Breach of confidentiality

43. 3. Performing a procedure on a client without informed consent can be grounds for charges of assault and battery. Fraud is to cheat, and harassment means to annoy or disturb. Breach of confidentiality refers to conveying information about the client.

CN: Safe, effective care environment; CNS: Coordinated care; CL: Comprehension

44. A surgical client newly diagnosed with cancer tells a nurse she knows the laboratory made a mistake about her diagnosis. Which term describes this reaction?

1. Denial
2. Intellectualization
3. Regression
4. Repression

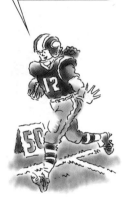

You've crossed the 50-yard line and you're headed for a touchdown!

44. 1. Cancer clients commonly deny this diagnosis when first made. Such a response may benefit the client in that it allows energy for surgical healing. Intellectualization describes speaking of the disease as if reading a textbook. Repression describes not remembering being diagnosed. Regression describes childlike behavior.

CN: Psychosocial integrity; CNS: None; CL: Comprehension

45. A client who's single and lives alone delivers a premature neonate. Which intervention would be included in her treatment plan?

1. An early postpartum physician visit
2. Referral to the health department
3. Request for a social service visit in the hospital
4. Request for a home health visit the day after discharge

45. 3. Because of the client's potential need for support and the premature condition of the neonate, a social service visit is appropriate. The social service visit will determine if there's a need for a referral to the health department. The mother has no physical indications for an early postpartum visit or need for an early home visit.

CN: Safe, effective care environment; CNS: Coordinated care; CL: Analysis

46. A nurse is reviewing principles of good body mechanics with a student practical nurse. Which of the following techniques should she emphasize?

1. Bending from the waist
2. Pulling rather than pushing
3. Stretching to reach an object
4. Using large muscles in the legs for leverage

46. 4. Keeping one's back straight and using the large muscles in the legs will help avoid back injury, as the muscles in one's back are relatively small compared with the larger muscles of the thighs. Bending from the waist can cause stress on the back muscles, causing a potential injury. Pulling isn't the best option and may cause straining. When feasible, one should push an object rather than pull it. Stretching to reach an object increases the risk of injury.

CN: Safe, effective care environment; CNS: Safety and infection control; CL: Application

CN: Client needs category   CNS: Client needs subcategory   CL: Cognitive level

47. A 6-year-old child needs diabetic teaching. Which factor is considered when the nurse plans the teaching?
1. Another child with diabetes can teach the client.
2. The child can teach his parents after the nurse teaches him.
3. The child and parents should be recipients of teaching.
4. Teaching should be directed to the parents, who then can teach the child.

48. A client who just gave birth is concerned about her neonate's Apgar scores of 7 and 8. She says she's been told scores lower than 9 are associated with learning difficulties in later life. Which response is best?
1. "You shouldn't worry so much, your infant is perfectly fine."
2. "You should ask about placing the infant in a follow-up diagnostic program."
3. "You're right in being concerned, but there are good special education programs available."
4. "Apgar scores are used to indicate a need for resuscitation at birth. Scores of 7 and above indicate no problem."

49. After delivering a neonate with a cleft palate and cleft lip, a client has minimal contact with her neonate. She asks the nurse to do most of the neonate's care. Which nursing diagnosis is appropriate?
1. *Anxiety related to fear of harming the neonate*
2. *Deficient knowledge related to neonate's health status*
3. *Risk for impaired parenting related to birth defect*
4. *Ineffective coping related to birth defect*

47. 3. The parents and child should participate in the nurse's teaching to ensure an understanding of teaching and that the child has adult caregivers who are knowledgeable. Another school-age child shouldn't be entrusted to teach this child, although his input would be valuable. The school-age child shouldn't be the sole provider of teaching to the parents. Parents should be included in the teaching plan but shouldn't be responsible for the teaching.
CN: Health promotion and maintenance; CNS: None; CL: Application

48. 4. Apgar scores don't indicate future learning difficulties; they're for rapid assessment of the need for resuscitation. Apgar scores of 7 and 8 are normal and don't indicate a need for intervention. It's inappropriate to simply tell a client not to worry.
CN: Health promotion and maintenance; CNS: None; CL: Application

49. 3. Neonates born with birth defects are at risk for impaired parenting. The parents must work through the issues and guilt associated with not producing a perfect child. There's nothing in the question that indicates the client felt anxious about caring for the neonate or had ineffective coping problems or knowledge deficit.
CN: Health promotion and maintenance; CNS: None; CL: Application

CN: Client needs category   CNS: Client needs subcategory   CL: Cognitive level

50. The care plan for an 89-year-old female who has had a stroke and is paraplegic indicates that the client should be turned at least every two hours. The nurse prepares to turn the client based on the understanding that:
1. turning provides needed physical and emotional stimulation.
2. immobility causes venous stasis that may lead to heart failure.
3. immobility can cause skin breakdown, pneumonia, and urinary tract infections (UTIs).
4. turning the client helps increase the client's level of comfort and safety.

51. A prenatal client says she can't believe she has such mixed feelings about being pregnant. She tried for 10 years to become pregnant and now she feels guilty for her conflicting reactions. Which response is best?
1. "You need to talk to your midwife about these feelings."
2. "You're experiencing the normal ambivalence pregnant mothers feel."
3. "These feelings are expected only in women who have had difficulty becoming pregnant."
4. "Let's make an appointment with a counselor."

52. A client with terminal cancer tells a nurse, "I've given up. I have no hope left. I'm ready to die." Which response is most therapeutic?
1. "You've given up hope?"
2. "We should talk about dying to a social worker."
3. "You should talk to your physician about your fears of dying so soon."
4. "Now, you shouldn't give up hope. There are cures for cancer found every day."

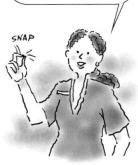

You've now finished 50 questions. The rest of the test should be a snap!

SNAP

50. 3. Immobility can lead to severe physiological problems such as skin breakdown, pressure ulcers, pneumonia, and UTIs. Therefore, frequent turning helps to minimize the effects of immobility. Immobility doesn't necessarily mean there's lack of stimuli. Although venous stasis can occur with immobility, heart failure doesn't develop as a result of venous stasis. Turning the client may improve how the client feels, but this isn't the primary rationale for this intervention.
CN: Physiological integrity; CNS: Basic care and comfort; CL: Analysis

51. 2. Conflicting, ambivalent feelings regarding pregnancy are normal for all pregnant women. These feelings don't call for counseling or other professional interventions. Ambivalence is felt by most pregnant women, not only mothers who had difficulty becoming pregnant.
CN: Psychosocial integrity; CNS: None; CL: Application

52. 1. The use of reflection invites the client to talk more about his concerns. Deferring the conversation to a social worker or physician closes the conversation. Telling the client the cure for cancer is right around the corner gives false hope.
CN: Psychosocial integrity; CNS: None; CL: Comprehension

CN: Client needs category   CNS: Client needs subcategory   CL: Cognitive level

53. Three days after discharge, a client bottle-feeding her neonate calls the postpartum floor, asking what she can do for breast engorgement. Which instruction is correct?
  1. Wear a supportive bra.
  2. Get under a warm shower and let the water flow on her breasts.
  3. Stop drinking milk because it contributes to breast engorgement.
  4. Contact the physician; she shouldn't be engorged at this late date.

54. A client complains of excessive flatulence. Which food, reported by the client as consumed regularly, may be responsible for this?
  1. Cauliflower
  2. Ice cream
  3. Meat
  4. Potatoes

55. A client is being treated for premature labor with ritodrine (Yutopar). After receiving this medication for 12 hours, her blood pressure is slightly elevated, her chest is clear, and her pulse is 120 beats/minute. She complains of a little nausea, and the fetal heart rate is 145 beats/minute. Which intervention is correct?
  1. Continue routine monitoring.
  2. Contact the physician immediately.
  3. Turn the client on her left side and give oxygen.
  4. Increase the flow rate of the I.V. and give oxygen.

56. At 6 cm of dilation, the client in labor receives a lumbar epidural for pain control. Which nursing diagnosis is possible?
  1. *Risk for injury related to rapid delivery*
  2. *Acute pain related to wearing off of anesthesia*
  3. *Hyperthermia related to effects of anesthesia*
  4. *Ineffective tissue perfusion related to effects of anesthesia*

53. 1. A supportive bra is recommended for the client bottle-feeding her neonate to reduce engorgement. A warm shower will stimulate milk production. It's normal to become engorged during the first few days after delivery; drinking milk isn't the cause. It isn't necessary to contact the physician.
CN: Physiological integrity; CNS: Basic care and comfort; CL: Application

54. 1. Cauliflower is the only food listed that commonly results in flatulence.
CN: Physiological integrity; CNS: Basic care and comfort; CL: Comprehension

55. 1. These findings are normal adverse reactions to the medication and don't call for interventions at this time except to continue routine monitoring. Contacting the physician, placing the client on her left side, changing the I.V. flow rate, and giving oxygen are all interventions for abnormal assessment findings.
CN: Physiological integrity; CNS: Pharmacological therapies; CL: Analysis

56. 4. A disadvantage of a lumbar epidural is the risk of hypotension. Epidurals are associated with a longer labor and hypothermia. There's no pain involved with the anesthesia wearing off.
CN: Physiological integrity; CNS: Basic care and comfort; CL: Application

57. When assessing a client who just gave birth, a nurse finds the following: blood pressure, 110/70 mm Hg; pulse, 60 beats/minute; respirations, 16 breaths/minute; lochia, moderate rubra; fundus, above the umbilicus to the right; and negative Homans' sign. Which intervention is correct?
1. Doing nothing; all findings are normal
2. Having the client void and recheck the fundus
3. Turning the client on her left side to decrease the blood pressure
4. Massaging the fundus to decrease lochia flow and prevent hemorrhage

58. A client with diabetes delivers a 9-lb, 6-oz neonate. The nurse should be alert for which condition in the neonate?
1. Hyperglycemia
2. Hypoglycemia
3. Hyperthermia
4. Hypothermia

59. A prenatal client, age 13, asks about getting fat while she's pregnant. A nurse tells her she needs to gain enough weight to be in the upper portions of her recommended weight due to her age to prevent which condition?
1. A premature neonate
2. A difficult delivery
3. A low-birth-weight neonate
4. Gestational hypertension

60. A nurse is preparing to bathe a client hospitalized for emphysema. Which nursing intervention is correct?
1. Removing the oxygen and proceeding with the bath
2. Increasing the flow of oxygen to 6 L/minute by nasal cannula
3. Keeping the head of the bed slightly elevated during the procedure
4. Lowering the head of the bed and rolling the client to his left side to increase oxygenation

57. 2. A fundus up and to the right indicates a full bladder. The client should empty her bladder and be rechecked. Lochia flow and blood pressure are normal. Placement of the uterus at the umbilicus and to the right isn't a normal finding.
CN: Physiological integrity; CNS: Reduction of risk potential; CL: Analysis

58. 2. Neonates of mothers with diabetes and large neonates are at risk for hypoglycemia related to increased production of insulin by the neonate in utero. Hyperglycemia, hyperthermia, and hypothermia aren't primary concerns.
CN: Physiological integrity; CNS: Reduction of risk potential; CL: Application

59. 3. Adolescent girls, especially those younger than age 15, are at higher risk for delivering low-birth-weight neonates unless they gain adequate weight during pregnancy. Gaining weight isn't associated with preventing a difficult delivery, risk of gestational hypertension, or a premature neonate.
CN: Physiological integrity; CNS: Reduction of risk potential; CL: Application

60. 3. The elasticity of the lungs is lost for clients with emphysema. Therefore, these clients can't tolerate lying flat because the abdominal organs compress the lungs. The best position is one with the head slightly elevated. Discontinuing oxygen or altering the oxygen delivery rate should never be done without an order from the physician. Increasing oxygen flow on a client with emphysema may also suppress the hypoxic drive to breathe. Positioning the client on his left side with the head of the bed flat would decrease oxygenation.
CN: Physiological integrity; CNS: Physiological adaptation; CL: Application

61. A client who's 36 weeks pregnant chokes on her food while eating at a restaurant. Which statement is correct about performing the Heimlich maneuver on a pregnant client?
  1. Chest thrusts are used when the client is pregnant.
  2. Only back thrusts are used when the client is pregnant.
  3. The Heimlich is performed the same as when not pregnant.
  4. The Heimlich maneuver can't be performed on a pregnant client.

61. 1. During pregnancy, chest thrusts are used instead of abdominal thrusts. Abdominal thrusts compress the abdomen, which would harm the fetus. Because of this, the Heimlich is adjusted for the pregnant woman. A fist is made with one hand, placing thumb side against the center of the breastbone. The fist is grabbed with the other hand and thrust inward. Avoid the lower tip of the breastbone. Back thrusts aren't done as they may result in dislodgment of the obstruction, further obstructing the airway.
CN: Physiological integrity; CNS: Reduction of risk potential; CL: Application

62. A nurse works in a mental health facility that uses a therapeutic community (milieu) approach to client care. Which statement describes the nurse's role in this facility?
  1. Primary caregiver
  2. Member of the milieu
  3. Supervision more than counseling
  4. Distinctly separate from the psychiatrist

62. 2. In a therapeutic community, everything focuses on the client's treatment. Staff and clients work together as a team or member of the milieu. The nurse wouldn't be a primary caregiver, but would work with the psychiatrist. The nurse's role could be that of supervision as well as counseling.
CN: Safe, effective care environment; CNS: Coordinated care; CL: Comprehension

63. A client with an alcohol abuse problem is being discharged from the state mental hospital. His discharge plans should include which intervention?
  1. Referral to Al-Anon
  2. Weekly urine testing for drug use
  3. Day hospital treatment for 6 months
  4. Participation in a support group like Alcoholics Anonymous (AA)

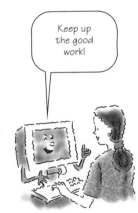

Keep up the good work!

63. 4. AA is a major support group for alcoholics after treatment. Membership in AA is associated with relapse prevention. Al-Anon is a support group for the family of the abuser of alcohol. Weekly urine testing or day hospital treatment isn't usual.
CN: Safe, effective care environment; CNS: Coordinated care; CL: Application

64. A nurse is removing an indwelling urinary catheter. Which of the following nursing actions reflects the best technique?
  1. Wear sterile gloves.
  2. Cut the lumen of the balloon.
  3. Document the time of removal.
  4. Position the client on his left side.

64. 3. The client should void within 8 hours of the removal of an indwelling urinary catheter. Documenting the time of removal allows the nurse and physician to verify the duration of elapsed time since removal, thus contributing to continuity of care. Clean, disposable gloves are required because it isn't a sterile procedure. The catheter may retrograde into the bladder, requiring surgical removal, if the balloon is cut from the lumen and the catheter isn't secured. The client should be positioned comfortably on his back, and privacy should be provided.
CN: Safe, effective care environment; CNS: Safety and infection control; CL: Application

CN: Client needs category   CNS: Client needs subcategory   CL: Cognitive level

65. A client is scheduled to retire in the next month. He phones his nurse therapist and says he can't cope; his whole world is falling apart. The therapist recognizes this reaction as which condition?
1. Panic reaction
2. Situational crisis
3. Normal separation anxiety
4. Maturational crisis

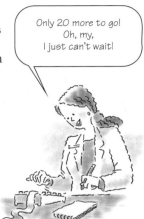

Only 20 more to go! Oh, my, I just can't wait!

66. A client with a phobic condition is being treated with behavior modification therapy. The client asks the nurse which treatment he should expect with this therapy. The nurse should tell the client to expect to receive which of the following treatments?
1. Dream analysis
2. Free association
3. Systematic desensitization
4. Electroconvulsive therapy (ECT)

67. A severely depressed client rarely leaves her chair. To prevent physiologic complications associated with psychomotor retardation, which step is appropriate?
1. Restricting coffee intake
2. Increasing calcium intake
3. Resting in bed three times per day
4. Emptying the bladder on a schedule

68. During the termination phase of a therapeutic nurse-client relationship, which intervention is most appropriate?
1. Tell the client there is no need for support groups now.
2. Address new issues with the client.
3. Review what has been accomplished during this relationship.
4. Avoid discussing the client's emotions.

69. The behavior of a client with borderline personality disorder causes a nurse to feel angry toward the client. Which response by the nurse is the most therapeutic?
1. Ignore the client's irritating behavior.
2. Restrict the client to her room until supper.
3. Report her feelings to the client's physician.
4. Tell the client how her behavior makes the nurse feel.

65. 4. A maturational (developmental) crisis is one that occurs at a predictable milestone during a life span; birth, marriage, and retirement are examples. A panic reaction would also involve physical symptoms. A situational crisis is caused by events such as an earthquake. Separation anxiety is a childhood disorder.
CN: Health promotion and maintenance; CNS: None; CL: Analysis

66. 3. Systematic desensitization is a behavior therapy used in the treatment of phobias. Dream analysis and free association are techniques used in psychoanalytic therapy. ECT is used with depression.
CN: Psychosocial integrity; CNS: None; CL: Application

67. 4. To prevent bladder infections associated with stasis of urine, the client should be encouraged to routinely empty her bladder. Neither calcium nor coffee intake are directly related to the psychological effects associated with this condition. Resting in bed is another form of psychomotor retardation.
CN: Health promotion and maintenance; CNS: None; CL: Application

68. 3. Reviewing what has been accomplished is a goal of this phase. It's appropriate to refer the client to support groups. During the termination phase, new issues shouldn't be explored. Discussing the client's emotions during this phase is appropriate.
CN: Psychosocial integrity; CNS: None; CL: Application

69. 4. A nursing intervention used with personality disorders is to help the client recognize how his behavior affects others. Ignoring the client, restricting the client, and reporting feelings to the physician aren't appropriate interventions at this time.
CN: Psychosocial integrity; CNS: None; CL: Application

CN: Client needs category   CNS: Client needs subcategory   CL: Cognitive level

70. During a manic state, a client paced around the dayroom for 3 days. He talked to the furniture, proclaimed he was a king, and refused to partake in unit activities. Which nursing diagnosis has priority?
1. *Hypertension related to hyperactivity*
2. *Risk for other-directed violence related to manic state*
3. *Imbalanced nutrition: Less than body requirements related to hyperactivity*
4. *Ineffective coping related to manic state*

71. A client with a panic disorder is having difficulty falling asleep. Which nursing intervention should be performed first?
1. Calling the client's psychotherapist
2. Teaching the client progressive relaxation
3. Allowing the client to stay up and watch television
4. Obtaining an order for a sleeping medication as needed

72. A 65-year-old client with major depression hasn't responded to antidepressants. Which intervention used to treat major depression might be added to the treatment plan?
1. Electroconvulsive therapy (ECT)
2. Electroencephalography (EEG)
3. Electromyography (EMG)
4. Tranquilizers

73. A client diagnosed with bipolar disease is receiving a maintenance dosage of lithium carbonate (Eskalith). His wife calls the community mental health nurse to report that her husband is hyperactive and hyperverbal. Which intervention is appropriate?
1. Performing a mental status examination
2. Measuring lithium blood levels
3. Evaluating him at the local emergency department
4. Admitting him to the hospital for observation

70. 3. During a manic state, clients are at risk for malnutrition due to not taking in enough calories for the energy they're expending. Hypertension isn't an approved nursing diagnosis. This client isn't showing violent behavior. Coping issues aren't the primary concern at this time.
CN: Physiological integrity; CNS: Basic care and comfort; CL: Application

71. 2. Relaxation techniques work very well with a client showing anxiety. If this doesn't work, then pharmacologic interventions, diversion activities, and contacting the psychotherapist would be in order.
CN: Psychosocial integrity; CNS: None; CL: Application

72. 1. ECT is commonly used for treatment of major depression for clients who haven't responded to antidepressants or who have medical problems that contraindicate the use of antidepressants. EEG is a tool used in the diagnosis and management of clients with anxiety, seizure disorder, sleep disorders, degenerative disorders, and others. EMG is used to assess muscles and the nerves that control them. Major tranquilizers are used to treat schizophrenia or anxiety disorders.
CN: Physiological integrity; CNS: Physiological adaptation; CL: Comprehension

73. 2. Hyperactive activity might indicate that the client's lithium levels are subtherapeutic; blood lithium levels will determine this. He doesn't need to have a mental status examination, go to the emergency department, or be admitted to the hospital at this time.
CN: Physiological integrity; CNS: Pharmacological therapies; CL: Analysis

CN: Client needs category   CNS: Client needs subcategory   CL: Cognitive level

74. After electroconvulsive therapy (ECT), which nursing intervention is correct?
1. Assessing the client's vital signs
2. Letting the client sleep undisturbed
3. Allowing the family to visit immediately
4. Restraining the client until completely awake

75. Which statement by a client who had nasal surgery indicates that the client needs further teaching about postoperative care?
1. "I'll do frequent mouth care."
2. "I'll eat two oranges per day."
3. "I'll eat two bananas per day."
4. "I'll drink at least 8 glasses of fluid per day."

76. A client recently placed on a cardiac monitor has a heart rate of 170 beats/minute, with frequent premature contractions. Which nursing action is best?
1. Call the client's physician immediately.
2. Check the client and make a full assessment.
3. Delegate one of the nursing assistants to take the client's vital signs.
4. Notify the supervisor about the change in the client's condition.

77. A client visits a physician's office and reports feelings of hopelessness, depression, poor appetite, insomnia, low self-esteem, and difficulty making decisions. The client tells the nurse that these symptoms began at least 2 years ago and have been ongoing. The nurse recognizes that the client's signs and symptoms are consistent with which disorder?
1. Major depression
2. Dysthymic disorder
3. Cyclothymic disorder
4. Atypical affective disorder

74. 1. Vital signs are monitored carefully for approximately 1 hour after ECT or until stable. The client shouldn't be restrained or left alone. Visitors should be allowed when the client is awake and ready.
CN: Physiological integrity; CNS: Reduction of risk potential; CL: Application

75. 3. After nasal surgery, the client shouldn't strain or bear down as this will increase the risk for bleeding. Bananas can cause severe constipation, which could lead to straining. The other interventions would be appropriate postoperative care for this client.
CN: Physiological integrity; CNS: Reduction of risk potential; CL: Comprehension

76. 2. Because a change has occurred in the client's status, the nurse must assess the client first. This shouldn't be delegated to unlicensed personnel. Before the physician or supervisor is notified, a full assessment must be made.
CN: Health promotion and maintenance; CNS: None; CL: Application

77. 2. Dysthymic disorder is marked by feelings of depression lasting at least 2 years, accompanied by at least two of the following symptoms: sleep disturbance, appetite disturbance, low energy or fatigue, low self-esteem, poor concentration, difficulty making decisions, and hopelessness. Major depression is a recurring, persistent sadness or loss of interest or pleasure in almost all activities, with signs and symptoms recurring for at least 2 weeks. Cyclothymic disorder is a chronic mood disturbance of at least 2 years' duration marked by numerous periods of depression and hypomania. Manic signs and symptoms characterize atypical affective disorder.
CN: Psychosocial integrity; CNS: None; CL: Analysis

78. Which technique is correct for postoperative coughing and deep-breathing exercises?
1. Splint the incision and cough.
2. Splint the incision, take a deep breath, and then cough.
3. Lie prone, splint the incision, take a deep breath, and then cough.
4. Lie supine, splint the incision, take a deep breath, and then cough.

78. 2. Splinting the incision with a pillow will protect the incision while the client coughs. Taking a deep breath will help open the alveoli, which promotes oxygen exchange and prevents atelectasis. Coughing and deep-breathing exercises are best accomplished in a sitting or semi-sitting position. Expectoration of secretions will be facilitated in a sitting position, as will splinting and taking deep breaths.
CN: Physiological integrity; CNS: Reduction of risk potential; CL: Application

79. The physician's order reads: 2 grams of cephalexin (Keflex) P.O. daily in equally divided doses of 500 mg each. The nurse would administer this medication at which frequency?
1. 3 times per day
2. 4 times per day
3. 6 times per day
4. 8 times per day

79. 2. 2 grams is equivalent to 2,000 mg. To give equally divided doses of 500 mg, divide the desired dose of 500 mg into the total daily dose of 2,000 mg. This gives an answer of 4 and is the number of times this dose of medication will be administered per day. This means you'll be giving 500 mg every 6 hours for a total of 4 times per day.
CN: Physiological integrity; CNS: Pharmacological therapies; CL: Analysis

80. A client on complete bed rest complains of excessive flatulence. Which position would be helpful to the client?
1. Fowler's
2. Knee-chest
3. Semi-Fowler's
4. Trendelenburg's

80. 2. Because gas rises, the knee-chest position facilitates the passage of flatus. Semi-Fowler's and Fowler's positions inhibit gas passage. In Trendelenburg's position the client lies flat with his head lower than his feet.
CN: Physiological integrity; CNS: Basic care and comfort; CL: Knowledge

81. A client had a laxative prescribed that acts by causing stool to absorb water and swell. Which term describes this type of laxative?
1. Bulk-forming
2. Emollient
3. Lubricant
4. Stimulant

81. 1. Bulk-forming laxatives cause stool to absorb water and swell. Emollients lubricate stool; lubricants soften stool, making it easier to pass; and stimulants promote peristalsis by irritating the intestinal mucosa or stimulating nerve endings in the intestinal wall.
CN: Physiological integrity; CNS: Pharmacological therapies; CL: Knowledge

82. A nurse encourages a client to avoid foods that have a constipating effect. Which food should the nurse recommend?
1. Wheat bread
2. Cheese
3. Eggs
4. White flour pasta

82. 1. All the foods listed except wheat bread have a constipating effect. Wheat bread contains fiber which promotes peristalsis and bowel elimination.
CN: Physiological integrity; CNS: Basic care and comfort; CL: Comprehension

83. A client is complaining of moderate pain. Which finding indicates a physiologic response to this pain?
1. Restlessness
2. Decreased pulse rate
3. Increased blood pressure
4. Protection of the painful area

84. Which symptoms reported by an adolescent's parents would suggest to the nurse that the adolescent is abusing amphetamines? Select all that apply:
1. Restlessness
2. Fatigue
3. Excessive perspiration
4. Talkativeness
5. Watery eyes
6. Excessive nasal drainage

85. The nurse suspects that a client is in cardiac arrest. According to the American Heart Association (AHA), the nurse would perform the following actions. Place the actions listed below in ascending chronological order. Use all the options.

1. Activate the emergency response system.
2. Assess responsiveness
3. Call for a defibrillator
4. Provide two slow breaths
5. Assess pulse
6. Assess breathing

83. 3. Increased blood pressure is a physiologic, or involuntary, response to moderate pain. Restlessness and protection of the painful area are behavioral responses. Decreased pulse rate occurs when pain is severe and deep.
CN: Physiological integrity; CNS: Physiological adaptation; CL: Comprehension

84. 1, 3, 4. Amphetamines are central nervous system stimulants. Symptoms of amphetamine abuse include marked nervousness, restlessness, excitability, talkativeness, and excessive perspiration.
CN: Health promotion and maintenance; CNS: None; CL: Analysis

85. Ordered response:

2. Assess responsiveness
1. Activate the emergency response system.
3. Call for a defibrillator
6. Assess breathing
4. Provide two slow breaths
5. Assess pulse

According to the AHA, the nurse should first assess responsiveness. If the client is unresponsive, she should activate the emergency response system, then call for a defibrillator. Next, she should assess breathing by opening the airway and then by looking, listening, and feeling for respirations. If respirations aren't present, she should administer two slow breaths, then assess the carotid pulse. If no pulse is present, she should start chest compressions.
CN: Physiological integrity; CNS: Physiological adaptation; CL: Application

I knew you could do it! Super job! You're well on your way to total confidence for the NCLEX.

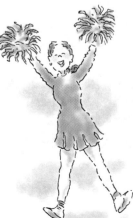

CN: Client needs category   CNS: Client needs subcategory   CL: Cognitive level

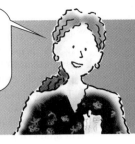

COMPREHENSIVE
Test 3

1. A client in the postoperative phase of abdominal surgery is to advance his diet as tolerated. The client has tolerated ice chips and a clear liquid diet. Which diet would the nurse anticipate giving next?
  1. Fluid restricted
  2. Full liquids
  3. House
  4. Soft

2. The following information is recorded on an intake and output record: milk, 180 ml; orange juice, 60 ml; 1 serving scrambled eggs; 1 slice toast; 1 can Ensure oral nutritional supplement, 240 ml; I.V. dextrose 5% in water at 100 ml/hour; 50 ml water after twice daily medications. Medications are given at 9 a.m. and 9 p.m. What's the client's total intake for the 7 a.m. to 3 p.m. shift?
  1. 1,000 ml
  2. 1,250 ml
  3. 1,330 ml
  4. 1,380 ml

3. A nurse is witnessing consent from a client before a cardiac catheterization. Which factor is a component of informed consent?
  1. Freedom from coercion
  2. Durable power of attorney
  3. Private insurance coverage
  4. Disclosure of previous answers given by the client

1. 2. Clear liquid diets are nutritionally inadequate but minimally irritating to the stomach. Clients are advanced to the full liquid diet next, adding bland and protein foods. A soft diet comes next, which omits foods that are hard to chew or digest. A regular, or house, diet has no limitations. A fluid restriction is ordered in addition to the diet order for clients in renal failure or heart failure.
CN: Physiological integrity; CNS: Basic care and comfort; CL: Comprehension

2. 3. The client's total intake is 1,330 ml. Use the following equation:
$$180 + 60 + 240 + 800 + 50 = 1,330 \text{ ml.}$$
CN: Physiological integrity; CNS: Basic care and comfort; CL: Analysis

3. 1. The client must give consent voluntarily without any type of outside influences from persons involved with the procedure or research. The client must also be of sound mind and not under the influence of types of medications that may interfere with reasoning. A durable power of attorney may be indicated if a client can't make decisions for himself. Private insurance coverage shouldn't be a factor in informed consent. All clients (or another appointed individual) have the right to make their own decisions regardless of type of insurance. Previous answers given by the individual shouldn't be an influencing factor in the informed consent process.
CN: Safe, effective care environment; CNS: Coordinated care; CL: Knowledge

CN: Client needs category CNS: Client needs subcategory CL: Cognitive level

4. In checking a client's chart, the nurse notes that there's no record of an opioid being given to her, even though the previous nurse signed for one. The client denies receiving anything for pain since the previous night. Which action should be taken next?

1. Notify the physician that an opioid is missing.
2. Notify the supervisor that the client didn't receive the prescribed pain medication.
3. Notify the pharmacist that the client didn't receive the prescribed pain medication.
4. Approach the nurse who signed out the opioid to seek clarification about the drug.

5. A client is seen in the emergency department with bruises on her face and back, common signs of a battered wife. Which community resource could provide assistance to the client?

1. Alcoholics Anonymous (AA)
2. Crime Task Force
3. Lifeline Emergency Aid
4. Women's shelter

6. Multidisciplinary team meetings are used frequently as a method of communication among health care disciplines. Which unit uses this method of communication?

1. Critical care units
2. Home health care services
3. Labor and delivery units
4. Outpatient surgical units

7. After maxillofacial surgery, a client, awake and alert, complains of pain, rating it as a 9 on a scale of 1 to 10. He receives meperidine (Demerol) 50 mg and hydroxyzine (Vistaril) 50 mg as ordered every 4 hours as needed. Twenty minutes after the first dose, he reports the pain as a 6; 2 hours later, it's an 8. What might the nurse suspect is occurring?

1. The hydroxyzine has interfered with the analgesic effect of the meperidine.
2. The client has been moving too much.
3. The client may need a higher dose.
4. The prescription should be changed.

4. 4. The nurse needs to seek clarification in a nonthreatening manner. If the nurse who signed out the opioid can't give a plausible explanation, the nurse who discovered the error must then notify the supervisor. The nurse who signed out the opioid may have a drug problem. The appropriate line of communication is to the hospital supervisor. The physician needs to be notified if the client didn't receive the prescribed medication. The pharmacist needs to be notified of discrepancies in the opioid count.
CN: Safe, effective care environment; CNS: Coordinated care; CL: Application

5. 4. A women's shelter can house women and children who need protection from an abusive partner or parent. AA is a support group for alcoholics and their families. The Crime Task Force and Lifeline Emergency Aid don't provide housing for women or children who want to leave an abusive relationship.
CN: Safe, effective care environment; CNS: Coordinated care; CL: Application

6. 2. Home health care services and restorative care services that use different disciplines are required by the Joint Commission on Accreditation of Healthcare Organizations or Medicare to hold multidisciplinary team meetings. This serves as a means of communicating the client's diagnosis, care plan, and discharge needs using all disciplines for input. Critical care units, outpatient surgical units, and labor and delivery units use between-shift reporting as a method of communicating.
CN: Safe, effective care environment; CNS: Coordinated care; CL: Application

7. 3. It's reasonable to assume that the dose is probably too low for the amount of pain, and it would be prudent to report the patient's response to the physician and inquire if he feels it's appropriate to increase the dose. The hydroxyzine potentiates the effects of meperidine and doesn't interfere with its effectiveness. There's no evidence to suggest that the client has been moving around too much. It's beyond the nurse's scope of practice to determine that the current medication should be changed.
CN: Physiological integrity; CNS: Pharmacological therapies; CL: Analysis

CN: Client needs category   CNS: Client needs subcategory   CL: Cognitive level

8. A client was admitted to a mental health unit for hyperexcitability, increasing agitation, and distractibility. Which nursing intervention has priority?

    1. Involving the client in a group activity

    2. Being direct and firm and setting rules for the client

    3. Using a quiet room for the client away from others

    4. Channeling the client's energy toward a planned activity

9. A client with type 2 diabetes tells the nurse in the clinic, "I keep gaining weight even though I'm not eating all that much. I can't exercise anymore because of these ulcers on my feet. I don't know what to do." Which response would be most appropriate?

    1. "Other types of exercises can be done even though you have ulcers on your feet."

    2. "Maybe you need to cut back on your eating even more."

    3. "Stop weighing yourself. You are only making it worse for yourself."

    4. "Walk anyway, even with the ulcers on your feet."

10. A public health nurse visiting a new postpartum client notices that the client has two children younger than age 4. The nurse notices one infant playing in the cabinet under the sink. Which instruction should the public health nurse give the client?

    1. Cover the infant's hands with gloves.

    2. Make sure all liquid cleaners are labeled.

    3. Tighten all cap tops on the bottles under the sink.

    4. Remove all liquid cleaners that could be ingested orally.

11. A nurse arrives at an automobile accident involving a school bus and a large truck. The school bus is lying on its side. Several people have been thrown from the windows of the school bus. Which victim needs priority care?

    1. A girl crying hysterically

    2. A boy who's unconscious

    3. A boy with a laceration of the scalp

    4. A girl with an obvious open fracture

8. 3. Being in a quiet environment away from stimuli facilitates helping the client regain a sense of control. The client can't focus on activity. If the nurse attempts to be firm and set rules for this client, it will most likely heighten the agitation. The client is too excited to focus at this time and group activities may worsen the client's situation.
CN: Psychosocial integrity; CNS: None; CL: Application

9. 1. The only appropriate response would be for the nurse to suggest other forms of exercise. Suggesting that the client change her eating pattern without consulting with the physician would be inappropriate. Instructing the client to not weigh herself is also not supportive to the care this client needs. Telling the client to ignore her foot ulcers and to walk anyway might be harmful to the healing of these ulcers.
CN: Physiological integrity; CNS: Basic care and comfort; CL: Application

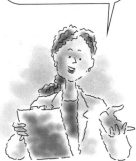

You're doing great so far! You studied hard and it shows.

10. 4. All liquid cleaners must be removed to reduce the risk of poisoning. Safety locks should be placed on cabinets to prevent young children from opening the cabinets or the bottles. Infants can't read danger labels.
CN: Safe, effective care environment; CNS: Safety and infection control; CL: Application

11. 2. An unconscious or unresponsive client always needs assistance first. The client's breathing and circulation status should be checked. When help arrives, the girl's fracture can be stabilized, pressure can be applied to the laceration of the scalp to stop the bleeding, and emotional support can be given to the girl crying hysterically.
CN: Safe, effective care environment; CNS: Safety and infection control; CL: Application

CN: Client needs category   CNS: Client needs subcategory   CL: Cognitive level

12. Which statement from a newly diagnosed client with diabetes mellitus indicates more instruction is needed?
   1. "I need to check my feet daily for sores."
   2. "I need to store my insulin in the refrigerator."
   3. "I can use my plastic insulin syringe more than once."
   4. "I need to see my physician for follow-up examinations."

12. 2. Insulin only needs to be stored in the refrigerator if it won't be used within 6 weeks after being opened; it should be at room temperature when given to decrease pain and prevent lipodystrophy. According to a poll by the Juvenile Diabetes Foundation, a high percentage of diabetics reuse their insulin syringes. However, it's recommended they be carefully recapped and placed in the refrigerator to prevent bacterial growth. The remaining statements show that the client understands his condition and the importance of preventing complications.
CN: Safe, effective care environment; CNS: Safety and infection control; CL: Analysis

13. A client with terminal cancer is receiving large doses of opioids for pain control. He becomes agitated and continues trying to get out of bed but can't stand without a two-person assistance. To reduce the risk of falling, which type of restraint is the most beneficial?
   1. Leg restraints
   2. Chemical restraints
   3. Mechanical restraints
   4. Tying him in bed with a sheet

13. 2. Chemical restraints are effective, especially with clients who are highly agitated and receiving large doses of opioids. For example, anxiety medications can be used to calm the client. Other forms of restraint will only increase the client's agitation and hostility, thus increasing the safety risk.
CN: Safe, effective care environment; CNS: Safety and infection control; CL: Application

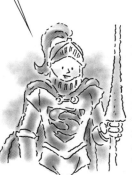

You're armed and ready. Keep up the good work!

14. A client who had a stem cell transplant is in protective isolation. Which explanation for this is correct?
   1. To protect the client from his own bacteria
   2. To protect the hospital staff from the client
   3. To protect the other clients on the nursing unit
   4. To protect the client from outside infections from others

14. 4. Immunosuppressed clients need to be protected from infections from others following stem cell transplants. Infections can occur if strict hand-washing techniques aren't observed, especially with hospital staff going from one room to the next. Protective isolation isn't used to protect the hospital staff and other clients from an infected client.
CN: Safe, effective care environment; CNS: Safety and infection control; CL: Application

15. A physician ordered a sterile dressing tray set up in a client's room to insert a subclavian central venous access device. Which step is done first to set up the sterile field?
   1. Open the tray toward the nurse.
   2. Use correct hand-washing technique.
   3. Put on sterile gloves before opening the tray.
   4. Place the sterile dressing tray on an overbed table.

15. 2. Use appropriate hand-washing technique before participating in a sterile procedure. Clean the area with an appropriate antiseptic, place the tray in the center of the clean area, and open it away from the nurse. After the dressing tray is opened, put on sterile gloves to assist the physician.
CN: Safe, effective care environment; CNS: Safety and infection control; CL: Application

CN: Client needs category   CNS: Client needs subcategory   CL: Cognitive level

16. The nurse is instructing a nursing assistant on safety precautions for biohazardous materials. Which color plastic bag is universally used for handling biohazardous waste?
1. Blue
2. Purple
3. Red
4. White

16. 3. Biohazardous waste products are placed in red biohazard bags. Blue bags are used for recycling plastics. Purple bags aren't used for biohazardous waste products. White bags are used for normal trash products.

CN: Safe, effective care environment; CNS: Safety and infection control; CL: Knowledge

17. While interviewing a young Pakistani client in her home, the public health nurse notices the client and the infant wear long skirts and coverings over their heads. The home isn't air-conditioned and the room is very warm. The nurse interprets the dress code as a component of the client's:
1. culture.
2. economic status.
3. race.
4. socialization.

17. 1. Many cultures have specific dress codes. The client's dress, as described, doesn't indicate economic status. Race refers to a group of people with similar physical characteristics such as skin color. Socialization is the process by which individuals learn the ways of a given society to function within that group.

CN: Health promotion and maintenance; CNS: None; CL: Application

18. Which action is included in the assessment step of the nursing process?
1. Identifying actual or potential health problems specific to the individual client
2. Judging the effectiveness of nursing interventions that have been implemented
3. Identifying goals and interventions specific to the individualized needs of the client
4. Systematically collecting subjective and objective data with the goal of making a clinical nursing judgment

18. 4. Assessment involves data collection, organization, and validation. Evaluation involves judging the effectiveness of nursing interventions and whether the goals of the care plan have been achieved. The nurse and client work together to identify goals, outcomes, and intervention strategies that will reduce identified client problems in the planning step. The diagnosis step of the nursing process involves the identification of actual or potential health problems.

CN: Safe, effective care environment; CNS: Coordinated care; CL: Knowledge

19. During an interdepartmental team meeting involving a hospice client, a nurse who practices Catholicism verbalizes concern for the spiritual needs of a terminally ill infant and her non-Catholic family. She suggests the infant be baptized before death. Which recommendation of the multidisciplinary team is most likely?
1. Insist the infant obtain baptism before death occurs.
2. Bathe the infant with special oil to prepare for death.
3. Schedule an appointment with a Catholic priest to see the family.
4. Recognize that not all religions practice infant baptism.

19. 4. Many religious organizations (for example, Baptist, Adventist, Buddhist, Quaker) don't practice baptism or only baptize adults. Hospice organizations use the family's religious leader as a choice for spiritual directions. Seventh Day Adventists believe in divine healing and anointing with oil. Deciding whether to baptize the infant isn't the nurse's responsibility. It's important to honor all customs and religious beliefs of families.

CN: Psychosocial integrity; CNS: None; CL: Application

CN: Client needs category   CNS: Client needs subcategory   CL: Cognitive level

20. A home health client asks a nurse for information on sources of financial support. The client's elderly parent is blind and living with her. To which program would it be appropriate for the nurse to refer the client?
1. Medicare
2. Meals On Wheels
3. Supplemental Security Income
4. Aid to Families with Dependent Children

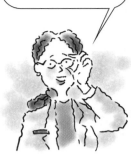

Stay focused, now. You're doing great.

20. 3. Supplemental Security Income is a governmental subsidy assisting the poor and medically disabled. Medicare is available to individuals age 65 and older and individuals younger than age 65 with long-term disabilities or end-stage renal disease. Meals On Wheels is a non-profit organization that delivers food to the poor. Aid to Families with Dependent Children is a state subsidy given to poor families with dependent children.
CN: Health promotion and maintenance; CNS: None; CL: Comprehension

21. Giving hearing and vision screening to elementary school children is an example of which type of prevention strategy?
1. Primary
2. Secondary
3. Tertiary
4. None of the above

21. 2. Screening is a major secondary prevention strategy. Secondary prevention is aimed at early detection and treatment of illness. Primary prevention strategies are aimed at preventing the disease from beginning by avoiding or modifying risk factors. Tertiary prevention strategies focus on rehabilitation and prevention of complications arising from advanced disease.
CN: Health promotion and maintenance; CNS: None; CL: Application

22. Which action would be the most appropriate one for the nurse to teach the nursing assistant when both are caring for a client with pain related to cancer?
1. Using heat or cold on painful areas
2. Keeping a hard bedroll behind the client's back
3. Allowing the client to stay in one position to prevent pain
4. Keeping bright lights on in the room so the nurse can assess the client more quickly

22. 1. Using either heat or cold can reduce inflammatory responses, which will reduce pain. Nurses should avoid pressure (such as bedrolls) on painful areas and change the client's position frequently. Activities should be coordinated with pain medication. Reducing bright lights and noise helps prevent anxiety, which can increase pain.
CN: Physiological integrity; CNS: Physiological adaptation; CL: Application

23. A new graduate is assigned to a nursing unit. A nurse manager assesses that the graduate's skills are deficient. Which action is most appropriate for the nurse manager to take?
1. Talk with the supervisor about terminating the new graduate.
2. Discuss with the graduate that a transfer to another unit is necessary.
3. Work with the graduate and develop a plan to improve the graduate's deficiencies.
4. Counsel the graduate that, if performance doesn't improve, the graduate will be terminated.

23. 3. A principle of leadership involves mastery over ignorance by working with people. The leader needs to work with the new graduate and provide opportunities for the graduate to grow and develop. The other responses wouldn't give the new graduate the opportunity and support needed for improvement.
CN: Safe, effective care environment; CNS: Coordinated care; CL: Application

CN: Client needs category CNS: Client needs subcategory CL: Cognitive level

24. A local community health nurse is asked to speak to a group of adolescent girls on the topic of preventing pregnancy. Which statement indicates the adolescents need more information on this topic?
1. "I can get pregnant even the first time we have sex."
2. "I can get pregnant even though I don't have sex regularly."
3. "I can't get pregnant because my menstrual cycle isn't regular yet."
4. "I can get pregnant even if my boyfriend withdraws before he comes."

25. Which nursing action is most appropriate in stimulating the appetite of a child with cancer?
1. Using food as a reward system
2. Serving large meals frequently
3. Preparing foods appropriate to the age of the child
4. Placing the child on a rigid time schedule for eating

26. While reviewing the food diary of a client with type 2 diabetes, the nurse learns the client skips breakfast and eats processed fast food for lunch 5 days per week. Which statement would be most helpful?
1. "Breakfast is the most important meal of the day."
2. "What suggestions can I make to help you plan breakfast at home before leaving for work?"
3. "Eating fast food is the only way to get a good lunch these days."
4. "A person with diabetes has to eat at least 2 meals per day."

27. A professional nurse should report positive tuberculosis (TB) smears or cultures to the health department within which time period?
1. 12 hours
2. 48 hours
3. 1 week
4. 10 to 14 days

24. 3. Many adolescents have misunderstandings related to risk periods and timing, including periods of susceptibility during the menstrual cycle, age-related susceptibility, and timing of male ejaculation.
CN: Health promotion and maintenance; CNS: None; CL: Analysis

25. 3. It's important to prepare foods appropriate to children in certain age-groups. Involve the child in food preparation and selection. Encourage parents to relax pressures placed on eating by stressing the legitimate nature of loss of appetite. Let the child eat all food that can be tolerated. Assess the family's beliefs about food habits. Take advantage of a hungry period and serve small snacks.
CN: Physiological integrity; CNS: Physiological adaptation; CL: Application

26. 2. The best statement would be to ask the client what can be done to help with meal planning so that breakfast can be eaten each day. Doing so individualizes the client's care and reinforces the need for a set eating pattern of meals and snacks. One meal isn't more important than another. Fast foods usually are highly processed with large amounts of fat and sodium; these might not be the best meals for this client. Two meals per day isn't enough for this client.
CN: Physiological integrity; CNS: Basic care and comfort; CL: Application

27. 2. A client is considered contagious if he has a positive TB smear or culture, so the results must be reported within 24 to 48 hours. The smear or culture may not have grown an organism in 12 hours. One week or 10 to 14 days is too long to wait.
CN: Health promotion and maintenance; CNS: None; CL: Application

CN: Client needs category   CNS: Client needs subcategory   CL: Cognitive level

28. A client is complaining about being unable to sleep because a roommate stays awake during the night and talks loudly to herself. Which response would be most appropriate?

   1. "I'll see if we can have the doctor order a sleeping pill for you tonight."

   2. "Perhaps medication will quiet the roommate at night."

   3. "It sounds like you're angry. Can you tell me more about what you're feeling?"

   4. "I'll see if we can transfer you or your roommate into another room."

29. A nurse must have expertise in many roles. In which nurse-client interaction is the nurse showing a secondary intervention as an advocate?

   1. Contacting the local church to borrow a walker for the client to use

   2. Listening to a client express feelings of frustration over the limitations imposed by his condition

   3. Giving I.V. antibiotic therapy every 12 hours with attention to sterile technique and prevention of complications

   4. Teaching a client with chronic obstructive pulmonary disease the effect of abdominal distention on breathing and ways to help bowel function

30. Which time would be ideal to begin discharge planning for a client admitted with an exacerbation of asthma?

   1. At the time of admission

   2. The day before discharge

   3. After the acute episode is resolved

   4. When the discharge order is written

28. 4. The most practical response would be to move the client or her roommate. Medicating the client or her roomate isn't the best course of action when less drastic measures can be implemented. It's always good nursing practice to create a therapeutic relationship with a client, but because the client has expressed her feelings, pursuing the issue further wouldn't accomplish anything. Although the client has complained, these complaints don't necessarily indicate anger.
CN: Physiological integrity; CNS: Basic care and comfort; CL: Analysis

29. 1. Referral to community agencies is an advocacy role for nurses. The role of the advocate implies the nurse can advise clients how to find alternative sources of care. Instructing clients about disease processes, giving emotional support, and giving therapies to clients are direct care activities.
CN: Safe, effective care environment; CNS: Coordinated care; CL: Application

30. 1. Discharge planning should begin as soon as the client is admitted. Client stays are increasingly shorter, giving the interdisciplinary team less time to accomplish care goals. Waiting for a discharge order or deferring planning until the end of the client's stay doesn't allow sufficient time. Waiting until the acute episode is resolved will greatly diminish the time available for discharge planning.
CN: Safe, effective care environment; CNS: Coordinated care; CL: Comprehension

31. A young pregnant client attending prenatal classes is concerned about her alcohol intake. Which statement indicates the client's child is at high risk for fetal alcohol syndrome (FAS)?
1. "I just snort once or twice per day."
2. "I don't feel like anyone loves me."
3. "I drink a six pack daily for my nerves."
4. "I smoke marijuana with my boyfriend."

31. 3. Ingestion of alcohol on a daily basis increases the risk of FAS. Although option 2 may reveal the patient's reason for her alcohol intake, it isn't an indication for the risk of her child's FAS. Other forms of addictive behavior, such as ingestion of cocaine and smoking marijuana, increase the risk of fetal abuse, not FAS.
CN: Health promotion and maintenance; CNS: None; CL: Comprehension

32. According to the Centers for Disease Control and Prevention, which group would most likely need preventive therapy for tuberculosis (TB)?
1. Clients with human immunodeficiency virus (HIV) infection
2. Clients wiith recent negative tuberculin skin tests and low-risk
3. People with no contact with infectious TB clients
4. Clients with abnormal chest X-rays

32. 1. Preventive therapy should be initiated for clients infected with HIV because latent TB can become active if the immune system is weakened. Clients with low risk and negative skin tests are unlikely to be infected with TB or to progress if infected. Clients with no contact with infectious TB cases aren't at high risk for developing TB. Although clients with active TB may have abnormal chest X-rays, many other conditions can cause such abnormalities.
CN: Health promotion and maintenance; CNS: None; CL: Application

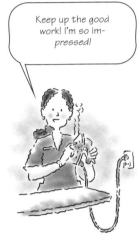

Keep up the good work! I'm so impressed!

33. A 62-year-old female client has been taking Vitamin C 500 mg by mouth (P.O.) daily, multi-vitamins 1 tablet P.O. every day, and aspirin 325 mg every 6 hours as needed for arthritic pain for 4 days. The nurse notices the client's stool is becoming darker and a test for occult blood is positive. What would the nurse most likely conclude?
1. The combination of vitamin C and multi-vitamins are irritating the lining of the intestine.
2. The aspirin should be withheld because it may be causing gastric bleeding.
3. Vitamin C is acidic in nature and may be irritating the GI tissues.
4. From the appearance of the stool, the nurse suspects the client has hemorrhoids.

33. 2. Aspirin is widely known for causing gastric irritation and bleeding. Vitamin C and multivitamins generally don't have an adverse effect in the GI tract. There may be hemorrhoids present, but bleeding from this source would generally be bright red.
CN: Physiological integrity; CNS: Pharmacological therapies; CL: Analysis

34. A concerned client called the school asking that the nurse assess her 13-year-old son for signs of depression. Which symptom would the nurse expect to see?
1. Becoming angry at peers easily
2. Seeking out support from peers
3. Eating several small meals daily
4. Feeling he can control everything in his life

34. 1. Adolescents experiencing depression may experience and express anger at peers. Adolescents feel a lack of control over their current situation, so they isolate from their peers. The adolescent commonly has an intake of nutrients insufficient to meet metabolic needs.
CN: Psychosocial integrity; CNS: None; CL: Analysis

CN: Client needs category   CNS: Client needs subcategory   CL: Cognitive level

35. The nurse is speaking to a 56-year-old client who has recently lost his 82-year-old father to lung cancer. Which signs of grief would the nurse expect to find when speaking with this client?
1. Decreased libido
2. Absence of anger and hostility
3. Difficulty crying or controlling crying
4. Clear dreams and imagery of the deceased

36. A 72-year-old client experienced the death of her husband 1 year ago. She now needs home health services due to severe osteoarthritis. Which statement indicates the client will need further bereavement counseling?
1. "I'm lucky my children live so close."
2. "I really don't have anything to live for."
3. "My health isn't very good, but I can live with it."
4. "I've always had trouble remembering where I placed things."

37. Which drug and route of administration is best to treat secondary syphilis?
1. Penicillin G orally
2. Penicillin G rectally
3. Cephalexin (Keflex) I.V.
4. Penicillin G I.M.

38. Your client must undergo an obstetric sonography. This test is typically indicated during the third trimester to rule out which disorder?
1. Adnexal mass
2. Blighted ovum
3. Molar pregnancy
4. Breech presentation

35. 4. A grieving client usually has vivid, clear dreams and fantasies. He also has a good capacity for imagery, particularly involving the loss. Decreased libido, absence of anger and hostility, and difficulty crying or controlling crying are signs of depression.
CN: Psychosocial integrity; CNS: None; CL: Analysis

36. 2. Wishing for death is a sign of depression. Usually after a year, most individuals accept the death of their loved ones and begin restoring their life. Being grateful for good health and close family ties is a sign of acceptance of a new life that one experiences after the loss of a loved one. Memory loss can be a sign of dementia or depression.
CN: Psychosocial integrity; CNS: None; CL: Analysis

37. 4. Penicillin is the drug of choice to treat syphilis. Because of the long-term consequences of inadequate treatment, penicillin is usually given either I.M. or I.V., especially for syphilis of the nervous system or secondary syphilis. Keflex isn't the drug of choice for syphilis.
CN: Physiological integrity; CNS: Pharmacological therapies; CL: Knowledge

38. 4. An obstetric sonography is indicated in the third trimester to assess presentation of the fetus. If the fetus is in breech position, external cephalic version or cesarean delivery may be considered. An adnexal mass or blighted ovum would have been ruled out during the first trimester. A molar pregnancy would have been ruled out during the first or second trimester.
CN: Health promotion and maintenance; CNS: None; CL: Comprehension

39. A client developed oral ulcerations secondary to chemotherapy agents. Which nursing action is most appropriate for reducing pain and irritation in the mouth?
1. Serving a high-fiber diet
2. Using a toothbrush to clean teeth
3. Avoiding oral temperatures
4. Rinsing the mouth with hydrogen peroxide and water

39. 3. If oral ulcers are present, taking oral temperatures will be painful. Use the axillary region, rectum, or ear as sites for temperature readings. A high-fiber diet won't reduce the patient's oral pain or irritation in his mouth. The high-fiber diet, depending on what high-fiber foods are chosen, may in fact irritate the patient's mouth even more. Use a soft-sponge toothbrush, cotton-tipped applicator, or gauze-wrapped finger to clean teeth. Give normal saline solution mouthwashes and rinses to reduce pain and inflammation. Hydrogen peroxide mixed with water is too irritating if oral ulcers are present.
CN: Physiological integrity; CNS: Physiological adaptation; CL: Application

40. A client is admitted to the emergency department after being sexually assaulted. Which of the following nursing interventions is the priority?
1. Assisting with medical treatment
2. Collecting and preparing evidence for the police
3. Attempting to reduce the client's anxiety from a panic to a moderate level
4. Providing anticipatory guidance to the client about normal responses to sexual assault

40. 3. Reducing anxiety will help the client participate in medical, forensic, and legal follow-up activities. Medical treatment should begin as soon as the client's anxiety decreases below the panic level. Collecting and preparing evidence and providing anticipatory guidance aren't high-priority interventions.
CN: Psychosocial integrity; CNS: None; CL: Analysis

41. The nurse is caring for an 8-year-old boy diagnosed with attention deficit hyperactivity disorder (ADHD). Which behavior is most common in children with ADHD?
1. Lethargy
2. Long attention span
3. Short attention span
4. Preoccupation with body parts

41. 3. Short attention span is a common characteristic of ADHD due to difficulty concentrating. These children show hyperexcitability, not lethargy. Children with this disorder are distracted by environmental stimuli, so they won't be concentrating on their body parts.
CN: Psychosocial integrity; CNS: None; CL: Comprehension

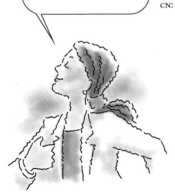

Excellent! You're nearly halfway to the end. You should feel proud—and motivated!

CN: Client needs category   CNS: Client needs subcategory   CL: Cognitive level

42. A client in the second stage of labor reports strong urges to bear down. The nurse interprets this reflex as:

1. Babinski's reflex.
2. Ferguson's reflex.
3. Moro's reflex.
4. Myerson's reflex.

43. A 35-year-old professional woman is admitted to an inpatient substance abuse unit with a diagnosis of alcohol dependence. Which comment by the client indicates that she's using rationalization to deal with her alcohol problem?

1. "I don't drink more than two beers when I'm out."
2. "I always remember what happens the next day."
3. "I always ask a friend to drive me home when I'm drinking."
4. "I've had four tickets for driving while intoxicated in the last month."

44. A nurse is working with a client with alcoholism in an acute care mental health unit. The client has been referred to Alcoholics Anonymous (AA). Which statement by the client indicates that the client is ready to begin the AA program?

1. "I know I'm powerless over alcohol and need help."
2. "I think it will be interesting and helpful to join AA."
3. "I'd like to sponsor another alcoholic with this same problem."
4. "My family is very supportive and will attend meetings with me."

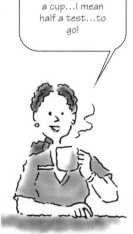

42. 2. Ferguson's reflex is characterized by the strong urge to bear down during the second stage of labor. Babinski's reflex results in dorsiflexion of the big toe and fanning of the other toes when the sole of the client's foot is scraped. Moro's reflex is a normal generalized reflex in an infant when he reacts to a sudden noise such as when a table is struck next to him. Myerson's reflex results in blinking when the client's forehead, bridge of the nose, or maxilla is tapped.
CN: Physiological integrity; CNS: Physiological adaptation; CL: Analysis

43. 3. By asking someone to drive them home, clients with alcohol dependence rationalize that it's okay to drink if they're responsible. The amount one drinks doesn't matter. An alcoholic experiences blackouts, which are periods of amnesia about experiences while intoxicated. Driving while intoxicated can be seen as a symptom of alcohol dependence. Designating drivers and limiting alcohol consumption are self-responsible actions, but don't address the underlying problem.
CN: Psychosocial integrity; CNS: None; CL: Analysis

44. 1. In step 1 of AA, a person admits their powerlessness over alcohol and is ready to accept help. This should occur before they begin AA. A supportive family and a desire to help others with the same problem are good for the client, but don't necessarily indicate readiness to participate in the program.
CN: Psychosocial integrity; CNS: None; CL: Analysis

45. In planning care for a client diagnosed with paranoid schizophrenia, which action is correct for the psychiatric nurse?
1. Confront the client about her hallucinations.
2. Ask the minister to provide spiritual direction.
3. Instruct family members to discourage delusions.
4. Affirm when client's perceptions and thinking are in touch with reality.

45. 4. The nursing care plan focuses on reinforcing perceptions and thinking that are in touch with reality. Confronting a client about her hallucinations and delusions isn't effective or therapeutic. Spiritual direction is important, but a client with paranoid schizophrenia may have issues surrounding her religious or spiritual orientation. Therefore, asking a minister to provide spiritual direction may not be effective or therapeutic. Using family members could create distrust between the client and the family.
CN: Psychosocial integrity; CNS: None; CL: Application

46. A psychiatric nurse finds a client with bipolar disorder sitting in the dayroom. The client is wearing a red polka dot dress, large yellow hat, and heavy makeup with large gold jewelry. Which phase of the illness is the client most likely in?
1. Delusional
2. Depressive
3. Manic
4. Suspicious

46. 3. Extreme labile moods are characteristic of clients in the manic phase of bipolar disorder. Hyperactivity, verbosity, and drawing attention to oneself through dress are typical of the manic phase. Delusions and suspiciousness may be seen in bipolar disorder, but are more commonly seen in schizophrenia. In the depressive phase, clients are withdrawn, cry, and may not eat. Visual or auditory hallucinations, delusional thoughts, and extreme suspiciousness are behaviors seen in clients diagnosed with paranoid schizophrenia.
CN: Psychosocial integrity; CNS: None; CL: Analysis

47. Which sign would the nurse expect to observe in a 4-week-old neonate in acute pain?
1. Whimpering
2. Eyes opened wide
3. Limp body posture
4. Desire to breast-feed frequently

47. 1. Crying, whimpering, and groaning are vocal expressions of acute pain in the neonate. Eyes tightly closed, decreased appetite, and fist clenching with rigidity are also signs of acute pain in the neonate.
CN: Health promotion and maintenance; CNS: None; CL: Application

48. Which position or equipment is needed to maintain posture for a child with juvenile rheumatoid arthritis?
1. Soft mattress
2. Prone position
3. Large fluffy pillows
4. Semi-Fowler's position

48. 2. Lying in the prone position is encouraged to straighten hips and knees. A firm mattress is needed to maintain good alignment of spine, hips, and knees, and no pillow or a very thin pillow should be used. Semi-Fowler's position increases pressure on the hip joints and should be avoided.
CN: Physiological integrity; CNS: Basic care and comfort; CL: Application

CN: Client needs category　CNS: Client needs subcategory　CL: Cognitive level

49. The health care provider determines that a fetus is in a complete breech presentation. The nurse understands this as:

1. a foot extending below the buttocks.
2. a knee extending below the buttocks.
3. the buttocks as the presenting part, with thighs and knees flexed.
4. the buttocks as the presenting part, with thighs flexed, and knees extended.

49. 3. In a complete breech, the buttocks are the presenting part and the thighs and knees are flexed. Two types of incomplete breech are footling breech, when a foot extends below the buttocks, and knee presentation, when a knee extends below the buttocks. A frank breech happens when the buttocks are the presenting part, the thighs are flexed, and the knees are extended.

CN: Physiological integrity; CNS: Physiological adaptation; CL: Comprehension

50. While putting an elderly client with an indwelling urinary catheter in bed, a nurse notices the tubing hanging below the bed. She places the tubing in a loop on the bed with the client and makes sure he won't lie on the tubing. Which rationale explains the nurse's action?

1. To inhibit drainage
2. To allow drainage to occur
3. To allow the urine to collect in the tubing
4. To have the client check the tubing for urine

50. 2. Catheter tubing shouldn't be allowed to develop dependent loops or kinks because this inhibits proper drainage by requiring the urine to travel against gravity to empty into the bag. Permitting the urine to collect in the tubing increases the risk of infection. Observing the catheter and tubing is the responsibility of the nurse.

CN: Physiological integrity; CNS: Reduction of risk potential; CL: Application

51. A client complains of severe burning on urination. Which instruction is best to give the client?

1. Wear only nylon panties.
2. Drink coffee to increase urination.
3. Soak in warm water with bubble bath.
4. Drink 2,500 to 3,000 ml of water per day.

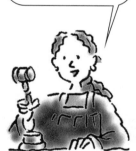

The verdict is in! You've finished 50 questions and you're doing fine.

51. 4. Drinking large amounts of water will help flush bacteria from the urinary tract. Avoid nylon underwear; wear only cotton undergarments to decrease the warm, moist environment. Avoid tea, coffee, carbonated drinks, and alcoholic beverages because of bladder irritation. Avoid using bubble baths, perfumed soaps, or bath powders in the perineal area. The scent in toiletries can be irritating to the urinary meatus.

CN: Physiological integrity; CNS: Basic care and comfort; CL: Application

52. Which instruction is given to a client with a hearing aid?

1. Clean the hearing aid with baby oil.
2. Wear the hearing aid while sleeping.
3. Keep the hearing aid out of direct sunlight.
4. Leave the hearing aid in place while showering.

52. 3. The hearing aid should be kept out of direct sunlight and away from high temperatures. Solvents or lubricants shouldn't be used on the aid. If there's a detachable ear mold, it can be washed in warm, soapy water and dried with a soft cloth. The hearing aid should be left in place while the client is awake, except when showering.

CN: Physiological integrity; CNS: Basic care and comfort; CL: Application

CN: Client needs category   CNS: Client needs subcategory   CL: Cognitive level

53. A 72-year-old client is being discharged from same-day surgery after having a cataract removed from her right eye. Which discharge instructions does the nurse give the client?
1. Sleep on the operative side.
2. Resume all activities as before.
3. Don't rub or place pressure on the eyes.
4. Wear an eye shield all day and remove it at night.

53. 3. Rubbing or placing pressure on the eyes increases the risk of accidental injury to ocular structures. The nurse should also caution against lifting objects, straining, strenuous exercise, and sexual activity because such activities can increase intraocular pressure. Glasses or shaded lenses should be worn to protect the eye during waking hours after the eye dressing is removed. Caution against sleeping on the operative side to reduce the risk of accidental injury to ocular structures. An eye shield should be worn at night.
CN: Physiological integrity; CNS: Reduction of risk potential; CL: Application

54. To ensure the safe administration of medications, which of the following actions should be performed first?
1. Make sure the client is in the right room.
2. Check for client allergies.
3. Have the client repeat his name.
4. Open the medications at the client's bedside.

54. 2. Checking for client's allergies is the first step in ensuring safe administration of medications. The other actions are important but are of less priority.
CN: Physiological integrity; CNS: Pharmacological therapies; CL: Analysis

55. Which instruction is correct for a client taking nortriptyline (Pamelor) for depression?
1. Be aware that this drug can cause a slow heart rate.
2. This drug will work immediately to treat depression.
3. Take this drug in the morning because it causes drowsiness.
4. Wear protective clothing and sunscreen when out in the sun.

55. 4. A common adverse effect of this drug is sensitivity to the sun. Protective clothing and sunscreen should be worn in the sun. This drug can cause an irregular heart rate. It doesn't work immediately, but takes 2 to 3 weeks to achieve the desired effect. Take this drug at bedtime if it causes drowsiness.
CN: Physiological integrity; CNS: Pharmacological therapies; CL: Application

56. Which instruction is correct for a client receiving lithium (Eskalith) for bipolar disorder?
1. Avoid drugs containing ibuprofen (Advil, Motrin, Nuprin).
2. Drink at least two cups of coffee daily.
3. Be aware that you may experience increased alertness.
4. It isn't necessary to monitor the blood level of this drug.

56. 1. Avoid drugs that alter the effect of lithium, such as ibuprofen and sodium bicarbonate or other antacids containing sodium. Lithium can decrease alertness and coordination. Avoid beverages with caffeine because they increase urination, which may alter the effect of lithium. Lithium levels may need to be monitored every 2 weeks, especially if adverse effects occur. The dose may need to be regulated.
CN: Physiological integrity; CNS: Pharmacological therapies; CL: Application

57. Which nursing intervention is correct for clients receiving I.V. therapy?
1. Changing the tubing every 8 hours
2. Monitoring the flow rate at least every hour
3. Changing the I.V. catheter and entry site daily
4. Increasing the rate to catch up if the correct amount hasn't been infused at the end of the shift

58. Which nursing intervention is correct for a client receiving total parenteral nutrition (TPN)?
1. Discard TPN solutions after 24 hours.
2. Teach the client to blow out during expiration when the tubing is disconnected.
3. Inspect the TPN solution for clearness and visibility.
4. Discard lipid emulsions after 20 hours.

59. Which drug form would the nurse expect to administer through a nasogastric (NG) tube?
1. Enteric coated
2. Oral
3. Parenteral
4. Sublingual

60. When preparing a client with suspected bacterial endocarditis for diagnostic testing, which test would the nurse anticipate the physician to order?
1. Electrolytes
2. Blood cultures
3. Prothrombin time (PT)
4. Venereal Disease Research Laboratory (VDRL)

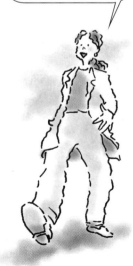

You're making great strides towards your goal. You should be so proud.

57. 2. Closely observing the rate of infusion prevents underhydration and overhydration. Tubing is changed according to facility policy but not at the frequency of every 8 hours. The I.V. catheter and entry site should be changed every 48 to 72 hours in most situations. Increasing the rate may lead to fluid overload.
CN: Physiological integrity; CNS: Pharmacological therapies; CL: Application

58. 1. TPN solutions are good media for fungi, so they should be discarded after 24 hours. The nurse should teach the client to perform Valsalva's maneuver, taking a deep breath and holding it, when the tubing is disconnected. Valsalva's maneuver increases intrathoracic pressure, which prevents air entry. Inspect TPN solutions for cloudiness, and the container for cracks or leaks before hanging. Lipid emulsions are also good media for fungi and should be discarded after 12 hours.
CN: Physiological integrity; CNS: Pharmacological therapies; CL: Application

59. 2. Most oral medications can be given via an NG tube because they're intended for passage into the stomach. Some oral drugs have special coatings intended to keep the pill intact until it passes into the small intestine; these enteric-coated pills shouldn't be crushed and put through an NG tube. Parenteral means I.V., I.M., and subcutaneous. Some parenteral medications, such as insulin, may be destroyed by gastric juices. Sublingual means under the tongue and the medication requires placement there for adequate absorption.
CN: Physiological integrity; CNS: Pharmacological therapies; CL: Comprehension

60. 2. Blood cultures are crucial in diagnosing bacterial endocarditis. Electrolyte levels indicate abnormalities that occur with drug therapy as well as with complications associated with heart failure. PT values are useful in monitoring anticoagulant therapy. A positive VDRL may be evidence of syphilitic heart disease.
CN: Physiological integrity; CNS: Reduction of risk potential; CL: Application

61. In preparing a client for cardiac catheterization, which statement or question is most appropriate?
1. "Are you allergic to contrast dyes or shellfish?"
2. "Have you ever had this kind of procedure before?"
3. "You'll need to fast 24 hours before the procedure."
4. "You'll be given medication to help you sleep during the procedure."

61. 1. The nurse must assess for allergies to iodine before the procedure because the contrast dye used during catheterization contains iodine, which shellfish also contains. Knowing the client's history and prior experience with this procedure would be helpful, but knowing the client's allergies is more important. The client needs to stay awake during the procedure to follow directions, such as taking a deep breath and holding it during injection of the dye, and to report chest, neck, or jaw discomfort. The client is instructed to fast for 6 hours before the procedure. The client will be asked to empty his bladder before the procedure.
CN: Physiological integrity; CNS: Reduction of risk potential; CL: Application

62. Which technique is considered a noninvasive diagnostic method to evaluate cardiac changes?
1. Cardiac biopsy
2. Cardiac catheterization
3. Magnetic resonance imaging (MRI)
4. Pericardiocentesis

62. 3. MRI is a noninvasive procedure that aids in the diagnosis and detection of thoracic aortic aneurysm and evaluation of coronary artery disease, pericardial disease, and cardiac masses. Cardiac biopsy, cardiac catheterization, and pericardiocentesis are invasive techniques used to evaluate cardiac changes.
CN: Health promotion and maintenance; CNS: None; CL: Knowledge

63. A client recovering from surgery tells a nurse, "I feel like I have to urinate more often than usual, and it burns when I urinate." Which of the following interventions would be most appropriate?
1. Obtain a urine culture.
2. Check the client's urine for glucose.
3. Check the client's urine for ketones.
4. Check the client's urine for specific gravity.

63. 1. The signs and symptoms of this client are those of a urinary tract infection, and a culture will probably show a bacterial infection. Ketones and glucose in the urine don't cause burning and frequency. Specific gravity is a measure of the concentration of the urine. A high or low specific gravity won't cause these symptoms.
CN: Physiological integrity; CNS: Reduction of risk potential; CL: Analysis

64. Which foods can alter results when stool is checked for occult blood?
1. Red meat
2. Dairy products, canned fruit, and pretzels
3. Horseradish, raw fruits, and vegetables
4. Potatoes, orange juice, and decaffeinated coffee

64. 1. Consumption of red meat has caused false-positive readings. Avoid foods that are high in iron. The other foods don't cause false-positive readings.
CN: Physiological integrity; CNS: Reduction of risk potential; CL: Comprehension

CN: Client needs category   CNS: Client needs subcategory   CL: Cognitive level

65. In caring for a client with arterial insufficiency, which instruction is most appropriate?
1. "You may leave your feet open to the air."
2. "Sit and rest for several hours per day."
3. "Avoid crossing your legs at the knees or ankles."
4. "Wear tight socks instead of no socks."

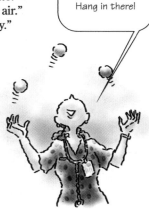

Only 20 left. Hang in there!

65. 3. Leg crossing should be avoided because it compresses the vessels in the legs. Although rest is important, it isn't as important as telling the patient he shouldn't cross his legs. Feet and extremities must be protected to reduce the risk of trauma. Avoid constrictive clothing, such as tight elastic on socks, to prevent compression of vessels in the legs. Injury to the extremity will require more blood to heal than to keep the tissue intact; an extremity with compromised circulation may not be able to provide the extra blood required.
CN: Physiological integrity; CNS: Reduction of risk potential; CL: Application

66. Which instruction would be appropriate for a client taking oral anticoagulants?
1. "Shave with a standard razor."
2. "Take ibuprofen (Advil, Motrin, Nuprin) or aspirin for pain."
3. "Take the anticoagulant at the same time each day."
4. "Eat a large quantity of green leafy vegetables several times per week."

66. 3. It's important to take the anticoagulant at the same time each day to maintain an adequate blood level. An electric razor reduces the risk of cutting the skin. Avoid the use of standard razors. Avoid taking aspirin or ibuprofen because these drugs decrease clotting time. Intermittently eating a large amount of green leafy vegetables, which contain vitamin K, increases the clotting time, thus requiring more anticoagulants.
CN: Physiological integrity; CNS: Pharmacological therapies; CL: Application

67. Which action is most appropriate to reduce sensory deprivation for a visually impaired elderly client in the hospital?
1. Keep the lights dimmed.
2. Close the curtains or blinds on windows to reduce glare.
3. Open the hospital door so bright light can shine in the room.
4. Open the curtains during the day so the sun can shine brightly.

67. 2. Closing curtains or blinds on windows can reduce glare and improve vision for the older client. Controlled lighting can help the older client see better in the hospital. Adequate background lighting helps the older client decrease visual accommodation when moving from brightly lit to dimly lit rooms and hallways.
CN: Physiological integrity; CNS: Reduction of risk potential; CL: Application

68. Which action is most appropriate to reduce sensory overload for a hearing-impaired elderly client?
1. Keep the overhead light on continuously.
2. Discuss the client's condition at the bedside.
3. Allow all family members to stay with the client.
4. Limit bedside conversation to that directed to the client.

68. 4. Limiting bedside conversation to that directed to the client creates fewer disturbances, thus reducing sensory overload. Turning off or dimming the overhead lights further reduces visual stimulation and facilitates day and night light fluctuations. Although fostering family interaction with the client is necessary, only one or two family members should be allowed to visit with the client at one time. Crowding of people in the client's room may precipitate a loss of privacy and control for the client.
CN: Physiological integrity; CNS: Reduction of risk potential; CL: Application

CN: Client needs category   CNS: Client needs subcategory   CL: Cognitive level

69. Which instruction is most appropriate for a client with osteoarthritis of the left knee?
1. Use cold on joints.
2. Keep the knee extended.
3. Develop a weight-reduction plan.
4. Have someone help the client in activities of daily living (ADLs).

70. A newly diagnosed client with diabetes is found semi-comatose with a rapid heart rate and low blood pressure. The client's skin is warm and dry. Which condition would the nurse suspect?
1. Hypoglycemia
2. Cardiogenic shock
3. Diabetic ketoacidosis (DKA)
4. Hyperosmolar hyperglycemic nonketotic syndrome (HHNS)

71. A nurse is standing next to a person eating fried shrimp at a parade. Suddenly, the man clutches at his throat and can't speak, cough, or breathe. The nurse asks the man if he's choking and he nods yes. Which response is most appropriate?
1. Attempt rescue breathing.
2. Perform abdominal thrusts.
3. Deliver external chest compressions.
4. Use the head tilt-chin lift maneuver to establish the airway.

72. Preparation is the key to successful resuscitation. Which response is most appropriate to prepare for a cardiopulmonary emergency?
1. Have nasal oxygen ready when needed.
2. Place an oropharyngeal airway at the bedside.
3. Keep the medication cart locked up for safety.
4. Don't start an I.V. line unless necessary.

69. 3. Reducing weight decreases joint stress. Local moist heat provides pain relief and will decrease stiffness. The client should perform muscle-strengthening exercises, which help prevent joint stiffness. The nurse should allow the client to perform ADLs as independently as possible.
CN: Physiological integrity; CNS: Reduction of risk potential; CL: Application

70. 3. DKA develops as a result of severe insulin deficiency. The incidence of DKA generally results from undiagnosed diabetes and inadequacy of prescribed medication and dietary therapies. Hypoglycemia involves episodes of low blood glucose levels caused by erratic or altered absorption of insulin. In cardiogenic shock, the client has pale, cool, and moist skin. HHNS is a deadly complication of diabetes distinguished by severe hyperglycemia, dehydration, and changed mental status.
CN: Physiological integrity; CNS: Physiological adaptation; CL: Application

71. 2. If a conscious victim acknowledges that he's choking, the best response is to perform abdominal thrusts to relieve the airway obstruction. The other options are used for an unresponsive victim with absent heart rate and breathing.
CN: Physiological integrity; CNS: Physiological adaptation; CL: Application

72. 2. A nurse should learn to anticipate clinical deterioration before overt signs and symptoms are apparent. If a client is having breathing difficulties, the nurse should place an oropharyngeal airway at the bedside while the client is monitored for deterioration. The emergency cart should be placed outside the client's room for easy access. If breathing stops, the client will need to be intubated and placed on a respirator, if necessary. The client should have a stable I.V. line for administration of emergency drugs.
CN: Physiological integrity; CNS: Physiological adaptation; CL: Analysis

CN: Client needs category   CNS: Client needs subcategory   CL: Cognitive level

73. Obtaining the dorsalis pedis and posterior or tibial pulses are helpful in monitoring which data?
1. Heart rate
2. Pulse rate
3. Lower extremity circulation
4. Evidence of tachycardia

74. A young client is admitted to the emergency department unconscious from an overdose of salicylates. The physician orders dialysis. Which dialysis method is most appropriate?
1. Hemodialysis
2. Peritoneal dialysis
3. Continuous hemofiltration
4. Continuous ambulatory peritoneal dialysis

75. Which nursing action is most appropriate for a low-birth-weight neonate?
1. Keeping the neonate's temperature cool
2. Gavage feeding the neonate if he has a weak sucking reflex
3. Keeping the neonate uncovered in the humidified incubator
4. Keeping the I.V. infusion at a keep-vein-open rate

76. A client's laboratory values are: calcium, 18 mg/dl; potassium, 3 mEq/L; and magnesium, 4 mEq/L. These values put this client most at risk for which complication?
1. Bleeding
2. Renal failure
3. Cardiac arrhythmia
4. Respiratory distress

73. 3. These pulses represent peripheral circulation and are rated by their quality from 0 (absent) to 4 (bounding). Heart rate and pulse rate are used interchangeably and established through examination of the radial or apical pulses. Tachycardia is a fast pulse rate best established by examination of the apical or radial locations.
CN: Physiological integrity; CNS: Physiological adaptation; CL: Knowledge

74. 1. Hemodialysis is a rapid method to correct fluid and electrolyte problems. It's also a fast way to treat accidental or intentional poisonings as a means of clearing drugs or toxins from the body. Peritoneal dialysis, continuous ambulatory peritoneal dialysis, and continuous hemofiltration are slower methods of removing toxins.
CN: Physiological integrity; CNS: Physiological adaptation; CL: Application

75. 2. To maintain adequate nutrition, a low-birth-weight neonate may need to be gavage fed. The neonate should be kept warm. The nurse should avoid situations that might predispose the neonate to chilling, such as exposure to cool air, and she should maintain adequate parenteral fluids to prevent dehydration.
CN: Physiological integrity; CNS: Physiological adaptation; CL: Application

76. 3. Low potassium, magnesium, and calcium levels cause the heart muscle to become irritable, resulting in arrhythmias. Bleeding is seen with a low calcium level. Renal failure isn't caused by low electrolyte levels. Respiratory weakness may occur with a low potassium level.
CN: Health promotion and maintenance; CNS: None; CL: Analysis

I'm quite impressed with your progress so far!

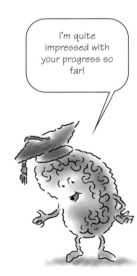

CN: Client needs category   CNS: Client needs subcategory   CL: Cognitive level

77. A client is 2 days postoperative from a left femoral popliteal bypass. The nurse's assessment finds the client's left leg cold, pale, and painful. Which action has priority?
1. Checking distal pulses
2. Notifying the physician
3. Elevating the foot of the bed
4. Wrapping the leg in a warm blanket

77. 1. The client has peripheral arterial disease and had vascular surgery. The nurse must assess the client for complications. A potential problem would be an obstruction at the surgical site, so the nurse must assess circulation by checking for distal pulses. Before the physician is notified, the nurse should determine if distal pulses are present. Elevating the foot of the bed would promote venous return but decrease arterial blood flow and shouldn't be done. The leg can be covered lightly after circulation is assessed.
CN: Physiological integrity; CNS: Physiological adaptation; CL: Application

78. A 40-year-old client is scheduled to have a repair of a deviated septum later in the morning. The nurse notes that the client's pulse rate is 130 beats/minute. Which physiological condition would best explain the tachycardia?
1. Age
2. Anxiety
3. Exercise
4. Pain

78. 2. Anxiety tends to increase heart rate, temperature, and respirations. Exercise will also increase the heart rate but most likely won't occur preoperatively. The normal heart rate for a client this age is 60 to 100 beats/minute. The client shouldn't be in any pain preoperatively.
CN: Physiological integrity; CNS: Physiological adaptation; CL: Analysis

79. Which statement is an example of a key element in the nursing care plan?
1. Advance diet to regular as tolerated.
2. Ambulate 30′ (9.1 m) with walker by discharge.
3. Give furosemide (Lasix) 40 mg I.V. now.
4. Discontinue I.V. fluids when tolerating oral fluids.

79. 2. Option 2 is a measurable expected outcome or goal, a key element of a nursing care plan. Other key elements include nursing diagnoses and interventions. The other options are physician's orders, not key elements of care plans.
CN: Safe, effective care environment; CNS: Coordinated care; CL: Application

80. A client had an appendectomy 24 hours ago. Which goal is appropriate for this client?
1. The client will be able to walk in the hallway.
2. The client will be able to attend physical therapy.
3. The client will be able to accomplish all activities of daily living (ADLs).
4. The client will be able to state the rationale for all postoperative medications.

80. 1. A 24-hour postoperative client is expected to be able to walk in the hallway. A client who just had an appendectomy shouldn't need physical therapy unless deconditioning was evident. At 24 hours, a client should begin to assume responsibility for ADLs, but shouldn't necessarily be responsible for all activities. It's too early to expect a client to state the rationale for all postoperative medications, especially if the client is elderly.
CN: Physiological integrity; CNS: Basic care and comfort; CL: Application

CN: Client needs category   CNS: Client needs subcategory   CL: Cognitive level

81. Which action is included in the principles of asepsis?
1. Maintaining a sterile environment
2. Keeping the environment as clean as possible
3. Testing for microorganisms in the environment
4. Cleaning an environment until it's free from germs

82. Two days after admission to a psychiatric unit, a client with bipolar disorder becomes verbally aggressive during a group therapy session. Which nursing response is best?
1. "You're behaving in an unacceptable manner, and you need to control yourself."
2. "You're scaring everyone in the group. You can't participate until you know how to act."
3. "This is why you have relationship troubles; you don't know how to talk to people."
4. "You're disturbing the other clients. Let's go to the exercise room to help you release some of your energy."

83. A client receiving thiothixene (Navane) has become restless and fidgety and has been pacing the hallway continuously for the past hour. Which of the following adverse reactions to phenothiazines best explains the client's behavior?
1. Dystonia
2. Akathisia
3. Parkinsonian effects
4. Tardive dyskinesia

81. 2. Asepsis is the process of avoiding contamination from outside sources by keeping the environment clean. A clean environment has a reduced number of microorganisms, but isn't necessarily sterile (the absence of all microorganisms). Testing for microorganisms or culturing isn't indicated in the promotion of asepsis.
CN: Safe, effective care environment; CNS: Safety and infection control; CL: Comprehension

82. 4. This response shows the nurse finds the client's behavior unacceptable, yet still regards the client as worthy of help. The third option is judgmental and not therapeutic. The other options give the false impression that the client is in control of the behavior; the client hasn't been in treatment long enough to control the behavior.
CN: Psychosocial integrity; CNS: None; CL: Analysis

83. 2. The client's behavior suggests akathisia—an adverse effect of phenothiazines such as Navane. Dystonia appears as excessive salivation, difficulty speaking, and involuntary movements of the face, neck, arms, and legs. Parkinsonian effects include a shuffling gait, hand tremors, drooling, rigidity, and loose arm movements. Tardive dyskinesia is characterized by involuntary jerky facial, tongue, trunk, and limb movements.
CN: Physiological integrity; CNS: Pharmacological therapies; CL: Analysis

84. An adolescent client seeks medical attention because of a sore throat and probable mononucleosis. The nurse palpates the client's submandibular lymph nodes for enlargement. Identify the area where the nurse should palpate to best feel these nodes.

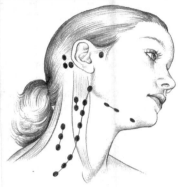

85. As a nurse is feeding an average-sized client, he begins choking on his food. According to the American Heart Association (AHA), the nurse should intervene using the actions listed below. Place the actions listed below in ascending chronological order. Use all the options.

1. Administer abdominal thrusts until effective, or until the client becomes unresponsive.
2. Activate the emergency response team.
3. Ask the client if he can speak.
4. Perform a tongue-jaw lift followed by a finger sweep.
5. Open the airway and attempt to ventilate the client.
6. Give up to five abdominal thrusts.

You've finished comprehensive test 3! Now grab some friends and celebrate!

84.

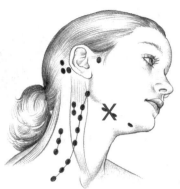

The submandibular lymph nodes are located beneath the mandible, or lower jaw, halfway to the chin. These nodes may be enlarged in a client with a throat infection or mononucleosis.
CN: Physiological integrity; CNS: Physiological adaptation; CL: Comprehension

85. Ordered response:

3. Ask the client if he can speak.
1. Administer abdominal thrusts until effective, or until the client becomes unresponsive.
2. Activate the emergency response team.
4. Perform a tongue-jaw lift followed by a finger sweep.
5. Open the airway and attempt to ventilate the client.
6. Give up to five abdominal thrusts.

According to the AHA, the nurse should ask the client if he can speak. Next, she should administer abdominal or chest thrusts (if the client is obese or pregnant) until they're effective or until the client becomes unresponsive. When the latter occurs, the nurse should activate the emergency response team, then perform a tongue-jaw lift followed by a finger sweep to clear visible food. Next, she should open the client's airway and try to ventilate him. If his airway still is obstructed, she should reposition his head and try to ventilate again. Then, she should give up to five abdominal thrusts.
CN: Physiological integrity; CNS: Physiological adaptation; CL: Application

CN: Client needs category   CNS: Client needs subcategory   CL: Cognitive level

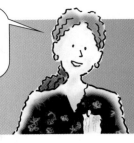

Here's the final comprehensive test to practice for the NCLEX. You'll do great!

COMPREHENSIVE
Test 4

1. You're caring for a neonate at 10 minutes after birth. Which finding would require you to notify the physician?
   1. Crackling noises during auscultation of breath sounds
   2. Respiratory rate of 50 breaths/minute
   3. Bluish gray pigmented nevi on the buttocks
   4. Shrill, high pitched cry that doesn't cease

2. A team leader notes increasing unrest among the staff members. Which action is best for the team leader to take?
   1. Discuss the problem with a coworker.
   2. Report the problem to the nurse-manager.
   3. Discuss the problem with the staff.
   4. Ignore the problem and hope it won't interfere with the functioning of the floor.

3. A physician orders a urine specimen for culture and sensitivity stat. Which approach is best for the nurse to use in delegating this task?
   1. "We need a stat urine culture on the client in room 101."
   2. "Please get the urine for culture from the client in room 101."
   3. "A stat urine was ordered for the client in room 101. Would you get it?"
   4. "We need a urine for culture stat on the client in room 101. Tell me when you send it to the lab."

1. 4. A shrill, high pitched cry that doesn't cease may indicate a central nervous system injury or abnormality. It's commonly found in neonates with genetic abnormalities, drug withdrawal, or fetal alcohol syndrome. Crackling noises heard during auscultation of breath sounds and a respiratory rate of 50 breaths/minute are normal. Bluish gray nevi on the buttocks (mongolian spots) are also common.
CN: Health promotion and maintenance; CNS: None; CL: Analysis

2. 3. The leader should comment to the group on the observed behavior. This is a firm approach but one that shows concern. Ignoring problems or discussing them with someone else doesn't confront the issue at hand.
CN: Safe, effective care environment; CNS: Coordinated care; CL: Application

3. 4. This option not only delegates the task, but also provides a checkpoint. To effectively delegate, you need to follow up on what someone else is doing. The other options don't provide for feedback, which is essential for communication and delegation.
CN: Safe, effective care environment; CNS: Coordinated care; CL: Application

Relax. You're up to the last test and you're doing swimmingly well.

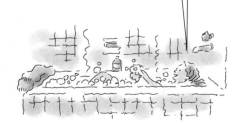

CN: Client needs category   CNS: Client needs subcategory   CL: Cognitive level

4. A female client is complaining of having difficulty urinating. When questioned, she states she doesn't have this difficulty at home. Which action would be most appropriate initially?
1. Offer the bedpan frequently and increase fluid intake.
2. Ensure the client has complete privacy when she uses the bathroom.
3. Find out if the client has a particular routine when she goes to the bathroom.
4. Pour warm water on her perineal area while she's attempting to void.

5. Which characteristics of the client goal in the care plan are correct?
1. Nurse-focused, flexible, measurable, and realistic
2. Client-focused, flexible, realistic, and measurable
3. Nurse-focused, time-limited, realistic, and measurable
4. Client-focused, time-limited, realistic, and measurable

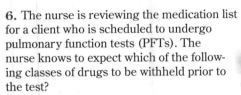

You're on a roll! Keep going!

6. The nurse is reviewing the medication list for a client who is scheduled to undergo pulmonary function tests (PFTs). The nurse knows to expect which of the following classes of drugs to be withheld prior to the test?
1. Antibiotics
2. Antitussives
3. Bronchodilators
4. Corticosteroids

7. After a liver transplant, a client develops ascites. Which procedure would the nurse expect to teach the client to do?
1. Increase the amount of water intake.
2. Brace the abdomen with a pillow during coughing.
3. Perform 10 leg raises every waking hour.
4. Reduce requests for pain medicine.

4. 3. The first and most appropriate course of action is to ask the client what her routine at home is and try to replicate this as much as possible, especially because the client reports not having this difficulty at home. After this is tried, other inventions may be used such as increasing fluid intake, offering the bedpan frequently, ensuring privacy, and using warm water to relax the meatus if the client is still having difficulty.
CN: Physiological integrity; CNS: Basic care and comfort; CL: Analysis

5. 4. All goals should be client focused, allowing the client to understand what needs to be accomplished. Specify a time limit for when this task should be achieved. Be realistic, so the client may be successful in reaching the goal. The goal must be measurable so all staff can evaluate the client's progress. Nurse flexibility is an important attribute and necessary for reassessing needs and approaches for the client's optimal recovery. However, in the actual goal, specific criteria must be identified to allow all staff to work from the same data for achieving client goals.
CN: Safe, effective care environment; CNS: Coordinated care; CL: Knowledge

6. 3. PFTs measure the volume and capacity of air. If a bronchodilator is given, it will improve the bronchial airflow and alter the test results. The other drugs would have no effect on the bronchial tree and PFT results.
CN: Physiological integrity; CNS: Pharmacological therapies; CL: Application

7. 2. Bracing the abdomen during coughing will reduce the risk of wound dehiscence after liver transplantation. Ascites is fluid retention in the abdomen; therefore, increasing water ingestion isn't indicated. Leg raises will put unwanted tension on the abdominal wound and suture line. Pain control is important in avoiding injury to the abdominal wound. Therefore, teaching the patient to reduce pain medicine requests is inappropriate.
CN: Physiological integrity; CNS: Reduction of risk potential; CL: Application

CN: Client needs category   CNS: Client needs subcategory   CL: Cognitive level

8. On the first day after undergoing a thoracotomy, a client exhibits a temperature of 100° F (37.8° C); heart rate, 96 beats/minute; blood pressure, 136/86 mm Hg; and shallow respirations at 24 breaths/minute with rhonchi at the bases. The client complains of incisional pain. Which nursing action has priority?
1. Medicating the client for pain
2. Helping the client get out of bed
3. Giving ibuprofen (Motrin) as ordered to reduce the fever
4. Encouraging the client to cough and deep-breathe

8. 1. Although all the interventions are incorporated in this client's care plan, the priority is to relieve pain and make the client comfortable. This would give the client the energy and stamina to achieve the other objectives.
CN: Physiological integrity; CNS: Basic care and comfort; CL: Application

9. A nurse is caring for a client who had abdominal surgery 2 days ago. The client reports slight dyspnea on exertion and the pulse oximetry reading is 93% on room air. The nurse receives the client's morning chest X-ray report and notes that it shows mild atelectasis at the bases of both lungs. Which nursing action would be most important to include in the client's care plan?
1. Giving oxygen continuously at 3 L/minute
2. Promoting coughing and deep breathing every 4 hours
3. Using the incentive spirometer every hour
4. Getting the client out of bed to a chair every day

9. 3. Incentive spirometry is used to prevent or treat atelectasis. Done every hour, it will produce deep inhalations that help open the collapsed alveoli. Oxygen use doesn't encourage deep inhalation, and the pulse oximetry reading is normal. Coughing and deep breathing is a good intervention, but rarely results in as deep an inspiratory effort as using an incentive spirometer and should be performed more frequently than every 4 hours. Getting the client out of bed will also help expand the lungs and stimulate deep breathing, but it's done less frequently than incentive spirometry.
CN: Safe, effective care environment; CNS: Coordinated care; CL: Application

10. Two hours after nasal surgery, the client's nostrils are packed and a drip pad is anchored under his nose. Which assessment alerts the nurse that the surgical site is bleeding?
1. Frequent swallowing
2. Dry mucous membranes
3. Decrease in urine output
4. Temperature elevation

10. 1. Frequent swallowing is a sign of hemorrhage in nasal surgery. Dry mucous membranes, decreased urine output, and temperature elevation are usually signs of dehydration.
CN: Safe effective care environment; CNS: Coordinated care; CL: Analysis

11. Which intervention is most important to reduce the risk of disuse osteoporosis in a bedridden client?
1. Turning, coughing, and deep breathing
2. Increasing fluids to 3,000 ml daily
3. Promoting venous return by elevating the legs
4. Providing active and passive range-of-motion (ROM) exercise

11. 4. All the interventions listed are good for a bedridden client. However, active and passive ROM exercises provide the mechanical stresses of weight bearing that are absent and lead to disuse osteoporosis.
CN: Health promotion and maintenance; CNS: None; CL: Application

CN: Client needs category   CNS: Client needs subcategory   CL: Cognitive level

12. An elderly client on bed rest for a week after a bout of pneumonia is in a negative nitrogen balance. Which complication has highest priority?
1. Constipation
2. Renal calculi
3. Muscle wasting
4. Vitamin B_6 deficiency

13. The nurse reviews the arterial blood gas results of a client with asthma. The nurse understands that the client's partial pressure of arterial oxygen (PaO_2) gives information on which factor?
1. Respiratory status
2. Degree of dyspnea
3. Efficiency of gas exchange
4. Effectiveness of ventilation

14. The nurse prepares to administer morphine to a client with an acute myocardial infarction for which reason?
1. To decrease cardiac output
2. To increase preload and afterload
3. To increase myocardial oxygen demand
4. To decrease myocardial oxygen demand

15. The mother of an 8-year-old boy admitted for a neurologic evaluation states that he used to take some pills when he had "bout of fits." She says she couldn't afford the medication and because he was doing well, she stopped giving it to him several months ago. She hands the nurse a bottle containing 10 small white tablets with a handwritten piece of tape on it labeled "barbital." Although precise identification of the medication is necessary, the nurse suspects that it's most likely:
1. pentobarbital (Nembutal).
2. bismuth subsalicylate (Pepto-Bismol).
3. phenobarbital (Solfoton).
4. secobarbital (Seconal).

12. 3. Negative nitrogen balance leads to muscle wasting. The body breaks down muscle tissue to use as energy. Renal calculi can be a complication of bed rest and demineralization of the bone but treating a negative nitrogen balance takes priority. Constipation and vitamin B_6 deficiency also need to be corrected but aren't the highest priority.
CN: Physiological integrity; CNS: Physiological adaptation; CL: Comprehension

13. 3. PaO_2 reflects the gas exchange ventilation and perfusion. It doesn't measure the respiratory status, degree of dyspnea, or the effectiveness of ventilation.
CN: Physiological integrity; CNS: Physiological adaptation; CL: Application

14. 4. Morphine will calm and relax the client and decrease respiratory rate, anxiety, and stress, decreasing the energy and oxygen demand of the heart. It doesn't have any affect on cardiac output or preload or afterload. It decreases myocardial oxygen demand.
CN: Physiological integrity; CNS: Pharmacological therapies; CL: Application

15. 3. The mother is a poor historian and it would definitely be worthwhile to ask her to describe what "bout of fits" means to her. The label on the bottle, "barbital," and the description of the pills would lead the nurse to think that the child may have experienced some sort of previous seizure activity and had been taking phenobarbital. Pentobarbital, supplied in capsules, elixirs, suppositories, and solution for injection, and secobarbital, supplied in capsule form, are used to induce sleep. Bismuth subsalicylate typically comes in caplets, chewable tablets, or oral solution that's pink and is used for indigestion and GI upset.
CN: Physiological integrity; CNS: Pharmacological therapies; CL: Analysis

16. A thin client is sitting up in bed talking on the phone and has a blood pressure of 96/60 mm Hg. Which nursing action is correct?
1. Increase fluids.
2. Call the physician.
3. Consider this a normal variation.
4. Suspect orthostatic hypotension.

16. 3. A thin client can have a blood pressure as low as 90/60 mm Hg and remain asymptomatic. Calling the physician with this information is inappropriate, as is increasing fluids. Orthostatic hypotension is a decrease in blood pressure and increase in heart rate that occur with a sudden change in position from lying to sitting. This condition could indicate some dehydration, but this client had been sitting up without symptoms for a while.
CN: Health promotion and maintenance; CNS: None; CL: Application

17. Which injury is least likely to become infected?
1. Contusion of the ankle in an 18-year-old
2. Laceration from glass in a 6-year-old
3. Stab wound in the leg of a 37-year-old
4. Cat bite to the left hand of an elderly client

17. 1. A contusion doesn't involve a break in the skin. The other options all involve a break in the skin that could lead to infection.
CN: Physiological integrity; CNS: Reduction of risk potential; CL: Comprehension

18. A client is hospitalized for 5 days with mononucleosis. Which finding indicates a possibly serious consequence?
1. Vomiting
2. Dark brown urine
3. Temperature of 101° F (38.3° C)
4. Cervical lymphadenopathy

18. 2. Dark brown urine could indicate the presence of bilirubin and implicate liver involvement. The other answers are typical findings for a client with this diagnosis.
CN: Physiological integrity; CNS: Physiological adaptation; CL: Analysis

19. A nurse is teaching a client about lifestyle changes that need to be made after a myocardial infarction (MI). The diagnosis of *Ineffective coping* is supported when the client is observed in which action?
1. Reading a book about meal planning
2. Pacing the floor of his room on occasion
3. Sitting quietly in his room for a short time
4. Telling his family he didn't have an MI

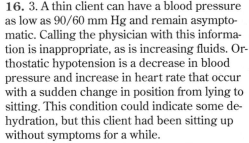

I'm impressed. You're really on your toes!

19. 4. When the client tells his family he didn't have an MI, he's showing the defense mechanism of denial. The client needs time to come to terms with his diagnosis. Reading a book on meal planning is a positive action. Pacing the floor on occasion is a form of anxiety that's normal for the client to experience. Sitting quietly is a normal behavior.
CN: Psychosocial integrity; CNS: None; CL: Comprehension

20. A client with a history of myasthenia gravis is admitted to the emergency department with complaints of respiratory distress and shallow respirations. The client's condition worsens and arterial blood gases are drawn. Which condition is expected?
1. Metabolic acidosis
2. Metabolic alkalosis
3. Respiratory acidosis
4. Respiratory alkalosis

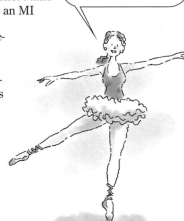

20. 3. The client has a restrictive lung problem because of myasthenia gravis. This is aggravated by respiratory distress. Because of the restrictive problem, the client won't be able to exhale efficiently and carbon dioxide will build up, causing respiratory acidosis. The client isn't at risk for developing a metabolic problem, and respiratory distress and shallow breathing would be evidenced by respiratory acidosis, not alkalosis, because shallow breathing causes acidosis and hyperventilation, not alkalosis.
CN: Physiological integrity; CNS: Physiological adaptation; CL: Analysis

CN: Client needs category   CNS: Client needs subcategory   CL: Cognitive level

21. Which food would the nurse allow a client receiving a full liquid diet?

1. Gelatin
2. Milkshake
3. Ice pops
4. Tea

22. A client who has recently had a myocardial infarction (MI) has begun to have symptoms of heart failure. The client voices a lack of understanding about the relationship between MI and heart failure. Which teaching statement by the nurse is most accurate?

1. "Due to the MI, your heart muscle is not able to pump your blood effectively."
2. "Your lungs are not working effectively due to the MI."
3. "This is just something that can happen after an MI."
4. "You are retaining fluid because the MI caused your kidneys to fail."

23. A client is admitted to the emergency department with severe epistaxis. The physician inserts posterior packing. Later, the client is anxious and says he doesn't feel he's breathing right. Which nursing action is appropriate?

1. Cutting the packing strings and removing the packing
2. Reassuring the client that what he's experiencing is normal
3. Asking the client to fully explain what he means by "right"
4. Using a flashlight and inspecting the posterior oral cavity of the client

21. 2. Full liquid diets contain milk, cereal, gruel, clear liquids, and plain frozen desserts. The clear liquid diet contains only foods that are clear and liquid at room or body temperature, such as gelatin; fat-free broth; bouillon; ice pops and similar frozen desserts; tea; and regular or decaffeinated coffee.
CN: Physiological integrity; CNS: Basic care and comfort; CL: Knowledge

22. 1. An MI causes damage to the heart muscle cells. Areas of scarred tissue and ischemia may decrease the heart's ability to contract normally and pump blood effectively. When blood flow to the rest of the body is inadequate due to diminished cardiac function, the client has heart failure. A client with heart failure may have respiratory symptoms as fluid backs up into the lungs but the problem is due to the heart's diminished pumping ability, not lung disease. Advising the client that this may "just happen" is incorrect and doesn't meet the client's need for information. Diminished blood flow to the kidneys may cause edema from sodium and water retention, but the ineffective heart function is a direct result of the MI.
CN: Physiological integrity; CNS: Physiological adaptation; CL: Application

23. 4. The nurse must assess the patency of the airway. The packing might have become dislodged. The nurse shouldn't remove the packing or give the client false reassurance. The client is too anxious to explain what he means.
CN: Physiological integrity; CNS: Reduction of risk potential; CL: Analysis

24. While performing nasopharyngeal suction, a nurse hears a client's pulse oximeter alarm. The pulse oximeter indicates the client's oxygen saturation reading is 86%. Which action should the nurse take?

1. Stop suctioning and give oxygen to the client.
2. Withdraw the suction catheter and tell the client to cough several times.
3. Continue suctioning for 10 to 15 more seconds and then withdraw the suction catheter.
4. Keep the suction catheter inserted and wait a few seconds before beginning suctioning.

25. Which action correctly explains the purpose of diaphragmatic breathing exercises for a client with chronic obstructive pulmonary disease (COPD)?

1. Dilate the bronchioles.
2. Decrease vital capacity.
3. Increase residual volume.
4. Decrease alveolar ventilation.

26. A client with chronic obstructive pulmonary disease (COPD) is being discharged from the hospital. The nurse provided teaching on medications, diet, and exercise. Which statement by the client indicates more teaching is needed?

1. "I'll eat six small meals per day."
2. "I'll get a flu shot every winter."
3. "I'll walk every morning before breakfast."
4. "I'll call my physician if I get cold symptoms."

27. A client is showing symptoms of bronchial obstruction. The client's nurse is teaching the nursing assistant about this condition. Which finding is expected?

1. Hacking cough
2. Diminished breath sounds
3. Production of rust-colored sputum
4. Decreased use of accessory muscles

24. 1. The pulse oximeter reading indicates the client isn't oxygenating well. The normal range for oxygen saturation is 90% to 100%. Suctioning draws air as well as secretions from the lungs, reducing oxygen saturation in the blood. The nurse must stop suctioning and give oxygen to increase the saturation. Withdrawing the suction catheter will stop the removal of oxygen, but coughing will delay an increase in saturation. The suction catheter occupies space in the airway, making it harder for the client to breathe when it's left in place. Further suctioning will reduce the oxygen level even further.
CN: Physiological integrity; CNS: Physiological adaptation; CL: Application

25. 1. In COPD, the bronchioles constrict during exhalation due to pressure changes in the lungs. Diaphragmatic breathing exercises keep the bronchioles open during exhalation. These exercises aren't performed for the other reasons stated.
CN: Physiological integrity; CNS: Reduction of risk potential; CL: Comprehension

26. 3. The worst time of the day for a client with COPD is morning. Exercise is important, but should be done later in the day. All other choices are appropriate for the client with COPD.
CN: Physiological integrity; CNS: Basic care and comfort; CL: Application

27. 2. Bronchial obstruction means no passage of air through the bronchi, so diminished or no breath sounds would be heard. A hacking cough is usually associated with upper respiratory infection and dryness in the upper airways. Rust-colored sputum is a sign of pneumococcal pneumonia. There would be increased use of accessory muscles.
CN: Safe, effective care environment; CNS: Coordinated care; CL: Knowledge

28. A client has just started treatment for tuberculosis. Rifampin (Rifadin) is the drug ordered by the physician. Which statement indicates the client has a good understanding of his medication?

    1. "I won't go to family gatherings for 6 months."

    2. "My urine will look orange because of the medication."

    3. "Now I don't need to cover my mouth or nose when I sneeze or cough."

    4. "I told my wife to throw away all the spoons and forks before I come home."

28. 2. Rifampin discolors body fluids, such as urine and tears. The client can go to family functions and eat with normal utensils. The client should cover his mouth and nose when coughing and sneezing.

CN: Physiological integrity; CNS: Pharmacological therapies; CL: Application

29. Before feeding a client with Parkinson's disease, which of the following nursing actions is most important?

    1. Sit the client upright.

    2. Have suction available.

    3. Order a clear liquid diet.

    4. Have a speech therapist evaluate the client.

29. 4. A speech therapist can evaluate the client's swallowing and make recommendations before the client is fed. Aspiration due to involuntary movement is common. Sitting the client upright and having suction available are helpful when feeding the client, but evaluation of the client's swallowing ability should come first. Clear liquids may be too difficult for the client; semisoft foods may be easier to swallow.

CN: Physiological integrity; CNS: Basic care and comfort; CL: Analysis

30. Management of a pregnant client with cardiovascular disease focuses on which treatment?

    1. Rest

    2. Hospitalization

    3. Therapeutic abortion

    4. Continuous cardiac monitoring

30. 1. The goal of antepartum management is to prevent complications and minimize the strain on the client. This is done with rest. Hospitalization may be required in older women or those with previous decompensation. Therapeutic abortion is considered in severe dysfunction, especially in the first trimester. Continuous cardiac monitoring isn't necessary.

CN: Physiological integrity; CNS: Reduction of risk potential; CL: Knowledge

31. Which finding most likely indicates a urinary tract infection (UTI) in a 5-year-old child?

    1. Incontinence

    2. Lack of thirst

    3. Concentrated urine

    4. Subnormal temperature

31. 1. Incontinence in a toilet-trained child is associated with UTI. Lack of thirst wouldn't be expected in a child with UTI. Concentrated urine is a sign of dehydration. Subnormal temperature isn't a sign of UTI.

CN: Physiological integrity; CNS: Physiological adaptation; CL: Application

32. A client has two prescriptions for fluid retention. One prescription reads "Lasix, 40 mg, one tablet daily." The other reads: "Furosemide, 40 mg, one tablet daily." Which instruction is given to the client?
1. Take both medications as ordered.
2. Lasix and furosemide are the same drug.
3. Use Lasix one day and furosemide the next day.
4. Throw away one of the drugs to not confuse the client.

33. A teacher tells the nurse that a preadolescent Vietnamese girl who's attending a new school in an affluent district sits in the back of the class and won't speak when spoken to, although her parents confirmed that the girl speaks English. Which finding is most likely?
1. The student is experiencing cultural shock.
2. The student is developing a peer support system.
3. The student is going through a socialization period.
4. The student is becoming acculturated to the new school.

34. A school nurse is screening for hearing and vision at a local middle school. Which technique is used to communicate effectively with this age-group?
1. Giving undivided attention to each student
2. Having the parents present during the screening
3. Having several adolescents listen to each other's health histories
4. Using puppets or dolls to show how the screening is going to take place

35. An 18-month-old infant is screened for developmental problems. Which screening test would the nurse expect to be used?
1. Goodenough draw-a-person test
2. Denver Developmental Screening test (DDST)
3. McCarthy Scales of Children's Abilities (MSCA)
4. Preschool readiness screening scales

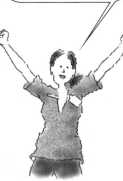

You're doing sensationally! So go ahead and shout about it!

32. 2. Using generic names for medications is common. It's the nurse's responsibility to teach the client both brand and generic names of drugs. Setting up medications in a medication tray, using only one pharmacy to dispense medications, and using all medications until the bottle is emptied will reduce medication errors.
CN: Physiological integrity; CNS: Pharmacological therapies; CL: Analysis

33. 1. Cultural shock is a feeling of helplessness, discomfort, and a state of disorientation when an outsider attempts to comprehend or adapt to a new cultural situation. Acculturation occurs when there's a blending of cultural or ethnic backgrounds. This process takes time to develop. Peer groups usually develop based on the background, interests, and capabilities of its members. Developing peer cultures is part of the socialization process.
CN: Health promotion and maintenance; CNS: None; CL: Application

34. 1. Give undivided attention to communicate effectively with adolescents. Respect their privacy. The presence of parents and use of puppets or dolls can be used to effectively communicate with younger children.
CN: Health promotion and maintenance; CNS: None; CL: Application

35. 2. The DDST is applicable for children from birth through age 6. The Goodenough draw-a-person test is used to assess intellectual ability in children ages 3 to 10. The MSCA is a developmental tool for children ages 2 to 8. Preschool readiness screening scales are designed for screening 5-year-old children's readiness for school.
CN: Health promotion and maintenance; CNS: None; CL: Application

CN: Client needs category   CNS: Client needs subcategory   CL: Cognitive level

36. In preparing educational intervention for college students, the nurse understands that drinking alcoholic beverages may be a behavior commonly associated with the relief of which problem?
1. Fatigue
2. Anxiety
3. Headache
4. Stomach pain

37. An educational program about relaxation techniques is provided for college students preparing for their final exams. Which relaxation technique is used to counteract anxiety?
1. Meditation
2. Music therapy
3. Dance therapy
4. Reality orientation

38. The parents of a 9-year-old child diagnosed with oppositional defiant disorder (ODD) are discussing treatment options with the nurse. Which action would the nurse expect to have the most positive impact on managing the child's behavior?
1. Daily administration of methylphenidate hydrochloride (Ritalin)
2. Providing praise to the child for positive behaviors
3. Group therapy with other children diagnosed with ODD
4. Assigning several household chores to the child for weekly completion

39. A 40-year-old client is admitted to the local women's shelter after being raped by her estranged husband. The client describes the traumatic event. Which response by the nurse is best?
1. Change the subject to prevent the client from crying.
2. Listen attentively while the client describes the event.
3. Arrange for the client to tell her story in group therapy.
4. Medicate the client with a tranquilizer to prevent hysteria.

36. 2. Drinking alcoholic beverages is commonly thought to alleviate anxiety. These beverages aren't commonly used to relieve fatigue, headache, or stomach pain.
CN: Psychosocial integrity; CNS: None; CL: Application

37. 1. Meditation is a relaxation therapy used to counteract anxiety related to stress-inducing internal and external stimuli. Music therapy, dance therapy, and reality orientation are used as adjuncts to psychiatric care.
CN: Psychosocial integrity; CNS: None; CL: Application

38. 2. Children with ODD consistently display negativity, defiance to authority, and hostility. ODD is best managed with consistent parenting and the establishment of a warm, positive home environment. Medication therapies aren't typically used for children with ODD. Methylphenidate is commonly used to manage attention deficit disorder. The focus of treatment for ODD is on the family unit, not on other children with similar problems. The child should be asked to participate in chores, but the parents need to be aware that overwhelming tasks may cause frustration and more defiance.
CN: Psychosocial integrity; CNS: None; CL: Analysis

39. 2. Retelling the event is part of the healing process. Giving medication and changing the subject don't allow the client to integrate the experience into her life. Group therapy may be helpful, but the best nursing response is to listen and convey empathy.
CN: Psychosocial integrity; CNS: None; CL: Application

CN: Client needs category CNS: Client needs subcategory CL: Cognitive level

40. The client with bipolar disorder tells the nurse that her family physician prescribed lithium (Eskalith). Which symptom indicates the client is developing lithium toxicity?
   1. Lethargy
   2. Hypertension
   3. Hyperexcitability
   4. Low urine output

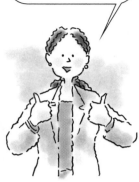

You're making great progress! Keep going!

40. 1. Nausea, vomiting, diarrhea, thirst, polyuria, lethargy, slurred speech, hypotension, muscle weakness, and fine hand tremors are signs of lithium toxicity. Hypertension, hyperexcitability, and low urine output aren't symptoms of lithium toxicity.
CN: Physiological integrity; CNS: Pharmacological therapies; CL: Application

41. Parents of a 10-year-old obese client ask the nurse how to encourage good eating habits in their child. Which response by the nurse is best?
   1. "You can begin by rewarding your child for not eating snacks between meals."
   2. "Take away a privilege whenever you discover your child eating junk food."
   3. "Don't permit your child to attend activities where junk food will be served."
   4. "Encourage your child to actively participate in meal planning and preparation."

41. 4. The nurse should instruct the parents to encourage their child to actively participate in meal planning and preparation. This gives the child a sense of control over his eating habits. Rewarding the child gives the parent control over the child's behavior. Taking away privileges causes resentment and promotes noncompliance. Keeping the child from activities with friends unnecessarily isolates the child from his peers.
CN: Physiological integrity; CNS: Basic care and comfort; CL: Application

42. A client states he's having arthritic pain and would like his medication. As you talk with him further you learn he isn't used to having such a firm mattress and this is aggravating his arthritic condition. Which action would be helpful in remedying his discomfort?
   1. Make sure the client receives a hypnotic and analgesic before bedtime.
   2. Place pillows behind his back and between his thighs.
   3. Request an order for a convoluted foam mattress.
   4. Call maintenance to see if they can locate a more comfortable bed.

42. 3. Requesting an order for a convoluted foam mattress or similar type cushion helps to provide a softer, more comfortable resting place for the client. Medicating the client is much too extreme when a simpler approach might be just as effective. Pillows might provide comfort, but they don't change the basic problem of a too firm mattress. Locating a more comfortable bed is highly unlikely.
CN: Physiological integrity; CNS: Basic care and comfort; CL: Analysis

43. Which nursing diagnosis is appropriate for a client with chronic obstructive pulmonary disease who's anxious, dyspneic, and hypoxic?
   1. *Ineffective breathing pattern related to anxiety*
   2. *Risk for aspiration related to absence of protective mechanisms*
   3. *Impaired gas exchange related to altered oxygen-carrying capacity of the blood*
   4. *Ineffective airway clearance related to presence of tracheobronchial secretions*

43. 3. The correct nursing diagnosis for this client is based on the impaired oxygenation at the cellular level. The first option applies to a client whose inhalation or exhalation pattern doesn't enable adequate pulmonary inflation or emptying. The second option applies if the client is at risk for aspirating gastric or pharyngeal secretions, food, or fluids into the tracheobronchial passages. The last option is appropriate for a client who can't clear secretions or obstructions from the respiratory tract.
CN: Physiological integrity; CNS: Reduction of risk potential; CL: Application

CN: Client needs category   CNS: Client needs subcategory   CL: Cognitive level

44. Which statement is a wellness nursing diagnosis?

1. *Readiness for enhanced spiritual well-being*
2. *Risk for activity intolerance related to prolonged bed rest*
3. *Grooming self-care deficit related to fatigue and muscle weakness*
4. *Constipation related to decreased activity and fluid intake as manifested by hard, formed stool every 3 days*

45. Which definition is correct for collaborative problems?

1. Unusual or unexpected human responses to pharmacological agents
2. Pathophysiological responses of body organs or systems for which physicians have ultimate responsibility
3. Human responses for which registered nurses are capable of intervening legally and independently of physicians
4. Certain physiological responses or complications of body organs or systems for which nurses intervene in association with physicians and other disciplines

46. An intake nurse at a local mental health facility is admitting a client with psychosis. Which technique is most valuable to use when planning this client's care?

1. Rorschach test
2. Interview with the client
3. Mental Status Examination (MSE)
4. Review old records of the client

47. Which action best describes the planning step of the nursing process?

1. Collecting client health data
2. Implementing the interventions identified in the care plan
3. Evaluating the client's progress toward attainment of the outcomes
4. Identifying the expected goals or outcomes individualized for the client and family

44. 1. Wellness diagnoses are one-part statements containing the label only and begin with "Readiness for enhanced," followed by the higher level of wellness desired for the individual or group. The second option is a "risk for" nursing diagnosis. The third option describes an existing problem for which additional data are needed for confirmation. The last option describes a manifested health problem validated by identifiable major defining characteristics.

CN: Psychosocial integrity; CNS: None; CL: Application

45. 4. This option describes a collaborative problem that requires physician and nurse prescribed actions. The first option describes an adverse reaction to a pharmacological agent. The second option describes the focus of a medical diagnosis. The third option describes a nursing diagnosis; interventions for nursing diagnoses fall within the scope of practice of registered nurses.

CN: Safe, effective care environment; CNS: Coordinated care; CL: Comprehension

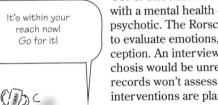

It's within your reach now! Go for it!

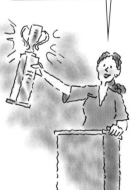

46. 3. The MSE is a basis for planning care with a mental health client, especially one who's psychotic. The Rorschach or inkblot test is used to evaluate emotions, intellect, affect, and perception. An interview with a client with psychosis would be unreliable. Reviewing old records won't assess the current state on which interventions are planned.

CN: Psychosocial integrity; CNS: None; CL: Comprehension

47. 4. Client goals or outcomes are identified in the planning step of the nursing process. Health data are collected in the assessment step of the nursing process. Planned interventions are done in the implementation step of the nursing process. A client's achievement of outcomes or goals is determined in the evaluation step of the nursing process.

CN: Safe, effective care environment; CNS: Coordinated care; CL: Knowledge

CN: Client needs category   CNS: Client needs subcategory   CL: Cognitive level

48. Which outcome is correct for a client with the nursing diagnosis *Risk for disuse syndrome*?
1. The client will be free from musculoskeletal complications.
2. The client will experience shorter periods of immobility and inactivity.
3. The nurse will stress the importance of maintaining adequate fluid intake.
4. The nurse will provide holistic care by collaborating with the health care team.

49. A 42-year-old client who underwent a right modified mastectomy with insertion of a closed drainage system will be hospitalized overnight because of minor complications. Which outcome statement is correct?
1. Teach proper care of the incision site and drain by postoperative day 1.
2. The client will know how to care for the incision site and drain by postoperative day 1.
3. The client will show the proper care of the incision site and drain by postoperative day 1.
4. The client will care for the incision site and contend with psychological loss by postoperative day 1.

50. Which expected outcome is correct for a client with the nursing diagnosis *Risk for injury* related to lack of awareness of environmental hazards?
1. Encourage the client to discuss safety rules with children.
2. Help the client learn safety precautions to take in the home.
3. The client will eliminate safety hazards in his surroundings.
4. Refer the client to community resources for more information.

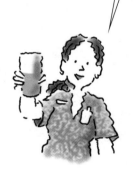

Halfway finished.
You can do it!

48. 2. Option 2 is an appropriate outcome for a client with this nursing diagnosis. Disuse syndrome, a result of prolonged or unavoidable immobility or inactivity, can be prevented. Musculoskeletal complications indicate actual disuse or complications of immobility. The last two options describe a nursing goal, not a client outcome.
CN: Physiological integrity; CNS: Reduction of risk potential; CL: Application

49. 3. This statement contains a specific measurable verb, clearly identifies the client behavior, and includes a date. The first option is a nursing goal as written, not a client-centered goal. The client goal of the second option isn't measurable as stated. The fourth option includes two goals that need to be addressed separately under the appropriate nursing diagnosis and it contains nonmeasurable verbs.
CN: Physiological integrity; CNS: Basic care and comfort; CL: Application

50. 3. This goal is appropriate and measurable as written and focuses on the client. The other options are nursing interventions as written.
CN: Health promotion and maintenance; CNS: None; CL: Application

CN: Client needs category   CNS: Client needs subcategory   CL: Cognitive level

51. The nurse is preparing a care plan for a client newly diagnosed with type 1 diabetes mellitus. Which goal statement will provide the greatest feedback to the nurse concerning the client's understanding of the nurse's teaching?
1. The client will state understanding of the material presented.
2. The nurse will complete medication teaching prior to discharge.
3. The client will demonstrate self-administration of insulin.
4. The client will be able to identify where the nurse should administer the next insulin injection.

51. 3. The goal statement should reflect the desired actions of the client, not the nurse. Therefore, a demonstration will enable the nurse to best assess the client's understanding of the teaching provided.
CN: Physiological integrity; CNS: Pharmacological therapies; CL: Analysis

52. A client with heart failure is given furosemide (Lasix) 40 mg I.V. daily. The morning serum potassium level is 2.8 mEq/L. Which action is the most appropriate?
1. Question the physician about the dosage.
2. Give 20 mg of the ordered dose and recheck the laboratory test results.
3. Notify the physician, give the potassium as ordered, then give the furosemide.
4. Give the furosemide and get an order for sodium polystyrene sulfonate.

52. 3. Furosemide is a diuretic. As water is lost, so is potassium. Diuresis is a treatment for heart failure. Notifying the physician of the low potassium level and getting an order for potassium chloride is the appropriate action before giving the furosemide. Furosemide, 40 mg, is an appropriate dose for the treatment of heart failure. The nurse shouldn't give half the dose without an order. Giving furosemide and sodium polystyrene sulfonate together would further lower the potassium level.
CN: Physiological integrity; CNS: Pharmacological therapies; CL: Application

53. Which client is at greatest risk for developing respiratory alkalosis?
1. A client in labor
2. A client with diabetes
3. A client with renal failure
4. An immediate postoperative client

53. 1. A client's respirations at certain stages of labor increase in volume, causing the partial pressure of arterial carbon dioxide to decrease, increasing the pH. Diabetes commonly causes a metabolic imbalance, resulting in metabolic acidosis. In renal failure, the inability of the kidneys to eliminate wastes increases the risk of developing metabolic acidosis. The respirations of a postoperative client are usually shallow after anesthesia and, because of pain, commonly cause respiratory acidosis.
CN: Physiological integrity; CNS: Physiological adaptation; CL: Application

54. Which condition should indicate to the nurse that the sterile field has been contaminated?
1. Sterile objects are held above the waist of the nurse.
2. Sterile packages are opened with the first edge away from the nurse.
3. The outer inch of the sterile towel hangs over the side of the table.
4. Wetness on the sterile cloth on top of the nonsterile table has been noted.

54. 4. Moisture outside the sterile package and field contaminates it because fluid can be wicked into the sterile field. The outer inch of the drape is considered contaminated but doesn't indicate that the sterile field itself has been contaminated. Bacteria tend to settle, so there's less contamination above waist level and away from the nurse.

CN: Safe, effective care environment; CNS: Safety and infection control; CL: Application

55. Which intervention should a nurse perform for a client with respiratory alkalosis?
1. Having the client breathe into a paper bag
2. Giving one ampule of bicarbonate as ordered
3. Giving oxygen at 3 L/minute through a nasal cannula
4. Repositioning the client and giving 75 mg of meperidine (Demerol) I.M. for pain

55. 1. By breathing into a paper bag, the client will rebreathe some of his own exhaled carbon dioxide and increase the carbon dioxide in his blood, which will correct his respiratory alkalosis. Giving one ampule of bicarbonate will worsen the alkalosis. Giving oxygen won't increase the carbon dioxide to correct the imbalance. Repositioning and giving meperidine are appropriate interventions for pain that may cause hyperventilation leading to respiratory alkalosis, but don't directly correct the problem.

CN: Physiological integrity; CNS: Physiological adaptation; CL: Analysis

56. The nurse is reviewing the laboratory results from a female diabetic client admitted to the acute care facility with dehydration. Which of the following laboratory results is consistent with a diagnosis of dehydration?
1. Serum hematocrit of 40%
2. Urine dipstick specific gravity of 1.035
3. Serum creatinine level of 0.8 mg/dl
4. HbA_{1C} level of 4%

56. 2. Urine specific gravity reflects the ability of the kidneys to concentrate urine. Normal urine specific gravity is 1.005 to 1.030. A higher urine specific gravity indicates that the urine is more concentrated, and this is consistent with dehydration. The normal hematocrit range for a female client is 36% to 48%, so this value is within normal limits. Dehydration would cause an increase in the hematocrit. Serum creatinine is used to assess kidney function; the normal range for women is 0.6 to 0.9 mg/dl. HbA_{1C} is used to monitor diabetes treatment and evaluates the average blood glucose over a period of months. The normal range for HbA_{1C} is 4% to 6.7%.

CN: Physiological integrity; CNS: Physiological adaptation; CL: Analysis

57. A client admitted with hypoparathyroidism is being monitored for hypocalcemia. Which sign is used to check for hypocalcemia?

1. Battle's sign
2. Brudzinski's sign
3. Chvostek's sign
4. Bonnet's sign

58. A client is complaining of pain 1 day after a colostomy. The nurse gives meperidine (Demerol) I.M. and, 30 minutes later, finds the client's respiratory rate at 8 breaths/minute, with the nasal cannula on the floor. Arterial blood gas (ABG) results are pH, 7.23; Pao_2, 58 mm Hg; $Paco_2$, 61 mm Hg; HCO_3^-, 24 mEq/L. Which group of factors contributes most to this client's ABG results?

1. Colostomy, pain, and meperidine (Demerol)
2. Meperidine, the nasal cannula on the floor, and the colostomy
3. Meperidine, respiratory rate of 8 breaths/minute, and the nasal cannula on the floor
4. Pain, respiratory rate of 8 breaths/minute, and the nasal cannula on the floor

57. 3. Hypocalcemia can cause Chvostek's sign, abnormal facial muscle and nerve spasms elicited when the facial nerve is tapped. Battle's sign is bruising over the temporal bone in the presence of a basilar skull fracture. A positive Brudzinski's sign is the flexion of the hips and knees in response to flexion of the head and neck toward the chest, indicating meningeal irritation. Bonnet's sign is pain on adduction of the thigh and is seen with sciatica.
CN: Physiological integrity; CNS: Reduction of risk potential; CL: Application

58. 3. This client has respiratory acidosis. Opioids can suppress respirations, causing retention of carbon dioxide. A partial pressure of arterial oxygen (Pao_2) of 58 mm Hg indicates hypoxemia, which is caused by the removal of the client's supplementary oxygen and the decreased respiratory rate. Pain increases—not decreases—the respiratory rate, which causes a decrease in partial pressure of arterial carbon dioxide ($Paco_2$). Colostomy drainage doesn't start until 2 to 3 days postoperatively, and this drainage would contribute to metabolic alkalosis.
CN: Physiological integrity; CNS: Physiological adaptation; CL: Analysis

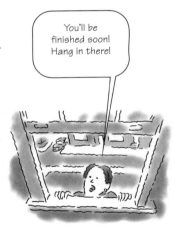

You'll be finished soon! Hang in there!

59. Which arterial blood gas (ABG) results are typical for a client with emphysema?
1. pH, 7.52; $Paco_2$, 18 mm Hg; HCO_3^-, 22 mEq/L
2. pH, 7.50; $Paco_2$, 38 mm Hg; HCO_3^-, 38 mEq/L
3. pH, 7.30; $Paco_2$, 52 mm Hg; HCO_3^-, 30 mEq/L
4. pH, 7.30; $Paco_2$, 40 mm Hg; HCO_3^-, 18 mEq/L

59. 3. Clients with emphysema retain carbon dioxide due to air trapping, causing an elevated partial pressure of arterial carbon dioxide ($Paco_2$) and respiratory acidosis. Because emphysema is a chronic disease, the kidneys compensate over time for the increased $Paco_2$ by retaining bicarbonate (HCO_3^-), thus attempting to normalize the pH. The other ABG results aren't consistent with results found in a client with emphysema.
CN: Physiological integrity; CNS: Physiological adaptation; CL: Comprehension

60. Which factor is a major cause of metabolic alkalosis in a client who had a colon resection?
1. Hyperventilation
2. Pain management
3. Nasogastric suction
4. I.V. therapy

60. 3. Removing acidic gastric secretions from the stomach is a metabolic cause of alkalinization of the blood pH. Hyperventilation decreases carbon dioxide and increases the pH, causing respiratory alkalosis. Pain management may further decrease the respiratory rate. Most I.V. fluids don't influence pH.
CN: Physiological integrity; CNS: Physiological adaptation; CL: Analysis

61. Which reason is correct for using a paper towel to turn off the faucet after hand washing?
1. To clean the faucet after use
2. To maintain sterility of the washed hands
3. To prevent contamination of the faucet handle
4. To prevent transmission of microorganisms from the faucet handle to the hands

61. 4. The faucet has microorganisms on it put there by all the "dirty" hands that touched it when turning it on. Although a paper towel isn't sterile, it's clean and protects the hands from becoming contaminated from the faucet after washing. Hand washing doesn't make the hands sterile. Wiping the faucet after use may make it look cleaner but isn't the reason for using a paper towel to turn off the faucet.
CN: Safe, effective care environment; CNS: Safety and infection control; CL: Comprehension

62. The nurse delegates to a nursing assistant the task of making an occupied bed for a 69-year-old client with dementia and problems with mobility. Which action would the nurse stress to the nursing assistant as the priority when the task is completed?
1. Placing the bed in the lowest position
2. Putting the call bell within the client's reach
3. Raising the top side rails to the upright position
4. Discarding soiled linen in a hamper or biohazard bag

62. 1. To reduce the risk of injury due to falls, the bed should be placed in the lowest position. The call bell should be in reach of the client, but the immediate safety of the client comes first. All four side rails should be up to prevent accidental falls and to remind clients to stay in bed. Soiled linens should be placed in a hamper or biohazard bag, but client safety is a priority.
CN: Safe, effective care environment; CNS: Coordinated care; CL: Comprehension

63. A client who underwent surgery to correct a bladder disorder is preparing to be discharged home with a Foley catheter for urinary drainage. After the nurse has performed discharge teaching, which statement by the client indicates a need for further instruction?

1. "I will empty the catheter bag before it becomes half full."
2. "I will lay the drainage bag on top of my bed at night so I won't trip on it."
3. "I will need to drink at least 6 to 8 glasses of water daily to ensure good urine output."
4. "If the catheter fails to drain, I will need to contact my physician's office."

64. Which client should be placed in an orthopneic position?

1. A client with edema of the lower legs and ankles
2. A client with a pressure ulcer on the coccyx and buttocks
3. An immobilized client with calf tenderness due to a deep vein thrombosis
4. An elderly client who has difficulty breathing unless in a sitting position

65. Two team members are helping a client transfer from the bed to a wheelchair. As the client rises from a supine to a sitting position, he complains of feeling light-headed and dizzy. Which action should the team members take next?

1. Lift the client quickly into the wheelchair.
2. Return the client to the supine position and apply a vest restraint.
3. Ask the client to dangle at the bedside while leaving the room for a few seconds to get additional assistance.
4. Have the client sit at the side of the bed for a few minutes while supporting his back and shoulders.

63. 2. Keeping the drainage bag below the level of the bladder is necessary to prevent reflux of urine into the bladder. In addition, placing the drainage bag on top of the bed may tangle the tubing and cause further problems. Frequent emptying of the urine drainage bag will ensure that the bag doesn't become too heavy for the client and will enable him to closely monitor his urine output. The client will need to consume at least 6 to 8 glasses of water daily. If the catheter doesn't drain, medical intervention will be needed to prevent complications.
CN: Health promotion and maintenance; CNS: None;
CL: Application

64. 4. The orthopneic position is a sitting position with the arms leaning on a bedside table. Sitting with the legs elevated to decrease edema is appropriate for clients with ankle and lower leg swelling. A client with a pressure ulcer will need to be positioned on his side and turned every 2 hours. Fowler's or semi-Fowler's positions are most appropriate for a client on complete bed rest.
CN: Physiological integrity; CNS: Physiological adaptation;
CL: Application

65. 4. A quick change in position will decrease blood pressure, causing momentary light-headedness and dizziness. An additional change in position may further reduce the client's blood pressure to a level that may require emergency assistance. This can be avoided by waiting with the client in the sitting position until the blood pressure stabilizes. Leaving the room may put the client in danger if the blood pressure decreases further and the client needs emergency assistance. If the client continues to complain of dizziness and light-headedness, then return him to bed. A vest restraint is inappropriate.
CN: Safe, effective care environment; CNS: Coordinated care;
CL: Application

CN: Client needs category   CNS: Client needs subcategory   CL: Cognitive level

66. Which action is the most effective infection-control measure for preventing the transmission of microorganisms?
1. Changing a client's bed linen daily
2. Washing hands before and after client contact
3. Wearing sterile gloves when touching a client's skin
4. Wearing a mask when in direct contact with infected clients

67. A client is admitted to the acute care facility with a diagnosis of meningococcal meningitis. When developing the care plan, the nurse knows to plan for which precaution?
1. The client must be in a private room, and the nurse must wear an N-95 respirator.
2. The client must be in a private room, and the door must be closed at all times.
3. The client must be in a private room, and the door may remain open.
4. The client must be in a private room equipped with negative air-pressure technology.

68. A team leader would instruct team members to wear a mask and protective eyewear or a face shield in which situation?
1. When strong odors are emitted from an infected wound
2. When the client has an oral temperature greater than 101° F (38.3° C)
3. If needles or other sharp instruments are to be used in the procedure
4. During a procedure where splashing of blood or body fluid is anticipated

69. A nurse is teaching a nursing assistant about standard precautions. Which statement by the nursing assistant indicates the need for further instruction?
1. "I must perform hand hygiene before I don gloves but not after I remove them."
2. "I must wear gloves to perform direct client care."
3. "I should never wash gloves and then reuse them."
4. "I should change gloves after I perform perineal care for a client."

66. 2. Most commonly, the transmission of microorganisms occurs when health care personnel don't wash their hands before and after touching a client or contaminated object. A daily linen change isn't the most effective method of controlling infection. Sterile gloves and a mask aren't needed during routine client care.
CN: Safe, effective care environment; CNS: Safety and infection control; CL: Comprehension

67. 3. A diagnosis of meningococcal meningitis requires the client to be put on droplet precautions. This type of infection can be transmitted only by close contact, so the door to the room may remain open. Because the infection is transmitted by droplets, masks should be worn by anyone entering the room; however, respirators and a negative-pressure environment are unnecessary.
CN: Safe, effective care environment; CNS: Safety and infection control; CL: Analysis

68. 4. Wearing eye goggles or face shields prevents blood or body-fluid splashes into the eyes. Odors don't transmit microorganisms. The use of needles or other sharp instruments doesn't mandate eye protection. A client with a fever isn't more likely to transmit microorganisms into the eyes than a client without a fever.
CN: Safe, effective care environment; CNS: Coordinated care; CL: Application

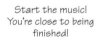

Start the music! You're close to being finished!

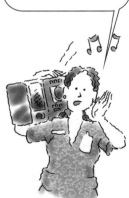

69. 1. Hand hygiene must be performed after removing gloves, as well as before. Gloves must be worn to perform direct client care and must never be reused. Gloves should be changed when moving from a contaminated body site, such as the perineal area, to a clean body site, such as the face.
CN: Safe, effective care environment; CNS: Safety and infection control; CL: Application

CN: Client needs category　CNS: Client needs subcategory　CL: Cognitive level

70. Which time frame is most appropriate for completing client teaching for a client undergoing an open cholecystectomy?
1. The day of discharge
2. A few weeks before the surgery
3. The first 12 hours after surgery
4. Before discharge, 1 to 2 days after the surgery

70. 4. Pain levels should have sufficiently subsided 1 to 2 days after the surgical procedure, allowing the client to concentrate on the information. The day of discharge is too late, because it doesn't give the client time to ask questions or practice procedures (such as syringe preparation) that may be necessary. Also, the individual may be anxious about returning home, which may interfere with learning. A few weeks before surgery is generally too early to retain information, and teaching within the first 12 hours after surgery isn't likely to produce retention of information, either.

CN: Physiological integrity; CNS: Basic care and comfort; CL: Application

71. For which individual is the use of an oral glass thermometer contraindicated?
1. A school-age client
2. An unconscious client
3. An alert, oriented client
4. An elderly client in no acute distress

71. 2. Oral glass thermometers can be broken by an unconscious client. Only a client who can follow directions to hold the thermometer in his mouth should be allowed to do so. The clients in the other three options should have no difficulty.

CN: Safe, effective care environment; CNS: Safety and infection control; CL: Knowledge

72. A nurse is preparing a client with a tracheostomy for discharge. Which of the following client statements indicates that he understands the teaching regarding his tracheostomy care?
1. "I will need to cover the opening when I shower."
2. "I can swim as long as I keep my head above water."
3. "I will need to wash my hands after caring for my tracheostomy."
4. "I will need to take antibiotics to prevent infections."

72. 1. The opening will require protection when bathing. Swimming isn't recommended; drowning can occur even if the client's head isn't submerged. It's necessary to wash hands before and after caring for the tracheostomy. Prophylactic antibiotics aren't required for the client with a tracheostomy.

CN: Safe, effective care environment; CNS: Safety and infection control; CL: Application

73. A 46-year-old single mother was concerned about her 15-year-old son's behavior. He suddenly decided his mother shouldn't date or have men in the house. He told his mother he was the "man of the house." Which disturbance was occurring in the internal dynamics of the family?
1. Age-appropriate behavior is occurring.
2. The son is powerful in the family system.
3. The son is trying to establish a role reversal.
4. It's culturally acceptable to be the man of the house at age 15.

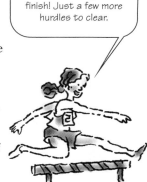

You're nearing the finish! Just a few more hurdles to clear.

73. 3. Role reversal occurs when the patterns of expected behavior aren't appropriate to age and ability. Males ages 13 to 17 are developing their identities, and separation from parents becomes necessary for individuation to occur. Males have a better understanding of their roles in relationships and families if they're raised around strong male role models. In healthy families, power is shared appropriate to age until the children are independent.

CN: Psychosocial integrity; CNS: None; CL: Analysis

CN: Client needs category   CNS: Client needs subcategory   CL: Cognitive level

74. Which behavior in a preschooler is a cause for concern?
1. Has nightmares
2. Cries and holds tightly to parents
3. Takes toys away from other children
4. Sits quietly and doesn't participate in play activities

74. 4. If a preschooler sits quietly and doesn't participate in play activities, it could be a sign of despair or hopelessness. During times of stress, it's typical for the preschooler to be frightened at night. It's normal for a child at this stage to show separation anxiety and play typical of preschoolers.
CN: Psychosocial integrity; CNS: None; CL: Knowledge

75. Which technique is appropriate for promoting proper breathing in a client experiencing pain or anxiety?
1. Rapid, light respirations
2. Rapid, deep respirations
3. In through the mouth and out through the nose
4. In through the nose and out through the mouth

75. 4. Air inhaled through the nose is warmed, humidified, and filtered for large particles with the nasal hairs, conditioning the air for delivery to the lungs. Exhaling through the mouth after inhaling through the nose requires some concentration and provides a focus to distract a client experiencing pain and anxiety. This method is used to control respiratory rates when clients are anxious or in pain and optimizes air exchange. Rapid, light, or deep respirations cause the client to lose oxygen exchange time while continuing to blow off carbon dioxide. This leads to hypoxemia and respiratory alkalosis.
CN: Physiological integrity; CNS: Physiological adaptation; CL: Application

76. A client with sinusitis comes to the ambulatory care clinic and admits using decongestant nasal spray and acetaminophen at home for the past several days to achieve comfort. After completing an examination, the physician prescribes amoxicillin. Which of the following interventions should also be included in the nurse's discharge teaching?
1. Continue use of the decongestant nasal spray while taking the antibiotics to promote maximum effectiveness.
2. Drink at least 6 to 8 glasses of water daily.
3. Lay flat at night to promote drainage of sinus passages.
4. Apply cold compresses to promote sinus comfort.

76. 2. Increasing fluid intake will aid in liquefying secretions. In addition, increasing fluid intake is recommended with antibiotic use. The excessive use of decongestant nasal sprays will result in a rebound effect and should be avoided. Lying flat won't promote nasal drainage. The client should be encouraged to rest with the head of the bed elevated 30 degrees. Application of cold compresses will promote vasoconstriction; heat is needed to achieve vasodilation and promote comfort.
CN: Physiological integrity; CNS: Physiological adaptation; CL: Application

77. Parents of a toddler are having problems putting him to bed at night. Which suggestion would be most appropriate?
    1. Stop the afternoon naps.
    2. Allow the toddler to have a tantrum for 30 minutes.
    3. Develop nighttime rituals.
    4. Allow the toddler to have some control over bedtime.

78. After abdominal surgery for repair of an aortic aneurysm, a client may show maladaptive coping behavior in response to body changes related to the surgery. Which nursing intervention is best?
    1. Letting the client express his feelings
    2. Explaining that a social service referral would be beneficial
    3. Instructing the client on how to use positive coping strategies
    4. Encouraging the client to participate in diversional activities

79. A nurse is reviewing treatment of hypercyanotic spells (tet spells) with the parents of a 4-month-old child being discharged from the hospital. Which discharge instruction is correct?
    1. "Calm the baby by holding her and placing her knees up to her chest."
    2. "Call 911 immediately and begin cardiopulmonary resuscitation (CPR) on the baby."
    3. "You'll need to administer four back blows to the baby if she begins having a tet spell."
    4. "You don't need to worry about these spells yet because the baby is too young. You'll need to watch for them when she becomes more mobile."

77. 3. Rituals are extremely important for toddlers to feel secure and relaxed. Allowing a toddler to make small decisions, such as choosing the order of the ritual and color of pajamas, will give him the feeling of some control but a nighttime ritual is more important. Stopping the naps may be helpful, depending on the toddler's needs. The toddler must clearly understand that tantrums won't get him what he wants.
CN: Psychosocial integrity; CNS: None; CL: Application

78. 1. Allowing verbalization of feelings is the most therapeutic nursing intervention. Making a referral may help, but initially the client should be allowed to express feelings. Giving advice may stop therapeutic communication. Providing diversional activities doesn't foster effective coping.
CN: Psychosocial integrity; CNS: None; CL: Application

79. 1. Tet spells are acute episodes of cyanosis and hypoxia that occur when the infant's oxygen demand exceeds the available supply. They may occur when the infant is crying or eating. Tet spells are emergency situations that require immediate intervention. Begin by calming the infant and placing her in the knee-chest position; this increases systemic vascular resistance by limiting venous return. This also decreases the right to left shunting and improves oxygenation. CPR won't calm the infant or improve oxygenation. Back blows are given to infants who have something lodged in their trachea. Telling the parents not to worry is incorrect because the spells can occur during periods of crying.
CN: Physiological integrity; CNS: Reduction of risk potential; CL: Application

80. Which nursing interventions treat gout?
1. Antibiotics, high fluid intake, opioids
2. Antihyperuricemic drugs, low-purine diet, opioids
3. High fluid intake, low-purine diet, antihyperuricemic drugs
4. High-purine diet, nonsteroidal anti-inflammatory drugs, prednisone (Deltasone)

80. 3. A low-purine diet decreases uric acid formation, and the high fluid intake increases urine output to flush out the uric acid. Drugs, such as antihyperuricemics, are used to reduce serum urate concentrations. Anti-inflammatory medications are used during acute phases, but because this is a long-term condition, opioids aren't generally given.
CN: Physiological integrity; CNS: Reduction of risk potential; CL: Application

81. A client with a fractured right tibia and fibula is hospitalized on the orthopedic care unit and has a newly applied plaster cast below the right knee. Which of the following assessment findings should be reported immediately?
1. The cast is slightly damp.
2. The client reports warmth beneath the cast.
3. The client reports poorly localized, progressive pain in the extremity.
4. Mild edema of the toes is visible beneath the cast.

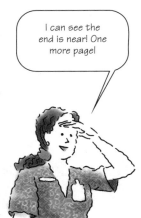

I can see the end is near! One more page!

81. 3. The presence of poorly localized, progressive pain in the extremity is consistent with impaired blood flow due to compartment syndrome and requires emergency treatment. Plaster casting may require a full day to dry, and the client may feel warmth beneath the cast. The presence of itching beneath the cast and mild edema are normal findings with casted fractures.
CN: Physiological integrity; CNS: Reduction of risk potential; CL: Application

82. A client with an arm cast complains of severe pain in the affected extremity and decreased sensation and motion are noted. Swelling in the fingers is also increased. Which intervention has priority?
1. Elevating the arm
2. Removing the cast
3. Giving an analgesic
4. Calling the physician

82. 4. The cast may be too tight and may need to be split or removed by the physician. Notify the physician when circulation, sensation, or motion is impaired. The arm should already be elevated. Giving analgesics wouldn't be the first step as it may mask the signs of a serious problem.
CN: Physiological integrity; CNS: Reduction of risk potential; CL: Application

CN: Client needs category   CNS: Client needs subcategory   CL: Cognitive level

83. The nurse receives a change-of-shift report for a 76-year-old client who had a total hip replacement. The client isn't oriented to time, place, or person and is attempting to get out of bed and pull out an I.V. line that's supplying hydration and antibiotics. The client has a vest restraint and bilateral soft wrist restraints. Which actions by the nurse would be appropriate? Select all that apply:

1. Assess and document the behavior that requires continued use of restraints.
2. Tie the restraints in quick-release knots.
3. Tie the restraints to the side rails of the bed.
4. Ask the client if he needs to go to the bathroom and provide range-of-motion (ROM) exercises every 2 hours.
5. Position the vest restraints so that the straps are crossed in the back.

84. A client with an I.V. line in place complains of pain at the insertion site. Assessment of the site reveals a vein that's red, warm, and hard. Which actions should the nurse take? Select all that apply:

1. Slow the infusion rate.
2. Discontinue the infusion.
3. Restart the infusion distal to the discontinued I.V. site.
4. Have the infusion restarted in the opposite arm.
5. Apply warm soaks to the I.V. site.
6. Document assessment of the I.V. site, the nurse's actions, and the client's response to the situation.

85. A toddler is ordered 350 mg of amoxicillin (Augmentin) by mouth, four times per day. The pharmacy supplies a bottle of amoxicillin with a concentration of 250 mg/5 ml. How many milliliters would the nurse give for each dose? Record the answer using a whole number.

_____ ml.

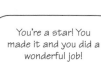

You're a star! You made it and you did a wonderful job!

83. 1, 2, 4. The client must be frequently reassessed to determine whether he's ready to have the restraints removed. The information should also be documented. Restraints should be tied in knots that can be released quickly and easily. Toileting and ROM exercises should be performed every 2 hours while a client is in restraints. Restraints should never be secured to side rails because doing so can cause injury if the side rail is lowered without untying the restraint. A vest restraint should be positioned so the straps cross in front of the client, not in the back.

CN: Safe, effective care environment; CNS: Safety and infection control; CL: Application

84. 2, 4, 5, 6. Redness, warmth, pain, and a hard, cordlike vein at the I.V. insertion site suggest that the client has phlebitis. The nurse should discontinue the I.V. line and insert a new I.V. catheter proximal to or above the discontinued I.V. site or in the other arm. Applying warm soaks to the site reduces inflammation. The nurse should document assessment of the I.V. site, actions taken, and the client's response to the situation. When phlebitis is present, slowing the infusion rate won't reduce the phlebitis. Restarting the infusion at a site distal to the phlebitis may contribute to the inflammation.

CN: Physiological integrity; CNS: Pharmacological therapies; CL: Application

85. 7. The nurse would give 7 milliliters for each dose. Use the following equation:

Dose on hand/Quantity on hand = Dose desired/X.

In this example, the equation is:

250 mg/5 ml = 350 mg/X;

X = 7 ml.

CN: Physiological integrity; CNS: Pharmacological therapies; CL: Analysis

CN: Client needs category   CNS: Client needs subcategory   CL: Cognitive level

Index

i refers to an illustration.

i refers to an illustration.

i refers to an illustration.

i refers to an illustration.

i refers to an illustration.

i refers to an illustration.

i refers to an illustration.

i refers to an illustration.

i refers to an illustration.